FLYNN'S PARASITES OF LABORATORY ANIMALS

SECOND EDITION

FLYNN'S PARASITES OF LABORATORY ANIMALS

SECOND EDITION

David G. Baker

DVM, MS, PHD, DACLAM (EDITOR-IN-CHIEF)

DIRECTOR AND PROFESSOR
DIVISION OF LABORATORY ANIMAL MEDICINE
SCHOOL OF VETERINARY MEDICINE
LOUISIANA STATE UNIVERSITY
BATON ROUGE, LA 70803

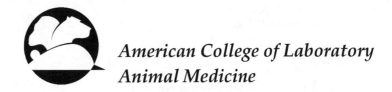

American College of Laboratory Animal Medicine

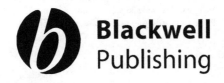

David G. Baker, DVM, MS, PhD, DACLAM, is Director and Professor, Division of Laboratory Animal Medicine, School of Veterinary Medicine at Louisiana State University, Baton Rouge.

Blackwell Publishing Professional
2121 State Avenue, Ames, Iowa 50014, USA

Orders: 1-800-862-6657
Office: 1-515-292-0140
Fax: 1-515-292-3348
Web site: www.blackwellprofessional.com

Blackwell Publishing Ltd
9600 Garsington Road, Oxford OX4 2DQ, UK
Tel.: +44 (0)1865 776868

Blackwell Publishing Asia
550 Swanston Street, Carlton, Victoria 3053, Australia
Tel.: +61 (0)3 8359 1011

First edition, ©1973 Iowa State University Press
Second edition, ©2007 Blackwell Publishing

Library of Congress Cataloging-in-Publication Data
Flynn's parasites of laboratory animals. – 2nd ed. / David G. Baker (editor-in-chief).
    p. ; cm.
Rev. ed. of: Parasites of laboratory animals / Robert J. Flynn. 1st ed. 1973.
Includes bibliographical references and index.
ISBN-13: 978-0-8138-1202-1 (alk. paper)
ISBN-10: 0-8138-1202-X (alk. paper)

1. Laboratory animals–Parasites. I. Flynn, Robert J., 1923—. @CRTXS:II. Baker, David G., 1956—. III. Flynn, Robert J., 1923—. Parasites of laboratory animals. IV. American College of Laboratory Animal Medicine. V. Title: Parasites of laboratory animals. [DNLM: 1. Animals, Laboratory. 2. Parasitic Diseases, Animal. 3. Parasites. SF 996.5 F648 2007]

SF996.5.F59 2007
636.088'5–dc22   2006033056

The last digit is the print number: 9 8 7 6 5 4 3 2

CONTENTS

*To Dr. Dale L. Brooks, mentor, colleague, and friend,
who envisioned this work fourteen years ago.*

PREFACE TO THE FIRST EDITION

ALTHOUGH much is known about the parasites of laboratory animals, information is often lacking and what is available is scattered. It is the purpose of this book to gather what is known in this field so that it is readily accessible to those who need it, and to point out what is not known.

Some of the stated deficiencies in our knowledge are probably incorrect in that the information is available but either has been overlooked or has not been published. It is hoped that these incorrect statements will stimulate persons with contrary information to point out the error or to divulge previously unpublished data.

It is also recognized that in a work of this sort, other errors are likely. It would be appreciated if these are pointed out so that they can be corrected in future editions, should the reception of this book warrant future revisions.

Many people helped write this book. A draft of each chapter was first prepared by the appropriate collaborator and then rewritten by me. The rewriting was done primarily to emphasize laboratory animals and secondarily to provide uniformity of style. The rewritten chapter was then reviewed by the collaborator and, in some cases, by others. Thus, each chapter in the book represents a joint effort of at least two people and, in some cases, of several.

Many people, besides the collaborators, assisted in the preparation of this volume. These include persons who reviewed chapters or parts of chapters, furnished illustrations, made literature searches and helped or advised in various ways.

The parasites described are those that occur spontaneously. Experimentally induced conditions are mentioned only if they are of special significance. No attempt is made to include the parasites of all domestic and wild animals. As a general rule, those of the common laboratory animals (mouse, rat, hamster, guinea pig, rabbit, dog, cat, rhesus monkey, and chicken) are all included, but for the less common species (such as other rodents, other primates, reptiles, amphibians, and fishes), only the commonest parasites of the animal species most likely to be used in the laboratory are described. Agents that occur only in domestic animals of agricultural importance are not described, even though these animals are sometimes used in the laboratory, as this information is readily available elsewhere.

Except for a few rare or uncommon animals, the common name only is used in the text. Although this may appear unscientific, the repeated use, for example, of *Mesocricetus auratus*, when one means the usual laboratory hamster, and *Oryctolagus cuniculus*, when one means the laboratory rabbit, is undesirable. Also, scientific names sometimes change, but common names tend to remain the same. Great care was taken to ensure that the scientific name is given for every common name that appears in the text, and that the common name is specific. Authorities used to determine the appropriate names are cited.

It is my sincere hope that the usefulness of this book will justify the efforts of all who helped prepare it.

ROBERT J. FLYNN

PREFACE TO THE SECOND EDITION

In the more than 30 years since publication of the first edition of this seminal text, dramatic changes have occurred in the fields of laboratory animal medicine and parasitology. Improvements in laboratory animal production, husbandry, transportation, veterinary care, diagnostics, and treatment, have resulted in dramatic declines in the prevalence of organisms causing parasitic diseases. Nowadays, commercially produced laboratory animals are free of nearly all unwanted organisms, including parasites. Modern facility design and husbandry practices preclude most infections or infestations. This is particularly true for parasites with indirect life cycles.

So, with all of these improvements, why is a new edition of this text warranted? Several reasons may be offered. First, in spite of the improvements in the components of animal care listed above, parasites continue to be found in and on laboratory animals. There are several possible reasons: infections or infestations were never completely eliminated from particular facilities; were inadvertently imported with incoming animals, either as a result of contamination during shipment or because parasitism was enzootic at the original location; entered the facility from feral animals in the local environment; or were carried in or on personnel and transferred to colony animals.

A second justification for revising the first edition is that animals in the wild are occasionally still collected and brought into the animal facility. While quarantine procedures should prevent transmission of parasites from wild to laboratory stock, transmission nevertheless occasionally occurs. Thirdly, the tremendous rise in the use of transgenic animals, some of which are immunologically compromised, provides opportunity for infections and/or infestations to take hold where such would not be the case with immunologically competent animals.

Finally, newer diagnostic and therapeutic approaches to controlling parasitism are available. These may facilitate discovery and elimination of unwanted pathogens. In addition to changes in the field of laboratory animal medicine, the field of parasitology has undergone radical changes. Here, changes have been most profound in the areas of diagnostics and treatment.

The stated purpose of the first edition was to gather into one source, what was known about the parasites of laboratory animals so that it was readily accessible to those who needed it, and to point out gaps in our knowledge of parasites and the diseases they cause. The purpose of this second edition is essentially the same, with the additional significant task of updating information in a field that has advanced substantially, parasitology of laboratory animals.

As with the first edition, many people contributed to this monumental work. Foremost among them are the chapter authors. Their efforts are greatly appreciated. In addition, all chapters were subjected to peer review. On behalf of the authors, I offer thanks to the reviewers for their many valuable suggestions for improving early drafts. Others contributed illustrations, photographs, or conducted literature searches. These too are greatly appreciated. Lastly, we want to give special thanks to Drs. P. Coan, R. Ermel, S. Feldman, and D. McClure. They constituted an advisory committee charged with assisting the Editor-in-Chief in critically evaluating the first edition, in an effort to identify, if possible, areas in which the second edition could be even more valuable than the first.

The breadth and scope of the original edition has been retained, thereby ensuring continued usefulness to the widest possible readership, including bonafide parasitologists. Introductory chapters have been added, beginning with a chapter on modern diagnostic techniques. The next five chapters present overviews of parasite biology. These should help the reader to better understand information presented in the host-specific chapters. Most significantly, the text has been entirely reformatted, in an attempt to improve utility and readability. The informational content has been reorganized into chapters based on vertebrate host. Parasites are presented phylogenetically within chapters. In addition, information included in comprehensive tables from the first edition has been updated, organized by host body system, and reformatted to coincide with host chapters. Finally, a formulary of drugs, uses, dosages, routes, and mechanisms of action, has been added as an appendix. It is hoped that these changes will increase the usefulness of an already highly valuable reference text.

DAVID G. BAKER

ACKNOWLEDGEMENTS

THE authors wish to acknowledge those who contributed to the high quality of this revision through their thoughtful reviews and comments. These include Drs. Judy Bell, Valerie K. Bergdall, Cory F. Brayton, Patricia N. Coan, Philip S. Craig, Richard W. Ermel, Craig S. Frisk, Nina E. Hahn, Fred W. Knapp, Michael R. Lappin, James E. Miller, Edward J. Noga, Thomas J. Nolan, Kevin O'Hair, Glen M. Otto, Sarah L. Poynton, Philip J. Richter, Jr., Yehia Mo Saif, Peter M. Schantz, Mark St.Clair, C. Dayton Steelman, Steven J. Upton, Mark T. Whary, Michael J. Yabsley, Thomas A. Yazwinski, and Anne M. Zajac.

LIST OF CONTRIBUTORS

DAVID G. BAKER, D.V.M., M.S., Ph.D., D.A.C.L.A.M.
Director and Professor
Division of Laboratory Animal Medicine
School of Veterinary Medicine
Louisiana State University
Baton Rouge, LA 70803
Tel: (225) 578-9643
Fax: (225) 578-9649
Email: dbaker@vetmed.lsu.edu

ROBERT A. BAKER, D.V.M.
Clinical Veterinarian
Animal Resources Program
University of Alabama at Birmingham
B10 Volker Hall
1717 7th Ave. South
Birmingham, AL 35294-0019
Tel: (205) 934-5530
Fax: (205) 934-1188
Email: bobbaker@uab.edu

LORA R. BALLWEBER, M.S., D.V.M., D.E.V.P.C.
Associate Professor
Department of Microbiology, Immunology, and Pathology
Colorado State University
1619 Campus Delivery
Ft. Collins, CO 80523-1619
Colorado State University
Tel: (970) 491-5015
Email: lora.ballweber@colostate.edu

DIANA M. PALILA BERGER, D.V.M., M.S.
Clinical Veterinarian and Assistant Director for Large Animal
    Clinical Medicine
Center for Comparative Medicine
Northwestern University
320 East Superior Street
Searle 13-507
Chicago, IL 60611-3010
Tel: (312) 503-7259

Fax: (312) 908-6428
Email: d-berger@northwestern.edu

DWIGHT D. BOWMAN, M.S., Ph.D.
Professor of Parasitology
Department of Microbiology & Immunology
College of Veterinary Medicine
Cornell University
C4-119 VMC Tower Road
Ithaca NY, 14853-6401
Tel: (607) 253-3406
Fax: (607) 253-4077
Email: ddb3@cornell.edu

RONNIE L. BYFORD, Ph.D.
Professor
Department of Entomology, Plant Pathology, and Weed Science
New Mexico State University
MSC 3BE
Skeen Hall Bldg, Room N141
Las Cruces, NM 88003
Tel: (505) 646-2458
Fax: (505) 646-8085
Email: rbyford@nmsu.edu

SAMUEL C. CARTNER, D.V.M., M.P.H., Ph.D.
Interim Director, Animal Resources Program
Associate Professor, Department of Genetics
University of Alabama at Birmingham
220A Research Support Bldg
1800 9th Ave. South
Birmingham, AL 35294-0019
Tel: (205) 934-8213
Fax: (205) 975-1188
Email: scartner@uab.edu

FRANK COGSWELL, Ph.D.
Director, Parasite Diagnostic Laboratory
Tulane National Primate Research Center
18703 Three Rivers Road

Covington, LA 70433
Tel: (985) 871-6224
Fax: (985) 871-1350
Email: cogswell@tulane.edu

MAURICE E. CRAIG, M.S.
Science Specialist
Department of Extension Plant Sciences
New Mexico State University
Las Cruces, NM 88003
Tel: (505) 646-3231
Fax: (505) 646-8085
Email: mcraig@nmsu.edu

THOMAS M. CRAIG, D.V.M., Ph.D.
Professor
Department of Veterinary Pathobiology
College of Veterinary Medicine
Texas A&M University
College Station, TX 77843-4467
Tel: (979) 845-9191
Fax: (979) 862-2344
Email: tcraig@cvm.tamu.edu

JOHN W. FOURNIE, M.S., Ph.D.
Fish Pathologist
U.S. Environmental Protection Agency
National Health and Environmental Effects Research Laboratory
Gulf Ecology Division
1 Sabine Island Drive
Gulf Breeze, FL 32561
Tel: (850) 934-9272
Fax: (850) 934-9201
Email: fournie.john@epa.gov

JAMES G. FOX, D.V.M., M.S., D.A.C.L.A.M.
Professor and Director
Division of Comparative Medicine
Massachusetts Institute of Technology
77 Mass Ave., Bldg 16-8th floor
Cambridge, MA 02139
Tel: (617) 253-9432
Fax: (617) 258-5708
Email: jgfox@mit.edu

LAURETTA W. GERRITY, D.V.M.
Associate Vice President for Research Operations and Compliance
Professor, Department of Genetics
University of Alabama at Birmingham
720 C Administration Bldg
701 20th St. South
Birmingham, AL 35294-0019
Tel: (205) 934-7677
Fax: (205) 975-7886
Email: lwgerrity@.uab.edu

F. CLAIRE HANKENSON, D.V.M., M.S., D.A.C.L.A.M.
Senior Associate Director, University Laboratory Animal Resources
Assistant Professor, Department of Pathobiology
School of Veterinary Medicine
3800 Spruce Street
177E Old Vet Quadrangle
Philadelphia, PA 19104-6009
Tel: (215) 573-3625
Fax: (215) 573-9998
fclaire@pobox.upenn.edu

JOHN E. HARKNESS, D.V.M., M.S., M.Ed., D.A.C.L.A.M.
Professor Emeritus
College of Veterinary Medicine
Mississippi State University
PO Box 6100
Mississippi State, MS 39762
Tel: (601) 325-1131
Fax: (601) 325-1498
Email: harkness@cvm.msstate.edu

AKIRA ITO, M.S., Ph.D., D.Med.Sci.
Director and Professor
Department of Parasitology
Asahikawa Medical College
Midorigaoka-Higashi 2-1-1-1
Asahikawa 078-8510
Hokkaido, Japan
Tel: +81-(0)166-68-2420
Fax: +81-(0)166-68-2429
Email: akiraito@asahikawa-med.ac.jp

MICHAEL L. KENT, M.S., Ph.D.
Director, Center for Fish Disease Research
Department of Microbiology
220 Nash Hall
Oregon State University
Corvallis, OR 97311-3804
Tel: (541) 737-8652
Fax: (541) 737-0496
Email: Michael.Kent@oregonstate.edu

CYNTHIA LANG, D.V.M., M.S.
Resident
Division of Laboratory Animal Medicine
School of Veterinary Medicine
Louisiana State University
Baton Rouge, LA 70803
Tel: (225) 578-9648
Fax: (225) 578-9649
Email: clang@vetmail.lsu.edu

STEPHANIE LEWIS, D.V.M.
Resident
Division of Laboratory Animal Medicine
School of Veterinary Medicine

Louisiana State University
Baton Rouge, LA 70803
Tel: (225) 578-9648
Fax: (225) 578-9649
Email: slewis@vetmed.lsu.edu

DAVID S. LINDSAY, Ph.D.
    Distinguished Veterinary Parasitologist
    Professor of Parasitology
    Center for Molecular Medicine and Infectious Diseases
    Department of Biomedical Sciences and Pathobiology
    Virginia-Maryland Regional College of Veterinary Medicine
    Duckpond Drive, Phase II
    Virginia Tech (0442)
    Blacksburg, VA 24061
    Tel: (540) 231-6302
    Fax: (540) 231-3426
    Email: lindsayd@vt.edu

JOHN. B. MALONE, JR., D.V.M., Ph.D.
    Professor
    Department of Pathobiological Sciences
    School of Veterinary Medicine
    Louisiana State University
    Baton Rouge, LA 70803
    Tel: (225) 578-9692
    Fax: (225) 578-9701
    Email: malone@vetmed.lsu.edu

MARK A. MITCHELL, D.V.M., M.S., Ph.D.
    Associate Professor
    Director, Wildlife Hospital of Louisiana
    Department of Veterinary Clinical Sciences
    School of Veterinary Medicine
    Louisiana State University
    Baton Rouge, LA 70803
    Tel: (225) 578-9525
    Fax: (225) 578-9559
    Email: mitchell@vetmed.lsu.edu

CLIFF M. MONAHAN, D.V.M., Ph.D.
    Department of Veterinary Preventive Medicine
    The Ohio State University
    1920 Coffey Road
    Columbus, OH 43212
    Tel: (614) 292-8335
    Fax: (614) 292-4142
    Email: monahan.19@osu.edu

TERESA Y. MORISHITA, D.V.M., M.P.V.M., M.S., Ph.D.,
D.A.C.P.V.
    Professor and Poultry Veterinarian
    College of Veterinary Medicine
    Western University of Health Sciences
    309 E. Second Street
    Pomona, California   91766

Tel: (909) 469-5512
Fax: (909) 469-5635
email: tmorishita@westernu.edu

MARY PATTERSON, M.S., D.V.M., D.A.C.L.A.M.
    Clinical Veterinarian
    Division of Comparative Medicine
    Massachusetts Institute of Technology
    77 Mass Ave., Bldg 16-8th floor
    Cambridge, MA 02139
    Tel: (617) 324-5403
    Fax: (617) 258-5708
    Email: mmpatt@mit.edu

JORDAN C. SCHAUL, M.S., Ph.D.
    Assistant Director, Laboratory for Wildlife and Environmental
        Health
    College of Veterinary Medicine
    Western University of Health Sciences
    309 E. Second Street
    Pomona, CA 91766
    Tel: (909) 469-5512
    Fax: (909) 469-5635
    Email: jschaul@westernu.edu

TRENTON R. SCHOEB, D.V.M., Ph.D.
    Professor, Department of Genetics
    Director, Comparative Pathology Laboratory
    University of Alabama at Birmingham
    724 Kaul Human Genetics Bldg.
    720 20th St. South
    Birmingham, AL 35294-0024
    Tel: (205) 934-2288
    Fax: (205) 975-4418
    Email: trs@uab.edu

PAT H. SMITH, B.S.
    Department of Pathobiological Sciences
    School of Veterinary Medicine
    Louisiana State University
    Baton Rouge, LA 70803
    Tel: (225) 578-9710
    Fax: (225) 578-9157
    Email: psmith@vetmed.lsu.edu

T. BONNER STEWART, Ph.D.
    Emeritus Professor
    Department of Pathobiological Sciences
    School of Veterinary Medicine
    Louisiana State University
    Baton Rouge, LA 70803
    Tel: (225) 578-9684
    Fax: (225) 578-9701

CHRISTINE A. SUNDERMANN, M.S., Ph.D.
   Professor of Biology
   Department of Biological Sciences
   131 Cary Hall
   Auburn University
   Auburn, AL 36849
   Tel: (334) 844-3929
   Fax: (334) 844-4065
   Email: sundeca@auburn.edu

GERALD L. VAN HOOSIER, JR., D.V.M., D.A.C.L.A.M.
   Emeritus Professor
   Department of Comparative Medicine
   Box 357190
   University of Washington
   Seattle, WA 98195-7190
   Tel: (206) 685-3261
   Fax: (206) 685-3006
   Email: gvanhoo@u.washington.edu

SEKLAU E. WILES, M.Sc.
   Research Associate
   Department of Pathobiological Sciences
   School of Veterinary Medicine
   Louisiana State University
   Baton Rouge, LA 70803
   Tel: (225) 578-9671
   Fax: (225) 578-9701
   Email: swiles@vetmed.lsu.edu

JAMES D. WILKERSON, J.D., D.V.M., D.A.C.L.A.M.
   Associate Director, Laboratory Animal Resource Center
   University of California
   Box 0564
   Medical Science 386D
   San Francisco, CA 94143-0564
   Tel: (415) 502-2729
   Fax: (415) 502-8252
   Email: james.wilkerson@ucsf.edu

FLYNN'S PARASITES OF LABORATORY ANIMALS

SECOND EDITION

CHAPTER

1

Collection, Preservation, and Diagnostic Methods

*Pat H. Smith, BS; Seklau E. Wiles, MSc; John B. Malone, Jr., DVM, PhD;
and Cliff M. Monahan, DVM, PhD*

INTRODUCTION

As the scope of this book indicates, the term "laboratory animal" can encompass virtually any animal species used in research. The parasite fauna of such a wide spectrum of hosts seems unlimited. However, within phyla, parasites share many traits. The purpose of this chapter is to describe diagnostic methods useful for parasite phyla likely to be encountered in the research animal environment.

Most laboratory animal facilities should be capable of performing most of the fundamental techniques outlined in this chapter. Performing any of these techniques correctly and reliably requires expertise developed through repetition. For uncommon techniques or obscure parasites, it is often more expedient to send samples to a laboratory with more extensive diagnostic capabilities. Several resources are available for more complete treatment of diagnostic techniques[1-3].

SAMPLE COLLECTION AND PRESERVATION

Feces

Number of Samples to Collect

The number of samples to be collected depends on several factors, including the source and health status of the animals, available financial resources, and the parasite phyla likely to be encountered. For routine screening of an asymptomatic animal, a single sample should suffice. For newly arrived animals with potential parasite exposure or questionable health history, or for symptomatic animals within the colony, sequential fecal examinations are warranted. These are typically performed over three days.

Most nematode infections are easily identified with a single fecal examination because the female worms pass hundreds to thousands of eggs per day. In contrast, low level trematode, cestode, or protozoal infections may not be detected with a single examination because eggs or oocysts may not be passed continuously or daily, or in great number. In these cases, collecting fecal specimens passed on three sequential days will increase diagnostic power. To assess the parasite status of a group of animals, 30 animals or 10% of the group, whichever is greater, should provide adequate sampling coverage.

Sample Collection

Proper collection and preservation methods are critical for finding fecal parasites. A fresh fecal sample, collected rectally or just dropped, is optimal. When feces must be collected from the ground, the specimen should be taken from the middle of the dropping. This will minimize contamination with organisms from the environment. When sampling a group of animals, individual samples should be collected and tested separately. Mixing samples may mask or underestimate the true extent of infection, because parasites are not evenly distributed within host populations. Collected specimens should be placed in clean, wide-mouth plastic containers with screw-top lids, or in sealable plastic bags. Using a permanent marker, specimens should be properly identified with animal identification, date of collection, and species of animal. Specimens should be refrigerated as soon as possible, unless direct smears are to be prepared for the detection of motile protozoa. If collections are made in the field, specimens may be placed among refrigeration packs.

Sample Preservation

Specimens which will not be immediately processed should be immersed in a suitable fixative. The choice of fixative depends on the tests to be performed (Table 1.1). Often, an initial fecal examination is performed on a fresh sample. Positive test results then direct the diagnostician to the appropriate fixation medium for additional testing of the remainder of the sample.

TABLE 1.1   Common fixatives and applications

Fixative	Applications
Formalin	2% in distilled water for modified Knott's recovery of microfilariae
	5–10% for concentration techniques (formalin-ethyl acetate; flotations and centrifugations)
	Cryptosporidium and *Giardia* antigen tests
	Not useful for making permanent mounts of most staining procedures
Schaudin's fluid	Permanent mounts of protozoa stained with trichrome or iron hematoxylin
Polyvinyl alcohol (PVA)	Permanent mounts of protozoa stained with trichrome or iron hematoxylin
Sodium acetate-acetic acid-formalin (SAF)	Concentration techniques (formalin-ethyl acetate; flotations and centrifugations)
	Permanent mounts of protozoa stained with trichrome or iron hematoxylin
Merthiolate-iodine-formalin	Wet mounts or direct smears
	Formalin-ethyl acetate sedimentation
	Limited use for staining of permanent mounts

Adapted from Ash and Orihel (1991) and Garcia (2001).

When sending samples to a commercial diagnostic laboratory, the protocol for preserving and shipping samples should be obtained prior to collection of samples. By adhering to these guidelines, the likelihood of an accurate diagnosis is maximized, and regulatory standards for shipping potential pathogens can be met. Pre-measured fixative vials are available for all of the fixatives described below, and simplify sample processing.

Regardless of the fixation method to be used, sample quality can be improved with centrifugation, or sieving followed by sedimentation. These methods remove water-soluble pigments and debris, and concentrate parasite forms. Diarrheic samples will benefit most by concentration. Ethyl acetate extraction is also useful for removing excess lipid. Once washed or cleaned, droplets of the unfixed sediment can be placed on slides for immediate examination or dried for staining and the remainder of the pellet fixed for shipment to a reference laboratory if necessary. Regardless of the fixative used, samples must be well mixed to ensure complete and uniform fixation of the specimen.

Formalin

Formalin is a readily available fixative that rapidly kills most pathogens, thus decreasing the zoonotic concerns of handling fecal samples. Formalin is not suitable for identifying whole helminths because it makes worms brittle and may interfere with special stains. Formalin fixation also may change the density of parasite structures such that recovery with flotation solutions is decreased. Flotation solutions of higher specific gravity (1.23–1.25) provide optimal recovery of formalin-fixed helminth eggs. Many fecal antigen tests are designed for use with formalin-fixed specimens, but this is not universal and must be verified before use. Also, formalin fixation results in cross-linking of many proteins associated with DNA. This may preclude using formalin-fixed specimens in polymerase chain reaction (PCR)-based assays. For fixation of fecal samples, 5% to 10% neutral buffered formalin solutions (NBF) are most commonly used.

Schaudin's fluid

Schaudin's fluid or fixative is used in-house and for fixing specimens in preparation for shipment. Droplets of a mixture of fresh feces and Schaudin's fluid can be applied directly to microscope slides for drying, then staining. Schaudin-fixed samples are not used in concentration procedures. Specimens can be fixed when passed, or can be prewashed as described below. The latter concentrates parasite forms. Schaudin's fixative provides excellent morphological preservation of trophozoites and amoebic cysts. Schaudin-fixed samples do not adhere well to glass slides, and so must be handled gently. Also, Schaudin's fixative contains mercury and therefore must be handled with caution. Newer preparations are available that employ zinc or copper as a substitute. While there may be a slight decline in the preservation of protozoal morphology, such as the chromatin pattern of amoebic cysts, handling and disposal of reagents with zinc or copper are less problematic than for reagents containing mercury.

Polyvinyl alcohol

Polyvinyl alcohol (PVA) was developed to overcome specimen adherence problems of Schaudin's fixative. While PVA fixation optimizes staining of some parasites, particularly intestinal protozoa, other fixatives are preferred for concentration procedures. Because PVA is carcinogenic, it must be handled with caution.

Merthiolate-iodine-formalin

Merthiolate-iodine-formalin (MIF) is commonly used for fecal specimens to be examined as direct wet mounts or following concentration techniques. It is not useful for preparing permanent mounts or for fixing specimens prior to staining. This fixative will also inactivate most pathogens.

Sodium acetate-acetic acid-formalin

Sodium acetate-acetic acid-formalin (SAF) is a good compromise fixative for shipment of samples destined to be processed either as permanent stains or concentration procedures. There may be a slight decline in protozoal integrity compared to the use of Schaudin's or PVA, but SAF does not contain mercury. Samples fixed with SAF can be stained with iron hematoxylin or trichrome stains.

Blood

Blood-borne parasites include the protozoan hemoparasites and the microfilariae (MF) of filarid nematodes, both of which benefit from collection of blood with an anticoagulant. Blood samples are also collected in tubes lacking anticoagulant, for use for antigen and antibody tests. Protozoan hemoparasites are typically identified by microscopic examination of stained blood smears. Thin films can be prepared immediately or from preserved whole blood. Most staining procedures can be performed on films that have been fixed with methanol. Although MF can often be found on blood films, adequate visualization is difficult for identification to genus or species. Samples of blood with an anticoagulant are necessary because the MF cannot be removed from a clot for staining.

Collecting adequate blood from small animals can be problematic. Following venipuncture, blood can be drawn into a single hematocrit tube from which a blood smear can immediately be made. The remainder can be centrifuged for determination of packed cell volume. The tube can then be scored and broken at the buffy coat for recovery of MF, and the small quantity of serum or plasma can be harvested for serology.

Urine

Urine samples can be collected and centrifuged to concentrate helminth eggs or microsporidia. These can be stored in saline and refrigerated for days if they cannot be examined immediately. For longer periods, fixation with 10% NBF or 70% ethanol and 5% glycerin are useful preservatives.

Tracheal Lavage Samples

Tracheal lavage samples should be collected from deep within the respiratory tract, using sterile saline. Lavage samples can be viscous in nature, and high viscosity can interfere with sample processing. Viscous samples should be mixed with a solution of 3% sodium hydroxide in saline, then centrifuged to concentrate parasite forms. Very thick mucus plugs can be subjected to ethyl acetate sedimentation as described for fatty fecal samples. Following centrifugation, samples can be preserved in 10% NBF, 70% ethanol (for helminths), or PVA fixative (for protozoa).

PARASITE COLLECTION AND PRESERVATION

Helminths

Helminths collected during necropsy examinations or passed directly by animals should be placed immediately into a container of 70% ethanol heated to 60°C to 63°C. This treatment will cause the helminths to straighten. Also, adult cestodes and acanthocephalans will protrude the rostellum or proboscis, respectively. Worms can then be transferred to 70% ethyl alcohol and 5% glycerin for long-term storage.

Arthropods

Macroscopically visible arthropods should be placed into 70%–90% ethanol. Formalin should not be used because fixation in NBF renders arthropods brittle. Skin scrapings can be collected directly onto microscope slides bearing a drop of mineral oil. However, initial processing with 10% potassium hydroxide (KOH) will facilitate visualization of arthropods by rendering the keratin more transparent. External parasites may frequently be recovered on clear adhesive tape that is brushed across the animal's fur, then adhered to a microscope slide.

FECAL EXAMINATION TECHNIQUES

Direct Smear Method

The direct smear is used only with samples in which motile trophozoites are suspected. The small quantity of sample employed is inadequate for other diagnostic procedures. The fecal sample should be either loose stool or diarrhea. Formed feces are unlikely sources of trophozoites, since under such conditions trophozoites either dehydrate and become distorted or form cysts during normal intestinal transit. Specimens must be examined immediately, before low external temperatures decrease trophozoite motility. Refrigeration of fecal samples renders trophozoites nonmotile and should not be used prior to preparing direct smears.

Materials
- Microscope slide and coverslip
- Saline
- Fecal loop or applicator stick
- Lugol's iodine

Method
1. Place a drop of saline on one end of a microscope slide and a drop of Lugol's iodine on the other.
2. Add a small quantity of fresh fecal specimen first to the saline drop and mix thoroughly, then transfer a small amount of the specimen to the Lugol's iodine drop.
3. Place a coverslip over each mixture.
4. Examine the saline/sample side first, with the light adjusted for ample contrast. Do not mistake Brownian motion for motility. Examine the entire coverslip using the 10 × objective, then 20 fields using the 40 × objective.
5. Examine the drop with Lugol's iodine for comparison.

Interpretation

The direct smear is a method for finding motile trophozoites. The quantity of sample used is so small that this method is not likely to accurately reflect the range of parasites which may be discovered using a concentration technique. Even when a direct smear is found to be positive, a concentration technique is still warranted to detect additional parasite forms. Not all protozoa observed in direct smears are parasitic, and therefore responsible for the clinical signs observed. During bouts of loose stool or diarrhea, intestinal or cecal protozoa can be expelled that are not normally seen during fecal examinations of asymptomatic animals. This is particularly true with herbivores, including reptiles and amphibians, because several ciliates and flagellates participate in digestion. Unwarranted treatment of these protozoa may alter the normal intestinal flora and prolong the symptoms.

Fecal Concentration Methods

The recovery of fecal parasites is enhanced by concentration procedures. These include flotation and sedimentation techniques, both of which depend on differences in specific gravity (sg) between the parasite form and the surrounding solution. Flotation techniques concentrate parasites by employing hypertonic solutions so that parasite forms rise to the surface of the flotation solution, while most debris fall (Table 1.2).

Sedimentation techniques employ solutions less dense than the parasites, so that parasite forms concentrate at the bottom of the collection vessel. Sedimentation methods generally allow for the recovery of more parasites than do flotation methods. With sedimentation, everything can be recovered, whereas with flotation techniques only those items of lower specific gravity than the flotation medium are recovered. Sedimentation techniques also are more easily performed in the field. In contrast, sedimentation has

TABLE 1.2   Common flotation solutions.

Solution	Specific Gravity	Ingredients/1 L H$_2$O
Sodium chloride	1.20	311 g sodium chloride
Sodium nitrate	1.20	338 g sodium nitrate
Sodium nitrate	1.30	616 g sodium nitrate
Sugar	1.20	1170 g sugar*
Sheather's sugar	1.27–1.30	1563 g sugar*
Zinc sulfate	1.20	493 g zinc sulfate

*Requires refrigeration of stock solution or addition of 9 ml phenol as preservative

the disadvantage of greater debris, which can complicate examination. Furthermore, when examining sediment, one must focus through multiple focal planes because parasite forms will drift at different levels within the solution between the slide and the coverslip. This results in longer examination time, versus flotations.

Passive Flotation

Passive flotation relies solely on gravity to separate parasites and debris, and is therefore much less sensitive than centrifugal flotation (discussed below). The densities of many parasite forms are too similar to those of the common flotation media to be recovered without the added force provided by centrifugation.

Although both zinc sulfate or sodium nitrate solutions can be used, zinc sulfate is preferable to sodium nitrate because the latter is more caustic and will degrade many helminth eggs, as well as protozoan cysts. Additionally, sodium nitrate solutions crystallize more quickly than zinc sulfate, and crystallization can distort parasitic structures.

Common mistakes in performing passive flotation include setting up multiple samples at one time and reading each sample as time permits. This results in nonuniformity in flotation time, and greater potential for crystallization to render slides unreadable. To minimize crystallization, slides may remain in place on top of the flotation apparatus until they are ready to be read. However, exceeding the recommended 15-minute flotation may result in salt solutions equilibrating with the internal milieu of the egg or oocyst, either by passive diffusion or by extraction of water into the hypertonic float solution through osmotic forces. As a result, eggs or oocysts will become distorted and no longer buoyant, and may fall away from the microscope slide. False negative results are more often obtained with the last slides to be read.

If zinc sulfate solution is used, all of the slides could be removed and coverslips applied at the 15 minute time point. Slides should then be placed on a rack in a simple humidified chamber to decrease the rate of crystal formation (Figure 1.1). These slides can be removed from the chamber and read as soon as possible, or the chamber placed in a refrigerator to be read later in the day. All salt solutions will crystallize, thus the timing of microscopy is very important.

Materials
- Pill vial or sputum jar
- Small petri dish or watch glass

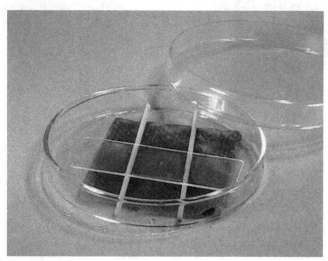

Fig. 1.1 A simple humidified chamber can be assembled to decrease the rate of crystal formation of flotation solutions.

- Disposable cup
- Applicator sticks
- Flotation medium (1.20 sg)
- Microscope slides and coverslips
- Tea strainer

Method

1. Place 2 to 3 g of fecal sample in the disposable plastic cup using the applicator sticks.
2. Add a small quantity of flotation medium and mix into a slurry.
3. Continue adding flotation medium, stirring to mix thoroughly.
4. Place the pill vial in the small petri dish as a guard against overflow.
5. Pour the mixture through the tea strainer into the pill vial, stirring with the applicator sticks to facilitate flow through the strainer.
6. Add drops of the float medium until a slight, bulging meniscus forms above the rim of the vial.
7. Place the microscope slide on top of the meniscus.
8. Allow 15 minutes for parasite forms to rise to the surface.
9. Gently lift the slide from the pill vial, invert the slide, and place a coverslip on the droplets of sample adhering to the slide.
10. Examine the entire coverslip using the 10 × objective, followed by 20 fields using the 40 × objective.

Interpretation

Passive flotation can be used effectively when the technician understands the limitations of the technique. Only a small subset of parasite forms will be recovered even when the technique is performed optimally. Strongyle-type eggs and coccidian oocysts are often passed in sufficient numbers that the poor sensitivity of passive flotation is overcome during routine fecal screening. Other parasite forms may not be sufficiently recovered. For this reason, passive flotation is not the diagnostic method of choice where accuracy is required.

Centrifugal Flotation

Centrifugal flotation is more sensitive than passive flotation because it magnifies gravitational forces, thereby accelerating the downward movement of more dense debris and the upward movement of less dense parasite forms.

The basic process of preparing a fecal sample for centrifugation is identical regardless of the flotation medium to be used. The sample should first be centrifuged with water to remove water-soluble pigments, free lipids, and other small debris.

Flotation solutions range from 1.20–1.30 sg (Table 1.2). The preferred salt solution for examination of fecal samples from carnivores is zinc sulfate at 1.20 sg. Zinc sulfate is sufficiently gentle to protozoal cysts that it enhances their recovery without distortion. Zinc sulfate at 1.20 is less effective at recovery of very dense parasite forms, such as *Physaloptera* eggs. For improved visualization of *Giardia* cysts, drops of Lugol's iodine can be added to the fecal pellet and mixed thoroughly for 30 seconds prior to addition of the zinc sulfate.

In general, sugar solutions are less sensitive than zinc sulfate. Sugar solutions are more viscous than salt solutions, and therefore are not very useful for passive flotation. Sugar solutions should be prepared with a preservative (e.g. formalin) to retard bacterial or yeast growth, since digestion of the sugar molecules will lower the specific gravity. Sheather's sugar is a more concentrated or super-saturated solution (1.30 sg) that is particularly suited for recovery of *Cryptosporidium* sp. oocysts.

Sugar solutions are superior to salt solutions in many ways. Sugar solutions are less expensive to make, do not distort eggs or oocysts to the same degree as salt solutions, and will not crystallize rapidly. The latter advantages mean that prepared slides may be refrigerated for days prior to examination, without loss of parasite structural integrity. Sugar solutions are particularly useful for processing herbivore fecal samples. Flotation solutions should be compared through side-by-side preparations using known positive samples.

Centrifuges with swinging bucket rotors are preferred because they allow each tube to be filled more than is possible with fixed-head rotors. Many diagnosticians prefer to place the coverslip on the sample tube during the centrifugation steps. This is not possible with fixed-head rotors. Because small vibrations can cause a coverslip to be lost during centrifugation, many laboratories perform the centrifugations with the fluid level in the tube at the maximum possible, then transfer the tube into a stationary rack before placing the coverslip on the sample to allow parasite stages to adhere to the coverslip. Sensitivities are equivalent for the two variations, and the difference in time required is negligible.

Materials
- Disposable plastic cups
- Applicator sticks
- Water or saline for washing
- Plastic centrifuge tubes and screens
- Centrifuge; swinging-bucket preferred, but fixed-head is also possible
- Test tube rack
- Flotation solution

Method
1. Place 2 to 3 g of feces in a disposable plastic cup. Mix very well with a small quantity of water and when mixed thoroughly, increase quantity of water to create a loose slurry. The quantity of water used should be approximately the volume of the centrifuge tube being used (approximately 15 ml).
2. Pour this mixture through a screen into a centrifuge tube and assist the passage through the screen by agitating with the applicator sticks.
3. Bring the volume of water in the sample tube to the top of the centrifuge tube, and equal to the volume in a second (balance) tube.
4. Centrifuge at 400 g for 3–5 minutes.
5. Remove sample tube from centrifuge and decant supernatant. If it is difficult to visualize the pellet apart from the supernatant, repeat this washing step by mixing the pellet thoroughly with water or saline a second or third time until the supernatant is clear.

6. Place a small drop of the washed pellet onto a microscope slide and examine as a sediment, or dry for staining.
7. Mix the remainder of the pellet thoroughly with a small volume of the flotation solution of choice, until a loose paste is achieved.
8. Bring the volume of the flotation solution to within millimeters of the rim of the centrifuge tube. Return the tube to the centrifuge. Place a balance tube opposite the sample tube. The specific gravity of water is only 1.00, thus a separate balance tube for flotation solutions is necessary.
9. Centrifuge for 5 minutes; 10 minutes if anticipating *Cryptosporidium* oocysts.
10. Transfer the tubes from the centrifuge to a test tube rack.
11. Add drops of the flotation solution to the top of the tube until a slightly bulging meniscus is formed. Do not overfill the tube because the floating parasite stages will be lost.
12. Place a coverslip on the slightly bulging meniscus and allow to stand 10 additional minutes.
13. Remove the coverslip to a microscope slide for examination.

Interpretation
Common mistakes in the performance of centrifugal flotation, which result in false negative results include:
1. Failure to thoroughly mix the sample with water prior to passage through the screen into the centrifuge tube, resulting in failure of parasite forms to pass through the screen. Often, too much water is added initially, so that the fecal sample drifts about without breaking apart.
2. Failure to stir or agitate the fecal slurry as it passes through the screen, rather than allowing it to simply drip through the tube, resulting in the buildup of debris on the screen that traps the suspended eggs or oocysts. This mat must be disrupted by stirring with the applicator sticks.
3. Failure to mix the pellet formed after centrifugation with a small quantity of flotation medium before filling the tube. The pellet is difficult to mix when the tube is too full with solution. Failure to mix adequately will trap any eggs or oocysts within the pellet, reducing sensitivity.
4. Overfilling the tube so that instead of forming a meniscus, parasite forms spill out of the tube and are lost.

Baermann Sedimentation

The Baermann technique uses simple gravity sedimentation to recover nematode larvae, either from a fecal culture or from tissue digests that liberate any larvae that may be present. The sample is placed into a funnel with warm water to facilitate nematode motility. Pulmonary tissues may be homogenized in a blender to recover lungworms, and diaphragm or other muscle tissues may be homogenized and placed in a Baermann apparatus for recovery of *Trichinella spiralis* larvae.

Materials
- Fine screen mesh or sieve, nylon coffee filter, or cheesecloth
- Funnel with latex tubing attached, with clamp
- Ring stand to hold funnel
- Collection tube
- Dish to collect spillage
- Petri plate for microscopic examination of the collected sediment
- Warm water to fill the Baermann apparatus

Method
1. Place clamp on latex tubing in open position and attach one end of the tubing to the funnel.
2. Insert collecting tube into the other end.
3. Place funnel assembly into a ring stand.
4. Add warm water to fill latex tubing and collecting tube until the funnel is half full.
5. Loosely wrap fecal or tissue sample in cheesecloth or place into sieve or coffee filter.
6. Place the sample into the funnel and gently fill with warm water until the sample is covered.
7. Leave the sample in the funnel for 12 to 18 hours.
8. Clamp the latex tube to prevent excess water from draining when the collecting tube is removed from the latex.
9. Decant the collected volume into a petri plate and examine this sediment for larvae.

Interpretation
The Baermann sedimentation is a technique often requested inappropriately due to a misunderstanding of its strengths and weaknesses. Historically, the Baermann has been used to recover cattle lungworm and strongylid larvae from feces. These larvae are very active and will swim free of the fecal sample. With parasitic infections that pass eggs or oocysts, or less active larvae, the Baermann sedimentation is far less sensitive than centrifugal flotation techniques. The first-stage larvae of most Metastrongyloidea are not active

enough to free themselves from the feces in which they were passed, since these nematodes use gastropods as intermediate hosts. Gastropods are drawn to feces for the nitrogenous meal that feces can provide, thus active larvae that leave the feces are less likely to be consumed by gastropods. This feature favors larvae that remain with the feces. In contrast, cattle lungworms and larvae of strongylid nematodes develop directly on pasture without an intermediate host. Larvae of these nematodes more actively extricate themselves from the fecal sample.

Simple Gravity Sedimentation

Simple gravity sedimentation can be performed without a centrifuge and is intended to collect parasite eggs too dense to recover with common flotation media, such as eggs of *Fasciola hepatica*. It also cleans some debris and water-soluble pigments in the process of decanting. The process involves a two-step sedimentation and decanting method whereby the first step follows a brief sedimentation that removes the densest debris while the parasite forms remain in the water column that is decanted into a second vessel for the second, longer sedimentation step. A pilsner glass or funnel-shaped vessel provides an advantage over a flat-bottom beaker in that the sediment is concentrated into the narrow bottom of the pilsner glass.

Materials
- Fecal sample and mixing container
- Water or saline
- Pilsner glasses or conical, round-bottomed vessels, approximately 250 ml capacity
- Petri dish for microscopic examination
- Methylene blue as an optional stain

Method
1. Mix the fecal sample in a container using water or saline of the approximate volume of the pilsner glass or other vessel.
2. Suspend the sample well and pour into the pilsner glass.
3. Allow the heaviest debris to sediment for about 2 minutes.
4. Decant the suspended sample into the second pilsner glass and allow this to sediment for at least 2 hours.
5. Decant the supernatant carefully so as to leave the sediment undisturbed.
6. Pour aliquots of the sediment into a petri dish and examine with a dissecting microscope. Several drops of methylene blue can add contrast to aid in visualization.

Interpretation

This sedimentation technique is applicable for heavy eggs, such as those of *Fasciola hepatica* or *Schistosoma* sp. It is readily applicable to field work.

Formalin-ethyl Acetate Sedimentation

Formalin-ethyl acetate sedimentation uses ethyl acetate as a non-miscible solvent to extract lipid from feces. Ethyl acetate forms a layer above the water or saline. The extracted portion of lipid is drawn into the ethyl acetate plug and can be discarded with the supernatant (Figure 1.2).

Formalin-ethyl acetate sedimentation is useful for cleaning steatorrhea or other diarrheic feces, thereby facilitating microscopic examination. The pellet can be examined directly, to prepare smears for staining, or for flotation procedures. Formalin-ethyl acetate sedimentation is highly efficient in recovering all parasite forms, including trophozoites, cysts, oocysts, eggs, and larvae. It is commonly used in human diagnostic laboratories. Formalin is used to kill any pathogens present, but water or saline can be employed to retain motility of protozoan trophozoites as an aid in identification. The use of formalin is most desirable where the concern of zoonotic disease is high, such as with non-human primates.

Most common intestinal parasites can be recovered using flotation techniques; however, sedimentation procedures are warranted where test sensitivity must be maximized. Viewing sediments can be tedious due to the range of focal planes that must be traversed. Formalin-ethyl acetate sedimentation, followed by centrifugal flotation, results in high sensitivity and economy of effort.

Materials

- Phosphate buffered saline (PBS) with or without 10% formalin (water can be used when trophozoites are not anticipated)
- Disposable plastic cup for mixing the fecal sample
- Applicator or stir sticks
- Polypropylene centrifuge tubes with caps
- Filter funnel
- Ethyl acetate
- Cotton swabs

Method

1. Place sample in a sealable container; add PBS with 10% NBF. Allow approximately 20 minutes for fixation.
2. Pour the sample through the filter screen into a polypropylene centrifuge tube to a volume of 10 ml.

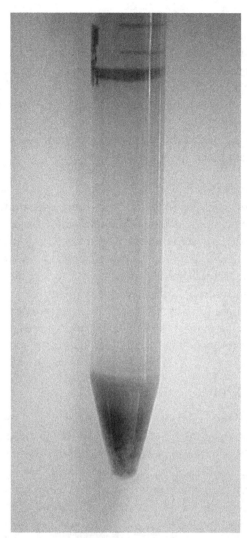

Fig. 1.2 Formalin–ethyl acetate sedimentation. Ethyl acetate forms a layer above the water or saline. The extracted portion of lipid is drawn into the ethyl acetate plug and can be discarded with the supernatant.

Polypropylene tubes are necessary due to the solvent activity of the ethyl acetate.
3. Add 3 ml of ethyl acetate to the sample; cap and shake vigorously to mix.
4. Centrifuge at 1,000 rpm for 5 to 10 minutes (10 minutes if *Cryptosporidium* is suspected).
5. Remove the tube from the centrifuge, remove the cap, and, using a stir stick, ring the plug of ethyl acetate and any trapped debris, freeing the plug from the wall of the centrifuge tube.
6. Decant the supernatant and ethyl acetate plug into a disposal container that will not be degraded by the ethyl acetate.

7. Using a cotton swab, remove residual ethyl acetate around the tube or perform another washing step to clean the pellet of any additional ethyl acetate droplets. These droplets can resemble amoebic cysts and confuse the microscopic interpretation.
8. Add a small amount of saline to the pellet and resuspend.
9. Place drops of this suspension on a microscope slide, place a coverslip on top, and examine.

Interpretation

The ethyl acetate plug can trap some eggs and cysts. Specific examples include *Alaria canis* and *Giardia intestinalis*. Ethyl acetate must not be discarded into municipal sewage systems but must be collected for disposal through an appropriate chemical processing system. For this reason alone, many laboratories may find it preferable to do several washing steps with saline or tap water to remove free lipid droplets and water-soluble pigments, instead of performing formalin-ethyl acetate sedimentation.

Fecal Stains

Preparation of slides for staining should be part of a routine diagnostic workup for symptomatic patients, but it serves little purpose for asymptomatic animals. Once prepared, the slides can be stained or held pending results of flotation or sedimentation procedures. Slides can also be prepared from the cleaned fecal pellet prior to the final centrifugation with the flotation medium.

Basic staining procedures adaptable to most laboratories include the Gram stain and the modified acid-fast stain. More specialized stains, such as Gomori's trichrome or Masson's trichrome stains, and the iron hematoxylin stain, can be included in the repertoire if consistent need dictates. Otherwise, it is generally more expedient and reliable to send fixed slides or samples to specialized laboratories that perform these techniques regularly. The shelf-life of reagents affects the decision whether to perform specialized stains in-house or to outsource them. Older reagents give unsatisfactory results. The Gram stain can be used for differentiating *Giardia* sp. from *Candida*-like, elliptical yeast, which stain Gram positive, whereas *Giardia* contain both positive and negative structures within the cyst. The method for performing the Gram stain is presented in microbiology laboratory manuals and will not be described here.

Modified Acid-fast Stain

The modified acid-fast stain can be used to detect *Cryptosporidium* sp. and fecal microsporidia. This procedure does not require heating of the slide or stain and uses a brilliant green counterstain, which facilitates visualization.

Materials

- Microscope slides, coverslip optional
- Absolute methanol
- Carbol fuchsin stain
- Acid alcohol decolorizer
- Brilliant green stain
- Immersion oil

Method

1. Air dry droplets of the fecal sample or smear on a clean glass slide.
2. Fix the dried slide in methanol for 2 minutes.
3. Cover the fecal smear with carbol fuchsin for 2 minutes.
4. Rinse gently with tap water.
5. Apply drops of the acid alcohol decolorizer for 1 to 6 seconds.
6. Rinse gently with tap water.
7. Cover the smear with brilliant green counterstain for 2 minutes.
8. Rinse gently with tap water, then blot or air dry until ready to examine microscopically.

Interpretation

The best results will be obtained when the fecal sample has been washed by centrifugations with water, or subjected to the ethyl acetate extraction process prior to placing droplets on slides. Smears must be uniformly thin and translucent for even decolorization, otherwise over-decolorization can result in false negatives.

The staining procedure is easy to perform but does require perfecting several steps in the process. Thin, homogeneous smears are very important because small particles of debris will leach carbol fuchsin during the decolorizing step and this may lead to excessive decolorizing time. A positive sample should be obtained and used to perfect the technique.

When the slide is dry it can be examined with oil immersion, but the red-stained oocysts are readily visible with lower power objectives. Place a drop of immersion oil on the stained sample before adding a coverslip. This compensates for light refraction from an otherwise irregular surface, and facilitates identification of stained oocysts.

Antigen and Fluorescent Antibody Diagnostics

Parasite antigens pass in feces and in some cases, are more readily identified using antigen tests than are parasite forms using microscopic examination. Test procedures include direct and indirect immunofluorescent antibodies directed at parasite antigens, enzyme immunoassays, and membrane chromatographic assays. Fluorescent antibodies directed against parasite antigens facilitate detection, but require use of a microscope with a UV light source. Enzyme immunoassays are labor intensive and are therefore most susceptible to operator error. Rapid chromatographic membrane assays are the most applicable to a typical diagnostic laboratory. They are very simple to perform but are more expensive per individual than enzyme immunoassay.

Antigen tests are not intended to replace microscopic examination, but to serve as useful adjuncts to microscopy. Eggs, oocysts, and larvae that do not react with the primary antibodies used in the assay will go undetected if an antigen test is used as the sole diagnostic procedure. However, some protozoan cysts or oocysts are not passed consistently, resulting in the need to perform multiple fecal examinations to ensure accurate diagnostic outcome. This is particularly true for the genera *Giardia, Cryptosporidium,* and *Entamoeba.* In these cases, antigen detection tests may facilitate diagnosis.

Most of the commercially available tests for fecal antigen detection are marketed for human diagnostics. The range of commercially available antigen detection kits applicable to laboratory animals is limited. Lists of currently available commercial human parasite antigen detection kits are available online through the Centers for Disease Control and Prevention.

DETECTION OF MICROFILARIA

Filarid nematodes produce MF that are ingested by biting arthropod intermediate hosts during a blood meal. Depending upon parasite species, blood or tissue samples may be collected and processed for the recovery and identification of MF. For select filarid infections of animals, antigen detection is possible using commercially available antigen detection kits such as for *Dirofilaria immitis.* These may be used regardless of host species. In contrast, detection kits that recognize host antibodies generated to parasite-specific antigens rarely have cross-species applications.

Blood

For large animals, a 1 ml venous blood sample provides sufficient sample for testing. For animals too small to provide this volume, a microhematocrit tube can be filled, and, following centrifugation, the tube placed on a microscope stage and the area of the buffy coat examined for MF. The interface between the buffy coat and the plasma fraction is most productive. The microhematocrit tube can be scored and broken at this junction to harvest any MF that may be present, saving the red cells for blood films and the serum or plasma for other tests.

Direct Smear or Wet Mount

The volume used in preparing a wet mount is so small that this is not intended to serve as a definitive diagnostic test, but merely as a quick screening tool for the presence of MF.

Materials
- Saline
- Applicator stick
- Microscope slides and coverslips

Method
1. Place a drop of saline on a microscope slide.
2. Mix a drop of the blood sample into the saline droplet.
3. Apply a coverslip and examine for MF.

Interpretation
A wet mount typically will not provide sufficient visualization to make identification of genus or species possible. Saline is important to dilute the red cells without rupturing them, as might a hypotonic solution. Samples that have been refrigerated may require brief warming for MF to resume activity.

Modified Knott's Test

The modified Knott's test uses a hypotonic solution to lyse red blood cells (RBC), leaving the white blood cells (WBC) and MF intact. A solution of 2% formalin in distilled water is often used to straighten the MF, facilitating identification. If visualization alone is desired, using distilled water without formalin allows the MF to continue moving, which can aid in detection. A centrifuge is most desirable for pelleting the lysate, but recovery of MF can be achieved by passive sedimentation.

Materials
- Centrifuge tubes, 12 to 15 ml
- Lysing and fixative solution (2% formalin/distilled water)
- 0.1% new methylene blue
- Microscope slides and coverslips

Method
1. Add 1 ml of blood to a centrifuge tube.
2. Add 9 ml of hypotonic lysing buffer (2% formalin/distilled water).
3. Invert the tube several times, causing the RBCs to rupture.
4. Centrifuge for 3–5 minutes at low speed.
5. Decant the supernatant carefully to retain the pellet in the bottom of the tube.
6. Add a drop of 0.1% new methylene blue and mix with the pellet.
7. Place a drop of this mixture on a microscope slide and coverslip for examination.

Polycarbonate Filter Technique

The polycarbonate filter technique uses a filter and filter housing unit as components of a commercially available kit. Therefore, this test is more expensive to perform than the Knott's test. However, the polycarbonate filter technique does not require a centrifuge. MF can be recovered, but it is not as easily visualized and identified to species as with the Knott's test. The polycarbonate filter technique is intended to detect only the presence of MF in animals known or suspected to be infected with adult filarid nematodes, such as dogs already determined to be antigen positive for *Dirofilaria immitis* infection.

Materials
- Syringe, 12 to 15 ml
- Filter housing and filters
- 0.1% methylene blue
- Lysing buffer (distilled water will suffice)
- Microscope slides and coverslips

Method
1. Draw 1 ml of blood into a 12 to 15 ml syringe.
2. Draw at least 9 ml lysing buffer into the syringe.
3. Invert for 2 minutes.

4. Place polycarbonate filter into filter holder, verifying that the gasket seal is in place.
5. Affix the filter apparatus to the syringe.
6. Slowly expel the lysed blood solution through the filter.
7. Remove the filter apparatus and refill the syringe with water.
8. Replace the filter apparatus onto the syringe.
9. Slowly expel the wash water through the filter to remove excess debris.
10. Remove the filter apparatus and refill the syringe with air.
11. Reattach the filter apparatus and flush the filter with air.
12. Remove the filter from the holder and place on a microscope slide with the side containing MF facing up.
13. Add a drop or two of methylene blue solution.
14. Place a coverslip on the liquid and examine for MF.

Interpretation
The polycarbonate filter technique is used when the genus or species of the MF, if present, is known. Clear visualization of MF, for identification of genus or species, requires the Knott's test.

Skin Samples

Some arthropods which transmit filarid nematodes feed on serum or plasma rather than whole blood. In these cases, MF are found within tissues such as the skin, rather than circulating in the blood stream. Skin biopsies must be processed to free the MF for visualization.

Materials
- Skin biopsy instruments
- Scalpel blades
- Pipettes
- Saline without preservative
- Microscope slides and coverslips
- Centrifuge tubes, 15 to 50 ml depending on sample size

Method
1. Macerate biopsy sample using a scalpel blade.
2. Place macerated material into a centrifuge tube with saline.
3. Incubate overnight at 37°C.
4. Remove tissue, then centrifuge for 3 to 5 minutes at low speed.
5. Carefully decant supernatant.

6. Using a pipette, place drops of the sediment on a microscope slide.
7. Place a coverslip on the drops and examine at low power (10 × objective).

Interpretation

The tissue sample does not need to be finely homogenized because the MF have motility and can extricate themselves from the macerated sample. The tube does need incubation near body temperature to facilitate motility.

MICROSCOPY TECHNIQUES

Standard Practice for Reading Microscope Slides

A standard approach to microscopic examinations of prepared specimens is essential for effective and efficient diagnoses of parasitic infections.

For fecal examinations, the 10 × objective is most commonly used, and the entire coverslip is examined systematically. Beginning at one corner of the coverslip, the slide is moved either vertically or horizontally in a direct line to the other corner of the coverslip. A mental notation is made of a small object just at the edge of the optical field, and the slide is moved just far enough to bring the object to the boundary of the new optical field. The objective is moved in a direct line back across the coverslip. The process is repeated until the entire coverslip has been examined with the 10 × objective. During these direct horizontal or vertical sweeps, the operator must learn to use the fine focus adjustment to change focal planes continuously because the smallest objects will be visible in different focal planes than those of larger diameter. Once the entire coverslip has been examined with the 10 × objective, 20 random fields should be examined with the 40 × objective, again, using the fine adjustment to compensate for changes in focal plane.

For blood films, or permanent mounts to be examined with the oil immersion lens (typically the 100 × objective), each laboratory must establish a standard number of fields to be examined, or a standard number of sweeps across the coverslip. The size of coverslip used should also be standardized. Coverslip dimensions of 22 × 22 mm are most commonly used. Larger sizes may have special application, but are too large for standard use.

Use of the Ocular Micrometer

An ocular micrometer is essential for accurate diagnoses. Measurements are often important for differentiating parasites from pseudoparasites, such as differentiating a grain mite egg from a parasitic strongyle-type egg. Differentiating larvae in a fecal sample or MF recovered from a Knott's test relies on measurements. A micrometer is placed in one of the ocular pieces of the microscope. The micrometer must be calibrated using a standardized, commercially available, etched microscope slide. Parasite eggs and oocysts are described in reference texts within a range of measurements because the area under the coverslip is three-dimensional, and eggs or oocysts can rotate within that space, so that objects may be viewed and measured while lying at different angles.

REFERENCES

1. Centers for Disease Control and Prevention. Division of Parasitic Diseases, Diagnostic Parasitology website: http://www.dpd.cdc.gov/dpdx/
2. Ash, L.R. and Orihel, T.C. (1991) *Parasites: A Guide to Laboratory Procedures and Identification.* American Society of Clinical Pathologists, Chicago.
3. Garcia, L.S. (2001) *Diagnostic Medical Parasitology,* 4th ed. American Society of Microbiology Press, Herndon, VA.

Biology of the Protozoa

David S. Lindsay, PhD, and Christine A. Sundermann, MS, PhD

INTRODUCTION

Protozoa are single-celled eukaryotes. They are a structurally and genetically diverse multiphyletic group of organisms (Figures 2.1, 2.2, 2.3, and 2.4)[1,2,3]. Many protozoa have features in common with fungi or algae, and the term "protist" is often used instead of "protozoa" to emphasize this fact.

FLAGELLATES: PHYLA EUGLENOZOA, PARABASALIA, RETORTAMONADA, AXOSTYLATA, CHROMISTA

Flagellated protozoans, sometimes referred to as "mastigophorans," can be either free-living or parasitic. The major groups which contain parasitic species are the kinetoplastid flagellates, parabasalians, and retortamonads;

these group names are sometimes elevated to class or phylum by various taxonomists[4].

Special Organelles

Whereas free-living flagellates typically possess a full complement of organelles, many parasitic flagellates lack one or more common organelles, and instead possess unique structures. For example, the trophozoite stage of most flagellates contains one nucleus, whereas *Giardia* spp. are binucleated (Figure 2.5)[5].

The kinetoplastid flagellates (e.g., *Leishmania* spp., *Trypanosoma* spp.) contain a unique structure, the kinetoplast. The kinetoplast is a large mass of mitochondrial DNA positioned near the flagellar basal body. Kinetoplast DNA exists as mini- and maxicircles and is located at one end of the cell's single mitochondrion[6], which is sometimes

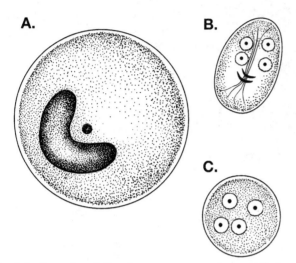

Fig. 2.1 Examples of diversity among protozoal cysts. (A) Cyst of a ciliate. (B) Cyst of a flagellate. (C) Cyst of an amoeba.

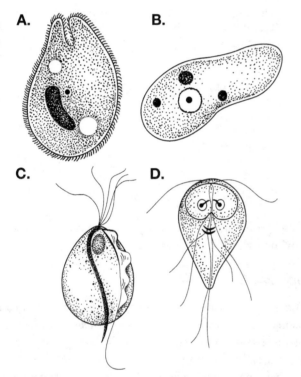

Fig. 2.2 Examples of diversity among protozoal trophozoites. (A) Trophozoite of a ciliate. (B) Trophozoite of an amoeba. (C) and (D) Trophozoites of flagellates.

referred to as the chondriome. Kinetoplast DNA readily stains with traditional DNA stains, and is easily observable under light microscopy. The glycosome is another organelle unique to some developmental stages of kinetoplastid flagellates. This membrane-bound organelle contains enzymes

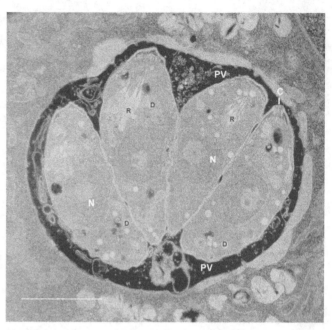

Fig. 2.3 A group of *Toxoplasma gondii* tachyzoites in a parasitophorous vacuole (PV) in a human fibroblast cell. The apical end (C) is clearly visible in 1 tachyzoite. The nucleus (N), rhoptries (R), and dense granules (D) are also readily visible in several tachyzoites. Transmission electron micrograph. Bar = 2 micrometers.

that function in the glycolytic pathway, and thus it is responsible for efficient, compartmentalized oxidation of glucose, resulting in high rates of glycolysis[7].

The parabasalians (e.g., *Tritrichomonas* spp., *Histomonas* spp.) possess an array of cellular features (e.g., nucleus, flagella, basal bodies, axostyle, costa, parabasal body, parabasal fiber) organized into a "karyomastigont system"[8] (Figure 2.6). The axostyle is a bundle of parallel, cross-linked microtubules extending from the anterior basal bodies of the flagella to the posterior end of the cell. The costa is a flexible rod-like structure with a striated appearance. It also originates near the anterior end of the cell and extends posteriorly. Functionally, the parabasal body is a large Golgi complex visible under light microscopy. It is associated with a parabasal fiber which originates near the anterior basal bodies. Trichomonad parabasalians lack mitochondria and instead possess hydrogenosomes. These are membrane-bound organelles that metabolize sugars and produce H_2 as an end product[9]. Ingestion of nutrients by many flagellates is typically by pinocytosis, although some use a cytostome (e.g., *Chilomastix* spp.).

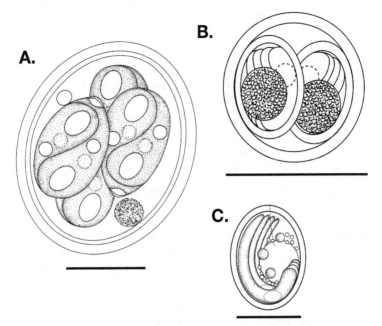

Fig. 2.4 Sporulated oocyst of coccidia. (A) *Eimeria* type. Bar = 10 μ. (B) *Cystoisospora* type. Bar = 10 μ. (C) *Cryptosporidium* type. Bar = 5 μ. (A) Reproduced from Lindsay, D.S., Upton, S.J., and Hildreth, M.B. (1999) with permission. (B) Reproduced from Lindsay, D.S., Upton, S.J., and Dubey, J.P. (1999) with permission. (C) Reproduced from Lindsay, D.S., Upton, S.J., Owens, D.S., Morgan, U.M., Mead, J.R., and Blagburn, B.L. (2000) with permission.

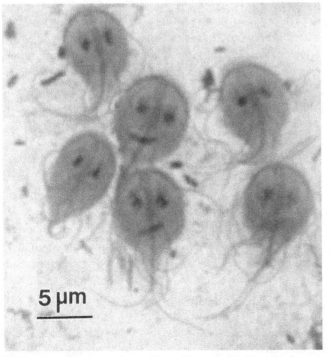

Fig. 2.5 Trophozoites of *Giardia* sp. Giemsa-stained intestinal smear from a hamster.

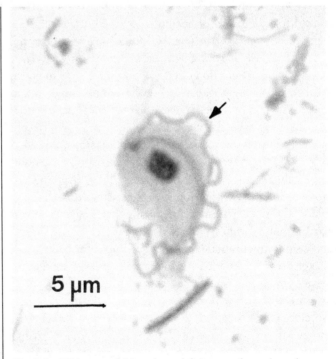

Fig. 2.6 Trichomonad. Note the undulating membrane (arrow).

Locomotion

Most flagellates possess one or more flagella; however, a few parasitic species have no visible external flagellum (e.g., *Dientamoeba* spp. and amastigotes of kinetoplastid flagellates)[10]. Flagella, although usually longer, are structurally similar to cilia in that they contain a 9 + 2 arrangement of microtubules. Most flagellates move by beating flagella in an undulating, whip-like, ATP-dependent manner. In some species, the flagellum is modified to form an "undulating membrane" such that an expanded membrane connects the flagellum to the cell surface. The result is a cell that appears to have a ruffled or curled area on one edge. A few flagellates have no external flagellum, although they retain basal bodies. Some species (e.g., *Dientamoeba fragilis* and *Histomonas meleagridis*) move in an amoeboid manner.

Life Cycles

The majority of flagellates reproduce by longitudinal binary fission. Sexual reproduction is practiced by very few species[11]. Intestinal dwellers are usually extracellular and are transmitted by the fecal-oral route. Most enteric flagellates encyst before exiting the host; and nuclear multiplication in the cyst may (e.g., *Giardia* spp.), or may not (e.g., *Chilomastix* spp.), occur. In one group, encystment is linked to production of hormones by the host so that the life cycles of protozoan (e.g., *Opalina* spp.) and host are linked. A few species (e.g., *Dientamoeba fragilis*, *Histomonas meleagridis*) do not encyst, and transfer to the next host relies on rapid transmission of trophozoites or other means, such as transfer via nematode eggs.

Kinetoplastid flagellates live in the extra- or intracellular environment, depending on the parasite species. Some (e.g., *Trypanosoma cruzi*, *Leishmania* spp.) have both intracellular (amastigote) and extracellular (trypomastigote, promastigote) stages in their life cycles. Most of these blood and tissue parasites rely on a hematophagous vector (arthropods, leeches) for transmission to a new host. In some kinetoplastid species, distinct developmental stages occur in the vector, while other species undergo no development but merely use the vector for mechanical transmission to the next host. Antigenic variation during developmental stages is a well known phenomenon[12]. A few important flagellated parasites, including *Tritrichomonas foetus* and *Trypanosoma equiperdum,* are venereally transmitted.

AMOEBA: PHYLUM HETEROLOBOSA

This phylum contains free-living, parasitic, and opportunistically parasitic amoebae, also commonly called "sarcodines." Phyla that contain species that are not parasitic in laboratory animals are not included here. Genera with the greatest medical and veterinary importance include *Acanthamoeba* spp., *Entamoeba* spp., and *Naegleria* spp. Many enteric amoebae are obligate commensals and not associated with disease.

Special Organelles

Amoebae are noted for possessing pseudopods for locomotion and food capture and ingestion, a single type of nucleus, and a lack of centrioles and cytoplasmic microtubules, though they do possess mitotic spindle microtubules. Pseudopods possessed by amoebae include (a) lobose pseudopods, which are transitory, cytoplasmic extensions with blunt or pointed ends, (b) actinopods, which are pointed and contain extrusomes and an inner core of microtubules, (c) filopods, which are very slender and filiform, and (d) reticulopods, which are web-like networks.

Many amoebae have two distinct regions of the cell. The ectoplasm is an outer, clearer, more viscous region surrounding the second distinct region, the endoplasm. The endoplasm is less viscous cytoplasm, and therefore appears denser. Some species have no identifiable anterior region of the cell unless the cell is moving; the anterior region then appears at the leading edge. The posterior region of the cell, the "uroid," is where myosin filaments are often concentrated. Actin microfilaments are found in the ectoplasmic regions. Most amoebae contain Golgi bodies, contractile vacuoles, food vacuoles, and mitochondria.

Amoebae obtain dissolved nutrients by pinocytosis, and larger particulate nutrients by phagocytosis. In both processes, invagination of the cell membrane occurs so that food enters the cell in a food vacuole that is completed when the membrane pinches off. Invagination of the membrane is accomplished through an actin-myosin system[13]. Several species of amoebae form a more prominent ingestion area, the amoebostome, which is large, rounded, and cup-shaped. Digestion in the food vacuole is initiated by hydrolytic enzymes, and waste products are released from the cell by exocytosis. Ingestion of prey is more complex for amoebae with axopods. Many species of parasitic amoebae contain a glycogen vacuole, which is a storage depot for carbohydrates.

Amoebae living in hypo-osmotic environments osmoregulate by use of a contractile vacuole. This organelle usually has no permanent position in the cell. The contractile vacuole can be visualized with light microscopy when it increases in size[14].

The nuclear structure of amoebae is diverse and species-specific. For example, *Entamoeba* spp. possess chromatin "granules" which may be circularly arranged adjacent to the inner nuclear membrane, or may be arranged in coarse clumps. This type of chromatin contains rRNA genes undergoing transcription, can be seen in stained slides, and the arrangement of the chromatin can be species-specific[15]. Additionally, some species possess a round, RNA-rich karyosome (endosome) which persists during mitosis and whose function is not known. The cysts of still other species possess a chromatoidal bar whose shape is of taxonomic importance. This bar is usually more noticeable in younger cysts and is formed from the crystallization of ribonucleoproteins arising from small, cytoplasmic helical bodies.

Locomotion

Most amoebae move by use of pseudopods, which are cytoplasmic extensions that can have a fixed or non-fixed position (Figure 2.7). Nearly all parasitic amoebae possess lobose pseudopods, which have a globular shape with rounded (e.g., *Entamoeba* spp., *Naegleria* spp.) or pointed (e.g., *Acanthamoeba* spp.) ends. Some species have only one pseudopod (monopodial) while others have two or more (polypodial).

During movement, a clear, hyaline, somewhat rigid cap forms at the leading edge of the lobose pseudopod. Endoplasm flows anteriorly and against the hyaline cap, then flows laterally until it is converted into the adjacent ectoplasm. Ectoplasm is converted back to endoplasm in the region of the uroid. Formation of, and movement by, pseudopods occurs by directed cytoplasmic streaming, or through a rolling motion. Force is provided by a system containing actin-myosin[16].

Actin microfilaments are located throughout the ectoplasm and are parallel to the cell membrane at the anterior end of a moving cell. Actin monomers are located in the endoplasm, and myosin filaments are concentrated near the uroid[17]. Amoeboflagellates such as *Naegleria fowleri* possess lobose pseudopods in both free-living and parasitic states, but can quickly form two flagella when food is limiting, enabling them to swim to more nutrient-rich areas.

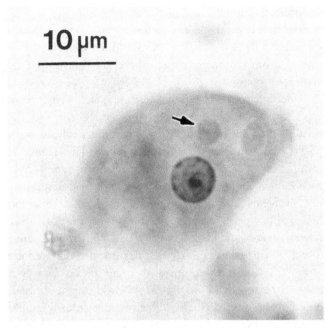

Fig. 2.7 Trophozoite of *Entamoeba histolytica*. An ingested red blood cell (arrow) is labeled. Iron-hematoxylin stain of human feces.

To do this, microtubules must be assembled *de novo,* and can be functional in little more than a hour[18].

Life Cycles

Intestinal amoebae have direct life cycles and transmission is fecal-oral. These species form cysts when they reach the lower large intestine. Multiplication may (e.g., *Entamoeba* spp.) or may not (e.g., *Iodamoeba* spp.) occur in the cyst. Amoeboflagellates normally are free-living in soil and water where they exist as trophozoites that ingest bacteria. Amoeboflagellates form environmentally resistant cysts under conditions of reduced environmental temperatures. Rarely, *Naegleria* spp., *Acanthamoeba* spp., and *Balamuthia mandrillaris* may enter a host and multiply as trophozoites[19]. It is assumed that this is a dead-end cycle and further transmission will not occur. *Acanthamoeba* spp. and *B. mandrillaris* also form cysts in host tissue, whereas *Naegleria* spp do not.

COCCIDIA AND COCCIDIA-LIKE PARASITES: PHYLUM APICOMPLEXA

Apicomplexan parasites include the coccidia, malaria and malaria-like parasites, and piroplasms of vertebrates.

Laboratory animals are important models for human infections caused by these parasites. Some apicomplexa have direct or two-host life cycles and are transmitted by the fecal-oral route, whereas others are transmitted by arthropod vectors.

Coccidian parasites with direct life cycles (*Cystoisospora* spp.) can be a chronic problem in kennels and catteries because they are transmitted by environmentally resistant oocyst stages and are difficult to eradicate. The tissue cyst forming coccidia that have two-host life cycles (*Toxoplasma gondii, Neospora caninum, Sarcocystis* spp., *Besnoitia* spp.) are not problems in modern animal facilities. Malaria and malaria-like blood parasites (*Plasmodium, Haemoproteus, Leucozytozoon*), and piroplasms (*Babesia, Theileria*) are rarely found in laboratory animal facilities because they require arthropod vectors to complete their life cycles. However, these parasites may be present in wild-caught animals brought into animal facilities. Wild-caught animals should be routinely examined for blood parasites as part of the quarantine program. Blood-borne apicomplexa may be found in zoos where animals are exposed to arthropod vectors.

Special Organelles

Motile stages of coccidian parasites possess an assemblage of organelles which form the apical complex. These include the polar rings, rhoptries, micronemes, dense granules, conoid, and subpellicular microtubules[20] (Figure 2.3). The apical complex is used for host cell penetration. Rhoptries, micronemes, and dense granules contain complex mixtures of proteins that, upon exocytosis, interact with host cell membranes during host cell invasion[21]. Rhoptries are osmiophilic, electron-dense, club-shaped structures originating in the conoidal end of sporozoites and merozoites. They usually are anteriorly positioned in the parasite and lay between the nucleus and conoid. In only a few instances have these structures been found in the posterior portion of the parasite. Rhoptry proteins are involved in parasitophorous vacuole formation. The number of rhoptries varies depending on the species of parasite. Micronemes are osmiophilic, electron-dense, rod-like bodies that are most numerous in the anterior one-half of the parasite. They are involved in host cell attachment by invasive stages[22]. Dense granules are electron-dense bodies that are primarily involved in modifying the host cell after invasion. The conoid is a hollow, truncated cone composed of spirally arranged microfibrillar elements[20]. The conoid usually is not present in merozoites of malarial and piroplasm parasites. The subpellicular microtubule cytoskeleton is important in locomotion and host cell invasion.

The body of coccidian parasites usually is enclosed by a trimembranous pellicle. Refractile bodies are osmiophilic, electron-dense, homogenous structures, present in sporozoites of many *Eimeria* species (Figure 2.4), and can sometimes be found in first-generation meronts and merozoites of some species[23]. Generally, two refractile bodies are present in sporozoites—one anterior and one posterior to the nucleus. Crystalloid bodies are accumulations of dense material resembling β-glycogen particles[24]. They are found in sporozoites and merozoites of some *Cystoisospora* species in the same location as eimerian refractile bodies. The functions of refractile bodies and crystalloid bodies are not completely known. They are believed to serve as energy reserves for the parasite. Refractile bodies may also play a role in host cell invasion. Lipid and amylopectin bodies may also be found in sporozoites and merozoites. Wall-forming bodies are specialized structures found in the macrogamonts of coccidial parasites, producing environmentally resistant oocyst walls. There are usually two types of wall-forming bodies. Oocyst wall formation represents a sequential release of the contents of wall-forming bodies types 1 and 2, and is probably controlled in the rough endoplasmic reticulum and/or Golgi bodies[25].

Locomotion

Apicomplexan invasive stages exhibit a unique form of actin-based gliding motility, which is essential for host cell invasion and spreading of parasites throughout the infected host[26]. Living sporozoites and merozoites undergo gliding, pivoting, and probing motions. Microgametes of most coccidia move by flagella. Macrogamonts and coccidial oocysts are usually non-motile.

Life Cycles

Coccidia

The typical coccidian life cycle (Figure 2.8) consists of three phases: sporogony, excystation and endogenous development. Sporogony, which occurs outside of the host in the environment, is the development of the unsporulated noninfectious oocyst into the sporulated infectious oocyst (Figure 2.4). Environmental temperature, oxygen levels, and moisture influence sporogony. Temperatures above 35°C

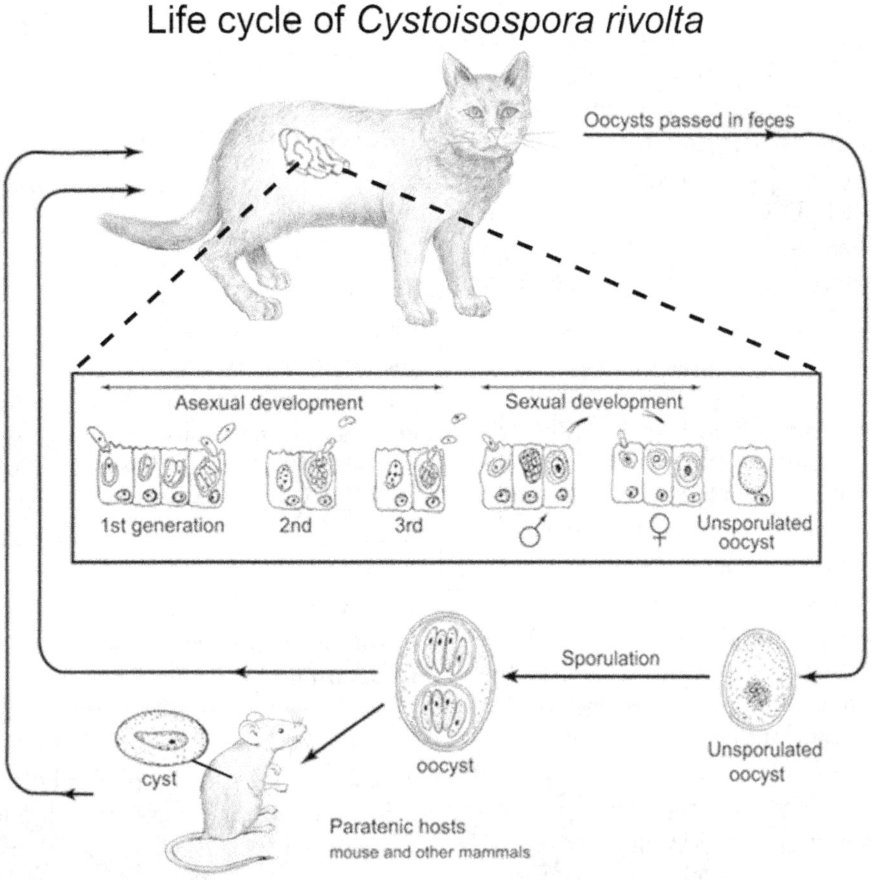

Fig. 2.8 Life cycle of *Cystoisospora rivolta* in the cat.

and below 10°C inhibit sporogony. Unsporulated oocysts may survive freezing to −7°C for nearly two months but can be killed after 24 hours at 40°C. Oocysts do not survive desiccation. Sporogony normally is an aerobic process.

Excystation occurs in the host and is the process by which sporozoites are released from sporocysts and eventually from the oocyst. Excystation of oocysts is not species-specific. Oocysts may excyst in nearly any host, but sporozoites fail to produce infections in abnormal hosts.

Endogenous development varies among coccidia, though the basic pattern is similar for all species. Intracellular developmental stages are located within a parasitophorous vacuole composed of the host cell plasma membrane. Sporozoites penetrate cells and undergo schizogony (merogony). In the process, the normally elongated sporozoites become spherical to form uninucleate trophozoites, which undergo multiple karyokinesis to form immature schizonts (meronts). Free merozoites are produced at the surface as the immature schizonts mature. The number of cycles of schizogony is characteristic of a species of coccidia. The terminal generation of merozoites penetrates cells and forms the sexual stages, microgamonts and macrogamonts (collectively, gamonts). Microgamonts undergo multiple karyokinesis and produce biflagellated microgametes that are actively motile and which fertilize the macrogamonts. The macrogamont is uninucleate and possesses a large nucleus and prominent nucleolus.

Eosinophilic wall-forming bodies are produced in the macrogamont cytoplasm as development progresses. These fuse with surface membranes of the macrogamont and produce the oocyst wall. The endogenous cycle is completed when oocysts are released from the host cells. The prepatent period is the time required from ingestion of sporulated oocysts to the release of unsporulated oocysts in the feces. The patent period is the length of time that oocysts are excreted in the feces.

Piroplasms

Piroplasms (*Babesia* spp., *Theileria* spp., *Cytauxzoon* spp.) are transmitted by ticks[27]. Depending on the species, sporozoites penetrate red blood cells, lymphocytes, or macrophages and undergo schizogony. It is still unclear whether sexual stages occur. Merozoites of all piroplasms develop in red blood cells. Development occurs in the tick after it feeds on infected red blood cells; oocysts are produced in ticks, and sporozoites are injected into appropriate hosts during tick feeding.

Malaria and Malaria-like Apicomplexans

The life cycles of protozoa-causing malaria begin when sporozoites are injected into the blood of the vertebrate host by a feeding female mosquito. Sporozoites travel to the liver where they penetrate hepatocytes. Here, they undergo pre-erythrocytic schizogony, producing merozoites, which enter red blood cells and transform into trophozoites (the feeding or ring stage). These undergo erythrocytic schizogony. Terminal generation merozoites enter red blood cells and develop into microgamonts or macrogamonts. These sexual stages are ingested by feeding female mosquitoes, and fertilization occurs in the gut of the mosquito. Motile ookinetes are produced. These penetrate the gut of the mosquito and develop into oocysts[28]. Oocysts sporulate, producing sporozoites. Sporozoites migrate to the salivary glands of the mosquito and are available to be transmitted to other vertebrate hosts.

The life cycles of malaria-like parasites are similar to those of *Plasmodium* spp., except they are transmitted by other blood-feeding arthropods. Malaria-like parasites also may undergo schizogony elsewhere in the vertebrate host body before infecting blood cells. *Haemoproteus* spp. are transmitted by midges, hippoboscid flies, or tabanids (horse flies), and undergo schizogony in the vascular endothelium of the lung, liver, kidney, and spleen. *Leucocytozoon* spp. are transmitted by midges and simuliid flies, and undergo schizogony in the liver and in phagocytic cells throughout the body of the vertebrate host.

CILIATES: PHYLUM CILIOPHORA

It is estimated that there are more than 10,000 species of ciliates[29]. The majority of ciliated protists are free-living, while others are important enteric commensals, that is, ciliates that live in the digestive tracts of ruminants, horses, some non-human primates, and other mammals. Still others are obligate internal or external parasites (e.g., *Balantidium coli* and *Ichthyophthirius multifiliis*). All parasitic ciliated protists have direct life cycles.

Special Organelles

Ciliates are unique among the protists in that most possess two different types of nuclei and, thus, display nuclear dimorphism. The usually large, polyploid macronucleus supports somatic functions, while one or more small, diploid micronuclei serve a genetic function and constitute the "germ line" of that cell[30]. Many ciliates are capable of sexual reproduction through conjugation, whereby two ciliated cells temporarily fuse and exchange an extra copy of their micronuclei, which are haploid at this time. After the cells separate, the newly acquired foreign micronucleus fuses with that cell's own micronucleus, giving rise to new genetic combinations[31].

Typically, ciliates possess one cytostome (mouth). The cytostome is an important taxonomic feature (Figure 2.2). It is surrounded by modified cilia (oral ciliature). Food passing the cytostome becomes surrounded by a membrane formed by cytoplasmic discoidal vesicles. A food vacuole is formed and is pinched off as the vacuole enters the cell, where digestion occurs through the action of acidosome vesicles and lysosomes[32]. Final waste products are released from the cell through a cytopyge (cytoproct). Much of the food vacuole membrane is recycled and incorporated back into discoidal vesicles.

Ciliate species living in hypotonic environments osmoregulate by collecting excess fluid into expandable contractile vacuoles. Excess water is released through a contractile vacuole pore. When distended, the contractile vacuole usually can be seen as a large, clear vacuole.

Locomotion

Most ciliates have two types of cilia. The first includes somatic cilia arranged in longitudinal rows (kineties) located over most of the cell surface. These primarily function in locomotion. The second type includes the oral ciliature which creates feeding currents and thereby facilitate ingestion of nutrients. Most ciliates move by beating their somatic cilia in a coordinated pattern such that metachronal waves pass over the cell surface. In some species, cilia may be arranged in intricate groupings (e.g., cirri, membranelles) to form structures with specialized functions. Each cilium has an internal axoneme with a typical 9+2 microtubule arrangement. Just below the cell surface, the cilium is anchored in a basal body, the kinetosome, which is composed of nine triplets of microtubules in a circle. A complex network of microfilamentous-like and microtubular structures extends between basal bodies, and this network is species-specific. One enteric species, *Allantosoma intestinalis,* has no cilia[33].

Life Cycles

As previously noted, some ciliates undergo sexual reproduction by conjugation of two cells and exchange of micronuclei, or by autogamy. Ciliates divide by transverse fission, or "homothetogenic" division, so that the cleavage furrow is equatorial instead of longitudinal. This process can be complex because a new cytostome must be formed for one of the daughter cells. Enteric commensal and parasitic ciliates are transmitted by the fecal-oral route. Some species form a cyst (e.g., *Balantidium* spp.) (Figure 2.1), whereas others, such as the commensal ciliates of horses, do not. Ectoparasitic parasites may (e.g., *Ichthyophthirius* sp.) or may not (e.g., *Trichodina* sp.) require a developmental period off the host.

MICROSPORIDIANS: PHYLUM MICROSPORA

Until recently, microsporidia were classified as protozoa in the phylum Microsporidia. Analysis of small subunit RNA has resulted in the reclassification of these pathogens to the fungi[34].

Special Organelles

Microsporidia (Figures 2.9, 2.10, and 2.11) are characterized by a resistant spore stage[35]. The microsporidial spore contains many special organelles. The coiled polar tube is used in host cell penetration and transfer of the sporoplasm to new host cells. It is also an important taxonomic structure. An anchoring disk is located in the anterior end of spores and serves as the site of attachment for the polar tube. The polaroplast is a lamellar organelle in the anterior end of spores and may act like a Golgi apparatus. A posterior vacuole is present in the posterior end of the spore and aids in expulsion of the sporoplasm.

Locomotion

Spores are non-motile. Motility of other stages has not been widely studied.

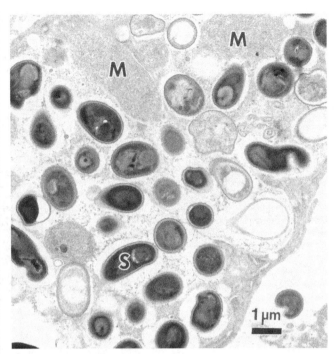

Fig. 2.9 Transmission electron micrograph of *Encephalitozoon intestinalis* in CV-1 cell culture. Spores (S) and meronts (M) are labeled. Courtesy of C.N. Jordan.

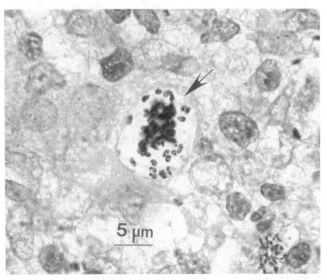

Fig. 2.10 Section of an adrenal gland from a mouse containing *Encephalitozoon cuniculi* (arrow). A Gram stain was used to demonstrate stages.

Life Cycles

Hosts are infected by ingestion or inhalation of spores, or by transplacental transmission (Figure 2.11). The spore penetrates a host cell via the polar tube. The polaroplast

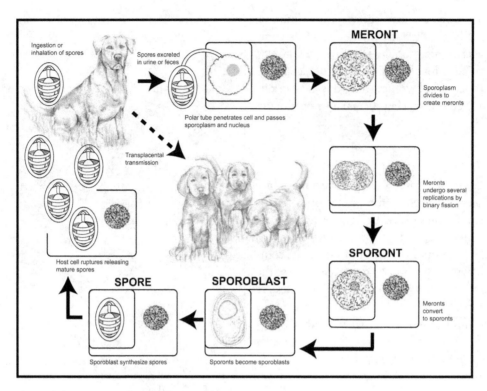

Fig. 2.11   Life cycle of *Encephalitozoon cuniculi* in dogs.

swells, and the anchoring disk stabilizes the polar tube. The polar tube is inverted while extruded, and membranes from the polaroplast connect with the tube to extend its length. Extrusion occurs with great force and allows penetration of the host cell without disturbance of the host cell membrane. The posterior vacuole swells and forces the sporoplasm and nucleus through the polar tube. The tip of the polar tube inside of the host cell envelopes the sporoplasm to become the parasite outer membrane.

The sporoplasm divides, creating meronts, which are proliferative stages that divide by binary fission. Meronts may be in direct contact with the host cell cytoplasm or in a parasitophorous vacuole lined by the host cell membrane, and may undergo several replications before converting into sporonts. In most species, sporonts exist within a parasitophorous vacuole. Sporonts convert to sporoblasts, either immediately or after one division.

Sporoblasts are the stages that synthesize the polar tube and its accessory organelles to become mature spores. Once a host cell is full of mature spores, the cell bursts and the spores are released. These spores are resistant to environmental stress and can remain viable for several years.

REFERENCES

1. Lindsay, D.S., Upton, S.J., and Hildreth, M.B. (1999) Descriptions of two new species of coccidia (Protozoa: Eimeriidae) and redescriptions of *Eimeria ivensae* and *Eimeria odocoilei* from captive white-tailed deer, *Odocoileus virginianus. J. Parasitol.* **85,** 1120–1125.
2. Lindsay, D.S., Upton, S.J., and Dubey, J.P. (1999) A structural study of the *Neospora caninum* oocyst. *Int. J. Parasitol.* **29,** 1521–1523.
3. Lindsay, D.S., Upton, S.J., Owens, D.S., Morgan, U.M., Mead, J.R., and Blagburn, B.L. (2000) *Cryptosporidium andersoni* n. sp. (Apicomplexa: Cryptosporiidae) from cattle, *Bos taurus. J. Euk. Microbiol.* **47,** 91–95.
4. Lee, J.J., Leedale, G.F., and Bradburn, P. (2000) *An Illustrated Guide to the Protozoa.* Society of Protozoologists, Lawrence, Kansas.
5. Yu, L.Z., Birky, W.C., and Adam, R.D. (2002) The two nuclei of *Giardia* each have complete copies of the genome and are partitioned equationally at cytokinesis. *Euk. Cell.* **1,** 191–199.
6. Vickerman, K. and Coombs, G.H. (1999) Protozoan paradigms for cell biology. *J. Cell Sci.* **112,** 2797–2798.
7. Hannert, V. and Michels, P.A.M. (1994) Structure, function and biogenesis of glycosomes in kinetoplastida. *J. Bioener. Biomem.* **26,** 205–212.
8. Honigberg, B.M., Mattern, C.F.T., and Daniel, W.A. (1971) Fine structure of the mastigont system in *Tritrichomonas foetus* (Riedmuller). *J. Protozool.* **18,** 183–198.
9. Muller, M. (1993) The hydrogenosome. *J. Gen. Microbiol.* **139,** 2879–2889.

10. Windsor, J.J. and Johnson, E.H. (1999) *Dientamoeba fragilis:* the unflagellated human flagellate. *Brit. J. Biomed. Sci.* **56,** 293–306.

11. Birky, C.W. (2005) Sex: Is *Giardia* doing it in the dark? *Current Biology* **15,** R56–58.

12. Barry, J.D. and McCullough, R. (2001) Antigenic variation in trypanosomes: enhanced phenotypic variation in a eukaryotic parasite. In: Baker, J.R., Muller, R. and Rollison, U.D. (eds), *Advances in Parasitology* vol. 49. Academic Press, New York.

13. Voigt, H. and Guillen, N. (1999) New insights into the role of the cytoskeleton in phagocytosis of *Entamoeba histolytica. Cell Microb.* **1,** 195–203.

14. Patterson, D.J. (1981) Contractile vacuole complex behavior as a diagnostic character for free-living amoebae. *Protistologica* **17,** 243–248.

15. Zurita, M., Alagon, A., Vargas-Villarreal, J., and Lizardi, P.M. (1991) The *Entamoeba histolytica* rDNA episome: nuclear localization, DNAase I sensitivity map, and specific DNA-protein interactions. *Mol. Microbiol.* **5,** 1843–51.

16. Pantaloni, D., Clainche, C.L., and Carlier, M.-F. (2001) Mechanism of actin-based motility. *Science* **292,** 1502–1506.

17. Allen, R.D. and Allen, N.S. (1978) Cytoplasmic streaming in amoeboid movement. *Ann. Rev. Biophys. Bioeng.* **7,** 469–495.

18. Walsh, C. (1984) Synthesis and assembly of the cytoskeleton of *Naegleria gruberi* flagellates. *J. Cell Biol.* **98,** 449–56.

19. Schuster, F.L., Dunnebacke, T.H., Booton, G.C., Yagi, S., Kohlmeier, C.K., Glaser, C., et al. (2003) Environmental isolation of *Balamuthia mandrillaris* associated with a case of amebic encephalitis. *J. Clin. Microbiol.* **41,** 3175–3180.

20. Dubey, J.P., Lindsay, D.S., and Speer, C.A. (1998) Structures of *Toxoplasma gondii* tachyzoites, bradyzoites, and sporozoites and biology and development of tissue cyst. *Clin. Microbiol. Rev.* **11,** 267–299.

21. Blackman, M.J. and Bannister, L.H. (2001) Apical organelles of Apicomplexa: biology and isolation by subcellular fractionation. *Mol. Biochem. Parasitol.* **117,** 11–25.

22. Carruthers, V.B. (2002) Host cell invasion by the opportunistic pathogen *Toxoplasma gondii. Acta Trop.* **81,** 111–122.

23. Hammond, D.M., Speer, C.A., and Roberts, W. (1970) Occurrence of refractile bodies in merozoites of *Eimeria* species. *J. Parasitol.* **56,** 189–191.

24. Lindsay, D.S., Blagburn, B.L., and Toivio-Kinnucan, M. (1991) Ultrastructure of developing *Isospora suis* in cultured cells. *Am. J. Vet. Res.* **52,** 471–473.

25. Ferguson D.J., Belli, S.I., Smith, N.C., and Wallach, M.G. (2003) The development of the macrogamete and oocyst wall in *Eimeria maxima:* immuno-light and electron microscopy. *Int. J. Parasitol.* **33,** 1329–1340.

26. Opitz, C. and Soldati, D. (2002) The glideosome: a dynamic complex powering gliding motion and host cell invasion by *Toxoplasma gondii. Mol. Microbiol.* **45,** 597–604.

27. Zintl, A., Mulcahy, G., Skerrett, H.E., Taylor, S.M., and Gray, J.S. (2003) *Babesia divergens,* a bovine blood parasite of veterinary and zoonotic importance. *Clin. Microbiol. Rev.* **16,** 622–636.

28. Shahabuddin, M. (1998) *Plasmodium* ookinete development in the mosquito midgut: a case of reciprocal manipulation. *Parasitology* **116,** S83–93.

29. Corliss, J.O. (2000) Biodiversity, classification, and numbers of species of protists. In: Raven, P. H. and Williams. T. (eds.), *Nature and Human Society: The Quest for a Sustainable World,* National Academy Press, Washington, DC, pp. 130–155.

30. Prescott, D.M. (1994) The DNA of ciliated protozoa. *Microbiol. Rev.* **58,** 233–267.

31. Jahn, C.L. and Klobutcher, L.A. (2002) Genome remodeling in ciliated protozoa. *Ann. Rev. Microbiol.* **56,** 489–520.

32. Allen, R.D. and Fok, A.K. (2000) Membrane trafficking and processing in *Paramecium: Int. Rev. Cytol.* **198,** 277–318.

33. Sundermann, C.A. and Paulin, J.J. (1981) Ultrastructural features of *Allantosoma intestinalis,* a suctorian ciliate isolated from the large intestine of the horse. *J. Protozool.* **28,** 400–404.

34. Vossbrinck, C.R., Andreadis, T.G., and Weiss, L.M. (2004) Phylogenetics: Taxonomy and the microsporidia as derived fungi. In: Lindsay, D.S. and Weiss, L.M. (eds.), Volume 9, *World Class Parasites: Opportunistic Infections: Toxoplasma, Sarcocystis,* and *Microsporidia,* Kluwer Academic Publishers, Boston, pp. 189–213.

35. Weiss, L.M. (2001) Microsporidia: emerging pathogenic protists. *Acta Tropica* **78,** 89–102.

Biology of Trematodes and Leeches

David G. Baker, DVM, MS, PhD, DACLAM

INTRODUCTION

Historically, it was not uncommon for animals—particularly wild-caught fish, birds, and primates—to be found infected with parasitic trematodes. However, with the advent of improved husbandry practices in laboratory animal facilities, the incidences of infection have declined markedly. This is due primarily to the interruption of indirect life cycles through elimination of obligate intermediate hosts, and also to the fact that laboratory-reared research animals have largely replaced those obtained from the wild. This chapter briefly describes the taxonomy, general life cycles, and morphology of the trematodes and leeches one may encounter in the laboratory setting. Specific parasite species are discussed in the chapters covering their hosts.

The phylum Platyhelminthes ("flatworms") includes the classes Trematoda ("flukes"), Cestoda ("tapeworms"), and Turbellaria ("planarians"). Worms in this phylum are dorsoventrally flattened, lack a body cavity, and instead contain organs embedded in a parenchyma. They reproduce by asexual and/or sexual means. Most are hermaphroditic. The life cycles are often complex and indirect. The

phylum Platyhelminthes has been further broken down according to diverse taxonomic schemes. For the purposes of this text, the class Trematoda includes three Orders: Monogenea, Aspidogastrea, and Digenea.

ORDER MONOGENEA

Trematodes in the order Monogenea are the most primitive of the flukes. The order includes several species identified as parasites of cold-blooded aquatic vertebrates including fish, amphibians, and reptiles. They are common in the wild, but extremely rare in the laboratory setting. Most members of the Monogenea are ectoparasites of the skin, gills, and fins. A few species occur in the mouth, esophagus, nose, urinary bladder, ureters, and lungs. Most species are nonpathogenic, though a few are significant pathogens of the gills and skin of fish. The most important genera are *Gyrodactylus* and *Dactylogyrus*[1]. Many Monogenea demonstrate considerable niche specificity, parasitizing specific anatomical locations on the host, or parasitizing hosts of specific ages. Niche specificity may be influenced by parasite nutritional requirements, worm motility, and by the physical attachment abilities of the worm[2].

The Monogenea have direct life cycles, requiring less than five days for completion. These short life cycles may facilitate the build-up of overwhelming populations in an aquarium or culture pond environment. Members of this class may be oviparous or viviparous. Eggs are usually operculated and have a filamentous structure at one or both ends[3]. This is used to anchor the egg to a host or other object. The ciliated larva (oncomiridium) swims freely until finding a suitable host. Unlike the other trematodes, the sexual and asexual generations do not alternate. Adults feed on mucus, epithelium, and blood[1–3].

Posteriorly, monogeneans have an "opisthaptor," a bulbous, disc-shaped adhesive organ which may bear suckers, clamps, and hooks used for attaching to a host. The morphology of these structures is of taxonomic significance (Figure 3.1). Physical trauma to gills, fins, and skin may result from the attaching structures of the opisthaptor. Resulting lesions may become secondarily infected and lead to color fading, weight loss, emaciation, and increased susceptibility to predation.

The worm surface is a living structure and is therefore referred to as the "tegument." The nervous system of the Monogenea consists of cerebral ganglia in the anterior region, with nerve trunks connected in a "ladder" pattern that extends the length of the body. The digestive system of the Monogenea includes the mouth, buccal funnel, prepharynx, pharynx, esophagus, and branched intestine. There is no anus. Indigestible material is regurgitated. Some monogeneans absorb nutrients through the tegument. The osmoregulatory system is typical of the platyhelminthes, and includes flame cells that connect to ducts and eventually, into two lateral excretory pores near the anterior of the worm. The reproductive system is hermaphroditic, and typical of the platyhelminthes in the inclusion of both male and female sex organs[1,2].

ORDER ASPIDOGASTREA

The Aspidogastrea comprise a relatively small group of several dozen species of trematodes which parasitize freshwater and/or marine mollusks, crustaceans, and fish, as well as freshwater turtles[4]. They are considered to be phylogenetically intermediate between the Monogenea and Digenea. All Aspidogastrea are aquatic and hermaphroditic.

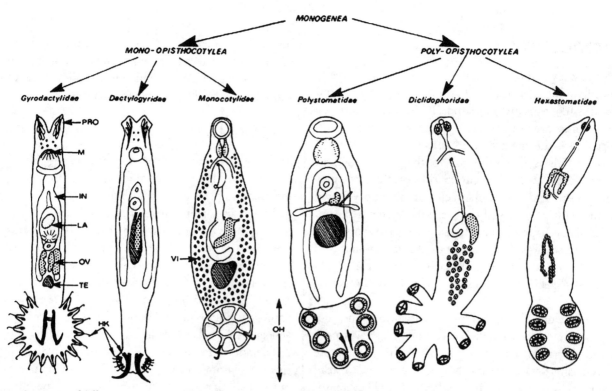

Fig. 3.1 Specimens of different monogenean families and their relations. HK, hooks; IN, intestine; LA, larva; M, mouth; OH, opisthaptor; OV, ovary; PRO, prohaptor; TE, testis; VI, vitellarium. Reproduced from Mehlhorn, H. (2001). Used with permission, courtesy of Springer-Verlag, Germany.

While not all of the life cycles are known, it appears that most of the Aspidogastrea have indirect life cycles, using a mollusk as an intermediate host and fish or turtles as definitive hosts[4]. For this reason, the Aspidogastrea may only be encountered when animals are collected in the wild or cultured in ponds. Four families of Aspidogastrea are recognized: Stichocotylidae, Rugogastridae, Aspidogastridae, and Multicalycidae (Figure 3.2).

The Stichocotylidae have an elongated, slender body. The ventral disc bears a single row of well-separated suckers. There are two testes, a single cecum, and follicular vitellaria in the lateral fields. These are parasites of rays and skates (Batoidea)[2,4].

The Rugogastridae have elongated bodies with a single row of transverse thickenings of the tegument, termed rugae. There is a weakly developed ventral sucker. There also is a pharynx, prepharynx, and esophagus; multiple testes; a pretesticular ovary; a Laurer's canal opening dorsally in the forebody; vitellaria distributed along the ceca; a uterus ventral to the testes; and numerous, operculated eggs. There is no seminal receptacle. These are parasites of rat fish, rabbit fish, and chimeras (Holocephali)[2,4].

Aspidogastridae have an oval or elongated body, an adhesive disc bearing four longitudinal rows of alveoli (Figure 3.3), one or two testes, and follicular vitellaria located laterally. These are parasites of mollusks, fishes, and turtles[2,4].

Multicalycidae bear a single row of deep alveoli separated by transverse septae and ventral, foot-like appendages. There is a single cecum and testis. The ovary is pretesticular, near the posterior end of the body. These are parasites of Holocephali and certain elasmobranchs[4].

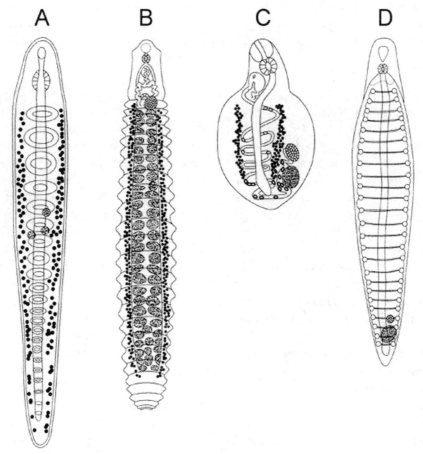

Fig. 3.2 Aspidogastrean trematodes. (A) *Stichocotyle nephropis* (Stichocotylidae). (B) *Rugogaster hydrolagi* (Rugogastridae). (C) *Aspidogaster piscicola* (Aspidogastridae). (D) *Multicalyx elegans* (Multicalycidae). Reproduced from Rohde, K. (2002). Used with permission, courtesy of CABI Publishing, Oxfordshire, UK.

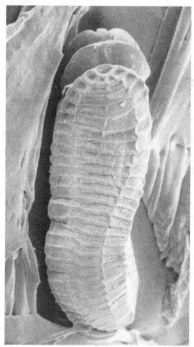

Fig. 3.3 Ventral surface of *Lobatostoma* sp. adult (Aspidogastridae). Courtesy of Dr. K. Rohde, University of New England, Armidale, Australia.

Important Aspidogastrean genera include *Aspidogaster, Cotylogaster, Lobatostoma,* and others.

The Aspidogastrean life cycle is comparatively simple. Unembryonated eggs released from the adult develop to the larval (cotylocidial) stage and then hatch in the environment. In other species, embryonated eggs are released when the larvae are nearly ready to hatch out. In still others, eggs do not hatch until they are consumed by a suitable intermediate host. One larva is released from each egg. The larva remains in the mollusk intermediate host until that host is eaten by the definitive host, wherein it undergoes further development to the adult stage. In some species, development to the adult stage occurs in the mollusk host[1].

The Aspidogastrea differ from other trematodes, whose life cycles include multiple developmental stages, most of which result in the asexual multiplication of the organism. Asexual multiplication of larval stages does not occur among the Aspidogastrea. Compared to other trematodes, the Aspidogastrea are relatively nonspecific in host range[4].

Aspidogastrea range in size from 2 mm to several centimeters in length[1]. Adults possess an attachment organ comprised of one to several ventral suckers, depending on the family. The morphology of the attachment organ is important in species identification[4]. As in the Monogenea, the worm surface is referred to as the tegument. Larval and adult Aspidogastreans possess a complex nervous system. The digestive system includes a mouth, pharynx, and single short cecum. The osmoregulatory system is typical of the platyhelminthes. The excretory ducts end in a posterior excretory bladder, and finally, exit the worm via an excretory pore. The reproductive system includes both male and female components, typical of the Trematoda[2].

ORDER DIGENEA

The Digenea comprise the largest and most diverse group of parasitic trematodes. As their name indicates, they have an asexual reproduction phase of their life cycle in a mollusk, and a sexual (usually hermaphroditic) reproduction phase in a vertebrate host. Concerning the latter, they may be found in virtually all species of vertebrates. Like other trematodes, they are common in the wild but rare in the laboratory setting. Most members of the Digenea are endoparasites of the gastrointestinal and pulmonary systems. Many species are pathogenic.

Given the size of the order, it is no wonder that species vary in some particulars of their life cycles. A generalized life cycle includes the egg, which is usually passed in the feces of the definitive host. Under suitable conditions, the egg hatches to release a ciliated, free-swimming miracidium, which actively penetrates a snail intermediate host. Within the snail, the miracidium loses its ciliated coat to become a sporocyst. From an individual sporocyst develop numerous rediae. From each rediae, many cercariae develop, and are released through a birth-pore. Cercariae actively or passively exit the snail intermediate host and swim until finding submerged vegetation on which to encyst.

During encystment, the tail is lost and other physiologic changes occur which lead to formation of the metacercaria, or infective stage. Infection of the definitive host is initiated with ingestion of the metacercaria, though in the family Schistosomatidae, cercariae actively penetrate the definitive host. Excystation occurs in the digestive tract and the immature fluke migrates to its predilection site. Because of asexual reproduction at the sporocyst and/or redia stages, tremendous amplification of trematode populations may result from a single miracidium. Adult flukes feed on blood, mucus, and host tissues[1,2].

Digenea vary in size from less than 1 mm to several centimeters in length. Like other trematodes, Digenea are dorsoventrally flattened, though body shapes range from long and narrow or leaf-shaped to thick and fleshy[3]. The body surface (cuticle or tegument) is a complex organ typical of the Trematoda, and is important in nutrient absorption. The Digenea possess an anterior (oral) sucker and, usually, a ventral sucker (acetabulum), often located in the anterior third of the ventral surface. The number and position of the suckers are important taxonomic keys. The anterior sucker surrounds the mouth, leading into the pharynx, esophagus, and intestine, which leads into two blind ceca. Some species possess an anus. The nervous system includes a circumesophageal ring of nerve fibers and paired ganglia. Nerves run anteriorly and posteriorly to the rest of the body in a typical ladder arrangement.

Like other flatworms, the osmoregulatory system consists of flame cells, which collect waste products from the parenchyma and expel them via an excretory bladder with an opening at the posterior end of the body. The reproductive system includes both male and female structures[1,2,3].

Regardless of the classification scheme used, there are several families of Digenean trematodes. The most important of those containing parasites noted in this text are briefly described here.

Family Dicrocoeliidae

Dicrocoeliids are small to medium-sized flukes which occur in the bile and pancreatic ducts and sometimes the intestine of mammals, birds, amphibians, and reptiles. These flukes have a flattened and elongated body. The cuticle usually lacks spines. The testes are located behind the ventral sucker, and the ovary is situated just posterior to the testes[3]. It is common for flukes in this family to include two intermediate hosts in their life cycle. Important genera include *Dicrocoelium*, *Eurytrema*, *Platynosomum*, and *Athesmia* (Figure 3.4).

Family Diplostomidae

Diplostomatid flukes have a flattened anterior region, whereas the posterior region is more cylindrical. Spatulate and ear-like processes may be present on the anterolateral parts of the body[3]. Diplostomatids usually occur in the intestine of mammals which have ingested infected amphibians or reptiles. The most important genus is *Alaria*.

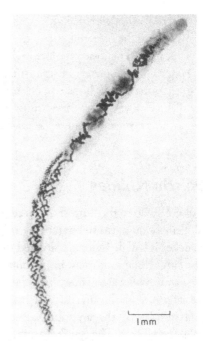

Fig. 3.4 *Athesmia foxi* adult. Courtesy of G.E. Cosgrove, Tulane National Primate Research Center.

Family Echinostomatidae

Echinostomatidae are elongated flukes with a pronounced ventral sucker. The body is usually spined. The testes lay in the posterior portion of the body and the ovary is anterior to the testes. Adults possess a distinctive "crown" of hooks surrounding the anterior—or oral—sucker[3]. Echinostomatids usually occur in the intestine of mammals and birds which have ingested infected raw mollusks, amphibians, or fish. The most important genus is *Echinostoma*.

Family Fasciolidae

Fasciolids are among the largest flukes. The body is broad, leaf-shaped, and usually spined. The anterior and ventral suckers are situated close to one another. Testes are posterior[3]. Fasciolids occur in the liver, intestine, and sometimes stomach of mammals which have fed on vegetation contaminated with metacercariae, as well as in animals obtained from their natural habitat. Important genera include *Fasciola*, *Fasciolopsis*, and *Fascioloides*.

Family Heterophyidae

Heterophyids are small flukes, typically less than 2 mm in length. The posterior region is wider than the anterior region. The body is covered with scale-like spines. These are more numerous toward the posterior end of the fluke, where the testes are located. The ovary is situated anterior to the testes[3]. Heterophyids occur in the small intestine of fish-eating mammals and birds which have ingested infected raw fish. These flukes have only rarely been reported. Important genera include *Metagonimus* and *Heterophyes*.

Family Opisthorchiidae

Opisthorchids are small to medium-sized flukes with a flattened, translucent body narrowed anteriorly (Figure 3.5)[5]. The ventral sucker is small. Testes are situated in the posterior portion of the fluke, and may be globular or highly branched. The ovary is located anterior to the testes[3]. The vitelllaria are lateral, and the uterus, which is filled with eggs, fills the middle of the anterior half of the body between the intestinal ceca. The eggs have a thick shell with a distinct, convex operculum, and contain an asymmetrical miracidium when passed in the feces. Opisthorchids occur in the gallbladder, bile duct, and sometimes the pancreatic duct and small intestine of mammals, birds, and reptiles

that have ingested infected raw fish. The most important genera include *Amphimerus, Chlonorchis, Metorchis,* and *Opisthorchis*.

Family Paramphistomatidae

Paramphistomid flukes are thick, typically appearing circular in transverse section. The ventral sucker lies at the extreme posterior of the fluke (Figure 3.6)[6]. The body lacks spines. The testes are situated in the middle portion of the body, with the ovary just posterior[3]. Paramphistomid flukes are common in the intestine of herbivorous mammals. Infection is usually by ingestion of contaminated vegetation. An important genus is *Gastrodiscoides*.

Family Plagiorchiidae

Plagiorchids are large flukes of varying shapes (Figure 3.7). The body is usually covered with small spines. The testes are located toward the posterior region, and the ovary lies anterior to the testes[3]. Plagiorchids include the oviduct flukes of the chicken and other birds. They occur only in animals that have ingested infected insects. Important genera include *Plagiorchis* and *Prosthogonimus*.

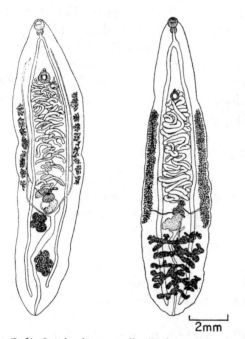

Fig. 3.5 (Left) *Opisthorchis tenuicollis.* (Right) *Opisthorchis sinensis.* Reproduced from Lapage, G. (1962). Used with permission, courtesy of Lippincott, Williams and Wilkins, Philadelphia.

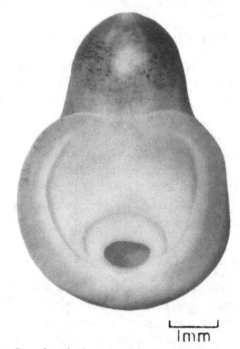

Fig. 3.6 *Gastrodiscoides hominis* adult. Reproduced from Graham, G.L. (1960). Used with permission, courtesy of New York Academy of Science.

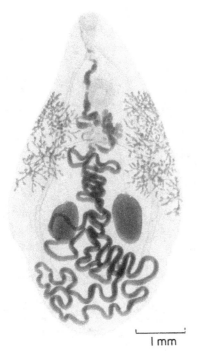

Fig. 3.7 *Prosthogonimus macrorchis* adult. Courtesy of Marietta Voge, University of California.

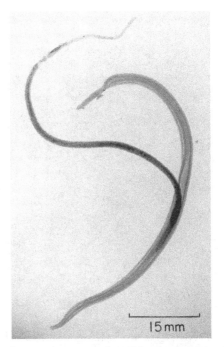

Fig. 3.8 *Schistosoma mansoni* male and female. Courtesy of Marietta Voge, University of California.

Family Schistosomatidae

In the Schistosomatidae, the sexes are separate and differ in appearance. The adults are long and slender (Figure 3.8). Both males and females have a small anterior sucker and a small ventral sucker that is about 10% of the length of the body, and is located behind the mouth. They occur in the blood vessels of their hosts and enter through the skin or are ingested in water. For many species, up to four of the more slender adult females may be carried in the gynecophoral canal of the male[3]. Some schistosome eggs bear distinctive morphologic features such as spines, which aid in identification (Figure 3.9). Schistosomes are found only in animals that have been permitted access to contaminated water. The most important genus is *Schistosoma*.

Family Troglotrematidae

Troglotrematids include some medically important flukes. These trematodes are flattened or concave ventrally and convex dorsally (Figure 3.10). The testes and ovary typically lay in the middle third of the body[3]. Troglotrematids occur in the lungs of carnivorous mammals and birds and are found only in animals that have ingested infected raw crustaceans or fishes. Important genera include *Paragonimus* and *Nanophyetus*.

LEECHES

Leeches are members of the phylum Annelida ("Segmented worms") and class Hirudinea. They are found in aquatic or tropical rain forest environments. They include scavengers that feed on nonliving material, predators that feed on tissues and fluids of soft-bodied invertebrates, and others that are blood-sucking ectoparasites of vertebrates. The soft, annulated body of a leech (2 to 16 external annuli per true internal segment) is usually flattened dorsoventrally. They are colorfully patterned in green, brown, or red.

The leech is characterized by great powers of distension and contraction, which enable it to penetrate extremely narrow body openings and to ingest and store relatively large volumes of blood. A pair of suckers—a large muscular hind sucker and a smaller anterior one surrounding the mouth—permits the looping movement and powerful adherence to prey or host during feeding (Figure 3.11)[7]. Leeches are hermaphroditic, but individual leeches usually cross-fertilize to produce eggs.

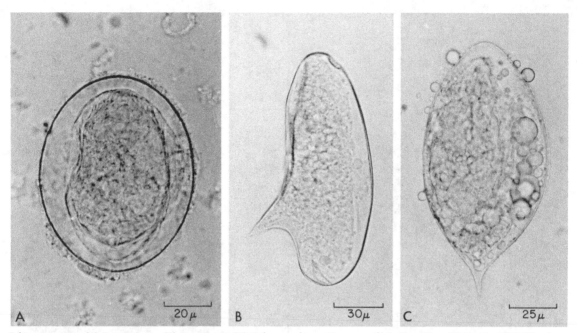

Fig. 3.9 *Schistosoma* eggs. (A) *S. japonicum.* (B) *S. mansoni.* (C) *S. haematobium.* Courtesy of Marietta Voge, University of California.

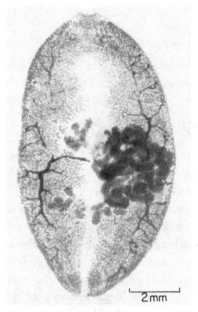

Fig. 3.10 *Paragonimus westermanii* adult. Courtesy of Marietta Voge, University of California.

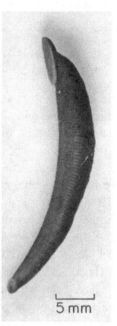

Fig. 3.11 *Dinobdella ferox.* Reproduced from Pryor, W.H. Jr., Bergner, J.F., and Raulston, G.L. (1970) with permission.

There are two orders of leeches: Gnathobdellidae and Rhynchobdellidae. The order Gnathobdellidae is characterized by the presence of cutting jaws. It includes the family Hirudinidae, which contains most leeches of medical and veterinary importance. The order Rhynchobdellidae is characterized by a penetrating proboscis rather than by cutting jaws. It includes a number of fish parasites, chiefly in the family Piscicolidae. The presence of a strong anticoagulant, capacious gut pouches which serve for long-term blood storage, and the extraordinary flexibility of the hardy body render leeches well adapted for a parasitic existence. Leeches are occasional parasites of certain endothermal laboratory animals in their natural habitats, but they are not normally found in colony-raised animals.

REFERENCES

1. Mehlhorn, H. (2001) *Encyclopedic Reference of Parasitology. Biology, Structure, Function,* 2nd Edition. Springer 2001, New York, 674 pages.
2. Roberts, L.S. and Janovy, J. Jr. (2004) *Foundations of Parasitology,* 7th Edition, The McGraw Hill Companies, New York, 702 pages.
3. Soulsby, E.J.L. (1982) *Helminths, Arthropods and Protozoa of Domesticated Animals,* 7th Edition, Lea and Febiger, Philadelphia.
4. Rohde, K. (2002) Subclass Aspidogastrea, Faust and Tang, 1936. In: *Keys to the Trematoda,* Volume 1. (Gibson, D.I., Jones, A., and Bray, R.A.), CABI Publishing, New York, pp. 5–14.
5. Lapage, G. (1962) *Mönnig's Veterinary Helminthology and Entomology.* 5th Edition. Lippincott, Williams and Wilkins, Philadelphia.
6. Graham, G.L. (1960) Parasitism in monkeys. *Ann. N.Y. Acad. Sci.* **85,** 735–992.
7. Pryor, W.H. Jr., Bergner, J.F., and Raulston, G.L. (1970) Leech (*Dinobdella ferox*) infection of a Taiwan monkey (*Macaca cyclopis*). *J. Am. Vet. Med. Assoc.* **157,** 1926–1927.

4

Biology of the Cestodes

Akira Ito, MS, PhD, DMedSci, and David G. Baker, DVM, MS, PhD, DACLAM

INTRODUCTION

Almost universally, cestode life cycles include both vertebrate and invertebrate hosts in complex, indirect life cycles[1]. Modern husbandry practices preclude the completion of such multiple-host life cycles; therefore, cestode infections have never been common in colony-raised laboratory animals. In contrast, wild-caught animals are commonly found infected with cestodes. Occasionally, these animals are brought into the animal facility. This chapter briefly describes the taxonomy, general life cycles, and morphology of the cestodes which may be encountered in the laboratory setting. Specific parasite species are discussed in the chapters covering their hosts.

CESTODE TAXONOMY

Several taxonomic schemes have been constructed for classifying the cestodes. The class Cestoda has been further divided into subclasses and orders. Cestodes discussed in this chapter comprise the subclass Eucestoda, class Cestoda, phylum Platyhelminthes. Though many other orders have been described, cestodes occurring in laboratory animals belong to two orders: Pseudophyllidea and Cyclophyllidea. Members of these two orders differ morphologically in all developmental stages, from egg to adult tapeworm.

BASIC CESTODE ANATOMY

Adult cestodes, or tapeworms, are flat, long, and ribbon-like. The body, or strobila, appears to be segmented and made up of a chain of a few to many rectangular units, or proglottids. Because parenchymal fluids move freely between proglottids, tapeworms are not truly segmented, but are pseudosegmented. The anterior end of the worm consists of a scolex, or hold-fast organ. The strobila grows throughout the life of the tapeworm by continuous proliferation of immature proglottids at the neck region behind the scolex. This process is termed "strobilation." More distal proglottids mature as new proglottids are added anteriorly. Mature proglottids contain one or two sets of both male and female reproductive organs[2]. Reproduction is through selfing and out-crossing[3], so that sexually mature proglottids contain eggs.

THE PSEUDOPHYLLIDEA

Morphology

Adult pseudophyllidean tapeworms typically bear two bothria—long, narrow, weakly muscular grooves—on the scolex[2]. In adult worms, segments appear uniform for much of the length of the tapeworm body and the genital pore is centrally located on each pseudosegment (Figure 4.1). Eggs differ from those of the cyclophyllidean tapeworms, and are operculated; therefore they must be distinguished from those of trematode parasites (Figure 4.2).

General Life Cycle

Sexually mature proglottids release individual eggs into the intestine of the definitive host. In the environment, eggs hatch and release the free-swimming larval form, or coracidium. Following ingestion by the first intermediate host, or copepod, the coracidium develops into a procercoid.

Second intermediate hosts in the life cycle of pseudophyllidean tapeworms include fish, amphibians, reptiles, or mammals, depending on the tapeworm species. After the

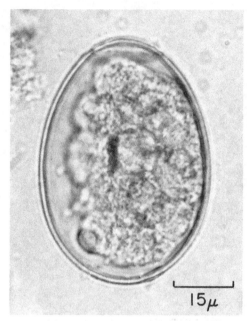

Fig. 4.2 *Diphyllobothrium latum*, egg. Note the faint, inconspicuous operculum (top). Courtesy of Marietta Voge, University of California.

second host ingests the infected copepod, the procercoid travels to the host's muscles, where it develops to a worm-like stage called a plerocercoid. When the second intermediate host is ingested by the mammalian definitive host, the plerocercoid attaches to the mucosal wall of the small intestine and grows into a sexually mature adult tapeworm (Figure 4.3).

THE CYCLOPHYLLIDEA

Morphology

Adult cyclophyllidean tapeworms bear four suckers, or acetabula, on the scolex. In some species, the scolex is "armed" with a ring of small hooklets encircling the anterior end of the scolex, or "rostellum" (Figure. 4.4). Maturing segments appear larger from the midpoint to the distal end of the worm, compared with the immature segments located more anteriorly. One or two genital pores are laterally located on each mature segment. As proglottids mature, the reproductive organs disintegrate, so that the proglottid becomes little more than a sack of eggs. In this condition, the proglottids are called gravid (Figure 4.5). Each egg contains a hexacanth embryo, or oncosphere. The eggs are thick-walled and can be distinguished by three pairs of refractile hooklets of the hexacanth in the center of each egg[2].

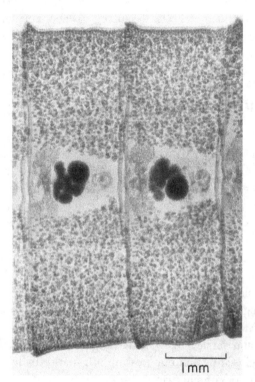

Fig. 4.1 *Diphyllobothrium latum*, mature proglottids. Note the centrally located, coiled uterus. Courtesy of Marietta Voge, University of California.

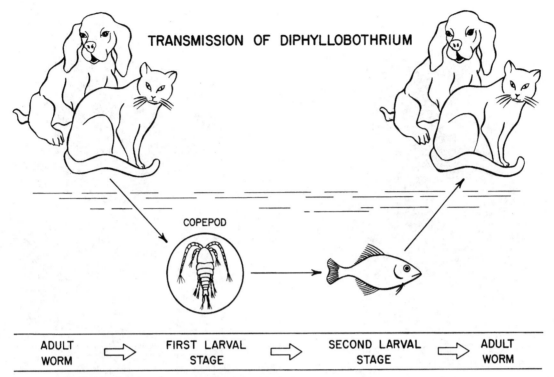

Fig. 4.3 *Diphyllobothrium latum*, diagram of life cycle. A coracidium is released from the egg, and, if ingested by a copepod, develops into a procercoid. When a fish consumes the infected copepod, the procercoid develops to a plerocercoid, which is infective to the definitive host. Courtesy of Marietta Voge, University of California.

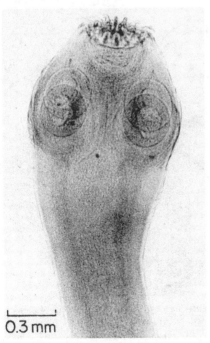

Fig. 4.4 *Taenia pisiformis* scolex. Note the armed rostellum and four acetabula. Courtesy of Marietta Voge, University of California.

General Life Cycle

Unlike the pseudophyllidean tapeworms, adult cyclophyllidean tapeworms do not release individual eggs into the intestine of the definitive host. Instead, they release gravid proglottids. These may rupture in transit, thereby releasing large numbers of eggs (Figure 4.6). Following ingestion by a suitable intermediate host, the oncosphere hatches in the intestine, invades the intestinal tissue, and is carried by the blood to the liver, lungs, brain, muscle or other sites, depending on the parasite species. There, the oncosphere develops to the second larval, or metacestode stage.

Several forms of metacestodes have been described from intermediate hosts (Figure 4.7). These include the cysticercoid in invertebrate hosts and the cysticercus, coenurus, strobilocercus, or hydatid in vertebrate hosts[2]. The specific metacestode form is characteristic of the cestode species. The cysticercoid is a solid-bodied larva with a noninvaginated scolex drawn into a small vesicle. The cysticercus is similar to the cysticercoid except that the body includes a fluid-filled bladder with one invaginated scolex attached to the bladder wall.

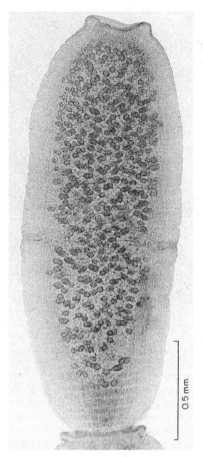

Fig. 4.5 *Dipylidium caninum*, gravid proglottids. Courtesy of Marietta Voge, University of California.

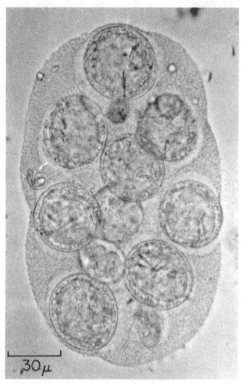

Fig. 4.6 *Dipylidium caninum*, intact egg capsule with eggs. Courtesy of R.R. Estes, U.S. Air Force School of Aerospace Medicine.

The coenurus is similar to the cysticercus except that several invaginated scolices are attached to the bladder wall. A strobilocercus resembles a cysticercus, except that the bladder is generally smaller, and the larval worm has begun to strobilate. A hydatid is a bladder, which, like the cysticercus, contains many scolices. However, unlike the cysticercus, there is usually internal budding of daughter cysts, each of which may contain many scolices (Figure 4.8)[4]. Typically hydatids are unilocular. Rarely, external budding may occur sparingly, resulting in multiple unilocular cysts, or may occur profusely, resulting in multilocular, or alveolar, cysts. These are highly invasive to surrounding host tissues.

Metacestodes may survive within the intermediate host for weeks to several years. Upon ingestion of an infected intermediate host by a suitable definitive host, metacestodes develop into adult tapeworms in the small intestine or bile duct of the definitive host (Figure 4.9).

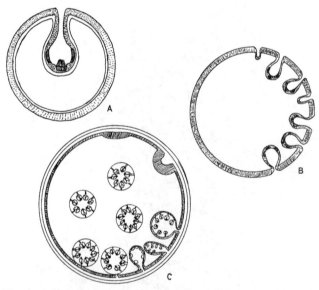

Fig. 4.7 Larval stages of taeniid cestodes: (A) Cysticercus. Note the single invagination and scolex. (B) Coenurus. Note the multiple invagination, each with a developing scolex. (C) Hydatid. Note the several buds or brood capsules, each with a number of developing scolices. Reproduced from Soulsby, E.J.L. (1965). Used with permission.

MURINE MODELS OF HUMAN CESTODE INFECTIONS

Much information has been published concerning the use of immune-deficient or immune-suppressed animals as models of human cestode infection[5]. In contrast, there are few reports on the effects of a host's genetic background on its susceptibility to infection. However, it is evident that susceptibility to cestode infection is to some extent genetically determined, not only in rodents[6], but also in arthropod intermediate hosts such as beetles[7].

Immune-deficient mice have proven useful as animal models of human cestode infection[8], and have facilitated development of systems for producing large numbers of metacestodes for experimental studies. For example, non-obese diabetic severe combined immunodeficiency (NOD/Shi-*scid*) mice have been used to produce metacestodes of *Taenia saginata*, *T. asiatica*, and *T. solium*[9,10,11].

Rodents have also been used to produce adult tapeworms for experimental studies. For example, in one study, researchers were able to grow adult *Rodentolepis nana* in rats, but only when rats were continuously administered corticosteroids. This work suggested that steroids might serve as direct stimulators of parasite growth[12]. Others have reported that *Echinococcus multilocularis* has insulin receptors[13], and that these receptors may function in worm growth.

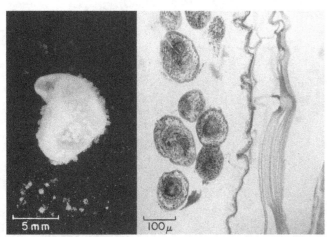

Fig. 4.8 *Echinococcus granulosus*. (Left) Hydatid cyst from the liver of a monkey. (Right) Microscopic section of hydatid cyst showing outer laminated membrane, thin germinative membrane, and several scolices. (Left) reproduced from Healy, G.R. and Hayes, N.R. (1963). Used with permission, courtesy of American Society of Parasitologists. (Right) courtesy of Marietta Voge, University of California.

REFERENCES

1. Andreassen, J., Ito, A., Ito, M., Nakao, M., and Nakaya, K. (2004) *Hymenolepis microstoma*: direct life cycle in immunodeficient mice. *J. Helminthol.* **77**, 1–5.
2. Soulsby, E.J.L. (1965) *Textbook of Veterinary Clinical Parasitology*, F.A. Davis, Philadelphia.
3. Nakao, M., Sako, Y., and Ito, A. (2003) Isolation of polymorphic microsatellite loci from the tapeworm *Echinococcus multilocularis*. *Infect. Genet. Evol.* **3**, 159–163.
4. Healy, G.R. and Hayes, N.R. (1963) Hydatid disease in rhesus monkeys. *J. Parasitol.* **49**, 837.

TRANSMISSION OF TAENIA PISIFORMIS

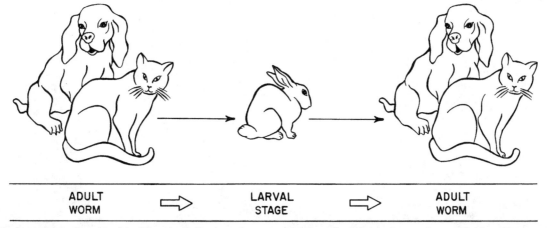

| ADULT WORM | ⇨ | LARVAL STAGE | ⇨ | ADULT WORM |

Fig. 4.9 *Taenia pisiformis*, diagram of the life cycle. Embryonated eggs excreted from the definitive host are ingested by the rabbit intermediate host. The resulting metacestode stage, in this case a cysticercus, is infective to the definitive host. Courtesy of Marietta Voge, University of California.

5. Ito, A. (1985). Thymus dependency of induced immune responses against *Hymenolepis nana* (cestode) using congenitally athymic nude mice. *Clin. Exp. Immunol.* **60**, 87–94.

6. Wassom, D.L., DeWitt, C.W., and Grundmann, A.W. (1974) Immunity to *Hymenolepis citelli* by *Peromyscus maniculatus*: genetic control and ecological implications. *J. Parasitol.* **60**, 47–52.

7. Zhong, D., Pai, A., and Yan, G. (2003) Quantitative trait loci for susceptibility to tapeworm infection in the red flour beetle. *Genetics* **165**, 1307–1315.

8. Ito, A. and Ito, M. (1999) Human *Taenia* in severe combined immunodeficiency (scid) mice. *Parasitol. Today* **15**, 64–67.

9. Ito, A., Ma, L., and Sato, Y. (1997) Cystic metacestodes of a rat-adapted *Taenia taeniaeformis* established in the peritoneal cavity of *scid* and nude mice. *Int. J. Parasitol.* **27**, 903–905.

10. Ito, A., Nakaya, K., Sako, Y., Nakao, M., and Ito, M. (2001) NOD-*scid* mouse as an experimental animal model for cysticercosis. *Southeast Asian J. Trop. Med. Public Health* **32** (Suppl 2), 85–89.

11. Ito, A., Wandra, T., Yamasaki, H., Nakao, M., Sako, Y., Nakaya, K., et al. (2004) Cysticercosis/taeniasis in Asia and the Pacific. *Vector Borne Zoonotic Dis.* **4**, 95–107.

12. Ito, A. (1984) *Hymenolepis nana*: worm recovery from congenitally athymic nude and phenotypically normal rats and mice. *Exp. Parasitol.* **58**, 132–137.

13. Konrad, C., Kroner, A., Spiliotis, M., Zavala-Gongora, R., and Brehm, K. (2002) Identification and molecular characterization of a gene encoding a member of the insulin receptor family in *Echinococcus multilocularis*. *Int. J. Parasitol.* **33**, 301–312.

5

Biology of Nematodes and Acanthocephalans

David G. Baker, DVM, MS, PhD, DACLAM

INTRODUCTION

Historically, infections with nematode parasites have been among the most common parasitisms affecting laboratory animals. Like other parasitisms, the range and number of nematode infections of laboratory animals have markedly decreased with improvements in animal husbandry and the predominating use of laboratory-raised animals. In spite of these improvements, some nematode infections, particularly those with direct life cycles, may still commonly be found in laboratory animals. In contrast, infection of laboratory animals with acanthocephalans has always been uncommon, and is even more so today. This chapter briefly describes the taxonomy, general life cycles, and morphology of the nematodes and acanthocephalans

one may encounter in the laboratory setting. Specific parasites are discussed in the relevant host chapters.

CLASS NEMATODA

The class Nematoda ("roundworms") contains the largest number of helminth parasites of endothermal animals. Worms in this class are cylindrical, unsegmented, and elongated. These worms have a pseudocoel (body cavity derived from the embryonic blastocoel) containing an alimentary canal. Histologically, this arrangement appears as "a tube within a tube." In most cases, the sexes are separate. The life cycles may be direct or indirect[1-3].

The class Nematoda is further divided into five orders and fourteen superfamilies. With relatively little training, nearly anyone can learn to differentiate worms by superfamily, and so facilitate arrival at parasite identification (Figure 5.1).

Order Rhabditida

Most members of the order Rhabditida are free-living, but a few are parasitic. Worms in the order are so named because of the shape of the esophagus, which in free-living forms includes a long, cylindrical portion that terminates in a posterior bulb with a valvular apparatus, which appears refractile under light microscopy. These worms are very small and have small lips and a reduced or absent buccal cavity. Spicules are of equal length. For parasitic species, parasitic and parthenogenetic females inhabit the small intestine. Eggs passed from the host can produce either parasitic female larvae (homogonic life cycle) or free-living male or female worms (heterogonic life cycle). The latter can produce either infectious parasitic or free-living forms.

Infection occurs when larvae enter the host either by ingestion or by penetration of the skin, after which they migrate into blood vessels and are carried to the lungs, where they enter the alveoli. They are then carried up the airways to the trachea and are swallowed. In the intestine the larvae develop into mature females within the intestinal crypts. Vertebrate parasites are found only in the superfamily Rhabditoidea.

Superfamily Rhabditoidea

Members of this superfamily are commonly associated with soiled living conditions. Vertebrate parasites are found in the families Rhabditidae and Strongyloididae.

PICTORIAL KEY TO NEMATODE SUPERFAMILIES
By HELEN E. JORDAN, D.V.M., Ph.D. and SANDRA SHERMAN, D.V.M.

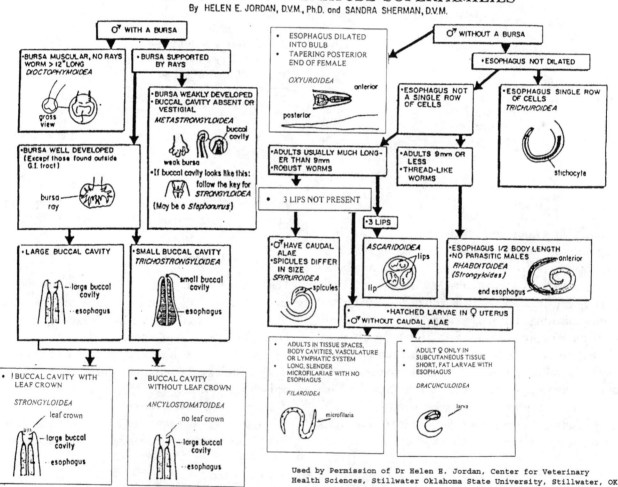

Used by Permission of Dr Helen E. Jordan, Center for Veterinary Health Sciences, Stillwater Oklahoma State University, Stillwater, OK

Fig. 5.1 Pictorial key to the Nematode superfamilies. Used with permission, courtesy of Dr. Helen Jordan, Oklahoma State University.

Order Ascaridida

Worms in this order possess three lips. Caudal alae may be present, and when so, are generally laterally placed. Adults are parasites of the gastrointestinal system. Parasites of vertebrates are found in three superfamilies.

Superfamily Ascaridoidea

Worms in this superfamily possess three prominent lips but lack a buccal capsule and, in most cases, an esophageal bulb. Ascarids are generally large, stout worms. The intestine may have ceca. The tail of the female is blunt, whereas that of the male is often coiled, and bears two spicules. The life cycle can be direct or indirect. Eggs are large and thick-shelled (Figure 5.2)[4]. The superfamily includes the families Ascarididae and Anisakidae.

Superfamily Heterakoidea

Worms in this superfamily are small to medium-sized, with poorly developed lips and a small buccal cavity. Lateral alae may be prominent and extend the length of the body. Male worms possess a preanal sucker. These are mostly parasites of birds, although the superfamily also includes a few species of rodent parasites. Parasite families of interest include Heterakidae and Ascaridiidae.

Superfamily Oxyuroidea

The oxyurids or "pinworms" are small to medium-sized worms. The three lips are inconspicuous. Males may have no, one, or two spicules. In general, the females are larger than the males, and the female tail is long and tapering. The esophagus ends in a posterior bulb (Figure 5.3)[5]. The eggs are often operculated. Life cycles are direct. The superfamily includes the families Oxyuridae and Kathlaniidae.

Order Strongylida

The order Strongylida includes some of the most common and pathogenic gastrointestinal or respiratory system parasites of vertebrates. There is considerable morphologic diversity within the order. Features shared by all are the general shape and appearance of the egg, and a well-developed copulatory bursa in the adult males. The number and arrangement of the bursal rays are useful for taxonomic identification. Equally important taxonomic features are the shape and length of the spicules. The order contains four superfamilies of importance.

Superfamily Strongyloidea

Many worms in this superfamily are characterized by having well-developed, capacious mouths, although this feature is not universal. For example, worms in the genus *Oesophagostomum* have a narrow buccal cavity. In many species, the mouth is surrounded by a corona radiata ("leaf-crown"), and contains cutting plates or teeth. The copulatory bursae of the males are well-developed and are supported by bursal rays. Males in the superfamily bear two spicules of equal length[1]. Important families include Strongylidae, Trichonematidae, Amidostomidae, Stephanuridae, and Syngamidae.

Superfamily Ancylostomatoidea

Worms in this superfamily are known as "hookworms." Adult worms lack a corona radiata. They possess large buccal cavities armed with either teeth or cutting plates. Most of the hookworms are voracious blood-suckers, and therefore highly pathogenic[1]. The eggs are thin-shelled and oval (Figure 5.4)[6]. The only family of veterinary importance is the Ancylostomatidae.

Superfamily Trichostrongyloidea

Trichostrongyloidea possess the prominent copulatory bursa typical of the order, but lack a corona radiata. Also lacking is the capacious buccal cavity characteristic of the Strongyloidea and Ancylostomatoidea. Instead, the buccal cavity is reduced or rudimentary. Lips are also inconspicuous. These worms are generally small, slender, and delicate in appearance. Key morphologic features include the shape and arrangement of the bursa, spicules, and cuticular

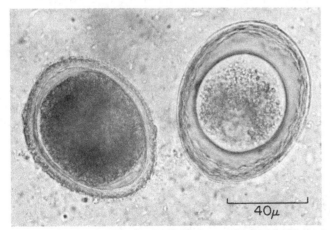

Fig. 5.2 Canine ascarid eggs. (Left) *Toxocara canis.* (Right) *Toxascaris leonina.* Reproduced from Ewing, S.A. (1967). Used with permission, courtesy of W.B. Saunders Co., Philadelphia.

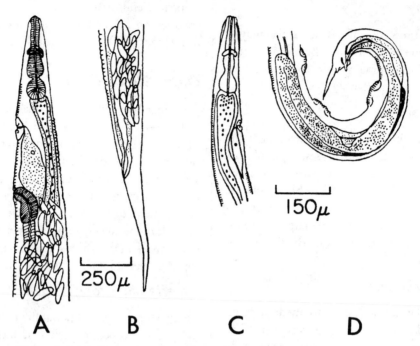

Fig. 5.3 *Syphacia obvelata.* (A) Female, head. (B) Female, tail. (C) Male, head. (D) Male, tail. Reproduced from Sasa, M., Tanaka, H., Fukui, M., and Takata, A. (1962). Used with permission, courtesy of Academic Press, New York.

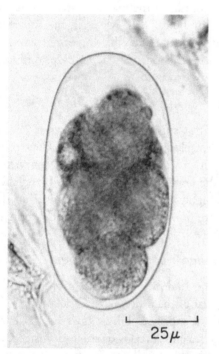

Fig. 5.4 *Ancylostoma braziliense* egg. Reproduced from Burrows, R.B. (1965). Used with permission, courtesy of Yale University Press, New Haven.

annulations or striations. Life cycles are direct. Free-living third-stage larvae are infective to susceptible hosts. Families of veterinary importance include Trichostrongylidae, Ollulanidae, and Dictyocaulidae.

Superfamily Metastrongyloidea

Worms in this superfamily are parasites of the respiratory system of mammals, and so are appropriately referred to as "lungworms." Like the Trichostrongylidae, worms in this superfamily have a much reduced or rudimentary buccal cavity and six inconspicuous lips. Likewise, these worms are small and slender. Unlike other members of the order, the copulatory bursa is reduced or absent. Lungworm life cycles usually, though not always, include obligatory intermediate hosts, typically terrestrial slugs and snails[1]. Families of veterinary importance include Metastrongylidae, Protostrongylidae, Filaroididae, Skrjabingylidae, and Crenosomatidae.

Order Spirurida

The order Spirurida is a biologically diverse group of parasitic nematodes, and contains some parasites of tremendous global importance to human and veterinary health. Adult worms are characterized by two well-developed lateral lips and a cylindrical buccal capsule and pharynx. The esophagus is divided into a muscular anterior portion and a glandular posterior portion, which is wider and longer than the muscular part. Cephalic ornamentation is common. Adult male worms typically have caudal alae and spicules of unequal length. The eggs have thick walls and are embryonated when laid. The life cycles of the Spirurida require development of larval stages within arthropod intermediate hosts. The order includes four superfamilies.

Superfamily Spiruroidea

The superfamily includes species that are commonly found parasitizing the stomach wall or lumen of vertebrate hosts. Others inhabit the periocular structures. The posterior end of the male is usually spirally coiled, with lateral alae and papillae. The eggs are thick-shelled and embryonated at the time of release from the female (Figure 5.5)[7]. Important families include Spiruridae, Thelaziidae, Acuariidae, and Tetrameridae.

Superfamily Physalopteroidea

The superfamily includes a small number of morphologically distinct gastric parasites. Worms in this superfamily are thick and muscular, and resemble ascarids. Adult worms have morphologically distinct lips bearing teeth or toothlike ridges[1]. Eggs are thick-shelled. Important families include the Physalopteridae and Gnathostomatidae.

Superfamily Filaroidea

The superfamily Filaroidea includes several species of human and veterinary parasites of tremendous medical importance. Stages found in vertebrate hosts often inhabit body cavities, connective tissues, or hemolymphatic vessels. Adult worms are long, thin, and delicate. The mouth is small. These worms lack lips, a buccal capsule, and a pharynx. The male is often smaller than the female (Figure 5.6), and bears spicules of dissimilar appearance. The vulva of the female is typically located near the anterior end of the worm. Larvae ("microfilariae") are released into lymph and connective tissue spaces, or into the blood stream of the definitive vertebrate host. Microfilariae are taken up by arthropod intermediate hosts during blood feeding. Morphologic features of the microfilariae are useful for species identification[1]. The most important families include the Filariidae, Setariidae, and Onchocercidae.

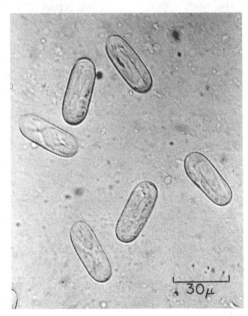

Fig. 5.5 *Spirocerca lupi* eggs. Reproduced from Bailey, W.S. (1963). Used with permission, courtesy of New York Academy of Science.

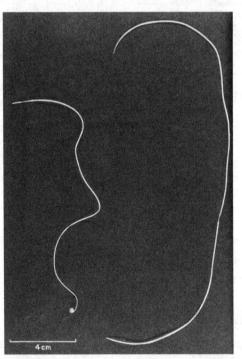

Fig. 5.6 *Dirofilaria immitis* adults. (Left) Male. (Right) Female. Courtesy of S.H. Abadie, Louisiana State University.

Superfamily Dracunculoidea

The superfamily contains a small number of medically important parasites. These have rudimentary mouths and readily observable cephalic papillae. Adult worms have been found inhabiting the subcutaneous tissues of vertebrate hosts of nearly all classes, while larval forms develop in invertebrates. In some cases, lower vertebrates such as fish and amphibians may serve as transport ("paratenic") hosts[1]. The only family of veterinary concern is Dracunculidae.

Order Enoplida

The Enoplida include a group of biologically diverse worms. Worms in this order may be found in a variety of host organ systems, including the gastrointestinal, musculoskeletal, urinary, and pulmonary systems. The order includes two superfamilies.

Superfamily Trichuroidea

The Trichuroidea are small to medium-sized worms. The lips and buccal cavity are absent or reduced. They are distinct in that the tissue of the worm esophagus is reduced, rendering the esophagus very slender. Also, the esophageal glands are on the outside of the esophagus in the form of a single row of cells ("stichocytes"). Males have one or no spicules. The eggs have a "polar plug" at each end (Figure 5.7). Life cycles of the Trichuroidea are usually direct. Parasite families of human and veterinary medical importance include Trichinellidae, Trichuridae, and Capillaridae.

Superfamily Dioctophymatoidea

The superfamily includes a small number of unusual but important nematode parasites. Adult worms are medium to large in size, and are typically found in the intestines, kidneys, or other organs of vertebrates. The lips and buccal cavity are reduced. Male worms possess one spicule and a prominent cup-, or trumpet-shaped copulatory bursa. Depending on the genus, there also may be a caudal or cephalic sucker present[1,2]. Only two relatively small families—the Dioctophymidae and Soboliphymidae—are of importance.

PHYLUM ACANTHOCEPHALA

The phylum Acanthocephala contains the "thorny-headed worms." These are so named because they possess a

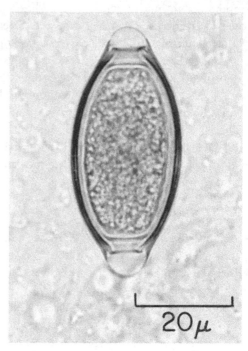

Fig. 5.7 *Trichuris trichiura* egg. Courtesy of R.R. Estes, U.S. Air Force School of Aerospace Medicine.

proboscis armed with rows of hooks, with which they attach to the intestinal wall of vertebrate hosts. These worms lack an alimentary canal, and instead absorb nutrients through the body surface. Sexes are separate, and adult males are much smaller than females (Figure 5.8)[8,9].

All Acanthocephalan life cycles are indirect, with arthropod or crustacean intermediate hosts. Each egg released from female worms contains an acanthor larva. Upon ingestion by a suitable intermediate host, the egg hatches, releasing the acanthor. The freed acanthor encysts in the intermediate host as a cystacanth. After a period of up to several months, the cystacanth reaches an infective stage, and, upon ingestion by a definitive host, develops to an adult worm. If consumed by an unsuitable host, the cystacanth may re-encyst. In this case, the infected host serves as a paratenic host. Acanthocephalans may be found in laboratory swine and in aquatic vertebrates such as fish and some birds. There are two orders of importance: Palaeacanthocephala and Archiacanthocephala. The former are relatively small worms with a retractable proboscis, while the latter are large worms with a non-retractable proboscis[1,3].

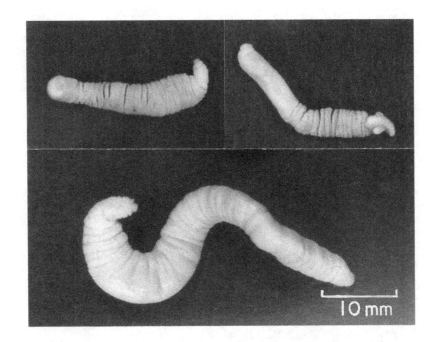

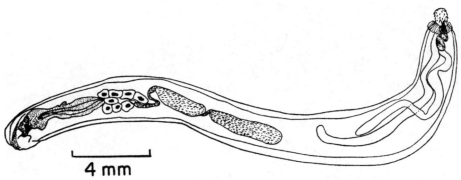

Fig. 5.8 *Prosthenorchis elegans.* (Top) Photograph of adult worms. (Bottom) Drawing of an adult male. (Top) reproduced from Worms, M.J. (1967). Used with permission, courtesy of Institute of Animal Technicians. (Bottom) reproduced from Machado Filho, D.A. (1950). Used with permission, courtesy of Memórias do Instituto Oswaldo Cruz.

REFERENCES

1. Soulsby, E.J.L. (1982) *Helminths, Arthropods and Protozoa of Domesticated Animals,* 7th Edition, Lea and Febiger, Philadelphia, 809 pp.

2. Roberts, L.S. and Janovy, J. Jr. (2004) *Foundations of Parasitology,* 7th Edition, The McGraw Hill Companies, New York, 702 pp.

3. Mehlhorn, H. (2001) *Encyclopedic Reference of Parasitology. Biology, Structure, Function,* 2nd Edition. Springer 2001, New York, 674 pp.

4. Ewing, S.A. (1967) Examinations for parasites. In: Coles, E.H. (ed.) *Veterinary Clinical Pathology.* W.B. Saunders Co., Philadelphia, pp. 331–391.

5. Sasa, M., Tanaka, H., Fukui, M., and Takata, A. (1962) Internal parasites of laboratory animals. In: Harris, R.J.C. (ed.) *The Problems of Laboratory Animal Disease.* Academic Press, Inc., Philadelphia.

6. Burrows, R.B. (1965) *Microscopic Diagnosis of the Parasites of Man.* Yale University Press, New Haven, 328 pp.

7. Bailey, W.S. (1963) Parasites and cancer: Sarcoma in dogs associated with *Spirocerca lupi. Ann. N.Y. Acad. Sci.* **108,** 890–923.

8. Worms, M.J. (1967) Parasites of newly imported animals. *J. Inst. Animal Technicians* **18,** 39–47.

9. Machado Filho, D.A. (1950) Revisáo do gênero *Prosthenorchis* Travassos, 1915 (Acanthocephala). *Mem. Inst. Oswaldo Cruz* **48,** 495–544.

Biology of Arthropods

Ronnie L. Byford, PhD, and Maurice E. Craig, MS

INTRODUCTION

The phylum Arthropoda includes the insects, and crustaceans, arachnids and spiders, along with several smaller and lesser-known groups. The word "Arthropoda" comes from the Greek "arthron" (jointed) and "podon" (foot). Thus, arthropods are animals that have joints in their external skeleton, including all of their appendages.

Arthropoda is, by far, the most successful phylum of animals, whether measured by diversity of habitat, extent of distribution, or number of species and individuals. About 80% of all known animal species are arthropods. They are

Tables are placed at the ends of chapters.

exceedingly diverse morphologically, developmentally, functionally, and behaviorally, and have adapted successfully to life in water, on land, and in the air.

This chapter provides an overview of the classification, morphology, and biology of arthropods, emphasizing parasites of laboratory animals. The reader interested in learning more about arthropods in general, or arthropod parasites specifically, is referred to several available references[1-6].

Arthropod parasites can be direct agents of disease. They cause damage by annoyance, stress, or blood loss; "fly worry" and "tick worry" are recognized conditions that reduce feed efficiency and weight gains in livestock. Ectoparasites can cause dermatoses and allergic reactions, and wounds or lesions offer entry to bacteria. Blood-feeding arthropods typically inject small quantities of saliva into the wound channel, which can result in envenomization or paralysis. Myiasis, which is the invasion of organs or tissues by fly larvae, is part of the normal life cycle of several species of Diptera.

Additionally, many arthropods are indirect agents of disease. Several arthropod species serve as intermediate hosts for parasites, or as vectors that transmit parasites, bacteria, rickettsia, and viruses to man and animals.

STRUCTURE AND FUNCTION

The first fundamental structural feature of the Arthropoda is that the body is divided longitudinally into discrete segments ("somites" or "metameres"). In nearly all adult arthropods, body segments and appendages are reduced in number, and retained appendages typically are highly modified into sensory, locomotory, reproductive, respiratory, and feeding structures.

A second fundamental feature is the grouping of adjacent body segments into distinct body regions or sections called "tagmata" (singular: tagma), that serve particular functions for the animal. The typical arthropod body consists of three distinct tagmata: the head, thorax, and abdomen. The head provides for neural integration, sensory perception, and food gathering; the thorax bears legs (and wings, in most insects) and serves locomotory functions; and the abdomen contains the organs that perform digestive, reproductive, and respiratory functions. Segmentation and tagmatization are expressed differently in various taxonomic groupings. In some taxa abdominal segmentation is minimal, and many groups have the head and thorax fused.

A third fundamental feature of arthropods is that they have a tough, insoluble, cuticular exoskeleton, which provides structural support and protection from predators and adverse environmental conditions. The exoskeleton contains chitin, a polysaccharide polymer of N-acetylglucosamine. Chitin occurs only in arthropods and in fungi and, after cellulose, is the second most abundant polysaccharide in nature. The cuticle is formed by the underlying epidermis, and is subdivided into the inner procuticle (endocuticle in crustaceans), composed primarily of chitin, and an outer epicuticle, composed primarily of sclerotized or "tanned" proteins. In most terrestrial arthropods the epicuticle has an external lipid layer, overlain by a "varnish," which serves to retard water loss.

The exoskeleton is not a uniformly hardened structure, but is composed of a series of relatively hard, inflexible plates, or sclerites, connected by thinner, flexible articular membranes that allow for movement of the body segments and appendages. The cuticle of each segment is divided into four primary sclerites: a dorsal tergite, two lateral pleurites, and a ventral sternite. Skeletal muscles are attached to cuticular ridges and spines arising from the inner surface of sclerites. Limb segments, or podomeres, are essentially hollow tubes articulating at condylar surfaces between adjacent sclerites and moved by internal muscles. In insects, podomeres of the leg (from proximal to distal) are: coxa, trochanter, femur, tibia, and tarsus. Legs in other taxa typically have a different number of podomeres and different nomenclature. The structure of the limbs varies greatly among groups and also among life stages in individual species. Often, different parts of the appendages bear highly developed processes and extensions.

Because their exoskeleton does not expand, to increase in mass, arthropods must undergo ecdysis (molting), in which the old cuticle is shed and a new one grown. The molting process is most studied in insects and crustaceans but is thought to be similar in other arthropod groups. In insects, neurosecretory cells in the brain produce prothoracicotrophic hormone that stimulates glands in the prothorax to secrete ecdysone (ecdysteroid), which mediates growth and development and initiates molting. The stage of the animal between molts is called an instar or intermolt. The length of each instar and the number of molts are variable, and depend on the species or external factors, such as nutrition or temperature. Ecdysis is a critical stage in arthropod development, and some of the drugs and pesticides used for controlling arthropods disrupt biochemical reactions in the molting process.

The arthropod coelom is much reduced, and most of the body cavity consists of a hemocoel in which tissues are bathed in hemolymph supplied by an open circulatory system comprising a dorsal heart and arteries. Nitrogenous wastes are removed from the hemolymph either by paired excretory glands (in crustaceans and others) or Malpighian tubules (in insects). The digestive system is complete and glandular, and the structures of the gut and associated digestive organs vary with different feeding strategies.

Respiration in very small arthropods is usually by direct diffusion across the body surface, while larger animals use respiratory structures. Most insects, mites, and ticks respire through a tracheal system—a series of intricately branched tubes (tracheae). Tracheae externally connect with openings in the exoskeleton (spiracles) and internally extend as very fine tubes (tracheoles) into all tissues of the body. All crustaceans and most aquatic immature insects use external gills, whereas most spiders and many arachnids respire through book lungs—sets of delicate, sheet-like tissues that function like internal gills.

The arthropod nervous system is capable of allowing complex behavior, including learned behavior, and consists of a dorsal brain that is connected to the subesophageal ganglia that innervate the mouthparts. Paired, ventral nerve cords originating from the subesophageal ganglia in turn connect with paired ganglia in each somite. Sensory organs are usually well developed; most arthropods have a pair of multifaceted compound eyes and one to many ocelli, or simple eyes. In addition, because most depend on chemical cues for finding food (or hosts) and for conspecific communication, they have sensitive chemoreceptors. The arthropod nervous system is the target of most pesticidal chemicals and antiparasitic drugs. Many of these are designed to interfere with synaptic or axonic processes, while others interfere with the chemical communication system.

DEVELOPMENT

With few exceptions, arthropods are dioecious and sexually dimorphic, and fertilization is internal. Most groups are oviparous or ovoviviparous. Embryonic development includes intralecithal cleavage and schizocoely.

Postembryonic development is highly variable. Some arthropods exhibit direct, or ametabolous, development, in which the egg hatches into a sexually immature juvenile that is essentially a miniature version of the adult, and simply grows larger with progressive molts until reaching sexual maturity. Usually, development is indirect; the egg hatches into a larval stage that is structurally dissimilar to the adult and occupies a different ecological niche. Larvae are highly variable in form and biology among the various arthropod taxa.

With indirect development, the larval stage must undergo structural reorganization, or "metamorphosis," before reaching the adult stage. Most crustaceans undergo anamorphic development (anamorphosis), in which a new terminal segment is added at each molt. Some arthropods exhibit gradual or incomplete metamorphosis, or hemimetabolous development, in which the immature instars gradually become more like the adult with each molt.

Most insect orders undergo complete metamorphosis, or holometabolous development. In this case, larvae do not resemble adults, even during late instars. After several molts, the larvae enter a quiescent stage, called a pupa, during which the entire animal is reorganized into the "imago," or adult.

Endocrine control of development in insects is mediated by juvenile hormone (JH), and the process is thought to be similar in other arthropod groups. In the insect, JH is produced by the corpus allatum, located behind the brain. Juvenile hormone impedes maturation, and when present at high levels, maintains larval or nymphal characteristics. As the immature arthropod continues to grow, the JH titer decreases, permitting development of adult characteristics. At some time during the last larval or nymphal instar, JH drops to undetectable levels, and the animal enters the next developmental stage—the adult in hemimetabolous taxa, the pupa in holometabolous insects. Because arthropods are exothermic, the time spent in each developmental stage varies considerably with temperature.

CLASSIFICATION

The systematics and phylogenetics associated with such an immense and diverse assemblage is complex and dynamic. Classical taxonomic status in the Arthropoda is in large part based on the morphology and function of appendages and on the characteristic tagmatization of a given group. However, scientific advances, particularly the development of nucleic acid sequence analysis, contribute new sources of data, which reorganize old taxonomic groupings. Authorities differ in classification schemes, particularly regarding higher taxonomic levels.

This text follows the U.S. Department of Agriculture Integrated Taxonomic Information System (USDA-ITIS) classification (Retrieved Aug. 9, 2004, from the Integrated Taxonomic Information System on-line database, http://www.itis.usda.gov), which divides the Arthropoda into four subphyla: Crustacea (crustaceans), Chelicerata (spiders, mites etc.), Hexapoda (insects), and Myriapoda (centipedes and kin). All but the Myriapoda contain species that are parasitic on animals.

Arthropods share some characteristics with the Annelida or segmented worms (leeches, earthworms, etc.), including external segmentation and a similar nervous system, and the two phyla once were considered to be closely related. However, this is no longer accepted, and the Arthropoda are now grouped along with the Nematoda and a few other small phyla into a group called the Ecdysozoa, all members of which have a cuticle that is periodically molted[6]. Legless arthropods, such as some insect larvae, may be confused with annelid worms, but in larval insects the body has fewer than 13 segments, while annelids generally have more than 13 segments.

CRUSTACEA

This large group of roughly 44,000 known species is composed of six classes: Branchiopoda (primarily fresh water crustaceans, including brine shrimp, water fleas, etc.), Malacostraca (crabs, shrimp, amphipods, pill bugs, etc.), Maxillipoda (copepods, fish lice, barnacles, etc.), Ostracoda (seed shrimp), Cephalocarida, and Remipedia. Sometimes referred to as "insects of the sea", crustaceans are the dominant arthropods in marine habitats, but are also found in large numbers in fresh water. A few taxa are terrestrial. There are comparatively few crustaceans that parasitize vertebrates, but from a practical standpoint, any arthropod parasite affecting fishes is probably a crustacean.

Crustacean appendages typically are biramous—that is, having two branches (the exopodite and endopodite)—but may be secondarily uniramous. Tagmata consist of a head (cephalon), thorax, and abdomen, or a cephalothorax (head fused with one or more thoracic segments) and abdomen. Most crustaceans have a dorsal carapace that covers the cephalothorax and sometimes the entire body. The crustacean head comprises five fused segments and their corresponding appendages, consisting of antennules (uniramous first antennae), antennae (second antennae), and three pairs of mouthparts—one pair of mandibles and two pairs of maxillae. One or more pairs of thoracic appendages may be modified for feeding and are called maxillepeds. In most crustacea, the coxae of at least some of the feeding appendages are modified for grinding food and passing it to the oral cavity. The remaining thoracic appendages are adapted for walking or swimming and are called pereiopods. Gills are always present on larger forms.

Development in most crustacean groups is anamorphic. The typical larva is a nauplius (plural: nauplii), which bears three pairs of swimming appendages (corresponding to the antennules, antennae and mandibles) and a single median eye, and shows little or no body segmentation. The nauplius goes through a series of instars, developing into a sexually immature juvenile stage that is structurally similar to the adult. With progressive molts, the juvenile crustacean increases in mass and adds segments, appendages, and other features until reaching the adult stage.

Two crustacean classes, Copepoda (copepods) and Branchiura (branchiurans), contain species that are parasitic on marine and freshwater fishes, and thus might be found on laboratory animals. An additional group, the Pentastomida (pentastomids or tongue worms), is composed entirely of unusual parasites of terrestrial vertebrates.

COPEPODS

Most copepods are free living, but as a group, they show great variation in exploiting symbiotic niches. Some free-living species serve as intermediate hosts for medically important parasites, including the broad fish tapeworm (*Diphyllobothrium latum*) and the guinea worm (*Dracunculus medinensis*). Parasitic copepod species feed on body fluids or skin secretions of fishes, and are important pests of many marine and freshwater species, sometimes causing severe damage to fisheries[4].

Copepods typically have elongated, segmented bodies consisting of a head, thorax, and abdomen. The carapace is reduced or absent. Most have a single, simple eye in the middle of the head. Female copepods retain their eggs in egg sacks, a pair of which protrudes finger-like from the posterior of the animal. Copepod development is anamorphic: the egg hatches into a nauplius that metamorphoses into a juvenile form called a copepodid. Some parasitic copepods (e.g., *Lernaea*, or anchor worms) are particularly suited to a permanent parasitic lifestyle, and thus are unrecognizable as copepods (or even as arthropods) except during early larval stages.

BRANCHIURANS

Branchiurans, or fish lice, are a small group of 130 known species, all of which are ectoparasites of fishes, although some can use frogs and tadpoles as hosts[7]. They are broadly oval, dorsoventrally flattened, have a broad carapace almost entirely covering the body, and have large, distinctive compound eyes. Appendages on the head are modified into hooks, spines and suckers for attaching to the host, and mouthparts are adapted for piercing the skin of the host and sucking blood and body fluids (Figure 6.1)[8]. Branchiurans are good swimmers. They can easily relocate to a different host, and female fish lice leave the host to lay their eggs on the substrate. When they locate a new host

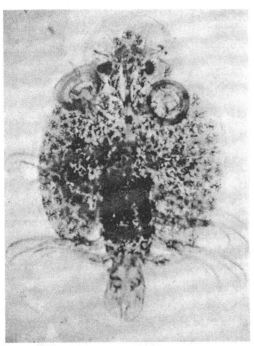 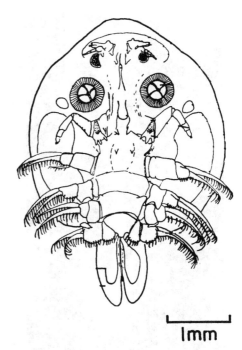

1mm

Fig. 6.1   (Left) *Argulus* from black bass. (Right) *Argulus japonicus* male, ventral view. (Left) courtesy of W.A. Rogers, Southeastern Cooperative Fish Disease Project, Auburn University. (Right) reproduced from Hoffman, G.L. (1967). Used with permission.

they typically attach behind the operculum or a fin, which reduces the likelihood they will be brushed or washed off of the host.

PENTASTOMIDS

The taxonomic status of the pentastomids (also called pentastomes or tongue worms) historically has been uncertain, but most evidence places them near the Branchiura in a class or subclass, the Pentastomida[9-11]. They are a small group (about 70 species) of mostly tropical to semitropical, hematophagous, pulmonary, or nasopharyngeal parasites, usually of snakes, lizards, amphibians, and crocodilians. A few species parasitize sea birds, canines, or felines. They are morphologically and biologically atypical of arthropods, and their phylogenic relationships have been problematic.

Superficially, pentastomids resemble annelids; they have wormlike, elongate, segmented bodies and lack antennae, eyes, obvious appendages, or other typical arthropodan features (Figure 6.2). A characteristic of all adult pentastomids is the presence of two pairs of retractable hooks, often at the end of stubby, leg-like appendages, adjacent to the mouth (Figure 6.3). Superficially, the two pairs of retracted hooks resemble four

additional mouths, hence the source of the subclass name (penta = five, stoma = mouth). The hooks serve to attach the worm to the host and to tear host tissues, releasing blood and fluids for ingestion by the parasite.

In the more evolved pentastomid species, the life cycle is heteroxenous and similar to that seen in many cestodes. The female lays eggs that pass up the trachea of the host, where they are expectorated or swallowed and passed out with the feces. A suitable intermediate host (including several species of fish, reptiles, amphibians, mammals, or insects) then ingests the eggs, which hatch in the intestine. Newly hatched larvae penetrate the gut wall and migrate through the body, eventually encysting in body tissues—usually in the viscera—and metamorphosing into quiescent nymphs. The definitive host is infected by eating animals or viscera containing nymphs.

Pentastomids have public health importance, because some species can use humans as either intermediate or definitive hosts. Human infection by *Linguatula serrata,* a parasite of dogs and other carnivores, causes nasopharyngeal pentastomiasis known as "halzoun" or "marrara" in parts of Asia, North Africa, and the Middle East. Infection occurs when nymphs are ingested with raw or undercooked viscera of ungulate animals.

CHELICERATA

The Chelicerata includes roughly 70,000 species distributed in three classes. The Merostomata (horseshoe crabs) and the Pycnogonida (sea spiders) are two small classes of marine arthropods. The Arachnida (arachnids), is by far the largest and most diverse class, and contains the parasitic mites and ticks.

Chelicerates typically have six pairs of appendages and do not have antennae. In most taxa, the body has two distinct divisions: the prosoma (cephalothorax), which is the fused head and thorax, and the opisthosoma (abdomen). The prosoma comprises six segments and their respective appendages. The chelicerae are post-oral feeding appendages, which may be chelate (pincer-like) or bear fangs. The second pair, the pedipalps, are variously modified for sensory, defensive, feeding, or reproductive functions. The remaining four pairs of appendages are walking legs. In most chelicerates, the coxae of one or more pairs of appendages are modified for grinding food and passing it to the oral cavity. The opisthosoma primitively comprises up to 12 segments, but abdominal segmentation is reduced or absent in many taxa. In several taxa the opisthosoma terminates in a tail, but appendages on the abdomen are usually absent.

Arachnida

The class Arachnida comprises the orders Acari (mites and ticks), Amblypygi (whipspiders), Araneae (spiders), Opiliones (daddy longlegs), Palpigradi (microscorpions), Pseudoscorpiones (pseudoscorpions), Ricinulei (ricinuleids), Schizomida (short-tailed whipscorpions), Scorpiones (scorpions), Solifugae (sun spiders), and Uropygi (whipscorpions)[6]. Spiders make up the majority of the more than 38,000 species in the class, followed by ticks and mites with more than 30,000 species. While there are some venomous spiders and scorpions that could potentially affect laboratory animals, by far the most medically important arachnids are the parasitic ticks and mites in the order Acari.

All species of ticks and several species of mites are cosmopolitan parasites of endothermic and exothermic animals. Ticks and mites are morphologically similar, yet they have distinct differences. Most notably, ticks are large and easily macroscopic, while most mites, especially those species that are animal parasites, are small to microscopic.

The classification of the Acari is unsettled, and can get somewhat complicated. Krantz[12] proposed two orders: Acariformes (acariform mites) and Parasitiformes (ticks

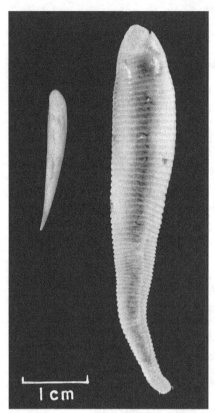

Fig. 6.2 *Linguatula serrata*. (Left) Male. (Right) Female. Courtesy of A. Fain, Institut de Médicine Tropicale Prince Léopold.

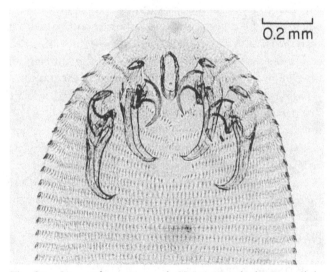

Fig. 6.3 *Linguatula serrata* nymph. Note spinous body rings and the two pairs of binate hooks. Courtesy of A. Fain, Institut de Médicine Tropicale Prince Léopold.

and parasitiform mites). Evans[13] elevates the Acari to subclass level and recognizes two superorders and seven orders. However, the primary difference between classification systems is the level (i.e., subclass, order, or suborder) assigned to the taxa. This text follows the classification of Barnes[3] as modified by Triplehorn and Johnson[6], in which the Acari form an order comprising six suborders. The suborder Ixodida contains the ticks, and the suborders Mesostigmata, Prostigmata, and Astigmata contain parasitic mites that might be encountered in laboratory situations. The suborders Opilioacariformes and Oribatida are composed entirely of free-living species, but some oribatid species are important as intermediate hosts of *Moniezia expansa,* a tapeworm of ruminants.

In the Acari, the prosoma and opisthosoma are fused, and there is no apparent segmentation. This situation has given rise to a special nomenclature for the body regions of this group. The capitulum, or gnathosoma, is the "head," composed of the segments of the mouth and its appendages. The rest of the body is the idiosoma.

Larval Acari have three pairs of legs and adults generally have four pairs; however, some adult mites have only one to three pairs. The mouthparts of the parasitic Acari are modified for specialized feeding. The feeding structures arise from a basal structure called the basis capitulum, the shape of which is taxonomically important. The pedipalps are modified for holding a fold of skin while the chelicerae lacerate the folded tissues. The hypostome, composed of the fused coxae of the pedipalps, is a rod-shaped structure that is inserted into the host during feeding to suck up the blood or lymph flowing into the wound. The hypostome of ticks is armed with recurved teeth, allowing for attachment to the host. In mites, the hypostome is smooth, and chelicerae are often modified to aid in attachment.

Suborder Ixodida (ticks)

The suborder Ixodida contains two subfamilies: the Ixodidae, or hard ticks, and the Argasidae, or soft ticks. All ticks have four stages in their life cycle: egg, a six-legged larval stage, and eight-legged nymphal and adult stages. Depending on species and availability of hosts, the life cycle may require from a few weeks to a few years to complete. Although some ticks are host-specific, most will feed on any suitable host. Many tick species can survive without feeding for several years.

Much of the behavior associated with ticks is under hormonal control. Tick pheromones have been recognized that influence aggregation, attachment, and reproduction. Mating behavior is typically species-specific, complex, and controlled at several stages by these chemicals.

Ticks can cause significant damage to their hosts. Heavy tick burdens cause dermatosis, secondary infections, debilitation, and anemia. Several tick species preferentially engorge in the ears of the host, a condition called otoacariasis, causing serious irritation, internal ear infections, or damage to external structures. A condition known as "tick paralysis" or "tick bite paralysis" affects man, cattle, dogs, and other mammals when certain tick species attach near the base of the skull. This apparently results from salivary secretions by the tick, and is quickly remedied when the tick is removed. In addition to directly harming hosts, ticks are excellent vectors for a large number of parasitic, bacterial, rickettsial, and viral diseases.

Family Ixodidae, the hard ticks, includes more than 800 species, and is divided into three subfamilies comprising ten genera: *Ixodes* (Figure 6.4); *Amblyomma* (Figure 6.5); *Haemaphysalis, Aponomma, and Dermacentor* (Figure 6.6); *Rhipicephalus; Anocentor; Hyalomma; Boophilu;* and *Margaropus.* Hard ticks usually inhabit environments with somewhat humid conditions.

In the ixodids, the capitulum projects anteriorly and can easily be seen when viewed dorsally. Other characteristics include a large sclerite (scutum) covering much of the idiosoma, eyes (when present) located on the scutum, sexual dimorphism (e.g., females are larger than males and the scutum of the female does not completely cover the idiosoma), and stigmatal (spiracular) plates behind the fourth pair of legs, and the posterior margin of the opisthosoma is often subdivided into sclerites called festoons (Figure 6.7). In addition, all Ixodidae have only one nymphal instar.

Depending on species, female ixodids lay 100 to 20,000 eggs that hatch into larvae ("seed" ticks) that then climb onto low vegetation and extend their front legs in response to a passing host—a behavior that is referred to as "questing." Once they attach to a host and obtain a blood meal, they molt to an eight-legged nymphal stage, then they must again feed and molt to the adult stage.

During the feeding process, ixodids secrete a salivary substance that cements them to the host, preventing them from being easily dislodged. The engorgement process in hard ticks may take several days to complete. Copulation occurs on the host with the male tick producing a spermatophore that is placed under the genital operculum of

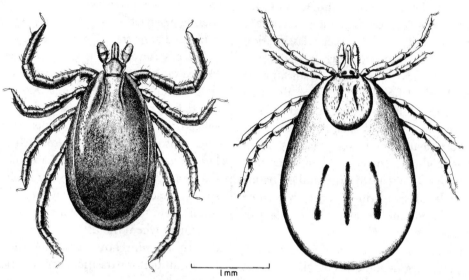

Fig. 6.4   *Ixodes scapularis.* (Left) Male. (Right) Female. Courtesy of U.S. Department of Agriculture.

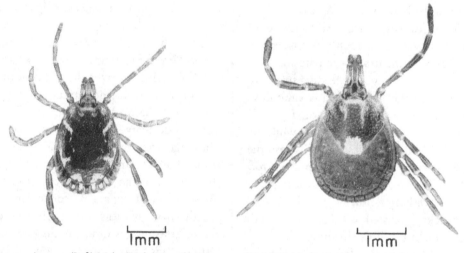

Fig. 6.5   *Amblyomma americanum.* (Left) Male. (Right) Female. Courtesy of G.M. Kohls, Rocky Mountain Laboratory.

the female. The engorged, fertilized female drops off the host and deposits her eggs in the soil or litter. The final blood meal is terminal, and after mating and oviposition, the adults die.

Hard ticks exhibit a variety of life histories, depending on the number of hosts on which they complete their life cycle. If the larval, nymphal, and adult stages of a tick species are completed on the same host, it is a one-host tick. If the larval and nymphal stages are completed on one host, and the nymph drops off to find and attach to another host on which it attains the adult stage, it is a two-host tick. However, most ixodids are three-host ticks, completing the

larval, nymphal, and adult stages on three different host animals.

The family of soft ticks, or Argasidae, includes more than 160 species in five genera, including *Argas, Ornithor-doros, Otobius, Nothoaspis,* and *Atricola. Nothoaspis* and *Atricola* spp. infest cave-dwelling bats in North and Central America and would not normally be encountered. In general, argasid ticks inhabit environments of extremely low relative humidity.

Argasid ticks have a capitulum that is subterminal and cannot be seen in dorsal view. The capitulum lies in a groove called the camerostome. Additionally, soft ticks do

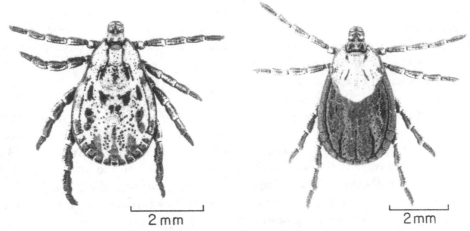

Fig. 6.6 *Dermacentor andersoni.* (Left) Male. (Right) Female. Courtesy of G.M. Kohls, Rocky Mountain Laboratory.

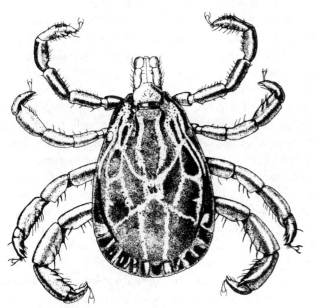

Fig. 6.7 *Amblyomma* male, dorsal view. Courtesy of U.S. Department of Agriculture.

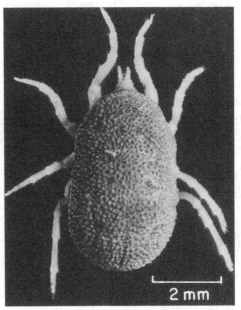

Fig. 6.8 *Ornithodoros turicata* adult male, dorsal view. Courtesy of U.S. Department of Agriculture.

not have festoons or a scutum, eyes are on the lateral margins of the body, stigmatal plates are behind the third pair of legs, and there is little sexual dimorphism (Figure. 6.8).

Some argasid ticks seek hosts by questing on low-lying vegetation, but most are nest parasites that rest in sheltered environments such as burrows, caves, or nests. Life stages of Argasids are not easily distinguishable. Larvae usually remain on the host until molting, but nymphs and larvae may leave the host between feedings. They typically feed quickly and hide nearby until the next feeding. Unlike ixodid ticks, many argasids go through multiple nymphal stages. Adult females deposit small batches of eggs in their hiding places between blood meals.

Suborder Mesostigmata

Mites of the suborder Mesostigmata are more closely related to the ticks than to other mites. They are characterized by having one or more sclerotized ventral plates, a large dorsal scutum, and a single pair of lateral stigmata on the idiosoma, located just behind and lateral to the third coxae[14]. A tracheal trunk (peritreme) usually extends anterior from each stigma, which makes it easy to recognize species belonging to this suborder. Although the majority are nonparasitic, numerous species are parasitic, some of which are capable of transmitting viruses, rickettsiae, bacteria, protozoans, and helminths.

Important families within this suborder are Laelaptidae, Halarachnidae, Dermanyssidae, and Rhinonyssidae. Laelaptidae is a cosmopolitan family that includes a large number of diverse genera. They are the most common ectoparasites of mammals, and some species parasitize invertebrates. Halarachnids are parasites of the respiratory systems of mammals. Dermanyssids are parasites on vertebrates and are of considerable economic and medical importance. Rhinonyssids are parasitic in the respiratory tracts of many species of birds.

Suborder Prostigmata

The Prostigmata are structurally and biologically diverse and include some of the most common parasites of animals. Important families with parasitic members include: Cheyletidae, Pyemotidae, Psorergatidae, Demodicidae, and Trombiculidae. Larvae of species in the Trombiculidae are called chiggers, which are cosmopolitan ectoparasites on a variety of wild and domestic vertebrates worldwide[15]. Larvae of some chigger species are vectors of *Rickettsia tsutsugamushi,* which causes scrub typhus in wild rats and man.

Suborder Astigmata

Mites of the suborder Astigmata are closely related to the Prostigmata. They are soft bodied in all life stages. Sexual dimorphism is common, and the males usually have prominent adanal suckers. Astigmatids lack a tracheal system and respire through the tegument. They lack tarsal claws and have sucker-like structures on their pretarsi. Some of the most important parasitic mites, the itch mites or mange mites, belong to this suborder. Important astigmatid families include Psoroptidae, Sarcoptidae, Knemidokoptidae, and Pyroglyphidae. Members of Psoroptidae feed on lymph produced by piercing the skin at the base of the hair, which causes severe inflammation and scabbing. Sarcoptids are morphologically similar to psoroptids. These mites burrow into the skin of the host, forming

tunnels within the subcutaneous layers of tissue and causing severe pruritus. Knemidokoptid mites are very similar in morphology and biology to the Sarcoptidae. Species of this family also burrow into the skin of the host.

HEXAPODA

The insects and their kin are the largest and most familiar group of arthropods, comprising more than 800,000 described species. Hexapoda includes 28 orders in the class Insecta, plus a group collectively called the Entognatha—three orders of primitively wingless hexapods exhibiting ametabolous development. Insecta is usually divided into the Apterygota, or wingless insects, consisting of two wingless orders, and the Pterygota, or winged insects, which comprises the remaining 26 orders and accounts for most hexapod species, including all taxa of veterinary interest. Parasitic insects that can affect laboratory animals are found in the orders Hemiptera (bugs), Pthiraptera (lice), Siphonaptera (fleas), and Diptera (flies).

All hexapods are characterized by having three pairs of legs; uniramous appendages; one pair of antennae; and tagmata consisting of head, thorax, and abdomen. The head is composed of five fused segments. Mouthparts consist of one pair of mandibles and one pair of maxillae, along with accessory structures: the labium (upper lip), labrum (lower lip) and hypopharynx (a tongue-like structure between the mandibles). There are two basic types of insect mouthparts: mandibulate and haustellate. In mandibulate mouthparts, the mandibles move in a transverse plane, and the insect bites off and chews solid food. Haustellate mouthparts are modified into an elongated proboscis, forming a tube through which liquid food is ingested.

There are three thoracic somites (prothoracic, mesothoracic, and metathoracic), each with a pair of legs. Most adult insects also have pairs of wings on the mesothoracic and metathoracic somites. Wings of insects are not typical arthropod appendages; they actually are outgrowths of the lateral wall of the thoracic segments. Insect wings typically are thin and membranous, and are supported and strengthened with hollow veins that may contain tracheae, nerves, and hemolymph. In groups that are entirely parasitic (e.g., lice and fleas), as well as some parasitic species in other orders, adults are secondarily apterous, an adaptation to life as permanent ectoparasites. The abdomen is made up of a maximum of 11 abdominal segments, with reproductive appendages on the terminal segments.

Insects exemplify all of the biological and ecological diversity previously described for the phylum Arthropoda with one notable exception: very few insects have exploited the marine environment. Most insects are terrestrial, but many are aquatic in fresh or brackish water for part or all of their life cycles.

Hemiptera

The hemimetabolous true bugs form the order Hemiptera, which contains about 35,000 species[6]. While morphologically and biologically diverse, the unifying characteristic of the order is unique; haustellate mouthparts composed of four piercing stylets (the mandibles and maxillae) enclosed in a slender, flexible sheath (the labium) that is usually segmented. The maxillae enclose a food channel, through which food is withdrawn, and a salivary channel, through which saliva is injected. The proboscis typically projects backwards under the head and thorax when at rest, and is only extended for feeding.

While most hemipterans are plant parasites or insect predators, using their mouthparts to suck plant sap or insect hemolymph, a few are parasites of vertebrates[4]. Polyctenidae are highly evolved parasites of bats. They are quite rare and it is unlikely they would be observed on laboratory animals. The Cimicidae and some of the Reduviidae are obligate, intermittent ectoparasites, sucking blood of vertebrate animals.

Cimicidae

The family Cimicidae contains more than 70 species in 22 genera[16]. Most genera are ectoparasites of bats, while others are pests of man, various mammals, chickens, and nesting birds. Many are local in distribution and of little medical or veterinary importance, but some species are extensively distributed. Most species will feed on other vertebrates when preferred hosts are unavailable.

Cimicids are dorsoventrally flattened, broadly oval, reddish brown bugs approximately 6 mm long. They have reduced wing pads but no actual wings. The integument is sparsely covered with short hairs or bristles (Figure 6.9). They have a distinctive, foul odor that is very noticeable, particularly with a large infestation.

Bed bugs hide in cracks and crevices near the hosts, feeding for 5- to 10-minute periods and then returning to their hiding places. Females lay up to 500 eggs in batches of 10 to 15 in their hiding places. Most species have five nymphal instars, each approximately one week long, with a blood meal required before each molt. A blood meal is also

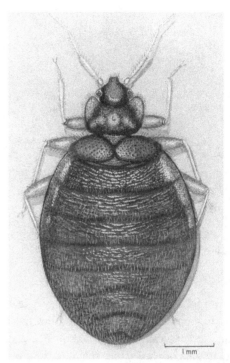

Fig. 6.9 *Cimex lectularius* female. Courtesy of M. Dorothy Cox and Loma Linda University.

required by females prior to oviposition and by males prior to mating. Bites by cimicids typically do not cause lesions when reared on animals under laboratory conditions. The most common pathologic effects are annoyance and loss of blood.

Reduviidae

Most reduviid bugs are predators on other arthropods, but those in the subfamily Triatominae, a group of about 110 species in 14 genera, are obligately hematophagous on vertebrates[17]. Commonly known as "kissing" bugs, blood sucking conenoses, cone-nosed bugs, or Mexican bedbugs, they are mainly tropical and subtropical, and are restricted to the Western Hemisphere and the Oriental region.

These are large insects, with some species exceeding 40 mm in length. They have a long, narrow, freely articulated, cone-shaped head with four-segmented antennae and a slender, three-segmented proboscis. Large, compound eyes are located midway or farther back on the sides of the head. The edges of the abdomen extend laterally beyond the folded wings and in many species are marked with orange or yellow spots (Figure 6.10).

Kissing bugs feed readily on a wide variety of mammalian hosts, including humans[4].

Triatomines tend to be specific in habitat preference, with several species favoring structures that provide cracks

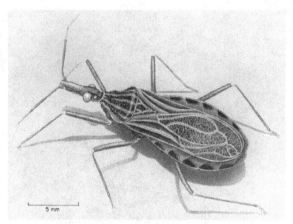

Fig. 6.10 *Rhodnius prolixus* male. Courtesy of M. Dorothy Cox and Loma Linda University.

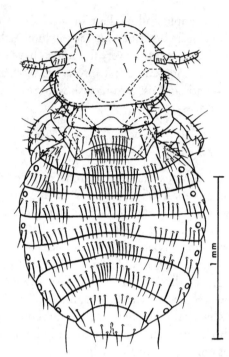

Fig. 6.11 *Trichodectes canis* female, dorsal view. Courtesy of R.D. Price, University of Minnesota.

and crannies for hiding places. Females lay a few dozen to 1,000 eggs in their preferred haunts. There are five instars per generation, and typically one generation per year. As with other hematophagous bugs, they spend most of their time in hiding, emerging at night to acquire a blood meal. Adults feed at least once per week, but can go without a blood meal for months at a time. The feeding bite is relatively painless.

The group is of great public health importance because several species are vectors of the protozoon parasite *Trypanosoma cruzi,* the causative agent of Chagas' disease, which affects man and other susceptible hosts throughout much of Central and South America. Dogs, cats, and rats are the most important reservoir hosts around human habitation.

Pthiraptera

The louse family comprises about 3,500 species and formerly was separated into two orders: Mallophaga (chewing lice) and Anoplura (sucking lice). Current classification places 18 families into four suborders: chewing lice in the Rhyncopthirina, Amblycera, and Ischnocera, and sucking lice in the Anoplura. Both chewing and sucking lice are important pests of many species of laboratory animals, including rats, mice, guinea pigs, dogs, cats, and birds.

Lice are small insects, 1 to 4 mm in length, and are yellowish to blue-black in color. All are well adapted for parasitism; they are apterous and dorsoventrally flattened, with eyes either reduced or absent. Lice typically have stout legs with claw-like tarsi for clinging to hair or feathers.

A simple feature used to separate chewing lice from sucking lice is that the head of chewing lice is short and

blunt and is typically broader than the prothorax (Figure 6.11). Chewing lice have mandibulate mouthparts and feed on bits of skin, fur, or feathers. However, some chewing lice of fowl bite through the feather shaft to feed on blood in the quill.

In contrast, the heads of sucking lice are often elongate and pointed, and are narrower than the prothorax (Figure 6.12). Sucking lice suck blood, and have mouthparts that are unlike any other arthropod group. The mouthparts are made up of three, unsegmented stylets, derived from the fused maxillae, the hypopharynx, and the labium[18]. When at rest, the stylets are retained in an eversible, saclike structure below the esophagus. During feeding, the stylets are everted through a haustellum at the anterior end of the head, penetrating the host tissues.

Lice are cosmopolitan, permanent, obligate ectoparasites of many species of endothermic animals. Chewing lice infest both mammals and birds, while sucking lice infest only mammals. They are highly host-specific and cannot complete a life cycle away from their preferred hosts, but will sometimes feed on an abnormal host. Many animals are hosts to more than one louse species, with each species tending to be found on a particular anatomical area on the host.

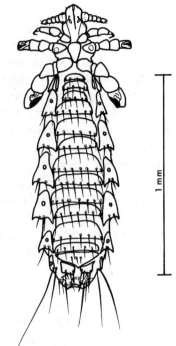

Fig. 6.12 *Polyplax serrata* female, ventral view. Courtesy of K.C. Kim, Pennsylvania State University.

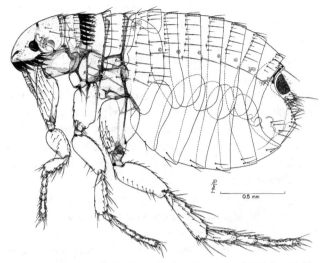

Fig. 6.13 *Ctenocephalides canis* female. Courtesy of R.E. Lewis, Iowa State University.

Louse eggs, called "nits," are glued to hairs or feathers and development is hemimetabolous with three nymphal instars. Generational times are two to four weeks under normal environmental conditions, but longer under hot or cold conditions. The number of lice on infested animals typically tends to increase in winter. Lice are transmitted mainly by direct contact between animals, but can be transmitted by sharing contaminated roosts, nesting areas, and similar sites.

Siphonaptera

More than 2,000 species of fleas are cosmopolitan, temporary, obligate ectoparasites of mammals and birds[1]. They are small, heavily sclerotized, bilaterally flattened, and secondarily apterous (Figure 6.13). Most fleas are reddish brown to black in color, but some species are tan or yellow, and all species feed exclusively on blood.

Adult fleas are 1 to 4 mm long, and males are characteristically shorter than females. Many of the morphological features of fleas are unique among the arthropods. The head has limited movement and is broadly joined to the thorax. Mouthparts are piercing sucking type. On the sides of the head capsule are grooves, containing the tiny

antennae. Eyes, if present, are located anteriorly to the antennae. Several species have a genal (or oral) ctenidium, a conspicuous comb-like structure composed of heavy spines, arising from the ventral margin of the head and surrounding the mouthparts. Some species also have a pronotal ctenidium arising from the posterior margin of the first thoracic segment. The body of the flea also has a number of caudally directed setae. Ctenidia and body setae are adaptations that assist the flea in retaining itself among the fur or feathers of its host. The metathoracic legs are highly developed for jumping.

Fleas undergo holometabolous development. The adult female produces about 15 to 20 eggs per day, up to a total of about 500, usually ovipositing while on the host. High humidity favors oviposition. The eggs drop from the host's body, typically into the nest or other area frequented by the host. Eggs are large (0.5 mm) compared to the adult flea. Larvae are white, legless, and eyeless, and have rows of stout hairs encircling the body. They have chewing mouthparts and feed on protein-rich organic detritus, especially the digested blood available in the feces of adult fleas. Larval fleas cannot close their spiracles, and therefore are sensitive to low humidity. There are usually three larval instars, at the end of which the fully developed larva pupates within a silken cocoon that it spins from salivary secretions. Under ideal environmental conditions, the life cycle of most species requires from 20 to 75 days to complete, but low temperatures can extend the larval period to more than 200 days and the pupal stage to nearly a year.

Depending on species, adult fleas can survive without a blood meal for up to 125 days, and periodically fed fleas have lived for more than three years under conditions of high humidity[1]. Such longevity allows flea-transmitted pathogens to survive long periods when vertebrate hosts are absent.

In general, fleas are not particularly host specific, although they have preferred hosts. Most are parasites of mammals, but about 100 species parasitize birds[19]. Most species easily transfer to other hosts, and are typical nest parasites; they are seldom on the host and spend most of their time in the host's lair. In some species, females attach permanently by their mouthparts to the host, while in a few other species, females penetrate the skin and are true intracutaneous parasites.

Families of fleas are separated principally by structure of the head and abdomen, and by the placement of various setae or bristles. Identification to species often requires dissection and examination of female genitalia. Siphonapteran families with medically important fleas that might be encountered on laboratory animals include Pulicidae, Ceratophyllidae, Letpopsyllidae, and Tungidae.

Diptera (true flies)

Diptera is one of the largest orders of insects, containing more than 150,000 species in approximately 140 families. Some flies, while not parasitic, breed and feed in filth and can cause significant irritation and mechanically transmit disease organisms to animals and man. Others are hematophagous as adults, while still others cause myiasis as larvae. Although many species of flies affect vertebrates, few are important pests of laboratory animals. Parasitism by flies is typically intermittent, and most likely encountered in animals collected from the wild, housed in outdoor facilities, or received from outside sources. Continued parasitism would be expected only in animals housed outdoors or subject to invasion from outside.

Adult diptera have only one pair of functional wings (di=two, ptera=wings) on the mesothorax. The metathoracic wings are reduced to knoblike structures, the halteres, which function to maintain stable flight. Some ectoparasitic species are secondarily apterous. Mouthparts of adult flies are haustellate, but their structure varies considerably. In the hematophagous groups, mouthparts are modified for piercing or lacerating tissues and for sucking or lapping blood. In other groups they are modified for sponging or lapping liquids, and, in a few species, they are vestigial or absent.

All Diptera are holometabolous. Most are oviparous, but some are ovoviparous (larviparous), with larvae being retained in the female after hatching. Retained larvae are usually deposited after the second instar, but in a few taxa, they are retained through complete larval development, with pupation taking place shortly after deposition. Dipteran larvae typically require a wet medium for development, and therefore are usually aquatic, semi-aquatic, or endoparasitic.

Identification of both the immature and adult stages of Diptera can be difficult and is best left to a specialist. Identification of larvae can involve dissection of mouthparts and examination of respiratory structures; whereas identification of adults is based on the structure of antennae and legs, on the pattern of wing venation, and on the distribution of setae and bristles on the body surface. In some groups, identification to the species level requires microscopic examination of reproductive structures or mouthparts.

Diptera is divided into two suborders, Nematocera and Brachycera, which are differentiated mainly by the general morphology of the larval and pupal stages and by the structure of antennae in the adult stage. In the Nematocera, the antennae are filamentous, usually longer than the head, and composed of many (more than three) relatively undifferentiated segments. Antennae of males are usually plumose. Nematoceran larvae have a well-developed head capsule with mandibulate mouthparts. In the pupal stage, appendages are not attached to the rest of the pupa, and, in many taxa, the pupae are free-swimming and capable of directed movement.

The Brachycera typically are robust flies, in which the antennae are reduced to three segments. The third segment is usually stylate or aristate, or it may be divided into a number of subsegments. In most brachycerans, particularly in the muscoid flies (a grouping of families sharing characteristics with the house fly), larvae are called maggots. They are cone-shaped and legless, and have a truncated posterior, on which is located a pair of respiratory spiracles. The head is vestigial, consisting primarily of a pair of mouth hooks that move in a vertical plane. Pupae of Brachycera are retained in a structure called a puparium that is formed by the cuticle of the last larval instar.

Blood-feeding Flies

Hematophagous flies are found in the nematoceran families Ceratopogonidae, Culicidae, Psychodidae, and Simuliidae, and in the brachyceran families Tabanidae, Hippoboscidae, and Muscidae. Only females of the ectoparasitic nematocerans are hematophagous, requiring blood protein for egg production. Males generally feed on nectar or plant juices. In hematophagous Brachycera, both males and females feed exclusively on blood.

Ceratopogonidae (biting midges)

Also called "punkies" or "no-see-ums," biting midges are minute (1 to 4 mm long) biting flies, typically with dark spotting on the thorax and wings. *Culicoides* is the most prevalent genus, with species distributed worldwide. Although their bite is irritating, species of *Culicoides* midges are important primarily as vectors of pathogens[1,20].

Culicidae (mosquitoes)

Mosquitoes are the most important insect vectors of human disease and the most common bloodsucking arthropods[4]. They are small flies, approximately 2.5 to 6 mm long, with long legs and wings and a long, slender abdomen and proboscis. Mosquitoes are found worldwide in practically any environment that provides developmental conditions that ensure completion of their life cycle.

There are four important genera affecting endothermic laboratory animals: *Culex, Aedes, Ochlerotatus,* and *Anopheles.* Most *Culex* mosquitoes are ornithophilic nocturnal feeders. *Aedes* and *Ochlerotatus* (formerly placed in the genus *Aedes*[21]) species are typically diurnal or crepuscular feeders. *Anopheles* spp. are nocturnal and crepuscular feeders.

Mosquitoes develop almost exclusively in standing water, and oviposition sites are somewhat species specific. Certain mosquito species are associated with floodwater (including flood irrigation), snowmelt, tree holes, artificial containers, or salt marsh pools. Some mosquitoes lay eggs either singly or in rafts on the water surface, while others (typically, floodwater species) oviposit on the ground in areas that will become flooded. Many species readily enter buildings and oviposit in standing water in drain traps, water bowls, and similar sites. Larvae feed actively on algae, small animals, and organic debris in the water, and respire air directly through modified spiracles or siphons on the posterior segments, spending most of the time suspended by these structures from the surface film. Pupae suspend and breathe through thoracic siphons and, if disturbed, will tumble quickly away from the surface (Figure 6.14).

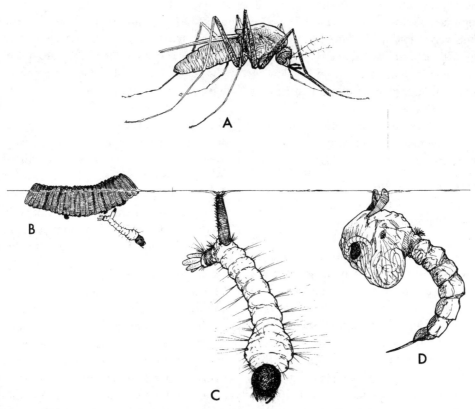

Fig. 6.14 General morphology of mosquitoes (Culicidae). (A) Adult female. (B) Eggs. (C) Larva. (D) Pupa. Courtesy of E.P. Catts, University of Delaware.

Psychodidae (sand flies)

The Psychodidae are a group of small, hirsute, moth-like flies. Most psychodids are not parasitic, but those in the subfamily Phlebotiminae, commonly called sand flies, are hematophagous, and occur in tropical and warm temperate regions worldwide. Hosts include several species of reptiles, amphibians, birds, and mammals. Sand flies are soft and delicate, and they are poor fliers, but are nonetheless good vectors of many disease agents[22]. Sand fly larvae are not aquatic, but require high humidity and a source of organic matter to develop. Typical breeding sites include animal burrows, hollow trees, around buttress roots, and under dead leaves on the forest floor[1].

Simuliidae (black flies)

Black flies are a morphologically homogeneous group of about 1,300 species in 24 genera, found worldwide wherever there is suitable developmental habitat[23]. Also known as turkey gnats or buffalo gnats, they are short (1 to 4 mm), robust flies, usually gray to black in color but sometimes brown to yellow. The prothoracic scutum is strongly pronounced, resulting in a prominent hump, and they have broad, strong wings with characteristically reduced venation. Immature stages are entirely aquatic in clean, well-oxygenated flowing water. Gravid females typically oviposit on rocks or trailing vegetation along the edges of rivers, streams, irrigation canals, and similar habitats. Larvae attach to the substrate and filter organic matter from the flowing water by means of labial fans. Females of most species are hematophagous, and are very persistent and bothersome, with a painful bite. Black flies are vectors of several species of parasitic protozoa and nematodes. *Simulium* and *Cnephia* are the most important genera in the Americas.

Tabanidae (horse flies and deer flies)

These are mostly medium to large (6 to 25 mm), heavy-bodied flies comprising about 4,000 species in up to 80 genera[1]. The eyes are very large, and often are striped with bands of bright colors. Females of most tabanid genera are hematophagous, with bladelike mouthparts adapted for slicing tissues, and labella adapted for sponging up the blood that flows from the wound. Tabanids typically develop in aquatic or semi aquatic conditions, such as in or along the edge of marshy ponds or in soil bordering streams, but some species develop in dry pastures or other areas that rarely hold free water. Eggs are laid on vegetation or other objects overhanging the preferred developmental habitat. Larvae are cylindrical, long, and maggot-like, and have a retractile head with powerful mouth hooks. Larvae move to drier areas of their habitat prior to pupation.

Tabanids are notorious biting pests of horses, cattle, deer, and other mammals, including man, but they are important primarily as vectors of a large number of parasitic protozoa and nematodes, as well as pathogenic bacteria.

Hippoboscidae (louse flies)

Louse flies are all semi-permanent to permanent ectoparasites of birds and some mammals, ranging in size from 2.5 to 10 mm. They are typically dark brown and dorsoventrally flattened, with tough, leathery bodies and strong, squat legs. Antennae are short and are inserted into depressions near the mouth. Some species are winged, while others are apterous for all or part of their life cycles. Larvae are retained within the female until shortly before pupation. The most important species of laboratory animals includes the sheep ked, *Melophagus ovinus,* and the pigeon fly, *Pseudolynchia canariensis.*

Muscidae (filth flies, tsetse flies, and stable flies)

This large, diverse family includes a number of usually dull-colored, small- to medium-sized flies, the best known of which is the house fly, *Musca domestica.* Most are non biting, but a few genera are hematophagous. Species in the genera *Musca, Fannia,* and *Muscina* are cosmopolitan, non-biting, synanthropic flies that oviposit on animal wastes or decaying organic matter. They are not obligately parasitic, but may occasionally cause accidental myiasis. They are most important as mechanical vectors of disease agents.

A few species of muscids are ectoparasites of endothermic animals. Tsetse (*Glossina* and other genera) are hematophagous flies native to tropical Africa. Most members of the genus *Stomoxys* are found in Asia or Africa, but the most common species, with worldwide distribution, is the stable fly, *S. calcitrans.* The stable fly superficially resembles the house fly, but is differentiated by its forward-projecting haustellum, as opposed to the subterminal, sponging mouthparts of the house fly.

Flies that cause Myiasis

Myiasis is the invasion of the organs or tissues of vertebrate animals by fly larvae that feed upon the tissues of the host or on the ingested food of the host[1]. Various terms are used to describe the location and type of myiasis—it may be enteric or gastrointestinal; dermal, sub-dermal, or cutaneous; nasopharyngeal; or urogenital. Myiasis is traumatic if it occurs on an open wound, and furuncular if a boil-like lesion is produced. If the path of larvae burrowing beneath the skin can be traced, it is described as creeping. Bloodsucking larvae of some calliphorid flies cause sanguinivorous myiasis.

Myiasis may also be accidental (pseudomyiasis), facultative, or obligatory. Accidental myiasis occurs when fly eggs or larvae are ingested, or when it is caused by a species that is not normally involved with myiasis. Facultative myiasis occurs when species that normally are carrion-feeders adapt to a parasitic existence on living vertebrates, and can be subdivided into primary and secondary facultative myiases. Species causing primary facultative myiasis are typically parasitic, but can develop saprophytically. This situation is reversed in secondary facultative myiasis. Obligatory myiasis occurs when a species is unable to complete its life cycle without a living host.

Important fly species that cause facultative or obligatory myiasis are in the muscoid families Calliphoridae, Sarcophagidae, and Oestridae. James[24] and Zumpt[25] review the literature and provide identification keys to immature and adult flies that cause myiasis in man, and Baumgartner[26] provides a review and host list of nearctic blow flies and flesh flies that cause myiasis in wild vertebrates.

Calliphoridae (blow flies)

This is a cosmopolitan family, most members of which are about the size of a housefly or slightly larger. They are generally metallic green, blue, or copper in color, and most species have dark stripes on the thorax. Adult calliphorids have mouthparts of the sponging-sucking type, and are omnivorous scavengers that feed on nectar, rotting animal matter, or excrement. In most species, masses of eggs (called "blow") are deposited on carrion, excrement, and similar materials. However, several genera contain species that could cause myiasis in animals that have been collected or housed outdoors.

Most calliphorids are involved in facultative myiasis, with larvae developing in necrotic wounds or on soiled pelage and only secondarily invading healthy tissue. In fact, larvae of some species are used for maggot debridement therapy to clean, disinfect, and stimulate healing in intractable wounds[27]. Important calliphorids include the screwworm fly, *Cochliomyia hominovorax,* endemic in tropical and warm temperate regions over much of the Americas; the Old World screwworm fly, *Chrysomyia bezziana,* which fulfills a similar niche in Africa, India, the Philippines and East Indies; toad flies in the genus *Bufolucilia;* and bird blow flies in the genus *Protocalliphora.*

Sarcophagidae (flesh flies)

Sarcophagids are widely distributed and common worldwide. They are morphologically similar to blow flies, and sometimes are placed with them in a single family, the Metopiidae[6]. However, unlike calliphorids, flesh flies are never metallic. Flesh flies are overall dull gray in color, and typically have a gray and black checkered abdomen and three, longitudinal, gray stripes on the dorsum of the thorax. Adults feed on sugar-containing materials, such as nectar and fruit juices, and larvae nearly all feed on some form of animal material, either as scavengers, as insect parasites, or as parasites of vertebrates. Important genera include *Wohlfahrtia* and *Sarcophaga.*

Oestridae (bot flies and warble flies)

This is a small family, all members of which are obligatory endoparasites of endothermic animals, causing dermal, nasopharyngeal, or enteric myiasis. Adults typically are large, hairy, and bee-like. They are non-feeding, and mouthparts are vestigial or lacking. Oestrids usually deposit eggs or first instar larvae on or near the host, and the mere presence of host-seeking adult flies often causes characteristic avoidance or escape behavior in potential host animals. First-instar larvae are very active, and enter the body of the host in various ways. Some species enter the host through natural body openings, while others work their way through intact skin. Bot fly larvae commonly are called grubs or bots, and typically are thick, short, and "C"-shaped, and variously armed with cuticular spines that aid in maintaining attachment in the host.

Wood[28] considers the oestridae to be a monophyletic group composed of four subfamilies: cuteribrinae (skin bots, rodent bots, and rabbit bots); oestrinae (nose bots, head maggots); hypodermatinae (cattle grubs, reindeer bots), and gasterophilinae (horse bots). These groups were formerly assigned family status, so, in the older literature, the group names end in the family suffix (–idae), rather than in the subfamily suffix (–inae).

All cuterebrines are endemic to the Western hemisphere, and include two important genera: *Cuterebra* and *Dermatobia*. *Cuterebra* includes 41 species of North American bot flies that cause dermal furuncular myiasis in rodents and lagomorphs, and rarely in other mammals, including humans. The female fly deposits eggs near a burrow or nest, and the newly hatched larvae attach to the first prospective host that brushes against them. The genus *Dermatobia* is comprised of one species, *D. hominis,* the human botfly or torsalo, which attacks a broad range of endothermal hosts from Mexico through most of South America (Figure 6.15).

Species of oestrinae cause either dermal or nasopharyngeal myiasis in sheep, cattle, deer, elephants, camels, and rodents. *Oestris ovis,* the sheep nose bot, is an economically important pest of domestic sheep and goats in the Americas.

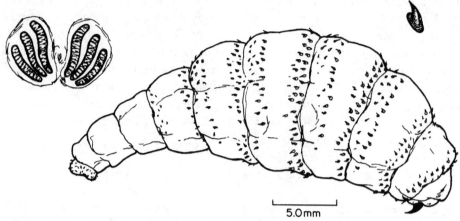

Fig. 6.15 *Dermatobia hominis*, third-stage larva. (Insets) Posterior spiracles (left) and typical spine (right). Courtesy of E.P. Catts, University of Delaware.

REFERENCES

1. Harwood, R.F. and James, M.T. (1979) *Entomology in Human and Animal Health*, 7th ed. Macmillan, New York.

2. Cheng, T.C. (1986) *General Parasitology*, 2nd ed. Academic Press, New York.

3. Barnes, R.D. (1987) *Invertebrate Zoology*, 5th ed. Saunders, Philadelphia.

4. Roberts, L.S. and Janovy, J. (2000) *Gerald D. Schmidt & Larry S. Roberts' Foundations of Parasitology*, 6th ed. McGraw-Hill, New York.

5. Mullen, G.L. and Durden, L.A. (2002). *Medical and Veterinary Entomology*. Academic Press, New York.

6. Triplehorn, C.A. and Johnson, N.F. (2005) *Borror and DeLong's Introduction to the Study of Insects*, 7th ed. Thomson Brooks/Cole, Belmont, California.

7. Tidd, W.M. (1963) Experimental infestations of frog tadpoles by *Lernaea cyprinacea*. *J. Parasitol.* **48**, 870.

8. Hoffman, G.L. (1967) *Parasites of North American freshwater fishes*. University of California Press, Berkeley.

9. Riley, J., Banaja, A.A., and James. J.L. (1978). The phylogenetic relationships of the Pentastomida: The case for their inclusion within the Crustacea. *Internat. J. Parasitol.* **8**, 245–254.

10. Abele, L.G., Kim, W., and Felgenhauer, B.E. (1989) Molecular evidence for inclusion of the phylum Pentastomida in the Crustacea. *Mol. Biol. Evol.* **6**, 685–691.

11. Martin, J.W. and Davis, G.E. (2001) *An Updated Classification of the Recent Crustacea*. Natural History Museum of Los Angeles, Science Series **39**, 1–124.

12. Krantz, G.W. (1978) *A Manual of Acarology*, 2nd ed. Oregon State University Bookstore, Corvallis.

13. Evans, G.O. (1992) *Principles of Acarology*. C.A.B. International, Wallingford, U.K.

14. Baker, E.W., and Wharton, G.H. (1952) *An Introduction to Acarology*. McMillan, New York.

15. Baker, E.W., Evans, T.M., Gould, D.J., Hull, W.B., and Keegan, H.L. (1956) *A Manual of Parasitic Mites of Medical or Economic Importance*. National Pest Control Association, New York.

16. Usinger, R.L. (1966) *Monograph of Cimicidae* (Hemiptera-Heteroptera). Entomological Society of America, College Park, Maryland.

17. Lent, H. and Wygodzinsky, P. (1979) Revision of the Triatominae (Hemiptera, Reduviidae) and their significance as vectors of Chagas' disease. *Bull. Am. Mus. Nat. Hist.* **163**, 123–520.

18. Kim, K.C., Pratt, H.D., and Stojanovich, S.J. (1986) *The Sucking Lice of North America*. The Pennsylvania State University Press, State College.

19. Holland, G.P. (1964) Evolution, classification and host relationships of Siphonaptera. *Annual Rev. Entomol.* **9**, 123–146.

20. Leathers, C.W. (1978) The prevalence of *Hepatocystis kochi* in African green monkeys. *Lab. Anim. Sci.* **28**, 186–189.

21. Reinert, J.F. (2000) New classification for the composite genus *Aedes* (Diptera: Culicidae: Aedini), elevation of subgenus *Ochlerotatus* to generic rank, reclassification of the other subgenera, and notes on certain subgenera and species. *J. Am. Mosq. Control Assoc.* **16**, 175–188.

22. Tesh, R.B. and Guzman, H. (1996) Sand flies and the agents they transmit. 117–127. In: Beaty, B.J. and Marquardt, W.C. (eds.) *The Biology of Disease Vectors*. University of Colorado Press, Boulder.

23. Adler, P.H., Currie, D.C., and Wood, D.M. (2004) *The black flies (Simuliidae) of North America*. Cornell University Press, Ithaca, N.Y.

24. James, M.T. (1947) The flies that cause myiasis in man. *U.S. Department of Agriculture, Misc. Publication No.* 631.

25. Zumpt, F. (1965) *Myiasis in Man and Animals in the Old World*. Butterworth and Co., London.

26. Baumgartner, D.L. (1988) Review of myiasis (Insecta: Diptera: Calliphoridae, Sarcophagidae) of Nearctic wildlife. *Wildlife Rehabilitation* **7**, 3–46.

27. Mumcuoglu, K.Y., Ingber, A., Gilead, L., et al., (1999) Maggot therapy for the treatment of intractable wounds. *Int. J. Dermatol.* **38**, 623–627.

28. Wood, D.M. (1987) Oestridae. In: J.F. McAlpine (ed.) *Manual of Nearctic Diptera*, Vol. 2, Monog. 28. Agriculture Canada, Ottawa, pages 1147–1158.

Michael L. Kent, MS, PhD, and John W. Fournie, MS, PhD

INTRODUCTION

The intent of this chapter is to describe the parasites of importance to fishes maintained and used in laboratory settings. In contrast to the first edition[1], the focus will be only on those parasites that pose a serious threat to or are common in fishes held in these confined environments. Parasites emphasized are those capable of spreading, proliferating, and causing significant disease in research facilities. For the most part, parasites that are contracted only in the wild are not addressed. Nevertheless, a few species of wild fishes are used extensively in laboratory research (e.g., stickleback, killifishes, sheepshead minnow),

and thus pathogenic parasites that are contracted in the wild and persist in these fishes after capture are included.

The use of aquatic animal models in research has significantly increased in recent years, as is exemplified by the dramatic increase in the use of zebrafish in genetic research[2]. Many fish species are used in laboratory research. However, coverage in this text is limited to the following fish species: zebrafish (*Danio rerio*), goldfish (*Carassius auratus*), rainbow trout (*Oncorhynchus mykiss*), stickleback (*Gasterosteus* spp.), mummichog (*Fundulus heteroclitus*), gulf killifish (*Fundulus grandis*), sheepshead minnow (*Cyprinodon variegatus*), fathead minnow (*Pimephales promelas*), and swordtails and platys (*Xiphophorus* spp.). Even though the Japanese medaka (*Oryzias latipes*) is widely used in aquatic toxicology, carcinogenicity testing, and biomedical research, this

------

Tables are placed at the ends of chapters.

species is not included because it appears to be resistant to infection by most of the common ectoparasites infesting captive fishes.

As in the previous edition[1], the material is organized by parasite taxa rather than hosts, because the most important parasites show very broad host specificity. However, when appropriate, sections addressing unique characteristics of specific host-parasite relationships are included.

GENERAL PREVENTION STRATEGIES

Parasites with direct life cycles can rapidly proliferate in confined research systems. Therefore, attention should be given to preventing the introduction of such pathogens. Avoidance of introduction of pathogens is accomplished by 1) using fishes from pathogen-free suppliers, 2) prophylactic treatment with formalin baths or other chemicals to remove external parasites, 3) holding fishes in quarantine for several weeks before introduction into the research facility, 4) avoidance of introducing water with new fishes into the holding systems, 5) disinfection of incoming water to the system by either ultraviolet sterilization or ozonation, and 6) using only eggs for new stock whenever possible. Eggs should be surface disinfected with either iodophors (for salmonid eggs) or chlorine (as used for zebrafish eggs) to remove external pathogens. Reviews on quarantine and prevention procedures are provided in several sources[3-6].

Avoidance of parasites begins with purchase of research fishes from reputable suppliers that can provide a general disease history of their stocks. It is generally better to obtain fishes that have been reared in enclosed systems, versus pond-reared or wild fishes. Aside from certain stocks of salmonids, most fish suppliers do not provide specific pathogen free (SPF) fish. Many healthy fish, particularly those from the wild or ponds, arrive with light infestations by external parasites.

The most common method to remove these monogeneans, ciliates, and flagellates is to immerse them in formalin at 125 to 250 ppm for 30 to 60 minutes[7]. The toxicity of formalin baths varies considerably among fish species, so it is important to test a few individuals before applying this treatment to large numbers of fish. Copper sulfate baths may also be used, particularly with marine systems[7]. These baths will not remove internal parasites, and thus careful observation of fish in separate quarantine systems is advised. In addition, researchers should consider complete necropsy and disease evaluations on representative specimens of new stocks of fish before introduction into large or valuable facilities.

Many facilities maintaining small fishes use dechlorinated city water, which will eliminate most fish parasites. In addition, sterilization of the incoming and recirculating water may be appropriate. The most common methods for disinfecting water entering fish systems are by either ultraviolet sterilization or ozonation. Certain fishes, such as salmonids, can be easily transported as eggs[5], and new stocks of those species should be obtained as eggs whenever possible. Another useful alternative is to obtain new fishes as brood stock, hold them in a separate facility, spawn the fish, and then disinfect the eggs before entry into the research facility[6].

Another important consideration in laboratories maintaining captive fishes is to prevent the spread of ectoparasites among aquaria, raceways, and large tanks in the facility. Because parasites can be spread between tanks by aerosol spray associated with water aeration[8], arrangement of holding tanks should be in a fashion that minimizes aerosol contamination. Designing and using fitted glass tops for aquaria and tanks is also an effective means of minimizing aerosol contamination. Parasites can also be spread among aquaria by contaminated nets. This type of contamination can be prevented by using a single net for each aquarium or by disinfecting nets between tanks.

An excellent method to monitor the overall health of captive fishes maintained for research is the incorporation of a sentinel animal program, similar to those used in mammalian research facilities, into the existing health monitoring activities. This is accomplished by placing fish in a location in the facility where they receive effluent from most tanks to optimize potential exposure to all pathogens in the facility. One effective practice that we use with zebrafish is to hold them for about three months and then examine them by histology. In this case, fishes are examined by only histology, because specific virus and bacterial pathogens (other than *Mycobacterium* spp.) are not well-described for zebrafish.

PROTOZOA
Phylum Dinoflagellata

Parasitic dinoflagellates infest both freshwater and marine fishes. The two most important species infesting captive fishes are *Piscinoodinium pillulare* and *Amyloodinium ocellatum*. These parasites are very similar morphologically and have the same life cycles. *Piscinoodinium pillulare* is a significant pathogen of both tropical and temperate freshwater fishes. *Amyloodinium ocellatum* is the marine analogue of *P. pillulare* and is one of the most important parasites infesting warm water marine fishes.

Piscinoodinium pillulare and Amyloodinium ocellatum

Morphology. The non-motile trophont of *Piscinoodinium pillulare* measures about 9 to 12 μ long by 40 to 90 μ wide, is pear-shaped (Figure 7.1), and possesses an attachment disc from which radiate numerous rod-like organelles called rhizocysts[9]. These structures penetrate into and are firmly embedded in host epithelial cells. The trophont is covered by a theca and contains well-developed chloroplasts and starch granules, but no digestive vacuoles. The disc-shaped chloroplasts are situated at the periphery of the cell. They also have a single, prominent, spherical nucleus that contains large dinoflagellate chromosomes. Trophonts of *A. ocellatum* are ovoid, mostly up to 150 μm long, and possess an attachment plate from which radiate filiform rhizoids and a stomopode[9]. The rhizoids embed in the host epithelial cells, and the stomopode is believed to produce lytic substances. Trophonts are covered by a theca which is reinforced by plates within thecal alveoli[9]. The trophont cytoplasm possesses a spherical nucleus, digestive vacuoles, and starch grains, but lacks chloroplasts.

Hosts. Virtually all freshwater fishes are susceptible to infestation with *P. pillulare* when maintained above 17°C to 20°C. Outbreaks of *P. pillulare* are occasionally seen in zebrafish research facilities. *A. ocellatum* is also nonspecific in its host range, infesting most marine teleosts, including both food and aquarium fishes. Even freshwater teleosts are susceptible to infestation when they are in brackish water[10].

Life Cycle. After approximately six days of growth at 25°C, the developed trophont of *P. pillulare* drops off the host, sinks to the substratum, rounds up, and becomes a tomont. It undergoes a series of successive divisions, resulting in the production of 256 tomites which differentiate into gymnospores[9]. Gymnospores possess a small stigma, are motile, and go on to infect other fish hosts. The life cycle of *A. ocellatum* is similar to that described for *P. pillulare*. Tomonts produce up to 256 infective

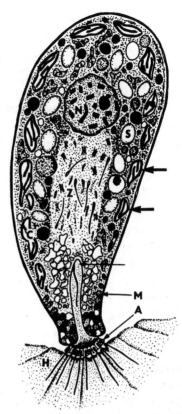

Fig. 7.1 *Piscinoodinium pillulare*. Line drawing of an attached trophont showing the characteristic morphological features. N = nucleus. S = starch granules. M = mucocyst. A = attachment disc. H = host cell. Thick arrows = chloroplasts. Long arrow = flagellar groove. Reproduced from Lom, J. and Dyková, I. (1992). Used with permission.

dinospores which attach to a host and differentiate into trophonts.

Pathologic Effects. Histopathologic changes in the gills of fishes infested with *P. pillulare* range from separation of the respiratory epithelium to lamellar fusion and prominent epithelial hyperplasia that may involve entire gill filaments. Eventually there is epithelial cell degeneration and necrosis. Similarly, skin infestations result in severe hyperplasia, petechial hemorrhages, and erosion of the epithelium. Fishes heavily infested with *A. ocellatum* exhibit widespread pathological changes to the gill epithelium. The gills are edematous and hyperplastic, showing inflammation and hemorrhage resulting in necrosis of gill filaments[9]. This severe gill damage together with anoxia is the apparent cause of death[11].

Clinical Disease. *Piscinoodinium* is the causative agent of velvet disease. Infested fishes may exhibit a golden, velvety hue on the body surface. Clinical signs include the appearance of discomfort, spreading opercula, and folding of fins. There may also be excess mucus, darkening of the skin, and petechial hemorrhages. Heavily infested fishes are lethargic, may hang near the surface of the water, and exhibit labored breathing. Some fish exhibit anorexia. *Amyloodinium* is the causative agent of marine velvet disease. Heavily infested skin may have a dusty appearance, but often fishes die without obvious skin lesions. Fishes with heavy infestations show typical signs of discomfort, including gasping for air, scratching against objects in the water, and loss of appetite.

Diagnosis. *Piscinoodinium* infestations are diagnosed by observation of the sac-shaped trophonts in either wet mounts or histological sections (Figure 7.2). For the former, *P. pillulare* is distinguished from many other surface-infesting protists by its lack of motility. *A. ocellatum* is diagnosed by finding the characteristic trophonts in wet mounts or histological sections of skin or gills. The highly vacuolated cytoplasm and large central nucleus are key identifying features.

Treatment. Prolonged immersion in salt at about 1 teaspoon/5 gallons is one of the safest and most effective treatments for *P. pillulare* infestations. However, very heavy, life-threatening infestations may require treatment with a one- to three-minute salt bath in full-strength sea water (35 ppt) to dislodge trophonts[7]. Note that not all freshwater fishes can tolerate saline baths. Raising water temperatures to 33°C to 34°C has also been reported to control infestations[12]. Copper has been suggested as a treatment[13], but its unpredictable toxicity in soft, acid freshwater often makes it dangerous to use in aquaria.

The most common treatments for *A. ocellatum* infestations are copper sulfate and formalin. Copper sulfate is used at 0.3 to 0.5 mg/l for ten days or formalin at 100 to 200 mg/l for 10 days. For these treatments, it is advisable to raise the water temperature to 24°C to 27°C to speed up the life cycle. The presence of off-host developmental stages should be considered when implementing a treatment regime. These increased temperatures shorten the time for trophont and tomont development, so the motile infective stages can be exposed to the chemicals. Both Noga[7] and Levy[14] show reviews of treatments for *Piscinoodinum* and *Amyloodinium*.

Prevention. Avoid exposure of fish and water systems to infected fish, water, nets, or any other items that have come in contact with infected systems. Quarantining fish and prophylactically treating them prior to their introduction into a laboratory system will also help prevent this parasitic dinoflagellate. Treatment of aquaria and other holding tanks with chlorine bleach followed by thorough washing with freshwater and then drying of the

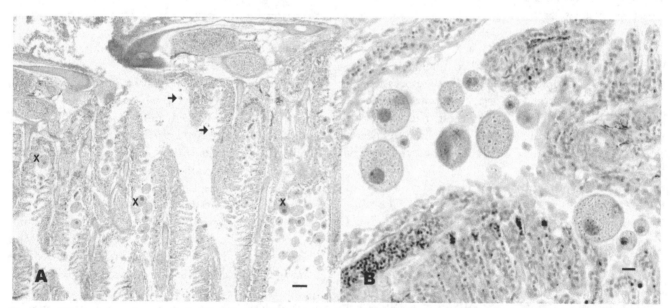

Fig. 7.2 Histological section of gills heavily infested with *Piscinoodinium pillulare* (X). Hematoxylin and eosin. Arrow = early, small stages. (A) Low magnification, bar = 50 μm. (B) High magnification showing large nucleus and refractile cytoplasmic granules. Bar = 10 μm.

systems for several days before reuse provides additional assurance for not spreading the parasite to newly introduced fishes.

Public Health Considerations. Neither of these parasites pose a threat to public health.

Phylum Euglenenozoa

Ichthyobodo necator

The bodonid flagellate *Ichthyobodo necator* (Syn. *Costia necatrix*) is a common ectoparasitic pathogen of fishes reared in fresh water[15]. The parasite exhibits very broad host and geographic distribution, infecting many species in freshwater and occasionally in seawater[16,17]. Cross-transmission studies[17] and recent molecular studies[18] indicate that the parasite actually represents an assemblage of morphologically indistinguishable species with narrower host specificities.

Morphology. *Ichthyobodo necator* is a small, actively swimming flagellate measuring about 10 μ long by 5 μ wide. It is one of the smallest ectoparasites that infests fishes. Two forms are observed: pyriform stages attached to the surface of gills and skin, and oval or bean-shaped free-swimming forms (Figures 7.3 and 7.4). The flagellate has a single, centrally located nucleus which contains a large nucleolus. It has two unequal flagella that extend from a deep flagellar pocket. These flagella are easily visualized by phase contrast microscopy.

Hosts. *Ichthyobodo necator sensulato* has very broad host specificity. It is a dangerous ectoparasite of practically all freshwater fishes. Goldfish and salmonids appear to be particularly susceptible, and if untreated, mass mortalities may occur within a few days. Although most infestations are reported from captive freshwater fishes, a marine form of the parasite causes disease in flatfish and salmonids in sea water[17,19].

Life Cycle. Reproduction is by binary division, which begins with a doubling of the flagellar number[9]. Transmission is direct from fish to fish, and no cyst stages have been detected. The duration that the parasite remains viable off its host has yet to be determined.

Pathologic Effects. *Ichthyobodo* attacks the whole surface of the host. Skin or gill infestations are often very intense, and the action of the flagellate results in disruption of the epithelial or epidermal cells, causing widespread pathological changes (Figure 7.5). Studies with salmonids have shown degenerative changes and severe hyperplasia in epidermal cells, exhaustion of goblet cells at the site of infestation, and hyperplasia of Malpighian cells[9].

Clinical Disease. Affected fish exhibit labored breathing and may be listless and position themselves at the surface, all signs of respiratory distress. Infestations of the body surface are associated with flashing behavior and a grayish cast

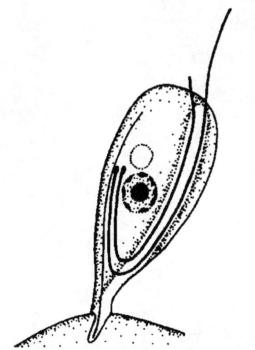

Fig. 7.3 *Ichthyobodo necator,* attached stage. Reproduced from Lom, J. and Dyková, I. (1992). Used with permission.

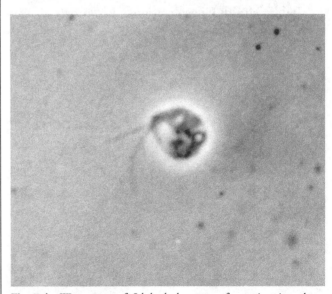

Fig. 7.4 Wet mount of *Ichthyobodo necator,* free swimming phase. Phase contrast microscopy.

on the skin. Heavily infested Atlantic salmon in Scotland were emaciated and anorexic, and swam near the surface[19].

Diagnosis. The infestation is identified by observing numerous flagellate parasites, with the morphology described above, in wet mounts of the skin or gills. *Ichthyobodo* can also be identified on gill surfaces in histological sections, but wet mounts are preferred because parasites may become dislodged from the gills during processing of tissues, and the small flagellates are more easily identified when they are actively motile.

Treatment. External treatments with formalin and malachite green have been used successfully to treat *Ichthyobodo* infections in fresh water[15,20]. Although bath treatments with formalin have long been the treatment of choice for *Ichthyobodo*, Tojo and Santamarina[21] reported that oral treatments with metronidazole, secnidazole, benzimidazole, or triclabendazole were each 100% effective. This approach should be considered when bath treatments are not practical.

Prevention. *Ichthyobodo necator* is ubiquitous in freshwater, and even well water may contain the organism. It can be prevented by incorporating ultraviolet disinfection for incoming water. As with other diseases, introduction of new fishes into a facility via disinfected eggs is a sound policy. If this cannot be achieved, fishes should be held in quarantine for about one month, external parasites removed with prophylactic formalin baths, and representative samples examined before the fishes are introduced into the main facility.

Public Health Considerations. *Ichthyobodo necator* is not a human pathogen.

Phylum Apicomplexa

Calyptospora funduli and Goussia carpelli

Coccidia are members of the phylum Apicomplexa and possess an apical set of organelles, called the apical complex, which facilitates invasion of host cells. Some coccidia are hemoparasites, but the most important fish pathogens infect solid tissues[7,22]. Eight genera infect fishes and belong in the families Eimeriidae, Calyptosporidae, and Cryptosporidiidae. Unlike those in endotherms, many piscine coccidians have oocyst walls of host origin, the site of infection is often extraintestinal, and the oocysts usually sporulate within the host. We discuss here two representatives of the group, *Calyptospora funduli* of killifishes and *Goussia carpelli* of cyprinids.

Morphology. Sporulated oocysts of *C. funduli* are thin-walled and measure about 25 μ in diameter (Figure 7.6). Each oocyst contains four ovoid sporocysts measuring 10 μ long by 6 μ wide. The sporocysts have approximately 15 sporopodia (Figure 7.7), projections of the sporocyst wall that appear to support a thin membranous veil that surrounds each sporocyst. There is a thickening of the posterior end of the sporocyst and an apical opening for sporozoite release at the anterior end[23,24].

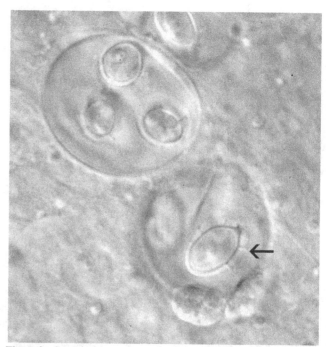

Fig. 7.6 Sporulated oocyst of *Calyptospora funduli.* Nomarski phase contrast. Arrow = sporocyst with sporopodia surrounded membranous veil.

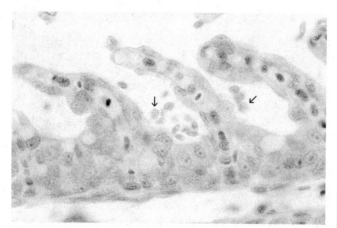

Fig. 7.5 Rainbow trout gill heavily infested with *Ichthyobodo necator* (arrows). Hematoxylin and eosin.

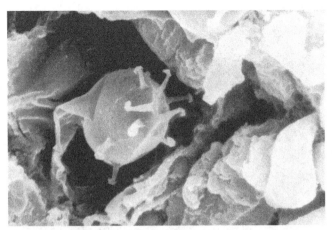

Fig. 7.7 Scanning electron micrograph of a sporocyst of *Calyptospora funduli* showing sporopodia.

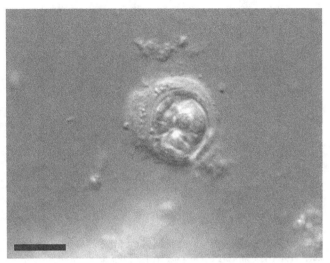

Fig. 7.8 Wet mount of sporulated oocyst of *Goussia carpelli* surrounded by "yellow body." Nomarski phase contrast. Bar = 10 μm.

Oocysts of *G. carpelli* are spherical, thin walled, and measure about 13 μ in diameter (Figure 7.8). Oocysts contain four centrally bulging, tapered oval sporocysts measuring approximately 8 μ long by 5 μ wide. Each sporocyst is composed of two valves adhering along a longitudinal suture line. Sporocysts contain two vermiform sporozoites and a granular residuum[25]. Oocysts are typically surrounded by ceroid or lipofuscin material of host origin, referred to as "yellow bodies"[26].

Hosts. Primary natural definitive hosts for *C. funduli* are the gulf killifish, *Fundulus grandis*, in the Gulf of Mexico and the mummichog, *Fundulus heteroclitus*, along the Atlantic coast. Fournie and Overstreet[27] indicated that *C. funduli* has broad host specificity, infecting at least seven natural and 10 additional experimental hosts. All are atheriniform and cyprinodontiform fishes within five families, but most are in the genus *Fundulus*.

Goussia carpelli occurs in the common carp (*Cyprinus carpio*), goldfish (*Carassius auratus*), and crucian carp, (*Carassius carassius*). Many additional species of cyprinids have also been reported to harbor infections[28].

Life Cycle. Coccidians infecting fishes may have direct or indirect life cycles. Direct life cycles are essentially as described in Chapter 2, Biology of the Protozoa. Steinhagen and Körting[29] demonstrated that direct infections of *Goussia carpelli* could occur by fecal contamination from fish to fish. Subsequently, Steinhagen and Körting[30] confirmed that tubificid oligochaete worms could serve as a paratenic host for *G. carpelli*, and that the sporozoites were located in the cytoplasm of the intestinal epithelial cells

of the oligochaete. No sporozoite development was noted, and the oligochaete was not needed to complete the life cycle. Coccidia with indirect life cycles include *Calyptospora funduli*, which uses a palaemonid grass shrimp intermediate host[31]. Asexual multiplication occurs in the grass shrimp, with sporozoite development occurring within about five days. These are infective to killifishes[32].

Pathologic Effects. Even though the liver is the primary site of infection and up to 85% of this organ can be replaced by the parasite, the host response to *Calyptospora funduli* by gulf killifish is minimal (Figure 7.9). Some inflammatory foci are seen, some oocysts are encapsulated by connective tissue, and lipofuscin and melanin accumulate around some oocysts. More extensive pathologic changes are seen in atypical hosts, such as freshwater cyprindontids, and mortality occurs only when fish are exposed to additional stressors, e.g., cold temperature.

Histopathologic changes in *G. carpelli*-infected goldfish include chronic enteritis with numerous sporulated oocysts surrounded by yellow bodies in the lamina propria of the intestine (Figure 7.10). Inflammatory and necrotic cells are abundant in the lamina propria, and the mucosal surface of large portions of the gut loses its villar structure[26].

Clinical Disease. Healthy fish infected with *Calyptospora funduli* exhibit no clinical signs. However, stressed fish may become lethargic and eventually die. For example, Fournie[33] showed that exposure of experimentally infected gulf killifish to temperatures of 3°C to 4°C resulted in mortality.

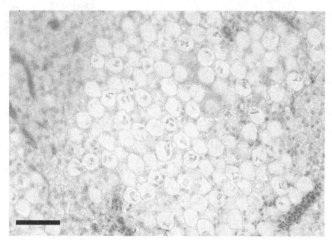

Fig. 7.9 *Calyptospora funduli.* Histological section of infected killifish liver with many sporulated oocysts. Bar=5 20 μm.

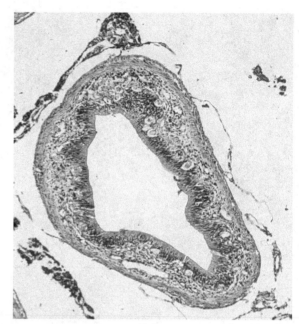

Fig. 7.10 Histological section of the intestine of a goldfish with heavy *G. carpelli* infection. Note complete loss of villar structure of gut.

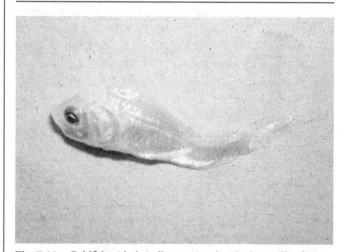

Fig. 7.11 Goldfish with dwindles associated with *G. carpelli* infection.

Goussia carpelli infections in goldfish cause a chronic disease in production ponds in several localities throughout the United States, including the southeast where the disease is commonly referred to as the "dwindles." Infected fish stop feeding, become lethargic, and eventually emaciated (Figure 7.11). Mortality rates of 50% to 75% can occur over two to three weeks.

Diagnosis. Definitive diagnosis requires identification of sporulated oocysts in wet mounts or histological sections of infected tissues. A non-specific diagnosis of coccidiosis can be made if other characteristic life cycle stages are observed, but species identification depends upon morphological features of sporulated oocysts.

Treatment. Treatment with the coccidiostat monensin significantly reduces infection burdens of *Calyptospora*. Solangi and Overstreet[34] reported a 50% to 70% reduction in oocysts within 20 days in infected fishes administered monensin orally. *Calyptospora funduli* has also been successfully treated with either the thiamine analog amprolium (0.63 ml/l of a 9.6% solution given over 2 days) in water, or the polyether antibiotic narasin (<0.005 g/moderate-sized *Fundulus*) in the food[35]. Treatment has been most successful when initiated soon after the fishes are infected. Chemotherapeutics in the feed have been used to control *Goussia carpelli* infections in carp in Europe[36], but control of infections in goldfish with this method is minimally effective because the fishes become infected almost immediately after hatching.

Prevention. The most reliable method of preventing infections with *Calyptospora funduli* is to eliminate the palaemonid grass shrimp intermediate hosts from the system. Prevention of *Goussia carpelli* coccidiosis could be accomplished by drying and disinfecting ponds between growing seasons for both carp and goldfish.

Public Health Considerations. Coccidiosis of fishes is not transmissible to humans.

Phylum Ciliophora

Class Oligohymenophora

Order Hymenostomatida
Ichthyophthirius multifiliis. **Morphology**. *Ichthyophthirius multifiliis* is a holotrichous ciliate, and is the largest parasitic protozoan that affects fishes. Adult trophonts are oval to

round, reach up to more than 1 mm in size, are uniformly ciliated, and possess a characteristic horseshoe-shaped macronucleus (Figure 7.12) as well as a subapically located buccal vestibulum with weakly developed buccal ciliary organelles[9].

Hosts. *Ichthyophthirius multifiliis* is the most important parasite affecting freshwater aquarium fishes. The parasite is also a problem in food fishes reared in captivity, such as catfish and salmonids, and has even caused epizootics in wild fishes[37]. Virtually all freshwater fishes are susceptible. In the laboratory setting, these include swordtails, platys, sticklebacks, and trout (when reared at warmer temperatures). Interestingly, epizootics of disease in zebrafish have not been reported.

Life Cycle. The life cycle of *I. multifiliis* is direct, but does include a free-living developmental stage (Figure 7.13)[38]. After a period of growth, large trophonts leave the host tissues, settle on the substratum, and secrete a gelatinous cyst. This non-motile tomont resorbs its buccal apparatus and divides successively by binary fission. One tomont may produce from 250 to 2,000 small tomites[9]. After the last division, the buccal apparatus is restored, and the tomites break through the cyst wall and become theronts. Susceptible fish are infected by free-swimming theronts. Theronts develop to the trophont stage under the epithelium of the skin or gills, where they expand in size (up to about 1 mm) and occasionally divide.

Pathologic Effects. *Ichthyophthirius multifiliis* is highly pathogenic, reproduces rapidly in confined systems, and shows broad host specificity. Because of these features, this parasite has the potential to cause serious disease in laboratory fishes[7,37]. Tissue irritation caused by *I. multifiliis* results in epithelial hyperplasia and excessive secretion of mucus on the body surfaces and gills. The epithelial erosion and ulceration that result from the ciliate's entrance into and exit from the host are probably as damaging as its feeding activity while on the host[7]. Lesions produced by *I. multifiliis* may lead to secondary bacterial or fungal microbial infections.

Clinical Disease. *Ichthyophthirius multifiliis* causes a condition known as "Ich," or "white spot disease." Infected fishes exhibit characteristic white spots on the body surfaces which result from the ciliates being encysted within the host's epithelium (Figures 7.14 and 7.15). Fishes with heavy infections also exhibit excessive mucus production, labored breathing, and lethargy.

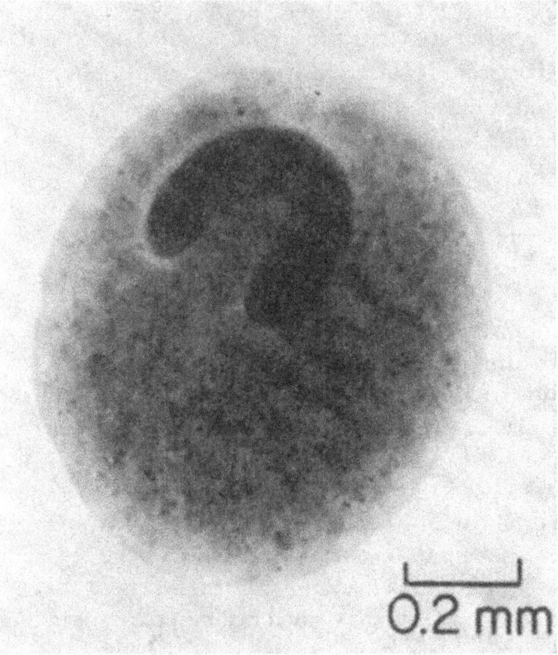

Fig. 7.12 *Ichthyophthirius multifiliis* trophozoite. Whole mount showing nucleus. Courtesy of Bureau of Sport Fisheries and Wildlife, U.S. Department of the Interior.

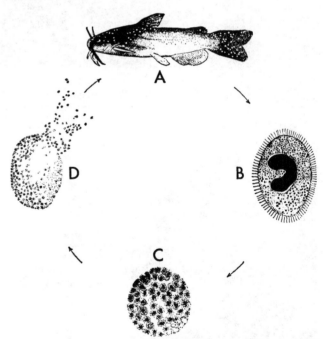

Fig. 7.13 Life cycle of *Ichthyophthirius multifiliis*. (A) Adult parasite on catfish. (B) Mature trophozoite after leaving fish. (C) Division of adult into many tomites after cyst formation. (D) Rupture of cyst-releasing theronts which re-infect fish. Reproduced from Davis, H.S. (1947). Used with permission.

Diagnosis. Identification of active ciliates of varying sizes in wet mounts of the skin or gills offers a good presumptive diagnosis. Definitive diagnosis is achieved by observing the distinctive horseshoe-shaped macronucleus, and by observing parasites under the epithelium of the gills or skin.

Treatment. Considerable information is available on control strategies for infection with *I. multifiliis.* The most common treatment is an external bath with formalin[7]. Usually fishes are treated with formalin at about 1:4,000 to 1:5,000 formalin for one hour. Each fish species responds differently to formalin, and thus a few fishes should be tested before applying the treatment to large numbers.

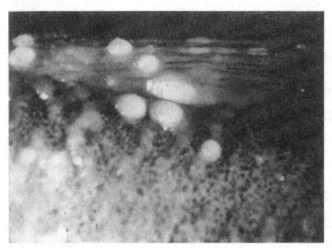

Fig. 7.14 Ichthyophthiriasis or white spot disease in a fish. Note typical white foci on skin. Courtesy of E. Elkan, London.

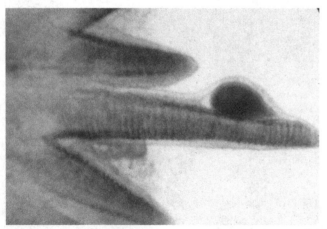

Fig. 7.15 Wet mount preparation of gill showing *Ichthyophthirius multifiliis* under the epithelium.

Multiple daily treatments are necessary to eliminate the stages under the skin, which are somewhat protected from external baths. The entire aquarium system should also be treated to destroy the free-living stages of the parasite. Unfortunately, treating the entire system may be detrimental to biological filters in recirculating systems.

The life cycle of *I. multifiliis* is affected by temperature, with warmer temperatures accelerating development. However, temperatures above 29°C to 30°C are lethal to theronts[39]. Therefore, if the host fishes can tolerate this regimen, raising water temperatures above 29°C for several days is an effective method for eradicating the infection. At higher temperatures, it is particularly important that the water is well aerated, because oxygen saturation in water is inversely correlated with temperature; fish at higher temperatures have higher oxygen demands, and the gills (and thus gas exchange) are impaired when they are infected. Sodium chloride may also be effective. Concentrations of NaCl at 7 to 20 ppt have been used in pond culture[40], so this option should be considered for euryhaline (salt tolerant) fishes such as salmonids and sticklebacks.

Prevention. Infections may be prevented by quarantine of new fish before introduction into a research system. This is particularly important because of the difficulty in eradicating free-living stages in recirculating systems. Strong water currents in flow-through systems will wash away free-swimming stages and thus reduce the severity of infections. There are no commercial vaccines against infection with *I. multifiliis,* but recovered fish are resistant. Dickerson and coworkers[41,42] have identified immobilizing ciliary antigens that can serve as a vaccine.

Public Health Considerations. *Ichthyophthirius multifiliis* is not infectious to humans.

Order Mobilida

Trichodina, Trichodinella, Tripartiella spp. **Morphology.** Trichodinids are peritrichous ciliates belonging to the family Trichodinidae. They have a saucer- to bell-shaped body, lack stalks, are motile, and have a highly developed adhesive disc on the aboral surface. A characteristic feature is the skeletal ring with radially arranged denticles that are readily apparent when viewed dorsoventrally (Figure 7.16). The number, arrangement, and shape of the teeth on the denticle are useful taxonomic features. These ciliates also have a large horseshoe-shaped macronucleus located in the endoplasm.

Hosts. These closely related ciliates infest a wide variety of marine and freshwater fishes. Trichodinids infest wild, cultured, and laboratory fishes in many parts of the world, and they occur on both freshwater and marine fishes. Five genera occur in fishes[9]. The most common genera include *Trichodina*, *Trichodinella*, and *Tripartiella*. Members of the genus *Trichodina* can be found both on the gills and body surface, and are the most frequently encountered ectoparasite in marine waters. *Trichodinella* and *Tripartiella* are only found on fish gills[7].

Life Cycle. All trichodinids have direct life cycles. Primary reproduction is asexual via binary fission; however, sexual reproduction via complicated conjugation of micro- and macro-conjugants does occur. Transmission is by direct contact with the ciliates in water.

Pathologic Effects. Light infestations probably have little pathologic effect, but heavy infestations can cause severe damage. These ciliates are capable of considerable tissue destruction, as evidenced by the presence of red blood cells in food vacuoles. Species that occur principally on the skin cause cutaneous hemorrhage, epithelial hyperplasia, and sloughing of the epidermis. Gill-infesting species can cause extensive epithelial hyperplasia.

Clinical Disease. All trichodinids are opportunists, and only cause disease in fishes debilitated by other factors. Examples of factors precipitating disease include poor nutrition, overcrowding, poor water quality, or other infectious agents. Dermal lesions, including epithelial erosion, loosened scales, and excess mucus production, often result in infested fishes having a grayish sheen. In severe infestations the fins may be frayed. Heavily infested fishes are also anorexic, lose condition, and occasionally die. Fishes with severe gill infestations exhibit dyspnea.

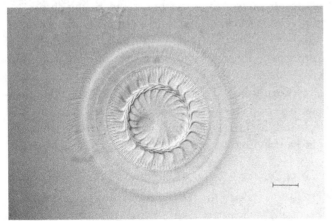

Fig. 7.16 *Trichodina* sp. Note radially arranged denticle ring. Bar = 10 μm.

Diagnosis. Trichodinids are easily identified in wet mounts of skin scrapings or gill filaments by their characteristic shape. The oral and aboral cilia and denticular ring with radially arranged denticles are readily apparent diagnostic features. These same features are seen in histological sections, as well as portions of the elongated macronucleus.

Treatment. Trichodinids are easily killed with a single application of an appropriate bath or drip treatment. The two most frequently used chemical treatments include copper sulfate (not in aquaria) and formalin.

Prevention. Good husbandry techniques are the most effective means of prevention. Maintaining good water quality in the culture systems, especially keeping organic loads low and water flow adequate, is essential to preventing outbreaks of trichodinosis.

Public Health Considerations. These parasites are not infective to humans.

Class Phyllopharyngea

Chilodonella spp.

Morphology. *Chilodonella* spp. are holotrichous ciliates that are typically heart-shaped, with the posterior end broader and slightly notched (Figures 7.17[43] and 7.18). They reach up to 80 μ in length, and the ventral surface is flat with parallel ciliary rows. These cilia move the parasite in a steady gliding manner over the epithelial cells of the skin and gills. There is a large oval macronucleus in the posterior third of the body.

Hosts. Most *Chilodonella* species are free living, but two species are pathogenic to fishes. *Chilodonella piscicola* infests the skin and gills of nearly all freshwater fishes. It is a particular problem in temperate climates at water temperatures of 5°C to 10°C and may be a serious pathogen in wintering carp. This ciliate is particularly pathogenic for fingerlings. *Chilodonella hexasticha* infests older fishes and causes epizootics at much higher water temperatures, up to 22°C, in species such as goldfish and channel catfish. Chilodonellosis has also been reported in wild fishes in Australia[44].

Life Cycle. The life cycles of *Chilodonella* spp. are direct. Reproduction is primarily by binary fission.

Pathologic Effects. *Chilodonella* can cause severe damage before any gross pathological changes are evident. As a result of feeding directly on epithelium, *Chilodonella* elicits a strong cellular response. Paperna and Van As[45] reported severe degeneration, necrosis, and subsequent

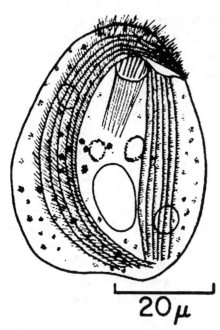

Fig. 7.17 *Chilodonella* trophozoites. Reproduced from Hoffman, G.L. (1999). Used with permission.

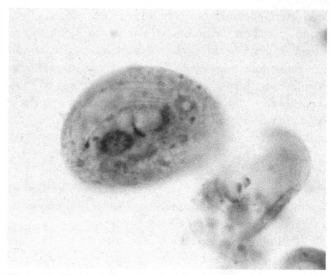

Fig. 7.18   Histological section of gill showing *Chilodonella.*

degradation of the branchial epithelium in infested cichlid fishes. Epithelial hyperplasia was focal, or occurred in an uneven pattern. Infestation also induced mucus and chloride cell proliferation. More extensive hyperplasia affecting entire arches was reported by Hoffman and coworkers[46] from channel catfish. Extensive hyperplasia of the lamellar epithelium resulted in severe fusion of lamellae. All these pathological changes in the gills drastically reduce the respiratory potential of the gills. Advanced infestations are sometimes associated with skin ulcers which can result in secondary bacterial infections.

Clinical Disease. Clinical signs of *Chilodonella* infestation include respiratory distress, clamped fins, and excessive mucus production. Heavily infested fishes exhibit a whitish or bluish sheen on the body, and there is sometimes a tattered appearance to the skin. Gills are also reddened and hemorrhagic. Because signs of infestation are less striking than white spot disease, chilodonellosis is much more insidious.

Diagnosis. *Chilodonella* spp. are easily recognized in wet mounts or histological sections. Members of this genus are identified by their oval, flattened shape and the characteristic bands of cilia on the ventral surface. The ciliate moves with a characteristic, slow circular movement and appears to glide.

Treatment. Identification to species is not necessary for proper treatment. A single application of formalin at 25 ppm, followed by a water change in four to eight hours, will kill ciliates on the fishes, as well as in the water.

Prevention. The most effective means of preventing infestation with *Chilodonella* spp. is to practice good husbandry techniques. Care must also be exercised not to introduce infested fishes into laboratory systems.

Public Health Considerations. *Chilodonella* spp. are not infective to humans.

PHYLUM MICROSPORIDIA

Microsporidians are common, intracellular, parasites that are related to fungi[47]. They cause disease in many species of invertebrates and vertebrates, including fishes[48,49]. We describe here three microsporidians that can be significant pathogens in research fishes: *Loma salmonae* of salmonids, *Pseudoloma neurophilia* of zebrafish, and *Glugea anomala* of sticklebacks.

Morphology. Many genera of microsporidia infecting fish form unique structures called xenomas. Infected host cells become transformed and hypertrophied, resulting in this unique, often macroscopic, host cell-parasite complex.

Hosts. Microsporidians of fish are usually host-specific, at least to the family level. *Loma salmonae* infects essentially all species of salmonids in the genus *Oncorhynchus,* including rainbow trout and Chinook and coho salmon. *Pseudoloma neurophilia* is a parasite of zebrafish. However, morphologically indistinguishable parasites have been detected in the brains of neon tetras (*Paracheirodon innesi*) (Authors' personal observations) and swordtails (*Xiphophorus helleri*) (P. Takvorkian, Rutgers University, Newark, N.J., personal communication). *Glugea anomala* infects the threespine stickleback, *Gasterosteus aculeatus,* and the ninespine stickleback, *Pungitius pungitius.*

Life Cycle. The general life cycle of microsporidia involves vegetative development within the host, culminating in the formation of spores. Spores are resistant to the external environment and represent the infectious stage. Fish-to-fish transmission by ingestion of spores or infected tissue occurs with *L. salmonae*[50], *P. neurophilia*[51], and *G. anomala*[52]. *Loma salmonae* can be easily transmitted by co-habitation with infected fishes[50]. Fishes exposed to either *P. neurophilia* or *L. salmonae* exhibit infections about six to eight weeks after exposure. *Glugea anomala* infections are seen about nine weeks post exposure.

Pseudoloma neurophilia is surprisingly common in research laboratories, in spite of the widespread use of dechlorinated city water in such facilities. It has been suggested that transovarial transmission may be another route of infection employed by this parasite[51,53], as documented for other microsporidia[54], including *L. salmonae*[55]. Transmission to progeny by sexual products (e.g., ovarian fluid and associated debris), in which the parasite is not within the egg itself, has also been suggested as a mode of transmission for *L. salmonae*[55] and *P. neurophilia*[51].

Pathologic Effects. *Loma salmonae* affects the gills and other vascularized tissues of salmonids reared in fresh water. All *Oncorhynchus* species are apparently susceptible to the infection, though Atlantic salmon are resistant[57]. Fish develop xenomas about four to six weeks after exposure (Figures 7.19 and 7.20).

A xenoma (parasite-infected host cell) is formed when the host cell alters its structure and size, becoming physiologically integrated with the parasite. The cytoplasmic contents are replaced by the parasite, and the surface of the host cell becomes modified for increased absorption. The host cell becomes extremely hypertrophied, so xenomas often appear as macroscopic, whitish cysts. Wet mount preparations reveal oval spores, usually about 5 μ long by 3 μ wide, with a distinctive posterior vacuole (Figure 7.21). There is usually minimal tissue reaction toward intact xenomas, but they can cause tissue damage because of their enormous size[49,58]. The associated lesions in the gills can become severe in salmon held in sea water[59,60].

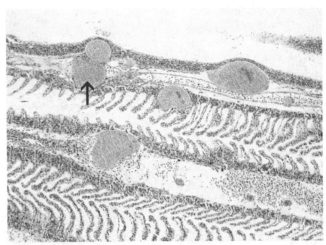

Fig. 7.19 *Loma salmonae* xenomas (arrow) in histological section of gill from a chinook salmon. Hematoxylin and eosin stain.

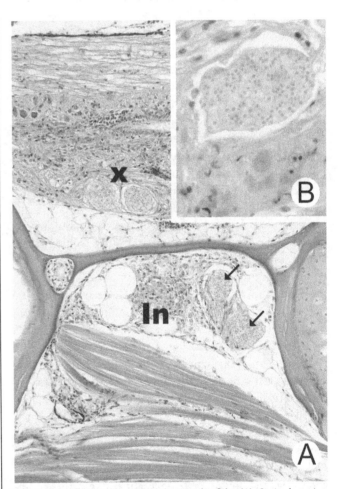

Fig. 7.20 *Pseudoloma neurophilia* in zebrafish. (A) Sagittal section through spinal cord and adjacent tissue. Xenomas in central nervous system (X). Xenomas in nerve root (arrows). Inflammation (In). (B) High magnification showing xenoma.

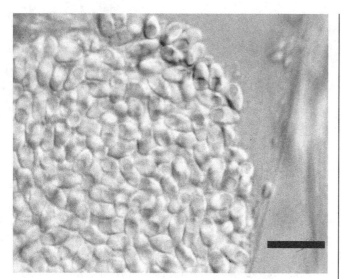

Fig. 7.21 Wet mount of spores, *Pseudoloma neurophilia*. Bar = 10 μm.

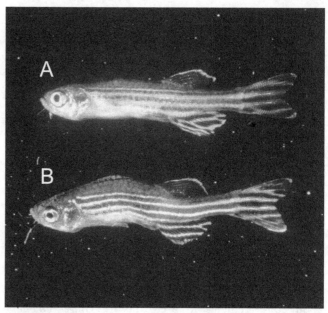

Fig. 7.22 *Pseudoloma neurophilia*. Heavily infected fish are often emaciated and lethargic, and may show curvature of the spine. (A) Emaciated fish. (B) Emaciated fish with scoliosis.

Although the gills are the primary site of infection, parasites and associated lesions can occur in the heart, spleen, kidney and pseudobranchs. Xenomas may rupture and release spores as the infection progresses. Free spores are found within macrophages and induce severe, chronic, multifocal vasculitis and perivasculitis in the gills.

The primary site of infection of *P. neurophilia* is the central nervous system. Histological examination of moribund zebrafish reveals microsporidia within multiple xenomas in the brain and spinal cord (Figure 7.20). Xenomas are commonly observed in axon-rich regions of the ventral spinal cord and the peripheral ventral roots projecting into the surrounding somatic muscle. Xenomas are also occasionally observed in the medial longitudinal fasciculus. Inflammation in the central nervous system is usually minimal and only occasionally seen surrounding xenomas or when dispersed spores are present in the central nervous system. In histological sections of heavily infected fishes, an associated tissue reaction extends through the meninges and into the skeletal muscle associated with the adjacent vertebrae. Emaciated fishes have a characteristic massive chronic inflammation of the skeletal muscle, in which free spores are found within phagocytes.

Glugea anomala forms massive xenomas, replete with spores in the skin, behind the eye and in other organs. Dyková and Lom[61] described the sequential development and tissue reaction to spores. Typical of xenomas, there is initially very little tissue reaction to intact xenomas. Eventually, a prominent, chronic inflammation is associated with fully-formed or ruptured xenomas.

Clinical Disease. Fishes mildly affected with *L. salmonae* may appear normal, but those with severely damaged gills may exhibit respiratory distress and become lethargic. Zebrafish heavily infected with *P. neurophilia* are often emaciated, or may be scoliotic (Figure 7.22). This condition is referred to as "skinny disease," and is one of the most prevalent clinical changes seen in zebrafish maintained in research facilities. *Glugea anomala* infections result in the formation of large xenomas, which are macroscopically visible on the skin (Figure 7.23). Heavily infected fish become emaciated and die.

Diagnosis. Microsporidia may be diagnosed by finding the characteristic spores in wet mounts or histological sections. Microsporidian spores are birefringent, oval, and usually have a prominent refractile vacuole. Most microsporidian spores of fish are about 3 μ long by 5 μ wide. Weber and coworkers[62] reviewed diagnostic methods for microsporidia. Spores are Gram positive in tissue smears or histological sections. Larger xenomas are easily seen with the naked eye or dissecting microscope (Figure 7.24), while smaller xenomas require histologic examination. Histology is also useful for demonstrating free spores within inflammatory lesions, and acid-fast stains may be used to enhance their detection. Xenomas caused by microsporidial infection must be differentiated from lesions caused by *Ichthyophthirius multifiliis*.

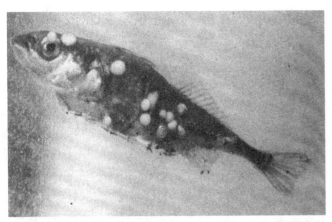

Fig. 7.23 *Glugea anomala* infection in a stickleback. Note subcutaneous cysts. Reproduced from Reichenbach-Klinke, H. and Elkan, E. (1965). Used with permission.

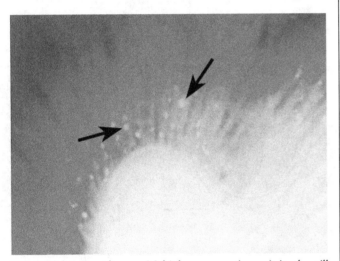

Fig. 7.24 *Loma salmonae*. Multiple xenomas (arrows) in the gill lameallae of chinook salmon.

Fluorescent stains (e.g., Fungi-Fluor, Polysciences, Warrington, PA) bind nonspecifically to β -linked polysaccharides found in cells containing chitin. Because chitin occurs in spore walls of microsporidia, these stains are excellent for demonstrating spores in either tissue smears or histological sections[8]. Weber and coworkers[62] described a related stain, Calcofluor, and other staining techniques for the identification of microsporidia.

Polymerase chain reaction (PCR)-based diagnostic tests have been developed for several microsporidia[55]. Such tests may be useful for screening fishes for subclinical infections before introducing them into research facilities.

Prevention. Spores of *L. salmonae* can survive iodine treatment at 100 ppm for 15 minutes, a dose typically used for disinfecting salmonid eggs after spawning. Therefore, the infection could enter a laboratory with infected or contaminated eggs or fry. Zebrafish eggs are usually disinfected with chlorine at 25 to 50 ppm. It has not been determined whether this will effectively eliminate spores of *P. neurophilia.* Moreover, eggs filled with spores of *Pseudoloma* have been observed by the authors. Spores within intact eggs could be protected from chlorine, even if this concentration is normally effective for killing free spores. It is recommended that all nonviable, unfertilized eggs be removed prior to bleaching.

Infected fishes should not be used for brood stock because vertical transmission of microsporidia may occur. Sensitive and specific PCR tests[55,63] are useful for screening fishes for subclinical infections. Because microsporidia are transmitted directly from fish to fish in aquaria, a good general practice is to remove fishes with obvious infections (xenomas for sticklebacks, emaciation for zebrafish) as soon as possible to prevent cannibalism and further transmission. Incorporation of ultraviolet sterilization units in recirculating systems will likely reduce infections. The ultraviolet dose required for a 3-log[10] or 99.9% reduction in the number of infective spores of *Encephalitozoon intestinalis* was determined to be 8.43 mW s/cm[64].

Treatment. Several drugs have been used experimentally to treat microsporidian infections in fishes. Fumagillin, an antimicrobial agent developed for treating *Nosema apis* infections in honey bees, is the most widely used drug for treating microsporidiosis in fishes[49], including *L. salmonae*[65]. Based on multiple reports, 3 to 10 mg fumagillin/kg fish/day is recommended for salmonids. Higher concentrations or prolonged treatment (e.g., 30 to 60 days) may cause anorexia, poor growth, anemia, renal tubule degeneration, and atrophy of hematopoietic tissues in salmonids. Fumagillin is heat labile; therefore, it is recommended that the feed be coated with the drug after processing, instead of incorporating it into the feed during milling. The drug is poorly soluble in water but is highly soluble in alcohol. In most studies, fumagillin was mixed with alcohol, sprayed on the feed, and then the feed was coated with oil.

Others have evaluated alternative therapies. Becker and coworkers[66] found that monensin was an effective prophylactic treatment; Speare and coworkers[67] reported that albendazole may be useful for treating the infection, and it has been reported that quinine hydrochloride delays xenoma formation[68]. The systemic triazinone, toltrazuril (Bayer AG), has been evaluated against *G. anomala* infections in stickleback[69,70]. Bath exposure of the drug caused destruction of all life stages of the parasite, but the overall effects of this drug for reducing prevalence or intensity of microsporidian infection in fishes have not been reported.

Public Health Considerations. Opportunistic microsporidial infections in humans are now a major concern with immune-compromised individuals. However, none of these infections have been linked to fish microsporidia.

PHYLUM MYXOZOA

Members of the phylum Myxozoa cause some of the most common and important parasitic diseases of fishes[9,48,71,72]. Hundreds of species have been described. Traditionally, the Myxozoa have been classified with the Protozoa. However, analysis of small subunit ribosomal DNA revealed that the Myxozoa belong within the kingdom Animalia[73]. Siddall[74] and others subsequently reported that, based on ribosomal DNA sequence and morphological features, the Myxozoa are most closely related to the Cnidaria. Affinities of the Myxozoa with the Cnidaria have been suggested for many years, particularly due to similarities of polar capsules with nematocysts. However, more recent data indicate that, although they are certainly primitive metazoans, they are not directly related to cnidarians[75].

Typically, myxosporeans are non-pathogenic. Histozoic species usually form small, well-defined, white cysts with little associated tissue damage. However, when numerous cysts occur in vital organs, such as the gills or heart, they can cause disease. Heavy infections of histozoic myxosporeans in the flesh may lower the market value of the affected fishes. Pathogenic histozoic species generally cause more diffuse infections without macroscopically visible cysts. Some myxozoans are very important causes of disease in wild and cultured fishes. They appear to be less problematic in confined research facilities, probably due to their requirement for an annelid worm (*Tubifex tubifex*) to complete their life cycle[72].

Many myxozoan diseases have been described from salmonids[65] and cyprinids, such as carp and goldfish[76]. Representative myxozoans described here include: *Tetracapsuloides bryosalmonae*, the PKX myxozoan of salmonids; *Myxobolus cerebralis*, the cause of "whirling disease" in salmonids; *Henneguya salminicola* from salmonids, an example of a histozoic species that causes macroscopic cyst-like structures; *Sphaerospora* spp. and *Hofferellus* spp., common pathogens of carp and goldfish; and *Myxidium* sp. from zebrafish.

Morphology. Myxozoans are characterized by the presence of multicellular spores (Figures 7.25 and 7.26).

Spores have two or more rigid valves, polar capsules with an internal coiled polar filament, and a sporoplasm (the infectious stage of the parasite for the invertebrate host). Spores develop within large, multicellular plasmodia comprised of vegetative nuclei and generative cells.

Hosts. Natural infections of fishes with *Tetracapsuloides bryosalmonae*, also known as the PKX agent, have been reported in rainbow trout and steelhead, *Oncorhynchus mykiss*; cutthroat trout, *O. clarki*; chinook salmon, *O. tshawytscha*; coho salmon, *O. kisutch*; Atlantic salmon, *Salmo salar*; brown trout, *S. trutta*; arctic char, *Salvelinus alpinus*; grayling, *Thymallus thymallus*; and pike, *Esox lucius*. Infections have been observed in captive and free-living populations. Kokanee salmon, *O. nerka*, and chum salmon, *O. keta*, have been experimentally infected. The rainbow

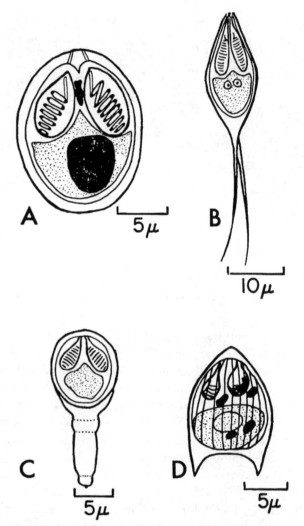

Fig. 7.25 Some myxozoans of fishes (spores). (A) *Myxobolus*. (B) *Henneguya*. (C) *Unicauda*. (D) *Hofferellus*. Reproduced from Hoffman, G.L. (1999). Used with permission.

trout is the primary host for this parasite. Essentially all members of the genus *Oncorhynchus* (Pacific salmon species) are susceptible; whereas the brown trout is considered a reservoir, and is more resistant to developing disease[77,78]. Numerous *Sphaerospora* spp. infect cyprinid fishes. Carp and goldfish are hosts for *S. renicola* and *S. molnari*, both of which are pathogenic. Two species of *Hoferellus* cause renal diseases in carp and goldfish: *H. cyprini* in carp and *H. carassii* in goldfish.

Life Cycle. The most complete information on the life cycle of a myxozoan is based on *Myxobolus cerebralis*[79,80]. The following is a description of a typical freshwater myxozoan life cycle. Multicellular myxospores are released from infected fish following death, or are discharged in body fluids. Oligochaetes (annelid worms), such as *Tubifex tubifex*, ingest the myxospores and serve as alternate hosts. In the oligochaete alternate host, asexual reproduction is followed by sporogony, resulting in the formation of actinospores. Actinospores are released from the oligochaete, and upon contacting the surface epithelium of a fish, release sporoplasms which penetrate the skin of the fish. Shortly thereafter, clusters of dividing myxosporean cells are found, sometimes intracelluarly, within the epithelium. The parasite then migrates to its final target tissue, where development continues. With *M. cerebralis,* the extrasporogonic (vegetative) forms migrate to the cartilage via peripheral nerves. These extrasporogonic forms continue to divide during migration to the target tissue. Some species (e.g., *Sphaerospora* spp. and *T. bryosalmonae*) exhibit prominent extrasporogonic multiplication in the circulatory system or vascular organs. The presporogonic organism becomes a multinucleated plasmodium containing free nuclei and internal generative cells. Sporogenesis is usually initiated by fusion of generative cells. The sporoblast divides and differentiates into the components of the spores.

Pathologic Effects. *Tetracapsuloides byrosalmonae* causes proliferative kidney disease (PKD) in salmonids. Histopathologic examination shows the kidney interstitium to be the primary site of infection, where *T. byrosalmonae* evokes a chronic interstitial nephritis. Coalescing whorls of inflammatory cells, primarily macrophages, surround the parasites (Figure 7.27). Parasites also infect blood vessels, where they adhere to vessel walls, occlude vessels, and evoke a necrotizing vasculitis. Well-vascularized extra-renal organs (e.g., gills, liver, spleen, and pancreas) also are infected and exhibit histologic changes similar to those found in the kidney.

Myxobolus cerebralis primarily infects bone and cartilage, resulting in necrosis and replacement of bone and cartilage with chronic inflammation.

Henneguya salminicola is typical of myxozoans which form large, whitish macroscopic cyst-like structures (plasmodia) in tissues. In general, there is minimal tissue reaction to intact plasmodia. Pathological changes are usually limited, unless infections are heavy, or when the parasite disrupts the function of vital organs.

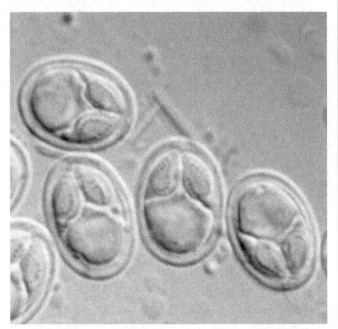

Fig. 7.26 Wet mount preparation of *Myxobolus* sp. spores. Nomarksi phase interference. Note: polar capsule with coiled polar filaments. Courtesy of S. Desser.

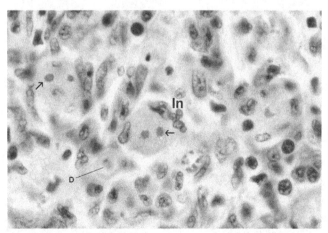

Fig. 7.27 *Tetracapsuloides bryosalmonae* extrasporogonic forms (trophozoites) in the renal interstitium of a rainbow trout. In = inflammatory cell surrounding parasites. Arrow = primary cell nucleus, D = internal daughter cell.

Numerous pathogenic *Sphaerospora* species have been described from carp and goldfish[48,76]. *Sphaerospora renicola* infects the renal tubules, where it causes atrophy and necrosis. Granulomas replace degenerated tubules. A more serious phase of the infection occurs in the swim bladder. Extrasporogonic stages proliferate in blood and in the swim bladder, and cause severe, chronic inflammation in the latter[9,81]. The swim bladder wall is thickened and hemorrhagic. Infections of the gill and skin by *S. molnari* may cause severe epithelial hyperplasia (Figure 7.28).

Two species of *Hoferellus* cause renal disease in carp and goldfish: *H. carassii* in goldfish and *H. cyprini* in carp. *Hoferellus carassii* causes "goldfish bloater disease" in the U.S.[65] and Japan[82]. *Hoferellus carassii* induces unusual histopathologic changes, where prespore stages infect the epithelium of renal tubules and cause massive cystic transformation of renal tubules (Figure 7.29). In *H. cyprini* infection, numerous trophozoites fill the renal epithelium and renal tubules of carp. This causes hyperplasia and syncytia formation, occluding the lumen of tubules[83,84]. Altered tubules may be replaced by chronic inflammation and fibroplasia[85].

An unidentified *Myxidium* species is usually confined to the lumen of the kidney tubules or collecting ducts of zebrafish, and is not associated with pathological changes. However, we have found kidney granulomas containing spores.

Clinical Disease. Myxozoan diseases in research fish are almost always due to pre-existing infections, especially if fish were previously reared in ponds (e.g., goldfish, carp), hatcheries (e.g., trout), or captured in the wild (e.g., sticklebacks). Infections can be initiated within a facility by introduction of oligochaete worms, perhaps accidentally with fish, snails, or aquatic plants. Oligochaete worms (e.g., *T. tubifex* or *Lumbriculus variegatus*) are often used as fish food, and this may also be a source of infection[86,87]. Once introduced, the worms can establish and replicate efficiently in aquarium gravel or in filters.

Fish infected with *T. bryosalmonae* are often lethargic and dark. They exhibit exophthalmos, lateral body swelling, and a distended abdomen. Gills are pale due to anemia. Fish infected with *M. cerebralis* exhibit spiral swimming, usually along a horizontal plane. Other changes include cranial deformities, scoliosis, lordosis, and darkening at the posterior region of the body ("black tail syndrome"). Fish infected with *H. salminicola* appear clinically normal. Large, whitish cysts are found in the muscle (Figure 7.30). Carp infected with *S. renicola* show swimming disorders and may swim in circles. Mortality in over wintering carp may reach 15%. *Sphaerospora molnari* causes respiratory distress due to gill damage and epithelial hyperplasia which reduces the respiratory surface. Infections have been associated with high mortality. Goldfish infected with *H. carassii* infections exhibit swollen abdomens (occasionally unilateral) due to greatly enlarged

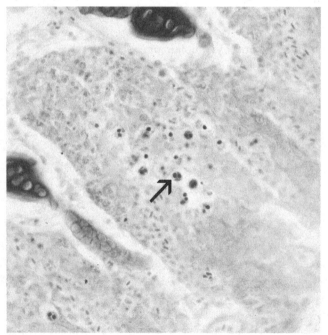

Fig. 7.28 *Sphaerospora molnari* spores (arrow) associated with prominent epithelial hyperplasia in histological sections of goldfish gills. Giemsa stain.

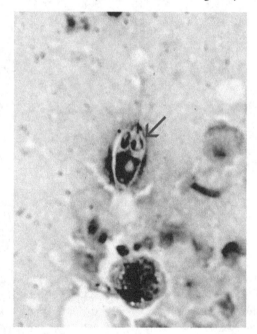

Fig. 7.29 *Hoferellus carassii*. Kidney imprint showing spore. Polar capsule (arrow). Giemsa stain.

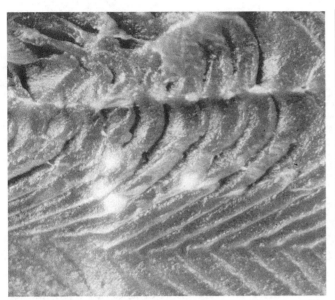

Fig. 7.30 *Henneguya salminicola* in sockeye salmon, characterized by whitish, oval cysts in the somatic muscle.

kidneys. Carp with *H. cyprini* show little clinical disease[9]. Zebrafish infected with *Myxidium* spp. are asymptomatic.

Diagnosis. Myxozoan infections are diagnosed by histology, tissue imprints, or wet mount preparations. In most cases, detection of the spore stage is essential for diagnosis. Wet mounts are most appropriate for precise observation of spore morphology (Figure 7.26), which is necessary for identification of species. Histology is useful for demonstrating organ locations, associated pathological changes, and for visualization of presporogonic stages. There are few spores in fish with *T. byrosalmonae* or *Hoferellus* spp. infections (Figure 7.29), and only presporogonic stages of *S. renicola* are found in the swim bladders of carp with associated inflammation. Tissue digest methods have been traditionally used to detect spores of *M. cerebralis*[88]. PCR tests have been developed for several myxozoans, including *M. cerebralis*[89] and *T. byrosalmonae*[90].

Treatment. Fumagillin is the most common drug used for treating myxozoan diseases of fishes[91]. Fumagillin has been used to treat fish infected with *S. renicola*[91,92] and *T. byrosalmonae*[78,93], but has been less successful in treating tissue myxozoans such as *M. cerebralis*. Based on several reports, the recommended dosage for treating salmonids is 3 to 10 mg fumagillin/kg fish/day. Higher concentrations or prolonged treatment (e.g., 30 to 60 days) may cause anorexia, poor growth, anemia, renal tubule degeneration, and atrophy of hematopoietic tissues in salmonids[94].

Prevention. Oligochaete worms (e.g., black worms, red worms) are commonly used as live food for ornamental fishes, and are sold through the pet fish industry. Lowers and Bartholomew[87] reported the presence of various actinosporeans in these worms, so this is a potential source of myxozoan infections. Moreover, oligochaete worms are ubiquitous in the aquatic environment and can easily establish themselves in aquarium systems, and thus provide a constant reservoir for these infections. Ultraviolet light and ozonation are effective for killing actinosporeans in water[95,96]. Myxospores are extremely resistant to disinfectants. For example, the myxospores of *M. cerebralis* require 1,600 ppm chlorine for 24 hours, or 5,000 ppm for 10 minutes, for effective killing of spores[97].

Public Health Considerations. The Myxozoa are not considered human pathogens.

PHYLUM PLATYHELMINTHES

Helminths of laboratory fishes include trematodes, cestodes, acanthocephalans, and nematodes. The majority of helminths are of little concern in fishes held in aquaria or other systems with controlled water sources. Usually, these helminths do not proliferate in these aquatic systems because most have indirect life cycles that require intermediate hosts. Indirect life cycles are easily disrupted by elimination of intermediate hosts. Wild-caught fish may occasionally arrive with such heavy infections that they may still cause disease, even if the parasites cannot reproduce or maintain their life cycle. However, some helminths, such as monogeneans, and certain capillarid nematodes have direct life cycles and thus are capable of causing disease in research systems.

Monogenea

Morphology. Monogenes are small parasitic flatworms. Two types of monogeneans may be identified based upon opisthaptor morphology. In the more common Monopisthocotylea, there is a single attachment organ with several large, centrally located, sclerotized anchors, and small marginal hooklets. In the Polyopisthocotylea, the opisthaptor consists of a group of small, muscular, adhesive suckers or clamps that are supported by cuticular sclerites. Two of the most common families of monopisthocotylid monogeneans infesting fishes are the Gyrodactylidae and Dactylogyridae. Gyrodactylids are small (1 mm or less), and are found on the skin and gills of freshwater and marine fishes (Figures 7.31 and 7.32). The opisthaptor is membranous with one pair of anchors, two transverse bars, and 16 marginal hooks. The developing young can be seen within the uterus. Dactylogyrids are also small (up to 2 mm) and are found on the gill filaments. The opisthaptor is membranous with one to two pairs of anchors, zero to three transverse bars, and 14 to 16 marginal hooks. The prohaptor has four prominent eyespots.

Hosts. Monogenes are common parasites of both marine and freshwater fish[98], and are of great economic importance as pathogens of captive fishes. *Gyrodactylus* causes disease in a variety of captive fish species, including goldfish, guppies, salmonids, sticklebacks, and others[99]. *Gyrodactylus* is also a continual problem in mummichogs maintained in laboratory holding facilities. *Dactylogyrus* occurs on the gills of goldfish, carp, gulf killifish, sheepshead minnows, and other species. There are numerous species of *Gyrodactylus* and *Dactylogyrus,* and most are host-specific[100]. For example, *D. vastator, D. anchoratus,* and *G. gurleyi* infect goldfish and carp, whereas *G. elegans* infects sticklebacks. These parasites are not usually identified to the species level when they cause disease, because the diseases that they cause and treatments for them are essentially the same.

Life Cycle. Members of both families have direct life cycles. Dactylogyrids are oviparous. Eggs settle to the bottom to develop. With hatching, eggs release free-swimming, infective, oncomiracidia, which seek out and attach to a new host. In contrast, gyrodactylids are viviparous. The young are retained in the uterus until they develop into functional subadults, and usually remain with the host on which they developed. Transmission of both families is greatly enhanced by overcrowding.

Pathologic Effects. Heavy gill infestations cause epithelial hyperplasia, destruction of gill epithelium, clubbing of gill filaments, and hypersecretion of mucus, resulting in death by asphyxiation. Heavy skin infestations can cause body and fin necrosis. Histologically, fins of infested trout have epidermal hyperplasia with zones of degeneration and necrosis[99]. High mortality is common in the crowded situations of aquaria, raceways, and fish culture ponds.

Clinical Disease. Captive fishes are often infested with heavy burdens of monogeneans, and frequently experience severe disease due to these infestations. Monogeneans feed on mucus, epithelium, and blood. Heavy infestations usually indicate poor sanitation, deteriorating water quality, or inadequate water flows. Clinical signs of dactylogyrid infestations include rapid respiratory movements, clamped fins, and flashing. Fish may become

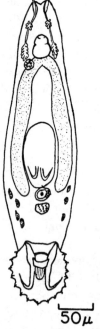

Fig. 7.31 *Gyrodactylus* adult. Note the absence of eye spots and presence of embryo or larva. Reproduced from Hoffman, G.L. (1999). Used with permission.

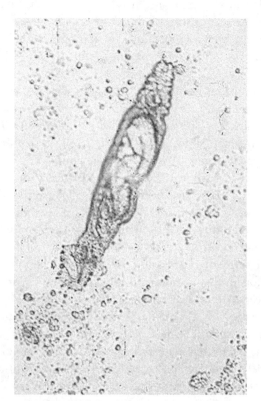

Fig. 7.32 Wet mount of *Gyrodactylus* sp. from a goldfish.

lethargic, swim near the surface, and refuse food. Heavy infestation with gyrodactylid skin flukes (Figure 7.33) results in white to grey-white areas of thick mucus on the body surface, localized hemorrhagic areas, and ragged-appearing fins. In both cases, infested fishes can be seen rubbing or scratching against the bottom or sides of the holding tank.

Diagnosis. Diagnosis of monogenean infestation is based on clinical signs, and is confirmed by identification of parasites in wet mounts or histological sections of skin or gills. In both cases, the characteristic morphological features are easily discernible, particularly the haptoral anchors and hooks.

Treatment. Designing an effective treatment depends on whether the monogenean is viviparous or oviparous, because the eggs of some monogeneans resist treatment, and thus several drug applications may be required for adequate control. Treatment with the organophosphate trichlorfon, at 0.25 mg/L, as a bath is very effective. Praziquantel baths (20 mg/L seawater for 2 hours), administered 48 hours apart, removed all skin and gill parasites from the yellow stripey *Lutjanus carponotatus.* Formalin is also an effective parasiticide for bath treatment of monogeneans. Treatment with 125 to 250 ppm formalin for up to 60 minutes eliminates infestations.

Prevention. Monogenean infestations are best prevented by not introducing wild-caught or hatchery-reared fishes or invertebrates into laboratory systems. Providing a rapid, continuous flow of water through systems will also aid in preventing heavy infestations. Because of their reproductive cycle, the offspring of viviparous monogeneans remain on the same host, so transmission can occur via fish-to-fish contact. Preventing overcrowding may reduce transmission by contact.

Public Health Considerations. Monogenean trematodes are not zoonotic.

Cestoidea

Cestodes are uncommon in cultured fishes because they have a complex life cycle that requires one or two intermediate hosts. Fishes can act as either intermediate or definitive hosts for several tapeworms. In the former, infections occur in extraintestinal sites, and, when massive, can cause disease. Adult tapeworms usually infect the lumen of the gut, and heavy infections may result in poor food conversation or, occasionally, obstruction of the intestinal tract.

Bothriocephalus Acheilognathi

Morphology. *Bothriocephalus acheilognathi* (Syn. *B. gowkongensis*) is a pseudophyllidean tapeworm known as the "Asian tapeworm." Adult worms are whitish, segmented, and may reach 50 cm. The scolex is flattened with two bothria, and the posterior is wider than the first few segments, even when contracted[101].

Hosts and Life Cycle. *Bothriocephalus acheilognathi* has an unusually wide host range. All fishes in the family Cyprinidae, with the exception of goldfish, are susceptible hosts[101]. This parasite has also been found in fishes of other families, including live bearers, killifishes, channel catfish, and perches. The life cycle is typical of pseudophyllidean tapeworms, and is described in Chapter 4, Biology of Cestodes. Adult worms mature in the anterior intestine[102].

Pathologic Effects and Clinical Disease. The intestinal tract may be chronically inflamed, greatly enlarged, stretched, and flaccid[101]. Heavy infections may cause blockage of the gastrointestinal tract, intestinal perforation, and destruction of the intestinal mucosa[103]. *Bothriocephalus acheilognathi* is one of the most serious cestodes of fishes. Infections may cause reduced growth, emaciation, suppressed swimming ability, "dropsy," and ultimately death[101,104,105].

Diagnosis. Intestinal cestodiasis is diagnosed from wet mounts of fecal contents, or by finding adult tapeworms in the intestinal tract. Speciation requires examination of the

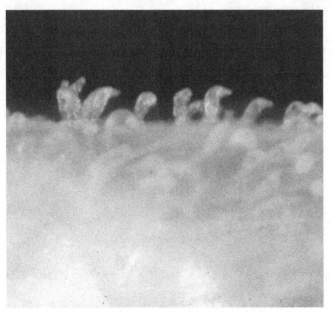

Fig. 7.33 Goldfish with heavy *Gyrodacytlus* infestation. Courtesy of G.L. Hoffman.

scolex and organization of the reproductive structures. *Bothriocephalus* may be distinguished from similar tapeworms because it lacks a neck and median and dorsal furrows, and has a scolex wider than the first few segments, even when contracted[101].

Treatment. Others have reviewed feed additive treatments that have been used successfully for treatment of infection with *B. acheilognathi*. These include Lintex (50 mg drug/kg fish); mebendazole at 100 mg drug/kg fish/day[104]; praziquantel at 30, 50, and 70 mg drug/kg fish; mebendazole at 10, 30, and 50 mg drug/kg fish; and nitroscanate at 2.0, 4.0, 6.0 mg drug/kg fish[106]. Of these, praziquantel was most effective.

Prevention. The most effective means to prevent *Bothriocephalus* infections in laboratory-held fishes is to eliminate copepod intermediate hosts from the system.

Public Health Considerations. *Bothriocephalus acheilognathi* is not infective to humans.

Schistocephalus Solidus

Morphology. Plerocercoid larvae are white and range from 20 to 76 mm long by about 6 mm wide. The cestode has a triangular scolex with shallow bothria and weakly muscular sucking grooves on the dorsal and ventral surfaces.

Hosts and Life Cycle. Fish-eating birds are the definitive hosts of *S. solidus*. Sticklebacks and other fishes in North America, Europe, and Asia serve as second intermediate hosts. The life cycle is typical of pseudophyllidean tapeworms, and is described in Chapter 4, Biology of Cestodes. Plerocercoid larvae are found in the abdominal cavity of infected fish.

Pathologic Effects and Clinical Disease. Heavy infections are pathogenic in fish. The plerocercoid larvae fill the abdominal cavity, causing compression of the visceral organs and obliteration of the gonads. Infected fish may develop severe abdominal distension, become sluggish, inhabit shallower water, and become more susceptible to predation[107].

Diagnosis, Treatment, and Prevention. Presumptive diagnosis is based on clinical signs and is confirmed by identification of the segmented plerocercoid larvae in the abdominal cavity. Treatments described for *Bothriocephalus acheilognathi* would likely also be effective against *S. solidus*. The most effective means to prevent *S. solidus* infections in laboratory-held sticklebacks is to eliminate copepod intermediate hosts from the system.

Public Health Considerations. *Schistocephalus solidus* is not infectious to humans.

PHYLUM NEMATODA

Nematodes are commonly recognized as important pathogens in aquaculture[102]. Only a few are considered significant fish pathogens in research environments because most require intermediate hosts to complete their life cycles. Among the most significant are the capillarids, members of the superfamily Trichuroidea.

Capillarids infect all classes of vertebrates, and are often pathogenic due to their invasive nature[108–110]. *Capillaria pterophylii* has been recognized for many years as a common pathogen of captive angelfish and discus fish, and *Capillostrongyloides ancistri* is highly pathogenic to the bushymouth catfish, *Ancistrus dolichopterus*[110]. However, the most important capillarid of laboratory fishes is *Pseudocapillaria tomentosa*[111–113].

Pseudocapillaria Tomentosa

Morphology. Females of *Pseudocapillaria tomentosa* are long, thin, white worms ranging from 7 to 12 mm long. Gravid worms are replete with the distinctive eggs bearing bipolar plugs. These characteristic eggs are easily visualized in wet mount preparations of the gut. Males are smaller, about 4 to 7 mm in length (Figure 7.34).

Hosts. *Pseudocapillaria tomentosa* has a broad host range, infecting many species of cyprinids. Fishes in the orders Anguilliformes (eels), Gadiformes (cod fish), Salmoniformes (salmon), and Siluriformes (catfish) are also susceptible[109].

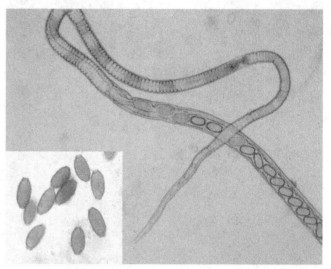

Fig. 7.34 Adult female *Pseudocapillaria tomentosa* from a zebrafish. Insert shows typical eggs with bipolar plugs.

Life Cycle. Lomankin and Trofimeno[114] showed that oligochaetes (e.g., *Tubifex tubifex*) can serve as paratenic hosts for *P. tomentosa* in laboratory transmission studies. They and others have demonstrated direct transmission in the absence of worms[112]. The latter observation explains why *P. tomentosa* can easily spread in zebrafish research facilities.

Pathologic Effects and Clinical Disease. Necropsy may reveal liver enlargement and anemia. Histological sections reveal the worms within the gut wall. Lesions include severe, diffuse cellulitis of the infected region, occasionally extending throughout the visceral cavity. The infection also seems to predispose fish to intestinal neoplasms[112]. Heavily infected fish are often dark, emaciated, and lethargic.

Diagnosis. Diagnosis is by observing the worms in wet mount preparations or histological sections of the intestine. Identification of capillarid nematodes is facilitated by the presences of eggs with distinctive, bi-polar plugs. Precise identification to the species level requires careful examination of the male sexual organs, which are rather diminutive in *Pseudocapillaria* spp. To date, the only nematode infection identified by the authors in zebrafish from research facilities is *P. tomentosa*.

Treatment. Ivermectin has been used for treating nematode infections in fishes[115], and may be useful for treating those infected with *P. tomentosa*. However, ivermectin has not been tested in zebrafish, and there appears to be great variability in the tolerance of the drug between closely related fish species[116,117].

Oral or bath treatments with levamisole and fenbendazole have also been used to treat nematode infections in fishes[7], but Hoffman[118] found that levamisole was not effective for treating capillarid infections in golden shiners. Brood stock zebrafish treated with levamisole have become sterile (D. Weaver, Scientific Hatcheries, Huntington Beach, California, personal communication). Pack and coworkers[113] reported that a mixture of trichlorfon and mebendazole ("Fluke-Tabs", Aquarium Products, Glen Burnie, MD) added to water eliminated the infection and resulted in weight gain in treated fish.

Prevention. Oligochaete worms may be a source of the infection, and thus should be avoided as food, particularly if their source is unknown. Direct transmission occurs between fish. The infection can spread within a population if not controlled. If fish are not highly valuable, the most appropriate choice would be to eliminate the infected population. At present, the infection is not widespread in research facilities, perhaps due to bleaching of fish eggs and quarantine procedures.

Public Health Considerations. *Pseudocapillaria tomentosa* does not infect humans, but freshwater fishes are an intermediate host for another capillarid (*Capillaria philippinensis*) that can be lethal to humans. It should be noted that fishes serve as intermediate or paratenic hosts for other nematodes that are pathogenic to humans. *Eustrongylides* in freshwater fishes and anisakine nematodes (*Anisakis, Psuedoterranova*) in marine fishes are examples. Humans should avoid eating raw fish that has not been previously frozen, particularly from fishes captured in the wild.

PHYLUM ARTHROPODA

Branchiurans (e.g., *Argulus* spp.) and copepods are crustaceans that parasitize both marine and freshwater fishes. The parasitic stages of these crustaceans are so morphologically specialized that they are often unrecognizable as arthropods. Some cause serious problems in captive fishes because of the pathological changes caused by their specialized feeding behavior. A few species are problems in research facilities and are discussed below.

Argulus spp.

Morphology. Branchiurans possess a flat, oval, dorsal shield which covers the majority of the appendages (Figure 7.35). Branchiurans are dorsoventrally flattened and thus adhere closely to the host's surface. Adults reach up to 12 mm in

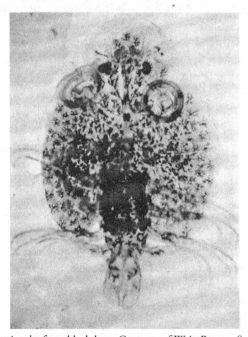

Fig. 7.35 *Argulus* from black bass. Courtesy of W.A. Rogers, Southeastern Cooperative Fish Disease Project, Auburn University.

length. *Argulus,* also known as the "fish louse," is the most widespread genus of this group. *Argulus* spp. possess compound eyes, a suctorial proboscis, two anterior-ventral prominent sucking discs that serve as attachment organs, four pairs of thoracic swimming legs, and a laterally expanded carapace that forms respiratory alae[119].

Hosts. *Argulus* spp. infest a wide range of both freshwater and marine fishes. Among captive laboratory fishes, the goldfish and carp are common freshwater hosts, and the sheepshead minnow, gulf killifish, and mummichog are common marine hosts.

Life Cycle. Mature female branchiurans leave their hosts to deposit eggs on vegetation or other objects. Eggs usually hatch and develop into juveniles within 10 to 50 days[120]. Juveniles range from 1 to 3 mm and look like adults without suckers. The juveniles must attach to a suitable host within two to three days or they will die. After attachment, they mature to the adult stage in about 30 days. Adults can survive without a host for several days.

Pathologic Effects. Areas of attachment of *Argulus* adults may leave abrasions on the skin from penetration of the stylet feeding organ. During feeding, the parasites are believed to elaborate toxic substances which are responsible for the severe local reaction[4]. The local mechanical injury results in hemorrhagic wounds that can serve as sites for secondary infections. The skin of infested fishes may also become erythemic, and excess mucus may be secreted. Heavy infestations can cause mass mortalities, especially of young fishes.

Clinical Disease. *Argulus* spp. can be seen moving around on the body surfaces of fishes. Slight to moderate infestations of argulids will cause fishes to rub against the sides and bottom of the aquarium or pond in an attempt to dislodge the irritating parasites. Heavy infestations may cause fishes to become lethargic, seek the sides of the aquarium or pond, and have difficulty maintaining equilibrium.

Diagnosis. The larger branchiuran crustaceans are easily recognizable grossly. Wet mounts of the skin or buccal cavity may be necessary for identification of smaller specimens. Diagnosis is easily made by identification of the distinctive features, including the flattened dorsal shield, the cuplike suckers, and the compound eyes.

Treatment. Small numbers of parasites can be removed with forceps, but this does not eliminate parasites in the environment. Two applications at weekly intervals of Masoten (0.25 mg/l) added to the water is reported to be effective at removing all life stages.

Prevention. Specific management practices may reduce or eliminate argulids. For example, increased water flow through ponds or enclosed systems may wash early parasite stages away before they can find a host. Removal of suitable habitat for egg-laying females may further reduce populations. Draining and drying ponds will destroy all stages of these parasitic crustaceans. We have seen several outbreaks of *Argulus* spp. on wild-caught sheepshead minnows held in flow-through aquaria. This infection could be prevented by using tank-reared sheepshead minnows, which are available from commercial suppliers, or by prophylactic treatment of wild-caught fish with formalin baths.

Public Health Considerations. *Argulus* spp. are not transmissible to humans.

Lernaea spp.

Morphology. *Lernaea* spp. (Copepoda) are commonly referred to as "anchor worms." Adult anchor worms are about 7 to 25 mm long, with the anterior end embedded under the skin of the fish (Figure 7.36). Two elongated egg sacs are seen at the posterior of the parasite. Careful dissection of the parasite from the skin reveals the anchor-like attachment structure. Copepodids can be easily visualized with a dissecting microscope. They are dark, actively moving, and resemble typical free-living copepods.

Hosts. *Lernaea cyprinacea* infests a wide variety of cyprinid fishes, and has also been found on fishes of other families, including salmonids such as rainbow trout reared in warm surface waters[43].

Life Cycle. Typical of many parasitic copepods, the adult female is the most pathogenic form. Eggs are released into the water, hatch, and release a larval stage, the nauplius. The nauplius develops through two additional free-living stages before locating a suitable host and maturing to the adult stage. Adults feed on skin mucus. Males die after mating. In temperate zones, the female overwinters as a larva, or as a juvenile adult attached to a fish. Females will attach to the skin and fins.

Pathologic Effects. Lester and Roubal[121] reviewed the pathogenesis of *L. cyprinacea* infestation. Infested fish may show hemorrhage, ulceration, hyperplasia, and fibrosis at the site of attachment[7]. Ulcers may serve as portals for secondary bacterial or fungal infections. Underlying muscles may become necrotic. A thick connective tissue encapsulation ultimately occurs around the portion of the parasite within the host[122].

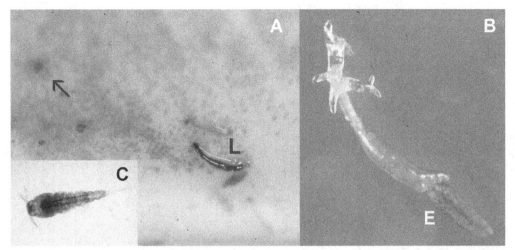

Fig. 7.36. *Lernaea* from koi carp. (A) Two attached females (L) and ulcer at site of previous attachment (arrow). (B) Adult females. Note anchor-like anterior end and egg sacs (E). (C) Copepodid.

Clinical Disease. *Lernaea cyprinacea* causes severe mortality in carp and goldfish reared in both ornamental and food fish ponds[121]. Heavy infestations can lead to anemia, debilitation, and death. Heavy infestations by copepodids on the gills may cause respiratory distress[121].

Diagnosis. Infestation is diagnosed by visualization of the females attached to the skin. This is best accomplished using a dissecting microscope.

Treatment. Organophosphate insecticides added to the water have been recommended for treating parasitic copepods, including anchor worms[7,20,40,121]. Dimilin (diflubenzuron) (UniRoyal Chemical Co.) applied in ponds at 0.01 to 0.03 ppm was effective at reducing *L. cyprinacea* infestations on golden shiners (*Notemigonus crysoleucas*)[121,123]. Incorporation of ivermectin and its analog, emamectin, into feed has been used successfully to treat another type of skin-parasitic copepod, caligid infestations in farmed salmon[124]. Emamectin is sold as Slice® (Schering-Plough Animal Health). *Salmincola californiensis,* a gill parasite, has been treated by oral intubation of ivermectin (0.2 mg/kg body weight)[125]. In light of these reports, oral administration of avermectins might also prove useful for *Lernaea* infestations.

Other commonly available chemicals used in aquaculture were evaluated for treating *Lernaea bhadraensis* infestations in the carp *Catla catla*[126]. Bath treatment twice per day over five consecutive days, with 30 ppm potassium permanganate ($KMnO_4$) for 20 minutes, was 100% effective in killing adult and larval parasites. Larval stages of *L. bhadraensis* were also highly sensitive to formalin at 150 and 250 ppm, while the adult parasites showed marked resistance, even up to 500 ppm at a water temperature of 25.5°C.

Prevention. Removal of adult females from fish before introduction into the animal facility will prevent the infestation.

Public Health Considerations. *Lernaea* spp. are not zoonotic.

ACKNOWLEDGEMENT

Support for preparation of this chapter was provided in part by National Institutes of Health grants NCRR P30 ES03850 and NCRR 5R24RR017386-03. The authors thank Denny Weber and Shawn Tucker for assistance with manuscript preparation.

Tables 7.1 through 7.6 were derived from the parasites covered in the first edition. That material included numerous hosts and parasites of fishes that are not common in laboratory settings and thus were not covered in the present chapter. Furthermore, this is not a complete list of parasites reported from the hosts listed. We have revised and updated the data where possible.

Mention of commercial or trade names does not imply endorsement by the U.S. Environmental Protection Agency.

TABLE 7.1 Parasites of fish—circulatory/lymphatic system.

Parasite	Geographic distribution	Hosts	Location in host	Method of infection	Pathologic effects	Reference
Flagellates						
Trypanoplasma (Cryptobia) cyprinid, T. borelli	Europe	Goldfish, carp, European minnow, others	Blood	Bite of intermediate host (leech)	Lethargy, anorexia, weight loss anemia, death	43, 128
Trypanoplasma (Cryptobia) gurneyorum, T. salmositica	North America	Salmonids, sticklebacks, others	Blood	Direct transmission or bite of intermediate host (leech)	Lethargy, anorexia, weight loss, anemia, death	43, 127
Trypanosoma spp.	North America	Brook trout, others	Blood	Bite of intermediate host (leech)	Not reported	43, 128, 129
Trypanosoma danilewski, T. granulosum,	Europe	Carp, eel, European minnow	Blood	Bite of intermediate host (leech)	Anemia, debilitation, death	128, 130
Apicomplexa						
Dactylosoma salvelini	Eastern Canada	Brook trout	Blood	Bite of unknown bloodsucking invertebrate	Not reported	43
Myxozoa						
Tetracapsuloides bryosamonae	Europe, North America	Salmonids	Blood, kidney, spleen, etc.	Actinosporean from bryozoans, penetration of skin and gills	Anemia, renosplenomegaly	247
Trematodes						
Sanguinicola armata, Sanguinicola spp.	Europe	Goldfish, carp, others	Blood vessels	Penetration of skin by cercaria released from snail	Ova and miracidia cause extensive gill damage, death	43, 132
Sanguinicola davisi, S. huronis	North America	Rainbow trout, black bass	Blood vessels	Penetration of skin by cercaria released from snail	Ova and miracidia cause extensive kidney and gill damage, death	43
Larval						
Ascocotyle leighi, A. tenuicollis	Southern United States	Topminnows, killfishes, mollies, others	Conus arteriosus	Penetration by cercaria released from snail of blood	Cysts in conus arteriosus which sometimes block flow	43, 133

TABLE 7.2 Parasites of fishes—enterohepatic system.

Parasite	Geographic distribution	Hosts	Location in host	Method of infection	Pathologic effects	References
Flagellates						
Spiromucleus (Hexamita) intestinalis	Europe	Goldfish, other aquarium fishes, salmonids, other fishes	Intestine	Ingestion of cyst passed in feces	Catarrhal enteritis, anorexia, listlessness, emaciation, retarded growth, death	9, 13, 43, 248
Spiromucleus (Hexamita) salmonis	North America	Salmonids, other fishes	Intestine	Ingestion of cyst passed in feces	Catarrhal enteritis, anorexia, listlessness, emaciation, retarded growth, death	9, 134, 248
Amoebae						
Schizamoeba salmonis	US	Trout, Pacific salmons	Stomach, intestine	Ingestion of organism passed in feces	Nonpathogenic	9, 43
Coccidia						
Calyptospora spp.	US	Fundulus spp.	Liver	Ingestion of shrimp intermediate host	Increased susceptibility to cold shock	27, 31, 32
Eimeria spp. and Goussia spp.	Europe, US	Goldfish, carp, salmonids, others	Various organs	Ingestion of oocyst passed in feces	Enteritis, anemia, emaciation, death	9, 25, 26 43, 135–137
Myxozoa						
Ceratomyxa shasta	Western US	Rainbow trout	Multiple organs	Actinosporeans from the aquatic polychaete Manayunkia speciosa	May cause high mortality in fry	138, 139
Chloromyxum spp.	Asia, Europe, North America	Carp, bluegill, sunfishes, salmonids	Gallbladder	Probably by actinosporeans released from oligochaete worms	May cause hypertrophy of gallbladder, anorexia, debilitation, diarrhea, anemia, death	13, 43
Myxidium spp.	Europe, North America	Sticklebacks, topminnows, killifishes, mosquitofish, salmonids, bass, others	Liver, gallbladder, kidney	Probably by actinosporeans released from oligochaete worms	Variable mortality, most nonpathogenic	13, 43, 140
Myxobolus capsulatis	Southern US	Topminnows	Viscera	Probably by actinosporeans released from oligochaete worms	Cysts in viscera	43
Myxobolus cyprini	Europe	Carp, others	Liver (also found in spleen, kidneys)	Probably by actinosporeans released from oligochaete worms	Inflammation of kidney and spleen	13
Myxobolus grandis	Northeastern US	Shiners, others	Liver	Probably by actinosporeans from oligochaete worms	Enlarged liver	43

(Continued)

TABLE 7.2 (*Continued*)

Parasite	Geographic distribution	hosts	Location in host	Method of infection	Pathologic effects	References
Trematodes						
Allocreadium spp.	US	Shiners, trout, catfish, goldfish, others	Stomach, intestine	Ingestion of metacercaria in arthropod, clam	Unknown	43
Alloglossidium corti	North America	Channel catfish, others	Intestine	Ingestion of intermediate host	Unknown	43, 147
Azygia spp.	Asia, Europe, North America	Bluegill, sunfish, catfish, salmonids, others	Intestine and/or stomach	Ingestion of cercaria in snail and/or in fish	Unknown	43, 144, 145
Bucephalus elegans	US	Bluegill, sunfish, others	Intestine	Ingestion of metacercaria in muscle or skin of fish	Unknown	43
Bucephalus polymorphus	Europe	Goldfish, carp, Atlantic salmon, eels, others	Intestine	Ingestion of metacercaria in gills or skin of fish	Unknown	43
Bunodera spp.	Europe, North America	Carp, black bass, brown trout, others	Intestine	Ingestion of intermediate host	Unknown	43
Centovarium lobotes	North America	Black bass, other centrarchids, channel catfish, eels, other fishes	Stomach, intestine	Ingestion of metacercaria in muscle	Unknown	43
Crepidostomum spp.	Europe, North America	Carp, catfish, sunfish, black bass, salmonids, others	Intestine	Ingestion of intermediate host	May cause enteritis and death	43, 148
Creptotrema funduli	US	Topminnows, sticklebacks, other fishes	Intestine	Ingestion of metacercaria in insect	Unknown	43
Cryptogonimus chyli	North America	Bluegill, sunfish, others	Stomach, intestine	Ingestion of metacercaria in muscle	Unknown	43
Homalometron armattum	Southern US	Sunfish, others	Intestine	Ingestion of metacercaria in muscle	Unknown	43, 149
Holostephanus ictaluri	US	Channel catfish	Intestine	Ingestion of cercaria released from mollusk	Unknown	43
Microphallus opacus	North America	Black bass, channel catfish, eels, other fishes	Stomach, intestine	Ingestion of metacercaria in crustacean	Unknown	43, 146
Plagioporus spp.	Europe, Middle East, North America	Sunfish, salmonids, shiners, chubs, others	Intestine	Ingestion of metacercaria in intermediate host (arthropod)	Unknown	43
Podocotyle spp.	Europe, North America	Salmonids, others	Intestine	Unknown	Unknown	43, 150
Proterometra macrostoma	US	Bluegill, sunfish, others	Esophagus	Ingestion of metacercaria in snail	Unknown	43, 141
Proterometra spp.	US	Bluegill, sunfish	Intestine	Ingestion of metacercaria in snail	Unknown	43, 142, 143
Rhipidocotyle septpapillata	US	Sunfish, others	Intestine	Ingestion of metacercaria in gills or skin of fish	Unknown	43
Sphaerostoma spp.	Europe	Carp, European minnow, chubs, eels, trout, others	Intestine	Ingestion of cercaria released from mollusk	Unknown	43
Vietosoma parvum	Eastern US	Channel catfish	Stomach, intestine	Ingestion of intermediate host (arthropod)	Unknown	43

	Geographic location	Host	Site	Mode of infection	Effect on host	References
Larval						
Acocotyle spp.	Southern US	Topminnows, mollies	Liver, intestinal wall, other organs	Penetration of surface by cercaria released from snail	Cysts in liver or intestinal wall	43
Petasiger nitidus	North America	Shiners, guppy, bluegill, other fishes	Esophagus	Penetration of surface by cercaria released from snail	Cysts in esophagus	43
Cestodes						
Adult						
Atractolytocestus huronensis	US	Carp	Intestine	Ingestion of intermediate host	Unknown	43, 161
Bothriocephalus spp.	Asia, Europe, North America	Bluegill, carp, sunfish, black bass, sticklebacks, eels, others	Intestine, pyloric ceca	Ingestion of intermediate host (copepod, small fish)	Enteritis, intestinal blockage	43, 152
Caryophyllaeus spp.	Europe, North America	Carp, others	Intestine	Ingestion of intermediate host (oligochaete)	Unknown	13, 43
Corallobothrium spp.	North America	Channel catfish, other ictalurids	Intestine	Ingestion of intermediate host (copepod, small fish)	Probably harmful to host	43, 151
Cyathocephalus truncatus	Europe, North America	Brown trout, other fishes	Intestine	Ingestion of intermediate host (small fish)	Unknown	43, 157
Eubothrium crassum, E. salvelini	Europe, North America	Salmonids, others	Pyloric ceca	Ingestion of intermediate host (copepod)	Reduced growth, swimming ability	43, 156
Khawia spp.	Central US	Carp, other cyprinids	Intestine	Ingestion of intermediate host	Unknown	43, 160
Ophiotaenia fragilis	North central US	Channel catfish	Intestine	Unknown	Unknown	43
Proteocephalus spp.	Europe, North America	Black bass, salmonids, catfish, sunfish, others	Intestine	Ingestion of intermediate host (copepod or small fish)	Unknown	43, 152–155
Triaenophorus spp.	Europe, North America	Carp, sunfish, black bass, rainbow trout, others	Intestine	Ingestion of intermediate host (small fish)	Unknown	43, 158, 159
Larval						
Corallobothrium imbriatum	North America	Shiners	Viscera	Ingestion of intermediate host (copepod)	Unknown	43
Diphyllobothrium spp.	Europe, North America	Salmonids, others	Viscera	Ingestion of intermediate host (copepod)	Zoonotic	43
Haplobothrium globuliforme	North America	Guppies, sunfish	Liver	Ingestion of intermediate host (copepod)	Unknown	43, 163
Proteocephalus spp.	North America	Chubs, shiners, topminnows, killfishes, bluegill, trout, catfish, others	Viscera (also found in gonads or muscle, depending on species)	Ingestion of intermediate host (copepod)	Migrating plerocercoids cause extensive damage to viscera, fibrosis adhesions, distortion of body, sterility	43, 153, 162
Triaenophorus nodulosus	North America, Europe	Goldfish, sunfish, salmonids, others	Liver	Ingestion of intermediate host (copepod)	Cysts in liver; massive infections cause destruction of liver, death	13, 43

(Continued)

TABLE 7.2 (*Continued*)

Parasite	Geographic distribution	hosts	Location in host	Method of infection	Pathologic effects	References
Nematodes						
Adult						
Camallanus spp.	Europe, North America	Carp, salmonids, sunfish, shiners, others	Intestine	Ingestion of intermediate host (copepod)	Unknown	13, 43
Capillaria catenata	North America	Bluegill, sunfish, catfish, others	Intestine	Probably by accidental ingestion of egg	Heavy infections cause enteritis	43
Capillaria eupomotis	Europe	European minnow, sunfish, others	Liver	Probably by accidental ingestion of egg	Extensive liver damage	43
Contracaecum aduncum	Europe	Salmonids, others	Stomach	Ingestion of second intermediate host (small fish)	Length: 18 to 36 mm. Unknown	56, 169
Contracaecum brachyurum	North America	Sunfish, others	Stomach, intestine	Ingestion of second intermediate host (small fish)	Length: up to 90 mm. Unknown	43
Dacnitoides cotylophora	North America	Chubs, sunfish, black bass, others	Intestine	Ingestion of copepod	Unknown	43
Dacnitoides robusta	North America	Channel catfish, other ictalurids	Intestine	Ingestion of copepod	Unknown	43
Haplonema aditum	North America	Eels	Intestine	Probably by ingestion of copepod	Unknown	43, 164
Metabronema salvelini	Northern US, Canada	Salmonids, others	Intestine	Ingestion of intermediate host (mayfly)	Unknown	43
Pseudocapillaria catostomi	US, Canada	Salmonids	Intestine	Unknown	Unknown	43, 108
Pseudocapillaria tomentosa	North America, Europe	Cyprinids	Intestine	Direct, ingestion of infective ova	Enteritis, neoplasia	109, 111–113
Rhabdochona denudata	Asia, Europe	Salmonids, others	Intestine	Ingestion of intermediate host	Unknown	165, 166
Spinitectus spp.	Europe, North America	Sunfish, black bass, catfish, others	Stomach, intestine	Ingestion of intermediate host (mayfly)	May cause enteritis and death	167, 168
Larval						
Contracaecum piculigerum	US, Canada	Shiners, sunfish, catfish, others	Viscera	Ingestion of copepod, amphipod	Migrating larvae cause extensive visceral damage	170
Spiroxys sp.	North America	Carp, shiners, catfish, sunfish, others	Viscera (also found in mesentery)	Ingestion of first intermediate host (copepod)	Cysts in mesentery; probably causes little damage except in heavy infections	171
Acanthocephala						
Acanthocephalus spp.	Europe, North America	Goldfish, carp, salmonids, catfish, others	Intestine	Ingestion of intermediate host (amphipod)	Enteritis, death	43
Echinorhynchus spp.	Europe, North America	Sunfish, salmonids, others	Intestine	Ingestion of intermediate host (amphipod)	Ulcerative enteritis	43, 152, 174

Species	Location	Hosts	Site in host	Transmission	Pathology	Reference
Leptorhynchoides thecatus	US, Canada	Carp, shiners, others	Adult: pyloric ceca Larva: mesentery, liver	Definitive: ingestion of intermediate host (amphipod, small fish) Intermediate: ingestion of intermediate host (amphipod)	Adult: extensive damage to cecal mucosa Larva: cysts in mesentery, liver	175
Neoechinorhynchus spp.	Asia, Europe, North America	Shiners, sunfish, salmonids, others	Adult: intestine Larva: liver	Definitive: ingestion of second intermediate host (small fish) Intermediate: ingestion of first intermediate host (ostracod)	Adult: local damage to intestinal mucosa Larva: cysts in liver	43, 172
Octospiniferoides chandleri	Southern US	Killifish, mosquitofish	Intestine	Ingestion of intermediate host (probably ostracod)	Unknown	43, 173
Pomphorhynchus bulbocolli	North America	Goldfish, carp, sunfish, salmonids, others	Adult: intestine Larva: mesentery, liver, spleen	Definitive: ingestion of second intermediate host (small fish) Intermediate: ingestion of first intermediate host (amphipod)	Adult: extensive damage to intestinal mucosa; sometimes perforation of intestine, trauma to liver Larva: cysts in mesentery, liver, spleen	43, 176
Pomphorhynchus laevis	Europe	Goldfish, carp, salmonids, sticklebacks, eels, others	Intestine	Ingestion of intermediate host (amphipod)	Extensive damage to intestinal mucosa; sometimes perforation of intestine, trauma to liver	43, 177

TABLE 7.3 Parasites of fishes—musculoskeletal system.

Parasite	Geographic distribution	hosts	Location in host	Method of infection	Pathologic effects	References
Myxozoa						
Myxobolus (Myxosoma) cerebralis	Asia, Europe, North America	Trout, other salmonids	Cartilage, spine	Ingestion of spores released from tissue	Destruction of cartilage of head, spine; deformation of head, spine; blackened tail; impaired locomotion ("whirling disease")	131, 178
Myxosoma spp.	North America	Bluegill, sticklebacks, sunfish, black bass	Cartilage, spine	Ingestion of spores released from tissue	Causes cysts in cartilage of head	43, 131
Myxobolus spp.	North America	Black bass, minnows, shiners, salmonids, others	Muscle	Probably by ingestion of spores released from tissue	Cysts in muscle	43, 179
Henneguya salmincola	Alaska, Siberia	Pacific salmon	Muscle, subcutis	Probably by ingestion of spores released from tissue	Cysts in muscle, subcutis ("tapioca disease")	180
Pleistophora spp.	Europe, North America	Topminnows, swordtails, tetras, others	Muscle released from tissue	Ingestion of spores	Cysts in muscle, emaciation, death ("neon tetra disease")	13, 56, 181
Trematodes						
Larval, digenetic						
Bolbophorus confusus	Africa, Europe, Northwestern US	Trout, others	Muscle	Penetration by cercaria released from snail	Cysts in muscle	43
Hysteromorpha triloba	Asia, Europe, Americas	Golden shiner, others	Muscle	Penetration by cercaria released from snail	Cysts in muscle	43
Prohemistomum ovatis	Europe	Carp, other cyprinids	Muscle	Penetration by cercaria released from snail	Cysts in muscle	182
Clinostomum marginatum	North America	Minnows, chubs, shiners, killifish, sunfish, others	Muscle, connective tissue, gills	Penetration by cercaria released from snail	Light yellow cysts in muscle, connective tissue, gills	13, 43, 183
Clinostomum complanatum	Eastern Europe, southern Asia	Goldfish, others	Muscle, connective tissue	Penetration by cercaria released from snail	Light yellow cysts in muscle, connective tissue, gills	13, 183
Bucephalus elegans	North America	Shiners, others	Muscle, skin	Penetration by cercaria released from snail	Cysts in muscle, skin	43
Macroderoides spinifera	North America	Killifish, mollies, mosquitofish	Muscle	Penetration by cercaria released from snail	Cysts in muscle	43
Paramacroderoides echinus	North America	Killifishes, mollies, mosquitofish	Muscle	Penetration by cercaria released from snail	Cysts in muscle	43, 184
Sellacotyle mustelae	North America	Fathead minnow, chubs, shiners, others	Muscle, mesentery	Penetration by cercaria released from snail	Small cysts in muscle, mesentery	43
Apophallus brevis	North America	Perch	Muscle	Penetration by cercaria released from snail	Bony ossicles	249
Apophallus donecius	North America	Cyprinids and salmonids	Bone, vertebrae	Penetration by cercaria released from snail	Vertebral deformities	250

Species	Region	Fish hosts	Site	Transmission	Effects	Ref.
Apophallus muelingi	Europe	Cyprinids	Muscle, gills	Penetration by cercaria released from snail	Cysts in muscle, gills	144
Centrovarium lobotes	North America	Bluntnose minnow, shiners, others	Muscle	Penetration by cercaria released from snail	Unpigmented cysts in muscle	43
Opisthorchis tenuicollis	Asia, Europe, North America	Carp, other cyprinids	Muscle, connective tissue	Penetration by cercaria released from snail	Cysts in muscle, connective tissue; may infect man	56
Opisthorchis tonkae	North America	Sunfish, others	Muscle	Penetration by cercaria released from snail	Cysts in muscle	185

Cestodes

Larval

Species	Region	Fish hosts	Site	Transmission	Effects	Ref.
Diphyllobothrium spp.	Worldwide	Salmonids, eels, others	Muscle, connective tissue, mesentery, liver, spleen	Ingestion of intermediate host (copepod)	Hemorrhage, fibrosis, adhesions, emaciation, reduces fertility, death	13, 43
Triaenophorus crassus	Europe, North America	Salmonids, others	Muscle, connective tissue	Ingestion of intermediate host (copepod)	Yellow cysts in muscle, connective tissue	43

Nematodes

Larval

Species	Region	Fish hosts	Site	Transmission	Effects	Ref.
Eustrongylides spp.	Europe, North America	Carp, sunfish, sticklebacks, trout, others	Muscle, viscera	Ingestion of intermediate host (oligochaete)	Large red cyst up to 10 mm in diameter in muscle, viscera	43

TABLE 7.4 Parasites of fishes—nervous system.

Parasite	Geographic distribution	Hosts	Location in host	Method of infection	Pathologic effects	Reference
Myxozoa						
Henneguya zikaweiensis	Europe	Goldfish	Eyes	Probably actinosporeans from oligochaetes	Cysts in cornea	13, 181
Myxobolus (Myxosoma) hoffmani, M. orbitalis	North America	Minnows, shiners	Eyes	Probably actinosporeans from oligochaetes	Cysts in sclera of eye	43
Myxobolus neurobius, M. kisutchi	Europe, North America	Salmonids	Spinal cord, nerves	Probably actinosporeans from oligochaetes	Cysts in nerves, spinal cord	13, 43, 180
Myxobolus spp.	North America	Minnows	Brain (also found in viscera)	Probably actinosporeans from oligochaetes	Cysts in brain, viscera	43, 180
Pseudoloma neurophilia	North America, Europe	Zebrafish, possibly neon tetras and swordtails	Hind brain, spinal cord, nerve roots, somatic muscle	Direct, ingestion of spores	Neuritis, meningitis, myositis, associated with emaciation and skeletal deformities	52, 53
Trematodes						
Larval digenetic						
Diplostomulum spp.	Europe, North America	Carp, goldfish, minnows, salmonids, shiners, sunfish, others	Vitreous body	Penetration by cercaria released from snail	Adults unknown; probably causes blindness	43
Diplostomum spp.	Europe, North America	Goldfish, carp, minnows, bass, salmonids, sunfish, others	Eye lens, vitreous body	Penetration by cercaria released from snail	Opacity of lens, blindness, increased intraocular pressure, rupture of cornea, death	43, 186–189
Ornitho-diplostomum ptychocheilus	North America	Cyprinids, fathead minnow	Brain	Penetration by cercaria released from snail	Behavior changes	43, 246
Tetracotyle lepomensis	North America	Shiners, bluegill	Vitreous body (also found in mesentery)	Penetration by cercaria released from snail	Probably causes blindness; cysts in mesentery	43

TABLE 7.5 Parasites of fishes—respiratory system/skin and connective tissue.

Parasite	Geographic distribution	Hosts	Location in host	Method of infection	Pathologic effects	Reference
Flagellates						
Amyloodinium ocellatum	Worldwide	Marine fishes		Direct contact with free-swimming dinospores	Hyperplasia, inflammation and necrosis of gill epithelium	9
Bodomonas concava	North America	Bluegills, other fishes	Gills	Direct contact with free-swimming stage	Unknown	43
Cryptobia spp.	North America	Goldfish, carp	Skin, gills	Unknown	Unknown, apparently a commensal	43, 127, 128
Colponema spp.	Americas	Bluegills, catfish, others	Gills	Direct contact with free-swimming stage	Unknown	43, 191
Ichthyobodo neactaor	Asia, Europe, North America	Salmonids, goldfish, guppies, platyfish, wordtail, tropical mouthbreeders, others	Skin, gills	Direct contact with free-swimming stage	Causes gray coating on skin, anorexia, debilitation, death	43, 190
Piscinoodinium pillulare	Europe, North America	Freshwater fishes	Skin, gills	Direct contact with free-swimming dinospores	Yellow-brown coating on skin, gills; debilitation; impaired respiration; sometimes death	9, 11–14, 43, 192
Myxozoa						
Chloromyxum externum	North America	Chubs, others	Gills	Probably infection of surface by actinosporeans from oligochaetes	Cysts in gills	43
Dermocystidium spp.	Asia, Europe, North America	Carp, goldfish, salmonids, sticklebacks	Gills and/or skin	Ingestion of spores	Cysts in gills or skin	13, 43, 196, 197
Glugea anomala	Alaska, Europe	Sticklebacks	Subcutaneous tissues, peritoneum, stomach, intestine, ovaries, cornea	Ingestion of spores released from tissue	Large thick-walled cysts in subcutaneous tissues, body deformation, death	13, 194, 195
Henneguya spp.	North America	Catfish, shiners, salmonids	Skin, subcutis, and gills (depending on parasite species)	Probably infection of surface by actinosporeans from oligochaetes	Cysts in skin, subcutis, gills	43, 180
Myxobolus spp.	North America	Salmonids, shiners, minnows, others	Skin and/or abdominal and cranial cavities	Probably infection of surface by actinosporeans from oligochaetes	Cysts in skin, cranial cavity, hepatic destruction, increased mortality	9, 43, 128
Myxobolus spp.	North America	Minnows, carp, others	Gills	Probably infection of surface by actinosporeans from oligochaetes	Cysts in gills, dyspnea, death	13, 43

103

(Continued)

TABLE 7-5 (Continued)

Parasite	Geographic distribution	Hosts	Location in host	Method of infection	Pathologic effects	Reference
Myxobolus spp.	Asia, Europe, North America	Carp, minnows, shiners, sunfish, others	Skin and/or gills, and viscera (depending on parasite species)	Probably infection of surface by actinosporeans from oligochaetes	Cysts in skin, gills, muscle, spleen, mesentery, intestine, ovaries	9, 13, 43, 179
Pleistophora salmonae	North America	Rainbow trout, Pacific salmon, other salmonids	Gills	Ingestion of spores released from tissue	Cysts in gills, anemia, inflammation of gills, proliferation of gill lamellae, death	43
Thelohanellus notatus	North America	Bluntnose minnow, shiners	Skin	Probably infection of surface by actinosporeans from oligochaetes	Cysts in skin	43
Unicauda brachyuran, U. fontinalis	North America	Shiners, trout	Skin, fins	Probably infection of surface by actinosporeans from oligochaetes	Cysts in fins	43, 193
Unicauda plasmodia	North America	Catfish	Gills	Probably infection of surface by actinosporeans from oligochaetes	Cysts in gills	43
Microsporidia						
Glugea anomala	Alaska, Europe	Sticklebacks	Subcutaneous tissues, peritoneum, stomach, intestine, ovaries, cornea	Direct, ingestions of spores	Large thick-walled cysts in subcutaneous tissues, body deformation, death	13, 61, 69, 194, 195
Loma salmonae	North America	Rainbow trout, Pacific salmon, other salmonids	Gills	Direct, ingestion of spores	Cysts in gills, anemia, inflammation of gills, proliferation of gill lamellae, death	43, 49, 57, 59
Choanoflagellate						
Dermocystidium spp.	Asia, Europe, North America	Carp, goldfish, salmonids, sticklebacks	Gills and/or skin	Unknown	Cysts in gills or skin	13, 43, 196, 197
Ciliates						
Ambiphrya ameiuri	North America	Catfish, bass, others	Gills	Direct contact with organism in water	Heavy infections may cause death	9, 43, 200
Amphileptus voracus	North America	Channel catfish, others	Gills	Direct contact with organism in water	Probably beneficial to host; ingests pathogenic protozoans	43
Apiosoma piscicola	Europe	Goldfish, sticklebacks, others	Gills	Direct contact with organism in water	Unknown	9, 13, 201
Chilodonella piscicola and	Worldwide	Freshwater fishes	Skin, gills	Direct contact with organism in water	Hyperplasia and necrosis of gill epithelium	13, 43, 45, 46

104

Organism	Distribution	Host	Location	Transmission	Signs	References
C. hexasticha Epistylis spp.	North America	Bluegills, black bass, trout, others	Skin	Direct contact with organism in water	Heavy infections sometimes cause erosion of scale, dermal ulcers	9, 13, 43
Ichthyophthirius multifiliis	Worldwide	All freshwater fishes; common on fishes in captivity	Skin, gills	Direct, infection of surface by free-swimming stage (theronts)	Irritation of skin, gray-white granulomatous dermal lesions, (ichthyophthiriasis, "ich," "white spot disease")	37, 41, 198
Ophryoglena spp.	North America	Chubs, bluegills, black bass, others	Skin	Direct contact with organism in water	Epithelial sloughing, lethargy, sometimes death	43, 199
Trichodina spp.	Asia, Europe, North America, Europe	Sunfish, catfish, goldfish, minnows, salmonids, others	Skin and/or gills	Direct contact with organism in water	Excess mucus production, skin blotches, loosened scales, frayed fins, epithelial hyperplasia, dyspnea, death	9, 202, 203
Trichodinella myakkae, T. subtilis	Europe, North America	Carp, goldfish, minnows, trout, others	Gills	Direct contact with organism in water	Hyperplasia of gill epithelium, dyspnea, death	9, 3, 202
Trichophrya spp.	North America	Black bass, catfish, salmonids, channel catfish	Gills	Direct contact with organism in water	Unknown	9, 43
Tripartiella spp.	Europe, North America	Chubs, catfish, minnows, others	Gills	Direct contact with organism in water	Heavy infections probably cause dyspnea, death	9, 43, 202
Trematodes						
Monogenetic						
Actinocleidus fusiformis	North America	Black bass	Gills	Direct contact	Heavy infections cause dyspnea, death	43
Anchoradiscoides serpentinus	North America	Sunfish	Skin, gills	Direct contact	Unknown	209
Clavunculus bursatus	North America	Bluegills, black bass	Gills	Direct contact	Heavy infections cause dyspnea, death	43
Cleidodiscus spp.	North America	Sunfish, catfish, others	Gills	Direct contact	Heavy infections cause dyspnea, death	43
Dactylogyrus spp.	Worldwide	Goldfish, carp, others	Gills	Direct contact	Hypertrophy of gill filaments, sometimes death	13, 43, 207
Diplozoon nipponicum	Asia	Carp, other cyprinids	Gills	Direct contact	Causes adhesions, edema of gills; dyspnea, death	56
Diplozoon paradoxum	Europe	Carp, European minnow, others	Gills	Direct contact	Adhesions, edema of gills; dyspnea, death	13
Discocotyle sagittata	Europe, North America	Trout, Atlantic salmon	Gills	Direct contact	Heavy infections cause dyspnea, death	43, 214
Gyrodactylus spp.	Asia, Europe, North America	Goldfish, carp, bluegills, catfish, minnows, shiners, trout, others	Skin, gills	Direct contact	Ingests blood; causes mucous coating on skin, gills; frayed fins; sometimes death	13, 43, 99, 100, 204–206
Lyrodiscus seminolensis, L. muricatus	North America	Bluegills	Skin, gills	Direct contact	Hypertrophy of gill filaments, sometimes death	209
Pseudacolpenteron pavlovskyi	Asia, Europe, North America	Carp, other cyprinids	Gills, fins	Direct contact	Hypertrophy of gill filaments, sometimes death	208

(Continued)

TABLE 7.5 (Continued)

Parasite	Geographic distribution	Hosts	Location in host	Method of infection	Pathologic effects	Reference
Urocleidoides spp.	Europe, North America, West Indies	Guppies, sunfish, others	Gills	Direct contact	Heavy infections cause dyspnea, death	210, 211
Urocleidus spp.	Europe, North America	Bluegills, sunfish, black bass	Gills	Direct contact	Heavy infections cause dyspnea, death	43, 212, 213
Larval, digenetic						
Apophallus brevis, A. venustus	Europe, North America	Carp, shiners, trout, others	Skin	Penetration by cercaria released from snail	Black cysts in skin	43
Ascocotyle angrense, A. coleostoma	Europe, North America	Topminnows, mollies, other fishes	Gills	Penetration by cercaria released from snail	Cysts in gills	43, 223
Ascocotyle mcintoshi	Southern US	Mollies, mosquitofish	Mesentery, viscera	Penetration by cercaria released from snail	Cysts in mesentery, viscera	43, 224
Bucephalus polymorphus	Europe	Cyprinids, eels, others	Gills, skin, fins	Penetration by cercaria released from snail	Cysts in gills, skin, fins; hemorrhagic necrosis in fins, eyes, mouth; sometimes death	220
Crassiphiala bulboglossa	North America	Fathead minnows, chubs, shiners, others	Skin, gills, muscle	Penetration by cercaria released from snail	Black cysts in skin, branchial arches, muscle; heavy infections cause death	43, 217
Echinochasmus donaldsoni, E. schwartzi	North America	Sticklebacks, others	Gills	Penetration by cercaria released from snail	Cysts in gills	43
Euparyphium melis	Asia, Europe, North America	Bluegills, other fishes	Nares, cloaca	Penetration by cercaria released from snail	Unknown	43, 221
Nanophyetus salmincola	Pacific coast of North America, Siberia	Goldfish, other cyprinids, mosquitofish, sunfish, salmonids, sticklebacks	Gills, eyes, tongue, muscle, heart, viscera	Penetration by cercaria released from snail	Cysts produce mechanical damage; heavy infections cause death; serious pathogen in some hatcheries; zoonotic vector for Neorickettsia helminthoeca	43
Neodiplostomum perlatum	Eastern Europe	Carp	Skin, muscle	Probably by penetration by cercaria released from snail	Cysts in skin, muscle	13
Ornithodiplostomum ptychocheilus	North America	Fathead minnows, chubs, shiners	Peritoneum, viscera, brain	Penetration by cercaria released from snail	Cysts in peritoneum, viscera, brain	43, 219
Posthodiplostomum cuticola	Europe	Goldfish, sticklebacks, others	Skin, gills, muscle, mouth	Penetration by cercaria released from snail	Black cysts in skin; heavy infections probably cause death	13, 218
Posthodiplostomum minimum	North America	Minnow, catfish, shiners, sunfish, others	Mesentery, kidneys, liver, spleen, pericardium	Penetration by cercaria released from snail	Cysts in mesentery, kidneys, liver, spleen, pericardium (white grub); heavy infections cause death	13, 219

Parasite	Geographic distribution	Hosts	Site	Mode of transmission	Effects	References
Ribeiroia ondatrae	North America	Bluegills, sunfish, black bass, others	Subcutis	Penetration by cercaria released from snail	Cysts in lateral line system	43, 222
Tetracotyle echinata, T. sogdiana	Asia, Europe	Carp, salmonids, others	Peritoneum	Penetration by cercaria released from snail	Cysts in peritoneum, adhesions, peritonitis	43, 215
Tetracotyle intermedia	Asia, North America	Brown trout, others	Pericardium	Penetration by cercaria released from snail	Cysts in pericardium	43
Uvulifer ambloplitis	North America	Minnows, shiners, sunfish, others	Skin, muscle	Penetration by cercaria released from snail	Black cysts in skin, muscle; heavy infections cause death	43, 216
Cestodes						
Larval						
Ligula intestinalis	Asia, Europe, North America	Goldfish, carp, minnows, shiners, black bass, trout, others	Abdominal cavity	Ingestion of intermediate host (copepod)	Abdominal distention, compression of viscera, excessive proliferation of connective tissue, obliteration of gonads, sterility, rupture of body wall, death	13, 43, 225
Schistocephalus solidus, S. thomasi	Asia, Europe, North America	Sticklebacks, other fishes	Abdominal cavity	Ingestion of intermediate host (copepod)	Heavy infections cause abdominal distention, compression of viscera, obliteration of gonads, decreased fertility	13, 43, 226
Nematodes						
Adult						
Cystidicola stigmatura, C. farionis	Europe, North America	Trout, other salmonids, sticklebacks	Swim bladder	Ingestion of intermediate host (shrimp)	None known	13, 43, 165
Philonema agubernaculum, P. oncorhynchi	North America	Trout, other salmonids	Abdominal cavity	Ingestion of intermediate host (copepod)	Abdominal adhesions	43, 227
Philometra carassii, P. sanguinea	Europe, North America	Goldfish, others	Caudal fin	Ingestion of intermediate host (copepod)	Fin lesions	43
Philometra cylindracea, P. abdominalis	Europe, North America	Black bass, cyprinids, others	Abdominal cavity	Ingestion of intermediate host (copepod)	Abdominal adhesions	13, 43, 228, 229
Rhabdochona cascadilla, R. decaturensis	Americas	Carp, catfish, chubs, shiners, black bass, salmonids, sticklebacks, others	Swimbladder, intestine	Ingestion of intermediate host (mayfly)	None known	43
Leeches						
Cystobranchus verrilli	North America	Bluegills, black bass, channel catfish, others	Skin	Direct contact	Ingests blood	43
Cystobranchus respirans	Europe	Atlantic salmon, other salmonids, others	Skin	Direct contact	Ingests blood	13, 43

(Continued)

TABLE 7.5 *(Continued)*

Parasite	Geographic distribution	Hosts	Location in host	Method of infection	Pathologic effects	Reference
Haementeria montifera, H. parasitica, Illinobdella spp.	North America	Carp, black bass, bluegills, others	Skin	Direct contact	Ingests blood	43
	North America	Golden shiner, bluegills, sunfish, black bass, catfish, others	Skin	Direct contact	Ingests blood	43
Piscicola spp.	Europe, North America	Goldfish, carp, trout, salmonids, sticklebacks, others	Skin	Direct contact	Ingests blood; causes weight loss; vector of *Crytobia*	43
Piscicolaria spp.	North America	Golden shiners, bluegills, channel catfish, others	Skin	Direct contact	Ingests blood	43
Mollusks						
Freshwater clams of unknown species	Worldwide	Goldfish, carp, shiners, sunfish, trout, others	Larva: gills, skin, fins	Direct contact	Cysts in gills; heavy infection sometimes cause death	43
Margaritifera margaritifera	Western North America	Trout, other salmonids	Larva: gills	Direct contact	Cysts in gills; heavy infection sometimes cause death	43, 230
Pisidium variable	North America	Rainbow trout, others	Adult: mouth	Direct contact	Attaches to mouth of young fishes; causes irritation	43
Crustaceans						
Achtheres spp.	North America salmonids	Black bass, catfish,	Gills	Direct contact	Damage to gills, impaired respiration, death	43
Argulus spp.	Worldwide	Goldfish, carp, bluegills, trout, sticklebacks, sunfish, eels, salmonids, others	Skin	Direct contact	Irritation of skin, loss of blood, sometimes death; possible vector of pathogens; Some species zoonotic	13, 43, 119, 120, 231
Ergasilus spp.	North America	Catfish, cyprinids, bluegill, sunfish, black bass, salmonids, others	Gills	Direct contact	Nodules on gills, anorexia, loss of weight, debilitation, fusion of gill lamellae, impaired respiration, death	43, 232
Lepeophtheirus spp.	Asia, Europe, North America	Salmonids	Perianal skin	Direct contact	Salmon louse. Cause damage to skin	43, 235
Lernaea spp.	Africa, Asia, Europe, North America	Goldfish, carp, catfish, shiners, tropical mouthbreeders, sunfish salmonids, others	Gills, fins, skin	Direct contact	Extensive damage to gills, fins, skin; debilitation; sometimes death	13, 43, 121, 122
Salmincola spp.	Asia, Greenland, Iceland, North America	Salmonids	Gills	Direct contact	Loss of blood, damage to gills, debilitation, death	233, 234

TABLE 7.6 Parasites of fishes—urogenital system.

Parasite	Geographic distribution	Hosts	Location in host	Method of infection	Pathologic effects	Reference
Myxozoa						
Chloromyxum spp.	North America	Killifishes, salmonids, others	Kidneys	Actinosporeans from oligochaetes	None known	43
Henneguya spp.	Europe	Sticklebacks	Kidneys, ovaries	Probably actinosporeans from oligochaetes	Ovarian cysts	13, 180, 240
Hoferellus cyprini	Europe	Carp	Kidneys	Actinosporeans from oligochaetes	May cause obstruction of renal tubules, ascites	13, 43, 241
Mitraspora spp.	Asia, North America	Carp, sunfish, others	Kidneys	Probably actinosporeans from oligochaetes	None known	43, 241, 242
Myxidium spp.	Europe, North America	Eels, minnows, salmonids, others	Kidneys. Also ovaries, gallbladder, liver, depending on species	Actinosporeans from oligochaetes	May cause renal tubule degeneration	13, 43, 140, 243
Myxobilatus spp.	North America	Sunfish, black bass	Urinary bladder	Probably actinosporeans from oligochaetes	None known	43
Myxobolus spp.	Europe, North America	Killifishes	Ovaries, testes	Actinosporeans from oligochaetes	Ovarian cysts	13, 43
Pleistophora ovariae	North America	Golden shiners	Ovaries, liver, kidneys	Ingestion of spores	Sterility in female	13, 43, 244
Sinuolinea gilsoni	Europe	eels	Urinary bladder	Probably actinosporeans from oligochaetes	None known	13, 236
Sphaerospora spp.	Europe, North America	Carp, goldfish, minnows, salmonids, sticklebacks, others	Kidneys, ovaries, swimbladder	Actinosporeans from oligochaetes	Swimbladder inflammation	13, 237–239
Wardia ovinocua	North America	Sunfish	Ovaries	Probably actinosporeans from oligochaetes	None known	43
Myxidium (Zschokkella) salvelini	North America	Brook trout	Kidneys	Actinosporeans from oligochaetes	None known	43
Trematodes						
Acetodextra amiuri	North America	Catfish	Ovaries	Ingestion of metacercaria in liver of fish	None known	43, 245
Phyllodistomum spp.	Europe, North America	Catfish, carp, goldfish, sunfish, salmonids, others	Ureters and/or urinary bladder	Ingestion of cercaria	None known	43, 152, 185

REFERENCES

1. Flynn, R.J. (1973) *Parasites of laboratory animals.* Iowa State University Press, Ames, Iowa, 884 pages.
2. Postlethwait, J.H. and Talbot, W.S. (1997) Zebrafish genomics: from mutants to genes. *Trends Genet* **13**(5), 183–190.
3. Stoskopf, M. (1992) *Fish Medicine.* W.B. Saunders Co., Philadelphia. 882 pages.
4. Gratzek, J.B. (1993) Parasites associated with freshwater tropical fishes: In: Stoskopf, M.K. (ed.) *Fish Medicine,* W.B. Saunders Co., Philadelphia. 573–590.
5. Kent, M.L. and Kieser, D. (2003) Avoidance of introduction of exotic pathogens with Atlantic salmon reared in British Columbia: In: Lee, C.S., O'Bryen, P.J. (ed.) *Biosecurity in Aquaculture Production Systems: Exclusion of Pathogens and Other Undesirables,* World Aquaculture Soc., Baton Rouge, Louisiana, 43–50.
6. Matthews, M., Trevarrow, B., and Matthews, J. (2002) A virtual tour of the guide for zebrafish users. *Lab. Anim.* **31**, 34–40.
7. Noga, E. (2000) *Fish Disease: diagnosis and treatment.* Blackwell Publishing, Malden, Massachusetts, 367 pages.
8. Bishop, T.M., Smalls, A., Wooster, G.A., and Bowser, P.R. (2003) Aerobiological (airborne) dissemination of the fish pathogen *Ichthyopthirus multifiliis* and implications in fish health management: In: Lee, C.S., O'Bryen, P.J. (ed.) *Biosecurity in Aquaculture Production Systems: Exclusion of Pathogens and Other Undesirables,* World Aquaculture Soc., Baton Rouge, Louisiana, 51–64.
9. Lom, J. and Dyková, I. (1992) *Protozoan parasites of fishes.* Elsevier, New York, 316 pages.
10. Lawler, A.R. (1980) Studies on *Amyloodinium ocellatum* (Dinoflagellata) in Mississippi Sound: Natural and Experimental Hosts. *Gulf Res. Rpts.* **6**, 403–413.
11. Paperna, I. (1980) *Amyloodinium ocellatum* (Brown, 1931) (Dinoflagellida) infestations in cultured marine fish at Eilat, Red Sea: epizootiology and pathology. *J. Fish Dis.* **3**, 363–372.
12. Untergasser, D. (1989) *Handbook of Fish Diseases.* Tropical Fish Hobbyist Publications, Neptune City, New Jersey, 160 pages.
13. Van Duijn Jr., C. (1973) *Diseases of Fishes.* 3rd ed. Betterworth and Co., London, 372 pages.
14. Noga, E.J. and Levy, M.G. (1995) Dinoflagellida (Phylum Sarcomastigophora): In: Woo, P.T.K. (ed.) *Fish Diseases and Disorders,* CAB Intl Pub, Wallingford, Oxon, UK, 1–25.
15. Becker, C.D. (1977) Flagellate Parasites of Fish: In: Kreier, J.P. (ed.) *Parasitic Protozoa,* Academic Press, New York, 358–416.
16. Roubal, F.R., Bullock, A.M., Robertson, D.A., and Roberts, R.J. (1987) Ultrastructural aspects of infestation by *Ichthyobodo necator* (Henneguy, 1883) on the skin and gills of the salmonids *Salmo salar* L. and *Salmo gairdneri* Richardson. *J. Fish Dis.* **10**, 181–192.
17. Urawa, S. and Kusakari, M. (1990) The survivability of the ectoparasitic flagellate *Ichthyobodo necator* on chum salmon fry (*Oncorhynchus keta*) in seawater and comparison to *Ichthyobodo* sp. on Japanese flounder (*Paralichthys olivaceus*). *J. Parasitol.* **76**, 33–40.
18. Todal, J.A., Karlsbakk, E., Isaksen, et al. (2004) *Ichthyobodo necator* (Kinetoplastida)—a complex of sibling species. *Dis. Aquat. Organ.* **58**, 9–16.
19. Ellis, A.E. and Wootten, R. (1978) Costiasis of Atlantic Salmon, *Salmo salar* L. smolts in seawater. *J. Fish Dis.* **1**, 389–393.
20. Hoffman, G.L. and Meyer, F.P. (1974) Parasites of freshwater fishes: A review of their control and treatment. J.C. Landolt (ed). *Tropical Fish Hobbyist Publication,* Neptune City, New Jersey, 224.
21. Tojo, J.L. and Santamarina, M.T. (1998) Oral pharmacological treatments for parasitic diseases of rainbow trout *Oncorhynchus mykiss.* III: *Ichthyobodo necator. Dis. Aquat. Organ.* **58**, 9–16.
22. Molnár, K. (1995) Phylum Apicomplexa: In: Woo, P.T.K. (ed.) *Fish diseases and disorders,* CAB International, Wallingford, Oxon, UK, 263–288.
23. Fournie, J.W., Hawkins, W.E., and Overstreet, R.M. (1985) *Calyptospora emprística* n.sp. (Eimeriorina: Calyptosporidae) from the liver of the starhead topminnow, *Fundulus notti. J. Eukaryot. Microbiol.* **32**, 542–547.
24. Hawkins, W.E., Solangi, M.A., and Overstreet, R.M. (1983) Ultrastructure of the macrogamont of *Eimeria funduli,* a coccidium parasitizing killifishes. *J. Fish Dis.* **6**, 45–57.
25. Steinhagen, D., Koerting, W., and van Muiswinkel, W.B. (1989) Morphology and biology of *Goussia carpelli* (Protozoa: Apicomplexa) from the intestine of experimentally infected common carp *Cyprinus carpio. Dis. Aquat. Organ.* **6**, 93–98.
26. Kent, M.L. and Hedrick, R.P. (1985) The biology and associated pathology of *Goussia carpelli* (Léger and Stankovitch) in goldfish *Carassius auratus* (Linnaeus). *Fish Pathol.* **20**, 485–494.
27. Fournie, J.W. and Overstreet, R.M. (1993) Host specificity of *Calyptospora funduli* (Apicomplexa: Calyptosporidae) in atheriniform fishes. *J. Parasitol.* **79**, 720–727.
28. Lukes, J., Steinhagen, D., and Körting, W. (1991) *Goussia carpelli* (Apicomplexa, Eimeriorina) from cyprinid fish: field observations and infection experiments. *Angew. Parasitol.* **32**, 149–153.
29. Steinhagen, D. and Körting, W. (1988) Experimental transmission of *Goussia carpelli* (Leger and Stankovitch, 1921; Protista: Apicomplexa) to common carp, *Cyprinus carpio* L. *Bull. Eur. Assoc. Fish Pathol.* **8**, 112–113.
30. Steinhagen, D. and Körting, W. (1990) The role of tubificid oligochaetes in the transmission of *Goussia carpelli. J. Parasitol.* **76**, 104–107.
31. Fournie, J.W. and Overstreet, R.M. (1983) True intermediate hosts for *Eimeria funduli* (Apicomplexa) from estuarine fishes. *J. Eukaryot. Microbiol.* **30**, 672–675.
32. Fournie, J.W., Vogelbein, W.K., Overstreet, R.M., and Hawkins, W.E. (2000) Life cycle of *Calyptospora funduli* (Apicomplexa: Calyptosporidae). *J. Parasitol.* **86**, 501–505.
33. Fournie, J.W. (1985) Biology of *Calyptospora funduli* (Apicomplexa) from Atheriniform fishes: University of Mississippi Press, p. 100.
34. Solangi, M.A. and Overstreet, R.M. (1980) Biology and pathogenesis of the coccidium *Eimeria funduli* infecting killifishes. *J. Parasitol.* **66**, 513–26.
35. Overstreet, R.M. (1988) Coccidiosis of killifishes: In: Sindermann, C.J., Lightner, D.V. (ed.) *Disease Diagnosis and Control in North American Marine Aquaculture,* Elsevier, New York, 373–376.
36. Kocylowski, B., Zelazny, J., Antychowicz, J., and Pancyk, J. (1976) Incidence of carp coccidiosis and its control. *Bull. Vet. Inst. Pulawy,* 20, 12–17.
37. Dickerson, H.W. and Dawe, D.L. (1995) *Ichthyophthirius multifiliis* and *Cryptocaryon irritans:* In: Woo, P.T.K. (ed.) *Fish diseases and disorders,* CAB International, Wallingford, Oxon, UK, 181–228.
38. Davis, H.S. (1947) Care and diseases of trout. *U.S. Fish and Wildlife Service Research Report #12,* 98 pages.
39. Brown, E.E. and Gratzek, J.B. (1980) *Fish farming handbook: food, bait, tropicals, and goldfish.* AVI Publishing Company, Westport, Connecticut, 391 pages.
40. Kabata, Z. (1985) *Parasites and diseases of fish cultured in the tropics.* Taylor and Francis, Philadelphia, 318 pages.

41. Dickerson, H. and Clark, T. (1998) *Ichthyophthirius multifiliis:* a model of cutaneous infection and immunity in fishes. *Immunol. Rev.* **166**, 377–384.

42. Maki, J.L. and Dickerson, H.W. (2003) Systemic and cutaneous mucus antibody responses of channel catfish immunized against the protozoan parasite *Ichthyophthirius multifiliis. Clin. Diagn. Lab. Immunol.* **10**, 876–881.

43. Hoffman, G.L. (1999) *Parasites of North American freshwater fishes.* Cornell University Press, Ithaca, New York, 414 pages.

44. Langdon, J.S., Gudovs, N., Humphrey, J.D., and Saxon, E.C. (1985) Death in Australian freshwater fishes associated with *Chilodonella hexasticha* infection. *Aus. Vet. J.* **62**, 409–413.

45. Paperna, I. and Van As, J.G. (1983) The pathology of *Chilodonella hexasticha* (Kiernik) infection in cichlid fishes. *J. Fish Biol.* **23**, 441–450.

46. Hoffman, G.L., Kazubski, S.L., Mitchell, A.J., and Smith, C.E. (1979) *Chilodonella hexasticha* (Kiernik, 1909) (Protozoa, Ciliata) from North American Warm Water fish. *J. Fish Dis.* **2**, 153–157.

47. Mathis, A. (2000) Microsporidia: emerging advances in understanding the basic biology of these unique organisms. *Int. J. Parasitol.* **30**, 795–804.

48. Dyková, I. (1995) Phylum Microspora: In: Woo, P.T.K. (ed.) *Fish Diseases and Disorders,* CAB International, Wallingford, Oxon, UK, pp. 149–179.

49. Shaw, R.W. and Kent, M.L. (1999) Fish Microsporidia: In: Wittner, M. (ed.) *Microsporidia and Microsporidiosis,* American Society for Microbiology Press, Washington, DC, 418–446.

50. Shaw, R.W., Kent, M.L., and Adamson, M.L. (1998) Modes of transmission of *Loma salmonae* (Microsporidia). *Dis. Aquat. Organ.* **33**, 151–156.

51. Kent, M.L. and Bishop-Stewart, J.K. (2003) Transmission and tissue distribution of *Pseudoloma neurophilia* (Microsporidia) of zebrafish, *Danio rerio* (Hamilton). *J. Fish Dis.* **26**, 423–426.

52. Kurtz, J., Kalbe, M., Aeschlimann, P.B., et al. (2004) Major histocompatibility complex diversity influences parasite resistance and innate immunity in sticklebacks. *Proc. Biol. Sci.* **271**, 197–204.

53. Summerfelt, R.C. (1972) Studies on the transmission of *Pleistophora ovariae,* the ovary parasite of the golden shiner (*Notemigonus crysoleucas*). National Marine Fisheries Service, Report No. 4–66-R., Washington, DC.

54. Dunn, A.M., Terry, R.S., and Smith, J.E. (2001) Transovarial transmission in the microsporidia. *Adv. Parasitol.* **48**, 57–100.

55. Docker, M.F., Devlin, R.H., Richard, J., Khattra, J., and Kent, M.L. (1997) Sensitive and specific polymerase chain reaction assay for detection of *Loma salmonae* (Microsporea). *Dis. Aquat. Organ.* **29**, 41–48.

56. Reichenbach-Klinke, H. and Elkan, E. (1965) *The Principal Diseases of Lower Vertebrates.* Academic Press, New York, 600 pages.

57. Shaw, R.W., Kent, M.L., Brown, A.M.V., Whipps, C.M., and Adamson, M.L. (2000) Experimental and natural host specificity of *Loma salmonae* (Microsporidia). *Dis. Aquat. Organ.* **40**, 131–136.

58. Lom, J. and Dyková, I. (2005) Microsporidian xenomas in fish seen in wider perspective. *Folia Parasitol. (Praha)* **52**, 69–81.

59. Kent, M.L., Elliott, D.G., Groff, J.M., and Hedrick, R.P. (1989) *Loma salmonae* (Protozoa: Microspora) infections in seawater reared coho salmon *Oncorhynchus kisutch. Aquaculture* **80**, 211–222.

60. Speare, D.J., Brackett, J., and Ferguson, H.W. (1989) Sequential pathology of the gills of coho salmon with a combined diatom and microsporidian gill infection. *Can. Vet. J.* **30**, 571–575.

61. Dyková, I. and Lom, J. (1978) Tissue reaction of the three-spined stickleback *Gasterosteus aculeatus* L. to infection with *Glugea anomala* (Moniez, 1887). *J. Fish Dis.* **1**, 83–90.

62. Weber, R., Schwartz, D.A., and Deplazes, P. (1999) Laboratory diagnosis of microsporidiosis: In: Wittner, M. (ed.) *The Microsporidia and Microsporidosis,* American Society for Microbiology Press, Washington, DC, 315–362.

63. Brown, A.M.V. and Kent, M.L. (2002) Molecular diagnostics for *Loma salmonae* and *Nucleospora salmonis* (Microsporidia): In: Cunningham, C. (ed.) *Molecular Diagnosis of Salmonid Diseases,* Kluwer Academic Publications, London, 267–283.

64. John, D.E., Nwachuku, N., Pepper, I.L., and Gerba, C.P. (2003) Development and optimization of a quantitative cell culture infectivity assay for the microsporidium *Encephalitozoon intestinalis* and application to ultraviolet light inactivation. *J. Microbiol. Methods* **52**, 183–196.

65. Kent, M.L. and Dawe, D.L. (1994) Efficacy of Fumagillin DCH against experimentally-induced *Loma salmonae* (Microsporea) infections in chinook salmon *Oncorhynchus tshawytscha. Dis. Aquat. Organ.* **20**, 231–233.

66. Becker, J.A., Speare, D.J., Daley, J., and Dick, P. (2002) Effects of monensin dose and treatment on xenoma reduction in microsporidial gill disease in rainbow trout, *Oncorhynchus mykiss* (Walbaum). *J. Fish Dis.* **25**, 673–680.

67. Speare, D.J., Athanassopoulou, F., Daley, J., and Sanchez, J.G. (1999) A preliminary investigation of alternatives to fumagillin for the treatment of *Loma salmonae* infection in rainbow trout. *J. Comp. Pathol.* **21**, 241–248.

68. Speare, D.J., Ritter, G., and Schmidt, H. (1998) Quinine hydrochloride treatment delays xenoma formation and dissolution in rainbow trout challenged with *Loma salmonae. J. Comp. Pathol.* **119**, 459–465.

69. Schmahl, G. and Mehlhorn, H. (1989) Treatment of fish parasites. 6. Effects of sym. triazinone (toltrazuril) on developmental stages of *Glugea anomale,* Moniez, 1887 (Microsporidia): A light and electron microscopic study. *Eur. J. Protistol.* **24**, 252–259.

70. Schmahl, G., Taraschewski, H., and Mehlhorn, H. (1989) Chemotherapy of fish parasites. *Parasitol. Res.* **75**, 503–511.

71. El-Matbouli, M., Fischer-Scherl, T., and Hoffmann, R.W. (1992) Present knowledge on the life cycle, taxonomy, pathology, and therapy of some *Myxosporea* spp. important for freshwater fish. *Ann. Rev. Fish Dis.* **3**, 367–402.

72. Kent, M.L., Andree, K.B., Bartholomew, J.L., et al. (2001) Recent advances in our knowledge of the Myxozoa. *J. Eukaryot. Microbiol.* **48**, 395–413.

73. Smothers, J.F., von Dohlen, C.D., Smith, L.H., Jr., and Spall, R.D. (1994) Molecular evidence that the myxozoan protists are metazoans. *Science* 111**265**, 1719–1721.

74. Siddall, M.E., Martin, D.S., Bridge, D., Desser, S.S., and Cone, D.K. (1995) The demise of a phylum of protists: phylogeny of Myxozoa and other parasitic cnidaria. *J. Parasitol.* **81**, 961–967.

75. Zrzavy, J. and Hypsa, V. (2003) Myxozoa, Polypodium, and the origin of the Bilateria: The phylogenetic position of "Endocinidozoa" in light of the rediscovery of the *Buddenbrockia. Cladistics* **19**, 164–169.

76. Dykova, I. and Lom, J. (1988) Review of pathogenic myxosporeans in intensive culture of carp (*Cyprinus carpio*) in Europe. *Folia Parasitol. (Praha)* **35**, 289–307.

77. Bartholomew, J.L. and Reno, P.W. (2002) The History and Dissemination of Whirling Disease. In: Bartholomew, J.L., Wilson, J.C., editors. 7. Ann. Whirling Disease Symposium, Salt Lake City, Utah, 8–9 Feb 2001, American Fisheries Society, 3–24.

78. Hedrick, R.P., El-Matbouli, M., Adkison, M.A., and MacConnell, E. (1998) Whirling disease: re-emergence among wild trout. *Immunol. Rev.* **166**, 365–376.

79. El-Matbouli, M. and Hoffmann, R.W. (1998) Light and electron microscopic studies on the chronological development of *Myxobolus cerebralis* to the actinosporean stage in *Tubifex tubifex* to the actinosporean stage triactinomyxon. *Int. J. Parasitol.* **28**, 195–217.

80. El-Matbouli, M., Hoffmann, R.W., and Mandok, C. (1995) Light and electron microscopic observations on the route of the triactinomyxon-sporoplasm of *Myxobolus cerebralis* from epidermis into rainbow trout cartilage. *J. Fish Biol.* **46**, 919–935.

81. Poimanska, T., Wlasow, T., and Gomulka, P. (1998) *Sphaerospora renicola* and *S. molnari* in Poland and spring sphaerosporosis of carp. *Acta Ichthyol. Pisc.* **28**, 25–31.

82. Molnár, K., Fischer-Scherl, T., Baska, F., and Hoffmann, R.W. (1989) Hoferellosis in goldfish *Carassius auratus* and gibel carp *Carassius auratus gibelio*. *Dis. Aquat. Organ.* **7**, 89–95.

83. Ahmed, A.T. (1973) Morphology and life history of *Mitraspora cyprini* Fujita, parasitic in the kidney of goldfish. *Jpn. J. Med. Sci. Biol.* **26**, 87–101.

84. Kovács-Gayer, E., Ratz, F., Baska, F., and Molnár, K. (1987) Light and electron microscopic studies on various developmental stages of *Hoferellus cyprini* (Doflein, 1898). *Eur. J. Protistol.* **23**, 185–192.

85. Molnár, K. and Kovács-Gayer, E. (1986) Observations on the intracellular and coelozoic developmental stages of *Hoferellus cyprini* (Doflein, 1898) (Myxosporea, Myxozoa). *Parasitol. Hungarica* **19**, 27–30.

86. Hallett, S.L. (2005) Dissemination of triactinomyxons (Myxozoa) via oligochaetes used as live food for aquarium fishes. *Dis. Aquat. Organ.* **65**, 137–152.

87. Lowers, J.M. and Bartholomew, J.L. (2003) Detection of myxozoan parasites in oligochaetes imported as food for ornamental fish. *J. Parasitol.* **89**, 84–91.

88. MacConnell, E. (2003) Whirling Disease of Salmonids. Chapter 3.6. In: *Suggested Procedures for the Detection and Identification of Certain Finfish and Shellfish Pathogens,* 5th. American Fisheries Society, Bethesda, Maryland.

89. Kelley, G.O., Zagmutt-Vergara, F.J., Leutenegger, C.M., et al. (2004) Evaluation of five diagnostic methods for the detection and quantification of *Myxobolus cerebralis*. *J. Vet. Diagn. Invest.* **16**, 202–211.

90. Kent, M.L., Khattra, J., Hervio, D.M.L., and Devlin, R.H. (1998) Ribosomal DNA sequence analysis of isolates of the PKX myxosporean and their relationship to members of the genus *Sphaerospora*. *J. Aquat. Anim. Health* **10**, 12–21.

91. Molnár, K., Baska, F., and Székely, C. (1987) Fumagillin, an efficacious drug against renal sphaerosporosis of the common carp *Cyprinus carpio*. *Dis. Aquat. Organ.* **2**, 187–190.

92. Molnár, K. (1993) Recent achievements in the chemotherapy of myxosporean infections of fish. *Acta Vet. Hung.* **41**, 51–58.

93. Higgins, M.J. and Kent, M.L. (1996) Field trials with fumagillin for the control of proliferative kidney disease in coho salmon. *Prog. Fish-Culturist* **58**, 268–272.

94. Wishkovsky, A., Groff, J.M., Lauren, D.J., Toth, R.J., and Hedrick, R.P. (1990) Efficacy of fumagillin against proliferative kidney disease and its toxic side effects in rainbow trout (*Oncorhynchus mykiss*) fingerlings. *Fish Pathol.* **25**, 141–146.

95. Hedrick, R.P., McDowell, T.S., Marty, G.D., et al. (2000) Ultraviolet irradiation inactivates the waterborne infective stages of *Myxobolus cerebralis:* a treatment for hatchery water supplies. *Dis. Aquat. Organ.* **42**, 53–59.

96. Jensen, J.O.T., McLean, W.E., Kent, M.L., et al. (1994) Determination of ozone efficacy against proliferative kidney disease (PKD). In: MacKinlay, D.D., editor. International Fish Physiology Symposium; 16–21 Jul 1994; Vancouver, BC (Canada): Fish Physiology Association, Vancouver, B.C., 485–488.

97. Wagner, E.J. (2002) Whirling Disease Prevention, Control, and Management: A Review. In: Bartholomew, J.L., Wilson, J.C., editors. 7. Ann. Whirling Disease Symposium, Salt Lake City, Utah: American Fisheries Society; 2002. 217–225.

98. Cone, D.K. (1995) Monogenea (Phylum Platyhelminthes): In: Woo, P.T.K. (ed.) *Fish diseases and disorders,* CAB International, Wallingford, Oxon, UK, pp. 289–328.

99. Cone, D.K. and Odense, P.H. (1984) Pathology of five species of *Gyrodactylus* Nordmann, 1832 (Monogenea). *Can. J. Zool.* **62**, 1084–1088.

100. Harris, P.D., Shinn, A.P., Cable, J., and Bakke, T.A. (2004) Nominal species of the genus Gyrodactylus von Nordmann 1832 (Monogenea: Gyrodactylidae), with a list of principal host species. *Syst. Parasitol.* **59**, 1–27.

101. Mitchell, A. (2003) Bothriocephalus chapter 3.12: In: *Am. Fish Soc. Fish Health Section Blue Book: Suggested procedures for the detection and identification of certain finfish and shellfish pathogens,* American Fisheries Society, Bethesda, Maryland.

102. Williams, H. and Jones, A. (1994) *Parasitic Worms of Fish.* London: Taylor and Francis, 593 pages.

103. Scott, A.L. and Grizzle, J.M. (1979) Pathology of cyprinid fishes caused by *Bothriocephalus gowkongensis* Yea, 1955 (Cestoda: Pseudophyllidea). *J. Fish Dis.* **2**, 69–73.

104. Dick, T.A. and Chodhury, A. (1995) Cestoidea (Phylum Platyhelminthes): In: Woo, P.T.K. (ed.) *Fish diseases and disorders,* CAB International, Wallingford, Oxon, UK, pp. 391–414.

105. Heckmann, R.A., Deacon, J.E., and Greger, P.D. (1986) Parasites of woundfin minnow, *Plagopterus argentissimus,* and other endemic fishes from the Virgin River. *Great Basin Nat.* **46**, 662–676.

106. Flores-Crespo, J., Flores-Crespo, R., Ibarra-Velarde, F., and Vera-Montenegro, Y. (1994) Evaluation of 4 vermifuges against *Bothriocephalus acheilognathi* in carp. *Rev. Latinoam Microbiol.* **36**, 197–203.

107. Lester, R.J. (1971) The influence of *Schistocephalus* plerocercoids on the respiration of *Gasterosteus* and a possible resulting effect on the behavior of the fish. *Can. J. Zool.* **49**, 361–366.

108. Moravec, F. (1982) Proposal of a new systematic arrangement of the family Capillariidae. *Folia Parasitol.* **29**, 119–132.

109. Moravec, F. (1987) *Revision of capillarid nematodes (subfamily Capillariinae) parasitic in fishes.* Praha: Academia Natkadatelství Ceskoslovenské Akademie V&ebreve;d. pp. 273.

110. Moravec, F., Gelnar, M., and Rehulka, J. (1987) *Capillostrongyloides Ancistri* sp. n. (Nematoda: Capillariidae) a new pathogenic parasite of aquarium fishes in Europe. *Folia Parasitol. (Praha)* **34**, 157–161.

111. Moravec, F., Ergens, R., and Repova, R. (1984) First record of the nematode *Pseudocapillaria brevispicula* (Linstow, 1873) from aquarium fishes. *Folia Parasitol. (Praha)* **31**, 241–245.

112. Kent, M.L., Bishop-Stewart, J.K., Matthews, J.L., and Spitsbergen, J.M. (2002) *Pseudocapillaria tomentosa,* a nematode pathogen, and associated neoplasms of zebrafish (*Danio rerio*) kept in research colonies. *Comp. Med.* **52**, 354–358.

113. Pack, M., Belak, J., Boggs, C., Fishman, M., and Driever, W. (1995) Intestinal capillariasis in zebrafish. *Zebrafish Sci. Mon.* **3**, 1–3.

114. Lomankin, V.V. and Trofimenko, V.Y. (1982) Capillarids (Nematoda: Capillariidae) of freshwater fish fauna of the USSR. *Tr. Gelan.* **31**, 60–87.

115. Heckmann, R. (1985) Ivermectin efficacy trials for nematodes parasitic in fish. *Am. Soc. Fish Health Sec. Newsletter* **13**, 6.

116. Johnson, S.C., Kent, M.L., Whitaker, D.J., and Margolis, L. (1993) Toxicity and pathological effects of orally administered ivermectin in Atlantic, chinook, and coho salmon and steelhead trout. *Dis. Aquat. Organ.* **17**, 107–112.

117. Toovey, J.P.G., Lyndon, A.R., and Duffus, J.H. (1999) Ivermectin inhibits respiration in isolated rainbow trout (*Oncorhynchus mykiss* Walbaum) gill tissue. *Bull. Eur. Assoc. Fish Pathol.* **19**, 149–152.

118. Hoffman, G.L. (1982) *Capillaria catostomi*, a new pathogenic nematode of golden shiners and other fishes. In: Catfish Farmers American Research Workshop, 49–50.

119. Roberts, L.S. and Janovy, J.J. (2004) *Foundations of Parasitology*, 7th Edition, Boston, MA: McGraw Hill, 720 pages.

120. Paperna, I. (1991) Diseases caused by parasites in the aquaculture of warm water fish. *Ann. Rev. Fish Dis.* **1**, 155–194.

121. Lester, R.J.G., and Roubal, F.R. (1995) Phylum Arthropoda. In: Woo, P.T.K. (ed.) *Fish Diseases and Disorders*, CAB International, Wallingford, Oxon, UK, 475–598.

122. Berry, C.R., Jr., Babey, G.J., and Shrader, T. (1991) Effect of *Lernaea cyprinacea* (Crustacea: Copepoda) on stocked rainbow trout (*Oncorhynchus mykiss*). *J. Wildl. Dis.* **27**, 206–213.

123. Burtle, G. and Morrison, J. (1987) Dimilin for control of *Lernaea* in golden shiner ponds. *Proc. Ark. Acad. Sci.* **41**, 17–19.

124. Pike, A.W. and Wadsworth, S.L. (1999) Sea lice on salmonids: their biology and control. *Adv. Parasitol.* **44**, 233–337.

125. Roberts, R.J., Johnson, K.A., and Casten, M.T. (2004) Control of *Salmincola californiensis* (Copepoda: Lernaeapodidae) in rainbow trout, *Oncorhynchus mykiss* (Walbaum): a clinical and histopathological study. *J. Fish Dis.* **27**, 273–279.

126. Tamuli, K.K. and Shanbhogue, S.L. (1996) Efficacy of some commonly available chemicals in the treatment of anchor worm (*Lernaea bhadraensis*) infection. *Environ. Ecol.* **14**, 259–267.

127. Woo, P.T. (2003) *Cryptobia* (*Trypanoplasma*) *salmositica* and salmonid cryptobiosis. *J. Fish Dis.* **26**, 627–646.

128. Schaperclaus, W. (1991) *Fish Diseases*. Oxonian Press Pvt. Ltd., New Delhi, 1,398 pages.

129. Bower, S.M. and Woo, P.T. (1979) The prevalence of *Trypanosoma catostomi* in white sucker (*Catostomus commersoni*). *J. Wildl. Dis.* **15**, 428–431.

130. Sures, B., Knopf, K., Wurtz, J., and Hirt, J. (1999) Richness and diversity of parasite communities in European eels *Anguilla anguilla* of the River Rhine, Germany, with special reference to helminth parasites. *Parasitology* **119**, 323–330.

131. Lom, J. and Hoffman, G.L. (2003) Morphology of the spores of *Myxosoma cerebralis* (Hofer, 1903) and *M. cartilaginis* (Hoffman, Putz, and Dunbar, 1965). *J. Parasitol.* **89**, 653–657.

132. Kirk, R.S. and Lewis, J.W. (1994) The distribution and host ranges of species of the blood fluke *Sanguinicola* in British freshwater fish. *J. Helminthol.* **68**, 315–318.

133. Armitage, M.H. (2000) Ultrastructure of metacercarial cysts of six heterophyid trematodes from fish. *Parasitol. Res.* **86**, 1003–1007.

134. McElwain, I.V., and G. Post. 1968. Efficacy of cyzine for trout hexamitiasis. Progressive Fish-Culturalist 30:84–91.

135. Hoffman, G.L. (1965) *Eimeria aurati* n. sp. (Protozoa: Eimeriidae) from goldfish (*Carassius auratus*) in North America. J. Protozool. 12:273–75.

136. Marinçk, M. 1965. Coccidial infection in carp. *Arch. Biol. Sci.* 17: 57–64.

137. Belova, L.M. and Krylov, M.V. (2000) Distribution of coccidians (Sporozoa: Coccidida) in various systematic groups of fishes. *Parazitologiia* **34**, 522–533.

138. Kent, M.L., Margolis, L., Whitaker, D.J., Hoskins, G.E., and McDonald, T.E. (1994) Review of Myxosporea of importance in salmonid fisheries and aquaculture in British Columbia. *Folia Parasitol. (Praha)* **41**, 27–37.

139. Bartholemew, J.L., Whipple, M.J., Stevens, D.G., and Fryer, J.L. (1997) The life cycle of *Ceratomyxa shasta*, a myxosporean parasite of salmonids requires a freshwater polychaete as an alternate host. *J. Parasitol.* **83**, 859–868.

140. Mitchell, L.G. 1967. *Myxidium macrocheili* n. sp. (Cnidospora: Myxidiidae) from the large scale sucker *Catostomus macrochelius* Girard, and a synopsis of the *Myxidium* of North American freshwater vertebrates. *J. Protozool.* 114: 415–24.

141. Riley, M.W. and Uglem, G.L. (1995) *Proterometra macrostoma* (Digenea: Azygiidae): variations in cercarial morphology and physiology. *Parasitology* 110, 429–436.

142. Anderson, M.G. and Anderson, F.M. (1962) Life history of *Proterometra dickermani* Anderson, 1962. *J. Parasitol.* **49**, 275–280.

143. Anderson, M.G. and Anderson, F.M. (1967) The life histories of *Proterometra albicauda* and *Proterometra septimae*, spp. n. (Trematoda: Azygiidae) and a redescriptions of *Proterometra catenaria* Smith, 1934. *J. Parasitol.* **53**, 31–37.

144. Yamaguti, S. 1958. The digenetic trematodes of vertebrates. Vol. I. 2 Parts. *In* S. Yamaguti. *Systema helminthum*. Interscience, New York.

145. Moravec, F. and Sey, O. (1989) Some trematodes of freshwater fishes from North Vietnam with a list of recorded endohelminths by fish hosts. *Folia Parasitol. (Praha)* **36**, 243–262.

146. Caveny, B.A. and Etges, F.J. (1971) Life history studies of *Microphallus opacus* (Trematoda: Microphallidae). *J. Parasitol.* **57**, 1215–1221.

147. Smythe, A.B. and Font, W.F. (2001) Phylogenetic analysis of *Alloglossidium* (Digenea: Macroderoididae) and related genera: life-cycle evolution and taxonomic revision. *J. Parasitol.* **87**, 386–391.

148. Moravec, F. (2002) External morphological differences between *Crepidostomum farionis* and *Crepidostomum metoecus* (Trematoda: Allocreadiidae), parasites of salmonids, as revealed by SEM. *Folia Parasitol. (Praha)* **49**, 211–217.

149. Cribb, T.H. and Bray, R.A. (1999) A review of the Apocreadiidae Skrjabin, 1942 (Trematoda: Digenea) and description of Australian species. *Syst. Parasitol.* **44**, 1–36.

150. Hanek, G., and W. Threlfall. 1969. Digenetic trematodes from Newfoundland, Canada. I. Three species from *Gasterosteus aculeatis* Linnaeus, 1758. *Can. J. Zool.* 47:793–94.

151. Rosas-Valdez, R., Choudhury, A., and de Leon, G.P. (2004) Phylogenetic analysis on genera of Corallobothriinae (Cestoda: Proteocephalidea) from North American ictalurid fishes, using partial sequences of the 28s ribosomal gene. *J. Parasitol.* **90**, 1123–1127.

152. Bykhovskaya-Pavlovskaya, I.E., Gusev, A.V., Dubina, M.N., et al. (1962) Key to parasites of freshwater fish of the USSR (in Russian). Zool. Inst. Akad. Nauk SSSR, Moscow-Leningrad. (Translated edition: 1964. U.S. Dept. Commerce, Office Tech. Serv. TT64-11040. 919 pp.)

153. Scholz, T. (1999) Life cycles of species of *Proteocephalus*, parasites of fishes in the Palearctic region: a review. *J. Helminthol.* **73**, 1–19.

154. Scholz, T. and Hanzelova, V. (1999) Species of *Proteocephalus* Weinland, 1858 (Cestoda: Proteocephalidae) from cyprinid fishes in North America. *J. Parasitol.* **85**, 150–154.

155. de Chambrier, A., Zehnder, M., Vaucher, C., and Mariaux, J. (2004) The evolution of the Proteocephalidea (Platyhelminthes, Eucestoda) based on an enlarged molecular phylogeny, with comments on their uterine development. *Syst. Parasitol.* **57**, 159–171.

156. Hanzelova, V., Kuchta, R., Scholz, T., and Shinn, A.P. (2005) Morphometric analysis of four species of *Eubothrium* (Cestoda: Pseudophyllidea) parasites of salmonid fish: an interspecific and intraspecific comparison. *Parasitol. Res.* **54**, 207–214.

157. Dezfuli, B.S., Capuano, S., and Conglu, L. (2002) Identification of life cycle stages of *Cyathocephalus truncatus* (Cestoda: Spathebothriidea) using molecular techniques. *J. Parasitol.* **88**, 632–634.

158. Yamaguti, S. (1959) The cestodes of vertebrates. Vol. II. In: Yamaguti, S. *Systema helminthum.* Interscience, New York.

159. Petkeviciute, R. and Ieshko, E.P. (1991) The karyotypes of *Triaenophorus nodulosus* and *T. crassus* (Cestoda: Pseudophyllidea). *Int. J. Parasitol.* **21**, 11–15.

160. Scholz, T. (1991) Development of *Khawia sinensis* Hsu, 1935 (Cestoda: Caryophyllidea) in the fish host. *Folia Parasitol. (Praha)* **38**, 225–234.

161. Oros, M., Hanzelova, V., and Scholz, T. (2004) The cestode *Atractolytocestus huronensis* (Caryophyllidea) continues to spread in Europe: new data on the helminth parasite of the common carp. *Dis. Aquat. Organ.* **23**, 115–119.

162. Fischer, H., and R.S. Freeman. (1969) Penetration of parenteral plerocercoids of *Proteocephalus ambloplitis* (Leidy) into the gut of smallmouth bass. *J. Parasitol.* **55**, 766–74.

163. Kodedova, I., Dolezel, D., Brouckova, M., et al. (2000) On the phylogenetic positions of the Caryophyllidea, Pseudophyllidea and Proteocephalidea (Eucestoda) inferred from 18s rRNA. *Int. J. Parasitol.* **30**, 1109–1113.

164. Arthur, J.R. and Margolis, L. (1975) Revision of the genus *Haplonema* Ward and Magath, 1917 (Nematoda: Seuratoidea). *Can. J. Zool.* **53**, 736–747.

165. Yamaguti, S. (1961) The nematodes of vertebrates. Vol. III. 2 Parts. In: Yamaguti, S. *Systema helminthum.* Interscience, New York.

166. Hirasawa, R., Urabe, M., and Yuma, M. (2004) Relationship between intermediate host taxon and infection by nematodes of the genus *Rhabdochona. Parasitol. Int.* **53**, 89–97.

167. Boomker, J. and Puylaert, F.A. (1994) Eight new Afrotropical *Spinitectus* spp. (Nematoda: Cystidicolidae) from freshwater fishes with a key to the members of the genus in the region. *Onderstepoort J. Vet. Res.* **61**, 127–142.

168. Jilek, R. and Crites, J.L. (1982) Comparative morphology of the North American species of *Spinitectus* (Nematoda: Spirurida) analyzed by scanning electron microscopy. *Trans. Am. Microsc. Soc.* **101**, 126–134.

169. Val'ter, E.D. (1973) Morphology of the cephalic end of *Contracaecum aduncum* (Ascaridata). *Parazitologiia* **7**, 275–279.

170. Kuiken, T., Leighton, F.A., Wobeser, G., and Wagner, B. (1999) Causes of morbidity and mortality and their effect on reproductive success in double-crested cormorants from Saskatchewan. *J. Wildl. Dis.* **35**, 331–346.

171. Moravec, F., Vivas-Rodriguez, C., Scholz, T., et al. (1995) Nematodes parasitic in fishes of cenotes (=sinkholes) of the Peninsula of Yucatan, Mexico. Part 2. Larvae. *Folia Parasitol. (Praha)* **42**, 199–210.

172. Amin, O.M. (2002) Revision of Neoechinorhynchus Stiles and Hassall, 1905 (Acanthocephala: Neoechinorhynchidae) with keys to 88 species in two subgenera. *Syst. Parasitol.* **53**, 1–18.

173. Bullock, W.L. (1966) A redescription of *Octospiniferoides chandleri* Bullock, 1957. *J. Parasitol.* **52**, 735–738.

174. Pichelin, S., Smales, L., and Bray, R.A. (2002) A discussion of the Heteracanthocephalidae Petrochenko, 1956 (Acanthocephala: Palaeacanthocephala). *Syst. Parasitol.* **52**, 145–152.

175. Fischthal, J.H. (1950) Additional hosts and geographical distribution records for the common fish acanthocephalan, *Leptorhynchoides thecatus. J. Parasitol.* **36**, 88.

176. Amin, O.M. (1987) Acanthocephala from lake fishes in Wisconsin: ecology and host relationships of *Pomphorhynchus bulbocolli* (Pomphorhynchidae). *J. Parasitol.* **73**, 278–289.

177. O'Mahony, E.M, Kennedy, C.R., and Holland, C.V. (2004) Comparison of morphological characteristics in Irish and English populations of the acanthocephalan *Pomphorhynchus laevis* (Muller, 1776). *Syst. Parasitol.* **59**, 147–157.

178. Roberts, R.J. and Elson, K.G.R. (1970) An outbreak of whirling disease in rainbow trout. *Vet. Record* **86**, 258–259.

179. Eiras, J.C., Molnar, K., and Lu, Y.S. (2005) Synopsis of the species of *Myxobolus* Butshli, 1882 (Myxozoa: Myxosporea: Myxobolidae). *Syst. Parasitol.* **61**, 1–46.

180. Eiras, J.C. (2002) Synopsis of the species of the genus *Henneguya* Thelohan, 1892 (Myxozoa: Myxosporea: Myxobolidae). *Syst. Parasitol.* **52**, 43–54.

181. Putz, R.E., Hoffman, G.L., and Dunbar, C.E. (1965) Two new species of *Pleistophora* (Microsporidea) from North American fish with a synopsis of Microsporidea of freshwater and euryhaline fishes. *J. Protozool.* **12**, 228–236.

182. Hoffman, G. L. (1960) Synopsis of Strigeoidea (Trematoda) of fishes and their life cycles. *U.S. Fish Wildlife Serv. Fishery Bull.* **175**, **60**, 439–469.

183. Dzikowski, R., Levy, M.G., Poore, M.F., Flowers, J.R., and Paperna, I. (2004) *Clinostomum complanatum* and *Clinostomum marginatum* (Rudolphi, 1819) (Digenea: Clinostomidae) are separate species based on differences in ribosomal DNA. *J. Parasitol.* **90**, 413–414.

184. Leigh, W.H. (1975) Observations on the life cycle of *Paramacroderoides pseudoechinus* sp. n. (Digenea: Plagiorchioidea) and *P. echinus* Venard 1941, trematodes from the Florida gar. *J. Parasitol.* **61**, 873–876.

185. Yamaguti, S. (1958) The digenetic trematodes of vertebrates. Vol. I, 2 Parts. In: Yamaguti, S. *Systema helminthum.* Interscience, New York.

186. Shigin, A.A. (1976) Metacercariae of the genus *Diplostomum* in the fauna of the USSR. *Parazitologiia* **10**, 346–351.

187. Palmieri, J.R., Van Dellen, A.F., Heckman, R.A. (1982) Diagnostic exercise. Diplostomatosis caused by *Diplostomum spathaceum. Lab. Anim. Sci.* **32**, 351–352.

188. Shigin, A.A. (1996) Morphological criteria of the species in cercariae of the genus *Diplostomum* (Trematoda: Diplostomidae) and methods for their study. *Parazitologiia* **30**, 425–439.

189. Rintamaki-Kinnunen, P., Karvonen, A., Anttila, P., and Valtonen, E.T. (2004) *Diplostomum spathecum* metacercarial infection and colour change in salmonid fish. *Parasitol. Res.* **93**, 51–55.

190. Schubert, G. (1968) The injurious effects of *Costia necatrix. Bull. Office Intern. Epizootiol.* **69**, 1171–1178.

191. Lee, R.E. and Kugrens, P. (1992) Relationship between the flagellates and the ciliates. *Microbiol. Rev.* **56**, 529–542.

192. Lom, J. (1981) Fish invading dinoflagellates: a synopsis of existing and newly proposed genera. *Folia Parasitol. (Praha)* **28**, 3–11.

193. Cone, D.K. and Melendy, J.S. (2000) Infections of *Unicauda clavicauda* (Kudo, 1934) (Myxozoa) in the skin of *Notropis hudsonius* (Cyprinidae) from Montana, with a synopsis of the genus *Unicauda* Davis, 1944. *Folia Parasitol. (Praha)* **47**, 273–278.

194. Voronin, V.N. (1976) Characteristics of the genus *Glugea* (Protozoa, Microsporidia) based on the example of the type *Glugea anomala* (Moniez, 1887) Gurley 1893 and its varieties. *Parazitologiia* **10**, 263–267.

195. Pomport-Castillion, C., Romestand, B., and De Jonchkheere, J.F. (1997) Identification and phylogenetic relationships of microsporidia by riboprinting. *J. Eukaryot. Microbiol.* **44**, 540–544.

196. Wildgoose, W.H. (1995) *Dermocystidium koi* found in skin lesions of koi carp (*Cyprinus carpio*). *Vet. Rec.* **23**, 317–318.

197. Zhang, Q. and Wang, Z. (2005) *Dermocystidium* sp. infection in cultured juvenile southern catfish *Silurus meridionalis* in China. *Dis. Aquat. Organ.* **65**, 245−250.

198. Maki, J.L., Brown, C.C., and Dickerson, H.W. (2001) Occurrence of *Ichthyophthirius multifiliis* within the peritoneal cavities of infected channel catfish *Ictalurus punctatus*. *Dis. Aquat. Organ.* **44**, 41−45.

199. Wright, A.D. and Lynn, D.H. (1995) Phylogeny of the fish parasite *Ichthyophthirius* and its relative *Ophryoglena* and *Tetrahymena* (Ciliophora, Hymenostomatia) inferred from 18S ribosomal RNA. *Mol. Biol. Evol.* **12**, 285−290.

200. Kuperman, B.I., Kolesnikova, I.Y., and Tiutin, A.V. (1994) *Ambiphrya ameiuri* (Ciliophora: Peritricha): its ultrastructure and distribution on the body of carp fry. *Parazitologiia* **28**, 214−221.

201. Chernysheva, N.B. (1976) Morphological characteristics and certain biological problems of the representatives of the genus *Apiosoma* (Infusoria, Peritricha) from the young of predatory fishes. *Parazitologiia* **10**, 170−177.

202. Lom, J. 1970. Observations on trichodinid ciliates from freshwater fishes. *Arch. Protistenk.* 112:153−77.

203. Xu, K., Song, W., and Warren, A. (2002) Taxonomy of Trichodinids from the gills of marine fishes in coastal regions of the Yellow Sea, with descriptions of two new species of *Trichodina* Ehrenberg, 1830 (Protozoa: Ciliophora: Peritrichia). *Syst. Parasitol.* **51**, 107−120.

204. Malmberg, G. (1970) The excretory systems and marginal hooks as basis for systematics of *Gyrodactylus* (Trematoda: Monogenea). *Arkiv. Zool. Ser. 2*, **23**, 1−192.

205. Rogers, W.A. (1967) Six new species of *Gyrodactylus* (Monogenea) from the Southeastern U.S. *J. Parasitol.* **53**, 747−751.

206. Rogers, W.A. (1968) Eight new species of *Gyrodactylus* (Monogenea) from Southeastern U.S. with redescription of *G. fairporti* Van Cleave, 1921, *G. cyprini* Diarova, 1964. *J. Parasitol.* **54**, 490−495.

207. Rogers, W.A. (1967) Studies on Dactylogyrinae (Monogenea) with descriptions of 24 new species of *Dactylogyrus*, 5 new species of *Pellucidhaptor*, and the proposal of *Aplodiscus* gen. n. *J. Parasitol.* **53**, 501−524.

208. Rogers, W.A. (1968) *Pseudocolpenteron pavlovskyi* Bychowsky and Gussev, 1955 (Monogenea), from North America, with notes on its taxonomic status. *J. Parasitol.* **54**, 339.

209. Rogers, W.A. (1967) New genera and species of Ancyrocephalinae (Trematoda: Monogenea) from centrarchids fishes of the Southern U.S. *J. Parasitol.* **53**, 501−524.

210. Jogunoori, W., Kritsky, D.C., and Venkatanarasaiah, J. (2004) Neotropical Monogenoidea. 46. Three new species from the gills of introduced fishes in India, the proposal of *Heterotylus* n. g. and *Diaphorocleidus* n.g., and the reassignment of some previously described species of *Urocleidoides* Mizelle and Price, 1964 (Polyonchoinea: Dactylogyridae). *Syst. Parasitol.* **58**, 115−124.

211. Mizelle, J.D., and Price, C.E. (1964) Studies of monogenetic trematodes: XXVII. Dactylogyrid species with the proposal of *Urocleidoides* gen. n. *J. Parasitol.* **50**, 579−584.

212. Maitland, P.S., and Price, C.E. (1969) *Urocleidus principalis* (Mizelle, 1936): A North American monogenetic trematode new to British Isles, probably introduced with the largemouth bass *Micropterus salmonoides* Lacépède, 1802. *J. Fish Biol.* **1**, 17−18.

213. Beverley-Burton, M., and Klassen, G.J. (1990) New approaches to the systematics of the ancyrocephalid Monogenea from Nearctic freshwater fishes. *J. Parasitol.* **76**, 1−21.

214. Rubio-Godoy, M. and Tinsley, R.C. (2004) Comparative susceptibility of brown trout and rainbow trout to *Discocotyle sagittata* (Monogenea). *J. Parasitol.* **90**, 900−901.

215. Shoop, W.L. (2001) Systematic analysis of the Diplostomidae and Strigeidae (Trematoda). *J. Parasitol.* **75**, 21−32.

216. Wittrock, D.D., Bruce, C.S., and Johnson, A.D. (1991) Histochemistry and ultrastructure of the metacercarial cysts of blackspot trematodes *Uvulifer ambloplitis* and *Neascus pyriformis*. **77**, 454−460.

217. Hoffman, G.L. (1956) The life cycle of *Crassiphiala bulboglossa* (Trematoda: Strigeidae); development of the metacercaria and cyst, and effect on the fish hosts. *J. Parasitol.* **42**, 435−444.

218. Ondrackova, M., Simkova, A., Gelnar, M., and Jurajda, P. (2004) *Posthodiplostomum cuticola* (Digenea: Diplostomatidae) in intermediate fish hosts: factors contributing to the parasite infection and prey selection by the definitive bird host. *Parasitology* **129**, 761−770.

219. Schleppe, J.L. and Goater, C.P. (2004) Comparative life histories of two diplostomatid trematodes *Ornithodiplostomum ptychocheilus* and *Posthodiplostumum minimum*. *J. Parasitol.* **90**, 1387−1390.

220. Hoffman, R.W., Korting, W., Fischer-Scherl, T., and Schafer, W. (1990) An outbreak of bucephalosis in fish of the Main river. *Angew. Parasitol.* **31**, 95−99.

221. Kostadinova, A. and Gibson, D.I. (2002) *Isthmiophora* Luhe, 1909 and *Euparyphium* Dietz, 1909 (Digenea: Echinostomatidae) re-defined, with comments on their nominal species. *Syst. Parasitol.* **52**, 205−217.

222. Johnson, P.T., Sutherland, D.R., Kinsella, J.M., and Lunde, K.B. (2004) Review of the trematode genus *Ribeiroia* (Psilostomidae): ecology, life history and pathogenesis with special emphasis on the amphibian malformation problem. *Adv. Parasitol.* **57**, 191−253.

223. Ostrowski de Nunez, M. (1992) Life history studies of heterophyid trematodes in the Neotropical region: *Ascocotyle* (Leighia) *hadra* sp. n. *Mem. Inst. Oswaldo Cruz* **87**, 539−543.

224. Leigh, W.H. (1974) Life history of *Ascocotyle mcintoshi* Price, 1936 (Trematoda: Heterophyidae). *J. Parasitol.* **60**, 768−772.

225. Arme, C. (2002) *Ligula intestinalis*—a tapeworm contraceptive. *Biologist (London)* **49**, 265−269.

226. Arme, C., and Owen, R.W. (1967) Infections of the three-spined stickleback, *Gasterosteus aculeatis* L., with the plerocercoid larvae of *Schistocephalus solidus* (Müller, 1776), with special reference to pathologic effects. *Parasitology* **57**, 301−314.

227. Moravec, F. and Nagasawa, K. (1999) New data on the morphology of *Philonema oncorhynchi* Kuitunen-Ekbaum, 1933 (Nematoda: Dracunuloidea) from the abdominal cavity of Pacific salmon (*Oncorhynchus* spp.). *Syst. Parasitol.* **43**, 67−74.

228. Moravec, F. (2004) The systematic status of *Philometra abdominalis* Nybelin, 1928 (Nematoda: Philmetridae) (a junior synonym of *P. ovata* (Zeder, 1803)). *Folia Parasitol. (Praha)* **51**, 75−76.

229. Molnár, K. and Fernando, C.H. (1975) Morphology and development of *Philometra cylindracea* (Ward and Magath, 1916) (Nematoda: Philometridae). *J. Helminthol.* **49**, 19−24.

230. Geist, J. and Kuehn, R. (2005) Genetic diversity and differentiation of central European freshwater pearl mussel (*Margaritifera margaritifera* L.) populations: implications for conservation and management. *Mol. Ecol.* **14**, 425−439.

231. Walker, P.D., Flik, G., and Bonga, S.E. (2005) The biology of parasites from the genus *Argulus* and a review of the interactions with its host. *Symp. Soc. Exp. Biol.* **55**, 107−129.

232. Roberts, L.S. (1970) *Ergasilus* (Copepoda: Cyclopoida): Revision and key to species in *North America. Trans. Am. Microscop. Soc.* **89**, 134−161.

233. Kabata, Z. (1969) Revision of the genus *Salmincola* Wilson, 1915 (Copepoda: Lernaeopodidae). *J. Fisheries Res. Board Can.* **26**, 2987−3041.

234. Roberts, R.J., Johnson, K.A., and Casten, M.T. (2004) Control of *Salmincola californiensis* (Copepoda: Lernaeapodidae) in rainbow trout, *Oncorhynchus mykiss*(Walbaum): a clinical and histopathological study. *J. Fish Dis.* **27**, 73–79.

235. Tully, O. and Nolan, D.T (2002) A review of the population biology and host-parasite interactions of the sea louse *Lepeophtheirus salmonis* (Copepoda: Caligidae). *Parasitology* **124**, S165–S182.

236. Zhao, Y. and Song, W. (2003) Studies on the morphology and taxonomy of three new myxosporeans of the genus *Sinuolinea* Davis, 1917 (Myxosporea: Sinuolineidae) infecting the urinary bladder of some marine fishes from the Shandong coast, China. *Syst. Parasitol.* **55**, 53–59.

237. McGeorge, J., Sommerville, C., and Wooten, R. (1996) Transmission experiments to determine the relationships between *Sphaerospora* sp. from Atlantic salmon, *Salmo salar,* and *Sphaerospora truttae:* a revised species description for *S. truttae. Folia Parasitol. (Praha)* **43**, 107–116.

238. Al-Samman, A., Molnár, K., Szekely, C., and Reiczigel, J. (2003) Reno-, hepato- and splenomegaly of common carp fingerlings (*Cyprinus carpio* L.) diseased in swimbladder inflammation caused by *Sphaerospora renicola* Dykova et Lom, 1982. *Acta Vet. Hung.* **51**, 321–329.

239. Eszterbauer, E. and Szekely, C. (2004) Molecular phylogeny of the kidney-parasitic *Sphaerospora renicola* from common carp (*Cyprinus carpio*) and *Sphaerospora* sp. from goldfish (*Carassius auratus auratus*). *Acta Vet. Hung.* **52**, 469–478.

240. Eiras, J.C., Malta, J.C., Varela, A., and Pavanelli, G.C. (2004) *Henneguya schizodon* n. sp. (Myxozoa, Myxobolidae), a parasite of the Amazonian teleost fish *Schizodon fasciatus* (Characiformes, Anostomidae). *Parasite* **11**, 169–173.

241. Molnár, K., Csaba, G., and Kovacs-Gayer, E. (1986) Study of the postulated identity of *Hoferellus cyprini* (Doflein, 1898) and *Mitraspora cyprini* Fujita, 1912. *Acta Vet. Hung.* **34**, 175–181.

242. Korting, W. and Hermanns, W. (1985) *Mitraspora cyprini* Fujita, 1912 (Protozoa Myxosporea Butschli, 1881) in the kidneys of carp from Lower Saxony pond farms. *Berl. Munch. Tierarztl. Wochenschr.* **98**, 63–64.

243. Sanders, J.E. and Fryer, J.L. (1970) Occurrence of the myxosporidan parasite *Myxidium minteri* in salmonid fish. *J. Protozool.* **17**, 354–357.

244. Nagel, M.L. and Hoffman, G.L. (1977) A new host for *Pleistophora ovariae* (Microsporida). *J. Parasitol.* **63**, 160–162.

245. Warner, M.C. and Hubert, W.A. (1975) Note on the occurrence of *Acetodextra amiuri* (Stafford) (Trematoda: Heterophidae) in channel catfish from the Tennessee River. *J. Wildl. Dis.* **11**, 37.

246. Shirakashi, S. and Goater, C.P. (2005) Chronology of parasite-induced alteration of fish behaviour: effects of parasite maturation and host experience. *Parasitology* **130**, 177–183.

247. Canning, E.U., Tops, S., Curry, A., Wood, T.S., and Okamura, B. (2002) Ecology, development, and pathogenicity of *Buddenbrockia plumatellae* Schroder 1910 (Myxozoa, Malacospora) (syn. *Tetracapsula bryozoides*) and establishment of *Tetracapsuloides* n. gen. for *Tetracapsula bryosalmonae. J. Eukaryot. Microbiol.* **49**, 280–295.

248. Poynton, S. L. and Sterud, E. (2002) Guidelines for species descriptions of diplomonad flagellates from fish. *J. Fish Dis.* **25**, 15–31.

249. Taylor, L.H., Hall, B.K., Miyake, T. and Cone, D.K. (1994) Ectopic ossicles associated with metacercariae of *Apophallus brevis* (Trematoda) in yellow perch, *Perca flavescens* (Teleostei): development and identification of bone and chondroid bone. *Anat. Embryol.* **190**, 29–46.

250. Kent, M.L., Watral, V., Whipps, C.M., Cunningham, M.E., Criscione, C.D., Heidel, J.R., et al. (2004) A digenean metacercaria (*Apophallus* sp.) and a myxozoan (*Myxobolus* sp.) associated with vertebral deformities in cyprinid fishes from the Willamette River, Oregon. *J. Aquat. Anim. Health* **16**, 116–129.

INTRODUCTION

Amphibians continue to serve as important animal models in science, and are commonly used in many disciplines of biomedical research and teaching, including toxicology, physiology, limb regeneration, evolutionary biology, and reproductive biology, to name just a few. Amphibians are readily available through vendors in both the United States and Europe, and may originate through captive breeding programs or through capture of animals in the wild. While the former are often free of parasites, the latter may harbor a wide range of commensal or parasitic organisms. Therefore, people involved in the care and/or use of amphibians in biomedical research or teaching should be familiar with the parasitic fauna of these important animal models.

PROTOZOA

Phylum Sarcomastigophora

Class Mastigophora (flagellates)

Hemoflagellates

Trypanosoma spp. **Morphology.** *Trypanosoma pipientis* measures 70 μ long by 4 μ wide[1] and has a round to elliptical nucleus located near the center of the body, a medium-sized kinetoplast, a narrow undulating membrane, and a long flagellum. *Trypanosoma ranarum* has two adult forms, one that measures 74 μ long by 5 μ wide and another that measures 71 μ long by 8 μ wide (Figure 8.1).

In the narrower form, the nucleus is located in the anterior one-third of the body, while in the wider form it is located in the middle third of the body. In both forms, the kinetoplast is large, the undulating membrane wide, and the flagellum less than one-half the body length.

Trypanosoma chattoni occurs in vertebrates, but only in a spherical form. It does not have an undulating

---

Tables are placed at the ends of chapters.

membrane, and the flagellum, when present, is very short. *Trypanosoma diemyctyli*, which has also been identified in reptiles and amphibians, is long and slender, measuring 45 to 116 μ long by 2 to 5 μ wide[2,3].

Hosts. All amphibians found in areas where trypanosomes are endemic are susceptible to infection. *Trypanosoma inopinatum* is common in Old World amphibians, *T. pipientis* in leopard frogs (*Rana pipiens*), *T. ranarum* in multiple species of frogs, and *T. diemyctyli* in newts[4].

Life Cycle. The life cycle of trypanosomes requires an invertebrate vector[3,5]. For most aquatic amphibians, the intermediate host for the trypanosome is probably a leech; for terrestrial amphibians it is probably a bloodsucking arthropod. Although anurans are usually thought to be infected during the tadpole stage by the bite of an infected leech, there is some evidence that adult frogs can be infected by the bite of an infected mosquito[6] and that adult toads can been infected by ingesting an infected sand fly (*Phlebotomus* sp.)[7].

Pathologic Effects. The pathogenicity of the species affecting frogs and toads varies[1]. *Trypanosoma inopinatum* is one of the most pathogenic species, causing either acute or chronic infections. In an acute infection, an excessive and continuous production of juvenile forms of the parasite is characteristic; in chronic infection, adult forms predominate. Acute infection can lead to necrotizing splenitis, which generally leads to the death of the amphibian host. *Trypanosoma pipientis* and *T. ranarum* can also cause splenitis, but death is uncommon. *Trypanosoma diemyctyli* can cause debilitation, anorexia, erythrocyte degeneration, and death. The degree of parasitemia and resultant pathologic effects are related to the environmental temperature, with pathogenicity greatest at 15°C and least at 20°C to 25°C[2,8].

Clinical Disease. Most captive amphibians with low-grade trypanosome infections are asymptomatic, and most cases are diagnosed as an incidental finding. Animals with

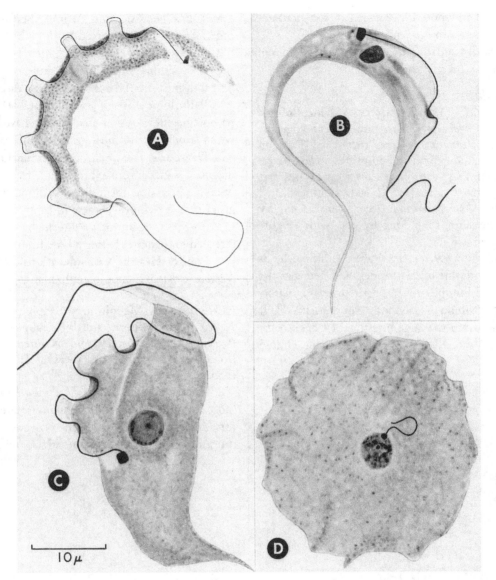

Fig. 8.1 Common trypanosomes of North American anurans. (A) *Trypanosoma pipientis* adult. (B) *T. ranarum* adult, narrow form. (C) *T. ranarum* adult, wide form. (D) *T. chattoni* adult. Reproduced from Diamond, L.S. (1965) with permission.

heavy burdens may become lethargic and depressed. In severe cases, anurans become anemic, with packed cell volumes of less than 20%.

Diagnosis. Antemortem diagnosis is based on identification of the parasite in the blood[1]. A blood sample can be collected from the ventral abdominal vein, femoral vein, heart, or lingual plexus to prepare a blood smear. Wright-Giemsa is the preferred stain when preparing slides. The living trypanosomes are usually readily recognized by their rapid, wavy motion. Postmortem diagnosis

can be made from identifying the parasites in affected tissues, such as the spleen.

Treatment. Quinine sulfate or bisulfate (30 mg/L, one-hour bath) may be used to treat trypanosomiasis. In severe cases, when animals have anemia, chloroquine (50 mg/kg administered orally once weekly) may be used[9].

Prevention. Because of the need for an invertebrate intermediate host, it is unlikely that the life cycle would be completed in the laboratory. However, infection may represent an unwanted research variable. To prevent this, wild-caught animals should be screened for parasites before being released into the general colony.

Public Health Considerations. The trypanosomes of amphibians do not infect humans.

Enteric flagellates

Hexamastix and Monocercomonas. Morphology. *Hexamastix* and *Monocercomonas* are morphologically similar to *Tritrichomonas*, except that they lack an undulating membrane and a costa[10,11]. *Hexamastix batrachorum* (Syn. *Polymastix batrachorum*) measures 7 μ to 15.5 μ long by 5 μ to 10.5 μ wide (Figure 8.2)[12]. *Monocercomonas batra chorum* (Syn. *Eutrichomastix batrachorum*) measures 15 μ long by 6 μ wide (Figure 8.3)[13].

Hosts and Life Cycle. *Hexamastix batrachorum* is common in the intestine of salamanders and newts in the United States and Europe[6,14,15,16]. *Monocercomonas batrachorum* is also common in laboratory amphibians[6,15]. It can be recovered from the large intestine of frogs, toads, salamanders, and the red-spotted newt from the United

States, Europe, Asia, and Africa. The prevalence of this organism has been reported to be as high as 77% in the red-spotted newt in the eastern United States[14]. Reproduction is by simple binary fission, and no cysts are formed. The transmission of these organisms is direct.

Pathologic Effects and Clinical Disease. Neither pathologic effects nor clinical disease have been associated with *Hexamastix* or *Monocercomonas* infections.

Diagnosis, Treatment, and Prevention. Antemortem diagnosis is made from a direct saline fecal smear. No treatment has been described. A course of metronidazole can be given if severe clinical disease in captive animals is attributed to these organisms. Wild-caught animals should be screened for parasites before release from quarantine.

Public Health Considerations. *Hexamastix* and *Monocercomonas* do not infect humans.

Hexamita spp. Morphology. Trophozoites of the genus *Hexamita* are pyriform and bilaterally symmetrical, with two nuclei, two axostyles, and six anterior and two posterior flagella[3]. Trophozoites measure 10 μ to 16 μ long (Figure 8.4).

Hosts and Life Cycle. *Hexamita batrachorum* is the most common species of *Hexamita* isolated from laboratory amphibians[6]. It has been recovered from the large intestine of frogs, toads, salamanders, and newts from the

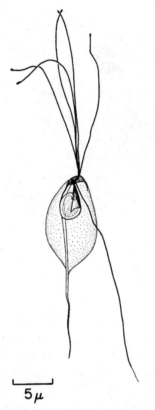

⌊___5μ___⌋

Fig. 8.2 *Hexamastix batrachorum.* Reproduced from Honigberg, B.M. and Christian, H.H. (1954) with permission.

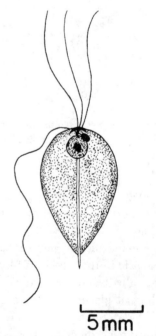

⌊___5mm___⌋

Fig. 8.3 *Monocercomonas.* Reproduced from Levine, N.D. (1961) with permission.

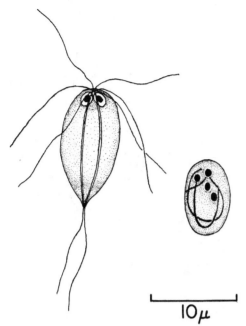

Fig. 8.4 *Hexamita intestinalis.* (Left) Trophozoite. (Right) Cyst. Reproduced from Cheng, T.C. (1964) with permission.

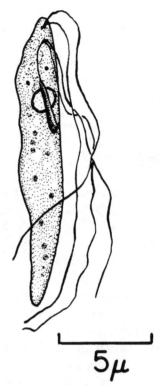

Fig. 8.5 *Karotomorpha bufonis.* Reproduced from Hughes, R.C. (1929) with permission.

United States. The prevalence of *H. batrachorum* in dusky salamanders from the eastern United States is 42%[14]. *Hexamita intestinalis* occurs in the large intestine of frogs, toads, salamanders, newts, and the axolotls from the United States, Europe, and Asia. The prevalence of *H. intestinalis* in marbled salamanders from the eastern United States has been estimated to be 38%[14]. Reproduction is by simple binary fission. Some species form cysts. The transmission of these organisms is direct.

Pathologic Effects and Clinical Disease. Heavy burdens of *Hexamita* may cause inflammatory bowel disease, resulting in diarrhea.

Diagnosis, Treatment, and Prevention. Antemortem diagnosis is made from a direct saline fecal smear. No treatment has been described. A course of metronidazole can be given if severe clinical disease in captive animals is attributed to these organisms. Wild-caught animals should be screened for *Hexamita* before release from quarantine.

Public Health Considerations. *Hexamita* does not infect humans.

Karotomorpha **spp. Morphology.** *Karotomorpha* spp. are elongated, spindle shaped, and measure 12 μ to 16 μ long by 2 μ to 6 μ wide[3]. There are two pairs of flagella at the anterior end (Figure 8.5).

Hosts and Life Cycle. *Karotomorpha bufonis* is the most common species isolated from laboratory amphibians[6,14] and can be recovered from the rectum of the leopard frog, European toad, tiger salamander, palmate newt, and axolotl from North America and Europe. *Karotomorpha swezyi* occurs in the rectum of the leopard frog, American toad, dusky salamanders, redspotted newt, and California newt in the United States. Reproduction is by simple binary fission. Transmission is direct.

Pathologic Effects and Clinical Disease. Neither pathologic effects nor clinical disease have been described in amphibians infected with *Karotomorpha* spp.

Diagnosis, Treatment, and Prevention. Ante-mortem diagnosis is made from a direct saline fecal smear. No treatment has been described. A course of metronidazole can be given if severe clinical disease in captive animals is attributed to these organisms. Wild-caught animals should be screened for *Karotomorpha* before release from quarantine.

Public Health Considerations. *Karotomorpha* does not infect humans.

Piscinoodinium spp. **Morphology, Hosts, and Life Cycle.** The morphology of *Piscinoodinium* spp., members of the phylum Dinoflagellata, is presented in Chapter 7, Parasites of Fishes. Natural hosts include larval amphibians[18]. The life cycle is direct. The trophont stage attaches to the skin or gill of the host and feeds via its attachment device. Eventually the trophont stage detaches from the host and forms a cyst with dinospores in the environment. When the cyst ruptures, the dinospores swim (via a flagellum) to an amphibian host, encyst, and develop into trophonts.

Pathologic Effects and Clinical Disease. *Piscinoodinium* can cause localized granuloma formation where the trophonts encyst. Affected amphibians may have a "velvet-like" or "gold-dust" appearance to their skin. Animals with skin lesions may rub their body against hard surfaces in an attempt to remove the parasites. In severe cases involving the ventral patch, amphibians may develop osmoregulatory problems. Larval amphibians with gill parasitic infestation of the gills may be dyspneic.

Diagnosis, Treatment, and Prevention. Antemortem diagnosis is based on identifying the protozoans from skin scrapings or gill biopsies. Postmortem diagnosis is based on identifying the parasites in skin and gill biopsies. Providing amphibians with water of high quality minimizes clinical outbreaks. Regular water changes are required in cases where high organic loads accumulate. Affected animals may be placed in distilled water baths for two to three hours, or in salt water baths (10 to 25 g/L, five to 30 minutes)[19]. Providing good quality water and adhering to quarantine and hygiene protocols reduces the likelihood of transmitting these organisms.

Public Health Considerations. *Piscinoodinium* does not infect humans.

Proteromonas spp. **Morphology.** Trophozoites in the genus *Proteromonas* are pyriform, but more elongated than those of other genera. They possess two flagella on the anterior end, one directed forward and the other trailing posteriorly (Figure 8.6)[3,20,21].

Hosts and Life Cycle. *Proteromonas longifila* is the most common species from the genus recovered from laboratory amphibians[6,15] and is found in the rectum of frogs, toads, salamanders, and newts from North America, South America, and Europe. This parasite is considered highly prevalent (89%) in the red-spotted newt from the eastern United States[14]. Reproduction is by simple binary fission. No cysts are formed[23]. Transmission is direct.

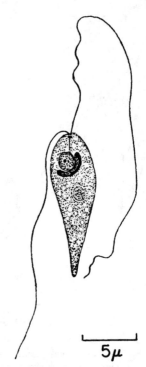

Fig. 8.6 *Proteromonas* sp. Reproduced from Kudo, R.R. (1966) with permission.

Pathologic Effects and Clinical Disease. Neither pathologic effects nor clinical disease have been described in amphibians infected with *Proteromonas* spp.

Diagnosis, Treatment, and Prevention. Antemortem diagnosis is made from a direct saline fecal smear. No treatment has been described. A course of metronidazole can be given if severe clinical disease in captive animals is attributed to these organisms. Wild-caught animals should be screened for *Proteromonas* before release from quarantine.

Public Health Considerations. *Proteromonas* does not infect humans.

Tetratrichomonas, Trichomitus, Tritrichomonas. **Morphology.** The trichomonads belong to the order Trichomonadida. *Tetratrichomonas* possesses four anterior flagella, whereas *Trichomitus* and *Tritrichomonas* possess three[11]. All have an oval to pyriform body, an undulating membrane, an axostyle that protrudes from the posterior end, and a costa. *Tetratrichomonas prowazeki* measures 5.5 μ to 22 μ long by 3.5 μ to 18.5 μ wide. *Trichomitus batrachorum* measures 6 μ to 21 μ long by 4 μ to 20 μ wide, is ovoid, and has an axostyle without granules and a V-shaped parabasal body (Figure 8.7). *Tritrichomonas augusta* measures 15 μ to 27 μ long by 5 μ to 13 μ wide.

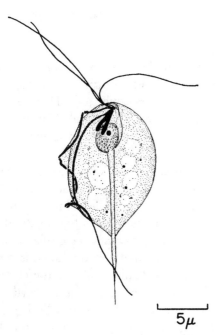

Fig. 8.7 *Trichomitus batrachorum.* Reproduced from Honigberg, B.M. (1953) with permission.

It is elongate and spindle-shaped, and has an axostyle that contains dark-staining granules and a rod- or sausage-shaped parabasal body[11,22,24].

Hosts. *Tetratrichomonas prowazeki* occurs in the large intestine of frogs, toads, salamanders, newts, and amphiumas from the United States, Europe, and South America[11,25]. *Trichomitus batrachorum* has been recovered from the large intestine of many species of frogs, toads, salamanders, newts, and the axolotl throughout the world[6,11,15,21,22,24]. *Tritrichomonas augusta* is common in the large intestine of frogs, toads, salamanders, newts, and lizards from North, Central, and South America; Europe; and Asia[6,15]. The prevalence of this parasite can be as high as 100% in salamanders from the eastern United States[14].

Life Cycle. Reproduction is by simple binary fission, and no cysts are formed. The transmission of these organisms is direct.

Pathologic Effects and Clinical Disease. The trichomonads are rarely associated with pathology or clinical disease. However, extremely heavy parasite burdens could alter the intestinal microflora, resulting in diarrhea. *Tritrichomonas augusta* has been associated with liver lesions in the leopard frog[6].

Diagnosis, Treatment, and Prevention. Antemortem diagnosis is by examining direct saline fecal smears. No treatment regimens have been described. A course of metronidazole (10 mg/kg SID, five to ten days) can be given if severe clinical disease in captive animals is attributed to these organisms. Wild-caught animals should be screened for parasites before being released from quarantine.

Public Health Considerations. Trichomonads of amphibians do not infect humans.

Class Sarcodina (amoebae)

Entamoeba ranarum

Morphology. *Trophozoites* of Entamoeba ranarum measure 10 μ to 50 μ in diameter. Cysts usually contain four nuclei, but may contain up to 16 nuclei[3,23].

Hosts. *Entamoeba ranarum* is found in the intestine of the leopard frog, green frog, bullfrog, grass frog, edible frog, European toad, red-spotted newt, common newt, and palmate newt from the United States, Europe, India, and the Philippine islands[6,16]. It may also be found in the liver and kidneys. This parasite can affect both adult and larval amphibians.

Life Cycle. Reproduction is by binary fission[26]. Before encysting, the trophozoite becomes round and small. It produces a cyst wall and the nucleus divides twice, producing four small nuclei. The quadrinucleate cyst is passed in the feces, and when it is ingested by a suitable host, an amoeba with four nuclei emerges. It divides several times and produces small uninucleate amebas, each of which develops into a trophozoite.

Pathologic Effects and Clinical Disease. Historically, *E. ranarum* has not been considered pathogenic in captive amphibians[3,26]. However, mucosal damage can occur with heavy infection. Renal infections have also been reported in *Bufo marinus*[27]. Affected amphibians develop anorexia, weight loss, dehydration, and diarrhea. Frank hemorrhage may be noted in the feces. When the kidneys are involved, ascites or anasarca may develop.

Diagnosis. Antemortem diagnosis is based on the microscopic demonstration of cysts and trophozoites in a fecal sample[28]. If erythrocytes and white blood cells are also observed in the sample, than it is likely that the *E. ranarum* is causing damage to the mucosal surface, and should be considered pathogenic.

Treatment. Cases of clinical amoebiasis should be treated with metronidazole. Recommended dosages include: 10 mg/kg orally once per day for five to ten days; 50 mg/kg orally once per day for three to five days; and 100 to 150 mg/kg orally once, repeated in two to three weeks. Care should be taken when using higher doses because these can cause hepatic encephalopathy. Affected amphibians should be maintained on a moistened paper towel substrate, to be changed daily, to reduce the likelihood of recontamination. Amphibians that become clinically dehydrated should be rehydrated.

Prevention. Infections can be prevented by strict attention to sanitation and by prophylactic treatment of new arrivals[29].

Public Health Considerations. *Entamoeba ranarum* does not infect humans.

Phylum Apicomplexa

Class Coccidia

Cryptosporidium spp.

The morphology of *Cryptosporidium* spp. is described in the Chapter 15, Parasites of Rabbits. It is likely that all amphibians are susceptible to infection with *Cryptosporidium*. The life cycle is presumed to be direct. Gastritis and enteritis were identified in a single case of cryptosporidiosis in an African clawed frog (*Xenopus laevis*)[30]. Affected amphibians may develop chronic weight loss, muscle atrophy, regurgitation, and diarrhea. At this time, there are no effective treatments for cryptosporidiosis in amphibians. Several chemotherapeutics have been used to control infections in reptiles, but they are not curative. The best method for preventing the introduction of *Cryptosporidium* spp. into an amphibian colony is to cull positive animals from quarantine. Once established, it is impossible to eliminate the infection. Animals should be quarantined for a minimum of four weeks, and four serial (weekly) negative fecal examinations should be required before releasing animals into the general colony. It is uncertain whether the *Cryptosporidium* isolated from amphibians is infectious to humans. Thus, animal workers should practice excellent personal hygiene when working with animals known or suspected to harbor *Cryptosporidium*.

Eimeria spp.

Morphology. Oocysts of *Eimeria* spp. are spherical to ovoid and measure 14 μ to 19 μ long by 14 μ to 17 μ wide[31].

Hosts. *Eimeria* spp. have been recovered from a number of different anurans and urodelans[6,9,15,31-34]. Most inhabit the intestine, although some may infect the kidneys and gall bladder.

Life Cycle. The life cycle is direct, and generally similar to the life cycles of mammalian *Eimeria*[3,10]. Oocysts may sporulate while still in the intestine of some anurans. When this occurs, animals within the same captive environment can be infected immediately upon being exposed to the parasite. In other cases, sporulation occurs in the environment.

Pathologic Effects. Coccidia undergo schizogony and gametogony in the epithelial cells of the intestine, gallbladder, bile duct, and kidneys. The damage associated with these parasites is generally mild. However, enteritis or nephritis may be noted histologically. The most severe disease would be expected to occur in juvenile or immunocompromised individuals.

Clinical Disease. Infection with *Eimeria* sp. is generally asymptomatic in adult amphibians. Clinical disease is more likely to occur in juvenile or immunocompromised animals. Affected animals may develop diarrhea or die acutely. Dehydration is a common sequella to the diarrhea.

Diagnosis. Antemortem diagnosis is by finding oocysts in the feces on a direct saline smear or a fecal flotation. For identification of genus, unsporulated oocysts can be sporulated in a 2.5% potassium dichromate solution. Sporulation is generally complete within seven days. Postmortem diagnosis is made histologically.

Treatment. Treating captive amphibians for coccidial infections can be difficult. Most available anticoccidials are only coccidiostats, and thus only temporarily suppress parasite reproduction. The author has used trimethoprim-sulfadimethoxine (15 mg/kg orally for 14 to 21 days) with good results. Other sulfa-based antibiotics may be equally effective.

Prevention. *Eimeria* may be excluded from the colony by culling animals that test positive in quarantine. Once established, *Eimeria* is difficult to eliminate. Animals should be quarantined for a minimum of four weeks, and four serial (weekly) negative fecal examinations should be required before introducing an animal into the colony.

Public Health Considerations. *Eimeria* of amphibians do not infect humans.

Isospora spp.

Oocysts of *Isospora* are ovoid and measure 18 μ to 23 μ long by 11 μ to 20 μ wide[31]. The host range, life cycle, and other aspects of the biology of *Isospora* in amphibians are similar to *Eimeria*[6,9,15,31,32]. Most inhabit the intestine, although some may infect the kidneys and gall bladder.

Erythrocytic coccidia

Morphology. Amphibians may become infected with several genera of coccidia found in the blood of the host, including hemogregarines (*Hemogregarina*, *Hepatozoon*), lankesterellids (*Lankesterella*, *Schellackia*), and dactylostomids (*Babesioma*, *Dactylosoma*). The forms found in the blood of laboratory amphibians vary with the stage of the life cycle and the species of the host[3,35], and range in size from 10 μ to 17 μ long by 2 μ to 4 μ wide. In the erythrocytes, hemogregarine and lankesterellid sporozoites are generally banana-shaped, whereas the dactylostomids are round.

Life Cycle. Reproduction for these parasites is both sexual and asexual. For hemogregarines, merogony occurs in the tissues and gametogony occurs in the erythrocytes. An invertebrate, such as a leech or arthropod, serves as the site for sporogony. Although the invertebrates may infect amphibians when collecting a blood meal, this is not always the case. *Hepatozoon catesbeiana* infects bullfrogs (*Rana catesbeiana*) after the frog ingests an infected mosquito (*Culex territans*) containing sporocysts[36]. In contrast, the entire life cycle of a lankesterellid occurs within the amphibian host[37]. Merogony generally occurs in the tissues (e.g., intestine, walls of the blood vessels) and sporogony in the erythrocytes. Amphibians become infected with lankesterellids when they ingest a sporozoite-infected invertebrate or are fed on by leeches. Dactylostomids are transferred to amphibians by leeches.

Pathologic Effects. Although usually considered nonpathogenic[28,37,38], heavy infections sometimes cause anemia[32]. The presence of a coccidian in an erythrocyte causes extreme distortion of the blood cell, including nuclear displacement and cytoplasmic attenuation[32]. The number of erythrocytes affected varies up to 80% or more[35].

Clinical Disease. Packed cell volumes (PCV) in amphibians are generally greater than 20%. Infection with erythrocytic coccidia may result in critically low PCV of less than 10%. Amphibians with high densities of parasites and anemia are clinically ill. Affected animals may also be lethargic, depressed, and have pale mucous membranes.

Diagnosis, Treatment, and Prevention. Diagnosis is based on detection of anemia and demonstration of the parasite in Wright-Giemsa-stained blood smears[32]. Treatment is not recommended unless severe anemia (<10%) is identified. Because of the potentially fragile nature of these animals, prognosis in severe cases is grave. Culling potentially infected animals during quarantine should prevent the need to manage severe cases. These apicomplexans should not be found in the modern animal facility because they require an intermediate host to complete their life cycle. Prescreening animals during quarantine may identify infected animals. Infected animals should be culled to eliminate an unwanted research variable.

Public Health Considerations. Erythrocytic coccidia are not infective for humans.

Phylum Microspora

Morphology. The morphology of the microsporidia varies with the stage of the life cycle[39]. Microsporidians measure 5 μ to 20μ, and are pyriform in shape with a posterior vacuole. Schizonts contain up to eight nuclei. Small sporonts have two to three nuclei but, when mature, may contain up to 100 nuclei. Genera found in amphibians include *Pleistophora* and *Alloglugea*. *Pleistophora myotropica* spores are oval and measure 3.5 μ to 6.7 μ long by 2 μ to 3 μ wide. On one side of the anterior pole of each spore is a small granule to which is attached a filament. When extended, this filament is 80 μ to 220 μ long.

Hosts. *Pleistophora myotropica* is a parasitic microsporidian that occurs in the skeletal muscle of the European toad[15,39] and has been reported in laboratory toads in Great Britain[39]. *Alloglugea bufonis* is a microsporidian that infects *Bufo marinus* tadpoles and toadlets[40].

Life Cycle. The life cycles of the microsporidia are direct. The life cycle of *Pleistophora myotropica* has been outlined (Figure 8.8[39]). The sporoplasm is thought to hatch in the gut and then migrate to the muscles by way of the vascular system. Eighteen days later, granular bodies are found in the muscle capillaries. The parasite multiplies between 18 and 23 days—first by binary fission, then by multiple fission, and finally by plasmotomy—until multinuclear sporonts are formed. Separation into sporoblasts precedes spore formation. Spores are released on the death and decomposition of the host[39,41]. Infection occurs by ingestion of a contaminated invertebrate that acts as a mechanical vector.

Pathologic Effects. Bufonids infected with *P. myotropica* may have white streaks in their striated muscles (Figure 8.9)[39]. Muscle atrophy may also occur. All stages of the parasite are seen in sections of muscle. Xenoma formation in the intestine, kidney, liver, and spleen may occur with *A. bufonis* infections[40].

Clinical Disease. Bufonids infected with *P. myotropica* or *A. bufonis* may be anorectic or emaciated, or may die suddenly. Atrophy of the muscles surrounding the long bones may occur with *P. myotropica* infection.

Diagnosis. Antemortem diagnosis is by identifying spores in the feces of infected animals. Electron microscopy is required to characterize the spores to the generic level. Postmortem diagnosis is based on identification of xenomas

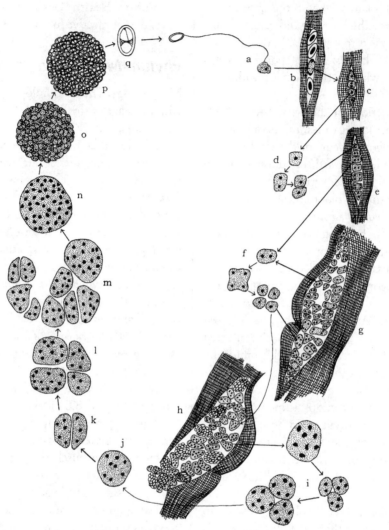

Fig. 8.8 *Pleistophora myotropica,* morphology and life cycle in skeletal muscle of a toad. (a) Sporoplasm hatches in the gut, (b) granular bodies form in muscular capillaries, (c, d) and multiply first by binary fission, (e-g) then by multiple fission, (h, i) and finally by plasmotomy (j-n) until multinuclear sporonts are formed. (o) Separation into sporoblasts precedes (p, q) spore formation. Reproduced from Canning, E.U., Elkan, E., and Trigg, P.I. (1964) with permission.

at the time of gross necropsy and spores within the tissues from histopathology.

Treatment. Microsporidian infections are difficult to treat. In the laboratory setting, it is probably best to cull infected animals. While animals are in quarantine, serial fecal samples should be collected and tested to reduce the likelihood of introducing these parasites into a colony. Chloramphenicol and topical oxytetracycline hydrochloric acid with polymyxin B have been used to suppress spore formation, but do not eliminate the parasite[42].

Prevention. Quarantining recently acquired animals, performing serial screening fecal samples, and obtaining animals from reputable breeders or wild populations where these parasites are not known to be endemic should be done to prevent the introduction of these parasites into captive amphibian colonies.

Public Health Considerations. Amphibian microsporidia do not infect humans.

Phylum Myxozoa

In some areas, amphibians are susceptible to myxosporidians in the genera *Chloromyxum* and *Myxidium.* The spores of these obligate parasites have polar capsules that are pyriform-shaped. The extent to which amphibians are exposed and infected to these parasites is unknown. While infections may be locally common in some anurans, in general, myxosporidial infections are not common in amphibians[43].

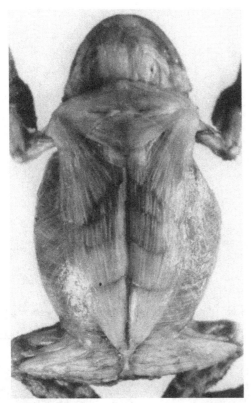

Fig. 8.9 *Pleistophora myotropica* infection in European toad. Spores packed between muscle fibers appear as white lines. Courtesy of E. Elkan, London.

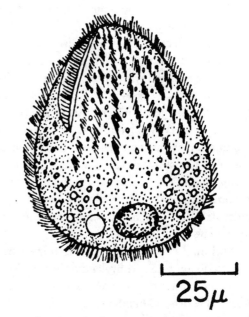

Fig. 8.10 *Balantidium duodeni.* Reproduced from Kudo, R.R. (1966) with permission.

The life cycles of the myxosporidians are indirect, typically involving invertebrate intermediate hosts. Infection with myxosporidians may cause severe, localized pathology in the intestines, muscles, kidneys, and gonads. Amphibians with heavy myxosporidian infections are generally anorectic, lethargic, and depressed. In some cases, the animals are found dead with no other history. Because the spores can be found in a variety of tissues, more specific clinical signs may occur based on the organ system involved.

Antemortem diagnosis can be made from squash preparations of affected tissues, urine, or bile. The spores have a polar capsule that is pyriform-shaped. Postmortem diagnosis is based on the presence of the spores in tissues. There is no known treatment for these parasites. Providing appropriate husbandry is considered an important method of reducing their spread. Disinfectants have been used to control infections in fish facilities. The effectiveness of these compounds for amphibian myxosporidian spores has not been tested. Until more is known regarding the life cycle of these parasites, it is difficult to make specific recommendations regarding prevention. Quarantining

animals and observing them for clinical signs consistent with the disease provide the best opportunities to reduce the likelihood of introducing these parasites. Myxosporidians from amphibians are not known to cause clinical disease in humans.

Phylum Ciliophora

Balantidium spp.

Morphology. The morphology of *Balantidium* spp. is typical of the phylum, and is described in Chapter 2, Biology of the Protozoa. Two stages occur in the life cycle, trophozoite and cyst. *Balantidium* spp. are oval, ellipsoidal, or subcylindrical, and possess longitudinally arranged rows of cilia. A peristome is located at or near the anterior end. *Balantidium entozoon, B. elongatum,* and *B. duodeni* are the species most likely to be encountered in laboratory amphibians[6,15]. *Balantidium entozoon* and *B. elongatum* measure 100 μ to 300 μ long, while *B. duodeni* measures only 70 μ to 80 μ long (Figure 8.10).

Hosts. *Balantidium entozoon* has been recovered from the intestine of the grass frog, edible frog, European toad, common newt, and crested newt from Europe. *Balantidium elongatum* occurs in the intestine of the grass frog, edible frog, alpine newt, common newt, and crested newt from both Europe and Asia. *Balantidium duodeni* occurs in the intestine of the grass frog and edible frog in Europe and Asia.

Life Cycle. The life cycle is direct. Reproduction is by conjugation and binary fission.

Pathologic Effects and Clinical Disease. *Balantidium* are not considered pathogenic. However, changes in the microbial flora associated with dietary changes, antibiotics, and stress could result in increased numbers of ciliates, possibly resulting in localized enteritis. Affected animals may be anorectic and develop diarrhea.

Diagnosis. Antemortem diagnosis is based on identifying the protozoans in a direct saline smear of the feces. *Balantidium* should not be confused with the opalinids.

Treatment. In cases where clinical disease is present, metronidazole (10 to 20 mg/kg orally once per day for seven to ten days) may be used.

Prevention. Infections may be minimized by strict adherence to quarantine and hygiene protocols. Minimizing stress in the captive environment is also important.

Public Health Considerations. *Balantidium* of amphibians do not infect humans.

Cepedietta spp.

Morphology. *Cepedietta* (Syn. *Haptophrya*) trophozoites possess an elongated, uniformly ciliated body with an anterior circular sucker and a long contractile canal[3,23,44]. No cyst is formed. *Cepedietta michiganensis* and *C. gigantean* are the species most likely to be encountered in laboratory amphibians[6,15]. *Cepedietta michiganensis* measures 1.1 mm to 1.6 mm long, while *C. gigantean* measures 1.3 to 1.6 mm long.

Hosts and Life Cycle. *Cepedietta michiganensis* has been recovered from the intestine of the leopard frog, wood frog, and American toad, and is also common in the Jefferson salamander, marbled salamander, dusky salamander, and axolotl in the United States. *Cepedietta gigantean* occurs in the intestine of the frogs and toads in Europe and Africa, and the slimy salamander (*Plethodon glutinosus*) in the United States[14]. The life cycle is direct. *Cepedietta* multiplies by budding, and often occurs as a chain of individuals.

Pathologic Effects and Clinical Disease. *Cepedietta* are not considered pathogenic. However, as for *Balantidium,* changes in the intestinal environment may result in overwhelming parasite burdens, which could cause localized enteritis. Thus, affected animals may be anorectic and develop diarrhea.

Diagnosis, Treatment, and Prevention. Diagnosis, treatment, and prevention are as described for *Balantidium*.

Public Health Considerations. *Cepedietta* do not infect humans.

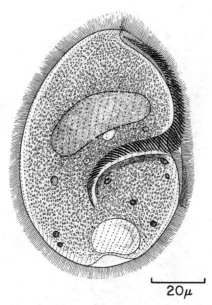

Fig. 8.11 *Nyctotheroides cordiformis.* Reproduced from Wenyon, C.M. (1926) with permission.

Nyctotheroides spp.

Morphology. *Nyctotheroides* (Syn. *Nyctotherus*) possess a flattened body, kidney-bean shaped macronucleus, small micronucleus, compound buccal cilia, long curved infundibulum, and a posterior contractile vacuole[3,23,45]. This protozoan measures 60 μ to 190 μ in length and 30 μ to 60 μ wide (Figure 8.11).

Hosts and Life Cycle. *Nyctotheroides cordiformis* has been recovered from the intestine of the leopard frog, green frog, bullfrog, grass frog, wood frog, pickerel frog, edible frog, cricket frog, European treefrog, green treefrog, spring peeper, chorus frog (*Pseudacris),* American toad, European toad, red-spotted newt, and California newt[6,15]. The life cycle is direct. Reproduction is by conjugation and binary fission. It is uncertain whether cysts are formed.

Pathologic Effects and Clinical Disease. *Nyctotheroides* are not considered pathogenic. However, as for *Balantidium,* changes in the intestinal environment may result in overwhelming parasite burdens, which could cause localized enteritis. Thus, affected animals may be anorectic and develop diarrhea.

Diagnosis, Treatment, and Prevention. Diagnosis, treatment, and prevention are as described for *Balantidium*.

Public Health Considerations. *Nyctotheroides* do not infect humans.

Trichodina spp.

Morphology. *Trichodina* possesses a bell-shaped body with a highly developed basal adhesive disc, a skeletal ring with radially arranged denticles, and an adoral zone of cilia arranged in a spiral[3,46–48]. Trophozoites measure 35 μ to 60 μ in diameter and 25 μ to 55 μ in height (Figure 8.12).

Hosts. *Trichodina urinicola, T. pediculus,* and *T. fultoni* are the species most likely to be encountered in laboratory amphibians[3,6,15,47,48]. *Trichodina urinicola* occurs in the urinary bladder of the edible frog, toads, and newts in North America, Europe, and Africa. *Trichodina pediculus* occurs on the skin of the edible frog and other frogs in North America, Europe, and Asia. *Trichodina fultoni* occurs on the gills of mudpuppies in the United States.

Life Cycle. The life cycle is direct. Asexual reproduction is by binary fission and sexual reproduction by conjugation[49].

Pathologic Effects. *Trichodina* are typically nonpathogenic. However, poor water quality, in combination with high densities of amphibians and protozoans, can result in disease. The pathology associated with this genus of protozoa in amphibians is similar to that described in fish. Affected animals may develop dermatitis. Larval amphibians may develop inflammatory changes at the levels of the gills.

Clinical Disease. Amphibians with dermatitis may rub their body against a hard surface in an attempt to remove the parasites. Excessive mucus production gives affected animals a white-gray appearance, and frequently occurs in response to the irritation caused by the parasites. Larval amphibians with parasites in the gills may be dyspneic.

Diagnosis. Antemortem diagnosis is based on identifying the protozoans from skin scrapings or gill biopsies. Postmortem diagnosis is based on identifying the parasites in skin and gill biopsies.

Treatment. Providing amphibians with good quality water is important for minimizing the risk of clinical disease. Regular water changes are required in cases in which high organic loads accumulate. Affected animals may be placed in distilled water for two to three hours, or in salt baths (10 to 25 g/L) for five to 30 minutes[19].

Prevention. Disease may be prevented by providing high quality water and adhering to quarantine and hygiene protocols.

Public Health Considerations. Trichodinids are not infectious to humans.

Opalina spp.

Morphology. *Opalina* spp. are flattened and oval and possess several nuclei. There is no cell mouth. The species most likely to be encountered in the laboratory are *O. obtrigonoidea* and *O. ranarum. Opalina obtrigonoidea* is the larger species, measuring 400 μ to 840 μ long by 175 μ to 180 μ wide; while *O. ranarum* measures approximately 300 μ long (Figure 8.13).

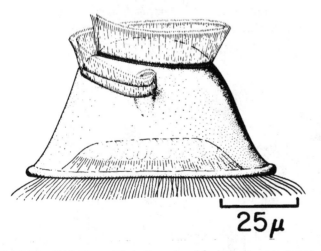

Fig. 8.12 *Trichodina urinicola.* Reproduced from Corliss, J.O. (1959) with permission.

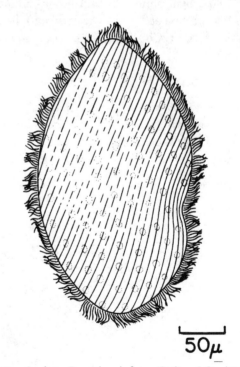

Fig. 8.13 *Opalina.* Reproduced from Corliss, J.O. (1959) with permission.

Hosts. *Opalina obtrigonoidea* has been recovered from the intestine of the leopard frog, wood frog, pickerel frog, green tree frog, spring peeper, cricket frog, chorus frog, and American toad from the United States. *Opalina ranarum* is also found in the intestine of anurans (grass frog, edible frog, European tree frog, European toad) and urodelans (alpine newt), but is only found in Europe.

Life Cycle. The life cycle is direct. The adult stage, or trophont, is located in the intestine of the amphibian, and reproduction is by simple binary fission. During the host's breeding cycle, some of the trophonts divide without growth, forming tomonts. These tomonts can encyst and pass with the feces. Larval amphibians, such as tadpoles, consume the tomonts. A sexual phase of reproduction can occur in the tadpole, eventually leading to the development of zygocysts. The zygocysts pass in the feces of the tadpole. If a metamorphosing tadpole consumes the zygocysts the life cycle is completed, and trophonts develop in the intestine of the adult frog.

Pathologic Effects and Clinical Disease. Neither pathologic lesions nor clinical signs have been described. *Opalina* feeds via pinocytosis, and is not considered to compete for nutrition with the host.

Diagnosis, Treatment, and Prevention. Diagnosis is by direct saline fecal smear. Treatment is generally not warranted. Wild-caught animals should be quarantined and screened for infection before being released into the colony.

Public Health Considerations. *Opalina* does not infect humans.

Protoopalina spp.

Morphology. *Protoopalina* spp. are cylindrical or spindle-shaped and have two nuclei. There is no cell mouth. The species most likely to be encountered in the laboratory are *P. intestinalis* and *P. mitotica*. *Protoopalina intestinalis* mea-sures 330 μ long by 68 μ wide (Figure 8.14), while *P. mitotica* measures 300 μ long by 37 μ wide.

Hosts and Life Cycle. *Protoopalina intestinalis* has been recovered from the intestine of the grass frog, edible frog, European treefrog, toads, common newt, and palmate newt from Europe, Africa, and Australia. *Protoopalina mitotica* has a narrower host distribution, and has been isolated from the intestine of the tiger salamander from the central United States. The life cycle is direct, and is similar to that of *Opalina*.

Pathologic Effects and Clinical Disease. Neither pathologic effects nor clinical disease have been reported in amphibians infected with *Protoopalina* spp.

Diagnosis, Treatment, and Prevention. These aspects are as described for *Opalina*.

Public Health Considerations. *Protoopalina* does not infect humans.

TREMATODES

Order Monogenea

Gyrodactylus spp.

Morphology. Adult *Gyrodactylus elegans* measures 500 μ to 800 μ long[51,52]. The anterior tip is bilobed. *Gyrodactylus* does not have eye spots, and an anterior sucker may or may not be present[9,53,54]. The posterior attachment organ, or haptor, often has two central hooks and is surrounded by 16 small hooklets (Figure 8.15).

Hosts. *Gyrodactylus* spp. is an important monogenetic trematode pathogen of fishes, but is also commonly found on the skin of adult aquatic amphibians and the gills of larval amphibians[9,51,56]. *Gyrodactylus* are generally host-specific, although *G. elegans* and *G. ensatus* may share hosts[54]. Some species of *Gyrodactylus* that are primary

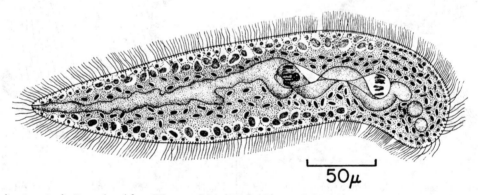

Fig. 8.14 *Protoopalina intestinalis.* Reproduced from Wenyon, C.M. (1926) with permission.

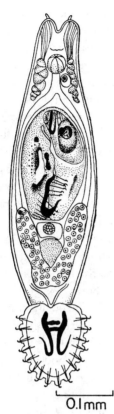

Fig. 8.15 *Gyrodactylus elegans* adult. Reproduced from Hoffman, G.L. (1967) with permission.

parasites of fishes may use amphibian larvae as paratenic hosts[9]. The incidence of *Gyrodactylus* in adult and larval captive anurans and urodelans is unknown, but may be high among wild populations or captive animals maintained at high density with poor water quality.

Life Cycle. The life cycle is direct. Adult *Gyrodactylus* are viviparous. Larvae develop within the uterus of the adult, and may themselves have larvae developing within them (serial polyembryony). Thus, large numbers of parasites may develop within the host. Larvae released into the environment swim until they locate a new host, where they attach to the skin or gills, and develop into adults[51]. *Gyrodactylus* is an obligate parasite and cannot survive more than 20 minutes unattached[51].

Pathologic Effects. Gyrodactylid flukes attach to the gills, fins, and skin of larval anurans and urodelans, and to the skin of adult anurans and urodelans. Heavy infestations on the gills can cause severe inflammation, reducing the surface area for respiratory exchange. In severe cases, larval tadpoles and urodelans may succumb to asphyxiation. Damage caused along the integument can lead to a failure of the innate immune system and allow opportunistic

bacterial and fungal pathogens to invade. Gyrodactylid flukes ingest blood from the superficial capillaries and epithelium lining the gills and skin[51,57].

Clinical Disease. Tadpoles and larval urodelans infested with gyrodactylids may be found gasping for air at the water surface because of an inability to transfer oxygen and excrete carbon dioxide at the gills. Because the gills of larval urodelans can be observed directly, they may appear swollen and covered with mucous. Increased mucous is often observed on the integument of amphibians with gyrodactylid infestations of the skin. Affected animals appear pruritic and may rub on hard surfaces within an enclosure in an attempt to dislodge the parasites.

Diagnosis. Gyrodactylid infestations can be diagnosed cytologically. A gill clip/biopsy can be collected from larval urodelans antemortem. A fine pair of iris scissors should be used to clip a sample of the gill. Internal gill samples from tadpoles are generally collected at postmortem. A glass slide can be used to perform a skin scrape in amphibians when a skin infestation is suspected. The glass slide should be placed cranial to the lesion and drawn caudally. Once collected, the samples should be placed on a glass slide with a drop of water from the enclosure from which the patient was removed. A coverslip is applied and the specimen examined under light microscopy.

Treatment. Because gyrodactylid trematodes are viviparous, both larval and adult forms of the parasite can be eliminated with water bath treatments. In addition, because this parasite can generally only survive off hosts for a short period of time, treatment may include water baths for the animals outside of the primary enclosure, with replacement into a new enclosure. Praziquantel is the treatment of choice. Bathing amphibians in a 10 mg/L water bath for three hours has been found to be effective[9]. Additional treatments can be given if a single treatment does not eliminate the parasites. Because these parasites commonly infest fishes, treatments used to eliminate them from fishes can also be considered for amphibians. Formalin baths are routinely used to eliminate these parasites from fishes (200 to 250 ppm for one hour), and have also been used by some to eliminate them from amphibians (formalin: 1.5 ml/L, 10 minutes, repeat weekly for three treatments)[9].

Prevention. To prevent the introduction of gyrodactylids into a laboratory colony, animals should only be accepted from approved, licensed breeders. New arrivals should be quarantined and skin scrapes evaluated to determine carrier status. Water samples can also be collected, centrifuged, the supernatant poured off, and the sediment evaluated for the presence of free-swimming gyrodactylids.

Public Health Considerations. Gyrodactylids do not affect humans.

Polystoma spp.

Morphology. Adult polystome trematodes vary in size and morphology, depending on whether they are located in the bladder or on the gills[58]. Those found in the bladder measure 250 to 450 μ long and 90 to 150 μ wide, while those found on the gills measure 160 μ to 500 μ long and 30 μ to 80 μ wide. The bladder form has a cordiform caudal disc with six cup-shaped, muscular suckers and two large hooks. The gill form has a caudal disc with six pedunculated suckers and only rudimentary hooks, if any (Figure 8.16). The larva is just slightly smaller than the adult is partly covered with cilia, and has four eye spots and a posterior sucker with 16 hooks. The eye spots are used to identify new hosts, and the cilia are used to assist the fluke in swimming to the tadpole. Eggs produced by both species of polystomes are ovoid and measure approximately 30 μ to 150 μ long.

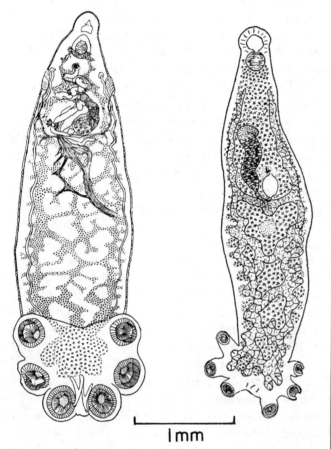

|1mm|

Fig. 8.16 *Polystoma nearticum.* (Left) Adult from bladder. (Right) Adult from gills. Reproduced from Paul, A.A. (1938) with permission.

Hosts. Polystome trematodes are the most common monogenetic trematodes of amphibians[15,59], and are primarily associated with anurans and less commonly with urodelans. Polystomes generally invade the gills of larval amphibians and the urinary bladders of adult amphibians. *Polystoma nearcticum* is found in North America and affects treefrogs[58]. *Polystoma integerrimum* is found in Europe, Asia, and Africa, and affects frogs, treefrogs, and toads[6,16,60]. The incidence of infections in anurans is generally considered low. In one survey of grassfrogs in Great Britain, 12.5% were found to be infected[61]. Young male frogs are most susceptible, and the rate of infection is highest in the autumn.

Life Cycle. Adult flukes are located in the urinary bladder. Egg laying coincides with the spawning period of the host to maximize the likelihood of providing a ready source of tadpole hosts for newly emerged larvae (oncomiracidium)[51,58]. The incubation period for the eggs is approximately two weeks. Egg development can be altered by exposure to both light and temperature[62]. Eggs exposed to alternating light and darkness only hatched in the light. This appears to be related to the need for the oncomiracidium to use their eyespots to identify potential hosts. Eggs hatched at 10°C required a longer incubation time (approximately one month) compared to those eggs hatched at 18°C. Once hatched, the free-swimming oncomiracidium attach to the gills of a tadpole. After a three-week maturation period, the flukes on the gills begin to lay eggs. The larvae produced from the gill stage infect the urinary bladder. It is not known how the larvae enter the bladder, but it is thought that they are ingested and passed through the gastrointestinal tract where they enter the bladder through the urodeum, or directly enter the vent and migrate through the urodeum to the bladder. Once in the bladder, the flukes remain with the host through metamorphosis and mature at the same time as the host. Thus, there is an alternation of generations, one requiring three weeks, one requiring three years.

Pathologic Effects and Clinical Disease. *Polystoma* feed on blood from the gills and urinary bladder[51]. However, they do not appear to cause significant disease.

Diagnosis. Polystomes, like gyrodactylids, can be diagnosed cytologically. Diagnosis is generally made at postmortem from a gill biopsy of a tadpole or from a biopsy of the urinary bladder from a tadpole or adult anuran.

Treatment. Although there are no reports of amphibians being treated for *Polystoma* infection, formalin (1.5 ml/L, ten minutes, repeat weekly for three treatments) or praziquantel water baths (10 mg/L, three hours) would likely be effective[9].

Prevention. The best method to prevent the introduction of these parasites into a laboratory colony of amphibians is to only accept animals from approved, licensed breeders. New arrivals should be quarantined. Water samples can also be collected, centrifuged, the supernatant poured off, and the sediment evaluated for the presence of free-swimming oncomiracidium.

Public Health Considerations. Humans are not susceptible to infection with polystomes.

Sphyranura spp.

Morphology. Adult *Sphyranura* measure 2.5 mm to 3 mm long[14,63]. The haptor is comprised of two large muscular suckers, two large hooks, seven small hooks on each side, and one hook in each sucker. Five to 23 testes are usually arranged linearly between the intestinal branches. The ovary is ovoid and is located just anterior to the center of the body (Figure 8.17).

Hosts. *Sphyranura oligorchis, S. polyorchis,* and *S. osleri* are common on the gills of the mudpuppy in North America[6,14,15]. Although there are no specific reports of these parasites in the laboratory, they are probably common on mudpuppies obtained from the wild.

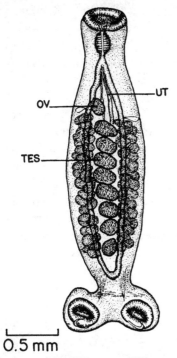

Fig. 8.17 *Sphyranura* adult. OV, ovary; TES, testes; UT, uterus. Reproduced from Cheng, T.C. (1964) with permission.

Life Cycle. Adult *Sphyranura* parasitize the gills of their host. The flukes are oviparous. After the eggs are laid, they settle in the substrate and hatch after 28 to 32 days[63]. The larvae have two different modes of locomotion: creeping or using their caudal disc to swim. Larvae must find a host within a few hours of hatching to survive. The larva, like the adult flukes, parasitize the gills. Once the larvae are attached to the gill, they require approximately two months for development to adults.

Pathologic Effects. *Sphyranura* ingest blood from the branchial circulation[63]. Heavy parasite burdens damage the gill filaments. In severe cases, excessive mucus production and mechanical damage lead to dyspnea and asphyxiation.

Clinical Disease. The clinical presentation for mudpuppies infested with *Sphyranura* spp. depends on parasite burden. Animals with low parasite burdens may be asymptomatic, while animals with heavy burdens develop respiratory distress. In severe cases, affected animals gasp at the surface of the water.

Diagnosis, Treatment, and Prevention. Diagnosis is by cytologic identification of parasites on gill biopsy. To date, no treatment methods have been described. Because praziquantel baths (10 mg/L for three hours) have been found to be effective against other monogenean flukes, this treatment may also be effective against *Sphyranura*[9]. No control methods have been described. The best method to prevent the introduction of these parasites into a laboratory colony of mudpuppies is to only accept animals from approved, licensed breeders. New arrivals should be quarantined. Gill biopsies can be performed to screen animals, although the sensitivity of this procedure may not be high with low parasite burdens. Water samples can also be collected, centrifuged, the supernatant poured off, and the sediment evaluated for the presence of the flukes.

Public Health Considerations. *Sphyranura* does not affect humans.

Order Digenea

Adult Trematodes

Brachycoelium salamandrae

Morphology. Adult *Brachycoelium salamandrae* measure 3 mm to 5 mm in length. Adults have short intestinal cecae that end at the level of the ventral sucker (Figure 8.18)[52,64]. The testes are rounded and symmetrical, while the ovary is anterior to the left testis. The uterus has long, folded, descending and ascending limbs and fills the posterior part

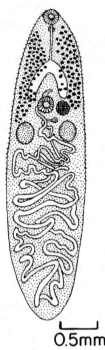

Fig. 8.18 *Brachycoelium salamandrae* adult. Reproduced from Dawes, B. (1946) with permission.

of the body. The genital pore is anterior to the ventral sucker. Vitellaria are confined to the anterior region. The eggs are light brown and measure 45 μ to 50 μ by 32 μ to 36 μ long.

Hosts. *Brachycoelium salamandrae* has a cosmopolitan distribution, and is one of the most common intestinal trematodes of amphibians[14,15,65,66]. Infections have also been reported in reptiles. *Brachycoelium salamandrae* has been isolated from wood frogs, pickerel frogs, cricket frogs, chorus frogs, green treefrogs, spring peepers, toads, mole salamanders, dusky salamanders, woodland salamanders (*Plethodon* spp.), red-spotted newts, and amphiumas from North America, and from grass frogs, European toads, European salamanders, and newts from Europe[6,16,66]. Terrestrial salamanders are more commonly infected than aquatic salamanders or frogs[14]. The prevalence of this parasite in amphibians from the eastern United States is variable and has been found to range from 11% to 100%[14,66,67,68].

Life Cycle. The life cycle requires a mollusk intermediate host[6,17]. The cercariae and metacercariae develop in the snail. The amphibian host becomes infected after ingesting an infected snail.

Pathologic Effects and Clinical Disease. Nothing is known of the pathologic effects of *B. salamandrae*. Infected

amphibians are asymptomatic. Animals with heavy burdens may become obstructed or develop diarrhea.

Diagnosis, Treatment, and Prevention. Antemortem diagnosis is by identifying eggs on a fecal flotation. Postmortem diagnosis is by demonstrating flukes in the intestines at necropsy. Although no treatment has been described, praziquantel (8 to 14 mg/kg orally every 14 days for three treatments) may be used. Because of the need for a mollusk intermediate host, it is unlikely that the life cycle would be completed in the laboratory.

Public Health Considerations. *Brachycoelium salamandrae* does not infect humans.

Diplodiscus spp.

Morphology. Adult trematodes measure 6 mm in length and 2.2 mm in thickness[15,17,63]. These flukes are conical rather than flat. All species have a well-developed oral sucker (which has a pair of posterior diverticula) and a large, terminal posterior sucker. Mature forms have only one testis[64].

Hosts. *Diplodiscus* spp. have been isolated from the large intestine of amphibians[6,66]. *Diplodiscus subclavatus* (Syn. *Opisthodiscus subclavatus*) is common in Europe, Africa, Asia, Australia, and New Zealand, and has been isolated from the large intestine of grass frogs, edible frogs, treefrogs, European toads, clawed toads, European salamanders, and newts[6,66]. *Diplodiscus japonicus* infects the large intestine and cloaca of frogs from Asia, and is the most common trematode of amphibians from Japan[6,15,66]. *Diplodiscus unguiculatus* infects the rectum of newts while *D. diplodiscoides* is found in the large intestine of edible frogs in Europe[6,66].

Life Cycle. The life cycle is indirect, and involves a snail intermediate host. In addition, the amphibian itself or another amphibian may serve as a second intermediate host[6,17,63,66,69]. Adult amphibians pass embryonated eggs in the feces. After hatching, larval flukes enter a snail and develop into cercariae. This stage of the life cycle requires approximately 90 days. Cercariae escape from the snail and encyst as metacercariae in the skin of larval or adult amphibians. Adult amphibians generally become infected from ingesting their sloughed epithelium. Larval amphibians, and possibly adults, can also become infected by ingesting cercariae. In these cases, cercariae encyst in the mouth, pass to the intestine, excyst, and remain there through metamorphosis. The prepatent period for those animals that ingest cercariae is approximately two to three months. Adult trematodes survive for about a year.

Pathologic Effects and Clinical Disease. Nothing is known of the pathologic effects of *Diplodiscus* spp. However, heavy burdens may cause localized inflammatory responses. Affected amphibians are asymptomatic.

Diagnosis, Treatment, and Prevention. Antemortem diagnosis is by identifying eggs on a fecal flotation or urine sample. Postmortem diagnosis is by demonstrating flukes at necropsy. Treatment recommendations are as described for *Brachycoelium salamandrae*. Because of the need for an intermediate host, the completion of the life cycle in the laboratory is unlikely.

Public Health Considerations. *Diplodiscus* spp. do not infect humans.

Dolichosaccus rastellus

Morphology. Adult *Dolichosaccus* are oval, wide, and measure 2 mm to 4 mm long and 0.8 mm to 1.2 mm wide[52]. The testes are at the posterior end of the body and the uterus anterior to them; the vitellaria extend beyond to level of the testes[64,66].

Hosts. *Dolichosaccus rastellus* (Syn. *Lecithopyge rastellum*) is a common intestinal trematode of European amphibians[15] including edible frogs, grass frogs, European toads, European salamanders, and several species of newts. It is the predominant species in Great Britain, where an 8% incidence has been observed in grass frogs obtained from their natural habitat[61].

Life Cycle. The life cycle requires two intermediate hosts[15]. A gastropod serves as the first intermediate host, while an insect or possibly a tadpole serves as the second intermediate host. The final host becomes infected by ingesting the insect or tadpole.

Pathologic Effects and Clinical Disease. Nothing is known of the pathologic effects of *D. rastellus*. Amphibians infected with *D. rastellus* are generally asymptomatic. Heavy burdens could result in intestinal obstruction or diarrhea.

Diagnosis, Treatment, and Prevention. Diagnosis is by demonstrating parasites in the intestine at necropsy. Although no treatment has been described, praziquantel (8 to 14 mg/kg orally every 14 days for three treatments) may be used. Because of the need for a mollusk and an insect as intermediate hosts, it is unlikely that the life cycle of these trematodes would be completed in captivity.

Public Health Considerations. *Dolichosaccus* spp. do not infect humans.

Glypthelmins spp.

Morphology. Adult *Glypthelmins pennsylvaniensis* measure 1.8 mm long by 0.6 mm wide[70]. The ovary is posterior to

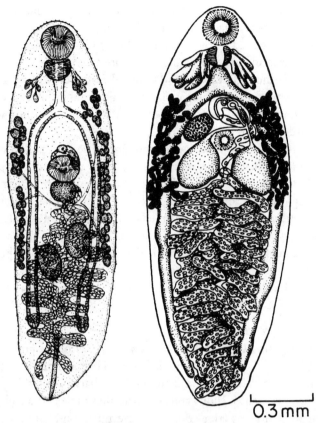

Fig. 8.19 (Left) *Glypthelmins pennsylvaniensis* adult. (Right) *G. quieta* adult. (Left) reproduced from Cheng, T.C. (1961) with permission. (Right) reproduced from Skrjabin, K.I. (1964) with permission.

the acetabulum, and the testes are arranged obliquely in the posterior half of the body. *Glypthelmins quieta* is similar in size and morphology, but the ovary is anterior to the acetabulum, and the testes are more anterior and are situated side by side (Figure 8.19).

Hosts. *Glypthelmins pennsylvaniensis* occurs in the intestine of spring peepers, bullfrogs, and chorus frogs (*Pseudacris*) in the United States; *G. quieta* occurs in the intestine of leopard frogs, green frogs, pickerel frogs, bullfrogs, chorus frogs, spring peepers, and toads in the United States, Mexico, South America, and Asia[6,66,68,71]. The prevalence of infection with *G. pennsylvaniensis* varies with species and range, with a 10% to 15% prevalence of infection in chorus frogs from the western United States, 30% prevalence in bullfrogs, and 18% prevalence in spring peepers from the northeastern United States.

Life Cycle. The life cycle is similar for both species and involves a snail intermediate host[70,72]. Free-swimming cercariae escape from the snail, penetrate the skin of the definitive host (anuran), encyst, and form metacercariae. The metacercariae are sloughed during ecdysis, the shed skin is ingested by the anuran, and the flukes complete the life cycle and become adults in the intestine.

Pathologic Effects and Clinical Disease. Nothing is known of the pathologic effects of these flukes. Affected anurans are generally asymptomatic. Animals with heavy burdens could develop diarrhea.

Diagnosis, Treatment, and Prevention. Fecal flotation or direct saline smear can be used to demonstrate fluke eggs in the feces of infected anurans. Postmortem diagnosis is by demonstration of the parasites in the skin or intestine at necropsy. Treatment options are as described for *Dolichosaccus rastellus*. Because of the need for a snail intermediate host, it is unlikely that the life cycle would be completed in the laboratory.

Public Health Considerations. *Glypthelmins* spp. do not infect humans.

Gorgodera spp.

Morphology. *Gorgodera amplicava* is typical of the genus. Adults measure about 4 mm in length. There is both an oral sucker and a large ventral sucker[73]. A pharynx is lacking, the esophagus is short, and the cecae are simple and terminate at the posterior end. Testes are numerous, round or irregular in shape, and arranged in two rows or one zigzag row. The genital pore is median or slightly submedian. The ovary is submedian, and the vitellaria are compact or lobed and paired (Figure 8.20). Eggs are non-operculated and embryonated when passed.

Hosts. *Gorgodera* spp. have a cosmopolitan distribution, and are found in the excretory systems of amphibians[6,73,74]. *Gorgodera amplicava* is commonly found (35%) in the bullfrog in the southern United States[75]. Infections are also common in urodelans.

Life Cycle. The life cycle is indirect[74]. Eggs passed by adults hatch upon reaching water. They are drawn into the mantel of a clam, enter through the gills, and develop into cercariae. Cercariae are ingested by frog tadpoles, salamander larvae, snails, or crayfish, and develop into metacercariae within 24 hours. In tadpoles, *Gorgodera* spp. generally encyst in the intestine[9]. The final host, an adult amphibian, becomes infected by ingesting the second intermediate host. After excysting in the stomach or intestine, larval flukes migrate down the alimentary tract into the cloaca, where they enter the urodeum and eventually the reproductive and excretory ducts. They remain in the ducts for approximately two weeks and then migrate to the urinary bladder and/or the kidneys, where they mature to adults in three weeks to two months.

Pathologic Effects and Clinical Disease. Generally, problems only arise with heavy trematode burdens[74]. Migrating larvae may cause tissue damage. Heavy renal fluke burdens result in renal tubule and duct occlusion and renal impairment. Most amphibians with low parasite burdens are asymptomatic. However, anorexia, listlessness, and death are common clinical findings in amphibians with heavy infections.

Diagnosis, Treatment, and Prevention. Diagnosis is by demonstration of flukes in the kidneys or urinary bladder at necropsy. Antemortem diagnosis can be made from a fecal examination or cloacal wash. While treatment may result in death in the flukes, the deteriorating parasites may cause vascular obstruction, leading to tissue necrosis. Anti-inflammatory drugs may be used to minimize harmful reactions to dying parasites. Some have suggested that digenetic flukes may be managed with praziquantel (8 to 14 mg/kg orally every 14 days for three treatments)[9]. However, this dosing regimen is empirical. Because of the need for a mollusk intermediate host, it is unlikely that the life cycle could be completed in the laboratory.

Public Health Considerations. *Gorgodera* spp. do not infect humans.

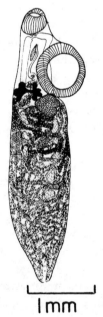

I mm

Fig. 8.20 *Gorgodera amplicava* adult. Reproduced from Goodchild, C.G. (1948) with permission.

Gorgoderina spp.

Flukes in the genus *Gorgoderina* are morphologically, biologically, and pathologically similar to *Gorgodera*[66]. *Gorgoderina vitelliloba* has been reported in 11.8% of grass frogs from Great Britain[61], while *G. bilobata* has been isolated from up to 16.5% of dusky salamanders and 7.3% of red-spotted newts in the southeastern United States[14]. *Gorgoderina* sp. encysts in the heart and liver of tadpoles[9]. Diagnosis, treatment, and prevention are as described for *Gorgodera*. These flukes do not affect humans.

Haematoloechus spp.

Morphology. Adult *Haematoloechus* spp. have a flattened body with a densely spined cuticle. Adult flukes measure 8 mm long by 1.2 mm wide[57,63,64]. The testes are oval and situated in the posterior one-third of the body. The ovary is elongate, smaller than the testes, and located in the middle third of the body. The genital pore is near the cecal bifurcation. Vitellaria are arranged in rosette-like configurations or clusters (Figure 8.21).

Hosts and Life Cycle. More than 40 species of *Haematoloechus* have been isolated from the lungs of anurans throughout the world[6,57,66]. The life cycle is indirect, and involves both snail and insect intermediate hosts[6,63]. Embryonated eggs deposited by the adult in the lung cavity pass up the respiratory tract to the mouth in the sputum, are swallowed, and are voided in the feces. The eggs do not hatch until they are ingested by a snail. Cercariae develop in the snail, are released, and are ingested by an insect. The frog or toad becomes infected by ingesting the insect.

Pathologic Effects and Clinical Disease. Little is known of pathologic effects induced by *Haematoloechus* spp. Heavy burdens may cause severe anemia[15], and are known to occur in anurans, with as many as 75 flukes being observed in a single frog[63]. Affected animals may become lethargic and weak due to anemia, and may die suddenly. Post-treatment mortality may be caused by pulmonary emboli.

Diagnosis, Treatment, and Prevention. Antemortem diagnosis can be made from identifying eggs on a fecal flotation. Postmortem diagnosis is based on demonstration and identification of the flukes in the lungs at necropsy. Treatment recommendations are as described for *Brachycoelium salamandrae*. Because of the need for two intermediate hosts, it is unlikely that the life cycle would be completed in the laboratory.

Public Health Considerations. *Haematoloechus* spp. does not infect humans.

Halipegus spp.

Morphology. Adult *Halipegus* measure 6 mm to 6.5 mm long and 1.8 mm wide[57,64]. The adult flukes are conical

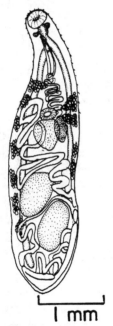

Fig. 8.21 *Haematoloechus* adult. Reproduced from Cheng, T.C. (1964) with permission.

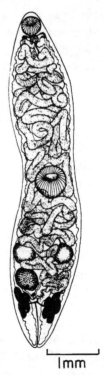

Fig. 8.22 *Halipegus* adult. Reproduced from Skrjabin, K.I. (1964) with permission.

rather than flat. The ventral sucker is near the middle of the body. The testes are in the posterior one-third of the body, and the ovaries are posterior to the testes. Two compact vitellaria are present and they are posterior to the ovary (Figure 8.22).

Hosts. *Halipegus* spp. inhabit the mouth, ear canals, pharynx, stomach, or intestine of frogs, toads, and occasionally reptiles[6,66]. *Halipegus eccentricus, H. occidualis,* and *H. amherstensis* occur in North America. *Halipegus eccentricus* is found in the ear canals of leopard frogs, green frogs, and bullfrogs; *H. occidualis* is found in the mouth, ear canals, and pharynx of leopard frogs, green frogs, and bullfrogs; and *H. amherstensis* is found in the mouth and ear canals of green frogs and bullfrogs. *Halipegus ovocaudatus* has been isolated from the mouth of edible frogs, grass frogs, and toads from Europe and southern Africa.

Life Cycle. The life cycle involves two intermediate hosts, a snail and a copepod or insect[63,68]. Eggs deposited by the adult trematode pass through the alimentary tract and are voided with the feces. The eggs are ingested by a snail, hatch, and then develop into cercariae. The cercariae are then ingested by a copepod or by an insect, and the amphibian becomes infected after ingesting the second intermediate host.

Pathologic Effects and Clinical Disease. Nothing is known of the pathologic effects of these trematodes; however, heavy burdens may cause local inflammation. Affected amphibians are generally asymptomatic.

Diagnosis, Treatment, and Prevention. Diagnosis, treatment, and prevention are as described for *Brachycoelium salamandrae.*

Public Health Considerations. *Halipegus* spp. do not infect humans.

Haplometra cylindracea

Morphology. The adult *Haplometra cylindracea* is elongate, cylindrical, and approximately 10 mm in length, although larger specimens of up to 20 mm have been described[52,66]. The ventral sucker is smaller than the oral sucker and posterior to it. The intestine bifurcates anterior to the ventral sucker. The testes are spherical, one behind the other, and located in the caudal third of the parasite; the ovary is anterior to the testes. The genital pore is located on the median and near the ventral sucker (Figure 8.23). Eggs are dark brown and measure 220 μ long by 40 μ wide.

Hosts. *Haplometra cylindracea* is a pulmonary trematode that has been isolated from edible frogs, grass frogs, treefrogs, and European toads[52,66]. In one study, *H. cylindracea*

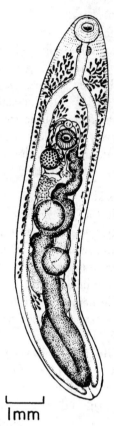

Fig. 8.23 *Haplometra cylindracea* adult. Reproduced from Skrjabin, K.I. (1964) with permission.

was found in 54% of grass frogs from Great Britain[61]. Parasite burdens vary widely, and range from five to 60 worms.

Life Cycle. The life cycle requires two intermediate hosts, a snail and a water beetle[6]. Adult anurans become infected with this parasite after consuming infected water beetles.

Pathologic Effects and Clinical Disease. Adult flukes attach to the pulmonary epithelium, where they ingest blood[76]. Affected anurans are generally asymptomatic. Although uncommon, heavy infestations could result in anemia.

Diagnosis, Treatment, and Prevention. Antemortem diagnosis is by identifying eggs in the sputum or feces of affected anurans. Postmortem diagnosis is made at necropsy by identifying the adult parasites in the lungs. Treatment attempts are as described for *Brachycoelium salamandrae.* Premedicating affected animals with an anti-inflammatory drug may diminish the risk of pulmonary emboli. Because of the need for two intermediate hosts, one of which is a water beetle, it is unlikely that the life cycle would be completed in the laboratory.

Public Health Considerations. *Haplometra cylindracea* does not infect humans.

Megalodiscus spp.

Megalodiscus spp. are morphologically similar to *Diplodiscus*, except that adult flukes have two testes (Figure 8.24)[64]. *Megalodiscus temperatus* is common in the Americas, and has been isolated from the large intestine of leopard frogs, green frogs, bullfrogs, green tree frogs, spring peepers, chorus frogs (*Pseudacris*), common toads, mole salamanders, dusky salamanders, water newts, and amphiumas[65,66]. The prevalence of *M. temperatus* in red-spotted newts in the eastern United States is 16% to 48%[14,65,68]. *Megalodiscus americanus* has been isolated from the intestine of leopard frogs, mole salamanders, dusky salamanders, California newts, and amphiuma from North America and Central America. *Megalodiscus intermedius* occurs in the rectum of bullfrogs and dusky salamanders; *M. microphagus* in the large intestine and urinary bladder of frogs, toads, and salamanders; and *M. rankini* in the intestine of red-spotted newts in the United States[66,69]. The life cycle and other aspects of the biology of *Megalodiscus* are similar to *Diplodiscus*.

Opisthioglyphe ranae

The genus *Opisthioglyphe* is morphologically, biologically, and pathologically similar to *Dolichosaccus* (Figure 8.25)[52,64,66]. *Opisthioglyphe ranae* (Syn. *Opisthioglyphe endoloba, Lecithopyge ranae*) is a common intestinal trematode of European amphibians[15,] occurring in edible frogs, grass frogs, treefrogs, European toads, clawed toads, European salamanders, and crested newts, and is the predominant species in continental Europe[15,66]. Diagnosis, treatment, and prevention are as described for *Brachycoelium salamandrae*. *Opisthioglyphe* spp. do not infect humans.

Pleurogenes spp.

Morphology. Adult *Pleurogenes claviger* are cylindrical and approximately 3 mm long, while adult *P. medians* are oval and approximately 1 mm long[15]. Vitellaria are restricted to the anterior half of the body, and the genital pore is anterior to the ventral sucker[64]. The intestinal ceca are long, extending beyond the ventral sucker, and the testes are posterior to the intestine (Figure 8.26).

Hosts. *Pleurogenes claviger* and *P. medians* occur in the small intestines of grass frogs, edible frogs, treefrogs, European toads, common newts, and crested newts from Europe (Walton 1964). *Pleurogenes medians* has also been reported in anurans and urodelans from Africa[6].

Life Cycle. The life cycle of *Pleurogenes* spp. involves two intermediate hosts, a snail and an arthropod. The cercariae develop in the snail, while the metacercariae develop

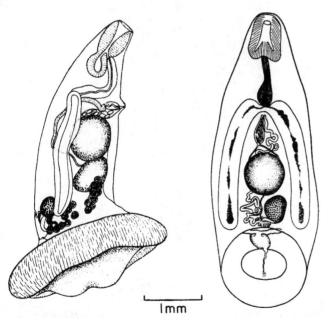

Fig. 8.24 (Left) *Megalodiscus* adult. (Right) *Diplodiscus* adult. Reproduced from Skrjabin, K.I. (1964) with permission.

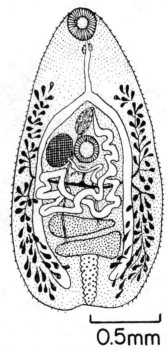

Fig. 8.25 *Opisthioglyphe ranae* adult. Reproduced from Dawes, B. (1946) with permission.

in the arthropod[6,15]. Adult anurans become infected after ingesting an infected arthropod.

Pathologic Effects and Clinical Disease. Nothing is known of the pathologic effects of these trematodes; however, heavy burdens may cause a localized inflammatory response. Affected amphibians are asymptomatic. Animals with heavy burdens may become obstructed or develop diarrhea.

Diagnosis, Treatment, and Prevention. Diagnosis, treatment, and prevention are as described for *Brachycoelium salamandrae*. *Pleurogenes* spp. do not infect humans.

Prosotocus confuses

Prosotocus confuses is morphologically similar to *Pleurogenes medians*, except that the intestinal ceca are short and the testes are located anterior to the intestine (Figure 8.26). *Prosotocus confuses* has been reported in grass frogs, edible frogs, and European toads from both Europe and southwestern Asia[6]. Other aspects of the biology of *P. confuses* are similar to *Pleurogenes* spp.

Larval Trematodes

Diplostomulum scheuringi

Morphology. Larval *Diplostomulum scheuringi* are unencysted and measure approximately 1 mm long and 0.2 mm wide[77]. The hindbody and lateral suckers are poorly differentiated. Numerous, small calcareous corpuscles are irregularly scattered throughout the parenchyma. Large, longitudinal muscle fibers give the body a striated appearance (Figure 8.27). The cercarial stage that occurs in the mollusk is typically strigeid[78]. An encysted form, the third intermediate stage, has been experimentally produced in rodents[78], but the adult and the egg are unknown[6].

Hosts. Amphibians serve as second intermediate hosts for larval diplostomulid flukes. *Diplostomulum scheuringi* occurs in the brain and eyes of red-spotted newts and greater sirens (*Siren lacertian*) in the United States[6,78]. Infections are common (12% to 100%) in the red-spotted newt and are likely to be encountered in laboratory specimens obtained from their natural habitat[78,79].

Life Cycle. The life cycle of *D. scheuringi* is not completely known[78]. The first larval stage, the cercariae, develops in a snail. The cercariae are shed by the snail and penetrate either the cornea of an adult newt or the cornea or skin of a larval newt. Cercariae that penetrate the skin of a larval newt usually migrate to the brain. It is also possible that those that enter the eye migrate through the optic stalk to the brain. These larval trematodes do not encyst in the urodelan intermediate host. Rodents experimentally infected with unencysted larvae develop encysted stages, suggesting that this parasite follows a four-host life cycle.

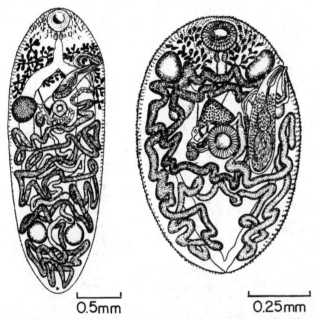

0.5mm   0.25mm

Fig. 8.26 (Left) *Pleurogenes claviger* adult. (Right) *Prosotocus confusus* adult. Reproduced from Skrjabin, K.I. (1964) with permission.

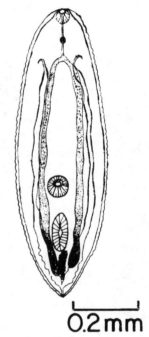

0.2mm

Fig. 8.27 *Diplostomulum scheuringi.* Fully developed, unencysted larva from the brain of a red-spotted newt. Reproduced from Etges, F.J. (1961) with permission.

The definitive host and the length of time required to complete the entire life cycle of this parasite are unknown.

Pathologic Effects and Clinical Disease. The cercariae produce small hemorrhages at the point of host penetration[78]. Those that enter the eye lodge chiefly in the vitreous body and may migrate along the optic stalk to the brain, but apparently never invade the lens[77]. Those that enter through the skin are carried by the circulatory system to the brain, leading to an increase in ventricular size, hyperplasia, and increased pigmentation of the meninges, and either hyperplasia of the choroids plexus or, when located intraventricularly, an absence of the plexus[79]. A relationship between the presence of the parasite and brain tumor formation has been suggested. Urodelans with low worm burdens may be asymptomatic, while animals with heavy burdens may be depressed, anorexic, or have difficulty navigating through their environment.

Diagnosis, Treatment, and Prevention. Postmortem diagnosis is by identification of larvae at necropsy. Because of the need for a snail intermediate host, and an unknown definitive host, it is unlikely that the life cycle would be completed in the laboratory. No treatment recommendations are available.

Public Health Considerations. *Diplostomulum scheuringi* does not infect humans.

Diplostomulum xenopi

Morphology. Larval *Diplostomulum xenopi* are unencysted and measure 0.5 mm long and 0.3 mm wide[80]. The cuticle is thin and lacks spines. The oral sucker is subterminal and has an auricular projection on either side (Figure 8.28). The lateral suckers are poorly developed and the acetabulum, which is located in the anterior part of the posterior half, is comparatively small and oval. Slightly posterior to the acetabulum is the tribocytic or holdfast organ. The latter is large, oval, and covered with proteolytic gland cells. Primordial gonads are immediately posterior to the tribocytic organ. The hindbody is poorly developed. Calcareous concretions are scattered throughout the body. Nothing is known of the morphology of the adult, egg, or cercarial forms.

Hosts. Larval flukes can be found in the pericardial cavity of the South African clawed frog[80,81]. The larvae have been found in imported clawed frogs from both the United States and Great Britain. These larval parasites appear to be common in this amphibian; the prevalence in laboratory specimens imported into the United States is 78%[80].

Life Cycle. The life cycle is unknown. It is presumed to involve a mollusk, probably a snail, as the first intermediate host, and a reptile as the definitive host[80].

Pathologic Effects and Clinical Disease. Motile larval flukes are readily observable in the pericardial cavity with the aid of a hand lens[80]. They are often present in large numbers, 25 to 150 per frog. These flukes do not encyst and, consequently, remain in the pericardial sac as long as the frog lives. The larvae can act as foreign bodies and cause an exudative pericarditis. The pericardial sac distends, encroaches on the lungs, and causes a reduced respiratory capacity. Concurrently, the increased intrapericardial pressure interferes with venous input and results in decreased cardiac output. These combine to produce hypoxia, respiratory failure, and death. Sudden death may occur in compromised animals.

Diagnosis, Treatment, and Prevention. Diagnosis is based on clinical signs and recovery of flukes in the pericardium. Currently, there is no treatment for this parasite.

Because of the probable need for a mollusk intermediate host, and an unknown definitive host, it unlikely that the life cycle would be completed in the laboratory.

Public Health Considerations. *Diplostomulum xenopi* does not infect humans.

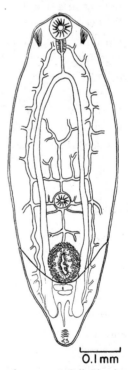

Fig. 8.28 *Diplostomulum xenopi.* Fully developed, unencysted larva from pericardial cavity of a South African clawed toad. Reproduced from Nigrelli, R.F. and Maraventano, L.W. (1944) with permission.

0.1 mm

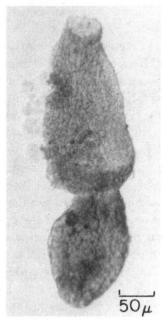

Fig. 8.29 *Neascus* sp. metacercaria from a cyst in the skin of a South African clawed toad. Reproduced from Elkan, E. and Murray, R.W. (1952) with permission.

Neascus sp.

A diplostomatid metacercaria (Figure 8.29) presumably of the larval genus *Neascus* has been reported once in Great Britain in a group of four imported South African clawed toads[82]. The metacercariae encyst in the skin below the lateral line system and cause a local proliferation of melanophores at the site of each neuromast (Figure 8.30). Affected toads die shortly after the infection becomes apparent. Nothing is known of the life cycle, control, or public health importance of this parasite.

CESTODES

Pseudophyllidea

Bothriocephalus Rarus

Morphology. The scolex of *Bothriocephalus rarus* is small and has two shallow, longitudinal bothria and a rectangular terminal disc[83]. Segmentation begins immediately posterior to the scolex, and there is no neck. The mature worm has 60 to 250 segments and is 67 mm to 300 mm in length. The reproductive organs generally appear in the 30th segment. The genital apertures are along the midline, the ovary is compact and bilobed, and the uterine sac is ventral. The egg is thick-shelled, operculated, and unembryonated when laid. Eggs measure 59 μ to 65 μ long by 41 μ to 56 μ wide.

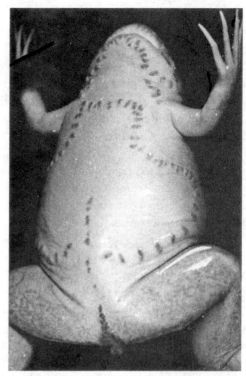

Fig. 8.30 *Neascus* sp. infection of a South African clawed toad. Metacercariae encysted in the skin below the lateral line system cause a local proliferation of melanophores at the site of each neuromast. Reproduced from Elkan, E. and Murray, R.W. (1952) with permission.

Hosts. The adult of this pseudophyllid cestode is common in the small intestine of red-spotted newts, California newts, and two-lined salamanders (*Eurycea bislineata*) in the United States[65,83,84]. Laboratory newts obtained from their natural habitats are likely to be infected. The prevalence of this parasite varies with locale, but as many as 30% of animals sampled in the north central and eastern United States have been found to be infested[14,65,83].

Life Cycle. The life cycle is typical of the Pseudophyllidea, and is described in Chapter 4, Biology of Cestodes. Adult newts can be infected directly by ingesting an infected copepod, but are usually infected after preying on an infected larval newt.

Pathologic Effects and Clinical Disease. Heavy infections cause enteritis in urodelans, which may appear weak and debilitated[83]. Severely debilitated animals may die.

Diagnosis, Treatment, and Prevention. Antemortem diagnosis is based on clinical signs and finding proglottids or eggs in the feces. Postmortem diagnosis is by finding adult worms in the small intestine at necropsy. Although no treatment has been described, praziquantel (8 to 14 mg/kg orally every 14 days for three treatments) may be used. Abrupt changes in water temperature have been found to cause newts in captivity to shed the tapeworms[83]. Because the life cycle cannot be completed in the absence of copepods, routine sanitation prevents the spread of the infection in the laboratory.

Public Health Considerations. *Bothriocephalus rarus* does not infect humans.

Cephalochlamys Namaquensis

Morphology. The scolex of *Cephalochlamys namaquensis* (Syn. *Chlamydocephalys xenopi*) has two large, oval bothridia that stand away from the body and give an arrowhead appearance[85–87]. Mature worms measure 16 mm to 36 mm long and 1.6 mm wide. Proglottids are wider than long (Figure 8.31). The ovary is located near the base of the segment. The uterus is narrow, and coiled, and extends almost to the anterior border. The genital aperture is medial and located on the anterior half of the segment. Eggs are oval, thin shelled, nonoperculated, and measure 37 μ long by 26 μ wide.

Hosts and Life Cycle. *Cephalochlamys namaquensis* is common in the small intestine of the South African clawed frog in the wild as well as in the laboratory[15,84,85]. Prevalence of infection in captive clawed frogs can be high[81]. The life cycle is unknown[85].

Pathologic Effects and Clinical Disease. Invasion of the jejunal mucosa by *C. namaquensis* has been observed (Figure 8.32). Although heavy infestations (more than 100 scolices in one toad) sometimes occur[15,85], no severe pathology has been reported. Affected clawed frogs may develop diarrhea; however, most animals are asymptomatic.

Diagnosis, Treatment, and Prevention. Antemortem diagnosis is by finding eggs in a fecal flotation. Postmortem diagnosis is by finding adult worms in the small intestine at necropsy. Bromphenol blue has been used effectively to treat infections with *C. namaquensis*[15,85]. Praziquantel may also be effective, as described for *Bothriocephalus rarus*. Because the complete life cycle is not known, recommendations for control cannot be made. Once freed of infection, frogs in captivity do not appear to become re-infected, thus indicating that the life cycle is not likely to be completed in the laboratory[85].

Public Health Considerations. *Cephalochlamys namaquensis* does not infect humans.

Cyclophyllidea

Nematotaenia Dispar

Morphology. Mature *Nematotaenia dispar* are cylindrical and can grow to 22 cm long and 0.5 to 0.6 mm wide[15,87]. The scolex is unarmed and bears four suckers. A rostellum is either poorly developed or absent. Segmentation is not apparent except in the last few proglottids. Each proglottid has two testes and numerous parauterine organs (Figure 8.33).

Hosts and Life Cycle. Adult *N. dispar* have been isolated from the small intestine of edible frogs, grass frogs, treefrogs, European toads, fire salamanders, other European salamanders, and alpine newts from Europe, Africa, and Asia[84]. Infections are common in southern Europe and northern Africa, and are likely to be encountered in laboratory amphibians obtained from these regions[15].

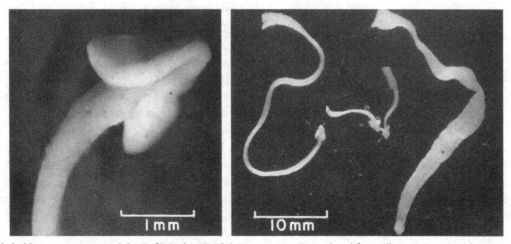

Fig. 8.31 *Cephalochlamys namaquensis* adult. (Left) Scolex. (Right) Entire worm. Reproduced from Elkan, E. (1960) with permission.

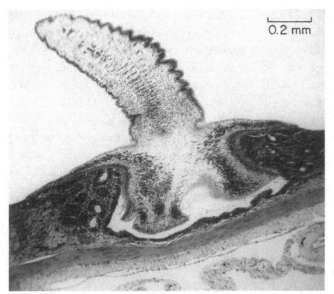

Fig. 8.32 *Cephalochlamys namaquensis* invading jejunal mucosa of a South African clawed toad. Reproduced from Reichenbach-Klinke, H. and Elkan, E. (1965) with permission.

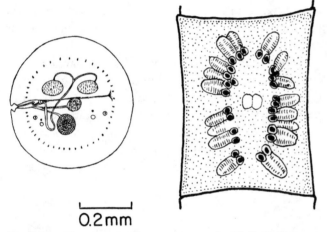

Fig. 8.33 *Nematotaenia dispar,* mature proglottid. (Left) Cross section. Note the cylindrical shape. (Right) Longitudinal view. Note the paruterine organs. (Left) reproduced from Wardle, R.A. and McLeod, J.A. (1952) with permission. (Right) reproduced from Cheng, T.C. (1964) with permission.

Nematotaenia dispar may also be found in leopard frogs, cricket frogs, American toads, common toads, and mud-puppies from North America[87]. The life cycle is unknown.

Pathologic Effects and Clinical Disease. *Nematotaenia dispar* does not appear to cause any significant pathology.

In small numbers, *N. dispar* is harmless, but in heavy infections may cause intestinal obstruction and death[85].

Diagnosis, Treatment, and Prevention. Antemortem diagnosis is by findings eggs in a fecal flotation. Postmortem diagnosis is by finding adult worms in the small intestine at necropsy. Treatment recommendations are as described for *Bothriocephalus rarus.* Because the life cycle of this parasite is unknown, it is difficult to determine what preventive methods should be taken to minimize the likelihood of transmitting the parasite. All new amphibians should be quarantined and serial fecal samples examined. Infected animals should be treated. Animals should not be released from quarantine until they have at least four negative fecals over a four-week period.

Public Health Considerations. *Nematotaenia dispar* does not infect humans. However, the life cycle is unknown and basic hygiene practices should be followed when handling amphibians infested with this parasite.

LARVAL CESTODES

Morphology. Larval *Diphyllobothrium erinacei* (Syn. *Diphyllobothrium mansoni, D. ranarum, D. reptans, Spirometra erinacei*) and *Spirometra mansonoides* (Syn. *Diphyllobothrium mansonoides*) have been recovered from amphibians. Plerocercoids are white, flattened, transversely wrinkled, and have a longitudinal medial groove on their ventral surface[55,88,89]. In amphibians, plerocercoids grow up to 30 mm in length and 0.7 mm in width.

Hosts. Pseudophyllidean larvae (sparganae) have been reported to encyst in the muscle and connective tissue of amphibians throughout the world[53,84,90]. Because of the controversy associated with the nomenclature of these parasites and the difficulty in precisely identifying the larvae, disagreement exists concerning specific names of sparganae in various geographic locations[88,91,92]. *Diphyllobothrium erinacei* is commonly applied to larval forms reported from Europe, Asia, Indonesia, Australia, and South America, while *Spirometra mansonoides* is applied to those reported from North America. *Diphyllobothrium erinacei* has been found in grass frogs, edible frogs, treefrogs, toads, fire salamanders, common newts, and other salamanders[53,90]; *S. mansonoides* has been reported in green frogs, bullfrogs, treefrogs, toads, tiger salamanders, and red-spotted newts[53,89]. *Diphyllobothrium erinacei* is most common in eastern Asia and Indonesia[88], with a prevalence of 82% reported in frogs (*Rana tigrina*) from southeastern Asia[90]. In a survey of several species of tadpoles and adult frogs from the south central United States, *S. mansonoides* was found in only 1% of animals tested[89]. Laboratory amphibians obtained from endemic regions are likely to be infected. The prevalence of these parasites in captive amphibians in other parts of the world is unknown.

Life Cycle. Carnivores (e.g., dogs and cats) serve as the definitive host for *D. erinacei* and *S. mansonoides*. The life cycle is typical of the pseudophyllidea, and is described in Chapter 4, Biology of Cestodes. Amphibians are usually infected in the immature stage (e.g., frog: tadpole; urodelan: newt larvae) after ingesting the infected copepod. Adult amphibians can become infected by ingesting an infected immature amphibian. The complete life cycle of *D. erinacei* requires about 54 days.

Pathologic Effects and Clinical Disease. The migration of plerocercoid larvae through the intestinal wall and body cavity may cause mechanical damage and adhesions in fishes[55], and presumably causes detrimental effects in amphibians. Rapidly growing cestode larvae may interfere with the nutrition and growth of the host[15]. Most affected amphibians are asymptomatic. Heavily infected frog tadpoles cease to grow[90]. Infected amphibians are generally diagnosed at necropsy as an incidental finding.

Diagnosis, Treatment, and Prevention. A tentative diagnosis is based on finding characteristic plerocercoid larva in the muscle[88]. A definitive diagnosis requires the experimental feeding of the immature parasite to a definitive host and the identification of the adult parasite. Because the parasites primarily encyst in the muscle and connective tissue, there is no effective treatment. Because the life cycle cannot be completed in the absence of copepods, routine sanitation prevents the spread of the infection in the laboratory.

Public Health Considerations. Although these parasites cause sparganosis in man, infected laboratory amphibians are unlikely to serve as a source of infection for animal workers.

LEECHES

Morphology, Hosts, and Life Cycle. Aquatic and terrestrial amphibians are susceptible to attack by leeches. Leeches have a direct life cycle. Mature forms are hermaphroditic and can therefore reproduce in captivity from a single adult. Most leeches are ectoparasitic and feed on amphibians by attaching themselves to an amphibian host.

However, there are also endoparasitic leeches[92–95] which have been found to parasitize anurans. The leeches gain entrance into the host via the cloaca, and feed on blood from the liver and heart.

Pathologic Effects and Clinical Disease. Although heavy leech burdens could result in significant blood loss in captive amphibians, the greater risk posed by these parasites is that they can serve as vectors for other diseases, including bacteria, viruses, and parasites[96]. Amphibians infested with leeches may become anemic, with packed cell volumes dropping below 20%. Anemic amphibians can become lethargic and depressed. Because leeches can serve as vectors for other infectious diseases, infested amphibians should also be closely monitored for clinical signs associated with bacterial, viral, and other parasitic infections.

Diagnosis. Ectoparasitic leeches can be observed grossly on the amphibian host or found in the aquatic environment. Endoparasitic leeches can be more difficult to identify. The amphibian should be trans-illuminated in cases where endoparasitic leeches are suspected. This can be done by placing a flashlight against the lateral body wall of the amphibian. In some cases it is only possible to identify endoparasitic leeches at necropsy.

Treatment. External leeches can be removed with forceps. The animal enclosure should also be cleaned to ensure that eggs are removed. Endoparasitic leeches are more difficult to control. Endoparasitic leeches may leave the host after feeding. It may be possible to control leeches by rotating the amphibian between enclosures and physically removing leeches from the animal enclosure.

Prevention. Newly acquired, wild amphibians should be closely inspected for leeches during quarantine. Leeches should be removed from the amphibian, and its enclosure changed to prevent later exposure to newly hatched leeches.

Public Health Considerations. Leeches that infest amphibians are not considered to pose an important human health risk.

NEMATODES

Hundreds of species of nematodes have been reported from amphibians[97,98]. In most cases the amphibian serves as the definitive host, although in a few cases it is the intermediate host. Nematode larvae are frequently reported encysted in the stomach and intestinal wall of green frogs, water newts, and other aquatic amphibians in eastern

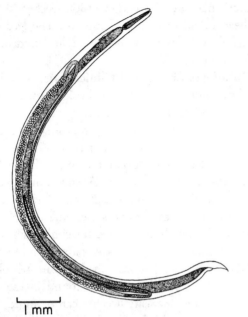

Fig. 8.34 *Rhabdias bufonis,* parthenogenic female. Reproduced from Yorke, W. and Maplestone, P.A. (1926) with permission.

United States[14,65,67,68]. Although they are called spirurid larvae, their exact identity is unknown.

Superfamily Rhabditoidea

Rhabdias spp.

Morphology. The parthenogenic female found in the lungs of anurans measures 11 mm to 13 mm long[15,98], and is characterized by a mouth with six insignificant lips, a short esophagus, a vulva located near the middle of the body, and a sharply tapered posterior extremity that ends in a finely conical point (Figure 8.34). The egg is thin-shelled and embryonated. The larval stage that occurs in the intestine of the frog or toad is typically rhabditiform. The free-living male and female are similar to the parthenogenic female; the infective larva is filariform.

Hosts. *Rhabdias* is common in the lungs of frogs and toads[15]. *Rhabdias ranae* occurs in the lungs of leopard frogs, bullfrogs, wood frogs, pickerel frogs, cricket frogs, chorus frogs, spring peepers, common toads, and other toads from North America[68,97]. *Rhabdias bufonis* occurs in Europe and Asia in the lungs of grass frogs, edible frogs, treefrogs, other frogs, European toads, and other toads[6,97]. The prevalence *R. ranae* in frogs from the northeastern United States is 31%[68], while the prevalence of *R. bufonis* in grass frogs from Great Britain is as high as 48%[61].

Reichenbach-Klinke and Elkan[15] suggest that most wild amphibians being brought into the laboratory should be considered positive.

Life Cycle. The life cycle is direct. Eggs passed by the parthenogenic female are carried up the bronchus to the mouth, swallowed, hatch, and pass in the feces as rhabditiform larvae[15,98]. Outside the host they transform either directly into infective larvae or indirectly by first passing through a bisexual generation. Frogs and toads become infected by ingestion of infective larvae or by penetration of the skin. Larvae migrate through the body tissues to the lungs, where they mature.

Pathologic Effects and Clinical Disease. Nothing is known of the pathologic effects of *Rhabdias*. Infections without pathologic changes are common[15,85], but heavy worm burdens may cause pneumonitis. Migrating nematode larvae sometimes cause cysts or are associated with tumors in amphibians[15]. Most amphibians are asymptomatic, but amphibians with heavy worm burdens may appear depressed or lethargic or die acutely.

Diagnosis, Treatment, and Prevention. Antemortem diagnosis is by finding rhabditiform larvae in a fecal flotation. Postmortem diagnosis is by finding the parthenogenic female in the lungs or the rhabditiform larvae in the intestine. Treatment is as described for *Aplectana*. Newly imported wild amphibians should be quarantined for a minimum of 30 days. Serial fecal samples should be collected to determine parasite status. Changing the enclosure substrate will minimize environmental contamination with *Rhabdias*. The author prefers to keep affected amphibians on a moistened paper towel substrate that can be changed daily.

Public Health Considerations. *Rhabdias* spp. do not infect humans.

Superfamily Cosmocercidae

Aplectana spp.

Morphology. Adult *Aplectana* measure 2 mm to 7 mm long, and possess a mouth bearing three lips, an esophagus which terminates in a bulb, and a simple intestine that has no diverticulum[98]. The males have two spicules of equal length; the females have a posterior extremity that is conical and pointed (Figure 8.35).

Hosts. *Aplectana* are common in the intestine of frogs, toads, and salamanders from North America and Europe[15,97]. The prevalence of *A. acuminata* has been

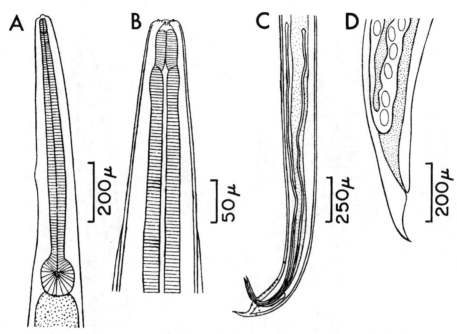

Fig. 8.35 *Aplectana.* (A) Anterior end, lateral view. (B) Anterior end, ventral view. (C) Posterior end of male. (D) Posterior end of female. Reproduced from Yorke, W. and Maplestone, P.A. (1926) with permission.

reported to be 23% for grass frogs from Great Britain[61]. Laboratory amphibians obtained from their natural habitat may be infected.

Life Cycle. The life cycle is unknown but is probably direct, with infection by ingestion of an embryonated egg or infective larva[57,98].

Pathologic Effects and Clinical Disease. Animals with low parasite burdens have minimal pathology, although enteritis may develop with heavy infections. Heavily infected amphibians may develop debilitation, intestinal obstruction, and peritonitis, and may die[15].

Diagnosis, Treatment, and Prevention. Antemortem diagnosis is by finding eggs in a fecal flotation. Postmortem diagnosis is by finding adult nematodes in the intestine. Infected animals may be treated with ivermectin (0.2 mg/kg orally or by injection) or fenbendazole (25 to 50 mg/kg orally). Newly imported wild amphibians should be quarantined for a minimum of 30 days. Serial fecal samples should be collected to determine parasite status. Animals should not be removed from quarantine until they have four serial negative fecals over a four-week period.

Public Health Considerations. Humans are not susceptible to infection with *Aplectana.*

Cosmocerca spp.

Adult *Cosmocerca* are morphologically similar to *Aplectana.* The prevalence of *Cosmocerca ornate* has been reported to be 81% in grass frogs from Great Britain[61]. Laboratory amphibians obtained from their natural habitat may be infected. The life cycle and other aspects of the biology and control of *Cosmocerca* are similar to those described for *Aplectana.*

Cosmocercoides spp.

Adult *Cosmocercoides* are morphologically similar to *Aplectana.* The prevalence of *Cosmocercoides dukae* in the red-spotted newt from the northeastern United States has been reported to vary from 2% to 16%[14,68]. The life cycle and other aspects of the biology and control of *Cosmocercoides* is similar to that described for *Aplectana.*

Oxysomatium spp.

Adult *Oxysomatium* are morphologically similar to *Aplectana.* The prevalence of *Oxysomatium americana* in salamanders from the northeastern United States has been reported to vary from 2% to 7%[65]. Laboratory amphibians obtained from their natural habitat may be infected. The life cycle and other aspects of the biology and control

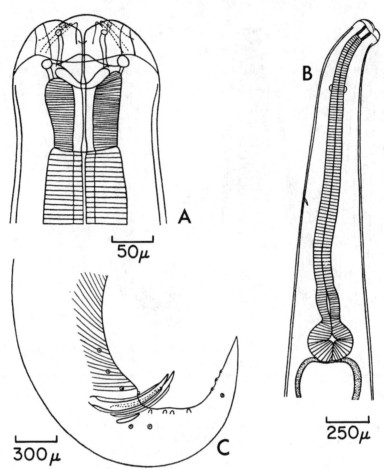

Fig. 8.36 *Falcaustra.* (A) Head, ventral view. (B) Anterior end, lateral view. (C) Posterior end of male, lateral view. Reproduced from Yorke, W. and Maplestone, P.A. (1926) with permission.

of *Oxysomatium* are similar to those described for *Aplectana.*

Superfamily Oxyuroidea

Falcaustra spp.

Morphology. Adult *Falcaustra* (Syn. *Spironoura*) measure 8 mm to 16 mm long and have an esophagus with a terminal bulb, a simple intestine without a diverticulum, and a pointed posterior extremity in both sexes[75,98]. The male has spicules of equal length and a gubernaculum, but no caudal alae (Figure 8.36).

Hosts and Life Cycle. *Falcaustra catesbeiana* is common in bullfrogs and also occurs in leopard frogs, chorus frogs, treefrogs, and other frogs[75,97]. The life cycle is unknown but is assumed to be direct, with infection occurring after ingestion of an embryonated egg[57,98].

Up to 50% of wild bullfrogs may be infected with this parasite. Thus, wild bullfrogs should be assumed to be infected.

Pathologic Effects and Clinical Disease. Pathologic effects have not been described for *F. catesbeiana.* Infections are asymptomatic. However, heavy burdens in captive amphibians might lead to enteritis or intestinal obstruction.

Diagnosis, Treatment, and Prevention. Diagnosis, treatment, and prevention are as described for *Aplectana.*

Public Health Considerations. *Falcaustra* does not infect humans.

Superfamily Trichostrongyloidea

Oswaldocruzia spp.

Morphology. Adult *Oswaldocruzia* are filiform worms measuring 6 mm to 14 mm long[75,98]. The buccal cavity is rudimentary or absent, the vulva is located in the posterior half of the body, and the spicules are short and stout and end in a number of processes (Figure 8.37).

Hosts and Life Cycle. *Oswaldocruzia* is a trichostrongylid nematode found in the intestine of amphibians throughout the world[15,97]. Approximately 18% of leopard frogs from the south central United States have been found to harbor *O. pipiens*[75]. The prevalence of *O. pipiens* is much higher (70%) in frogs from the northeastern United States[68]. A single report on salamanders stated that approximately 23% of dusky salamanders from the northeastern United States were infected[68]. The prevalence of *O. pipiens* in Great Britain is similar (63%) to that reported for frogs from the northeastern U.S. All anurans and urodelans should be considered susceptible to infection. The life cycle is unknown but is probably direct, with infection by ingestion of an infective larva[57,98].

Pathologic Effects and Clinical Disease. Nothing is known of the specific pathologic effects of *Oswaldocruzia*. Animals with heavy worm burdens could develop enteritis. Infected animals are generally asymptomatic, but heavily infected animals may become debilitated and develop intestinal obstruction, and may die[15].

Diagnosis, Treatment, and Prevention. Diagnosis, treatment, and prevention are as described for *Aplectana*.

Public Health Considerations. *Oswaldocruzia* does not infect humans.

Superfamily Filaroidea

Foleyella spp.

Morphology. Adult *Foleyella* spp. are white, fragile, filiform worms[98–100]. Males measure 15 mm to 25 mm long and females measure 60 mm to 72 mm long. The mouth of *Foleyella* is simple with no lips or teeth. The esophagus is short and is divided into two parts, a muscular portion and a glandular portion. The male has long caudal alae, anal papillae, and unequal spicules (Figure 8.38). The vulva of the female is near the posterior end of the esophagus. The microfilariae are sheathed and vary in length with species. The microfilaria of *F. brachyoptera* measures 120 μ to 168 μ long; that of *F. dolichoptera* measures 263 μ to 295 μ long; and that of *F. ranae* measures 114 μ to 163 μ long.

Hosts. *Foleyella* is common in frogs[99,100]. Adults are found in the abdominal cavity in mesenteric and subcutaneous tissues. Microfilariae are found in the blood, lymph, and tissue fluids. *Foleyella brachyoptera* and *F. dolichoptera* occur in leopard frogs in the southeastern United States; *F. americana* in leopard frogs and green frogs from the United States and Canada; *F. ranae* in leopard frogs, green frogs, and

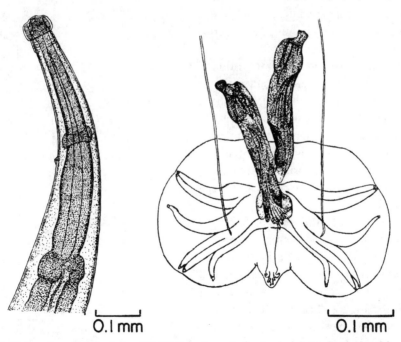

Fig. 8.37 *Oswaldocruzia*. (Left) Anterior end, lateral view. (Right) Posterior end of male, dorsal view. Reproduced from Yorke, W. and Maplestone, P.A. (1926) with permission.

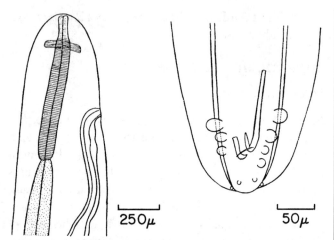

Fig. 8.38 *Foleyella.* (Left) Anterior end of female, lateral view. (Right) Posterior end of male, ventral view. Reproduced from Yorke, W. and Maplestone, P.A. (1926) with permission.

bullfrogs from the United States and Canada; and *F. duboisi* in edible frog from Israel. Infections may be encountered in laboratory frogs obtained from endemic areas[99,100].

Life Cycle. Adult worms occur in the body cavity of the frog, usually in the mesentery, but sometimes in the subcutis[15,63]. Fertilized eggs develop into sheathed microfilariae in the female, pass out into the tissues, and enter the lymph and blood vessels[99,100]. Here they can survive about two years awaiting ingestion by a mosquito intermediate host. In the mosquito, larvae become infective for the vertebrate host in about 18 days. Frogs are infected when bitten by an infected mosquito.

Pathologic Effects and Clinical Disease. Adult worms can stimulate the formation of dermal, subcuticular, or mesenteric cysts, depending on the species. The cysts are well-delineated in these cases. Microfilariae have been associated with the formation of dermal tumors[6,15]. Amphibians with low burdens are generally asymptomatic. Animals with dermal cysts may appear pruritic, rubbing the mass against solid objects. Death can occur in animals with heavy filarid burdens[15].

Diagnosis, Treatment, and Prevention. Antemortem diagnosis is by identification of microfilaria on a blood smear. Postmortem diagnosis is by identification of the adult worm in the body cavity[15]. No clinical trials have been performed to determine an effective treatment. Empirically, ivermectin (0.2 mg/kg once, repeated in 10 days for two to three treatments) may be used. In captivity, the absence of the intermediate host will prevent the life cycle of the parasite from being completed.

Public Health Considerations. *Foleyella* does not infect humans.

Icosiella spp.

Adult *Icosiella* are morphologically similar to *Foleyella*, except that the mouth of *Icosiella* is surrounded by four small spinose teeth and the esophagus is longer. Also, male *Icosiella* lack caudal alae and papillae. *Icosiella quadrituberculata* occurs in the leopard frog, bullfrog, and amphiuma in the United States, and *I. neglecta* in the grass frog and edible frog from Europe, Asia, and Africa. *Icosiella* may be encountered in laboratory frogs obtained from endemic areas[99]. The life cycle and other aspects of the biology of *Icosiella* are similar to those of *Foleyella*.

ACANTHOCEPHALA

Acanthocephalus ranae

Morphology. Adult *Acanthocephalus ranae* (Syn. *A. falcatus*) are cylindrical and have an elongated proboscis, with six to 28 longitudinal rows of four to 15 hooks each (Figure 8.39)[54]. The male measures approximately 3.2 mm in length and has two tandem, oval testes in the midregion of the body[101]. The female is longer, measuring approximately 6 mm in length.

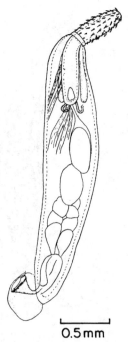

Fig. 8.39 *Acanthocephalus ranae* male. Reproduced from Van Cleave, H.J. (1915) with permission.

Hosts. *Acanthocephalus ranae* has been found in the stomach and intestine of grass frogs, edible frogs, and toads from Europe[15,61]. It also occurs in other European frogs, toads, salamanders, newts, and water snakes[6]. The prevalence of *A. ranae* in grass frogs from Great Britain has been reported to be 18%[61], while as many as 50% of the edible frogs from the European continent may be infected[101].

Life Cycle. An aquatic crustacean (isopod) serves as the intermediate host for *A. ranae*[6]. Eggs passed in the feces of the definitive host are ingested by a crustacean, and the amphibian is infected by ingesting the crustacean. Snakes, which normally do not feed on isopods, become infected by ingesting an infected amphibian[15]. Animals obtained from endemic areas should be screened for this parasite.

Pathologic Effects and Clinical Disease. The elongated proboscis of *A. ranae* can penetrate deep into the gastric or intestinal wall, causing severe tissue reaction and mechanical damage to the mucosa and submucosa at the point of attachment (Figure 18.40)[15,85,102]. Animals with low parasite burdens are generally asymptomatic. Amphibians with heavy burdens may become anorexic and emaciated. Severe burdens may also result in anemia. Untreated animals may die.

Diagnosis, Treatment, and Prevention. Antemortem diagnosis is by identification of the eggs in a fecal sample. Postmortem diagnosis is by identification of the parasite in the stomach or intestine. No clinical trials have been performed to determine an effective treatment. Empirically, ivermectin (0.2 mg/kg once, repeated in 10 days for two to three treatments) may be used. Because of the need for an isopod intermediate host, it is unlikely that the life cycle would be completed in the laboratory. Newly acquired animals should be quarantined prior to being introduced into a colony and screened (eg., fecal exams) for the parasite.

Public Health Considerations. *Acanthocephalus ranae* does not infect humans.

ARTHROPODS

Class Branchiura

Argulus sp.

Morphology. *Argulus* sp., the fish louse, is a branchiuran crustacean. The body is flattened and covered with an oval-shaped carapace. *Argulus* have compound eyes, a pair of large suckers, four pairs of swimming limbs, and they measure 5 mm to 20 mm in diameter (see Figure 6.1 in Chapter 6, Biology of Arthropods).

Hosts and Life Cycle. *Argulus* sp. can parasitize any aquatic amphibian. They are most commonly found on newts and tadpoles sold through the pet retail market. The life cycle of *Argulus* sp. is direct. Unlike other crustaceans which carry their eggs on their body, *Argulus* sp. deposit their eggs in the environment.

Pathologic Effects and Clinical Disease. *Argulus* sp. can induce pathology when it attaches and feeds on an

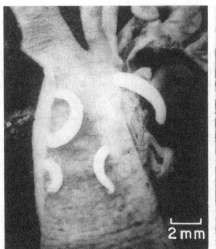
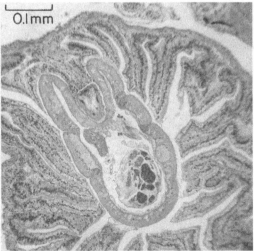

Fig. 8.40 *Acanthocephalus ranae* in European toad. (Left) Adult worms attached to the intestinal mucosa. (Right) Section of small intestine containing a worm. Courtesy of E. Elkan, London.

amphibian. During attachment, these parasites can cause damage to the epithelium. The break in the epithelial barrier increases the susceptibility of the host to opportunistic infections and osmoregulatory disorders. Amphibians infested with *Argulus* sp. rub against rough surfaces to remove parasites.

Diagnosis, Treatment, and Prevention. *Argulus* sp. can be observed grossly on an infested amphibian. The parasites typically leave an amphibian or fish once it is removed from the water. For mild infestations, the parasites can be removed manually with forceps. The amphibians should be placed into a new enclosure to prevent re-infestation by recently hatched *Argulus*. Salt (10 to 25 g/L for five to 10 minutes) and ivermectin (10 mg/L, 30 to 60 minutes) baths may be used to eliminate *Argulus* in the aquatic environment[9]. Amphibians should be examined closely during quarantine to ensure that they are not infested with *Argulus* sp.

Public Health Considerations. *Argulus* does not infest humans.

Class Insecta

Order Diptera

Family Calliphoridae

Bufolucilia spp. Morphology. Larvae of *Bufolucilia bufonivora* (Syn. *Lucilia bufonivora*) and *B. silvarum* (Syn. *L. silvarum*) (toad flies) are typically calliphorid[103]. Larvae are white, measure 10 mm to 18 mm long, and have several bands of microspines around their body. The head is retractile and bears paired mouth hooks. Adults resemble houseflies, but are larger, measuring 6 mm to 11 mm long. The body is metallic green, the legs are black, and the arista of the antenna is plumose.

Hosts. The larvae of *Bufolucilia* sp. cause severe and often fatal myiasis of toads and frogs[103,104]. *Bufolucilia bufonivora* occurs in Europe, Asia, northern Africa, and possibly North America[103]. It is common in European toads and sometimes affects other toads, grass frogs, edible frogs, treefrogs, European salamanders, and crested newts[103]. *Bufolucilia silvarum* occurs in North America and possibly Europe and northern Africa[105]. In North America, it has been recovered from bullfrogs and American toads[104], but is considered rare. Infection with larvae of these flies would not be expected in laboratories with proper fly control, but it could be present in specimens recently obtained from their natural environment.

Life Cycle. *Bufolucilia bufonivora* is an obligate parasite of amphibians, while *B. silvarum* is a facultative parasite[103]. Eggs usually hatch in one to three days, but sometimes remain unhatched for many days. Larvae pupate in two to seven days and metamorphose to adults in 10 to 21 days. The entire life cycle requires two to four weeks.

Pathologic Effects and Clinical Disease. The eggs are laid on the skin of the host. Following hatching, larvae migrate to the nasal passages[103] where they cause erosion of the mucous membranes and occasionally penetrate the underlying bone and enter the orbit or brain[106,107]. Affected amphibians may be anorexic, lethargic, and depressed. Infected toads generally succumb.

Diagnosis, Treatment, and Prevention. Diagnosis is based on the clinical signs and the presence of the larvae in the lesions. The maggots can be manually removed. Ivermectin (0.2 to 0.4 mg/kg topically or intramuscularly, repeated in seven to 10 days) may kill the maggots. Bathing frogs in ivermectin (10 mg/L, 30 to 60 minutes) may also prove larvicidal[9]. Treating affected anurans with an organophosphate (diclorvos, <60-minute exposure) has been suggested, but may also be toxic to the amphibian[19]. Newly acquired specimens should be examined and, if infected, culled. Amphibians maintained in laboratory colonies should not be exposed to these flies. However, proper fly control prevents infection.

Public Health Considerations. *Bufolucilia* have not been reported to affect humans.

Class Arachnida

Suborder Prostigmata

Trombiculids

Morphology. Trombiculid mites appear reddish-orange. *Hannemania* sp. larvae have six legs and an ovoid body, and measure approximately 0.6 to 1.0 mm long and 0.3 mm to 0.6 mm wide[108]. As the larvae approach the nymphal stage, rudiments of the fourth pair of legs become apparent. The nymphal and adult stages both have eight legs.

Hosts. The larvae of *Hannemania* mites embed beneath the skin of various amphibians in North and South America[108,109]. The most common species, *H. dunni,* is prevalent in the eastern United States[108,110,111], and has been reported to infest pickerel frogs, spotted salamanders, marbled salamanders, and dusky salamanders[111]. The prevalence of this mite in salamanders has been reported to vary from 7% to 33%[14]. *Hannemania penetrans* is another common trombiculid mite from the eastern United States and has been recovered from leopard frogs, green frogs, bullfrogs, and toads[108]. Laboratory specimens obtained from areas where the mites are endemic may be infested.

Eutrombicula sp. and *Neotrombicula* sp. mites are primarily found on reptiles and occasionally found on amphibians obtained from their natural habitat[15,108,112]. The most common species in North America is *E. alfreddugesi,* the common chigger. It is prevalent throughout the Western Hemisphere and has been reported to affect toads[108,113]. Another common species occurring in the southeastern United States is *E. splendens.* This mite has been recovered from treefrogs[114]. Only the larvae of these genera are parasitic; the nymphs and adults are free-living[115]. The larvae feed on tissue fluids from a single host until engorged.

Life Cycle. The life cycle is direct, and involves larval, nymph, and adult stages[110]. Although most trombiculid mites are ectoparasites, the larva of this genus is usually found beneath the skin of the host. Unengorged larvae penetrate the skin and become completely embedded in about two hours. The length of time spent under the skin varies, sometimes lasting six months. The nymph and adults are free-living and feed on small arthropods or arthropod eggs. The life cycle cannot be completed in the laboratory.

Pathologic Effects and Clinical Disease. Embedded larvae cause the formation of orange-to-red vesicles less than 1 mm in diameter on the ventral surface of the rear legs and in the cloacal region[108,116]. Encysted mites are seen in the vesicles in microscopic sections. Animals with severe mite infestations may develop generalized vesicles, and appear listless. Amphibians can become anemic with chronic infestations. The mites can also serve as vectors for bacterial and viral diseases.

Diagnosis, Treatment, and Prevention. Diagnosis is by identifying the skin lesions and the mites on the surface of the amphibian. Because the mites are highly contagious, infested animals should be removed from the colony and housed separately. Treatment is as described for *Bufolucilia* sp. Newly acquired amphibians should be carefully examined upon arrival and culled if infested.

Public Health Considerations. Trombiculids cause dermatitis in humans[115]. Special precautions, such as wearing gloves and laboratory coats, should be followed to minimize the likelihood of contact between animal caretakers and infested amphibians.

MOLLUSKS

Morphology. Amphibians may become parasitized by larval clams, including *Anodonta cygnaea, Megalonaeas gigantean,* and *Simpsonichoncha ambigua.* Larval mollusks typically measure up to 0.5 mm in length.

Hosts. During dispersal, freshwater clam larvae sometimes embed in the gills of amphibian larvae[15,115]. Larvae of *S. ambigua* and *M. gigantean* have been found in the gills of the mudpuppy (*Necturus*) from the United States[117,118], and *A. cygnaea* from the gills of axolotl from Europe[15].

Life Cycle. Little is known regarding the life cycle of these parasites in amphibians. In fishes, glochidia attach to the gills and become encysted as a result of the host immune response. The larvae have phagocytizing cells in their mantle that derive nutrition from the host. The life cycle is approximately 10 to 30 days. Eventually the larvae excyst and start a benthic life cycle. *Simpsonichoncha ambigua* may parasitize *Necturus* or develop in the adult clam's gills.

Pathologic Effects and Clinical Disease. Larval clams generate a mild, localized inflammatory response in the gill. Affected amphibians would not be expected to develop severe disease because the burdens are generally low.

Diagnosis, Treatment, and Prevention. Antemortem or postmortem diagnosis can be made based on the identification of the parasitic larvae from a gill biopsy. No treatments have been described. The parasitic larvae eventually excyst from the amphibian and the lesion generated by the parasite heals. Larval clams would not be expected to be a concern in captive amphibians, unless amphibians were maintained in a mixed species exhibit with mollusks.

Public Health Considerations. Larval clams are not known to infest humans.

TABLE 8.1 Parasites of amphibians—circulatory/lymphatic system.

Parasite	Geographic distribution	Hosts	Location in host	Method of infection	Pathologic effects	Reference
Flagellates						
Cryptobia sp.	North America	Newts, salamanders	Blood	Unknown	Unknown	6
Trypanosoma inopinatum	India, southern Europe, northern Africa	Frogs	Blood	Bite of leech	Spleen destruction, death	121
Trypanosoma pipientis	North America	Frogs	Blood	Bite of leech	Spleen enlargement	122
Trypanosoma schmidti	Southeastern US	Leopard frogs	Blood	Probably by bite of leech or arthropod	Unknown	123
Trypanosoma sp.	North America	Newts, salamanders	Blood	Probably by bite of leech or arthropod	Usually none; some species may cause debilitation, anorexia, erythrocyte degeneration	3, 119, 120
Trypanosoma sp.	Worldwide	Frogs, toads	Blood	Probably by bite of leech or arthropod	None	1,3
Coccidia						
Cytamoeba bacterifera	Europe, US	Axolotl, frogs, newts, salamanders	Blood	Unknown	Unknown	141
Cytamoeba grassi	Europe	Treefrogs	Blood	Unknown	Unknown	6
Haemogregarina sp.	Africa, Europe, US	Toads, bullfrogs, other frogs	Blood	Unknown	None	6, 139
Haemohormidium stableri	US	Leopard frogs	Blood	Unknown	Unknown	141
Haemohormidium jahni	US	Red-spotted newts	Blood	Unknown	Degeneration of erythrocytes	141
Hepatozoon catesbeiana	Unknown	Bullfrogs	Blood	Ingestion of mosquito containing sporocysts	Variable anemia	36
Lankesterella bufonis	Africa	Toads	Blood	Bite of leech	None	142
Lankesterella canadensis	Canada	Bullfrogs	Blood	Bite of leech	Unknown	6
Lankesterella minima	Worldwide	Frogs, toads	Blood	Bite of leech	Unknown	3, 143
Leeches						
Batrachobdella picta	US	Bullfrogs	Dorsal lymph sac	Direct contact	Unknown	15

TABLE 8.2 Parasites of amphibians—enterohepatic system.

Parasite	Geographic distribution	Hosts	Location in host	Method of infection	Pathologic effects	Reference
Flagellates						
Chilomastix caulleryi	North America, Europe	Axolotl, frogs, newts, salamanders, toads	Intestine	Ingestion of organism passed in feces	None	6
Giardia agilis	Worldwide	Frogs, toads	Small intestine	Ingestion of organism passed in feces	None	15, 125
Hexamastix batrachorum	Europe, North America	Newts, salamanders	Intestine	Ingestion of organism passed in feces	None	6, 12, 15
Hexamita batrachorum	North America	Frogs, newts, salamanders, toads	Large intestine	Ingestion of organism passed in feces	Enteritis	6, 14
Karotomorpha bufonis	Europe, North America	Frogs, newts, salamanders, toads	Rectum	Ingestion of organism passed in feces	None	6, 14
Karotomorpha suezyi	US	Frogs, toads, salamanders, newts	Rectum	Ingestion of organism passed in feces	None	6, 14
Monocercomonas batrachorum	Worldwide	Frogs, newts, salamanders, toads	Large intestine	Ingestion of organism passed in feces	None	6, 15
Monocercomonoides rotunda	Europe	European toads, European salamanders	Intestine	Ingestion of organism passed in feces	None	15
Octomitus sp.	US	Frogs, dusky salamanders	Large intestine	Ingestion of organism passed in feces	None	20
Opalina sp.	Worldwide	Frogs, newts, toads	Intestine	Ingestion of organism passed in feces	None	3, 6, 15
Proteromonas longifila	Americas, Europe	Axolotl, frogs, newts, salamanders, toads	Rectum	Ingestion of organism passed in feces	None	15
Protoopalina sp.	Worldwide	Frogs, newts, salamanders, toads	Intestine	Ingestion of organism passed in feces	None	3, 6
Retortamonas dobelli	Europe, US	Frogs, newts, salamanders, toads	Intestine	Ingestion of organism passed in feces	None	127
Tetratrichomonas prowazeki	Americas, Europe	Frogs, newts, salamanders, snakes, toads, salamanders	Large intestine	Ingestion of organism passed in feces	None	11, 25
Treponema agilis	Europe	Frogs, newts	Intestine	Ingestion of organism passed in feces	None	6
Treponema sp.	US	Leopard frogs, salamanders	Intestine	Ingestion of organism passed in feces	None	6
Trichomitus batrachorum	Worldwide	Axolotl, frogs, lizards, newts, salamanders, snakes, toads	Large intestine	Ingestion of organism passed in feces	None	22
Trimitus parvus	Europe, US	European toads, frogs, garter snakes, red-spotted newts	Intestine	Ingestion of organism passed in feces	None	60
Tritrichomonas augusta	Americas, Asia, Europe	Frogs, lizards, newts, salamanders, toads	Large intestine	Ingestion of organism passed in feces	Hepatitis	15, 124
Amoebae						
Copramoeba salamandrae	US	Red-spotted newts	Intestine	Ingestion of organism passed in feces	None	15

(Continued)

155

TABLE 8.2 (*Continued*)

Parasite	Geographic distribution	Hosts	Location in host	Method of infection	Pathologic effects	Reference
Entamoeba cyrrens	Europe	Edible frogs, toads	Intestine	Ingestion of organism passed in feces	None	6
Entamoeba pyrrhogaster	US	Red-spotted newts	Intestine	Ingestion of organism passed in feces	None	15
Entamoeba ranarum	Europe, India, Philippine Islands, US	Frogs, newts, toads	Intestine	Ingestion of organism passed in feces	Enteritis, hepatitis, nephritis	27
Mastigamoeba hylae	Americas, Europe	Frogs, newts, toads	Intestine	Ingestion of organism passed in feces	None	60
Vahlkampfia sp.	Europe	Frogs	Intestine	Ingestion of organism passed in feces	None	6, 15
Vahlkampfia salamandrae	US	Newts	Intestine	Ingestion of organism passed in feces	None	15
Coccidia						
Cryptosporidium sp.	Unknown	Clawed frogs	Stomach	Ingestion of sporulated oocyst in feces	Gastritis, enteritis	30
Eimeria sp.	Asia, Europe, US	Frogs, newts, salamanders, toads	Intestine	Ingestion of sporulated oocyst in feces	None	6, 15, 127
Isospora jeffersonianum	US	Jefferson salamanders	Intestine	Ingestion of sporulated oocyst in feces	None	6
Ciliates						
Balantidium sp.	Africa, Asia, Europe, North America	Frogs, newts, salamanders, toads	Intestine	Ingestion of organism passed in feces	None	3, 6, 15
Cepedietta sp.	Africa, Europe, North America	Axolotl, frogs, salamanders, toads	Intestine	Ingestion of organism passed in feces	None	44
Nyctotheroides cordiformis	Worldwide	Frogs, newts, toads	Intestine	Ingestion of organism passed in feces	None	45, 129
Opalina obtrigonoidea	US	Frogs, toads	Intestine	Ingestion of zygocysts in feces of tadpole	None	144
Opalina ranarum	Europe	Frogs, newts, toads	Intestine	Ingestion of zygocysts in feces of tadpole	None	144
Protoopalina sp.	Africa, Australia, Europe	Frogs, newts, salamanders, toads	Intestine	Ingestion of zygocysts in feces of tadpole	None	145
Microspora						
Alloglugea bufonis	South America	Toads	Intestine, liver, kidney, spleen	Probably ingestion of spores released from tissue	Xenoma formation	40
Myxozoa						

156

Myxidium serotinum	US	Frogs, salamanders, toads	Gallbladder	Probably by actinosporeans released from oligochaete worms	None	128

Trematodes

Adult Digenetic

Brachycoelium ambystomae	Southeastern US	Marbled salamanders	Small intestine	Ingestion of metacercaria in tissues of intermediate host (snail)	None	130
Brachycoelium salamandrae	Worldwide	Amphiumas, frogs, newts, salamanders, toads, reptiles	Intestine	Ingestion of metacercaria in tissues of intermediate host (snail)	None	131
Brachycoelium stablefordi	Eastern US	Dusky salamanders	Small intestine	Ingestion of metacercaria in tissues of intermediate host (snail)	None	132
Cephalogonimus amphiumae	US	Amphiumas	Intestine	Probably by ingestion of metacercaria in arthropod or skin of amphibian	None	6
Cephalogonimus sp.	Europe, North America	Frogs	Intestine	Ingestion of metacercaria in skin of amphibian, possibly by ingestion of arthropod	None	133
Crepidostomum sp.	Europe, North America	Amphiumas, frogs, mudpuppies, salamanders	Intestine	Ingestion of second intermediate host (arthropod)	None	55
Diplodiscus subclavatus	Africa, Australasia, Europe	Frogs, newts, salamanders, toads	Large intestine	Ingestion of metacercaria in skin of amphibian	None	15, 134
Diplodiscus unguiculatus	Europe	Newts	Rectum	Ingestion of metacercaria in skin of amphibian	None	6
Diplodiscus sp.	Asia	Frogs	Large intestine, cloaca	Ingestion of metacercaria in skin of amphibian	None	6, 15, 64
Dolichosaccus rastellus	Europe	Frogs, newts, salamanders, toads	Intestine	Ingestion of second intermediate host (insect, tadpole)	None	15, 61
Glypthelmins sp.	Americas, Asia	Frogs, toads	Intestine	Ingestion of metacercaria formed in skin after penetration by cercaria	None	6, 135
Haplometrana intestinalis	Western US	Frogs, toads	Intestine	Ingestion of metacercaria formed in skin of frog after penetration by cercaria	None	63
Halipegus amherstensis	North America	Frogs	Mouth, ear canal	Ingestion of second intermediate host (arthropod)	None	63

(Continued)

TABLE 8.2 (*Continued*)

Parasite	Geographic distribution	Hosts	Location in host	Method of infection	Pathologic effects	Reference
Halipegus eccentricus	US	Frogs	Mouth, ear canal	Ingestion of second intermediate host (arthropod)	Unknown	63
Halipegus eschi	Costa Rica	Frogs	Esophagus	Ingestion of second intermediate host (arthropod)	None	136
Halipegus occidualis	North America	Frogs	Mouth, ear canals, pharynx	Ingestion of second intermediate host (arthropod)	None	137
Halipegus ovocaudatus	Europe, southern Africa	Frogs	Mouth	Ingestion of second intermediate host (arthropod)	None	138
Loxogenes arcanum	North America	Frogs	Intestine, viscera	Ingestion of metacercaria encysted in second intermediate host	Cysts in viscera (insect)	6
Megalodiscus americanus	North and Central America	Amphiuma, frogs, newts, salamanders	Intestine	Ingestion of metacercaria in skin of amphibian	None	6, 64
Megalodiscus intermedius	US	Bullfrogs, dusky salamanders	Rectum	Ingestion of metacercaria in skin of amphibian	None	6, 64
Megalodiscus microphagus	US	Frogs, salamanders, toads	Large intestine, urinary bladder	Ingestion of metacercaria in skin of amphibian	None	69
Megalodiscus rankini	US	Red-spotted newts	Intestine	Ingestion of metacercaria in skin of amphibian	None	6
Megalodiscus temperatus	Americas	Amphiumas, frogs, newts, salamanders, toads	Large intestine	Ingestion of metacercaria in skin of amphibian	None	15, 153
Opisthioglyphe ranae	Africa, Europe	Frogs, newts, salamanders, toads	Intestine	Ingestion of second intermediate host (arthropod)	None	15, 66, 154
Plagitura parva	Eastern US	Red-spotted newts	Small intestine	Ingestion of metacercaria in tissue of second intermediate host (snail, insect)	None	158
Plagitura salamandra	Eastern US	Red-spotted newts, salamanders	Small intestine	Ingestion of metacercaria in tissue of second intermediate host (snail, insect)	None	159
Pleurogenes claviger	Europe	Frogs, newts, toads	Small intestine	Ingestion of second intermediate host (arthropod)	None	15
Pleurogenes medians	Europe, Africa	Frogs, newts, toads	Small intestine	Ingestion of metacercaria encysted in second intermediate host (insect) or in skin of tadpole	None	6, 155

Species	Distribution	Host	Site	Mode of infection	Effects	Ref
Prosotocus confusus	Asia, Europe	Frogs, toads	Small intestine	Ingestion of second intermediate host (arthropod)	None	156
Telorchis sp.	North America	Amphiuma, mudpuppies	Intestine	Ingestion of second intermediate host (arthropod)	Unknown	160
Larval digenetic						
Cotylurus variegatus	Europe	Frogs	Liver	Unknown	Unknown	161
Echinoparyphium recurvatum	Worldwide	Frogs, newts, toads	Liver, kidneys	Penetration by cercaria released from snail	Unknown	162
Gorgodera amplicava	North America	Tadpoles of frogs, larvae of spotted salamanders	Intestinal wall	Ingestion of cercaria released from snail	Unknown	73
Cestodes						
Adult						
Bothriocephalus rarus	US	Newts, two-lined salamanders (*Eurycea bislineata*)	Small intestine	Ingestion of intermediate host (copepod) or newt larva	Weakness, debilitation, death	83
Cephalochlamys namaquensis	Great Britain, southern Africa	South African clawed toads	Small intestine	Unknown	Unknown	86
Cylindrotaenia americana	Americas	Frogs, salamanders, toads, lizards, softshell turtles, snakes	Small intestine	Unknown	Unknown	163
Cylindrotaenia quadrijugosa	North central US	Leopard frogs	Small intestine	Unknown	Unknown	15
Distoichometra bufonis	Southeastern US	Toads	Small intestine	Unknown	Unknown	15
Nematotaenia dispar	Africa, Asia, Europe	Frogs, newts, salamanders, toads	Small intestine	Unknown	Intestinal obstruction, death	16
Ophiotaenia perspicua	Americas	Leopard frogs, garter snakes, water snakes	Intestine	Ingestion of intermediate host (copepod) or frog tadpole or fish	Unknown	15
Ophiotaenia saphena	North central US	Frogs	Small intestine	Ingestion of intermediate host (copepod)	Unknown	15
Ophiotaenia sp.	North America	Amphiumas, frogs, mudpuppies, salamanders, toads	Small intestine	Unknown	Unknown	6, 15
Larval						
Ligula intestinalis	Asia, Europe, North America	Tiger salamanders	Intestine	Ingestion of first intermediate host (copepod)	Unknown	6
Ophiotaenia perspicua	US	Frogs	Liver	Ingestion of first intermediate host (copepod)	Unknown	6

(Continued)

TABLE 8.2 (*Continued*)

Parasite	Geographic distribution	Hosts	Location in host	Method of infection	Pathologic effects	Reference
Nematodes						
Camallanidae						
Procamallanus slomei	Southern Africa	South African clawed toads	Stomach	Ingestion of copepod	Embeds head deeply in stomach wall, apparently ingests blood, causes trauma	6
Cosmocercidae						
Aplectana acuminata	Africa, Americas, Europe	Frogs, newts, salamanders, toads	Intestine	Probable ingestion of embryonated eggs or infective larva	Possible debilitation, intestinal obstruction, peritonitis, death	16
Cosmocerca commutata	Europe, South America	Frogs, newts, salamanders, toads	Intestine	Probable ingestion of embryonated eggs or infective larva	Debilitation, intestinal obstruction, death	6
Cosmocerca ornata	Europe	Frogs, newts, toads	Intestine	Probable ingestion of embryonated eggs or infective larva	Possible debilitation, intestinal obstruction, peritonitis, death	164
Cosmocercoides dukae	North America	Frogs, newts, salamanders, toads, box turtles, hognose snakes	Intestine	Probable ingestion of embryonated eggs or infective larva	Possible debilitation intestinal obstruction, peritonitis, death	165
Oxysomatium americana	US	Frogs, salamanders, toads	Large intestine	Probable ingestion of embryonated eggs or infective larva	Possible debilitation, intestinal obstruction, peritonitis, death	6
Oxysomatium brevicaudatum	Europe	Frogs, toads, European salamanders, newts	Large intestine	Probable ingestion of embryonated egg or infective larva	Possibly causes debilitation, intestinal obstruction, peritonitis, death	166
Oxyuroidea						
Falcaustra catesbeianae	US	Frogs	Large intestine	Probable ingestion of embryonated egg	Unknown	6
Thelandros magnavulvaris	US	Red-spotted newts, salamanders	Intestine	Ingestion of embryonated egg	Unknown	6
Trichostrongyloidea						

160

	Geographic location	Host	Location in host	Mode of infection	Effects	Reference
Oswaldocruzia leidyi	North America	Frogs, salamanders, toads, box turtles, geckoes	Small intestine	Ingestion of infective larva	Possible debilitation, intestinal obstruction, peritonitis, death	168
Oswaldocruzia subauricularis	Americas	Frogs, mudpuppies, toads	Small intestine	Ingestion of infective larva	Possible debilitation, intestinal obstruction, death	15
Oswaldocruzia goezi	Asia, Europe	Frogs, toads, European salamanders, common newts	Small intestine	Ingestion of infective larva	Possible debilitation, intestinal obstruction, death	6
Oswaldocruzia bialata	Africa, Asia, Europe	Frogs, toads	Small intestine	Ingestion of infective larva	Possible debilitation, intestinal obstruction, death	6
Oswaldocruzia sp.	Asia, Europe	Frogs, newts, salamanders, toads, European lizards	Small intestine	Ingestion of infective larva	Possible debilitation, intestinal obstruction, death	6
Pharyngodonidae						
Pharyngodon sp.	Africa, Asia, Europe	Salamanders, newts (also found in European lizards)	Intestine	Probably by ingestion of embryonated egg	Unknown	169
Spiruroidea						
Spiroxys contortus	Africa, Europe, North America	Red spotted newts, turtles	Stomach	Ingestion of copepod or transport host (fish, amphibian)	Penetrates mucosa, causes abscess formation in stomach, duodenal wall	170
Trichuroidea						
Amphibiocapillaria tritonispunctati	Worldwide	Amphiumas, frogs, newts	Intestine	Probably by ingestion of embryonated egg or earthworm	Unknown	171
Acanthocephala						
Acanthocephalus sp.	Worldwide	Frogs, newts, salamanders, toads, turtles, water snakes	Intestine	Probably by ingestion of isopod or amphipod	Enteritis	6
Acanthocephalus ranae	Europe	Frogs, newts, salamanders, toads	Stomach, intestine	Ingestion of intermediate host (isopod)	Traumatic gastritis, enteritis, sometimes death	101, 172
Centrorhynchus aluconis	Asia, Europe	Frogs, toads	Intestine	Ingestion of insect larva	Unknown	173
Corynosoma semerme	Europe	Edible frogs	Intestine	Ingestion of aquatic crustacean (amphipod)	Unknown	6
Leptorhynchoides thecatus	US	Amphiumas, mudpuppies, fishes	Intestine	Probably by ingestion of amphipod	Unknown	174
Neoechinorhynchus rutili	Europe	Edible frogs, fishes, turtles	Stomach, intestine	Ingestion of intermediate host (ostracod)	Intestinal occlusion, gastritis, enteritis	175
Pomphorhynchus bulbocolli	Eastern US	Red-spotted newts, fishes	Intestine	Ingestion of amphipod	Enteritis	55

161

TABLE 8.3 Parasites of amphibians—skin, connective tissue, musculoskeletal system.

Parasite	Geographic distribution	Hosts	Location in host	Method of infection	Pathologic effects	Reference
Flagellates						
Oodinium pillularis	Europe	Axolotl, frogs, newts	Skin, gills	Direct contact with free-living stage in water	Heavy infections cause gray coating on skin, gills; debilitation; impaired respiration; sometimes death	15
Piscinoodinium sp.	Worldwide	Larval amphibians	Skin, gills	Direct contact with free-living stage (trophont) in water	Localized granuloma	18
Microsporidia						
Pleistophora myotropica	Europe	European toads	Muscle	Ingestion of invertebrate mechanical vector	Anorexia, emaciation, death	39
Myxozoa						
Glugea danilewskyi	Europe	Grass frogs, European pond terrapins, water snakes	Muscle	Unknown	Intramuscular cysts	15
Myxobolus conspicuous	US	Red-spotted newts	Muscle	Probably ingestion of spores released from tissue	Unknown	15
Ciliates						
Trichodina fultoni	US	Mudpuppies	Gills	Direct contact with organism in water	Unknown	48
Trichodina pediculus	North America, Europe, Asia	Frogs	Skin	Direct contact with organism in water	Unknown	48
Trematodes						
Adult Monogenetic						
Gyrodactylus sp.	Europe, North America	Frogs, fishes	Skin, gills	Direct transmission of infective larvae	Asphyxiation	56
Sphyranura sp.	North America	Mudpuppies	Gills	Direct contact	Ingests blood, causes frayed gills, sometimes asphyxiation	63, 146
Larval digenetic						
Alaria alata	Europe	Frogs, European toads, snakes	Skin, subcutis, muscle	Penetration by cercaria released from snail	None	6
Alaria intermedia	US	Leopard frogs, garter snakes	Muscle, kidneys, pericardium	Penetration by cercaria released from snail	Unknown	6

Species	Location	Host(s)	Site in host	Mode of infection	Clinical signs	Reference
Alaria sp.	North America	Tadpoles, occasionally adult frogs, toads, salamander larvae	Skin, subcutis, muscle	Penetration by cercaria released from snail	None	6, 63
Allassostomoides parvum	North America	Tadpoles of leopard frogs	Skin	Penetration by cercaria released from snail	Unknown	6
Cercaria vesiculosa	Canada	Frogs	Throat muscle	Unknown	Unknown	6
Clinostomum attenuatum	North America	Frogs, salamanders (also found in snakes)	Muscle	Penetration by cercaria released from snail	Unknown	192
Clinostomum complanatum	Asia, Eastern Europe	Frogs, humans	Muscle	Penetration by cercaria released from snail	Unknown	193
Codonocephalus urnigerus	Europe	Frogs, snakes	Skin, subcutis, muscle	Penetration by cercaria released from snail	Unknown	194
Dasymetra conferta	North America	Tadpoles of frogs	Muscle	Ingestion of cercaria released from snail	Unknown	195
Dasymetra villicaeca	US	Tadpoles of frogs	Muscle	Ingestion of cercaria released from snail	Unknown	6
Diplostomulum vegrandis	US	Tadpole of leopard frogs, snakes	Muscle	Ingestion of cercaria released from snail	Unknown	6
Diplostomulum xenopi	Africa, Britain, North America	South African clawed toads	Pericardial sac	Ingestion of cercaria released from snail	Exudative pericarditis	196
Diplostomulum sp.	North America	Salamanders	Body cavity	Ingestion of cercaria released from snail	Unknown	6
Encyclometra colubrimurorum	Europe, Asia	Frogs	Muscle	Ingestion of cercaria released from snail	Unknown	197
Euparyphium melis	Asia, Europe, North America	Tadpoles of frogs	Tail	Penetration by cercaria released from snail	Unknown	6
Euryhelmis monorchis	North America	Frogs	Skin, subcutis	Penetration by cercaria released from snail	Skin vesicles, cysts	198
Euryhelmis squamula	Europe	Frogs, toads, newts	Skin	Penetration by cercaria released from snail	Unknown	199
Fibricola cratera	North America	Frogs	Skin, muscle, body cavity	Penetration by cercaria released from snail	Unknown	200
Glypthelmins pennsylvaniensis	US	Frogs	Skin	Penetration by cercaria released from snail	Unknown	70
Glypthelmins quieta	Americas, Asia	Frogs	Skin, intestine	Penetration by cercaria released from snail	Unknown	72
Lechriorchis sp.	North America	Frogs	Muscle	Ingestion of cercaria released from snail	Unknown	201
Ochetosoma sp.	North America	Tadpoles of frogs	Muscle	Ingestion of cercaria released from snail	Unknown	6
Opisthioglyphe xenopi	Southern Africa	South African clawed toads	Skin	Ingestion of cercaria released from snail	Unknown	6
Pleurogenes medians	Africa, Europe	Frogs	Skin	Penetration by cercaria released from snail	Unknown	155
Ratzia parva	Africa, Europe	Edible frogs	Muscle	Unknown	Unknown	202
Tetracotyle crystallina	North America	Leopard frogs	Muscle	Unknown	Unknown	6

(Continued)

TABLE 8.3 *(Continued)*

Parasite	Geographic distribution	Hosts	Location in host	Method of infection	Pathologic effects	Reference
Zeugorchis eurinus	US	Tadpoles of frogs	Muscle	Ingestion of cercaria released from snail	Unknown	6
Zeugorchis signatus	Europe	Tadpoles of frogs	Muscle	Ingestion of cercaria released from snail	Unknown	6
Cestodes						
Larval						
Diphyllobothrium erinacei	Australasia, Europe, South America	Frogs, newts, salamanders, toads, snakes, turtles	Muscle, connective tissue	Ingestion of first intermediate host (copepod) or immature amphibian	Larval migration causes mechanical damage	90
Diphyllobothrium latum	Americas, Asia, Europe	Frogs	Various tissues	Ingestion of first intermediate host (copepod)	Unknown	60
Schistocephalus solidus	Europe	Edible frogs, fishes	Body cavity	Ingestion of first intermediate host (copepod)	Unknown	6
Spirometra mansonoides	US	Frogs, newts, salamanders, toads, snakes, turtles	Muscle	Ingestion of first intermediate host (copepod) or amphibian or reptile	Unknown	89
Leeches						
Batrachobdella algira	Eastern Europe	Frogs	Skin	Direct contact	Unknown	6
Haementeria costata	Asia, Europe	Edible frogs, European pond terrapins	Skin	Direct contact	Vector of *Haemogregarina*	15, 176
Hemiclepsis marginata	Asia, Europe	Frogs, turtles	Skin	Direct contact	Unknown	15, 177
Limnatis nilotica	Africa, Europe	Edible frogs	Skin	Direct contact	Unknown	178
Macrobdella sp.	US	Frogs	Skin	Direct contact	Unknown	6
Oligobdella biannulata	US	Dusky salamanders	Skin	Direct contact	Unknown	6
Placobdella montifera	US	Frogs, toads	Skin	Direct contact	Unknown	55
Nematodes						
Filaroidea						
Foleyella duboisi	Israel	Edible frogs	Body cavity, mesentery	Bite of mosquito	Mesenteric cysts	15
Foleyella sp.	North America	Frogs	Body cavity, mesentery	Bite of mosquito	Mesenteric cysts	99, 182
Icosiella neglecta	Africa, Asia, Europe	Frogs	Subcutis	Bite of mosquito or midge	Subcuticular cysts	15, 99
Icosiella quadrituberculata	US	Amphiumas, frogs	Body cavity, mesentery	Probably bite of mosquito	Mesenteric cysts	16
Arthropods						
Insecta						

	Geographic location	Host	Site	Transmission	Effect	Reference
Diptera (Flies)						
Aedes sp.	Worldwide	Frogs, other vertebrates	Skin	Direct contact	Ingests blood, transmits pathogens	183
Anolisimyia blakeae	US	Green anoles	Skin	Direct contact	Myiasis	6
Batrachomyia mertensi (larva)	Australia	Treefrogs, toads	Skin	Direct contact	Myiasis	60
Bufolucilia bufonivora	Worldwide	Toads, frogs, newts, salamanders	Nostrils, deeper tissues	Direct contact	Myiasis	106
Bufolucilia sylvarum	Africa, Europe, North America	Toads, frogs	Nostrils, deeper tissues	Direct contact	Myiasis	190
Culex sp.	Worldwide	Frogs, snakes	Skin	Direct contact	Ingests blood, transmits pathogens	183, 184
Forcipomyia fairfaxensis (midge)	North America	Leopard frogs	Skin	Direct contact	Ingests blood, transmits pathogens	184
Lucilia porphyrina (larva)	Asia	Toads	Skin, orbit	Direct contact	Myiasis, death	185
Phlebotomus squamirostris	China	Toads	Skin	Direct contact	Ingests blood, transmits trypanosomes	186
Phlebotomus sp.	US	Frogs, toads	Skin	Direct contact	Ingests blood, transmits pathogens	6
Sarcophaga ruralis	Europe	European toads	Skin	Direct contact	Myiasis	6
Arachnida						
Ticks (Hard)						
Amblyomma dissimile	Americas	Toads, reptiles	Skin	Direct contact	Irritation	187
Amblyomma rotundatum	Americas	Toads, reptiles	Skin	Direct contact	Irritation	6
Ticks (Soft)						
Ornithodoros erraticus	Africa, Asia, Europe	Toads, reptiles	Skin	Direct contact	Probably causes irritation, trauma	16
Mites						
Prostigmates						
Eutrombicula alfreddugesi	Americas	Toads, reptiles, humans, other vertebrates	Skin	Direct contact	None	188
Eutrombicula insularis	West Indies	Anoles	Skin	Direct contact	Unknown	15
Eutrombicula splendens	Southeastern US	Treefrogs, lizards, snakes	Skin	Direct contact	None	189
Hannemania sp.	Worldwide	Frogs, salamanders, toads	Skin	Direct contact	Dermal vesicles	109, 110
Mollusks (Larval clams)						
Anodonta cygnaea	Europe	Axolotl	Gills	Direct contact	Local inflammation	115

(Continued)

165

TABLE 8.3 (*Continued*)

Parasite	Geographic distribution	Hosts	Location in host	Method of infection	Pathologic effects	Reference
Megalonaeas gigantean	US	Mudpuppies	Gills	Direct contact	Local inflammation	115
Simpsonichoncha ambigua	US	Mudpuppies	Gills	Direct contact	Local inflammation	115
Crustaceans						
Argulus americanus	US	Frogs, newts, salamanders, fishes	Skin	Direct contact	Anemia, dermatitis	55
Argulus japonicus	Worldwide	Tadpoles of leopard frogs	Skin	Direct contact	Anemia, dermatitis	55, 16
Lernaea cyprinacea	Worldwide	Frogs, newts, salamanders	Gills, skin	Direct contact	Trauma of gills, skin	55
Lernaea ranae	US	Tadpoles of green frogs	Gills	Direct contact	Trauma of gills, skin	55

166

TABLE 8.4 Parasites of amphibians—Respiratory, nervous, urogenital systems, and miscellaneous tissues.

Parasite	Geographic distribution	Hosts	Location in host	Method of infection	Pathologic effects	Reference
Coccidia						
Isospora lieberkuehni	Europe	Frogs, toads	Kidneys	Ingestion of sporulated oocyst passed in urine	Nephritis	203, 204
Leptotheca ohlmacheri	Europe, North America	Frogs, toads	Kidneys	Ingestion of organism passed in urine	Renal hypertrophy, congestion	204
Pleistophora bufonis	Europe, North America	Toads	Bidder's organ	Unknown	Unknown	6
Trichodina urinicola	Africa, Europe, North America	Edible frogs, newts, toads	Urinary bladder	Direct contact with organism in water	Unknown	3
Ciliates						
Glaucoma sp.	US	Axolotl	Brain, spinal cord	Unknown	Unknown	15
Trichodina urinicola	Africa, Europe, North America	Frogs, newts, toads	Urinary bladder	Ingestion of organism passed in urine	None	47
Microsporidia						
Myxosoma ranae	Australia, Europe	Grass frogs, treefrogs	Various tissues	Probably ingestion of spores released from tissue	Unknown	15
Trematodes						
Adult Monogenetic						
Polystoma sp.	Worldwide	Frogs, toads	Urinary bladder, gills	Direct transmission of infective larvae	Ingests blood; pathologic effects slight	15, 58, 146
Adult Digenetic						
Gorgodera amplicava	North America	Frogs, salamanders, toads	Kidneys, urinary bladder	Ingestion of second intermediate host (frog tadpole, salamander larva, snail, crayfish)	Heavy infections cause listlessness, anorexia, uremia, death	73
Gorgodera cygnoides	Europe, North America	Frogs, salamanders, toads	Urinary bladder	Ingestion of second intermediate host (frog tadpole, salamander larva, snail, crayfish)	Heavy infections cause listlessness, anorexia, uremia, death	147

(Continued)

TABLE 8.4 (Continued)

Parasite	Geographic distribution	Hosts	Location in host	Method of infection	Pathologic effects	Reference
Gorgoderina attenuata	Americas	Frogs, newts, snakes	Kidneys, urinary bladder	Ingestion of second intermediate host (frog tadpole, salamander larva, snail, crayfish)	Heavy infections cause listlessness, anorexia, uremia, death	147
Gorgoderina vitelliloba	Africa, Asia, Europe	Frogs, toads	Urinary bladder	Ingestion of second intermediate host (frog tadpole, salamander larva, snail, crayfish)	Heavy infections cause listlessness, anorexia, uremia, death	60, 148
Gorgoderina sp.	Americas	Frogs, newts, salamanders, toads	Urinary bladder	Ingestion of second intermediate host (frog tadpole, salamander larva, snail, crayfish)	Anorexia, uremia, death	6, 60, 149
Phyllodistomum americanum	North America	Toads, salamanders	Urinary bladder	Ingestion of second intermediate host (arthropod)	Unknown	6
Phyllodistomum solidum	Eastern US	Dusky salamanders	Urinary bladder	Ingestion of second intermediate host (arthropod)	Unknown	6
Larval Digenetic						
Allocreadium anguisticolle	Europe	Grass frogs	Various tissues	Penetration by cercaria released from snail	Unknown	6
Apharyngostrigea pipientis	US	Tadpoles of leopard frogs, treefrogs	Various tissues	Penetration by cercaria released from snail	Unknown	6
Cercaria elodes	US	Tadpoles of leopard frogs	Notochord	Unknown	Unknown	6
Diplostomum flexicaudum	US	Tadpoles of frogs, American toads	Eye lens	Penetration by cercaria released from snail	Unknown	157
Diplostomulum scheuringi	US	Red-spotted newts, greater sirens (Siren lacertina)	Eyes, brain	Penetration by cercaria released from snail	Local hemorrhages	78
Echinoparyphium flexum	North America	Frogs	Kidneys	Penetration by cercaria released from snail	Unknown	205
Echinoparyphium spinigerum	Europe	Edible frogs	Various tissues	Penetration by cercaria released from snail	Unknown	6
Echinostoma revolutum	Worldwide	Amphibians	Various tissues	Penetration by cercaria released from snail	Unknown	210

Species	Geographic location	Host	Site	Mode of infection	Effects	References
Echinostoma xenopi	Southern Africa	South African clawed toads	Brain, subcutis	Penetration by cercaria released from snail	Unknown	6
Gorgodera cygnoides	North America, Europe	Frogs, toads	Urinary bladder	Penetration by cercaria released from clam	Unknown	206
Haematoloechus asper	Africa, Europe	Frogs, toads	Lungs	Ingestion of second intermediate host (arthropod)	Anemia	6, 15, 150
Haematoloechus sp.	Americas	Frogs	Lungs	Infection of second intermediate host (arthropod)	Anemia	6, 63, 151
Haplometra cylindracea	Europe	Frogs, European toads	Lungs	Ingestion of second intermediate host (water beetle)	None	15, 61, 76, 152
Hypoderaeum conoideum	Asia, Europe, North America	Edible frogs	Various tissues	Penetration by cercaria released from snail	Unknown	211
Leptophallus nigrovenosus	Africa, Europe	Tadpoles of frogs, newts, toads, lizards	Various tissues	Penetration by cercaria released from snail	Unknown	6
Neascus sp.	Great Britain, southern Africa	South African clawed frogs	Lateral line system	Unknown	Local proliferation of melanophores, death	82
Sphaerostoma bramae	Europe	Treefrogs	Various tissues	Penetration by cercaria released from snail	Unknown	6
Strigea elegans	US	Tadpoles of frogs, American toads, larva of marbled salamander; snakes	Various tissues	Penetration by cercaria released from snail or ingestion of tadpole	Unknown	209
Cestodes						
Larval						
Mesocestoides sp.	US	Leopard frogs, toads, lizards, snakes	Kidneys, liver, intestinal wall, mesentery	Ingestion of unknown first intermediate host	Unknown	207
Nematodes						
Rhabditoidea						
Rhabdias bufonis	Asia, Europe	Frogs, toads	Lungs	Ingestion of infective larva or penetration of skin by larva	Unknown	179

(Continued)

169

TABLE 8.4 (*Continued*)

Parasite	Geographic distribution	Hosts	Location in host	Method of infection	Pathologic effects	Reference
Rhabdias entomelas	US	Frogs	Lungs	Ingestion of infective larva or penetration of skin by larva	Unknown	6
Rhabdias ranae	North America	Frogs, toads, snakes	Lungs	Ingestion of larva or penetration of skin by larva	Unknown	180
Rhabdias rubrovenosa	Europe	Frogs, toads	Lungs	Ingestion of infective larva or penetration of skin by larva	Unknown	6
Rhabdias sphaerocephala	Central America, Europe	Toads	Lungs	Ingestion of infective larva or penetration of skin by larva	Unknown	181
Arthropods						
Arachnida						
Mites						
Lawrencarus sp.	Worldwide	Toads	Nasal passages	Direct contact	Unknown	16
Xenopacarus africanus	Southern Africa	South African clawed toads	Nasal passages	Direct contact	Unknown	208

REFERENCES

1. Diamond, L.S. (1965) A study of the morphology, biology and taxonomy of the trypanosomes of anura. *Wildl. Dis.* **44,** 1–85.

2. Barrow, Jr., J.H. (1958) The biology of *Trypanosoma diemyctyli,* Tobey: III. Factors influencing the cycle of *Trypanosoma diemyctyli* in the vertebrate host *Triturus v. viridescens. J. Protozool.* **5,** 161–170.

3. Kudo, R.R. (1966) *Protozoology.* 5th ed. Charles C. Thomas, Springfield, Illinois. 1174 pages.

4. Marcus, L.C. (1981) *Veterinary Biology and Medicine of Captive Amphibians and Reptiles.* Lea and Febiger, Philadelphia, Pennsylvania, 239 pages.

5. Woo, P.T.K. (1969) The life cycle of *Trypanosoma chrysemydis. Can. J. Zool.* **47,** 1139–1151.

6. Walton, A.C. (1964) The parasites of amphibia. *Wildl. Dis.* **40,** 28 pages.

7. Anderson, J.R. and Ayala, S.A. (1968) Trypanosome transmitted by *Phlebotomus:* First report from the Americas. *Science* **161,** 1023–1025.

8. Nigrelli, R.F. (1929) Atypical etythrocyctes and erythroplastids in the blood of *Triturus viridescens. Anat. Record* **43,** 257–270.

9. Poynton, S.L. and Whitaker, B.R. (2001) Protozoa and Metazoa infecting amphibians. In: Wright, K.M. and Whitaker, B.R (eds.) *Amphibian Medicine and Captive Husbandry.* Krieger Publishing Co., Malabar, Florida, 193–221.

10. Levine, N.D. (1961) *Protozoan Parasites of Domestic Animals and of Man.* Burgess, Minneapolis, Minnesota, 412 pages.

11. Honigberg, B.M. (1963). Evolutionary and systematic relationships in the flagellate order Trichomonadida Kirby. *J. Protozool.* **10,** 20–63.

12. Honigberg, B.M. and Christian, H.H. (1954) Characteristics of *Hexamastix batrachorum* (Alexeieff). *J. Parasitol.* **40,** 508–514.

13. Dobell, C.C. (1909) Research on the intestinal protozoa of frogs and toads. *Quart. J. Microscop. Sci.* **53,** 201– 277.

14. Rankin, J.S., Jr. (1937) An ecological study of parasites of some North Carolina salamanders. *Ecol. Monographs* **7,** 170–269.

15. Reichenbach-Klinke, H. and Elkan, E. (1965) The principal diseases of lower vertebrates. Academic Press, New York. 600 pages.

16. Walton, A.C. (1966) Supplemental catalog of the parasites of amphibia. *Wildl. Dis.* **48,** 58 pp.

17. Cheng, T.C. (1964) *The Biology of Animal Parasites.* W.B. Saunders, Philadelphia. 727 pages.

18. Woo, P.T.K. and Poynton, S.L. (1994) Flagellate Parasites of Fish. In: Krieier, J.P. (ed.) *Parasitic Protozoa,* (2nd ed., vol. 8.) Academic Press, San Diego, California, 1–80.

19. Wright, K.M. and Whitaker, B.R. (2001) Pharmacotherapeutics. In: Wright, K.M. and Whitaker, B.R. (eds.) *Amphibian Medicine and Captive Husbandry.* Krieger Publishing, Malabar, Florida, 309–330.

20. Honigberg, B.M. (1950) Intestinal flagellates of amphibians and reptiles. I. Survey of intestinal flagellates of reptiles. II. Structure and morphogenesis of the members of the genus *Trichomonas* Donne, 1836 from amphibians and reptiles. Doctoral dissertation, University of California, Berkeley. 260 pages.

21. Moskowitz, N. (1951) Observations on some intestinal flagellates from reptilian host (Squamata). *J. Morphol.* **89,** 257–321.

22. Honigberg, B.M. (1953) Structure, taxonomic status, and host list of *Tritrichomonas batrachorum* (Perty). *J. Parasitol.* **39,** 191–208.

23. Wenyon, C.M. (1926) *Protozoology.* Hafner, New York, New York.

24. Honigberg, B.M.(1950). On the structure of the parabasal body in *Tritrichomonas batrachorum* (Perty) and *Tritrichomonas augusta* (Alexeieff) of amphibians and reptiles. *J. Parasitol.* **36,** 89.

25. Honigberg, B.M. (1951) Structure and morphogenesis of *Trichomonas prowazeki* Alexeieff and *Trichomonas brumpti* Alexeieff. *Univ. Calif. Publ. Zool.* **55,** 337–394.

26. Geiman, Q.M. and Ratcliffe, H.L. (1936) Morphology and the life-cycle of an amoeba producing amoebiasis in reptiles. *Parasitology* **28,** 208–228.

27. Valentine, B.A. and Stoskopff, M.K. (1984) Amebiasis in a neotropical toad. *J. Am. Vet. Med. Assoc.* **185,** 1418–1419.

28. Marcus, L.C. (1968) Diseases of snakes and turtles. In: Kirk, R.W. (ed.) *Current Veterinary Therapy III: Small Animal Practice.* W.B. Saunders, Philadelphia, Pennsylvania, 435–442.

29. Cowan, D.F. (1968) Diseases of captive reptiles. *J. Am. Vet. Med. Assoc.* **153,** 848–859.

30. Green S.L., Bouley, D.M., Josling, C.A., and Fayer, R. (2003) Cryptosporidiosis associated with emaciation and proliferative gastritis in a laboratory reared South African clawed frog (*Xenopus laevis*). *Comp Med* **53,** 81–84.

31. Bolek, M.G., Janovy, J. Jr., and Irizarry-Rovira, A.R. (2003) Observations on the life history and descriptions of coccidia (Apicomplexa) from the western chorus frog, *Pseudacris triseriata triseriata,* from eastern Nebraska. *J. Parasitol.* **89,** 522–528.

32. Fantham, H.B. and Porter, A. (1954) The endoparasites of some North American snakes and their effects on the Ophidia. *Proc. Zool. Soc. London* **123,** 867–898.

33. Pellerdy, L.P. (1963) *Catalogue of Eimeriidea (Protozoa: Sporozoa).* Akademiai Kiado, Budapest, 160 pages.

34. Saxe, L.H. (1955) Observations on *Eimeria* from *Ambystoma tigrinum,* with descriptions of four new species. *Proc. Iowa Acad. Sci.* **62,** 663–673.

35. Hull, R.W. and Camin, J.H. (1960) Haemogregarines in snakes: The incidence and identity of the erythrocytic stages. *J. Parasitol.* **46,** 515–523.

36. Desser, S.S., Hong, H., and Martin, D.S. (1995) The life history, ultrastructure and experimental transmission of *Hepatozoon catesbianae* n. comb., an apicomplexa parasite of the bullfrog, *Rana catesbeiana* and the mosquito, *Culex territans* in Algonquin Park, Ontario. *J. Parasitol.* **81,** 212–222.

37. Desser, S.S., Hong, H., Siddall, M.F., and Barta, J.R. (1993) An ultrastructural study *Brugerolleia algonquinensis* gen. nov., sp. nov. (Diplomonadina; Diplomonadida) a flagellate parasite in the blood of frogs from Ontario, Canada. *J. Protistol.* **29,** 72–80.

38. O'Connor, P. (1966) Diseases of snakes. In: Kirk, R.W. (ed.) *Current Veterinary Therapy: Small Animal Practice.* W.B. Saunders, Philadelphia, Pennsylvania, 582–585.

39. Canning, E.U., Elkan, E., and Trigg, P.I. (1964) *Pleistophora myotropica* spec. nov., causing high mortality in the common toad *Bufo bufo* L., with notes on the maintenance of *Bufo* and *Xenopus* in the laboratory. *J. Protozool.* **11,** 157–166.

40. Paperna, I. and Lainson, R. (1995) *Allogugea bufonis* nov. gen., nov. sp. (Microsporidia: Glugeidae), a microsporidian of *Bufo marinus* tadpoles and metamorphosing toads (Amphibian: Anura) from Amazon Brazil. *Dis. Aq. Organ.* **23,** 7–16.

41. Canning, E.U. (1966) The transmission of *Pleistophora myotropica,* a microsporidian infecting the voluntary muscles of the common toad. In: Corradetti, A. (ed.) *Proceedings of the First International Congress on Parasitology.* Pergamon Press, New York, 446–447.

42. Graczyk, T.K., Cranfield, M.R., Bicknese, E.J., and Wisnieski, A.P. (1996) Progressive ulcerative dermatitis in a captive, wild-caught, South American giant tree frog (*Phyllomedusa bicolor*) with microsporidial septicemia. *J. Zoo Wild. Med.* **27,** 522–527.

43. McAllister, C.T. and Trauth, S.E. (1995) New host records for *Myxidium serotinum* (Protozoa: Myxosporea) from North American amphibians. *J. Parasitol.* **81,** 485–488.

44. Woodhead, A.E. (1928) *Haptophrya michiganensis* sp. nov., a protozoan parasite of the four-toed salamander. *J. Parasitol.* **14,** 177–182.

45. Golikova, M.N. (1963) Morphological and cytochemical study of the life cycle of *Nyctotherus cordiformis* Stein (in Russian). *Acta Protozool.* **1,** 31–42.

46. Corliss, J.O. (1959) An illustrated key to the higher groups of the ciliated protozoa with definition of terms. *J. Protozool.* **6,** 265–281.

47. Lom, J. (1958) A contribution to the systematics and morphology of endoparasitic trichodinids from amphibians, with a proposal of uniform specific characteristics. *J. Protozool.* **5,** 251–263.

48. Lom, J. (1970) Observations on trichodinid ciliates from freshwater fishes. *Arch. Protistenk.* **112,** 153–177.

49. Davis, H.S. (1947) Studies of the protozoan parasites of fresh-water fishes. *U.S. Fish Wildlife Serv. Fishery Bull.* **41,** 29 pages.

50. Corliss, J.O. (1959) Comments on the systematics and phylogeny of the protozoa. *Syst. Zool.* **8,** 169–190.

51. Cameron, T.W.M. (1956) *Parasites and Parasitism.* John Wiley, New York, 322 pages.

52. Dawes, B. (1946) *The Trematoda, with Special Reference to British and Other European Forms.* Cambridge University Press, Cambridge, England, 644 pages.

53. Noble, E.R. and Noble, G.A. (1961) *Parasitology: The Biology of Animal Parasites.* Lea and Febiger, Philadelphia, Pennsylvania, 767 pages.

54. Dogiel, V.A., Polyanski, Y.I., and Kheisin, E.M. (1964) *General Parasitology.* Oliver and Boyd, Edinburgh and London, 516 pages.

55. Hoffman, G.L. (1967) *Parasites of North American Freshwater Fishes.* University of California Press, Berkeley, 486 pages.

56. Hoffman, G.L. and Putz, R.E. (1964) Studies on *Gyrodactylus macrochiri* n. sp. *(Trematoda: Monogenea)* from *Lepomis macrochirus.* *Proc. Helminthol. Soc. Wash. D.C.* **31,** 76–82.

57. Cheng, T.C. (1964) *The Biology of Animal Parasites.* W.B. Saunders, Philadelphia, Pennsylvania, 727 pages.

58. Paul, A.A. (1938) Life history studies of North American fresh-water polystomes. *J. Parasitol.* **24,** 489–510.

59. Savage, R.M. (1962) *The Ecology and Life History of the Common Frog (Rana temporaria temporaria).* Hafner, New York, 221 pages.

60. Walton, A.C. (1967) Supplemental catalog of the parasites of amphibia. *Wildl. Dis.* **50,** 38 pages.

61. Lees, E. (1962) The incidence of helminth parasites in a particular frog population. *Parasitology* **52,** 95– 102.

62. MacDonald, S. and Combes, C. (1978) The hatching rhythm of *Polystoma integerrimum,* a monogenean from the frog *Rana temporaria. Chronobiologia* **5,** 277–285.

63. Olsen, O.W. (1967) *Animal Parasites: Their Biology and Life Cycles.* 2nd ed. Burgess, Minneapolis, Minnesota, 431 pages.

64. Skrjabin, K.I. (1964) *Keys to the Trematodes of Animals and Man.* Arai, H.P. (ed.) University of Illinois Press, Urbana, Illinois, 351 pages.

65. Fischthal, J.H. (1955) Ecology of worm parasites in south-central New York salamanders. *Am. Midland Naturalist* **53,** 176–183.

66. Yamaguti, S. (1958) The Digenetic Trematodes of Vertebrates. Vol. I. 2 Parts. In: Yamaguti, S. *Systema Helminthum.* Interscience, New York.

67. Fischthal, J.H. (1955) Helminths of salamanders from Promised Land State Forest Park, Pennsylvania. *Proc. Helminthol. Soc. Wash. D.C.* **22,** 46–48.

68. Rankin, J.S., Jr. (1945) An ecological study of the helminth parasites of amphibians and reptiles of western Massachusetts and vicinity. *J. Parasitol.* **31,** 142–150.

69. Efford, I.E. and Tsumura, K. (1969) Observations on the biology of the trematode *Megalodiscus microphagus* in amphibians from Marion Lake, British Columbia. *Am. Midland Naturalist* **82,** 197–203.

70. Cheng, T.C. (1961) Description, life history, and developmental pattern of *Glypthelmins pennsylvaniensis* n. sp. (Trematoda: Brachycoeliidae), new parasite of frogs. *J. Parasitol.* **47,** 469–477.

71. Ubelaker, J.E., Duszynski, D.W., and Beaver, D.L. (1967) Occurrence of the trematode, *Glypthelmins pennsylvaniensis* Cheng, 1961, in chorus frogs, *Pesudacris triseriata,* in Colorado. *Bull. Wildlife Dis. Assoc.* **3,** 177.

72. Schell, S.C. (1962) Development of the sporocyst generations of *Glypthelmins quieta* (Stafford, 1900) (Trematoda: Plagiorchioidea), a parasite of frogs. *J. Parasitol.* **48,** 387–394.

73. Goodchild, C.G. (1948) Additional observations on the bionomics and life history of *Gorgodera amplicava* Loos, 1899 (Trematoda: Gorgoderidae). *J. Parasitol.* **34,** 407–427.

74. Goodchild, C.G. (1950) Establishment and pathology of gorgoderid infections in anuran kidneys. *J. Parasitol.* **36,** 439–446.

75. Harwood, P.D. (1932) The helminths parasitic in the amphibia and reptilia of Houston, Texas, and vicinity. *Proc. U.S. Natl. Museum* **81,** 1–71.

76. Arvy, L. (1950). Donees cytologiques et histochimiques sur l'hematophagie chez *Haplometra cylindracea* Zader 1800. *Ann. Parasitol. Humaine Comparee* **25,** 27–36.

77. Hughes, R.C. (1929) Studies on the trematode family Strigeidae (Holostomidae) No. XIX: *Diplostomulum scheuringi* sp. nov. and *D. vegrandis* (La Rue). *J. Parasitol.* **15,** 267–271.

78. Etges, F.J. (1961) Contributions to the life history of the brain fluke of newts and fish, *Diplostomulum scheuringi* Hughes, 1929 (Trematoda: Diplostomatidae). *J. Parasitol.* **47,** 453–458.

79. Lautenschlager, E.W. (1959) Meningeal tumors of the newt associated with trematode infection of the brain. *Proc. Helminthol. Soc. Wash. D.C.* **26,** 11–14.

80. Nigrelli, R.F. and Maraventano, L.W. (1944) Pericarditis in *Xenopus laevis* caused by *Diplostomulum xenopi* sp. nov., a larval strigeid. *J. Parasitol.* **30,** 184–190.

81. Southwell, T. and Kirshner, A. (1937) On some parasitic worms found in *Xenopus laevis,* the South African clawed toad. *Ann. Trop. Med. Parasitol.* **31,** 245–265.

82. Elkan, E. and Murray, R.W. (1952) A larval trematode infection of the lateral line system of the toad, *Xenopus laevis* (Daudin). *Proc. Zool. Soc. London* **122,** 121–126.

83. Thomas, L.J. (1937) Environmental relations of life history of the tapeworm *Bothriocephalus rarus* Thomas. *J. Parasitol.* **23,** 133–152.

84. Yamaguti, S. (1959) The cestodes of vertebrates. Vol. II. In: Yamaguti, S. *Systema helminthum.* Interscience, New York.

85. Elkan, E. (1960) Some interesting pathological cases in amphibians. *Proc. Zool. Soc. London* **134,** 275–296.

86. Ortlepp, R.J. (1926) On a collection of helminthes from a South African farm. *J. Helminthol.* **4,** 127–142.

87. Wardle, R.A. and McLeod, J.A. (1952) *The Zoology of Tapeworms.* University of Minnesota Press, Minneapolis, Minnesota, 780 pages.

88. Belding, D.L. (1965) *Textbook of Parasitology* 3rd ed. Appleton-Century-Crofts, New York, 1374 pages.

89. Corkum, K.C. (1966) Sparganosis in some vertebrates of Louisiana and observations on a human infection. *J. Parasitol.* **52,** 444–448.

90. Galliard, H. and Ngu, D.V. (1946) Particularites du cycle evolutif de *Diphyllobothrium mansoni* au Tonkin. *Ann. Parasitol. Humaine Comparee* **21,** 246–253.

91. Witenberg, G.G. (1964) Zooparasitic diseases: A. Helminthozoonoses In: van der Hoeden, J. (ed.) *Zoonoses.* Elsevier, New York, pages 529–719.

92. Burrows, R.B. (1965) *Microscopic Diagnosis of the Parasites of Man.* Yale Univ. Press, New Haven, Connecticut, 328 pages.

93. Mann, K.H. and Tyler, M.J. (1963) Leeches as endoparasites of frogs. *Nature* **190,** 1224–1225.

94. Richardson, L.R. (1974) A contribution to the general zoology of the land leeches (Hirudinea: Haemadypsoidea superfam. Nov.). *Acta. Zoologica Acad. Scien. Hungary* **21,** 119–152.

95. Tyler M.J., Parker, F., and Bulmer, R.N.H. (1966) Observations on endoparasite leeches infesting frogs in New Guinea. *Rec. South Austral. Museum* **1592,** 356–359.

96. Burreson, E.M. (1995) Phylum Annelida: Hirudinea as vectors and disease agents, in Woo, P.T.K. (ed.). *Fish Diseases and Disorders. Volume 1. Protozoa and Metazoan Infections.* CAB International, Wallingford, UK, 529–629 pages.

97. Yamaguti, S. (1961) The nematodes of vertebrates. Vol. III. 2 Parts. In Yamaguti, S. *Systema helminthum.* Interscience, New York.

98. Yorke, W. and Maplestone, P.A. (1926) The nematode parasites of vertebrates. Blakeston, Philadelphia, Pennsylvania, 536 pages.

99. Crans, W.J. (1969) Preliminary observations of frog filariasis in New Jersey. *Bull. Wildlife Dis. Assoc.* **5,** 342–347.

100. Kotcher, E. (1941) Studies on the development of frog filariae. *Am. J. Hyg.* **34,** 36–65.

101. Van Cleave, H.J. (1915) Acanthocephala in North American amphibia. *J. Parasitol.* **1,** 175–178.

102. Bullock, W.L. (1961) A preliminary study of the histopathology of Acanthocephala in the vertebrate intestine. *J. Parasitol.* **47,** 31.

103. Zumpt, F. (1965) *Myiasis in Man and Animals in the Old World: A Textbook for Physicians, Veterinarians and Zoologists.* Butterworth, London, 267 pages.

104. Bleakney, J.S. (1963) First North American record of *Bufolucilia silvarum* (Meigen) (Diptera: Calliphoridae) parasitizing *Bufo terrestris americanus* Holbrook. *Can. Entomol.* 95, 107.

105. Stone, A., Sabrosky, C.W., Wirth, W.W., Foote, R.H., and Coulson, J.R. (1965) *A Catalog of the Diptera of America North of Mexico.* U.S. Dept. Agr. Handbook 276, 1696 pages.

106. Sandner, H. (1955) *Lucilia bufonivora* Moniez, 1876 (Diptera) Polsce. *Acta Parasitol. Pol.* **2,** 319–329.

107. Stadler, H. (1930) Uber de Befag einer Krote (*Bufo vulgaris* Laur.) durch die Larven von *Lucilia sylvarum* Meig; Krankheitsgeschiche und Sektionsbefund. *Z. Parasitenk.* **2,** 360–367.

108. Sambon, L.W. (1928) The parasitic acarians of animals and the part they play in the causation of the eruptive fevers and other diseases of man: Preliminary considerations based upon an ecological study of typhus fever. *Ann. Trop. Med.* **22,** 67–132.

109. Hyland, Jr., K.E. (1956) A new species of chigger mite, *Hannemania hegeneri* (Acarina: Trombiculidae). *J. Parasitol.* **42,** 176–179.

110. Hyland, Jr., K.E. (1950) The life cycle and parasitic habit of the chigger mite *Hannemania dunni* Sambon, 1928, a parasite of amphibians. *J. Parasitol.* **36,** 32–33.

111. Murphy, T.D. (1965) High incidence of two parasitic infestations and two morphological abnormalities in a population of the frog, *Rana pulustris* Le Conte. *Am. Midland Naturalist* **74,** 233–239.

112. Feider, Z. (1958) Sur une larve du genre *Trombicula* (Acari) parasite sur les lizards de la roumanie. *Z. Parasitenk.* **18,** 441–456.

113. Ewing, H.E. (1926) The common box-turtle, a natural host for chiggers. *Proc. Biol. Soc.,* Washington, D.C. **39,** 19–20.

114. Chandler, A.C. and Read, C.P. (1961) *Introduction to Parasitology.* 10th ed. John Wiley, New York, 822 pages.

115. Faust, E.C., Beaver, P.C., and Jung, R.C. (1968) *Animal Agents and Vectors of Human Disease.* 3rd ed. Lea and Febiger, Philadelphia, Pennsylvania, 461 pages.

116. Worms, M.J. (1967) Parasites in newly imported animals. *J. Inst. Animal Tech.* **18,** 1839–1847.

117. Howard, A.D. (1951) A river mussel parasitic on a salamander. *Chicago Acad. Sci. Nat. Hist. Mus.* **77,** 1–6.

118. Harris, Jr., J.P. (1954) The parasites of amphibia. *Field Lab.* **22,** 52–58.

119. Woo, P.T., Bogart, J.P., and Servage, D.L. (1980) *Trypanosoma ambystomae* in *Ambystoma* spp. (order Caudata) in southern Ontario. *Can. J. Zool.* **58,** 466–469.

120. Lehmann, D.L. (1952) Notes on the life cycle and infectivity of *Trypanosoma barbari. J. Parasitol.* **38,** 550–553.

121. Buttner, A. and Bourcart, N. (1955) Some biological particulars of a trypanosome in the green frog, *Trypanosoma inopinatum* Sergent, 1904. *Ann. Parasitol. Hum. Comp.* **30,** 431–445.

122. Siddall, M.E and Desser, S.S. (1992) Alternative leech vectors for frog and turtle trypanosomes. *J. Parasitol.* **78,** 562–563.

123. Werner, J.K., Davis, J.S., and Slaght, K.S. (1988) Trypanosomes of *Bufo americanus* from northern Michigan. *J. Wildl. Dis.* **24,** 647–649.

124. Borges, F.P., Wiltuschnig, R.C., Tasca, T., and De Carli, G.A. (2004) Scanning electron microscopy study of *Tritrichomonas augusta. Parasitol. Res.* **94,** 158–161.

125. Feely, D.E. and Erlandsen, S.L. (1985) Morphology of *Giardia agilis:* observation by scanning electron microscopy and interference reflexion microscopy. *J. Protozool.* **32,** 691–693.

126. Delvinquier, B.L.J. and Freeland, W.J. (1988) Protozoan parasites of the Cane toad, *Bufo marinus,* in Australia. *Aus. J. Zool.* **36,** 301–316.

127. Bolek, M.G., Janovy, J. Jr., and Irizarry-Rovira, A.R. (2003) Observations on the life history and descriptions of coccidia (Apicomplexa) from the western chorus frog, *Pseudacris triseriata triseriata,* from eastern Nebraska. *J. Parasitol.* **89,** 522–528.

128. McAllister, C.T. and Trauth, S.E. (1995) New host records for *Myxidium serotinum* (Protozoa: Myxosporea) from North American amphibians. *J. Parasitol.* **81,** 485–488.

129. Paulin, J.J. (1967) The fine structure of *Nyctotherus cordiformis* (Ehrenberg). *J. Protozool.* **14,** 183– 196.

130. Couch, J.A. (1966) *Brachycoelium ambystomae* sp. n. (Trematoda: brachycoelidae) from *Ambystoma opacum. J. Parasitol.* **52,** 46–49.

131. Bertman, M. (1986) *Brachycoelium salamandrae* (Frolich, 1789) (Trematoda, Brachycoeliidae) in *Salamandra salamandra* L. *Wiad. Parazytol.* **32,** 173–175.

132. Cheng, T.C. and Chase, Jr., R.S. (1961) *Brachycoelium stablefordi,* a new parasite of salamanders; and a case of abnormal polylobation of the testes of *Brachycoelium storerliae* Harwood, 1932 (Trematoda: Brachycoeliidae). *Trans. Am. Microscop. Soc.* **80,** 33–38.

133. Goldberg, S.R., Bursey, C.R., and Cheam, H. (1998) Helminths of two native frog species (*Rana chiricahuensis, Rana yavapaiensis*) and one introduced frog species (*Rana catesbeiana*) (Ranidae) from Arizona. *J. Parasitol.* **84,** 175–177.

134. Bertman, M. (1993) *Diplodiscus subclavatus* (Pallas, 1760) (Trematoda) and *Acanthocephalus ranae* (Schrank, 1788) (Acanthocephala) in grass snake—*Natrix natrix* (L.). *Wiad. Parazytol.* **39,** 405–406.

135. Razo-Mendivil, U.J., Leon-Regagnon, V., and Perez-Ponce de Leon, G. (2004) Description of two new species of *Glypthelmins* Stafford, 1905

(Digenea: Macroderoididae) in *Rana* spp. from Mexico, based on morphology and mtDNA and rDNA sequences. *Syst Parasitol.* **59**, 199–210.

136. Zelmer, D.A. and Brooks, D.R. (2000) *Halipegus eschi* n. sp. (Digenea: Hemiuridae) in *Rana vaillanti* from Guanacaste Province, Costa Rica. *J. Parasitol.* **86**, 1114–1117.

137. Zelmer, D.A. and Esch, G.W. (1999) Reevaluation of the taxonomic status of *Halipegus occidualis* Stafford, 1905 (Digenea: Hemiuridae). *J. Parasitol.* **85**, 157–160.

138. Kechemir, N. (1978) Demonstration of life cycle with four obligatory hosts of the Hemiurid Trematodes. *Ann. Parasitol. Hum. Comp.* **53**, 75–92.

139. Davies, A.J. and Johnston, M.R. (2000) The biology of some intraerythrocytic parasites of fishes, amphibia and reptiles. *Adv. Parasitol.* **45**, 1–107.

140. Lehman, D.L. (1964) Cytological and cytochemical studies on *Cytamoeba bacterifera* Labb'e, 1894. *Parasitology* **54**, 121–124.

141. Laird, M. and Bullock, W.L. (1969) Marine fish haematozoa from New Brunswick and New England. *J. Fisheries Res. Board Can.* **26**, 1075–1102.

142. Mansour, N.S. and Mohammed, A.H. (1962) *Lankesterella bufonis* sp. nov. parasitizing toads, *Bufo regularis* Reuss, in Egypt. *J. Protozool.* **9**, 243–248.

143. Desser, S.S., Siddall, M.E., and Barta, J.R. (1990) Ultrastructural observations on the developmental stages of *Lankesterella minima* (Apicomplexa) in experimentally infected *Rana catesbeiana* tadpoles. *J. Parasitol.* **76**, 97–103.

144. Kretschmar, W. (1963) Studies on the cellular structure of Opalina ranarum for the taxonomy of opalinids. *Z. Parasitenkd.* 4, 274–308.

145. Kostka, M., Hampl, V., Cepicka, I., and Flegr, J. (2004) Phylogenetic position of *Protoopalina intestinalis* based on SSU rRNA gene sequence. *Mol. Phylogenet. Evol.* **33**, 220–224.

146. Williams, J.B. (1995) Phylogeny of the Polystomatidae (Platyhelminthes, Monogenea), with particular reference to *Polystoma integerrimum.* *Int. J. Parasitol.* **25**, 437–441.

147. Kim, K.H., Joo, K.H., and Rim, H.J. (1995) Gorgoderid trematodes (Digenea: Gorgoderidae) from the urinary bladder of frogs in Korea. *Korean J. Parasitol.* **33**, 75–83.

148. Lees, E. (1953) Life history of *Gorgoderina vitelliloba* (Olsson). Nature **171**, 485.

149. Mata-Lopez, R. and Leon-Regagnon, V. (2005) *Gorgoderina festoni* n. sp. (Digenea: Gorgoderidae) in Anurans (Amphibia) from Mexico. *Syst. Parasitol.* **62**, 185–190.

150. Snyder, S.D. and Tkach, V.V. (2001) Phylogenetic and biogeographical relationships among some holarctic frog lung flukes (Digenea: Haematoloechidae). *J. Parasitol.* **87**, 1433–1440.

151. Leon-Regagnon, V. and Paredes-Calderon, E.L. (2002) *Haematoloechus danbrooksi* n. sp. (Digenea: Plagiorchioidea) from *Rana vaillanti* from Los Tuxtlas, Veracruz, Mexico. *J. Parasitol.* **88**, 1215–1221.

152. Goumghar, M.D., Abrous, M., Ferdonnet, D., Dreyfuss, G., and Rondelaud, D. (2000) Prevalence of *Haplometra cylindracea* infection in three species of *Lymnaea* snails in central France. *Parasitol. Res.* **86**, 337–339.

153. Nollen, P.M. and Nadakavukaren, M.J. (1974) *Megalodiscus temperatus:* scanning electron microscopy of the tegumental surfaces. *Exp. Parasitol.* **36**, 123–130.

154. Panin, V.I. and Nesterenko, L.T. (1987) Tegumental ultrastructure of *Opisthioglyphe ranae* (Trematoda, Plagiorchidae). *Parazitologiia* **21**, 677–680.

155. Buttner, A. (1951) Progenesis of digenetic trematodes. Personal study of two already known progenetic species: *Ratzia joyeuxi* (E. Brumpt, 1922) and *Pleurogenes medians* (Olsson, 1876). *Ann. Parasitol. Hum. Comp.* **26**, 138–189.

156. Baianov, M.G. (1975) The progenesis of the trematode *Prosotocus confusus* (Loss, 1894)—an amphibian parasite. *Parazitologiia* **9**, 122–126.

157. Cort, W.W., Hussey, K.L., and Ameel, D.J. (1957) Variations in infections of *Diplostomum flexicaudum* (Cort and Brooks, 1928) in snail intermediate hosts of different sizes. *J. Parasitol.* **43**, 221–232.

158. Mead, R.W. and Cordero, K.P. (1967) Encysted cercaria of *Plagitura parva* (Trematoda: Plagiorchiidae) in the snail *Helisoma antrosa.* *J. Parasitol.* **53**, 1287.

159. Russell, C.M. (1954) The effects of various environmental factors on the hatching of eggs of *Plagitura salamandra* Holl (Trematoda: Plagiorchiidae). *J. Parasitol.* **40**, 461–464.

160. Radtke, A., McLennan, D.A., and Brooks, D.R. (2002) Resource tracking in North American *Telorchis* spp. (Digenea: Plagiorchiformes: Telorchidae). *J. Parasitol.* **88**, 874–879.

161. Faulkner, M., Halton, D.W., and Montgomery, W.I. (1989) Sexual, seasonal and tissue variation in the encystment of *Cotylurus variegatus* metacercariae in perch, *Perca fluviatilis.* *Int. J. Parasitol.* **19**, 285–290.

162. Moravec, F., Barus, V., Rysavy, B., and Yousif, F. (1974) Observations on the development of two echinostomes, *Echinoparyphium recurvatum* and *Echinostoma revolutum,* the antagonists of human schistosomes in Egypt. *Folia Parasitol.* **21**, 107–126.

163. Goldberg, S.R., Bursey, C.R., Gergus, E.W., Sullivan, B.K., and Truong Q.A. (1996) Helminths from three treefrogs *Hyla arenicolor, Hyla wrightorum,* and *Pseudacris triseriata* (Hylidae) from Arizona. *J. Parasitol.* **82**, 833–845.

164. Galli, P., Crosa, G., Gentilli, A., and Santagostino, M. (2001) New geographical records of parasitic nematodes from *Bufo bufo* in Italy. *Parassitologia* **43**, 147–149.

165. Lewis, Jr., P.D. (1973) Helminths from terrestrial molluscs in Nebraska. I. New host and locality records for *Cosmocercoides dukae* (Holl, 1928) Travassos, 1931 (Nematoda: Cosmocercidae). *Trans. Am. Microsc. Soc.* **92**, 286–287.

166. Galli, P., Crosa, G., Gentilli, A., and Santagostino, M. (2001) New geographical records of parasitic nematodes from *Bufo bufo* in Italy. *Parassitologia* **43**, 147–149.

167. Bursey, C.R. and Goldberg, S.R. (1998) Helminths of the Canadian toad, *Bufo hemiophrys* (Amphibia: Anura), from Alberta, Canada. *J. Parasitol.* **84**, 617–618.

168. Criscione, C.D. and Font, W.F. (2001) The guest playing host: colonization of the introduced Mediterranean gecko, *Hemidactylus turcicus,* by helminth parasites in southeastern Louisiana. *J. Parasitol.* **87**, 1273–1278.

169. Hasegawa, H. (2005) Two new genera of the pharyngodonidae (Nematoda: Oxyuroidea) found in rhacophorid frogs of the Ryukyu Archipelago, Japan. *J. Parasitol.* **91**, 111–116.

170. Mishra, G.S. and Gonzalez, J.P. (1978) Parasites of fresh water turtles in Tunisia. *Arch. Inst. Pasteur Tunis.* **55**, 303–326.

171. Yildirimhan, H.S., Bursey, C.R., and Goldberg, S.R. (2005) Helminth parasites of the Caucasian salamander, *Mertensiella caucasica,* from Turkey. *Comp. Parasitol.* **72**, 75–87.

172. Bertman, M. (1993) *Diplodiscus subclavatus* (Pallas, 1760) (Trematoda) and *Acanthocephalus ranae* (Schrank, 1788) (Acanthocephala) in grass snake—*Natrix natrix* (L.). *Wiad. Parazytol.* **39**, 405–406.

173. Ewald, J.A. and Crompton, D.W. (1993) *Centrorhynchus aluconis* (Acanthocephala) and other helminth species in tawny owls (*Strix aluco*) in Great Britain. *J. Parasitol.* **79**, 952–954.

174. Fischthal, J.H. (1950) Additional hosts and geographical distribution records for the common fish acanthocephalan, *Leptorhynchoides thecatus.* *J. Parasitol.* **36**, 88.

175. Merritt, S.V. and Pratt, I. (1964) The life history of *Neoechinorhynchus rutili* and its development in the intermediate host (Acanthocephala: Neoechinorhynchidae). *J. Parasitol.* **50**, 394–400.

176. Hajduk, D. (1980) Leeches: *haementeria costata* (Fr. Muller) and *Hirudo medicinalis* L. (Hirudinea) in the Kopan lake. *Wiad. Parazytol.* **26**, 721–726.

177. Kikuchi, Y. and Fukatsu, T. (2005) *Rickettsia* infection in natural leech populations. *Microb. Ecol.* **49**, 265–271.

178. Alcelik, T., Cekic, O., and Totan, Y. (1997) Ocular leech infestation in a child. *Am. J. Ophthalmol.* **124**, 110–112.

179. Tinsley, R.C. (1995) Parasitic disease in amphibians: control by the regulation of worm burdens. *Parasitology* **111**, S153–178.

180. Goldberg, S.R., Bursey, C.R., and Cheam, H. (1998) Helminths of two native frog species (*Rana chiricahuensis, Rana yavapaiensis*) and one introduced frog species (*Rana catesbeiana*) (Ranidae) from Arizona. *J. Parasitol.* **84**, 175–177.

181. Williams, R.W. (1960) Observations on the life history of *Rhabdias sphaerocephala* Goodey, 1924 from *Bufo marinus* L., in the Bermuda Islands. *J. Helminthol.* **34**, 93–98.

182. Levine, N.D. and Nye, R.R. (1977) A survey of blood and other tissue parasites of leopard frogs *Rana pipiens* in the United States. *J. Wildl. Dis.* **13**, 17–23.

183. Ramos, B. and Urdaneta-Morales, S. (1977) Hematophagous insects as vectors for frog trypanosomes. *Rev. Biol. Trop.* **25**, 209–217.

184. Gruia-Gray, J. and Desser, S.S. (1992) Cytopathological observations and epizootiology of frog erythrocytic virus in bullfrogs (*Rana catesbeiana*). *J. Wildl. Dis.* **28**, 34–41.

185. Tumrasvin, W., Kurahashi, H., and Kano, R. (1977) Studies on medically important flies in Thailand II. Record of four species of Lucilia Robineau-Desvoidy (Diptera: Calliphoridae). *Bull. Tokyo Med. Dent. Univ.* **24**, 1–8.

186. Leng, Y.J., Wang, H.B., and Ge, N.L. (1991) A survey of phlebotomine sandflies (Diptera: Psychodidae) in Hubei Province, China. *Parassitologia* **33**, 377–379.

187. Schumaker, T.T. and Barros, D.M. (1994) Notes on the biology of *Amblyomma dissimile* Koch, 1844 (Acari:Ixodida) on *Bufo marinus* (Linnaeus, 1758) from Brazil. *Mem. Inst. Oswaldo Cruz.* **89**, 29–31.

188. Ulbrich, A.P. (1969) Chiggers, with special reference to occurrence in Michigan and to *Eutrombicula alfreddugesi*. *J. Am. Osteopath. Assoc.* **68**, 913–923.

189. Johnston, D.E. and Wacker, R.R. (1967) Observations on postembryonic development in *Eutrombicula splendens* (Acari-Acariformes). *J. Med. Entomol.* **4**, 306–310.

190. Bolek, M.G. and Janovy, Jr., J. (2004) Observations on myiasis by the calliphorids, *Bufolucilia silvarum* and *Bufolucilia elongata*, in wood frogs, *Rana sylvatica,* from southeastern Wisconsin. *J. Parasitol.* **90**, 1169–1171.

191. Wetzel, E.J. and Esch, G.W. (1997) Infrapopulation dynamics of *Halipegus occidualis* and *Halipegus eccentricus* (Digenea: Hemiuridae): temporal changes within individual hosts. *J. Parasitol.* **83**, 1019–1024.

192. Miller, D.L., Bursey, C.R., Gray, M.J., and Smith, L.M. (2004) Metacercariae of *Clinostomum attenuatum* in *Ambystoma tigrinum mavortium, Bufo cognatus* and *Spea multiplicata* from west Texas. *J. Helminthol.* **78**, 373–376.

193. Dias, M.L., Eiras, J.C., Machado, M.H., Souza, G.T., and Pavanelli, G.C. (2003) The life cycle of *Clinostomum complanatum* Rudolphi, 1814 (Digenea, Clinostomidae) on the floodplain of the high Parana river, Brazil. *Parasitol. Res.* **89**, 506–508.

194. Grabda, B. (1958) Development of *Codonocephalus urnigerus* (Rus., 1918). *Wiad. Parazytol.* **4**, 625–626.

195. Byrd, E.E. and Maples, W.P. (1969) Intramolluscan stages of *Dasymetra conferta* Nicoll, 1911 (Trematoda: Plagiorchiidae). *J. Parasitol.* **55**, 509–526.

196. King, P.H. and Van As, J.G. (1997) Description of the adult and larval stages of *Tylodelphys xenopi* (Trematoda: Diplostomidae) from southern Africa. *J. Parasitol.* **83**, 287–295.

197. Liang-Sheng, Y. (1958) A review of the trematode genus *Encyclometra* Baylis and Cannon, 1924. *J. Helminthol.* **32**, 99–114.

198. Ameel, D.J., Cort, W.W., and Van der Woude, A. (1950) Germinal development in the heterophyid, *Euryhelmis monorchis* Ameel, 1938. J. Parasitol. **36**, 427–432.

199. Anerson, G.A. and Pratt, I. (1965) Cercaria and first intermediate host of *Euryhelmins squamula*. *J. Parasitol.* **51**, 13–15.

200. Ulmer, M.J. (1955) Notes on the morphology and host-parasite specificity of *Fibricola cratera* (Barker and Noll, 1915) Dubois 1932 (Trematoda: Diplostomatidae). *J. Parasitol.* **41**, 460–466.

201. Cort, W.W., Ameel, D.J., and Van der Woude, A. (1952) Development of the mother and daughter sporocysts of a snake Plagiorchioid, *Lechriorchis primus* (Trematoda: Reniferidae). *J. Parasitol.* **38**, 187–202.

202. Timon-David, J. (1961) *Ratzia parva* (M. Stossich 1904) is among the fauna of France (Trematoda, Digenea, Opisthorchiidae). *Ann. Parasitol. Hum. Comp.* **36**, 166–167.

203. Modry, D., Slapeta, J.R., Jirku, M., Obornik, M., Lukes, J., and Koudela, B. (2001) Phylogenetic position of a renal coccidium of the European green frogs, '*Isospora*' *lieberkuehni* Labbe, 1894 (Apicomplexa: Sarcocystidae) and its taxonomic implications. *Int. J. Syst. Evol. Microbiol.* **51**, 767–772.

204. Levine, N.D. and Nye, R.R. (1977) A survey of blood and other tissue parasites of leopard frogs *Rana pipiens* in the United States. *J. Wildl. Dis.* **13**, 17–23.

205. Najarian, H.H. (1961) The identity of *Echinoparyphium flexum* (Linton, 1892) Dietz, 1910 (Trematoda: Echinostomatidae). *J. Parasitol.* **47**, 635–636.

206. Kim, K.H., Joo, K.H., and Rim, H.J. (1995) Gorgoderid trematodes (Digenea: Gorgoderidae) from the urinary bladder of frogs in Korea. *Korean J. Parasitol.* **33**, 75–83.

207. McAllister, C.T. and Conn, D.B. (1990) Occurrence of tetrathyridia of *Mesocestoides* sp. (Cestoidea: Cyclophyllidea) in North American anurans (Amphibia). *J. Wildl. Dis.* **26**, 540–543.

208. Baker, R.A. (1971) Observations on aspects of nutrition in *Xenopacarus africanus* (Ereynetidae: Trombidiformes). *J. Med. Entomol.* **8**, 307–313.

209. Miller, G.C., Harkema, R., and Harris, A. (1965) Notes on the life history of *Strigea elegans* Chandler and Rausch, 1947 (Trematoda: Strigeidae). *Parasitol.* **51**, 894–895.

210. Fried, B. and Graczyk, T.K. (2004) Recent advances in the biology of *Echinostoma* species in the "*revolutum*" group. *Adv. Parasitol.* **58**, 139–195.

211. Munoz-Antoli, C., Toledo, R., and Esteban, J.G. (2000) The life cycle and transmission dynamics of the larval stages of *Hypoderaeum conoideum*. *J. Helminthol.* **74**, 165–172.

INTRODUCTION

Reptiles are used as animal models in biomedical research for studies involving cardiovascular physiology, environmental toxicology, evolutionary and reproductive biology, vector-borne diseases, and others; and as sources of snake venoms important in human medicine. Reptiles are readily available through vendors in both the United States and Europe, and may originate through captive breeding programs or through capture of wild animals. While the former are often free of parasites, the latter may harbor a wide range of commensal or parasitic organisms. Therefore, people involved in the care and/or use of reptiles in biomedical research or teaching should be familiar with the parasitic fauna of these important animal models.

PROTOZOA

Phylum Sarcomastigophora

Class Mastigophora (flagellates)

Giardia, Hexamita, Trichomonas

Morphology. *The flagellates identified in reptiles are morphologically similar to those observed in other vertebrates. The interested reader is directed to Chapter 8, Parasites of Amphibians, for morphologic descriptions.*

Hosts and Life Cycle. Flagellates may be found in snakes, lizards, chelonians, and crocodilians. Reproduction is by simple binary fission. Some species form cysts. The transmission of these organisms is direct. These organisms can be found in both the urogenital and gastrointestinal systems of reptiles.

Pathologic Effects and Clinical Disease. The intestinal flagellates of reptiles are often found in asymptomatic animals, typically during routine fecal examinations, but have also been implicated in primary enteric disease. Heavy burdens of intestinal flagellates may cause inflammatory bowel disease or nephritis. Affected reptiles may be anorexic and lose weight. Diarrhea is a common finding, and melena may be observed with small bowel disease. Frank hemorrhage may also be noted with large bowel infection or chronic straining. Severe dehydration may result without treatment.

Diagnosis, Treatment, and Prevention. Antemortem diagnosis is made from a direct saline fecal or urine smear. Postmortem diagnosis is made from histopathologic findings of inflammatory bowel disease and the presence of the organisms. Reptiles with flagellated protozoa that are not

Tables are placed at the ends of chapters.

experiencing clinical disease should not be treated. Treating animals based purely on the presence of the organisms could lead to alterations in the microflora, allowing certain opportunistic pathogens (e.g., bacterial or protozoal) an opportunity to exploit the host. In cases where clinical disease is associated with the presence of the flagellates, the treatment of choice is metronidazole given orally (50 to 100 mg/kg) for seven to 10 days. Avoid using high doses (>100 to 150 mg/kg), because these can be associated with hepatic encephalopathy or death. Wild-caught animals under quarantine should be screened for parasites before being released into the colony. At least four consecutive weekly fecal examinations should be done before newly arrived animals are released from quarantine.

Public Health Considerations. Flagellates of reptiles are not likely to infect humans. However, caretakers should always practice good hygiene by wearing disposable gloves and washing their hands thoroughly after handling infected animals.

Class Sarcodina (amoebae)

Entamoeba invadens

Morphology. *Entamoeba invadens* (Syn. *Entamoeba serpentis*) closely resembles *E. histolytica.* Trophozoites are amoeboid, actively motile, can vary their shape and size, and typically measure 16 μ in diameter (Figure 9.1). The endoplasm is dense and contains a nucleus and food vacuoles filled with host-cell debris, leucocytes, or bacteria. Cysts are indistinguishable from those of *E. histolytica,* and measure 11 μ to 20 μ in diameter and contain one to four nuclei, a glycogen vacuole, and chromatoid bodies.

Hosts. *Entamoeba invadens* is one of the most important pathogens of captive snakes and lizards worldwide[1].

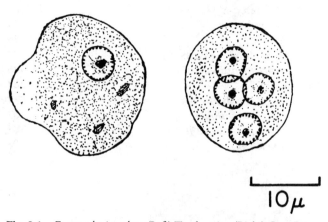

Fig. 9.1 *Entamoeba invadens.* (Left) Trophozoite. (Right) Cyst. Reproduced from Fantham, H.B. and Porter, A. (1953–1954) with permission.

Infections occur primarily in the intestines, although gastric and hepatic infections also occur.

Life Cycle. Reproduction is by binary fission and the infective stage is the cyst[2]. Trophozoites become round and small before encysting. A cyst wall is produced and the nucleus divides twice, producing four small nuclei. The quadrinucleate cyst is passed in the feces, and when ingested by a suitable host, emerges as an amoeba with four nuclei. This amoeba divides several times and produces small uninucleate amoebas, each of which develops into a trophozoite.

Pathologic Effects. Most snakes and lizards are susceptible to infection with *E. invadens,* where infection often results in significant morbidity and mortality[3]. Chelonians can harbor *E. invadens* but typically only serve as asymptomatic carriers or reservoirs of the parasite. This can pose a problem in multispecies exhibits where chelonians are mixed with lizards and snakes. Crocodilians also appear relatively unaffected by this parasite.

Although the organisms may cause minor damage in the lungs, spleen, pancreas, and kidneys[4], the most severe lesions occur in the gastrointestinal tract and liver[3]. Lesions in the colon and liver are typical and appear to be primary; those in the small intestine and stomach appear to be secondary. In the colon, discrete, irregular ulcers develop in the mucosa and measure 1 mm to 5 mm in width. Adjacent tissues are first congested and edematous and later necrotic. The initial lesions rapidly extend to the entire colonic mucosa, and the wall becomes thickened, intensely congested, and inelastic. The submucosa and muscularis become involved, and the organism enters the blood and lymph vessels. Lesions in the small intestine (ileum) appear to be extensions of those in the large intestine. They are often as widespread as those in the colon, but the necrosis usually involves only the mucosa and superficial submucosa. Blood-stained mucus containing large numbers of cysts and trophozoites fills the lumen.

Initial lesions in the stomach consist of cone-shaped ulcers, measuring approximately 2 mm in diameter and 1 mm in depth. The ulcers can extend into the submucosa, and be filled with a soft friable, blood-stained mass of exudates and debris containing many trophozoites. Although the ulcers increase in size and number, they rarely coalesce. The liver is mottled, pale brown to dark red, and usually swollen and friable. Focal necrosis of the hepatic parenchyma occurs but is often obscured by thromboembolic disease caused by obstruction of the portal vein. Macroscopically, hepatic lesions appear as necrotic foci that measure 1 cm to 4 cm in diameter.

Clinical Disease. Signs of infection are usually nonspecific and localized to the gastrointestinal tract. Affected animals may develop anorexia, weight loss, dehydration, diarrhea, and frank hemorrhage in the feces[3]. Death usually occurs in two to 10 weeks. Animals that survive for extended periods often become severely dehydrated and cachexic.

Diagnosis. Diagnosis is based on the microscopic demonstration of cysts and trophozoites in the feces of the living animal or in the lesions at necropsy. Saline enemas may be given to reptiles to collect samples for screening[1].

Treatment. Effective treatment consists of metronidazole (125 mg/kg repeated twice at 72 and 96 hours[3] or 275 mg/kg given once[5]). Infections may also be ameliorated with gentamicin (2.2 to 4.4 mg/kg every 72 hours for five treatments) or chloramphenicol (50 mg/kg twice daily for 14 days)[5]. It is important to consider the animal's environmental temperature when treating affected animals with these compounds. Temperatures above 37°C and below 13°C reduce pathogen survival and/or virulence[6].

Prevention. Control is based on sanitation and prophylactic treatment. All newly acquired reptiles should be screened for infection with *E. invadens.* Animals should not be released from quarantine until they have been shown to be parasite-free following at least three fecal examinations over a 60-day period. Because turtles may serve as reservoirs of infection for snakes and lizards, these should not be housed together. Further, water from turtle enclosures should be prevented from reaching snakes, and separate cleaning and feeding utensils should be used for these different reptiles.

Public Health Considerations. Humans have not been shown to be susceptible to infection with *E. invadens.*

Phylum Apicomplexa

Class Coccidia

Cryptosporidium sp.
Morphology. *Cryptosporiduim* sp. found in reptiles include *C. serpentis* and *C. saurophilum. Cryptosporidium serpentis* oocysts measure 5.6 μ to 6.6 μ long by 4.8 μ to 5.6 μ wide. *Cryptosporidium saurophilum* oocysts are slightly more narrow, measuring 4.4 μ to 5.6 μ long by 4.2 μ to 5.2 μ wide[7].

Hosts. *Cryptosporidium serpentis* is most commonly found in the stomach of snakes, while *C. saurophilum* is primarily found in the intestinal tract of lizards. Chelonians can also become infected, but less commonly.

Life Cycle. The life cycles of *Cryptosporidium* found in reptiles are assumed to be similar to those of others in the genus. Typical of the genus, sporulation occurs in the host cells, ensuring that the oocysts are infective when passed with the feces. Transmission occurs via the fecal-oral route. In the captive setting, oocysts can be easily disseminated within an enclosed environment.

Pathologic Effects and Clinical Disease. Infection with *C. serpentis* results in loss of the brush border, flattening of the epithelial cells, and proliferation of gastric mucous cells[8]. Infections with *C. saurophilum* can lead to similar epithelial changes in the intestines, resulting in enteritis[9]. Affected animals may be asymptomatic. However, most cases presented to veterinarians present with clinical disease. In snakes, the clinical course may include anorexia or a voracious appetite, vomiting/regurgitation of recently eaten meals, weight loss, dehydration, and gastric swelling. Infections with *C. saurophilum* can lead to similar clinical findings, including anorexia, weight loss, and diarrhea; however, the stomach is not usually involved. An unusual presentation for cryptosporidiosis may also occur in green iguanas, where the animals develop aural abscesses.

Diagnosis. Diagnosis is by examination of direct smears, acid-fast staining of feces, or examination of gastric lavage samples from infected animals. An immunofluorescent antibody stain (IFA) (Merifluor, Meridian Diagnostic, Cincinnati, OH) can also be used, and increases the likelihood of confirming a diagnosis. Diagnosis by fecal examination is complicated by the intermittent shedding of oocysts. Gastric or intestinal biopsies with histopathological review of the samples may confirm the diagnosis. For large collections, diagnostic necropsies may be warranted.

Treatment and Prevention. There is no effective treatment for cryptosporidiosis in any host species. Antibiotics, bovine hyperimmune bovine colostrum, altering environmental temperature, and immunization with oocyst wall antigens have all been attempted and found to provide some relief, but do not consistently eliminate the organism. At this time, culling infected animals is recommended. Strict hygiene and quarantine are essential to controlling cryptosporidiosis. Animals should be quarantined prior to admission into the collection. Serial fecal samples should be examined weekly using an acid-fast stain. Prior to release from quarantine it is advisable to test a pooled fecal sample with the Merifluor IFA test.

Public Health Considerations. Reptilian cryptosporidial organisms do not appear to be zoonotic.

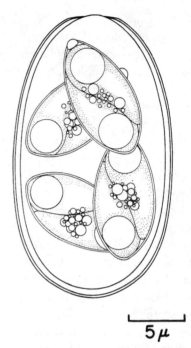

Fig. 9.2 *Eimeria scriptae* oocyst. Reproduced from Sampson, J.R. and Ernst, J.V. (1969) with permission.

Eimeria spp.

Morphology. The morphology and biology of the *Eimeria* spp. are presented in the chapters on parasites of birds, rabbits, and others. Briefly, *Eimeria* oocysts, when sporulated, contain four sporocysts, each with two sporozoites (Figure 9.2)[9].

Hosts. Several species of *Eimeria* may be found in captive reptiles, including snakes, lizards, chelonians, and crocodilians[1,11]. Most *Eimeria* inhabit the intestine, but some of those occurring in snakes are found in the gallbladder and bile duct, and rarely, in the kidneys.

Life Cycle. The life cycles of the *Eimeria* are as described in other chapters. Briefly, reptiles become infected after ingesting oocysts. Schizogony occurs in the epithelial lining of various organ systems, depending on parasite species. Oocysts are shed with the feces following gametogony.

Pathologic Effects. The pathologic effects of coccidia appear mild for most reptiles; however, more severe cases resulting in epithelial ulceration and fibrosis, and septicemia from the loss of epithelial integrity, may occur. For example, *E. bitis* infections in garter snakes have been found to cause denuding of the mucosa and extensive fibrosis of the submucosa of the gallbladder[1].

Clinical Disease. Reptiles infected with *Eimeria* may be asymptomatic, or show clinical signs consistent with gastrointestinal disease. Clinically affected reptiles may be anorexic, dehydrated, and have diarrhea. Regurgitation and vomiting can occur but are rare.

Diagnosis, Treatment, and Prevention. Antemortem diagnosis is by direct saline fecal smear or fecal flotation. Biliary and renal coccidial infections are generally diagnosed at necropsy. Several antibiotics and antiprotozoal agents have been suggested as possible treatments for coccidial infections in reptiles, though few controlled studies have been reported. Sodium sulfamethazine in the drinking water at a level of 7 g/L has been suggested as a treatment for reptiles, but its effectiveness is unknown[12]. Recommendations using trimethoprim-sulfadiazine in both parenteral (30 mg/kg intramuscularly once a day for two days, then every 48 hours for five days) and oral forms (30 mg/kg once, then 15 mg/kg once per day for 14 to 21 days) have also been published[13]. Because sulfonamides are coccidiostatic, most infections are only controlled and not eliminated with these drugs. Control is based on sanitation and prophylactic treatment.

All newly acquired reptiles should be screened for infection with *Eimeria*. Animals should not be removed from quarantine until they have been shown to be parasite-free on at least three fecal examinations over a 60-day period. In cases where a colony is positive, it is generally prudent to prophylactically treat the animals during times of high stress to reduce the likelihood of overwhelming infections.

Public Health Considerations. None of the species of *Eimeria* of reptiles are known to infect humans.

Isospora spp.

The morphology, biology, and clinical effects of *Isospora* are generally similar to those of *Eimeria*. *Isospora* spp. can be differentiated from *Eimeria* spp. by the fact that its oocyst produces two sporocysts, each with four sporozoites (Figure 9.3)[14]. *Isospora* spp. have been reported in snakes, lizards, and crocodilians. Infections are found in the intestine. *Isospora amphiboluri*, a coccidian parasite of bearded dragons, causes severe pathologic changes in juvenile dragons. Diagnosis, treatment, and prevention are as described for *Eimeria* of reptiles. Humans are not susceptible to infection with *Isospora* spp.

Hemogregarines

Morphology. The forms found in the blood of captive reptiles (Figure 9.4) vary with the stage of the life cycle and

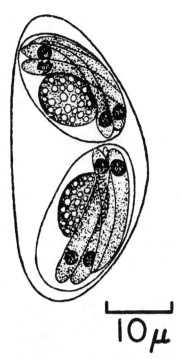

Fig. 9.3 *Isospora lieberkühni* oocyst. Reproduced from Wenyon, C.M. (1926) with permission.

species of host[9,15]. The most common genera of hemogregarines found in reptiles include *Haemogregarina*, *Hepatozoon*, *Karyolyses*, *Lainsonia*, and *Schellackia*. Intracellular gamonts range in size from 10 to 17 μ long by 2 μ to 4 μ wide.

Hosts. Hemogregarines are the most common blood protozoa of wild-caught snakes and turtles. Classification schemes differ from author to author. For this text, classification of reptilian hemogregarines is based on features of the life cycle. There are two suborders of importance: Eimeriorina and Adeleorina. *Lainsonia* and *Schellackia* are included among the Eimeriorina. These parasites are usually found in lizards and snakes. The Adeleorina include *Haemogregarina*, *Hepatozoon*, and *Karyolysus*, which have been found in snakes, lizards, chelonians, and crocodilians.

Relatively little is known of the biology and life cycles of the reptilian hemogregarines. Among the best studied are the *Haemogregarina* spp. *Haemogregarina stepanowi* is found in turtles, including snapping turtles, painted turtles, red-eared slider turtles, cooters, box turtles, softshell turtles, European pond terrapins, and other turtles from the United States and Europe[16–19]. Prevalence rates are often high, with 45% to 75% of animals tested found to be positive in the central and southern United States[17,19,20]. *Haemogregarina* spp. have also been identified in racers, rat snakes, kingsnakes, water snakes, bullsnakes, garter snakes, and other snakes from North America. In a cross-sectional study evaluating the prevalence of the parasite in snakes, 40% (20/50) of snakes (nine species) from the central United Snakes and 31% (186/600) of snakes from the central and southwestern United States were found infected with this hemoparasites[15,17].

Life Cycle. Hemogregarines are intracellular parasites, commonly found in erythrocytes, leukocytes, and other cells within the body (e.g., spleen, liver) (Figure 9.4)[9]. In the Eimeriorina, merogony, sporogony, and gametogony all occur in the definitive host. Invertebrates serve only as vectors. Transmission occurs after an invertebrate consumes a blood meal from an infected reptile and is then ingested by another reptile. In Adeleorina, merogony occurs in the

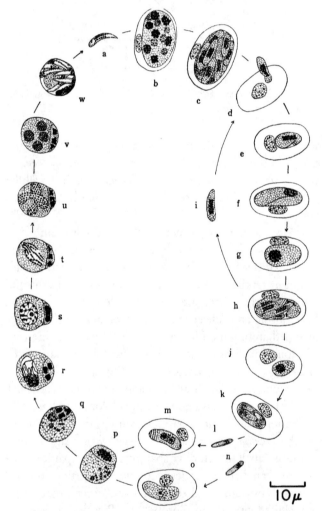

Fig. 9.4 *Haemogregarina stepanowi,* morphology and life cycle: a–o, schizogony and gametogony in turtle; p–w, sexual reproduction in bloodsucking invertebrate. Reproduced from Kudo, R.R. (1966) with permission.

reptilian definitive host, gametogony occurs in reptilian blood cells, and sporogony occurs in arthropod intermediate hosts.

Pathologic Effects and Clinical Disease. Although usually considered nonpathogenic, heavy infections may cause anemia[1]. The presence of a hemogregarine in an erythrocyte causes distortion of the blood cell, including nuclear displacement and cytoplasmic attenuation[1]. The number of erythrocytes affected by these parasites can approach 80%[15]. Heavily infected reptiles become anemic[1]. Reptiles generally have packed cell volumes (PCV) > 20%; however, it is not uncommon to have reptiles present with PCV between 10% to 20%. The author does not become concerned until the PCV falls below 8%. Regardless, most affected reptiles are asymptomatic.

Diagnosis, Treatment, and Prevention. Diagnosis is based on the demonstration of the parasite in stained (Diff-Quik or Wright-Giemsa) blood smears[1]. A diagnosis of secondary anemia is based on a PCV < 20%. No effective treatment regimens have been reported. In severe cases, treatment with doxycycline, chloroquine, or pyrimethramine may be attempted. A dosing schedule should be extrapolated from the mammalian and avian literature. Hemogregarines should not be found in captive, indoor reptiles. During quarantine, reptiles should be closely inspected for the presence of potential vectors. An insecticide can be applied to minimize the likelihood of introducing vectors to a colony. Insecticides should also be applied to the environment if flying vectors (e.g., mosquitoes) are a concern.

Public Health Considerations. Hemogregarines do not infect humans.

Class Haemosporidia

Important Haemosporidia found in reptiles include those of the genera *Fallisia, Haemoproteus, Plasmodium,* and *Saurocytozoon.* These hemoparasites are morphologically similar to related protozoa of other vertebrates. The Haemosporidia may be found in lizards, snakes, and chelonians; lizards are most commonly infected. The life cycles of the Haemosporidia are poorly known but all require arthropod vectors. While most infections are asymptomatic, heavy infections result in anemia.

Diagnosis is by demonstrating parasites in stained (Diff-Quik or Wright-Giemsa) blood smears[1]. No effective treatments have been reported. In severe cases, treatment with doxycycline, chloroquine, or pyrimethramine may be instituted, with dosing schedules extrapolated from the mammalian and avian literature. Infection with hemoparasites should not occur in captivity where arthropod vectors are excluded. During quarantine, reptiles should be closely inspected for the presence of potential vectors and infested reptiles treated with insecticide. Insecticides should also be applied to the environment if flying vectors (e.g., mosquitoes) are a concern. The Haemosporidia of reptiles do not infect humans.

Phylum Microspora

Morphology. As noted in Chapter 15, Parasites of Rabbits, the Microspora have been reclassified as fungi. They are included here for historical reasons. The morphology of the microspordia varies with the stage of the life cycles. Microsporidians measure 5 μ to 20 μ in length. They are pyriform in shape and have a posterior vacuole. Schizonts contain up to eight nuclei. Small sporonts have two to three nuclei when immature and up to 100 nuclei when mature. *Pleistophora* spp. spores are oval and measure 3.5 μ to 6.7 μ long by 2 μ to 3 μ wide. On one side of the anterior pole of each spore is a small granule to which is attached a filament. When extended, this filament measures 80 μ to 220 μ long. A microsporidian recently isolated from African skinks (*Mabuya perrotetii*) was found to have slightly curved spores. The spores measured 2.9 μ long by 1.2 μ wide, and were identical to those of *Encephalitozoon lacertae*[21].

Hosts and Life Cycle. *Pleistophora* is the most common microsporidian associated with reptiles. Encysted spores have been found in snakes, lizards, and chelonians. An unidentified microsporidian was recently identified in inland bearded dragons (*Pogona vitticeps*)[22], and unidentified microsporidia have been identified in snakes[8]. These organisms are probably more prevalent than is currently recognized. The life cycles of the microsporidia are direct, and though incompletely known, are likely similar to those of other members of the phylum. These are discussed in Chapter 7, Parasites of Fishes, and Chapter 15, Parasites of Rabbits.

Pathologic Effects. Encysted microsporidia may appear as non-specific granulomas in muscle or other tissues. Severe hepatic necrosis with clusters of light basophilic, intracytoplasmic microorganisms was found in bearded dragons. The disease appeared well disseminated, with similar microorganisms found within cytoplasmic vacuoles in distended renal epithelial cells, pulmonary epithelial cells, gastric mucosal epithelial cells, enterocytes, and capillary endothelial cells and ventricular ependymal cells in the brain. The microsporidium isolated in the bearded dragons

was Gram-positive and acid-fast, and stained positive using the periodic acid-Schiff reaction. In the African skinks, the histopathological changes were found in the large intestine and included villous atrophy, blunting of mucosa, and flattening of individual epithelial cells[21].

Clinical Disease. Reptiles infected with microsporidia frequently develop clinical signs consistent with gastrointestinal disease. African skinks with microsporidiosis had decreased appetite, diarrhea, and weight loss. Systemic disease might also be expected in cases of widespread disseminated microsporidiosis, as described in the bearded dragon.

Diagnosis. Antemortem diagnosis is by identifying spores in the feces of infected animals. Electron microscopy is required to characterize the spores to the generic level. Postmortem diagnosis is by gross identification of xenomas and microscopic identification of tissue spores.

Treatment and Prevention. Microsporidial infections are difficult to treat. In the laboratory setting, it is probably best to cull infected animals. Quarantine and examining serial fecal samples may be used to reduce the likelihood of introducing these parasites into a colony. Chloramphenicol and topical oxytetracycline hydrochloric acid with polymyxin B have been used to suppress spore formation, but did not eliminate the parasite[23]. Quarantining recently acquired animals, serially screening fecal samples, and obtaining animals from reputable breeders or wild populations where these parasites are not known to be endemic should be done to prevent the introduction of these parasites into captive amphibian colonies.

Public Health Considerations. The microsporidia of reptiles do not infect humans.

Phylum Ciliophora

Balantidium spp.

Morphology. *Balantidium* spp. are among the most common ciliates of reptiles. The reader is directed to Chapter 8, Parasites of Amphibians, for a description of their morphology.

Hosts and Life Cycle. *Balantidium* spp. are commonly found in the intestines of chelonians, where they are considered commensals. Reproduction is by conjugation and binary fission. Trophozoites inhabit the intestinal tract, while the cyst stage is released into the fecal stream as the environmentally resistant infective stage.

Pathologic Effects and Clinical Disease. *Balantidium* are not considered pathogenic. However, changes in the microbial flora associated with dietary changes, antibiotics, and stress could result in increased populations of ciliates, leading to localized enteritis, anorexia, and diarrhea. However, clinical balantidiasis is rare.

Diagnosis, Treatment, and Prevention. Antemortem diagnosis is based on identifying ciliates in a direct saline smear of the feces. In cases where clinical disease is present, metronidazole may be administered (10 to 20 mg/kg orally once daily for seven to 10 days). Strict adherence to quarantine and hygiene protocols will reduce the likelihood of transmitting *Balantidium*. Minimizing stress in the captive environment is also important.

Public Health Considerations. *Balantidium* spp. from reptiles are not infectious to humans.

Nyctotheroides spp.

The morphology, biology, and clinical effects of *Nyctotheroides* (Syn. *Nyctotherus* spp.) are presented in Chapter 8, Parasites of Amphibians. Like *Balantidium* spp., *Nyctotheroides* spp. are among the most common ciliates of reptiles. *Nyctotheroides* spp. are commonly found in the intestine of chelonians, where they are considered to be commensals. Reproduction is by conjugation and binary fission. Cysts are only sometimes formed. As described for *Balantidium* spp., changes in the microbial flora may be associated with increased enteric burdens of *Nyctotheroides*, leading to localized enteritis. Diagnosis, treatment, and prevention are as described for *Balantidium*. *Nyctotheroides* spp. do not infect humans.

TREMATODES

Dasymetra, Lechriorchis, Ochetosoma, Zeugorchis

Morphology. Adult digenean trematodes share certain morphologic features. These are described in Chapter 3, Biology of Trematodes and Leeches. The adult of *Dasymetra conferta* measures 3.8 mm to 1.1 mm long[24]. The adult of *Lechriorchis primus* measures 1.8 mm to 5.7 mm long and 0.6 mm to 1.3 mm wide; the egg is oval, has an operculum, and measures 48 μ to 50 μ long by 23 μ to 25 μ wide[25]. The adult of *L. tygarti* measures 2.2 mm to 6.9 mm long by 0.6 mm to 1.6 mm wide; its eggs are also oval and operculate and measure 43 μ to 53 μ long by 20 μ to 34 μ wide. The adult of *Ochetosoma aniarum* (Syn. *Neorenifer aniarum*) measures 1.8 mm to 3.5 mm long by 0.7 mm to 1.1 mm wide; the eggs measure 32 μ to 4 2 μ long by 20 μ to 25 μ wide[26]. The adult of *Zeugorchis eurinus* measures 1.9 mm to

3.3 mm long by 0.6 mm to 0.8 mm wide. Its eggs are similar to those of *Lechriorchis* and measure 42 μ to 46 μ long by 18 μ to 23 μ wide.

Hosts. These flukes, often called renifers, inhabit the lung, mouth, and digestive tract of snakes[27]. Although common throughout the world, little is known of the epidemiology of these parasites[28]. In a single study evaluating garter snakes from the north-central United States, the prevalence *L. primus* was 25%, suggesting that this parasite is common in some populations of snakes[25].

Life Cycle. The life cycles of the renifers are similar to one another[25]. Eggs are deposited by the adult flukes into the lung, swallowed, and passed in the feces. The eggs hatch after being ingested by a gastropod such as a snail and, after four to five weeks, leave the snail as cercariae. The cercariae are ingested by tadpoles and encyst in the muscles. Snakes become infected after ingesting infected tadpoles. The metacercariae excyst in the stomach and develop into young worms in the small intestine. After approximately seven months, the young worms migrate through the stomach into the esophagus. Once in the esophagus the parasites remain for another three months, after which they pass through the mouth to the lung. Another year is required for maturation to the adult stage.

Pathologic Effects and Clinical Disease. Although most infections appear harmless, heavy infections have been shown to cause pulmonary irritation, dyspnea, and weight loss[29]. Additional signs may include nervousness and irritability, though there is disagreement on this issue[30].

Diagnosis, Treatment, and Prevention. Diagnosis is by finding eggs in the feces or parasites in the mouth of living animals, or in the digestive tract or lung at necropsy. Trematodes identified in the oral cavity can be removed using forceps. Endoscopic removal of the adult nematodes from the lungs may be possible in larger reptiles. Praziquantel (8 mg/kg, subcutaneously, intramuscularly or per os)[31] effectively eliminates trematodes in reptiles, although dosing is anecdotal. The oral administration of tetrachlorethylene (0.2 ml per kg of body weight by capsule) has been reported to be an effective treatment for the immature flukes in the intestine[29]. The drug is given four days after feeding to avoid its absorption by residual fats in the stomach. Because of the need for mollusk and tadpole intermediate hosts, it is unlikely that the life cycles of these flukes would be completed in the laboratory.

Public Health Considerations. Aspidogastrean trematodes of reptiles do not pose a health risk to humans.

Gyrodactylus spp.

The morphology and biology of *Gyrodactylus* spp. are presented in Chapter 7, Parasites of Fishes. While *Gyrodactylus* spp. are important monogenean pathogens of fishes, they are also commonly found on the skin, in the oral cavity, and in the urinary bladder of aquatic turtles[32]. Monogenean trematodes are not considered significant parasites of turtles. In most cases, these organisms are incidental findings. In the rare cases where heavy infestations occur, mild, localized enteritis may occur at the sites of attachment of the trematode hooks.

Monogenean infestations can be diagnosed cytologically. A skin scrape can be collected antemortem and examined under light microscopy. Treatment is not generally warranted. However, if treatment is pursued, praziquantel is the treatment of choice. Bathing an animal in a 10 mg/L water bath for three hours has been found to be effective. Additional treatments may be required. *Gyrodactylus* may be excluded from the animal colony by only accepting animals from approved, licensed breeders. New arrivals should be quarantined and skin scrapes collected to determine carrier status. Water samples can also be collected, centrifuged, the supernatant poured off, and the sediment evaluated for the presence of free-swimming gyrodactylids. These parasites do not affect humans.

Other Trematodes

Spirorchis spp.

Morphology. Taxonomists classify trematodes under different taxonomic schemes. Many consider the spirorchids to be members of the order Strigeatida and family Spirorchiidae. Adult spirorchids are thin, transparent, measure 1 mm to 2 mm long, and do not possess a ventral sucker (Figure 9.5)[24,33]. The esophagus is long and the two ceca extend almost to the posterior end of the body. The testes are arranged in a linear series anterior to the ovary. The ovary and the genital pore are located near the posterior end of the body. Vitellaria are follicular and usually occupy all available space in the body not occupied by reproductive organs, from the esophagus to beyond the ends of the ceca. Eggs are large, measure 55 μ to 140 μ long, and may or may not have an operculum.

Hosts. Species of this genus inhabit the cardiovascular system of turtles from North America[27,33]. *Spirorchis parvus* and *S. elephantis* occur in painted turtles, *S. artericola* and *S. innominata* infect pond turtles and other turtles, and *S. haematobium* is found in the snapping

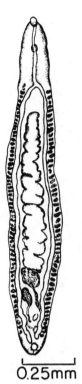

0.25mm

Fig. 9.5 *Spirorchis* adult. Reproduced from Skrjabin, K.I. (1964) with permission.

turtle[33–35]. All are common. The prevalence of *S. parvus* has been reported to be 18% in painted turtles obtained from their natural habitat in the north central United States[33], while as many as 70% of snapping turtles from the central Unites States have been found infected with *S. haematobium*[35].

Life Cycle. Adults of *S. parvus* occur in the mesenteric arterioles in the wall of the stomach and intestine[33]. Adults of other species are found in the heart or in the arteries of the lungs and other organs. Eggs are deposited in the blood vessels, collect in the gut wall, pass into the lumen, and are voided in the feces. Eggs hatch in water in four to six days, and the miracidia penetrate a snail and eventually develop into cercariae. The cercariae, when released from the snail, penetrate the thin epithelial membranes of a turtle, migrate through the tissues to the blood vessels, and circulate until they reach the heart or arteries. Once in the cardiovascular system of the reptile, these parasites become adults. The time of development in the snail is about 18 days, while the time to maturity in the turtle is about three months. Once the eggs are laid, it takes approximately two weeks for them to reach the lumen of the intestine.

Pathologic Effects and Clinical Disease. Turtles infected with *Spirorchis* spp. are frequently asymptomatic. *Spirorchis parvus* cercariae cause irritation while entering the turtle host. Ischemic necrosis is a common finding in tissues when the trematode eggs lodge in the capillary beds, and may lead to organ failure. In massive infections, the fluke eggs can become lodged in the intestinal wall, forming granulomas. Inflammatory responses can be fatal[33].

Diagnosis, Treatment, and Prevention. Diagnosis is by identification of the eggs on an antemortem fecal examination, or in the tissues at necropsy. Adult parasites may also be identified in the blood vessels or heart at necropsy. Ischemia may result in alterations in serum biochemistry panels indicative of specific organ failure.

Treatment recommendations for spirorchids are limited to treatment of sea turtles. Adnyana and coworkers[36] found that three treatments of praziquantel (50 mg/kg) in one day effectively eliminated spirorchids in naturally infected green sea turtles (*Chelonia mydas*). Jacobson and coworkers[37] also found praziquantel (25 mg/kg, three times, using a three-hour dosing interval) to be effective against spirorchids in loggerhead sea turtles (*Caretta caretta*). Because of the need for a snail intermediate host, completion of the life cycle in the laboratory is unlikely.

Public Health Considerations. Humans are not susceptible to infection with *Spirorchis* spp.

CESTODES

Diphyllobothrium erinacei

The morphology and biology of *Diphyllobothrium erinacei* are discussed in Chapter 8, Parasites of Amphibians, and Chapter 4, Biology of Cestodes. *Diphyllobothrium erinacei* has been found in both snakes and turtles[38]. Snakes from South America, Australia, and Eastern Asia commonly serve as second intermediate or paratenic hosts after consuming infected amphibians[13]. Plerocercoid larvae encysted in the muscle or subcutaneous tissues do not appear to cause overt clinical disease. However, when the larvae are encysted in the subcutaneous tissues, it may be disconcerting to reptile handlers to observe the movement of the parasites under the skin.

A tentative diagnosis is based on the demonstration of the characteristic plerocercoid larva in the muscle at necropsy or after surgical removal of subcutaneous larvae.

Larvae located in the subcutaneous can generally be surgically removed using local anesthesia. An incision should be made near the location of the parasite, and the worm retrieved using thumb forceps. General anesthesia may be required for animals requiring the removal of numerous larvae. A definitive diagnosis requires the experimental feeding of the immature parasite to a definitive host and subsequent identification of the adult parasite.

Because the life cycle cannot be completed in the absence of copepods or a mammal (e.g., definitive host), routine sanitation prevents the spread of the infection in the laboratory. Reptiles should not be offered wild-caught larval amphibians. No treatment is known. Infected laboratory reptiles are unlikely to be a public health hazard because humans are infected only after ingesting uncooked flesh from infected animals.

Spirometra mansonoides

Morphology and Hosts. *Spirometra mansonoides* is biologically similar to *Diphyllobothrium erinacei*, but is found in North America. The morphology and biology of *S. mansonoides* is presented in Chapter 8, Parasites of Amphibians, and Chapter 4, Biology of Cestodes. *Spirometra mansonoides* has been reported in kingsnakes, racers, water snakes, garter snakes, and turtles[39]. In a cross-sectional study of snakes from the south central United States, *S. mansonoides* was found in 18% of the animals surveyed[39]. Thus, wild-caught snakes and turtles from North America are commonly infected and should be screened for these parasites during quarantine.

Life Cycle. The life cycle of *S. mansonoides* generally includes both terrestrial and aquatic systems. Eggs are passed in the feces of a definitive host (e.g., dog, cat, or other carnivores), and hatch after reaching water. A copepod ingests the coracidium, which develops into a procercoid larva in the invertebrate host[38,39]. Amphibians are usually infected in the immature stage (e.g., frog tadpole, newt larva) after ingesting the infected copepod. Adult reptiles serve as secondary intermediate or paratenic hosts and become infected after ingesting an infected immature amphibian. The definitive host becomes infected after ingesting an infected reptile.

Pathologic Effects and Clinical Disease. The pathologic effects and clinical diseases caused by larval *S. mansonoides* are similar to those of *D. erinacei*.

Diagnosis, Treatment, Prevention, and Public Health Considerations. These aspects are similar to those of *D. erinacei*.

NEMATODES

Superfamily Rhabditoidea

Morphology. Reptiles are known to harbor three important genera of rhabditids: *Entomelas*, *Rhabdias*, and *Strongyloides*. *Rhabdias* spp. are characterized by a mouth that has six insignificant lips, a short esophagus, a vulva near the middle of the body, and a sharply tapered posterior extremity that ends in a finely conical point. The major difference between *Rhabdias* and *Entomelas* is that *Rhabdias* has a small buccal capsule, whereas that of *Entomelas* is large. The size of adult *Rhabdias* spp can vary depending on life stage. For example, parasitic adult stages of *Rhabdias agkistrodonis* measure 4.1 mm to 6.4 mm, while saprophytic forms measured <1.5 mm. Variability in length may occur between species and genera, too. For example, *Entomelas ophisauri* is slightly larger than *R. agkistrodonis*, measuring 6.4 mm to 9.8 mm long, as well as being larger than *Entomelas dujardini*, which measures 2.7 mm to 8.5 mm long.

Hosts. *Rhabdias* and *Strongyloides* primarily infect snakes, with *Rhabdias* infecting the respiratory tract and *Strongyloides* the intestinal tract. *Entomelas* primarily infects the respiratory tract of lizards.

Life Cycle. The life cycles of the rhabditids of reptiles are similar to those of other members of the superfamily. All genera have two different life cycles: a free-living cycle and a parthenogenic or parasitic cycle. In the case of *Rhabdias* and *Entomelas,* the parthenogenic female releases eggs or larvae in the lung. First-stage larvae migrate out of the lung via the trachea and into the oral cavity, where they are either swallowed and passed with the feces or released out of the oral cavity. The larvae continue to develop, and it is the third-stage larvae that are infective to reptiles. These larvae can infect reptiles either through the oral cavity or by penetrating the integument. *Strongyloides* is shed via the feces.

Pathologic Effects. The pathologic lesions associated with *Rhabdias* and *Entomelas* infections can be mild to severe, depending on the density of parasites, general health status of the host, and presence or absence of opportunistic infections. Animals that succumb to the infections generally have a severe inflammatory response and pneumonia. *Strongyloides* infections can result in numerous ulcerations in the intestine.

Clinical Disease. Reptiles infected with these parasites can be asymptomatic or develop severe clinical disease. Snakes and lizards infected with *Rhabdias* and *Entomelas* may present with open-mouth breathing, dyspnea, and collapse. In severe cases, the infections can be fatal. Snakes with *Strongyloides* infections may present with diarrhea and weight loss.

Diagnosis. Antemortem diagnosis of *Rhabdias* and *Entomelas* is based on identification of the egg or rhabditiform larvae in the oral cavity or feces of snakes and lizards. Postmortem diagnosis is based on identification of the adult worms in the respiratory tract. Antemortem and postmortem diagnoses for *Strongyloides* are based on the identification of eggs/larvae or adult worms in the feces or intestine, respectively.

Treatment and Prevention. Dosing regimens for reptilian parasites are subjective. Fenbendazole (25 to 100 mg/kg) and ivermectin (0.2 mg/kg) are generally considered the most effective anthelminthics for nematodes, including rhabditids. Recommended dosing frequencies vary, with most redosing every 10 to 14 days for two to three treatments. Fenbendazole can also be administered over a three- to five-day period and repeated in 14 days. All recently acquired reptiles should be screened for rhabditids during quarantine. Prophylactic treatment may be considered. Because these parasites can infect reptiles percutaneously, it is important to regularly remove and disinfect the substrate.

Public Health Considerations. Rhabditids of reptiles do not infect humans.

Superfamily Oxyuroidea

Alaeuris spp. and Ozolaimus spp.

Morphology. Oxyurids, or pinworms, are small to medium-size nematodes (2 mm to 7 mm in length), with a mouth bearing three lips, an esophagus which terminates in a bulb, and a simple intestine that lacks a diverticulum. The males have spicules which are used as taxonomic keys. Female pinworms have a posterior extremity that is conical and pointed. The eggs are large and smooth.

Hosts. Oxyurid infections are common among lizards and chelonians, especially herbivorous species. It is common to visualize adult pinworms in the colon of herbivorous lizards or chelonians during exploratory surgery. Pinworms are rarely observed in snakes, and have not been reported in crocodilians. The two most common genera found in captive reptiles are *Alaeuris* and *Ozolaimus.*

Life Cycle. The life cycles of parasites in the genera *Alaeuris* and *Ozolaimus* are direct, with infection occurring by ingestion of an embryonated egg[40]. The eggs hatch and the larvae develop in the anterior intestine, but eventually migrate to the large intestine.

Pathologic Effects and Clinical Disease. Many authors consider pinworms that feed on digesta in the colon of reptiles to be commensals[41]. In fact, reptiles with oxyurid infections are generally asymptomatic. Pathologic changes are rare, but possible. McGuire and coworkers[42] reported intestinal intussusception in a green iguana with a severe oxyurid infection. The nematodes were found throughout the alimentary tract from the stomach to the colon, and were considered to play a role in the iguana's condition.

Diagnosis, Treatment, and Prevention. Antemortem diagnosis is by identification of eggs or adult worms in the feces. Postmortem diagnosis can be made based on identification of adult worms in the alimentary tract. Infections can be controlled with administration of fenbendazole (25 to 100 mg/kg orally for five days, repeated 10 and 20 days later). Complete elimination of infection is often not possible. It is advisable to use a low dosage of fenbendazole when treating

entire colonies because toxicity is a rare but possible outcome. Routine prophylactic treatment with anthelminthics may be used to control pinworm infections in reptiles.

Public Health Considerations. Members of the genera *Alaeuris* and *Ozolaimus* are not infective to humans.

Falcaustra spp.

Morphology. Adult *Falcaustra* spp. (Syn. *Spironoura* spp.) measure 8 mm to 16 mm long and have an esophagus with a terminal bulb, a simple intestine without a diverticulum, and a pointed posterior extremity in both sexes (Figure 9.6)[26,43]. The male has spicules of equal length and a gubernaculum, but no caudal alae.

Hosts and Life Cycle. The genus includes some of the most common intestinal nematodes found in turtles from the United States[27,44]. *Falcaustra affinis* occurs in box turtles, map turtles, spotted turtles, and Blanding's turtles;

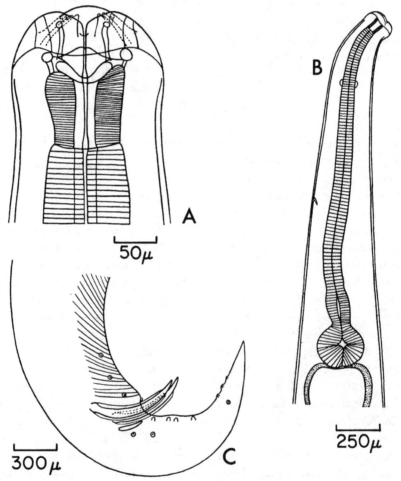

Fig. 9.6 *Falcaustra* (*Spironoura*). (A) Head, ventral view. (B) Anterior end, lateral view. (C) Posterior end of male, lateral view. Reproduced from Yorke, W. and Maplestone, P.A. (1926) with permission.

F. procera occurs in painted turtles, cooters, and sliders; *F. wardi* occurs in map turtles and snapping turtles; and *F. chelydrae* occurs in snapping turtles, red-eared turtles, and other aquatic turtles. Infections are common, and have been noted in 19% to 97% of turtles examined[26,35]. The life cycle is unknown but is probably direct, with infection occurring by ingestion of an embryonated egg[43].

Pathologic Effects and Clinical Disease. Nothing is known of the pathologic effects of the *Falcaustra* spp. In captive situations it is possible that heavy burdens may develop in closed systems, and that in these cases a mild enteritis response occurs. However, infections are not generally associated with clinical disease.

Diagnosis, Treatment, and Prevention. Antemortem diagnosis is by identification of the eggs in the feces, while postmortem diagnosis is by identification of the parasite in the intestine. Because these parasites do not generally cause disease, treatment is not necessary. If clinical disease does occur, fenbendazole (25 to 100 mg/kg orally for five days, repeated in 10 days) would be recommended. Reptiles should be screened for infection with *Falcaustra* during quarantine. To reduce the likelihood of introducing the parasite, prophylactic treatment with fenbendazole can be considered.

Public Health Considerations. Humans are not susceptible to infection with *Falcaustra* spp.

Tachygonetria spp.

Morphology. Adults worms measure 1.5 mm to 4.6 mm in length (Figure 9.7)[43,45]. They possess a mouth with six small lips, a long esophagus with a terminal bulb, and a simple intestine. The female has a short conical tail, and the vulva is posterior to the middle of the body. The male has a single, short spicule and a gubernaculum.

Hosts and Life Cycle. The genus includes the nematodes that are common to European and African tortoises[27,46]. Wild-caught tortoises are frequently infected, often with several different species and hundreds of worms[46]. The life cycle is direct, with infection by ingestion of an embryonated egg[43,46].

Pathologic Effects and Clinical Disease. Although heavy infections are common and usually cause no apparent ill effects, intestinal impaction and death have been reported[47].

Diagnosis, Treatment, and Prevention. These aspects are as described for *Falcaustra* spp.

Public Health Considerations. *Tachygonetria* is not known to infect humans.

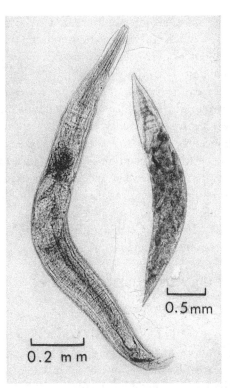

Fig. 9.7 *Tachygonetria longicollis.* (Left) Male. (Right) Female. Reproduced from Forstner, M.J. (1960) with permission.

Superfamily Strongyloidea

Diaphanocephalus spp. *and* Kalicephalus *spp.*

Morphology, Hosts, and Life Cycle. *Diaphanocephalus* spp. and *Kalicephalus* spp. are hookworms inhabiting the alimentary tracts of snakes, and less commonly, lizards. Adult worms measure 7 mm to 9 mm long. The life cycles are direct. Eggs are shed in the feces or can be expelled out of the oral cavity if infections are located in the cranial alimentary tract (e.g., esophagus).

Pathologic Effects and Clinical Disease. Susceptible hosts become infected through ingestion or percutaneous passage of larvae. These parasites ingest blood, and can cause significant ulceration in the alimentary tract. Gastrointestinal impactions may occur with heavy burdens. Reptiles may be asymptomatic or develop severe gastrointestinal disease. Anorexia, weight loss, anemia, intestinal impaction, and diarrhea may occur. Severe infections can be fatal.

Diagnosis, Treatment, and Prevention. Antemortem diagnosis of *Kalicephalus* and *Diaphanocephalus* is by identification of the egg or adult worm in the feces or oral cavity. Postmortem diagnosis is based on identification of the adult worms in the intestinal tract.

Dosing regimens for reptilian parasites are subjective. Fenbendazole (25 to 100 mg/kg) and ivermectin (0.2 mg/kg) are generally considered the most effective anthelmintics for nematodes. Recommended dosing frequencies are variable. Repeat treatments are often given every 10 to 14 days for two to three treatments. Fenbendazole can also be dosed over a three- to five-day period and repeated in 14 days. All recently acquired reptiles should be screened for hookworms while in quarantine. Prophylactic treatment may be warranted. Because percutaneous transmission occurs, it is important to regularly remove and disinfect the substrate.

Public Health Considerations. Reptilian hookworms do not infect humans.

Superfamily Trichostrongyloidea

Oswaldocruzia spp.

Morphology. Adult *Oswaldocruzia* spp. are filiform worms measuring 6 mm to 14 mm long[26,43]. The buccal cavity is rudimentary or absent, the vulva of the female is in the posterior half of the body, and the spicules of the male are short and stout and end in a number of processes (Figure 9.8).

Hosts and Life Cycle. This relatively nonpathogenic trichostrongylid nematode occurs in the intestine of reptiles throughout the world. It is most common in turtles and occurs primarily in aquatic species[48]. The life cycle is direct, with infection by ingestion of infective larvae[43].

Pathologic Effects and Clinical Disease. Infections are asymptomatic. While it is possible that extremely heavy infections could lead to enteritis, such cases have not been reported.

Diagnosis, Treatment, and Prevention. Diagnosis is by demonstration and identification of the parasite in the intestine at necropsy. Because these parasites do not generally cause disease, treatment is not necessary. In the research setting however, it may be desirable to eliminate all pathogens. In these cases, treatment may be administered as described for strongylid infections. Reptiles should be screened for infection during quarantine. Prophylactic treatment can be administered to reduce the likelihood of introducing the parasite.

Public Health Considerations. *Oswaldocruzia* does not infect humans.

Superfamily Spiruroidea

Camallanus spp.

Morphology. Adults of *Camallanus microcephalus* and *C. trispinosus* have a filiform body measuring 5 mm to 10 mm long, a slit-like mouth with two lateral chitinous valves, and an esophagus comprised of a short anterior

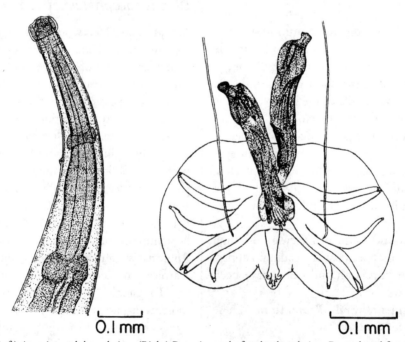

Fig. 9.8 *Oswaldocruzia.* (Left) Anterior end, lateral view. (Right) Posterior end of male, dorsal view. Reproduced from Yorke, W. and Maplestone, P.A. (1926) with permission.

muscular portion and a long posterior glandular portion (Figure 9.9)[43]. The posterior extremity of the male is rolled ventrally and bears small caudal alae, dissimilar and unequal spicules, and no gubernaculum. The vulva of the female is near the middle of the body.

Hosts. *Camallanus microcephalus* and *C. trispinosus* are common gastric and duodenal worms of turtles from the United States[49,50]. *Camallanus microcephalus* is common in painted turtles, map turtles, Blanding's turtles, and snapping turtles. The prevalence of this parasite can be high in wild populations, with as many as 54% of painted turtles in the north central U.S. found to be positive and 83% of snapping turtles from the south central U.S. found to be positive[35,49]. *Camallanus trispinosus* is common in painted turtles, snapping turtles, and other turtles. Again, the prevalence of these parasites in wild turtles from the south central U.S. can be very high (87% to 100%)[26]. Wild-caught turtles acquired for the laboratory are likely to be positive[50].

Life Cycle. The life cycle is indirect and requires a copepod as a first intermediate host and sometimes an amphibian or fish as a paratenic host[51]. The reptilian definitive host is infected by ingestion of an infected copepod, amphibian, or fish.

Pathologic Effects and Clinical Signs. *Camallanus* spp. embed deeply in the stomach and duodenal wall and sometimes form abscesses. Heavy worm burdens could result in gastric ulceration and bacteremia. Most infected reptiles are asymptomatic. Animals with heavy burdens may become anorexic, lose weight, and develop melena and diarrhea.

Diagnosis, Treatment, and Prevention. Diagnosis is based on the identification of the eggs in the feces or the adult parasite in the stomach or duodenum. Because of the need for a copepod intermediate host, it is unlikely that the life cycle would be completed in the laboratory, and no special control procedures should be required. However, treatment is warranted if newly acquired animals have heavy burdens, and consists of fenbendazole (25 to 100 mg/kg orally for five days, repeated in 10 days). Reptiles should be screened for infection during quarantine.

Public Health Considerations. *Camallanus* spp. do not infect humans.

Spiroxys contortus

Morphology. *Spiroxys contortus* is biologically similar to *Camallanus* spp. Adults of *S. contortus* measure 15 mm to 30 mm long, and have a mouth with two large, distinctly trilobed lips and an esophagus that has a short anterior muscular portion and a longer posterior glandular portion (Figure 9.10)[43]. The male has well-developed caudal alae,

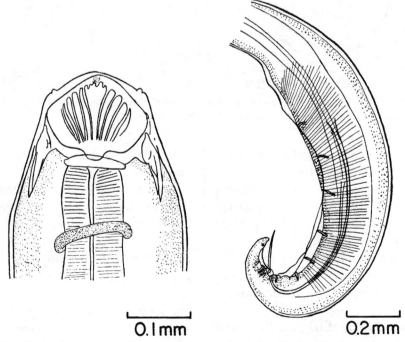

0.1mm   0.2mm

Fig. 9.9 *Camallanus.* (Left) Anterior end, lateral view. (Right) Posterior end of male, lateral view. Reproduced from Yorke, W. and Maplestone, P.A. (1926) with permission.

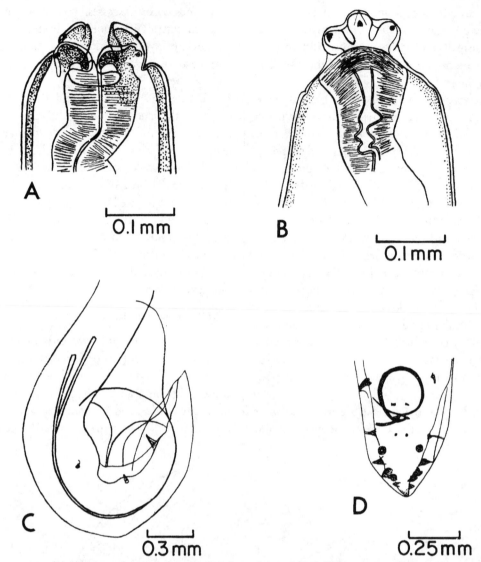

Fig. 9.10 *Spiroxys contortus.* (A) Anterior end, ventral view. (B) Anterior end, lateral view. (C) Posterior end of male, lateral view. (D) Posterior end of male, ventral view. Reproduced from Yorke, W. and Maplestone, P.A. (1926) with permission.

delicate and subequal spicules, and no gubernaculum. The vulva of the female is near the middle of the body.

Hosts and Life Cycle. *Spiroxys contortus* is common in the stomach and duodenum of painted turtles, map turtles, and snapping turtles[52]. The prevalence of this parasite in turtles from the south central U.S. is approximately 25% in painted turtles and 38% in snapping turtles[26,35]. Wild caught turtles acquired for the laboratory are likely to be positive[50]. The life cycle is similar to that described for *Camallanus.*

Pathologic Effects and Clinical Disease. Pathologic effects and clinical disease are as described for *Camallanus.* Most infections are asymptomatic, but animals with heavy burdens may become anorexic, lose weight, and develop melena and diarrhea.

Diagnosis, Treatment, Prevention, and Public Health Considerations. These aspects are as described for *Camallanus.*

Superfamily Filaroidea

Foleyella spp.

The morphology and biology of *Foleyella* spp. are presented in Chapter 8, Parasites of Amphibians. *Foleyella* are primarily associated with infections of lacertid lizards and Old World chameleons[13]. *Foleyella furcata, F. brevicauda,* and *F. candezei* are the filarids most often found in chameleons[53,54]. Reptiles are infected when bitten by an infected mosquito. Most infections are asymptomatic. Heavy infections may result in anorexia, weight loss, weakness, lethargy, and collapse. Heavy microfilarial burdens could lead to thromboembolic disease. Diagnosis is by identification of the adult worm in the body cavity or microfilariae in the blood. No treatment has been described. Adult worms may be removed surgically. Anti-inflammatory drugs may minimize the likelihood of thromboembolic disease. The life cycle is not easily completed in the animal facility environment because of the lack of suitable arthropod intermediate hosts. *Foleyella* do not infect humans.

ACANTHOCEPHALA

Neoechinorhynchus spp.

Morphology. Adults are small worms with cylindrical, unspined, and usually curved bodies (Figure 9.11)[55]. Adult males measure 4.7 mm to 26.4 mm long by 0.4 mm to 1.0 mm wide, depending on the species. Adult females measure 7 mm to 39.2 mm long by 0.4 to 1.5 mm wide[56,57]. The proboscis is short and globular and contains three circles of six hooks each. Eggs are generally oval to elliptical but vary greatly in size and shape, depending on the species.

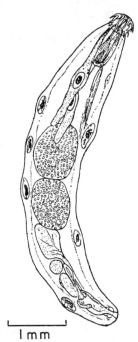

l mm

Fig. 9.11 *Neoechinorhynchus* male. Reproduced from Borradaile, L.A. and Potts, F.A. (1958) with permission.

Hosts. Several species of *Neoechinorhynchus* occur in the intestine of turtles from North America. *Neoechinorhynchus emydis* is found in map turtles, false map turtles, Blanding's turtles, and red-eared turtles[49,56]. *Neoechinorhynchus pseudemydis* occurs in painted turtles, Blanding's turtles, and red-eared turtles[57,58]. *Neoechinorhynchus chrysemydis* is found in painted turtles, red-eared turtles, and other cooters and sliders[57,58]. *Neoechinorhynchus emyditoides* occurs in painted turtles, Blanding's turtles, and red-eared turtles[58]. *N. stunkardi* occurs in false map turtles[56]. All are common and likely to be encountered in laboratory turtles obtained from their natural habitats.

Life Cycle. The life cycles of the North American species are not completely known. Eggs passed in the feces of a turtle hatch when ingested by an ostracod (a bivalved arthropod), in which an unencysted immature worm develops. Ostracods are ingested by snails, which in turn are ingested by turtles[59,60]. It is uncertain whether snails are obligatory or facultative intermediate hosts. *Neoechinorhynchus rutili,* which infects turtles in Europe, does not require a snail intermediate host but is infective while in the ostracod.

Pathologic Effects and Clinical Disease. Most infections are asymptomatic. Heavy infections of 200 to 700 worms occur[49,50,60]. Worm populations may become high enough to cause intestinal blockage, rupture, and bacteremia[26]. The worms have a short proboscis and penetrate only the intestinal mucosa and a small amount of the lamina propria[61]. Although they cause inflammation and thickening of the mucosa[49], tissue damage apparently is not severe[60]. They have also been associated with benign neoplastic lesions of the intestine[49] and benign granulomatous lesions of the pancreatic duct[50]. When present, clinical signs may include anorexia, regurgitation, listlessness, lethargy, weakness, diarrhea, an absence of feces, and death from intestinal rupture.

Diagnosis, Treatment, and Prevention. Diagnosis is by identification of the eggs in the feces or adult parasite in the intestine. Elimination of infection may be attempted by the administration of fenbendazole (25 to 100 mg/kg orally for five days, repeated in 10 days). However, there are no entirely effective anthelmintic therapies for infections with acanthocephala. The requirements of the life cycle generally preclude establishment within the environment of the animal facility. Animals should be screened for infection upon arrival.

Public Health Considerations. *Neoechinorhynchus* is not known to affect humans.

ARTHROPODS

Class Insecta

Order Diptera (flies)

Cistudinomyia cistudinis

Morphology. Larvae of *Cistudinomyia cistudinis* (Syn. *Sarcophaga cistudinis*) are heavily spined (Figure 9.12). The first instar measures about 2 mm long when newly deposited and about 4 mm long at the time of molting. The second instar measures 4 mm to 10 mm long and the third instar measures 10 mm to 15 mm long. Adults are typically sarcophagid and resemble the housefly.

Hosts and Life Cycle. Larvae of this sarcophagid fly parasitize turtles and tortoises in the eastern and southern United States[62,63]. The parasite affects several species of land turtles, including box turtles (*Terrapene* spp.), painted turtles (*Trachemys scripta elegans*), and gopher tortoises (*Gopherus polyphemus*). Infection with larvae of this fly is particularly common in the southeastern United States.

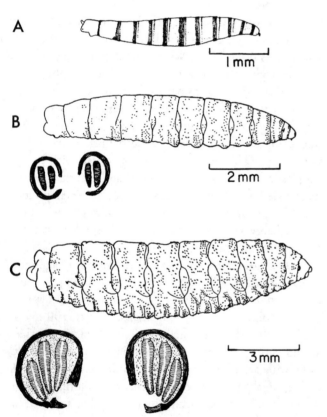

Fig. 9.12 *Cistudinomyia cistudinis* larvae. (A) First instar larva. (B) Second instar larva and posterior spiracles. (C) Third instar larva and posterior spiracles. Reproduced from Knipling, E.F. (1937) with permission.

A gravid female deposits first instar larvae in an open wound, often in lesions produced by the gopher-tortoise tick, *Amblyomma tuberculatum*[63]. Larval development requires about 50 to 60 days, pupation takes 14 to 21 days, and the entire life cycle requires 69 to 81 days.

Pathologic Effects and Clinical Disease. *Cistudinomyia cistudinis* larvae cause a serious and sometimes fatal myiasis in suitable hosts. Feeding larvae congregate in closely packed groups with their posterior ends toward the wound opening[63]. Larvae destroy tissue and produce a fetid odor and a dark discharge from the wound. Opportunistic bacterial infections are common sequellae. Larval invasion is usually contained by the formation of a fibrous wall. Only occasionally is the infection heavy enough to cause death[63,64].

Diagnosis, Treatment, and Prevention. Diagnosis is by demonstration of the characteristic larvae in the wounds. Newly acquired animals should be examined and, if infected, treated. Treatment requires removal of the maggots and aggressive wound debridement[47]. This author prefers to disinfect the wound with chlorhexidine or an iodine solution, followed by a hypertonic solution (50% dextrose) and saline. Systemic antibiotics should be given for large, infected wounds. Ivermectin should not be used to eliminate these maggots, because it can be fatal in chelonians. Infection with *C. cistudinis* is unlikely to occur in the laboratory setting. For outdoor facilities, proper fly control prevents infection.

Public Health Considerations. Humans are not suitable hosts for *C. cistudinis*.

Class Arachnida

Ticks

Reptiles may serve as hosts to a vast array of hard and soft ticks. Only the most common are mentioned here.

Family Argasidae

Ornithodoros turicata, the relapsing fever tick (Figure 9.13), is native to the United States and Mexico[65]. It is commonly found on endothermic animals, and is usually uncommon on ectotherms. However, heavy infections occasionally occur on the box turtle in its natural habitat, and it was reported to have become established in captive reptiles in the United States[65].

Adult and nymphal tick stages are considered most important because they can actively feed on reptilian hosts, for which they serve as vectors for bacteria, viruses, and

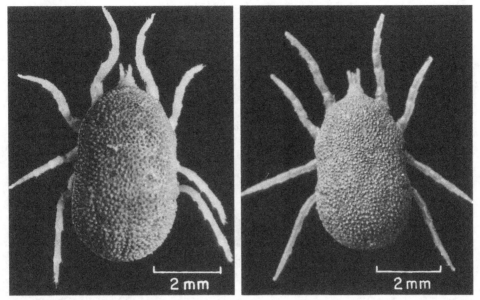

Fig. 9.13   *Ornithodoros turicata* (Left) Adult male, dorsal view. (Right) Nymph, dorsal view. Courtesy of U.S. Department of Agriculture.

protozoal infections. For the most part, individual ticks are of little clinical significance. Ticks are generally located in those areas where they can easily burrow, including the conjunctiva, skin folds, gular area, and inguinal and axillary regions. Treatment consists of manual removal. Provent-a-mite can be used topically to treat the reptile and its environment. Reptiles should be closely inspected during quarantine, and treated accordingly.

Ornithodoros turicata can transmit the agent of relapsing fever in man, and may be a vector of *Leptospira pomona*[65]. All ticks removed from reptiles should be considered potential vectors for zoonotic infectious diseases and disposed of properly.

Family Ixodidae
Amblyomma spp.   The morphology of *Amblyomma* spp. is described in Chapter 6, Biology of Arthropods, and Chapter 10, Parasites of Birds. *Amblyomma tuberculatum*, the Gopher-tortoise tick (Figure 9.14), is one of the largest of the reptilian ticks[67]. The male measures 6.2 mm long by 5.5 mm wide. The unengorged female measures up to 7.5 mm long and 5.5 mm to 6 mm wide[66]. Engorged females can attain a length of 18 mm to 24 mm.

Amblyomma dissimile, the iguana tick (Figure 9.14), is native to the southeastern United States, Mexico, West Indies, Central America, and South America. This tick is commonly found on ectotherms (both reptiles and amphibians) from these regions[67]. Although the principal host is the iguana, gopher snakes, rattlesnakes, eastern fence lizards, and several other reptiles are occasionally affected[66,67]. The larvae

of *Amblyomma tuberculatum* occur on mammals and birds. The adults and nymph occur almost exclusively on the gopher tortoise (*Gopherus polyphemus*)[66,67]. Treatment and prevention are as described for *Ornithodoros,* with the added note that care must be taken to remove embedded mouthparts.

Hyalomma spp. *Hyalomma aegyptium* (Figure 9.15), is commonly found on European chelonians, including Greek tortoises and European pond terrapins[47,68]. It occurs in southern Europe and southwestern Asia and, although originally described from a tortoise in Egypt, may be extinct in Africa[69]. Treatment and prevention are as described for *Amblyomma.*

Mites

Suborder Mesostigmata
Entonyssus spp. and Entophionyssus spp.   Entonyssid mites are common parasites of the trachea and lungs of snakes[70]. The genera most likely to be encountered in laboratory snakes are *Entonyssus* and *Entophionyssus* (Figure 9.16). Although these parasites are frequently found in snakes that have died of pulmonary disease, no evidence exists of a causal relationship or the production of any harmful effects by the mites.

Ophionyssus natricis
Morphology. Adult *Ophionyssus natricis* (Syn. *Ophionyssus serpentium, Serpenticola serpentium*) measure 0.6 mm to 1.3 mm long (Figure 9.17)[71,72]. Unfed females are yellow-brown in color, while engorged females are dark red or black.

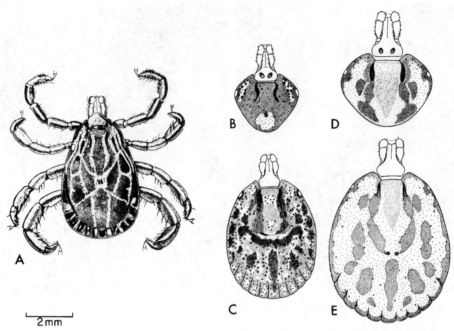

Fig. 9.14 (A) *Amblyomma* male, dorsal view. (B) Scutum of *A. dissimile* female. (C) Scutum of *A. dissimile* male. (D) Scutum of *A. tuberculatum* female. (E) Scutum of *A. tuberculatum* male. (A) courtesy of U.S. Department of Agriculture. (B),(C),(D), and (E) reproduced from Cooley, R.A. and Kohls, G.M. (1944) with permission.

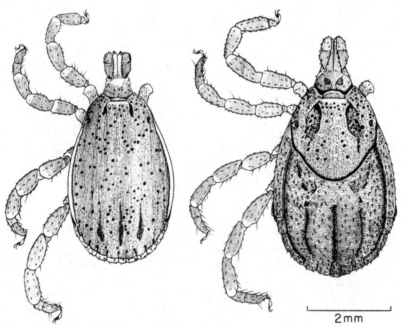

Fig. 9.15 *Hyalomma aegyptium.* (Left) Adult male, dorsal view. (Right) Adult female, dorsal view. Courtesy of H. Hoogstraal, U.S. Naval Medical Research Unit.

Hosts and Life Cycle. This hematophagous mite is the most common ectoparasite found on captive snakes[73]. All snakes should be considered susceptible to infection. Mites are found on the skin or under the scales. Lizards can also be infested[73]. Although common in captivity, it is seldom found on wild specimens. Female mites take a blood meal and then leave the host to deposit her eggs in the cage crevices or substrate[72]. The eggs hatch in one to four days, and the parasite goes through larval protonymphal and deutonymphal stages before reaching

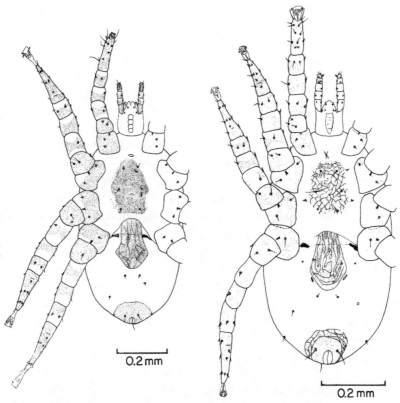

Fig. 9.16 Entonyssid mites. (Left) *Entonyssus colubri* female, ventral view. (Right) *Entophionyssus glasmacheri* female, ventral view. Reproduced from Fain, A. (1961) with permission.

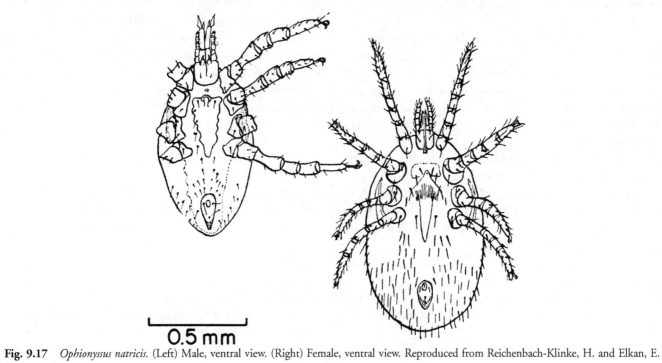

Fig. 9.17 *Ophionyssus natricis.* (Left) Male, ventral view. (Right) Female, ventral view. Reproduced from Reichenbach-Klinke, H. and Elkan, E. (1965) with permission.

the adult stage. Larvae do not feed, but nymphs must feed before molting to the next stage. The entire life cycle requires 13 to 19 days. Some mites live as long as 40 days. The source of infection is usually infested animals that have been added to a colony without quarantine or treatment.

Pathologic Effects. The number of mites that present on captive snakes can vary from a few to hundreds. Infestations may become generalized, with mites feeding between scales over the entire body or focal, with mites found near the eyes and the gular fold[74]. Heavy infestations are characterized by irritation, severe anemia, and death. *Ophionyssus natricis* is a mechanical vector of *Aeromonas hydrophila*, an important bacterial pathogen of snakes[75], and has been implicated in the transmission of inclusion body disease, a potentially devastating viral disease of snakes.

Clinical Disease. Snakes infested with mites may appear listless, irritated, and lethargic. It is not uncommon for mite-infested snakes to produce serial sheds in an attempt to rid their body of the mites. Affected snakes may also be found regularly soaking in water in an attempt to obtain some relief.

Diagnosis. Infestation with *O. natricis* is often first recognized by the appearance of small white deposits of mite feces on the body. Clinical signs aid in diagnosis[73]. Definitive diagnosis is by identification of the mite. A cotton-tipped applicator soaked in mineral oil can be used to collect mites from the snake for microscopic examination.

Treatment. Newly acquired snakes should be carefully inspected and, if infested, isolated, treated, and placed in clean, sterilized cages. Affected animals can be soaked in lukewarm water daily to drown mites. Ivermectin (0.2 mg/kg, repeated in two weeks for three treatments) can be used to treat mites on the snakes, but provides no effect on larval stages. Provent-a-mite (0.5% permethrin)(Pro Products Mahopac, NY) has excellent efficacy against mites on snakes and mites in the environment.

In addition to treating with Provent-a-mite, the enclosure substrate should be replaced daily. The author prefers to use newspaper or paper towels because of the ease of daily replacement.

Biological control methods using predatory mites (*Hypoaspis* sp.) can also be used. These mites seek out and prey on *Ophionyssus*. Once the predatory mites have contained the snake mite infestation, they may feed on detritus in the vivarium or simply expire.

Prevention. Preventing the introduction of *Ophionyssus* into a snake colony is critical, and can be accomplished using strict hygiene and quarantine procedures. Prophylactic spraying of newly acquired snakes with Provent-a-mite prior to entering and exiting quarantine is highly recommended.

Public Health Considerations. Infestation of laboratory personnel has been reported[71].

Suborder Prostigmata
Trombiculids **Morphology.** Often classified as "chigger mites," these six-legged mites are common on wild reptiles from North America and farm-raised iguanas from Central and South America. These mites often have a red to orange color, and are similar in size to *Ophionyssus* mites.

Hosts. Important genera include *Eutrombicula*, *Hirstiella*, and *Neotrombicula*. Larvae are often found on reptiles and sometimes on amphibians obtained from their natural habitats[71]. The most common species found on North American reptiles is *E. alfreddugesi*, the common chigger (Figure 9.18)[76]. It is prevalent throughout the Western Hemisphere and has been reported to affect box turtles, other turtles, racers, hognose snakes, kingsnakes, garter snakes, other snakes, and lizards[77,78]. Another common species found in the southeastern United States is *E. splendens*, which infests snakes and lizards. *Hirstiella* is the most common genus isolated from green iguanas in Central America. The common harvest mite of Europe, *N. autumnalis*, also parasitizes reptiles and has been found on the viviparous lizard and possibly on snakes[78].

Life Cycle. The life cycle is typical of Trombiculid mites. Only the larvae are parasitic. Nymphs and adults are free-living. Larvae feed to engorgement. The life cycle has not been completed in the laboratory.

Pathologic Effects and Clinical Disease. Mites are generally found in the skin folds surrounding the axillary and inguinal regions, although infestations may become generalized. The pathologic effects and clinical presentation are similar to those of *O. natricis*.

Diagnosis, Treatment, and Prevention. Infestation with chigger mites is often first recognized by the appearance of clusters of red-orange mites. A cotton-tipped applicator soaked in mineral oil or thumb forceps can be used to collect mites for microscopic examination. Recommendations for treatment and prevention of mite infestation are as described for *Ophionyssus*.

Public Health Considerations. Trombiculids cause severe dermatitis in humans. Infested laboratory animals

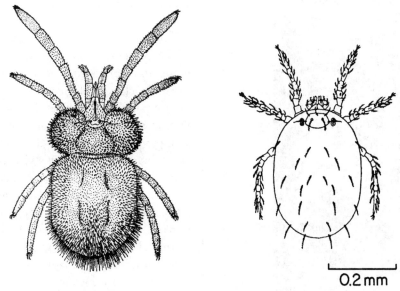

0.2 mm

Fig. 9.18 *Eutrombicula alfreddugesi.* (Left) Adult female, dorsal view. (Right) Larva, dorsal view. Reproduced from Ewing, H.E. (1929) with permission.

are not considered a major risk for human infestation because larvae feed only once, and the life cycle has not been completed in the laboratory.

Class *Pentastomida*

Morphology. Adult pentastomes are vermiform arthropods common in tropical snakes and lizards.

Hosts. Snakes and lizards commonly serve as hosts to a variety of pentastomes. Among the most important genera are *Armillifer, Kiricephalus, Porocephalus, Raillietiella,* and *Sebekia.*

Armillifer spp. has been found in vipers and African pythons (*Python sebae*). *Kiricephalus* spp. are generally associated with non-venomous snakes. *Kiricephalus coarctatus* is common in North, Central, and South American colubrid snakes[79]. Immature stages are found in the subcutaneous muscles of racers, rat snakes, garter snakes, and other snakes. Adults occur in the lungs of rat snakes, garter snakes, and other snakes. *Kiricephalus pattoni* occurs in colubrid and boid snakes from Asia, Indonesia, Australia, and Madagascar[80]. Immature stages have been found in the subcutaneous tissues or the stomach wall of snakes[81]. Adults occur in the lungs of racers and other snakes.

Adults of the genus *Porocephalus* (Figure 9.19) occur in the lungs of crotalid, boid, and some colubrid snakes in North and South America and Africa[80,81]. *Porocephalus crotali* is particularly common in rattlesnakes (*Crotalus*

spp.) in the United States. Prevalence rates have been estimated to be >50% in some areas[82]. Although *Porocephalus* is uncommon in laboratory snakes, members of the genus are important because immature stages occur in certain laboratory rodents and primates. These are discussed in the chapters covering those host species.

Raillietiella has a cosmopolitan distribution among lizards and snakes[80,81]. Only one species, *Raillietiella bicaudata,* occurs in North America. It is found in the lungs of rat snakes and other snakes[81]. The most common species from Europe, *R. orientalis,* occurs in the lungs of racers, rat snakes, and other snakes[81]. *Raillietiella boulengeri* is the most common species in Africa[81]. Immature stages of this species are found in various tissues of snakes and lizards, and adults occur in colubrid, boid, viperid, and other snakes[83]. Only one species, *R. furcocerca,* occurs in South America[81]. Larvae and nymphs of this species are found in various tissues of racers and rat snakes, and adults occur in the lungs of colubrid, boid, crotalid, and other snakes. *Sebekia* spp. are primarily found in crocodilians. Adults of *S. oxycephala* occur in the lungs, trachea, and pharynx of crocodiles, alligators, and spectacled caimans in North and South America[80,81]. Immature stages are frequently encountered in hognose snakes and occasionally in lizards. They also occur in fishes[51].

Life Cycle. Adult pentastomes usually live in the lungs, bronchi, trachea, pharynx, and oral or coelomic cavities. Larvae and nymphs occur in the lungs or other

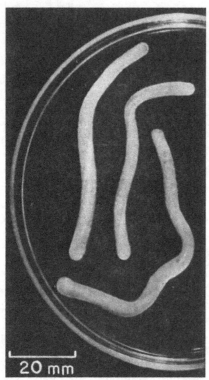

Fig. 9.19 *Porocephalus* females. Reproduced from Fain, A. (1961) with permission.

organs and tissues. Eggs shed by the adult stage are coughed up, swallowed, and passed with the feces. The eggs are ingested by an intermediate host, where they develop into infective nymphs. The life cycle is continued after a reptile consumes an infected intermediate host. Once ingested, the infective larva penetrates the intestinal wall and migrates to specific locations in the body, depending on parasite species, where it develops into an adult.

Pathologic Effects and Clinical Disease. The majority of the pathology associated with pentastomid infections is localized. Commonly there is localized inflammation at the site of attachment of the adult stages. Larval stages can also induce pathologic changes during the migration from the intestines to the site of adult development. Most cases are asymptomatic. Respiratory distress and dyspnea occur with heavy burdens. The most severe clinical disease occurs in crocodilians, where pulmonary changes can be more severe.

Diagnosis. Antemortem diagnosis is by finding pentastomid eggs on fecal flotation or by endoscopic examination of the respiratory tract and visualization of adult worms. Postmortem diagnosis can be made from the demonstration of the adult worms at the time of gross necropsy, or by histologic evidence of migrating larvae from the intestine.

Treatment. Ivermectin (0.2 to 1.0 mg/kg, repeated in two and four weeks) may be used to reduce egg production by pentastomids, but may not be eliminate the infection. Anthelmintic treatment may secondarily result in thromboembolic disease if the adult parasites succumb to the treatment, though this sequella appears to be rare. Adult worms can also be removed endoscopically.

Prevention. Reptiles should be screened for patent pentastome infections during quarantine. Laboratory reptiles represent "dead end" hosts because the life cycle cannot be completed without suitable intermediate hosts.

Public Health Considerations. Humans can become incidentally infected with pentastomids.

TABLE 9.1 Parasites of reptiles—circulatory/lymphatic system.

Parasite	Geographic distribution	Hosts	Location in host	Method of infection	Pathologic effects	Reference
Flagellates						
Trypanosoma chrysemydis	North America	Turtle	Blood	Leech transmission	None	100
Trypanosoma thamnophis	North America	Garter snakes	Blood	Probably bite of arthropod	Unknown	101
Coccidia						
Haemogregarina spp.	North America	Snakes	Blood	Leech transmission	Anemia	15, 98
Haemogregarina ibera	Europe	Tortoises	Blood	Leech or tick transmission	Anemia	98
Haemogregarina stepanowi	Europe, North America	Turtles	Blood	Leech or tick transmission	Anemia	16, 98
Hepatozoon mauritanicum	Africa, Europe	Tortoises	Blood	Ingestion of tick	None	99
Karyolysus lacertae	Europe	Lizards	Blood	Ingestion of mite	None	103
Plasmodium floridense	Central and North America	Anoles, spiny lizards	Blood	Bite of bloodsucking arthropod	Heavy infections sometimes cause death	102
Plasmodium mexicanum	North America	Spiny lizards	Blood	Bite of sandfly	None	104
Tunetella emydis	Europe	Pond turtles	Blood	Bite of bloodsucking arthropod	None	71
Trematodes						
Spirorchis spp.	North America	Turtles	Heart, blood vessels	Penetration of skin by cercaria released from snail	Massive infections probably cause death	27, 105

TABLE 9.2 Parasites of reptiles—enterohepatic system.

Parasite	Geographic distribution	Hosts	Location in host	Method of infection	Pathologic effects	Reference
Flagellates						
Chilomastix bursa	North America	Lizards	Intestine	Ingestion of organism passed in feces	None	108
Chilomastix sp.	North America	Tortoises, turtles	Intestine	Ingestion of organism passed in feces	None	84
Giardia sp.	Europe, North America	European pond terrapins, snakes	Small intestine	Ingestion of organism passed in feces	None	1
Greponemas spp.	North America	Turtles	Intestine	Ingestion of organism passed in feces	None	84
Hexamastix spp.	North America	Lizards	Intestine	Ingestion of organism passed in feces	None	108
Hexamita natrix	Asia	Water snakes	Stomach, small intestine	Ingestion of organism passed in feces	None	84
Hexamita parvus	Worldwide	Turtles	Large intestine	Ingestion of organism passed in feces	None	85
Hypotrichomonas acosta	Worldwide	Snakes, lizards	Large intestine	Ingestion of organism passed in feces	None	109
Leishmania chamaeleonis	Africa	Chameleons	Intestine	Probably by ingestion of invertebrate	None	84
Leishmania spp.	Western US	Desert night lizards	Intestine	Probably by ingestion of invertebrate	None	110
Monocercomonas spp.	Worldwide	Snakes, lizards	Intestine	Ingestion of organism passed in feces	None	111
Monocercomonoides lacertae	Asia, North America	Snakes, lizards	Intestine	Ingestion of organism passed in feces	None	112
Octomitus spp.	Worldwide	Lizards	Large intestine	Ingestion of organism passed in feces	None	113
Proteromonas lacertaeviridis	Worldwide	Lizards, snakes	Rectum	Ingestion of organism passed in feces	None	112
Proteromonas regnardi	Europe	European pond terrapins	Rectum	Ingestion of organism passed in feces	None	114
Retortamonas saurarum	Europe, North America	Snakes, lizards	Intestine	Ingestion of organism passed in feces	None	112
Retortamonas spp.	South America	Tortoises	Intestine	Ingestion of organism passed in feces	None	112
Tritrichomonas nonconforma	North America, West Indies	Green anoles	Intestine	Ingestion of organism passed in feces	None	86
Amoebae						
Endolimax clevelandi	North America	Turtles	Intestine	Ingestion of organism passed in feces	None	116
Entamoeba barreti	North America	Snapping turtles	Intestine	Ingestion of organism passed in feces	Unknown	9

Organism	Distribution	Host	Location	Transmission	Pathology	Reference
Entamoeba invadens	Worldwide	Snakes, lizards, turtles	Intestine, stomach, liver	Igestion of organism passed in feces	Gastrointestinal ulceration, hepatitis	87
Entamoeba terrapinae	North America	Red-eared turtles	Intestine	Ingestion of organism passed in feces	None	9
Entamoeba testudinis	Europe, North America	Turtles	Intestine	Ingestion of organism passed in feces	None	9
Entamoeba spp.	Great Britain, North America	Garter snakes	Intestine	Ingestion of organism passed in feces	None	1
Vahlkampfia dobelli	Europe	Lizards	Intestine	Ingestion of organism passed in feces	None	71
Vahlkampfia reynoldsi	North America	Eastern fence lizards	Intestine	Ingestion of organism passed in feces	None	116
Coccidia						
Caryospora spp.	Americas	Snakes	Intestine	Ingestion of oocyst passed in feces or tissue forms in mice	None	117
Caryospora simplex	Europe	Snakes	Intestine	Ingestion of oocyst passed in feces or tissue forms in mice	None	118
Cryptosporidium saurophilum	Worldwide	Lizards	Intestine	Ingestion of sporulated oocyst	Enteritis	88
Cryptosporidium serpentis	Worldwide	Snakes	Stomach	Ingestion of sporulated oocyst	Gastritis	88
Eimeria crocodyli	Central America	American crocodiles	Intestine	Ingestion of sporulated oocyst	None	91
Eimeria spp.	Worldwide	Lizards	Intestine	Ingestion of sporulated oocyst	None	89
Eimeria spp.	Worldwide	Snakes	Gallbladder, bile duct, intestine	Ingestion of sporulated oocyst	None	90
Eimeria spp.	Europe	Tortoises	Intestine	Ingestion of sporulated oocyst	None	95
Eimeria spp.	Worldwide	Turtles	Intestine	Ingestion of sporulated oocyst	None	92, 93, 94
Isospora spp.	Worldwide	Snakes	Intestine	Ingestion of sporulated oocyst	None	96
Sarcocystis lacertae	Europe	Snakes	Intestine	Ingestion of intermediate host (lizard)	None	149
Myxozoa						
Myxidium chelonarum	North America	Turtles	Bile duct, gallbladder	Probably by ingestion of organism passed in feces	None	97

(Continued)

TABLE 9.2 *(Continued)*

Parasite	Geographic distribution	Hosts	Location in host	Method of infection	Pathologic effects	Reference
Ciliates						
Balantidium spp.	Worldwide	Tortoises, turtles, lizards	Intestine	Ingestion of organism passed in feces	None	119
Nyctotheroides spp.	Worldwide	Tortoises, turtles, lizards	Intestine	Ingestion of organism passed in feces	None	119
Trematodes						
Monogenetic and Aspidobothretic						
Aspidogaster conchicola	Worldwide	Turtles	Stomach, intestine	Ingestion of infected clam	None	120
Cotylaspis cokeri	North America	Turtles	Stomach, intestine	Ingestion of infected clam	None	71
Cotylaspis spp.	Asia	Turtles	Stomach, intestine	Ingestion of infected clam	None	121
Cotylaspis stunkardi	North America	Snapping turtles	Stomach, intestine	Ingestion of infected clam	None	71
Gyrodactylus spp.	Worldwide	Turtles	Oral cavity (also skin, urinary bladder)	Direct contact	Enteritis	32
Polystomoides spp.	Asia, North America	Turtles	Mouth	Direct contact	None	122
Adult Digenetic						
Allassostoma magnum	North America	Turtles	Large intestine	Ingestion of metacercaria	None	123
Allassostomoides spp.	North America	Turtles, frogs	Colon (also found in urinary bladder, cloaca)	Ingestion of metacercaria	None	124
Encyclometra colubrimurorum	Asia, Europe	Snakes	Intestine	Ingestion of frog tadpole	None	125
Leptophallus nigrovenosus	Africa, Europe	Snakes, lizards	Esophagus, intestine	Ingestion of second intermediate host (arthropod)	Esophagitis, enteritis	126
Microphallus spp.	North America	Turtles	Intestine	Ingestion of second intermediate host (crustacean)	None	49
Paradistomum mutabile	Asia, Europe	Lizards	Gallbladder	Ingestion of second intermediate host (arthropod)	Cholecystitis	127
Protenes chapmani	North America	Red-eared turtles	Intestine	Ingestion of second intermediate host (arthropod)	None	128
Telorchis spp.	North America	Turtles, snakes	Intestine	Ingestion of second intermediate host (arthropod)	None	129
Larval digenetic						

	Americas	Anoles, cats	Bile duct	Ingestion of isopod	None	130
Platynosomum fastosum	Americas	Anoles, cats	Bile duct	Ingestion of isopod	None	130
Cestodes						
Acanthotaenia spp.	Africa	Reptiles	Small intestine	Ingestion of intermediate host	Inflammation at site of attachment	149
Baerietta spp.	Australia	Lizards	Small intestine	Ingestion of intermediate host	None	154
Crepidobothrium spp.	South America	Snakes	Small intestine	Ingestion of intermediate host	Inflammation at site of attachment	150
Ophiotaenia spp.	Africa, North America	Snakes, turtles	Small intestine	Ingestion of intermediate host	Inflammation at site of attachment	151, 152
Oochoristica spp.	North America	Anoles, snakes, lizards, turtles	Intestine	Ingestion of intermediate host	None	131, 132
Proteocephalus testudo	North America	Turtles	Intestine	Ingestion of intermediate host	Inflammation at site of attachment	133
Proteocephalus spp.	South America	Lizards, snakes	Intestine	Ingestion of intermediate host	Inflammation at site of attachment	153
Nematodes						
Rhabditoidea						
Strongyloides spp.	Worldwide	Snakes	Esophagus, Intestine	Ingestion of infective larva or penetration of skin by larva	Enteritis	136
Ascaridoidea						
Ophidascaris labiatopapillosa	North America	Snakes	Stomach	Ingestion of intermediate host (amphibian)	Gastritis	138
Strongyloidea						
Atractis carolinea	North America, Carribean	Box turtles, anoles	Intestine	Ingestion of infective larva	None	137
Atractis dactyluris	Europe, northern Africa	Tortoises	Large intestine	Ingestion of infective larva	None	137
Diaphanocephalus spp.	South America	Snakes	Stomach, intestine	Probably by ingestion of arthropod	Gastroenteritis, anemia	137
Kalicephalus spp.	North America	Snakes	Stomach, intestine	Probably by ingestion of arthropod	Gastroenteritis, anemia	137
Oxyuroidea						
Alaeuris spp.	Worldwide	Lizards, tortoises, turtles	Large intestine	Ingestion of embryonated egg	Potential intussusception	141
Falcaustra spp.	Americas	Turtles	Large intestine	Ingestion of embryonated egg	None	44, 137
Ozolaimus spp.	Worldwide	Lizards, tortoises, turtles	Large intestine	Ingestion of embryonated egg	Potential intussusception	141
Tachygonetria spp.	Worldwide	Tortoises	Large intestine	Ingestion of embryonated egg	Intestinal obstruction	139

(Continued)

TABLE 9.2 (continued)

Parasite	Geographic distribution	Hosts	Location in host	Method of infection	Pathologic effects	Reference
Trichostrongyloidea						
Oswaldocruzia spp.	Worldwide	Reptiles	Intestine	Ingestion of infective larvae	None	141
Spiruroidea						
Camallanus microcephalus, *C. trispinosus*	North America	Turtles, frogs	Stomach, duodenum	Ingestion of copepod	Gastritis, enteritis	49, 50
Spiroxys contortus	Africa, Europe, North America	Turtles	Stomach, duodenum	Ingestion of copepod	Gastritis, enteritis	35
Trichuroidea						
Capillaria serpentina	North America	Turtles	Intestine	Ingestion of embryonated egg or earthworm	None	142
Capillaria spp.	Worldwide	Snakes	Intestine	Ingestion of embryonated egg or earthworm	None	143
Acanthocephalans						
Neoechinorhynchus spp.	Europe, North America	Turtles	Intestine	Ingestion of first intermediate host (ostracod) or second intermediate host (snail)	Intestinal obstruction	144
Arachnida						
Mites						
Prostigmates						
Caminacarus spp.	Israel, North America	Pond turtles	Rectum	Direct contact	None	145
Chelonacarus spp.	Asia, North America	Turtles	Rectum	Direct contact	None	146
Theodoracarus testudinis	Israel	Tortoises	Rectum (also found in muscle)	Direct contact	None	147
Pentastomids						
Subtriquetra shipleyi	Asia	Crocodilians	Pharynx	Ingestion of intermediate host (fish)	None	148
Subtriquetra subtriquetra	Africa, South America	Crocodilians	Mouth, pharynx	Ingestion of intermediate host (fish)	None	148

TABLE 9.3 Parasites of reptiles—skin and connective tissue and musculoskeletal system.

Parasite	Geographic distribution	Hosts	Location in host	Method of infection	Pathologic effects	Reference
Coccidia						
Sarcocystis lacertae	Europe	Lizards	Muscle	Ingestion of sporocysts from definitive host (snake)	None	149
Nematodes						
Dracunculoidea						
Chelonidracunculus globocephalus	North America	Snapping turtles	Body cavity	Ingestion of intermediate host (copepod)	None	137
Ophiodracunculus ophidensis	North America	Garter snakes	Subcutis or body cavity	Ingestion of intermediate host (copepod)	None	137
Filaroidea						
Foleyella spp.	Worldwide	Lizards	Subcutaneous tissue, abdominal cavity	Mosquito transmission	Debilitation	150
Cestodes						
Larval						
Diphyllobothrium erinacei	Asia, Australia, South America	Snakes, turtles	Subcutaneous tissues	Ingestion of first intermediate host (amphibians)	None	38
Spirometra mansonoides	North America	Snakes, turtles	Subcutaneous tissues	Ingestion of first intermediate host (amphibians)	None	39
Leeches						
Actinobdella annectens	North America	Snapping turtles	Skin	Direct contact	None	71
Ozobranchus branchiatus	North America	Green turtles	Skin of neck, eyelids	Direct contact	Associated with skin tumors	151
Diptera (flies)						
Anolisimyia blakeae (Sarcophagidae)	North America	Green anoles	Skin	Eggs deposited by female fly	Myiasis	152
Calliphoridae	Europe	Tortoises, turtles	Skin wounds	Eggs deposited by female fly	Myiasis	71
Cistudinomyia cistudinis (Sarcophagidae)	North America	Turtles, gopher tortoises (*Gopherus polyphemus*)	Skin wounds	Eggs deposited by female fly	Myiasis	63
Ceratopogonidae (midges)	Worldwide	Reptiles	Skin	Direct contact	Irritation, pathogen transmission	153

(Continued)

207

TABLE 9.3 *(Continued)*

Parasite	Geographic distribution	Hosts	Location in host	Method of infection	Pathologic effects	Reference
Culicidae (mosquitoes)	Worldwide	Reptiles	Skin	Direct contact	Irritation, pathogen transmission	154
Psychodidae (sand flies)	Worldwide	Reptiles	Skin	Direct contact	Pathogen transmission	155
Arachnida						
Ticks (Hard)						
Amblyomma testudinis	South America	Reptiles	Skin	Direct contact	Probably causes irritation	164
Amblyomma tuberculatum	North America	Gopher tortoises (*Gopherus polyphemus*), box turtles, Eastern fence lizards	Skin	Direct contact	Irritation, pathogen transmission	165
Amblyomma spp.	Africa, Americas	Reptiles	Skin	Direct contact	Irritation, pathogen transmission	166
Aponomma elaphense	North America	Rat snakes	Skin	Direct contact	Irritation, pathogen transmission	167
Aponomma spp.	Africa	Reptiles	Skin	Direct contact	Irritation, pathogen transmission	166
Haemaphysalis concinna	Asia, Europe	Reptiles	Skin	Direct contact	Irritation, pathogen transmission	168
Haemaphysalis punctata	Africa, Asia, Europe	Lizards, snakes, mammals	Skin	Direct contact	Irritation, pathogen transmission	169
Hyalomma aegyptium	Asia, Europe	Tortoises, turtles, lizards	Skin	Direct contact	Irritation, pathogen transmission	170
Ixodes pacificus	North America	Garter snakes, lizards	Skin	Direct contact	Irritation, pathogen transmission	171
Ixodes ricinus	Europe	Lizards	Skin	Direct contact	Irritation, pathogen transmission	172
Ticks (Soft)						
Ornithodoros moubata complex	Southern Africa	Tortoises	Skin	Direct contact	Irritation, pathogen transmission	69
Ornithodoros turicata	North America	Box turtles, gopher tortoises (*Gopherus polyphemus*), rattlesnakes (*Crotalus*)	Skin	Direct contact	Irritation, pathogen transmission	65
Mites						
Mesostigmata						
Asiatolaelaps spp.	Asia	Snakes	Skin	Direct contact	None	157
Haemilaelaps spp.	Worldwide	Snakes	Skin	Direct contact	None	157

Ixobiodes butantanensis	South America	Colubrid snakes	Skin	Direct contact	None	157
Ixodorhynchus spp.	Asia, North America	Snakes	Skin	Direct contact	None	157, 158
Neoliponyssus spp.	Asia, Europe	Lizards	Skin	Direct contact	None	156
Ophionyssus natricis	Worldwide	Snakes, lizards	Skin	Direct contact	Irritation, anemia, mechanical vector of *Aeromonas hydrophila*	74
Strandtibbettsia gordoni	Asia	Water snakes	Skin	Direct contact	None	157
Prostigmata						
Eutrombicula hirsti	Asia	Snakes	Skin	Direct contact	None	71, 78
Eutrombicula insularis	West Indies	Anoles	Skin	Direct contact	None	71
Geckobiella texana	North America	Lizards	Skin	Direct contact	None	159
Hirstiella spp.	North America	Lizards	Skin	Direct contact	None	160
Neotrombicula spp.	Worldwide	Lizards	Skin	Direct contact	None	78, 161
Ophioptes spp.	Americas	Snakes	Skin	Direct contact	None	162
Trombicula hasei	Europe	Lizards	Skin	Direct contact	None	163
Trombicula agamae	Asia	Starred lizards (*Agamo stellio*)	Skin	Direct contact	None	71

209

TABLE 9.4 Parasites of reptiles—respiratory, nervous, and urogenital systems.

Parasite	Geographic distribution	Hosts	Location in host	Method of infection	Pathologic effects	Reference
Myxozoa						
Myxidium americanum	North America	Softshell turtles	Kidneys	Ingestion of organism passed in urine	None	97
Trematodes						
Monogenetic and Aspidobothretic						
Polystomoides spp.	Asia, Europe, North America	Turtles	Urinary bladder	Direct contact	None	174
Adult digenetic						
Dasymetra conferta	North America	Water snakes	Lungs (also found in mouth, esophagus, intestine)	Ingestion of second intermediate host (frog tadpole)	Pneumonitis	175
Heronimus chelydrae	North America	Turtles	Lungs	Ingestion of intermediate host (snail)	None	176
Lechriorchis spp.	North America	Garter snakes	Lungs (also found in mouth, esophagus, intestine)	Ingestion of second intermediate host (frog tadpole)	Pneumonitis	177
Ochetosoma spp.	North America	Snakes	Lungs (also found in mouth, esophagus, intestine)	Ingestion of second intermediate host (frog tadpole)	Pneumonitis	178
Zeugorchis spp.	North America	Garter snakes	Lungs (also found in mouth, esophagus, intestine)	Ingestion of second intermediate host (frog tadpole)	Pneumonitis	175
Larval digenetic						
Alaria marcianae	North America	Snakes, frogs, birds (Paratenic hosts)	Subcutaneous tissues	Ingestion of intermediate host (frog tadpole)	None	85, 113
Nematodes						
Rhabditoidea						
Entomelas spp.	Europe	Lizards	Lungs	Ingestion of infective larva or penetration of skin by larva	Pneumonitis	134
Rhabdias spp.	Worldwide	Snakes, anoles, chameleons	Lungs	Ingestion of infective larva or penetration of skin by larva	Pneumonitis	135

210

Arachnida

Mites

Mesostigmata

	Geographic distribution	Host	Location	Transmission	Pathology	Reference
Entonyssus spp.	Asia, North America	Snakes	Trachea, lungs	Direct contact	None	70
Viperacarus europaeus	Europe	European vipers	Trachea, lungs	Direct contact	None	70

Pentastomids

	Geographic distribution	Host	Location	Transmission	Pathology	Reference
Alofia spp.	Africa, Asia, South America	Crocodilians	Lungs, trachea	Ingestion of intermediate or paratenic host	None	80, 179
Armillifer armillatus	Africa	Snakes	Lungs, trachea	Ingestion of intermediate host (primates, rodents, others)	Usually none	173
Armillifer moniliformis	Africa, Asia, Australia	Snakes	Lungs, trachea	Ingestion of intermediate host (rodents)	Usually none	81
Kiricephalus spp.	Worldwide	Snakes	Lungs, subcutaneous tissues, stomach wall	Ingestion of intermediate or paratenic host	Usually none	180
Leiperia cincinnalis	Africa	Nile crocodiles	Lungs (also found in heart, aorta)	Ingestion of intermediate or paratenic host	Usually none	181
Leiperia gracilis	South America	Crocodilians	Lungs	Ingestion of intermediate or paratenic host	Usually none	106
Porocephalus spp.	Africa, Americas	Snakes	Lungs, subcutaneous tissues	Ingestion of intermediate or paratenic host	None	81
Raillietiella spp.	Worldwide	Snakes	Lungs	Ingestion of intermediate or paratenic host	None	81, 83
Sebekia spp.	Americas, Asia, South America	Crocodilians	Lungs	Ingestion of intermediate or paratenic host	None	80
Subtriquetra megacephala	Africa	Crocodiles	Cephalic tissues	Ingestion of intermediate or paratenic host	None	80
Waddycephalus teretiusculus	Asia, Australia	Snakes	Lungs	Ingestion of intermediate or paratenic host	None	81

REFERENCES

1. Fantham, H.B. and Porter, A. (1953–1954) The endoparasites of some North American snakes and their effects on the Ophidia. *Proc. Zool. Soc. London* **123**, 867–898.

2. Geiman, Q.M. and Ratcliffe, H.L. (1936) Morphology and the life-cycle of an amoeba producing amoebiasis in reptiles. *Parasitology* **28**, 208–228.

3. Donaldson, M., Heyneman, D., Dempster, R., and Garcia, L. (1975) Epizootic of fatal amebiasis among exhibited snakes: epidemiologic, pathologic, and chemotherapeutic considerations. *Am. J. Vet. Res.* **36**, 807–817.

4. Zwart, P. (1964) Studies on renal pathology in reptiles. *Pathol. Vet.* **1**, 542–556.

5. Jacobson, E.R. (1983) Parasitic diseases of reptiles. In: Kirk, R.W. (ed.) *Current Veterinary Therapy 8: Small Animal Practice,* W.B. Saunders, Philadelphia, p. 601.

6. Gillin, F.D. and Diamond, L.S. (1980) *Entamoeba histolytica* and *Entamoeba invadens:* effects of temperature and oxygen tension on growth and survival. *Exp. Parasitol.* **49**, 328–338.

7. Xiao, L., Fayer, R., Ryan, U., and Upton, S.J. (2004) *Cryptosporidium* taxonomy: recent advances and implications for public health. *Clin. Microbiol. Rev.* **17**, 72–97.

8. Graczyk, T.K. and Cranfield, M.R. (2000) *Cryptosporidium serpentis* oocysts and microsporidian spores in feces of captive snakes. *J. Parasitol.* **86**, 413–414.

9. Kudo, R.R. (1966) *Protozoology.* 5th ed. Charles C. Thomas, Springfield, Illinois. 1174 pp.

10. Sampson, J.R. and Ernst, J.V. (1969) *Eimeria scriptae* n. sp. (Sporozoa: Eimeriidae) from the red-eared turtle *Pseudemys scripta elegans. J. Protozool.* **16**, 444–445.

11. Saxe, L.H. (1955) Observations on *Eimeria* from *Ambystoma tigrinum,* with descriptions of four new species. *Proc. Iowa Acad. Sci.* **62**, 663–673.

12. Wallach, J.D. (1969) Medical care of reptiles. *J. Am. Vet. Med. Assoc.* **155**, 1017–1034.

13. Lane, T.J. and Mader, D.R. (1996) Parasitology. In: Mader, D.R. (ed.) *Reptile Medicine and Surgery,* Saunders, Philadelphia, pages 185–203.

14. Wenyon, C.M. (1926) *Protozoology.* Vol. 2. Hafner, New York.

15. Hull, R.W. and Camin, J.H. (1960) Haemogregarines in snakes: The incidence and identity of the erythrocytic stages. *J. Parasitol.* **46**, 515–523.

16. Acholonu, A.D. (1966) Occurrences of *Haemogregarina* (protozoa) in Louisiana turtles. *J. Protozool.* **13**, 20.

17. Marquardt, W.C. (1966) Haemogregarines and Haemoproteus in some reptiles in southern Illinois. *J. Parasitol.* **52**, 823–824.

18. Roudabush, R.L. and Coatney, G.R. (1937) On some blood protozoa of reptiles and amphibians. *Trans. Am. Micro. Soc.* **56**, 291–297.

19. Wang, C.C. and Hopkins, S.H. (1965) Haemogregarina and Haemoproteus (Protozoa, Sporozoa) in blood of Texas freshwater turtle. *J. Parasitol.* **51**, 682–683.

20. Herban, N.L. and Yaeger, R.G. (1969) Blood parasites of certain Louisiana reptiles and amphibians. *Am. Midland Naturalist* **82**, 600–601.

21. Koudela, B., Didier, E.S., Rogers, L.B., Modry, D., and Kucerova, S. (1998) Intestinal microsporidiosis in African skink *Mabuya perrotetii. Folia Parasitol.* 45, 149–155.

22. Jacobson, E.R., Green, D.E., Undeen, A.H., Cranfield, M., and Vaughn, K.L. (1998) Systemic microsporidiosis in inland bearded dragons (*Pogona vitticeps*). *J. Zoo Wild. Med.* **29**, 315–323.

23. Graczyk, T.K., Owens, R., and Cranfield, M.R. (1996) Diagnosis of subclinical cryptosporidiosis in captive snakes based on stomach lavage and cloacal sampling. *Vet. Parasitol.* **67**, 143–151.

24. Skrjabin, K.I. (1964) *Keys to the Trematodes of Animals and Man* (English translation). Arai, H.P. (ed.) University of Illinois Press, Urbana. 351 pages.

25. Talbot, S.B. (1933) Life history studies on trematodes of the subfamily Reniferinae. *Parasitology* **25**, 518–545.

26. Harwood, P.D. (1932) The helminthes parasitic in the amphibia and reptilia of Houston, Texas, and vicinity. *Proc. U.S. Natl. Museum* **81**, 1–71.

27. Yamaguti, S. (1958) The digenetic trematodes of vertebrates. Vol. I., 2 Parts. In: Yamaguti, S. (ed.). *Systema helminthum.* Interscience, New York.

28. Stewart, P.L. (1960). Lung-flukes of snakes, genera *Thamnophis* and *Coluber,* in Kansas. *Univ. Kansas Sci. Bull.* **41**, 877–890.

29. Nelson, D.J. (1950) A treatment for helminthiasis in Ophidia. *Herpetologica* **6**, 57–59.

30. Goodman, J.D. (1951) Some aspects of the role of parasitology in herpetology. *Herpetologica* **7**, 65–67.

31. Carpenter, J.W., Mashima, T.Y., and Rupiper, D.J., In: *Exotic Animal Formulary,* 2nd edition, Saunders, Philadelphia, p. 55.

32. Harris, P.D., Shinn, A.P., Cable, J., and Bakke, T.A. (2004) Nominal species of the genus *Gyrodactylus* von Nordmann 1832 (Monogenea: Gyrodactylidae), with a list of principal host species. *Syst. Parasitol.* **59**, 1–27.

33. Wall, L.D. (1941) *Spirorchis parvus* (Stunkard) its life history and the development of its excretory system (Trematoda: Spirorchiidae). *Trans. Am. Microscop. Soc.* **60**, 221–260.

34. Thatcher, V.E. (1954) Some helminthes parasitic in *Clemmys marmorata. J. Parasitol.* **40**, 481–482.

35. Williams, R.W. (1953) Helminths of the snapping turtle, *Chelydra serpentina,* from Oklahoma, including the first report and description of the male of *Capillaria serpentina* Harwood, 1932. *Trans. Am. Microscop. Soc.* **72**, 175–178.

36. Adnyanna, W., Ladds, P.W., and Blair, D. (1997) Efficacy of Praziquantel in the treatment of green sea turtles with spontaneous infections of cardiovascular flukes. *Aust. Vet. J.* **76**, 405–407.

37. Jacobson, E.R., Harman, G.R., Maxwell, L.K., and Laille, E.J. (2003) Plasma concentrations of praziquantel after oral administration of single and multiple doses in loggerhead sea turtles (*Caretta caretta*). *Am. J. Vet. Res.* **64**, 304–309.

38. Galliard, H. and Ngu, D.V. (1946) Particularites du cycle evolutif de *Diphyllobothrium mansoni* au Tonkin. *Ann. Parasitol. Humaine Comparee* **21**, 246–253.

39. Corkum, K.C. (1966) Sparganosis in some vertebrates of Louisiana and observations on a human infection. *J. Parasitol.* **52**, 444–448.

40. Moravec, F., Salgado-Maldonado, G., and Mayen-Pena, E. (1996) Two pharyngodonid nematodes, *Alaeuris mexicana* n. sp. and *Ozolaimus ctenosauri,* from the iguanid lizard *Ctenosaura pectinata* from Nayarit, Mexico. *J. Parasitol.* **82**, 1011–1016.

41. Telford, S.R. and Campbell, H.W. (1981) Parasites of the American alligator, their importance to husbandry and suggestions towards their prevention and control. In: Cardeilac, P., Lane, T., and Larsen, R.(eds) *Proceedings of the First Annual Alligator Production Conference.* University of Florida, Gainesville.

42. McGuire, N., Mitchell, M.A., Tully, T.N., Mark, S.L., Pechman, R., Kim, D.Y., et al. What's Your Diagnosis? (1999) *Bull. Reptile Amphib. Vet.* **9**, 47–49.

43. Yorke, W. and Maplestone, P.A. (1926) The nematode parasites of vertebrates. Blakeston, Philadelphia. 536 pages.

44. Hidalgo-Vila, J., Ribas, A., Florencio, M., Perez-Santigosa, N., and Casanova, J.C. (2006) *Falcaustra donanaensis* sp. nov. (Nematoda: Kathlaniidae) a parasite of *Mauremys leprosa* (Testudines, Bataguridae) in Spain. *Parasitol Res.* (E-pub ahead of printing).

45. Forstner, M.J. (1960) Ein Beitrag zur Kenntnis parasitischer Nematoden aus griechischen Landschildkröten. *Z. Parasitenk.* **20**, 1–22.

46. Traversa, D., Capelli, G., Iorio, R., Bouamer, S., Cameli, A., and Giangaspero, A. (2005) Epidemiology and biology of nematode fauna affecting *Testudo hermanni*, *Testudo graeca* and *Testudo marginata* in Italy. *Parasitol. Res.* **98**, 14–20.

47. Graham-Jones, O. (1961) Some clinical conditions affecting the North African tortoise ("Greek" tortoise), *Testudo graeca*. *Vet. Record* **73**, 317–321.

48. Rankin, Jr., J.S. (1945) An ecological study of the helminth parasites of amphibians and reptiles of western Massachusetts and vicinity. *J. Parasitol.* **31**, 142–150.

49. Rausch, R. (1947) Observations on some helminths parasitic in Ohio turtles. *Am. Midland Naturalist* **38**, 434–442.

50. Wieczorowski, E. (1939) Parasitic lesions in turtles. *J. Parasitol.* **25**, 395–399.

51. Hoffman, G.L. (1967) *Parasites of North American Fishes*. University of California Press, Berkeley. 486 pages.

52. Mishra, G.S. and Gonzalez, J.P. (1978) Parasites of fresh water turtles in Tunisia. *Arch. Inst. Pasteur Tunis.* **55**, 303–326.

53. Brygoo, E.R. (1963) Contribution a la connaissance de la parasitologie des cameleons malgaches. *Ann. Parasitol. Hum. Comp.* **38**, 149–334, 525–739.

54. Irizarry-Rovira, A., Wolf, A., Bolek, M., Christian, J.A., and DeNicola, D.B. (2002) Blood smear from a wild-caught panther chameleon (*Furcifer pardalis*) *Vet. Clin. Path.* **31**, 129–132.

55. Borradaile, L.A. and Potts, F.A. (1958) The invertebrate: A manual for the use of students. 3rd ed. Cambridge University Press, Cambridge, England. 739 pages.

56. Cable, R.M. and Fisher, Jr., F.M. (1961) A fifth species of *Neoechinorhynchus* (Acanthocephala) in turtles. *J. Parasitol.* **47**, 666–667.

57. Cable, R.M. and Hopp, W.B. (1954) Acanthocephalan parasites of the genus Neoechinorhynchus in North American turtles with the description of two new species. *J. Parasitol.* **40**, 674–680.

58. Acholonu, A.D. (1967) Studies on the acanthocephalan parasites of Louisiana turtles. *Bull. Wildlife Dis. Assoc.* **3**, 40.

59. Lincicome, D.R. (1948) Observations on *Neoechinorhynchus emydis* (Leidy), an acanthocephalan parasite of turtles. *J. Parasitol.* **34**, 51–54.

60. Van Cleave, H.J. and Bullock, W.L. (1950) Morphology of *Neoechinorhynchus emydis*, a typical representative of the Eoacanthocephala: I. The praesoma. *Trans. Am. Microscop. Soc.* **69**, 288–308.

61. Bullock, W.L. (1961) A preliminary study of the histopathology of Acanthocephala in the vertebrate intestine. *J. Parasitol.* **47** (Suppl.), 31.

62. Knipling, E.F. (1937) The biology of *Sarcophaga cistudinis* Aldrich (Diptera), a species of Sarcophagidae parasitic on turtles and tortoises. *Proc. Entomol. Soc. Wash. D.C.* **39**, 91–101.

63. Jackson, Jr., G.G., Jackson, M.M., and Davis, J.D. (1969) Cutaneous myiasis in the three-toed box turtle, *Terrapene carolina triunguis*. *Bull. Wildlife Dis. Assoc.* **5**, 114.

64. King, W. and Griffo, Jr., J.V. (1958) A box turtle fatality apparently caused by *Sarcophaga cistudinis* larvae. *Florida Entomologist* **41**, 44.

65. Cooley, R.A. and Kohls, G.M. (1944) The Argasidae of North America, Central America, and Cuba. *Am. Midland Naturalist Monograph 1.* 152 pp.

66. Cooley, R.A. and Kohls, G.M. (1944) The genus *Amblyomma* (Ixodidae) in the United States. *J. Parasitol.* **30**, 77–111.

67. Bishopp, F.C. and Trembley, H.L. (1945) Distribution and hosts of certain North American ticks. *J. Parasitol.* **31**, 1–54.

68. Worms, M.J. (1967) Parasites in newly imported animals. *J. Inst. Animal Tech.* **18**, 39–47.

69. Hoogstraal, H. (1956) African Ixodoidea: I. Ticks of the Sudan (with special reference to Equatoria Province and with preliminary review of the genera *Boophilus*, *Margaropus*, and *Hyalomma*). U.S. Navy Dept. Washington, D.C. Res. Rept. N.M 005 050.29.07. 1101 pages.

70. Fain, A. (1961) Les acariens parasites endopulmonaires des serpents (Entonyssidae: Mesostigmata). *Inst. Roy. Sci. Nat. Belg. Bull.* **37**, 1–135.

71. Reichenbach-Klinke, H. and Elkan, E. (1965) *The Principal Diseases of Lower Vertebrates*. Academic Press, New York. 600 pages.

72. Camin, J.H. (1953) Observations on the life-history and sensory behavior of the snake mite, *Ophionyssus natricis* (Gervais). *Chicago Acad. Sci. Spec. Publ. 10.* 75 pp.

73. Page, L.A. (1966) Diseases and infections of snakes: A review. *Bull. Wildlife Dis. Assoc.* **2**, 111–126.

74. Yunker, C.E. (1956) Studies on the snake mite, *Ophionyssus natricis*, in nature. *Science* **124**, 979–980.

75. Heywood, R. (1968) *Aeromonas* infection in snakes. *Cornell Vet.* **58**, 236–241.

76. Ewing, H.E. (1929) *A Manual of External Parasites*. Charles C. Thomas, Springfield, Ill. 225 pages.

77. Ewing, H.E. (1926) The common box-turtle, a natural host for chiggers. *Proc. Biol. Soc. Wash. D.C.* **39**, 19–20.

78. Sambon, L.W. (1928) The parasitic acarians of animals and the part they play in the causation of the eruptive fevers and other diseases of man: Preliminary considerations based upon an ecological study of typhus fever. *Ann. Trop. Med.* **22**, 67–132.

79. Self, J.T. and Cosgrove, G.E. (1968) Pentastome larvae in laboratory primates. *J. Parasitol.* **54**, 969.

80. Fain, A. (1961) Les pentastomidés de l'Afrique Centrale. *Ann. Musee Roy. Afrique Centrale, Ser. 8, Sci. Zool.* **92**, 1–115.

81. Fain, A. (1966) Pentastomida of snakes—their parasitological role in man and animals. *Mem. Inst. Butantan (São Paulo)* **33**, 167–174.

82. Self, J.T. and McCurry, F.B. (1948) *Porocephalus crotali* Humboldt (Pentastomida) in Oklahoma. *J. Parasitol.* **34**, 21–23.

83. Fain, A. (1964) Observations sur le cycle évolutif du genre *Raillietiella* (Pentastomida). *Bull. Acad. Roy. Belg.* **50**, 1036–1060.

84. Honigberg, B.M. (1950) Intestinal flagellates of amphibians and reptiles. I. Survey of intestinal flagellates of reptiles. II. Structure and morphogenesis of the members of the genus *Trichomonas* Donné, 1836 from amphibian and reptiles. Doctoral dissertation, University of California, Berkeley. 260 pages.

85. Walton, A.C. (1964) *The Parasites of Amphibia. Wildlife Diseases 40.* Wildlife Disease Association.

86. Honigberg, B.M. (1963) Evolutionary and systematic relationships in the flagellate order Trichomonadida Kirb. *J. Protozool.* **10**, 20–63.

87. Donaldson, M., Heyneman, D., Dempster, R., and Garcia, L. (1975) Epizootic of fatal amebiasis among exhibited snakes: epidemiologic, pathologic, and chemotherapeutic considerations. *Am. J. Vet. Res.* **36**, 807–817.

88. Xiao, L., Ryan, U.M., Graczyk, T.K., Limor, J., Li, L., Kombert, M., et al. (2004) Genetic diversity of *Cryptosporidium* spp. in captive reptiles. *Appl. Environ. Microbiol.* **70**, 891–899.

89. Duszynski, D.W. 1969. Two new coccidian (Protozoa: Eimeriidae) from Costa Rican lizards with a review of the *Eimeria* from lizards. *J. Protozool.* **16**, 581–585.

90. Vetterling, J.M. and Widmer, E.A. (1968) *Eimeria cascabeli* sp. n. (Eimeriidae: Sporozoa) from rattlesnakes, with a review of the species of *Eimeria* from snakes. *J. Parasitol.* **54**, 569–576.

91. Lainson, R. (1968) Parasitologic studies in British Honduras: IV. Some coccidial parasites of reptiles. *Ann. Trop. Med. Parasitol.* **62**, 260–266.

92. Segade, P., Crespo, C., Ayres, C., Cordero, A., Arias, M.C., Garcia-Estevez J.M., et al. (2006) *Eimeria* species from the European pond turtle, *Emys orbicularis* (Reptilia: Testudines), in Galicia (NW Spain), with description of two new species. *J. Parasitol.* **92**, 69–72.

93. Bone, L.W. (1975) *Eimeria pseudemdis* Lainson, 1968, from the redeared turtle, *Pseudemys scripta elegans,* in Arkansas. *J. Wildl. Dis.* **11**, 290–291.

94. Sampson, J.R. and Ernst, J.V. (1969) *Eimeria scriptae* n. sp. (Sporozoa: Eimeriidae) from the red-eared turtle *Pseudemys scripta elegans. J. Protozool.* **16**, 444–445.

95. Hurkova, L., Modry, D., Koudela, B., and Slapeta, J. (2000) Description of *Eimeria motelo* sp. n. (Apicomplexa: Eimeriidae) from the yellow footed tortoise, *Geochelone denticulata* (Chelonia: Testudinidae), and replacement of *Eimeria carinii* Lainson, Costa and Shaw, 1990 by *Eimeria lainsoni* nom. nov. *Mem. Inst. Oswaldo Cruz.* **95**, 829–832.

96. Asmundsson, I.M., Upton, S.J., and Freed, P.S. (2001) Five new species of Coccidia (Apicomplexa: Eimeriidae) from colubrid snakes of Ecuador. *J. Parasitol.* **87**, 1077–1081.

97. Eiras, J.C. (2005) An overview on the myxosporean parasites in amphibians and reptiles. *Acta Parasitologica* **50**, 267–275.

98. Davies, A.J. and Johnston, M.R. (2000) The biology of some intraerythrocytic parasites of fishes, amphibia and reptiles. *Adv. Parasitol.* **45**, 1–107.

99. Michel, J.C. (1973) *Hepatozoon mauritanicum* (Et. and Ed. Sergent, 1904) n. comb., a parasite of *Testude graeca:* a new description of sporogony in *Hyalomma aegyptium* and of tissular schizogony drawn from the material of E. Brumpt *Ann. Parasitol. Hum. Comp.* **48**, 11–21.

100. Woo, P.T.K. (1969) The life cycle of *Trypanosoma chrysemydis. Can. J. Zool.* **47**, 1139–1151.

101. Woo, P.T.K. (1969) Trypanosomes in amphibians and reptiles in southern Ontario. *Can. J. Zool.* **47**, 981–988.

102. Telford, S.R. Jr., Johnson, R.N., and Young, D.G. (1989) Additional *Plasmodium* species from Anolis lizards of Hispaniola and Panama. *Int. J. Parasitol.* **19**, 275–284.

103. Smith, T.G. and Desser, S.S. (1997) Phylogenetic analysis of the genus *Hepatozoon* Miller, 1908 (Apicomplexa: Adeleorina). *Syst. Parasitol.* **36**, 213–221.

104. Schall, J.J. and Smith, T.C. (2006) Detection of a malaria parasite (*Plasmodium mexicanum*) in ectoparasites (mites and ticks), and possible significance for transmission. *J. Parasitol.* **92**, 413–415.

105. Skrjabin, K.I. (1964) Keys to the Trematodes of Animals and Man. Arai, H.P. (ed.) University of Illinois Press, Urbana, 351 pages.

106. Riley, J. and Huchzermeyer, F.W. (1996) A reassessment of the pentastomid genus *Leiperia* Sambon, 1922, with a description of a new species from both the Indopacific crocodile *Crododylus porosus* and Johnston's crocodile *C. johnsoni* in Australia. *Syst. Parasitol.* **34**, 53–66.

107. Moskowitz, N. (1951) Observations on some intestinal flagellates from reptilian host (Squamata). *J. Morphol.* **89**, 257–321.

108. Janakidevi, K. (1961) A new species of *Hexamastix* (protozoa) parasitic in the spiny-tailed lizard, *Uromastix hardwickii. Z. Parasitenkd.* **21**, 151–154.

109. Mattern, C.F., Daniel, W.A., and Honigberg, B.M. (1969) Structure of *Hypotrichomonas acosta* (Moskowitz) (Monocercomonadidae, Trichomonadida) as revealed by electron microscopy. *J. Protozool.* **16**, 668–685.

110. Noyes, H.A., Arana, B.A., Chance, M.L., and Maingon, R. (1997) The *Leishmania hertigi* (Kinetoplastida; Trypanosomatidae) complex and the lizard *Leishmania:* their classification and evidence for a neotropical origin of the *Leishmania-Endotrypanum* clade. *J. Eukaryot. Microbiol.* **44**, 511–517.

111. Krishnamurthy, R. (1967) A new flagellate of the genus *Monocercomonas* Grassi, 1879 from the green snake in India. *Riv. Parassitol.* **28**, 161–164.

112. Moskowitz, N. (1951) Observations on some intestinal flagellates from reptilian host (Squamata). *J. Morphol.* **89**, 257–321.

113. Muzzall, P.M. (2005) Parasites of amphibians and reptiles from Michigan: A review of the literature 1916–2003. Michigan Department of Natural Resources. Fisheries research report #2077. 33 pages.

114. Telford, S.R. and Bursey, C.R. (2003) Comparative parasitology of squamate reptiles endemic to scrub and sandhills communities of north-central Florida, U.S.A. *Comp. Parasitol.* **70**, 172–181.

115. Gutierrez-Ballesteros, E. and Wenrich, D.H. (1950) *Endolimax clevelandi*, n. sp., from turtles. *J. Parasitol.* **36**, 489–493.

116. Ettinger, M.R., Webb, S.R., Harris, S.A., McIninch, S.P.C., Garman, G., and Brown, B.L. (2003) Distribution of free-living amoebae in James River, Virginia, USA. *Parasitol. Res.* **89**, 6–15.

117. Seville, R.S., Asmundsson, I.M., and Campbell, J.A. (2005) Descriptions of six new species of *Caryospora* (Apicomplexa: Eimeriidae) from Guatemalan snakes (Serpentes: Colubridae and Viperidae). *J. Parasitol.* **91**, 1452–1458.

118. Modry, D., Koudela, B., Volf, J., Necas, P., and Hudcovic, T. (1997) *Vipera berus* and *V. ammodytes* (Serpentes: Viperidae) represent new host for *Caryospora simplex* (Apicomplexa: Eimeriidae) in Europe. *Folia Parasitol.* **44**, 99–102.

119. Geiman, Q.M. and Wichterman, R. (1937) Intestinal protozoa from Galapagos tortoises (with description of three new species). *J. Parasitol.* **23**, 331–347.

120. Hendrix, S.S. (1968) New host and locality records for two aspidogastrid trematodes, *Aspidogaster conchicola* and *Cotylaspis insignis. J. Parasitol.* **54**, 179–80.

121. Cho, S.Y. and Seo, B.S. (1977) Studies on the parasitic helminths of Korea: IV. Intestinal trematodes from freshwater mud-turtle (*Amyda sinensis* Wiegmann) with description of new species, *Cotylaspis coreensis. Kisaengchunghak Chapchi.* **15**, 1–10.

122. Euzet, L. and Combes, C. (1965) *Polystomoides chabaudi* n. sp. (Monogenea) in the fresh water turtle *Pelomedusa subrufa* Lacepede 1788. *Ann. Parasitol. Hum. Comp.* **40**, 445–450.

123. Johnson, C.A. III. (1968) New host for *Allassostoma* (Trematoda: Digenea) and *Neoechinorhynchus* (Acanthocephala) from *Pseudemys concinna* (Le Conte) (Chelonia). *Bull. Wildl. Dis.* **4**, 129.

124. Platt, T.R. (2000) Helminth parasites of the western painted turtle, *Chrysemys picta belli* (Gray), including *Neopolystoma elizabethae* n. sp. (Monogenea: Polystomatidae), a parasite of the conjunctival sac. *J. Parasitol.* **86**, 815–818.

125. Liang-Sheng, Y. (1998) A review of the trematode genus *Encyclometra* Baylis and Cannon, 1924. *J. Helminthol.* **32**, 99–114.

126. Biserkov, V.V. and Kostadinova, A. (1998) Intestinal helminth communities in the green lizard, *Lacerta viridis,* from Bulgaria. *J. Helminthol.* **72**, 267–271.

127. Timon-David, J. and Timon-David, P. (1967) Contribution to the knowledge of the biology of the Dicrocoeliidae (Trematoda, Digenea). Experimental studies on the life cycle of *Paradistomum mutabile* (Molin), parasite of the biliary tract of *Lacerta muralis* (Laurenti). *Ann. Parasitol. Hum. Comp.* **42**, 187–206.

128. Mayberry, L.F., Canaris, A.G., Bristol, J.R., and Gardner, S.L. (2000) Bibliography of parasites and vertebrate hosts in Arizona, New Mexico, and Texas (1893–1984). http://hwml.unl.edu/UTEP-UNL/utep.

129. Radtke, A., McLennan, D.A., and Brooks, D.R. (2002) Resource tracking in North American *Telorchis* spp. (Digenea: Plagiorchiformes: Telorchidae). *J. Parasitol.* **88,** 874–879.

130. Goldberg, S.R. and Bursey, C.R. (2000) Transport of helminths to Hawaii via the brown anole, *Anolis sagrei* (Polychrotidae). *J. Parasitol.* **86,** 750–755.

131. Yamaguti, S. (1959) The cestodes of vertebrates. In: Yamaguti, S. (ed.) *Systema Helminthum.* Vol. 2. Interscience, New York.

132. Arizmendi-Espinosa, M.A., Garcia-Prieto, L., and Guillen-Hernandez, S. (2005) A new species of *Oochoristica* (Eucestoda: Cyclophyllidea) parasite of *Ctenosaura pectinata* (Reptilia: Iguanidae) from Oaxaca, Mexico. *J. Parasitol.* **91,** 99–101.

133. Acholonu, A.D. (1970) Studies of the acanthocephalan parasites in Louisiana turtles. *Bull. Wildl. Dis. Assoc.* **3,** 40.

134. Bertman, M. and Okulewicz, A. (1984) *Entomelas dujardini* (Maupas, 1916), (Nematoda) in the lizard *Anguis fragilis* L. *Wiad. Parazytol.* **30,** 341–343.

135. Grego, K.F., Gardiner, C.H., and Catao-Dias, J.L. (2004) Comparative pathology of parasitic infections in free-ranging and captive pit vipers (*Bothrops jararaca*). *Vet. Rec.* **154,** 559–562.

136. Holt, P.E., Cooper, J.E., and Needham, J.R. (1979) *Strongyloides* infection in snakes: three case reports. *Vet. Rec.* **104,** 213–214.

137. Yamaguti, S. (1961) The nematodes of vertebrates. In: Yamaguti, S. (ed.) *Systema Helminthum.* Vol. 3. Interscience, New York.

138. Ash, L.R. and Beaver, P.C. (1963) Redescription of *Ophidascaris labiatopapillosa* Walton, 1927, an ascarid parasite of North American snakes. *J. Parasitol.* **49,** 765–770.

139. Bouamer, S. and Morand, S. (2004) Descriptions of *Tachygonetria africana* n. sp. and *T. pretoriensis* n. sp. and redescriptions of two other species of *Tachygonetria* Wedl, 1862 (Nematoda: Pharyngodonidae), all parasitic in *Geochelone pardalis* (Testudinidae) from South Africa. *Syst. Parasitol.* **58,** 199–208.

140. Moravec, F., Salgado-Maldonado, G., and Mayen-Pena, E. (1996) Two pharyngodonid nematodes, *Alaeuris mexicana* n. sp. and *Ozolaimus ctenosauri,* from the iguanid lizard *Ctenosaura pectinata* from Nayarit, Mexico. *J. Parasitol.* **82,** 1011–1016.

141. Badreddine, B.S. and Durette-Desset, M.C. (1996) Four New Species of *Oswaldocruzia* (Nematoda: Trichostrongylina, Molineoidea) Parasitizing Amphibians and Lizards from Ecuador. *Mem. Inst. Oswaldo Cruz.* **91,** 317–328.

142. Platt, T.R. (1983) Redescription of *Capillaria serpentina* Harwood, 1932, (Nematoda: Trichuroidea) from freshwater turtles in Virginia. *Canadian Journal of Zoology* **61:** 2185–2189.

143. Akinboade, O.A. and Dipeolu, O.O. (1982) Studies on parasites of African snakes. *Int. J. Zoonoses.* **9,** 87–89.

144. Amin, O.M. (2002) Revision of *Neoechinorhynchus* Stiles and Hassall, 1905 (Acanthocephala: Neoechinorhynchidae) with keys to 88 species in two subgenera. *Syst. Parasitol.* **53,** 1–18.

145. Pence, D.B. and Casto, S.D. (1975) Two new species of the genus *Caminacarus* (Acarina: Cloacaridae) from turtles in Louisiana. *J. Parasitol.* **61,** 133–139.

146. Pence, D.B. and Wright, S.D. (1998) *Chelonacarus elongatus* n. gen., n. sp. (Acari: Cloacaridae) from the cloaca of the green turtle *Chelonia mydas* (Cheloniidae). *J. Parasitol.* **84,** 835–839.

147. Fain, A. (1968) Notes sur les acariens de la famille Cloacaridae Camin et al. Parasites du cloaque et des tissus profonds des tortues (Cheyletoidea: Trombidiformes). *Inst. Roy. Sci. Natl. Belg. Bull.* **44,** 1–33.

148. Junker, K. and Boomker, J. (2006) Check-list of the pentastomid parasites crocodilians and freshwater chelonians. *Onderstepoort J. Vet. Res.* **73,** 27–36.

149. Volf, J., Modry, D., Koudela, B., and Slapeta, J.R. (1999) Discovery of the life cycle of *Sarcocystis lacertae* Babudieri, 1932 (Apicomplexa: Sarcocystidae), with a species redescription. *Folia Parasitologica* **46,** 257–262.

150. Szell, Z., Sreter, T., and Varga, I. (2001) Ivermectin toxicosis in a chameleon (*Chamaeleo senegalensis*) infected with *Foleyella furcata. J. Zoo Wildl. Med.* **32,** 115–117.

151. Greenblatt, R.J., Work, T.M., Balazs, G.H., Sutton, C.A., Casey, R.N., and Casey, J.W. (2004) The Ozobranchus leech is a candidate mechanical vector for the fibropapilloma-associated turtle herpesvirus found latently infecting skin tumors on Hawaiian green turtles (*Chelonia mydas*). *Virology* **321,** 101–110.

152. Gunter, G. (1958) A sarcophagid fly larva parasitic in *Anolis carolinensis. Copeia* **4,** 336.

153. Mullens, B.A., Barrows, C., and Borkent, A. (1997) Lizard feeding by *Leptoconops* (*Brachyconops*) *californiensis* (Diptera: Ceratopogonidae) on desert sand dunes. *J. Med. Entomol.* **34,** 735–737.

154. Ebraheem, M.H., Rashdan, N.A., Fayed, H.M., and Galal, F.H. (2006) Influence of amphibian and reptile on the feeding preference, longevity and reproductive capacity of Egyptian *Culex pipiens* Linneaus (Diptera-Culicidae). *J. Egypt. Soc. Parasitol.* **36,** 33–39.

155. Dyce, A.L. and Wellings, G. (1991) Phlebotomine sandflies (Diptera: Psychodidae) from caves in Australia. *Parassitologia.* **33,** 193–198.

156. Till, W.M. (1957) Mesostigmatic mites living as parasites of reptiles in the Ethiopian region (Acarina: Laelaptidae). *J. Entomol. Soc. S. Afr.* **20,** 120–143.

157. Fain, A. (1962) Les acariens mesostigmatiques ectoparasites des serpents. *Inst. Roy. Sci. Nat. Belg. Bull.* **38,** 1–149.

158. Voss, W.J. (1967) First ixodorhynchid mite from Philippine snakes. *J. Med. Entomol.* **4,** 387–390.

159. Lane, J.E. (1954) A redescription of the American lizard mite, *Geckobiella texana* (Banks) 1904, with notes on systematics of the species (Acarina: Pterygosomidae). *J. Parasitol.* **40,** 93–99.

160. Newell, I.M. and Ryckman, R.E. (1964) *Hirstiella pyriformis* sp. n. (Acari, Pterygosomidae), a new parasite of lizards from Baja California. *J. Parasitol.* **50,** 163–171.

161. Reardon, J.T. and Norbury, G. (2004) Ectoparasite and hemoparasite infection in a diverse temperate lizard assemblage at Macraes Flat, South Island, New Zealand. *J. Parasitol.* **90,** 1274–1278.

162. Fain, A. (1964). Les Ophioptidae, acariens parasites des ecailles des serpents (Trombidiformes). *Inst. Roy. Sci. Nat. Belg. Bull.* **40,** 1–57.

163. Feider, Z. (1958) Sur une larve du genre *Trombicula* (Acari) parasites sur les lizards de la roumanie. *Z. Parasitenk.* **18,** 441–456.

164. Lehmann, H.D., Roth, B., and Schneider, C.C. (1969) The tick *Amblyomma testudinis* (Conil 1877): its development and effect on the host. *Z. Tropenmed. Parasitol.* **20,** 247–259.

165. Keirans, J.E. and Durden, L.A. (1998) Illustrated key to nymphs of the tick genus *Amblyomma* (Acari: Ixodidae) found in the United States. *J. Med. Entomol.* **35,** 489–495.

166. Burridge, M.J. and Simmons, L.A. (2003) Exotic ticks introduced into the United States on imported reptiles from 1962 to 2001 and their potential roles in international dissemination of diseases. *Vet. Parasitol.* **113,** 289–320.

167. Keirans, J.E. and Degenhardt, W.G. (1985) *Aponomma elaphense* Price, 1959 (Acari: Ixodidae): Diagnosis of the adults and nymph with first description of the larva. *Proc. Biol. Soc. Wash.* **98,** 711–717.

168. Nosek J. (1971) The ecology, bionomics and behaviour of *Haemaphysalis* (*Haemaphysalis*) *concinna* tick. *Z. Parasitenkd.* **36,** 233–241.

169. Sixl, W. and Nosek, J. (1974) Morphology of *Haemaphysalis* (*Aboimisalis*) *punctata* Can. et Franz. ticks in relation to its behaviour and ecology. *Rev. Suisse Zool.* **81,** 971–974.

170. Apanaskevich, D.A. (2003) Towards a diagnostic view of *Hyalomma aegyptium* (Acari, Ixodidae). *Parazitologiia* **37,** 47–59.

171. Eisen, L., Eisen, R.J., and Lane, R.S. (2004) The roles of birds, lizards, and rodents as hosts for the western black-legged tick Ixodes pacificus. *J. Vector Ecol.* **29,** 295–308.

172. Matuschka, F.R., Fischer, P., Musgrave, K., Richter, D., and Spielman, A. (1991) Hosts on which nymphal Ixodes ricinus most abundantly feed. *Am. J. Trop. Med. Hyg.* **44,** 100– 107.

173. De Meneghi, D. (1999) Pentastomes (Pentastomida, *Armillifer armillatus* Wyman, 1848) in snakes from Zambia. *Parassitologia* 41, 573–574.

174. Allen, K.M. and Tinsley, R.C. (1989) The diet and gastrodermal ultrastructure of polystomatid monogeneans infecting chelonians. *Parasitology* 98, 265–273.

175. Talbot, S.B. (1934) A description of four new trematodes of the subfamily Reniferinae with a discussion of the systematics of the subfamily. *Trans. Am. Microscop. Soc.* **53,** 40–56.

176. Crandall, R.B. (1960) The life history and affinities of the turtle lung fluke, *Heronimus chelydrae* Maccallum, 1902. *J. Parasitol.* **46,** 289–307.

177. Cort, W.W., Ameel, D.J., and Van Der Woude, A. (1952) Development of the mother and daughter sporocysts of a snake Plagiorchioid, *Lechriorchis primus* (Trematoda: Reniferidae). *J. Parasitol.* **38,** 187–202.

178. Stewart, P.L. (1960) Lung flukes of snakes, genera *Thamnophis* and *Coluber,* in Kansas. *Univ. Kansas Sci. Bull.* **41,** 877–890.

179. Junker, K., Boomker, J., and Bolton, L.A. (1999) Pentastomid infections in Nile crocodiles (*Crocodylus niloticus*) in the Kruger National Park, South Africa, with a description of the males of *Alofia simpsoni. Onderstepoort. J. Vet. Res.* **66,** 65–71.

180. Riley, J. and Self, J.T. (1980) On the systemics and life-cycle of the pentastomid genus *Kiricephalus* Sambon, 1922 with descriptions of three new species. *Syst. Parasitol* **1,** 127–140.

181. Junker, K., Boomker, J., Swanepoel, D., and Taraschewski, H. (2000) *Leiperia cincinnalis* Sambon, 1922 (Pentastomida) from Nile crocodiles *Crocodylus niloticus* in the Kruger National Park, South Africa, with a description of the male. *Syst. Parasitol.* **47,** 29–41.

CHAPTER

10

Parasites of Birds

Teresa Y. Morishita, DVM, MPVM, MS, PhD, DACPV; and Jordan C. Schaul, MS, PhD

Tables are placed at the ends of chapters.

INTRODUCTION

Several species of birds are used as subjects in biomedical research. Many of these, especially those collected from the wild, are infected or infested with parasites. This chapter covers the major parasites in those orders of birds commonly housed in laboratory settings. These include birds in the following orders: Galliformes (chickens, turkeys, and related species), Anseriformes (waterfowl), Passeriformes (perching songbirds), Columbiformes (pigeons, doves, and related species), and Psittaciformes (parrots and related species).

PROTOZOA

Phylum Sarcomastigophora

Class Mastigophora (Flagellates)

Chilomastix gallinarum

Morphology. *Chilomastix gallinarum* is pear- or carrot-shaped and measures 11 μ to 20 μ long by 5 μ to 12 μ wide[1]. It is a cyst-forming flagellate with a large, 8-shaped cytostomal cleft and lacks an undulating membrane[1,2]. Cysts are lemon-shaped and measure 7 μ to 9 μ long by 4 μ to 6 μ wide, and have a single nucleus[1].

Hosts and Life Cycle. *Chilomastix gallinarum* has been reported in the ceca of Galliformes (chickens, turkeys, pheasants, quail, chukar partridges) and Anseriformes (ducks and geese)[3,4]. In one study, up to 40% of chickens surveyed in the eastern U.S. harbored *C. gallinarum*[3]. The life cycle is direct. Multiplication is via binary fission. Transmission is via ingestion.

Pathologic Effects and Clinical Disease. While some report that *C. gallinarum* is nonpathogenic[2], in quail, gross lesions include distension of the lower digestive tract. The contents are green, watery, and foamy. Microscopic examination demonstrated superficial necrosis of the intestinal mucosal[5]. Birds with *C. gallinarum* infection have watery, foamy, and/or bloody feces in the absence of other detectable pathogens[6].

Diagnosis. Diagnosis requires fresh, warm feces. Detection is not possible with refrigerated feces or dead carcasses[6].

Treatment. Metronidizole (100 mg/kg body weight [BW] daily for five days) improved growth of experimentally infected chickens, but did not eliminate the parasite[6]. However, Spartrix (carnidazole; 3 tablets/kg BW for two consecutive days) given to individually caged birds eliminated the infection. Fecal consistency and frequency returned to normal[6].

Prevention. It was recommended that nitroimidazole be added to the food for at least three weeks to protect birds under field conditions[6]. The prevention or control of *C. gallinarum* infection in chickens requires improved hygiene[7].

Public Health Considerations. *Chilomastix gallinarum* does not infect humans.

Cochlsosoma anatis

Morphology. Trophozoites of *Cochlosoma anatis* possess an adhesive disk similar to that of *Giardia* sp., suggesting a phylogenetic relationship[8]. Trophozoites of *C. anatis* measure 8.4 μ to 10.3 μ long by 5 to 6.1 μ wide. Some have considered *C. anatis* synonymous with *C. rostratum*. However, trophozoites of *C. rostratum* measure 6 μ to 10 μ long by 3.9 μ to 6.7 μ wide. The anterior end of the *C. anatis* trophozoite bears a conspicuous adhesive disk measuring 4.6 μ to 5.6 μ long by 4.6 μ to 5.3 μ wide[8]. The adhesive disk covers half of the surface of the cell.

Hosts. *Cochlosoma anatis* has been found in Anseriformes (geese) and Galliformes[9]. Besides *C. anatis,* there are four other *Cochlosoma* species: *C. picae* from a magpie (*Pica pica hudsonia*)[10], *C. turdi* from an American robin (*Turdus migratorius*)[10], *C. striatum* from a ruffled grouse (*Bonasa umbelus*)[11], and *C. scolopacis* from a woodcock (*Scolopax rusticola*). In addition, a *Cochlosoma* sp. was found in the blue-faced parrot-finch, zebra finch, painted finch, nutmeg mannikin, and double-barred finch[12], while *C. anatis*-like protozoans have been found in red-headed parrot-finches, Bengalese finches, and Lady Gould finches[12].

Life Cycle. The life cycle is direct. Transmission is via the fecal-oral route. Reproduction occurs by binary longitudinal fission.

Pathologic Effects. *Cochlosoma anatis* has been isolated from turkeys with enteritis[9,13]. Histological lesions in these cases were characterized by blunting and fusion of the intestinal villi. Moreover, there was a cellular infiltration of the lamina propria with lymphocytes, plasma cells, histiocytes, and heterophils. An increased number of mitotic figures was also noted in the crypt epithelium. Although pathological lesions were not noted in adult finches, there were numerous flagellates between the colorectal villi and the cloacal mucosal folds[12]. Experimental inoculations of ducklings with *C. anatis* resulted in increased villus length and crypt depth, but without clinical signs[14].

Clinical Disease. Infection of *Cochlosoma* species in adult finches is usually subclinical[12], though runting has been reported in ducklings[15].

Diagnosis, Treatment, and Prevention. Diagnosis is via observation of the parasite on wet mounts or direct smears. Metronidazole and ronidazole were found to be effective against *Cochlosoma* species[12]. Prevention is achieved by reducing environmental contamination.

Public Health Considerations. *Cochlosoma anatis* does not infect humans.

Giardia psittaci

Morphology. *Giardia psittaci* trophozoites are dorsoventrally flattened, possess eight flagella, and have an adhesive disc on the ventral surface. They possess a claw-hammer-shaped median body, similar to other members of the genus. *Giardia psittaci* differs from *G. duodenalis* of mammals by lacking a ventrolateral flange and thus having no marginal groove bordering the anterior and lateral borders of the adhesive disc[16]. Box[17] described *Giardia* in budgerigars as *Giardia duodenalis* race *psittaci* because the trophozoites were of the *G. duodenalis*-type with elongated median bodies, which were pointed on one or both ends and that were perpendicular to the long axis. These trophozoites were 10 μ to 18 μ long by 4.5 μ to 11 μ wide, with a length-to-width ratio of 2:1.

Hosts. *Giardia psittaci* has been reported in a variety of bird species, including Anseriformes (Canada geese)[18] and Psittaciformes (budgerigars)[19]. *Giardia* trophozoites have been observed in the duodenum of the budgerigar[20]. Unidentified *Giardia* have been reported in free-living passerines with the following prevalences: 35% blackbirds (*Turdus merula*), 50% thrushes (*Turdus philomelos*), 15.4% sparrows (*Passer domesticus*), 60% chaffinches (*Fringilla coelebs*), and 14.3% hedge sparrows (*Prunella modularis*)[21].

Life Cycle. The life cycle is direct. Transmission is via the fecal-oral route. Reproduction occurs by binary longitudinal fission.

Pathologic Effects and Clinical Disease. Enteritis has been reported in budgerigars[19]. *Giardia psittaci* may cause diarrhea, retarded growth, and dehydration in budgerigars[19]. Clinical signs do not always accompany infection. For example, *G. psittaci* has also been isolated from clinically healthy geese and songbirds[18,21].

Diagnosis, Treatment, and Prevention. Diagnosis is confirmed by observing the protozoa on direct smears and wet mounts. Metronidazole in the drinking water resulted in budgerigars being negative for *G. psittaci* five days after treatment[19]. Reduction of fecal contamination reduces potential transmission.

Public Health Considerations. *Giardia psittaci* does not infect humans.

Hexamita columbae

Hexamita columbae (Syn. *Spironucleus columbae, Octomitus columbae*) measures 5 μ to 9 μ long by 2.5 μ to 7 μ wide, is piriform-shaped, and has two nuclei near the anterior end. It has six anterior and two posterior flagella[1]. *Hexamita columbae* has been reported in the pigeon, and has been found in the duodenum, jejunum, ileum, and large intestine[1]. It has been reported to cause catarrhal enteritis[1]. The duodenum can be dilated[22]. In young pigeons, *Hexamita* has been associated with weight loss, diarrhea, and unthriftiness. Racing pigeons also demonstrated reduced flight performance, emaciation, changes in posture, and slow crop emptying. Pigeons aged seven to 10 weeks are most commonly affected[22].

Diagnosis is through observation of the protozoa in fresh fecal material via a wet mount. Observation of clinical signs aids in diagnosis. The nitroimidazole family of drugs has been effective. Carnidazole at 20 mg/kg BW works effectively in individual birds[23]. Proper hygiene and sanitation are important to reduce transmission among birds. There are no known reports of *Hexamita columbae* causing disease in humans. In addition to *H. columbae*, an unidentified *Hexamita* species was reported in the small intestines and cecum of a finch (*Poephila gouldiae gouldiae*)[20].

Hexamita meleagridis

Morphology. *Hexamita meleagridis* (Syn. *Spironucleus meleagridis*) trophozoites are piriform-shaped, bilaterally symmetrical, and measure 6 μ to12 μ long by 2 μ to 5 μ wide with binucleate large endosomes[24]. Trophozoites have two anterior nuclei, four anterior flagella, two anterolateral flagella, two posterior flagella, and two separate axostyles. The four anterior flagella recurve along the body[2].

Hosts. *Hexamita meleagridis* is found in pheasants, quail, chukar partridges, peafowl, and turkeys[1]. An unidentified species of *Hexamita* has also been reported in psittacines and young pigeons[23]. In young birds, *Hexamita* is primarily found in the duodenum and small intestines[1]. In adults, the cecum and bursa of Fabricius are also colonized[1].

Life Cycle. The life cycle is direct. Transmission is via ingestion of contaminated food and/or water. Multiplication is by longitudinal binary fission[1]. Recovered birds can serve as carriers[1].

Pathologic Effects. Pathologic changes occur in the small intestine, and include catarrhal inflammation and a lack of intestinal tone[1]. The intestinal contents are watery and foamy. The cecum also contains fluid and the cecal tonsils are congested[1]. Petechial hemorrhages may be observed on the serosal surface of the duodenum. Histologically, one finds lymphocytic, plasmacytic inflammation in the mucosa of the duodenum and cecum, with numerous flagellated protozoa present[25].

Clinical Disease. *Hexamita meleagridis* has been reported to cause clinical disease in four- to 14-week-old turkeys[25]. Emaciation and intestinal distension with watery contents have been noted in affected turkeys, pigeons, and parrots. Affected turkeys are depressed and huddled, and they vocalize, have diarrhea, and may eat their litter (pica). Mortality may reach 12%[25]. In young pigeons, signs of weight loss, diarrhea, and unthriftiness have been reported[23].

Diagnosis. Diagnosis is by examination of wet mounts made from fresh intestinal scrapings, especially from the duodenum and jejunum, and/or from histological sections containing this protozoan. *Hexamita* may also be recognized by their rapid, straight motion[22]. In pigeons, highly motile flagellates on fresh direct fecal smears are diagnostic[23].

Treatment. The nitroimidazole antiprotozoal drugs are the most effective and include carnidazole (Spartrix), dimetridazole (Emtryl), ronidazole (Ridzol-S), and metronidazole. Carnidazole is the drug of choice for pigeons at 20 mg/kg BW[23].

Prevention. Proper sanitation and management can reduce transmission among birds. Prevention of fecal-oral contact is important to control hexamitiasis in pigeon flocks.

Public Health Considerations. *Hexamita meleagridis* is not zoonotic.

Histomonas meleagridis

Morphology. *Histomonas meleagridis* is an intestinal protozoan parasite[3]. It is pleomorphic, with the shape depending on its location in the body[3]. In the intestine, it appears flagellated and ranges in size from 6 μ to 18 μ in diameter. There is a clear outer zone of cytoplasm with an inner granular zone. One to two flagella originate from a basal granule near the nucleus (Figure 10.1)[26]. Within the cecal wall and liver, *H. meleagridis* appears to lose its flagella, and becomes more amoeboid. Size also varies depending upon tissue location. Invasive ameboid forms measure 8 μ to 17 μ in diameter, vegetative forms measure 12 μ to 21 μm long by 12 μ to 15 μ wide, and compact forms measure 4 μ

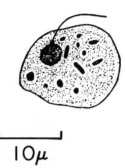

Fig. 10.1 *Histomonas meleagridis.* Trophozoite from cecum of chicken. Reproduced from Wenrich, D.H. (1943) with permission.

to 11 μ in diameter. Bacteria and food particles may be found within the organism.

Hosts. *Histomonas meleagridis* has been reported in most gallinaceous birds. However, clinical disease has been more frequently reported in turkeys, game birds (i.e. pheasants), and peafowl. Chickens are also susceptible but most often develop unapparent infections.

Life Cycle. The primary means of transmission of *H. meleagridis* is through ingestion of the ova of the cecal worm, *Heterakis gallinarum*. Direct transmission may occur if feces containing *H. meleagridis* is consumed immediately after defecation, but this is probably not a significant source of infection[27]. Mechanical transmission via insect vectors has also been reported. Norton and co-workers[28] reported a case of histomoniasis in the absence of *Heterakis gallinarum*, but in the presence of *Ascaridia dissimilis*.

Pathologic Effects. The livers of affected birds have crater-like lesions that can measure up to 1 cm in diameter. These depressed circular lesions represent necrotic areas and appear yellow to white in color. Ulcerations also occur on the cecal mucosa. Cecal cores, consisting of hardened yellow caseated plugs, fill the cecal lumen. In severe cases, the cecum may rupture. Histomonads may be observed microscopically in liver and cecal lesions.

Clinical Disease. Histomoniasis is also referred to as "blackhead." The incubation period is 14 days[29]. Clinical disease may be severe in turkeys, game birds (i.e. pheasants), and peafowl. Affected birds appear listless, have ruffled feathers, and have yellow (sulfur-colored) diarrhea. In turkeys, mortality may reach 100%. The disease is less severe in chickens, where mortality is limited to 5% to 20%[30]. Young chickens are more susceptible to clinical disease[3]. Concurrent infection of chickens with *Eimeria tenella* may result in more severe clinical signs of histomoniasis[31].

Diagnosis. A presumptive diagnosis of histomoniasis is based on finding yellow diarrhea and increased mortality in the flock. Circular, depressed lesions on the liver, and ulcers with cecal cores in the cecum, are also presumptive for histomoniasis. Confirmation is based on finding *H. meleagridis* in histological sections or in cecal scrapings.

Treatment. There are no products available for the treatment of *H. meleagridis* in food-producing animals in the United States[30]. For non-food-producing birds, metronidazole has been effective for the control of histomoniasis. Experimentally challenged birds had significantly greater body weights during treatment and two weeks post-treatment as well as lower lesion scores when compared to untreated controls[29]. Albendazole (100 mg/kg) and fenbendazole (10 mg/kg) given orally twice a day for five consecutive days were ineffective for treating clinical disease. However, prophylactic use of either drug increased mean body weight gains and reduced liver and cecal lesion scores. It was suggested that the flagellated form of *H. meleagridis* may be more sensitive to chemotherapeutic agents than the amoeboid form found in tissues[29]. The nitroimidazoles, dimetridazole, metronidazole, ornidazole, and tinidazole, were effective at 200 ppm in the feed[32]. Levamisole given subcutaneously at a dose of 2.5 mg/100 g BW has been used successfully in pheasants and quail[33].

Prevention. Good management and sanitation can help reduce the incidence of histomoniasis. In addition, elimination of the cecal worm must be a component of an overall control program.

Public Health Considerations. *Histomonas meleagridis* does not infect humans.

Pentatrichomonas gallinarum

Pentatrichomonas gallinarum is piriform-shaped, with five anterior flagella, four of which are of equal length and the remaining flagellum shorter. An undulating membrane traverses the length of the cell, with a free flagellum at its end[1]. *Pentatrichomonas gallinarum* has been found in the liver and ceca of chickens, turkeys, and guinea fowl[1]. Transmission is via oral ingestion. *Pentatrichomonas gallinarum* is nonpathogenic[1]. Diagnosis is via examination of direct smears. As for other nonpathogenic trichomonads, treatment is not warranted. Good hygiene can reduce transmission among birds. *Pentatrichomonas gallinarum* does not infect humans.

Spironucleus sp.

An unidentified *Spironucleus* species was reported in Australian king parrot (*Alisterus scapularis*) intestines[26].

Specific details on the morphology and life cycle of this organism are lacking. In the single case report, wasting and diarrhea were observed in affected birds. Yellow-green, foamy, and liquid contents were found in the intestines. *Spironucleus* was seen in the crypts of Lieberkuhn and associated with mucus exudation. Catarrhal and lymphoplasmacytic enteritis were also evident. Clinically affected birds were emaciated, and had diarrhea, with fecal debris adhered to their vents[26]. A definitive diagnosis may be made by identifying *Spironucleus* on wet mounts that are prepared from feces or intestinal contents. Specific treatment regimens for *Spironucleus* are lacking. Proper sanitation and good management practices will prevent re-infection. The *Spironucleus* found in birds has not been reported in humans.

Tetratrichomonas anatis

Tetratrichomonas anatis (Syn. *Trichomonas anatis*) measures 13 μ to 27 μ long by 8 μ to18 μ wide and possesses four anterior flagella and an undulating membrane that extends most of its length[1]. The parasite inhabits the ceca of ducks[1]. The life cycle is direct, with transmission occurring through ingestion of contaminated food and water. *Tetratrichomonas anatis* does not cause clinical disease or pathologic changes in birds. Diagnosis can be made through examination of wet mounts. Good hygiene will reduce contamination among birds. *Tetratrichomonas anatis* does not infect humans.

Tetratrichomonas anseris

Tetratrichomonas anseris (Syn. *Trichomonas anseris*) measures 8 μ long by 5 μ wide. Four anterior flagella are present, and an undulating membrane extends the length of the cell. A free trailing flagellum is also present[1]. *Tetratrichomonas anseris* has been reported in the ceca of geese. Transmission is via ingestion. There are no pathologic effects or clinical signs associated with this infection. Diagnosis is via examination of direct smears. Treatment is not warranted. Good hygiene will reduce transmission among birds. *Tetratrichomonas anseris* does not infect humans.

Tetratrichomonas gallinarum

Morphology. *Tetratrichomonas gallinarum* (Syn. *Trichomonas gallinarum*, *Trichomonas pullorum*)[1] is piriform-shaped and measures 7 μ to 15 μ long by 3 μ to 9 μ wide. There are four anterior flagella and one posterior flagellum which runs along its undulating membrane[1].

Hosts and Life Cycle. Several avian species may serve as host to *T. gallinarum,* including chickens, turkeys, guinea fowl, quail, pheasants, and chukar partridges[1]. This parasite is usually found in the cecum[1]. Infection is direct, through ingestion of contaminated water and feed.

Pathologic Effects and Clinical Disease. No pathologic changes or clinical disease are noted in the cecal mucosa although there can be numerous organisms in the villi crypts[34].

Diagnosis, Treatment, and Prevention. Diagnosis can be confirmed with wet mounts. Moreover, this parasite can be cultivated using trichomonal media[1]. Infections with this parasite are not normally treated. Good hygiene will prevent infection.

Public Health Considerations. *Tetratrichomonas gallinarum* does not infect humans.

Trichomonas gallinae

Morphology. The trophozoites of *Trichomonas gallinae* are piriform-shaped and measure 6 μ to 19 μ long and 2 μ to 9 μ wide. They also have four anterior flagella and an axostyle[3] (Figure 10.2)[35]. *Trichomonas gallinae* is not found in the cyst form[3].

Hosts. *Trichomonas gallinae* has been reported in many bird species. It is most commonly reported in birds belonging to the Order Columbiformes[3], but also occurs in Galliformes, Passeriformes, and Psittaciformes[3,36]. McKeon and co-workers reported finding *T. gallinae* in zero to 11.4% of budgerigars, 46% of wild Senegal doves, and 59% of a flock of racing pigeons[36].

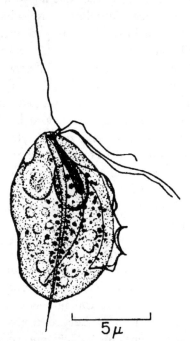

Fig. 10.2 *Trichomonas gallinae* trophozoite. Reproduced from Wenrich, D.H. (1930) with permission.

Life Cycle. Transmission is via ingestion of contaminated feed and water. In addition, pigeons can transmit *T. gallinae* to offspring via the crop milk ("pigeon milk")[2]. *Trichomonas gallinae* reproduces via binary fission.

Pathologic Effects and Clinical Disease. Lesions consisting of caseous, necrotic nodules, plaques, or ulcers are commonly reported in the upper digestive tract, e.g. oropharynx, esophagus, and crop[3]. Based on the appearance of the lesions, clinical trichomoniasis is often referred to as "canker." Affected birds are listless and reluctant to eat. Acute mortality has been reported in pigeons.

Diagnosis. A diagnosis of *T. gallinae* infection can be made by identification of organisms on direct smear, or in stained tissue sections. Experimental studies have demonstrated that viable *T. gallinae* can be obtained from dove carcasses at least eight hours, and possibly up to 24 hours, after the death of the host[37]. Besides direct examination, oropharynx and crop samples can be incubated in Diamond's medium until the *T. gallinae* are numerous enough to be easily found in aliquots examined under a microscope. Commercially available kits (In-Pouch TF) for *T. gallinae* culture are also available[38].

Treatment. Oral treatment with 2-amino-5-nitrothiazole (Aminonitrothiazole) at 28 to 45 mg/kg daily for seven days, or 0.16% in the drinking water for seven to 14 days, has been reported to be effective. Inghelbrecht and co-workers[39] reported that dimetridazole (400 mg/L) for three days in water was effective to suppress *T. gallinae* infection, while a two-day treatment with a dimetridazole tablet (20 mg/tablet) was not effective in homing pigeons. Likewise, McLoughlin[40] found dimetridazole useful at a concentration of 0.05% in the drinking water for pigeons. However, this drug is no longer available in the U.S.[2]. There have been reports of drug resistance among various pigeon isolates[41,42]. For example, 45% of pigeon strains have demonstrated resistance to ronidazole, though in one study, ronidazole at 100 to 150 mg/L water for five to seven days was reported to be effective in pigeons[41]. Infected birds should be removed from the flock.

Prevention. The most effective control strategy for *T. gallinae* is to eliminate the parasite in the adults and to prevent spread to the offspring via the crop milk[3].

Public Health Considerations. *Trichomonas gallinae* does not infect humans.

Tritrichomonas eberthi

Morphology. *Tritrichomonas eberthi* (Syn. *Trichomonas eberthi*) is carrot-shaped, measures 8 μ to 14 μ long by 4 μ to 7 μ wide and has three anterior flagella and a prominent undulating membrane, which extends the full length of the body. A posterior flagellum extends beyond the undulating membrane, about half the body length beyond the undulating membrane[1].

Hosts and Life Cycle. *Tritrichomonas eberthi* has been found in chickens, turkeys, and ducks[1,43]. Reproduction is by longitudinal binary fission. There are no known sexual stages and cysts are not formed[1]. *Tritrichomonas eberthi* is directly transmitted from bird to bird through fecal-oral contamination. Infection is primarily established in the ceca[43].

Pathologic Effects and Clinical Disease. *Tritrichomonas eberthi* is considered nonpathogenic. It is often found in association with *Tetratrichomonas gallinarum* and *Chilomastix gallinarum*[43]. *Tritrichomonas eberthi* does not cause clinical disease.

Diagnosis, Treatment, and Prevention. Diagnosis is through microscopic examination of fecal or cecal material in wet mount. Treatment is not necessary because *T. eberthi* is nonpathogenic. Good hygiene will reduce transmission among birds.

Public Health Considerations. *Tritrichomonas eberthi* does not infect humans.

Trypanosoma avium

Morphology. Avian trypanosomes are pleomorphic and usually measure 26 µ to 69 µ long. The kinetoplast is distant from the posterior end. They possess a free flagellum and appear striated[1].

Hosts. Trypanosomes have been reported in Galliformes, Anseriformes, and Passeriformes. Besides *T. avium*, *T. calmettei* has been reported in chickens in Southeast Asia; *T. gallinarum* has been reported in chickens in central Africa; and *T. hannai* has been reported in pigeons[1]. In addition, *T. dafilae* has been recovered from a pintail duck[1] and from American crows[44].

Life Cycle. Transmission is via blood-sucking insects such as mosquitoes, simuliids, and hippoboscid flies[1,45]. Desser[46] reported *Simulium rugglesi* as a potential vector of *T. avium*.

Pathologic Effects and Clinical Disease. Most species of avian trypanosomes are nonpathgenic[1]. Because avian trypanosomes are considered nonpathogenic, clinical disease has not been described[1].

Diagnosis, Treatment, and Prevention. A diagnosis can be made by identifying trypanosomes in stained, thin blood smears. No treatment is necessary because there is no clinical disease associated with avian trypanosomiasis.

Control of biting arthropods can reduce the transmission of *Trypanosoma* species.

Public Health Considerations. Avian trypanosomes are not zoonotic, and therefore are not considered a public health concern.

Class Sarcodina

Endolimax gregariniformis

Endolimax gregariniformis trophozoites measure 4 µ to 13 µ long. Cysts measure 7 µ by 10 µ. *Endolimax gregariniformis* has been found in chickens, turkeys, guinea fowl, pheasants, geese, ducks, and other wild birds, including herons and owls. The life cycle is direct. Multiplication is via binary fission[1]. Transmission is via ingestion of infectious cysts. *Endolimax gregariniformis* is not pathogenic and is not associated with clinical disease[1]. Fecal smears stained with hematoxylin aid in diagnosis. Cysts can be detected with a zinc sulfate flotation solution[1]. Treatment is not warranted. Good hygiene and management can reduce transmission among species. *Endolimax gregariniformis* is not zoonotic.

Entamoeba anatis

Entamoeba anatis trophozoites measure 20 µ to 30 µ in diameter. Red blood cells may be observed within the trophozoites. Cysts are spherical and measure 13 µ to14 µ in diameter, and contain one to four nuclei[1]. *Entamoeba anatis* has been reported in the large intestine of a duck[1]. The life cycle is direct. Multiplication is via binary fission. Prior to passing out in the feces, trophozoites round up, become smaller, eliminate food vacuoles, and transform to the environmentally resistant and infective cyst stage. Transmission is via ingestion of cysts. No pathological effects have been described in birds infected with *E. anatis*. Thus, clinical disease has not been reported.

Fecal smears stained with hematoxylin will aid in diagnosis. Cysts can be detected with a zinc sulfate flotation solution[1]. Because infection is asymptomatic, treatment is not warranted. Good hygiene and sanitation can reduce transmission among species. *Entamoeba anatis* does not infect humans.

Entamoeba gallinarum

Trophozoites of *Entamoeba gallinarum* measure 9 µ to 25 µ long with most measuring 16 µ to 18 µ long. Cysts measure 12 µ to 15 µ long and contain eight nuclei[1]. *Entamoeba gallinarum* has been isolated from the ceca of chickens, turkeys, guinea fowl, ducks, and geese[1]. The life cycle is direct. Multiplication is via binary fission.

Transmission is via ingestion of infective cysts. *Entamoeba gallinarum* is considered nonpathogenic[1]. There have been no reports of *E. gallinarum* causing clinical disease in avian species. Fecal smears stained with hematoxylin aid in diagnosis, and zinc sulfate flotation concentrates cysts for diagnosis. Treatment is not warranted. Good hygiene and sanitation help to reduce transmission. *Entamoeba gallinarum* does not infect humans.

Entamoeba struthionis

Entamoeba struthionis has been reported in ostriches (*Struthio camelus*) and rheas (*Rhea americana*)[47]. Trophozoites measure 8 μ to 35 μ long. The nucleus measures 4 μ to 7 μ in diameter. Cysts measure 8 μ to 20 μ in diameter, but are usually 11 μ to 16 μ in diameter, and contain one nucleus that is 2 μ to 7 μ in diameter[47]. *Entamoeba struthionis* has a direct life cycle, with cysts serving as the infective stage. These are directly transmitted by fecal-oral contamination[47]. Pathologic effects have not been reported[47]. Thus, infection with *E. struthionis* is not associated with clinical disease[47]. Diagnosis is via identification of *E. struthionis* on a wet mount. Because *E. struthionis* is nonpathogenic, treatment is not warranted. Good sanitation and hygiene reduce transmission between birds. *Entamoeba struthionis* does not infect humans.

Phylum Apicomplexa

The Phylum Apicomplexa is composed of a wide variety of parasites, including the coccidian and malarial parasites, the toxoplasmids, and the piroplasmasids.

Class Coccidia

Common enteric coccidial genera of birds include *Eimeria*, *Isospora*, and *Cryptosporidium*. These are monoxenous; that is, they require only one host to complete their life cycle. The most important enteric avian coccidia belong to the genus *Eimeria*. It should be noted that oocysts of *Eimeria* sp. are commonly found on fecal flotation examinations of asymptomatic birds. This alone does not warrant a diagnosis of clinical coccidiosis. Clinical signs and/or intestinal lesions must also be present. Speciation based only on morphological characteristics is difficult. The location of the lesions within the intestines will also aid in speciation.

In general, *Eimeria* remain viable in the soil for at least a year, but may be killed by subfreezing temperatures. Oocysts are also destroyed by ultraviolet light, heat, and desiccation. Younger birds should be raised separately from older birds which can serve as a source of infection. It appears that live attenuated anti-coccidial vaccines have been protective and can reduce the negative effects of coccidiosis in chickens[48].

Arthrocystis galli

Arthrocystis galli has been reported in the skeletal and cardiac muscles of chickens. Meronts measure 1,400 μ by 126 μ[1]. No details are available on the morphology of *A. galli* sporocysts. The definitive host of *A. galli* is unknown. Likewise, specific details on the life cycle of *A. galli* are lacking. *Arthrocystis galli* meronts appear to be aligned end-to-end, taking on the appearance of bamboo in the muscle tissue[1]. Some mortality was noted in a flock of affected chickens. *Arthrocystis galli* can be diagnosed in the chicken by histological examination. There is no effective treatment for this disease. Prevention is through elimination of carnivore feces, as described for *Sarcocystis*. Human infections with *A. galli* have not been reported.

Atoxoplasma sp.

Atoxoplasma (Syn. *Lankesterella*) species have been reported in the mononuclear leukocytes (lymphocytes, macrophages, and monocytes) of passerines. Specific details on the morphology of *Atoxoplasma* are lacking. However, merozoites, macrogametes, and microgamonts are present in the epithelial cells of the intestines. *Atoxoplasma* species have been reported in passerines, including the greenfinch (*Carduelis chloris*)[49] and canary[50].

Specific details on the life cycle of *Atoxoplasma* species are lacking, but it is transmitted by blood-feeding mites (i.e. *Dermanyssus gallinae*). Mortality has been noted in infected nestlings. Affected birds may die suddenly. Diagnosis is by identifying *Atoxoplasma* sporozoites in the mononuclear leukocytes of peripheral blood smears, or on cytological examination of the liver, spleen, or lung impression smear. Specific treatment regimens for *Atoxoplasma* species are lacking. Mite control is an important aspect of preventing transmission. *Atoxoplasma* species occurring in birds have not been reported in humans.

Cryptosporidium meleagridis and Cryptosporidium baileyi

Cryptosporidium meleagridis (Syn. *C. anserinum*, *C. tyzzeri*) and *C. baileyi* have been reported in the intestines, respiratory tract, and kidneys of a variety of bird species. In a recent review of *Cryptosporidium* in birds, Sreter and Varga suggested that *C. meleagridis* may be closely related or identical to *C. parvum*, a parasite of mammals[51]. Further studies are needed to clarify this issue.

Morphology. *Cryptosporidium meleagridis* oocysts measure 5.1 μ long by 4.5 μ wide, while those of *C. baileyi* are larger and more ovoid, and measure 6.5 μ long by 4.25 μ wide[52].

Hosts. Turkeys are the natural hosts of *C. meleagridis*. In addition, *C. meleagridis* has been reported in chickens, partridges, peafowl, pheasants, quail (*Coturnix coturnix*), geese, Indian ring-necked parrots (*Psittacula krameri*), and red-lored parrots (*Amazona autumnalis*)[52]. *Cryptosporidium baileyi* has been found in many bird species. Both *C. meleagridis* and *C. baileyi* have been reported in cockatiels[53]. An unidentified *Cryptosporidium* has been isolated in finches and a black duck[54].

Life Cycle. Details on the life cycle of *C. meleagridis* and *C. baileyi* are sparse. It is assumed that their life cycles are direct, and similar to other members of the genus.

Pathologic Effects. *Cryptosporidium meleagridis* and *C. baileyi* are usually nonpathogenic. However, Trampel and co-workers reported developing stages in the epithelial cells lining the renal collecting tubules and ureters such that lymphoplasmacytic infiltrates in the ureters and hyperplasia of parasitized epithelial cells partially obstructed the ureters[55]. The bursa was affected in pheasants[56].

Clinical Disease. *Cryptosporidium meleagridis* and *C. baileyi* have been associated with diarrhea or respiratory disease. In addition, visceral gout may be exacerbated by urinary cryptosporidiosis[55]. Birds affected with *C. baileyi* shed two to three times more oocysts than those infected with *C. meleagridis*[57].

Diagnosis, Treatment, and Prevention. Diagnosis is by identification of organisms, along with clinical signs and lesions. A semi-quantitative microscopic slide flotation method using modified Sheather's sugar solution is a rapid, specific, and sensitive low-cost test[58]. Although not registered for use in birds, paromomycin reduced oocyst shedding by 67% to 82%[59]. Proper sanitation and good management practices can reduce re-infection in the flock. A 50% bleach solution to disinfect premises has been recommended to prevent future outbreaks.

Public Health Considerations. *Cryptosporidium bailey* does not infect humans, while *C. meleagridis* has been reported from immune-suppressed people. Personnel working with birds infected with *C. meleagridis* should use personal protective equipment and practice hygienic techniques. Immune-suppressed people should not work with or around birds infected with *C. meleagridis*.

Cryptosporidium spp.

Unidentified *Cryptosporidium* species have been reported in cockatiels, white-lored euphonias, bronze mannikin finches, and Australian diamond fire tailed finches[60]. Infections in cockatiels occurred mostly in the small intestine, although *Cryptosporidium* has been noted in the esophageal glands, air sacs, and proventriculus[60]. In the white-lored euphonias, infection was documented in either the small intestine or the proventriculus[60]. *Cryptosporidium* was documented in the proventriculus of bronze mannikin finches and Australian diamond fire tailed finches[60]. Tsai and co-workers reported *Cryptosporidium* in the small intestine of Amazon parrots (*Amazona aestiva aestiva*), African grey parrots (*Psittacus erithacus*), and budgerigars (*Melopsittacus undulatus*)[20]. Moreover, *Cryptosporidium* was reported in the bulbar and palpebral conjunctiva of a lovebird (*Agapornis roseicollis*)[20].

Eimeria acervulina

Morphology. *Eimeria acervulina* oocysts are ovoid and measure 12 μ to 23 μ by 9 μ to 17 μ. The oocyst has a smooth two-layered wall and no micropyle[1]. Oocysts sporulate within one day.

Hosts and Life Cycle. Chickens are the hosts of *Eimeria acervulina*. The life cycle is typical of the genus. The prepatent period is four days and the patent period lasts for several days.

Pathologic Effects. *Eimeria acervulina* is found in the anterior small intestine of the chicken (Figure 10.3). *Eimeria acervulina* occasionally causes inflammation of the anterior small intestine but is usually nonpathogenic. Inoculation of a large dose (more than 1 million oocysts) causes intestinal wall thickening and catarrhal enteritis. White or gray spots or streaks are observed on the intestinal mucosa[1].

Clinical Disease. Clinical signs are only observed following exposure to massive numbers of sporulated oocysts. Unlike other *Eimeria* species, bloody diarrhea is rarely observed, even in severe infections.

Diagnosis, Treatment, Prevention, and Public Health Considerations. These aspects are as described for *E. tenella*.

Eimeria dispersa

Morphology. *Eimeria dispersa* oocysts measure 22 μ to 31 μ by 18 μ to 24 μ, with an average of 26 μ by 21 μ.

Hosts and Life Cycle. *Eimeria dispersa* infects the upper intestinal tract of turkeys, bobwhite quail, ringnecked pheasants, chukar partridges, ruffed grouse and

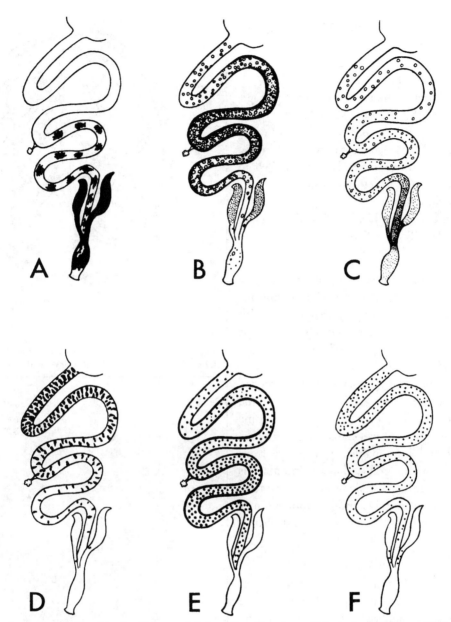

Fig. 10.3 *Eimeria* species commonly found in the chicken and their preferred locations within the intestinal tract. (A) *E. tenella*. (B) *E. necatrix*. (C) *E. brunetti*. (D) *E. acervulina*. (E) *E. maxima*. (F) *E. mitis*. Reproduced from Levine, N.D. (1961) with permission.

sharp-tailed grouse[1]. The life cycle is direct, and typical of the genus. The prepatent period is approximately five to six days[1].

Pathologic Effects and Clinical Disease. *Eimeria dispersa* is only mildly pathogenic. Affected birds have markedly dilated and edematous intestines that contain a cream-colored mucoid exudate. Clinical disease is usually not observed.

Diagnosis. Diagnosis is as described for *E. tenella*.

Treatment. Because *Eimeria dispersa* is generally non-pathogenic, treatment is often not needed. However, diclazuril (0.5, 1, or 2 ppm in the feed) was effective in suppressing lesions, abnormal droppings, and oocyst shedding[61]. Likewise, maduramicin ammonium (5 to 7 ppm in the feed) was effective and reduced oocyst shedding[62]. Watkins and co-workers reported that 60 ppm of monensin was effective[63]. Others have reported that feeding halofugione (3 mg/kg) and monensin (60 mg/kg or 100 mg/kg) were most effective while amprolium (125 mg/kg), zoalene (125 mg/kg), and sulfadimethoxine plus ormetoprim (62.5 mg/kg and 37.5 mg/kg, respectively) were least effective in reducing the severity of the intestinal lesions[64].

While all coccidiostats tested reduced oocyst passage, halofugione produced the fewest oocysts[64]. For quail, monensin (90 g/ton of feed) has been effective[33]. For pheasants, amprolium (9.6% solution) in the drinking water (1 ml/liter water for three to five days or 0.0175% in the feed) was effective. Salinomycin was also effective for bobwhite quail and pheasants[33].

Prevention and Public Health Considerations. These aspects are as described for *E. tenella*.

Eimeria maxima

Eimeria maxima commonly affects the small intestine, primarily the jejunum, of chickens (Figure 10.3). *Eimeria maxima* oocysts measure 21 μ to 42 μ by 16 μ to 30 μ, with an average of 29 μ to 31 μ by 21 μ to 23 μ. The life cycle is typical of the genus. The prepatent period is five to six days and the patent period is a few days[1].

The pathologic effects of *E. maxima* depend on the strain involved. Generally, there are hemorrhages in the wall of the small intestine. The intestinal wall may become thickened, dilated, and lose its tone. Catarrhal enteritis has also been reported and intestinal contents range from brown to orange, although blood within the intestines is uncommon[1]. Affected birds appear depressed and can have gray to orange mucoid diarrhea. Diagnosis, treatment, prevention, and public health considerations are as described for *E. tenella*.

Eimeria tenella

Morphology. Oocysts of *Eimeria tenella* are oval-shaped, and measures 14 μ to 31 μ long by 9 μ to 25 μ wide. The oocyst has a smooth wall and lacks a micropyle (Figure 10.4)[3,65]. Oocysts sporulate within a few days and subsequently contain four sporocysts, each with two sporozoites.

Hosts and Life Cycle. Chickens are the hosts of *Eimeria tenella*. The life cycle is direct, and is described in Chapter 2, Biology of the Protozoa. The prepatent period is seven days[66].

Pathologic Effects. *Eimeria tenella* is the most pathogenic coccidian of chickens[3]. It is the causative agent of a classical coccidiosis reported in chickens, which occurs primarily in the cecum (Figure 10.3). Early lesions include hemorrhagic cecal mucosae which subsequently become fibrinonecrotic. The cecal wall becomes thickened and the lumen fills with blood (Figure 10.5). Finally, cecal cores often form.

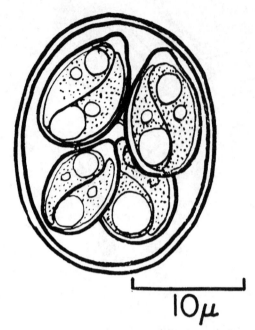

Fig. 10.4 Sporulated oocysts of *Eimeria tenella*. Reproduced from Chandler, A.C. and Read, P.R. (1961) with permission.

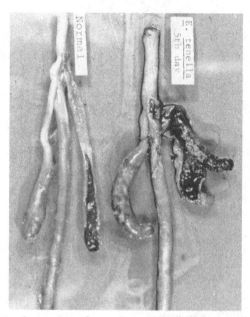

Fig. 10.5 Comparison of normal ceca (left) with diseased ceca (right) due to *Eimeria tenella*. Courtesy of W.M. Reid, University of Georgia.

Clinical Disease. Depending on the age and infectious dose, birds may have an unapparent infection, or demonstrate severe clinical signs. Affected chickens are listless, anorexic, have bloody diarrhea, and may die. Mortality may vary from 32% to 90%. Young chickens around four weeks of age are most susceptible, whereas older birds are more resistant. Resistance is most likely related to partial immunity resulting from previous exposure.

Diagnosis. A definitive diagnosis is made by demonstration of fecal oocysts, characteristic histologic lesions, and clinical signs. A two-step polymerase chain reaction can differentiate the eight species of *Eimeria* in chickens[67].

Treatment. Several treatment regimens have been described for avian coccidiosis. These include conventional treatments such as lasalocid (75 mg/kg) in the feed, or toltrazuril in the drinking water (7 mg/kg BW for two consecutive days between days 10 and 14 of placement)[68]. Toltrazuril can also be used for supplemental control with in-feed anticoccidials, or as a primary anticoccidial with nonmedicated feed[68]. Effective alternative treatments have included oregano essential oil (300 mg/kg)[69] and sugar cane extract[70]. Shuttle treatments (starter to grower) have also proven effective[71].

Coccidiosis can also be affected by dietary modifications. Dietary n-3 fatty acids, such as those found in menhaden oil or flaxseed oil, can induce oxidative stress and can inhibit coccidial development[72]. By these and other mechanisms, artemisinin from *Artemisia annua,* tumeric, and betaine (from sugar beets) have reduced the effects of coccidiosis[72].

Prevention. Coccidial infection is self-limiting. However, re-infection with less severe manifestations is common if proper sanitation and management are not practiced. Live vaccines can reduce clinical disease[73].

Public Health Considerations. Avian coccidia are not infective to humans.

Eimeria spp.

Several additional *Eimeria* species have been reported in quail and pheasants. *Eimeria coturnicis, E. bateri, E. taldykurganica, E. tsunodai,* and *E. uzura* has been reported in Coturnix or Japanese quail (*Coturnix japonica*). *Eimeria colini, E. dispersa,* and *E. lettyae* has been reported in bobwhite quail (*Colinus virginianus*). *Eimeria phasianus* has been reported in pheasants. Most of these *Eimeria* species are nonpathogenic, except *Eimeria tsunodai,* which causes hemorrhagic typhlitis and reduced growth and weight gains in Coturnix quail[33]. Domestic birds are likewise susceptible to many species of coccidia of the genus *Eimeria.* While some of these are pathogenic, many are not. The species found in these birds are summarized in the tables at the end of the chapter. Where treatment is warranted, treatments used to eliminate *E. tenella* are likely to also be effective against other *Eimeria* species.

Isospora spp.

Additional *Isospora* sp. have been reported in the intestines of a variety of bird species. Species isolated include *Isospora lacazei, I. gryphoni., I. serini,* and *I. canaria.*

Morphology. For *Isospora gryphoni,* oocysts measure 25 μ to 33 μ by 28 μ to 34 μ, with an average of 29.2 μ by 30.7 μ. *Isospora serini* have spheroid oocysts which have an average measurement of 19.2 μ by 20.1 μ[74]. *Isospora canaria* have elliptical oocysts that measure 21.8 μ by 24.6 μ[74].

Hosts. *Isospora lacazei* was reported in a domestic sparrow[75]. *Isospora gryphoni* has been recovered from an American goldfinch[76]. *Isospora serini* and *Isospora canaria* have been reported in canaries[74].

Life Cycle. Specific details on the life cycle of these *Isospora* species are lacking. However, colonization of mononuclear leukocytes is evident in birds infected with *I. serini,* while *I. canaria* colonizes the intestinal epithelium.

Pathologic Effects and Clinical Disease. Specific details on these aspects are lacking.

Diagnosis, Treatment, and Prevention. Diagnosis is by identification of *Isospora* oocysts in the feces. In the case of *I. serini,* a diagnosis is made by identifying the asexual stages in the mononuclear leukocytes of a peripheral blood smear. Specific treatment regimens are lacking. Proper sanitation and good management practices can reduce exposure in the flock.

Public Health Considerations. Avian *Isospora* do not infect humans.

Sarcocystis falcatula

Sarcocystis falcatula schizonts measured 24 μ by 6.8 μ and contained 24 to 96 merozoites, and are found in the pulmonary air passages and capillaries[77]. Several avian species, such as canaries, are intermediate hosts for *S. falcatula.* Specific details on the life cycle of *S. falcatula* are lacking. The Virginia opossum (*Didelphis virginiana*) is the definitive host. In birds, infection leads to pulmonary edema, interstitial pneumonitis, and hepatitis[78,79]. Affected birds often die prior to exhibiting clinical signs. Some birds can exhibit respiratory distress.

Sarcocystis falcatula can be diagnosed by histological examination. However, because there are no clinical signs associated with this disease, the parasite is often an incidental finding at necropsy. There is no effective treatment for this disease. Infection can be prevented by eliminating sources of opossum feces. *Sarcocystis falcatula* does not infect humans.

Sarcocystis horvathi

Sarcocystis horvathi (Syn. *Sarcocystis gallinarum*) cysts have been found in the muscles of the chicken intermediate host. Definitive hosts include dogs and cats[1]. The sporocysts found in dog feces measure 10 μ to 13 μ by 7 μ to 9 μ.

The genus *Sarcocystis* is considered heteroxenous; one host (usually a predator species) is required for the sexual stages and another host (prey species) is required for the asexual stages[1]. The life cycle is perpetuated when the intermediate host ingests the sporocysts shed by the definitive host. In the definitive host, the prepatent period is six to 10 days and the patent period in the dog is 21 to 23 days[1]. The asexual stages can be found in the striated muscle of the chicken, where they may cause severe myositis. Sarcocystosis can be diagnosed in the intermediate host by histological examination. However, because clinical signs are rare in birds, this disease is often diagnosed post-mortem.

There has been little success in treating sarcocystosis in intermediate hosts. Infection can be prevented by preventing birds from ingesting contaminated feces from definitive hosts. *Sarcocystis horvathi* does not infect humans.

Sarcocystis rileyi

Sarcocystis rileyi (Syn. *Balbiania rileyi*, *Sarcocystis anatina*) has been found in the muscles of the duck intermediate host. The sporocysts recovered from skunks measured 10 μ to 14 μ by 5 μ to 10 μ[1]. *Sarcocystis rileyi* is common in dabbling ducks, but is also found in diving ducks and domestic ducks. Definitive hosts include striped skunks, opossums, dogs, and cats.

The life cycle is similar to those of other members of the genus. Sarcocysts may be observed microscopically in skeletal muscles 85 days post-infection, and can be seen macroscopically 154 days post-infection, when they measure 2 mm to 8 mm long by 1 mm wide[1]. Individual sarcocysts can reach several centimeters in length[80]. The sarcocysts in the duck muscle are not pathogenic. Therefore, clinical disease is not noted in the duck.

Sarcocystis rileyi can be diagnosed in the duck by a histological examination. However, because there are no clinical signs associated with this disease, a diagnosis is often made at necropsy. There is no effective treatment for this disease. Infection may be prevented by eliminating sources of feces excreted by definitive hosts. *Sarcocystis rileyi* does not infect humans.

Sarcocystis spp.

Unidentified *Sarcocystis* species have been recovered from the breast and thigh muscles of African grey parrots (*Psittacus erithacus*), Amazon parrots (*Amazona aestiva aestiva*), and budgerigars (*Melopsittacus undulatus*)[20].

Toxoplasma gondii

Toxoplasma gondii infects nearly all mammalian and many avian species. Susceptible bird species include chickens, pigeons, and canaries. The budgerigar is resistant to *T. gondii* infection[81]. The biology of *T. gondii* in the definitive host is discussed in Chapter 18, Parasites of Cats.

Avian intermediate hosts become infected by ingesting sporulated oocysts or contaminated tissues. Following ingestion, *T. gondii* disseminates via the blood and lymph to cause generalized infection and bradyzoite cyst formation. Commonly affected tissues include the spleen, lungs, liver, heart, and brain. *Toxoplasma gondii* is not pathogenic for chickens, but infected canaries develop nonsuppurative chorioretinitis, blindness, and torticollis[82,83]. Dubey and co-workers found that 16.9% of backyard chickens had antibodies to *T. gondii*, and viable *T. gondii* were recovered from 55% of seropositive chickens[83].

Diagnosis is by immunostaining of affected tissues, or by inoculation of experimental animals. There is no effective treatment for toxoplasmosis of birds. In canaries, trimethoprim (0.08 g/ml water) and sulfadiazine (0.04 g/ml water) for two weeks followed by a second treatment regimen given for three weeks was effective in relieving clinical signs[82]. To prevent infection in birds, food stocks must be protected from contamination with cat feces. *Toxoplasma gondii* is a common zoonosis. However, people working with infected birds would have to consume bird tissues to become infected.

Tyzzeria parvula

Tyzzeria parvula (Syn. *Eimeria anseris*, *E. parvula*, *T. anseris*) has been reported in the small intestines of geese. *Tyzzeria anseris* oocysts measure 10 μ to 16 μ by 9 μ to 14 μ. The sporozoites are banana-shaped. *Tyzzeria parvula* has been reported in domestic geese, white-fronted geese, snow geese (*Chen caerulescens*), Ross' geese (*Chen rossii*), Brant (Atlantic) geese (*Branta bernicla*), Canada geese (*Branta canadensis*), and possibly the whistling swan[1].

There is a lack of information on the life cycle of *T. parvula*. However, its prepatent period is four days[1]. *Tyzzeria parvula* is not pathogenic; therefore, clinical disease has not been observed. A definitive diagnosis can be made by identification of *T. parvula* in the feces. Treatment is not warranted. Proper sanitation and good management practices can reduce re-infection in the flock. *Tyzzeria parvula* does not infect humans.

Tyzzeria perniciosa

Tyzzeria perniciosa has been reported in the small intestines of ducks. *Tyzzeria perniciosa* oocysts measure 10 μ to 13 μ by 9 μ to 11 μ. *Tyzzeria perniciosa* has been reported in domestic ducks, pintails, lesser scaups (*Aythya affinis*) and another diving duck (*Aythya erythropus*).

The prepatent period is five days. *Tyzzeria perniciosa* is highly pathogenic. A common histopathologic finding is hemorrhagic enteritis. The intestinal wall is often thickened and white spots can be observed on the serosal surface. The intestinal lumen is filled with blood and can contain a yellowish exudate. The intestinal lumen is often sloughed in long strips. *Tyzzeria perniciosa* is especially pathogenic for young ducklings. Affected ducks stop eating, lose weight, become lethargic, and continuously emit vocalizations.

Diagnosis is by identification of *T. perniciosa* along with clinical signs and lesions. Specific treatment regimens for *T. perniciosa* are lacking. Proper sanitation and good management practices can reduce re-infection in the flock. *Tyzzeria perniciosa* does not infect humans.

Wenyonella anatis

Wenyonella anatis is found in the intestinal tract of ducks. Oocysts measure 11 μ to 17 μ by 7 μ to 10 μ. There is a lack of information on the life cycle of *W. anatis*. *Wenyonella anatis* is not pathogenic. Thus, clinical disease does not occur. Diagnosis is by identifying *W. anatis* in the feces. Treatment is not warranted. Proper sanitation and good management practices can reduce re-infection in the flock. *Weyonella anatis* does not infect humans.

Wenyonella columbae

Wenyonella columbae occurs in the small intestine of the pigeon. *Wenyonella columbae* oocysts measure 21 μ to 27 μ by 21 μ to 26 μ. Specific details on the life cycle of *Wenyonella columbae* are lacking. *Wenyonella columbae* is not pathogenic. Thus, clinical signs are not observed. Diagnosis is made by identifying *W. columbae* in the feces. Treatment is not warranted. Proper sanitation and good management practices can reduce re-infection in the flock. *Wenyonella columbae* does not infect humans.

Wenyonella gallinae

Wenyonella gallinae has been reported in the lower intestine of chickens. *Wenyonella gallinae* oocysts measure 29 μ to 34 μ by 20 μ to 23 μ. Specific details on the life cycle of *W. gallinae* are lacking. The intestines of infected birds are thickened and congested. Pinpoint hemorrhages are noted in the mucosa. Affected birds have greenish diarrhea.

Diagnosis is through identification of *W. gallinae* in the feces, along with clinical disease and lesions. Specific treatment regimens for *W. gallinae* are lacking. Proper sanitation and good management practices can reduce re-infection of the flock. *Wenyonella gallinae* does not infect humans.

Class Piroplasmidia

Babesia moshkovskii

Babesia moshkovskii (Syn. *Sogdianella moshkovskii*, *Babesia ardeae*, *Nuttallia shortti*, *Aegyptianella moshkovskii*) has been found in erythrocytes of chickens, turkeys, pheasants, and other wild birds[1]. The form in chickens measures 0.2 μ by 2.5 μ, while the form found in turkeys measures 0.5 μ by 2 μ[1]. Details on the life cycle of *B. moshkovskii* are lacking. Ticks have been reported to serve as vectors of *Babesia*. *Babesia moshkovskii* is not pathogenic. Thus, clinical disease has not been reported. Diagnosis is via identification of *B. moshkovskii* on stained blood smears. Treatment is not warranted. The elimination and control of ticks will aid in the prevention of *B. moshkovskii* infection. *Babesia moshkovskii* does not infect humans.

Class Haemosporidia

Haemoproteus columbae

Haemoproteus columbae is a haemosporidian found in the pigeon and other Columbiformes. Mature macrogametes and microgamonts are elongated and banana-shaped[1]. Birds become infected when they are bitten by the hippoboscid fly (*Pseudolynchia canariensis*)[1]. Merogony occurs in the endothelial cells of the blood vessels of the lungs, liver, and spleen. Merozoites undergo gametogony in erythrocytes. Oocyst formation occurs in the hippoboscid vector. Sporozoites migrate to the salivary gland, where they can be injected into a new host[1].

Haemoproteus columbae is not pathogenic. Thus, clinical disease is not observed. Diagnosis is by finding organisms in stained blood smears. Treatment is generally not warranted. However, in one study, dexamethasone lowered the level of parasitemia, the packed cell volume and the heterophil:lymphocyte ratio[84]. In addition, buparvaquone was effective, while diminazene aceturate was ineffective and triquine was toxic[85]. Prevention of *Haemoproteus* infections is accomplished through control of insect vectors. *Haemoproteus columbae* does not infect humans.

Haemoproteus spp.

Additional species of *Haemoproteus* infecting birds include *Haemoproteus coatneyi* in white-crowned sparrows[86];

H. handai in lesser sulphur-crested cockatoos[87]; *H. lophortyx* in bobwhite quail[88]; *H. meleagridis* in turkeys[89]; *H. nettionis* (Syn. *Parahaemoproteus nettionis, Haemoproteus anatis, H. hermani, H. anseris, Halteridium nettionis*) in waterfowl such as ducks, geese, and swans[1]; *H. picae* and *H. danilewskii* in American crows[44]; and *H. sacharovi* in Columbiformes such as doves and pigeons[1]. Most of these species are nonpathogenic in their avian hosts. Diagnosis is accomplished through microscopic examination of stained blood smears.

Leucocytozoon caulleryi

Morphology. Gamonts of *Leucocytozoon caulleryi* (Syn. *L. schueffneri, Akiba caulleryi*) are round and measure 15.5 μ by 15 μ in diameter.

Hosts and Life Cycle. *Leucocytozoon caulleryi* has been reported in chickens, guinea fowl, and pheasants. Mosquitoes become infected with *L. caulleryi* during ingestion of a blood meal. Gametogony occurs in the arthropod host. Following transmission of sporozoites to a susceptible bird, schizogony occurs in the kidney, liver, lungs, heart, spleen, pancreas, thymus, muscles, intestines, trachea, ovaries, adrenals, and brain[1].

Pathologic Effects. Pathogenicity varies with parasite strain. Mortality can be high. Pathologic changes include hemorrhages in the lung, liver, and kidneys, due to lysis of infected cells. Schizonts of *L. caulleryi* have been reported in the ovary and oviducts of chickens, and were associated with granulomatous and lymphocytic inflammation, edema, and pressure atrophy associated with these schizonts[90].

Clinical Disease. Affected chickens are anemic, lethargic, and have pale combs and diarrhea. Reduced egg production and soft-shelled eggs have been reported in chickens[90]. Chickens appear to be resistant to re-infection with *L. caulleryi*[91].

Diagnosis, Treatment, and Prevention. *Leucocytozoon* can be diagnosed on a stained blood smear. Specific treatment regimens for *L. caulleryi* are lacking. Control of *Culicoides* effectively prevents infection. A recombinant protein used as an antigen in an oil-in-water vaccine has been documented to be effective[92].

Public Health Considerations. *Leucocytozoon caulleryi* does not infect humans.

Leucocytozoon spp.

Additional species of *Leucocytozoon* infecting birds include *L. andrewsi* (Syn. *L. schoutedeni*) in chickens and pheasants; *L. lovati* (Syn. *L. bonasae, L. jakamowi, L. mansoni*) in grouse; *L. marchouxi* (Syn. *L. turtur*) in Columbiformes such as the turtle dove and mourning dove; *L. naevei* (Syn. *L. costai, L. numidae*) in guinea fowl; *L. sabrazesi* (Syn. *L. francolini, L. kerandeli, L. martini, L. macleani, L. mesnili, L. schuffneri*) in chickens, pheasants, and jungle fowl; *L. simondi* (Syn. *L. anatis, L. anseris*) in ducks and geese; and *L. smithi* in turkeys[1,93–96]. Several of these species are pathogenic in their avian hosts. Diagnosis is accomplished through microscopic examination of stained blood smears.

Plasmodium cathemerium

Morphology. Gamonts and meronts of *Plasmodium cathemerium* (Syn. *Haemamoeba cathemerium*) are round. The meronts produce six to 24 merozoites[1].

Hosts and Life Cycle. Passerines are the natural hosts of *P. cathemerium*. The life cycle is described in Chapter 2, Biology of the Protozoa. Briefly, sporozoites enter the blood through a mosquito bite and penetrate hepatic parenchymal cells, where they undergo schizogony[1]. Later, gametogony occurs in erythrocytes. Mosquitoes are infected while taking a blood meal. Oocysts form in the mosquito midgut. Sporozoites migrate to the mosquito salivary glands. Mosquito genera which can serve as hosts include *Culex, Aedes, Anopheles,* and *Culiseta*[1].

Pathologic Effects and Clinical Disease. *Plasmodium cathemerium* is highly pathogenic for canaries. Capillary abnormalities include endothelial degeneration and penetration of the endothelial cells by the parasites, with subsequent necrosis[97]. The skeletal muscle can also be a target tissue for *P. cathemerium*. Affected canaries have subcutaneous hemorrhages, anemia, splenomegaly, and hepatomegaly.

Diagnosis, Treatment, and Prevention. *Plasmodium cathemerium* is diagnosed by finding and identifying it on blood smears that are stained with a Romanowsky stain such as Giemsa. Treatment with chloroquine or pyrimethamine has been successful in some birds. Reinfection often occurs. Control of *P. cathemerium* is achieved through vector control.

Public Health Considerations. *Plasmodium cathemerium* is not zoonotic.

Plasmodium circumflexum

Plasmodium circumflexum (*Giovannolaia circumflexum*) has been found in birds in temperate zones[1]. The type host of *P. circumflexum* is the German thrush (*Turdus pilaris*). Other susceptible species include ruffed grouse, woodcocks, Canada geese, and ducks[1]. The gamonts and trophozoites are elongated. The life cycle of *P. circumflexum* is similar to those of other species in the genus. Vector mosquitoes include *Culex tarsalis, Culiseta annulata, Culiseta melaneura, Culiseta morsitans,* and *Mansonia crassipes*[1,98]. Clinical disease has not been reported with this parasite.

Diagnosis is by identifying blood smears stained with a Romanowsky stain, such as Giemsa. Treatment with chloroquine or pyrimethamine is sometimes successful. Re-infection often occurs. Infection with *P. circumflexum* can be prevented with the use of mosquito (vector) control strategies. *Plasmodium circumflexum* does not infect humans

Plasmodium spp.

Several other species of *Plasmodium* have been found in birds. These include *Plasmodium durae* (*Giovannolaia durae*) in turkeys; *P. fallax* in guinea fowl; *P. gallinaceum* (Syn. *Haemamoeba gallinaceum*) in jungle fowl and other gallinaceous birds; *P. hermani* (Syn. *Huffia hermani*) in turkeys and bobwhite quail; *P. juxtanucleare* (Syn. *P. japonicum, Novyella juxtanucleare*) in chickens and other gallinaceous birds; *P. matutinum* (Syn. *Haemamoeba matutinum, P. relictum matutinum*) in wild bird species; and *P. relictum* (Syn. *Haemamoeba relictum, P. praecox*) in pigeons, doves, ducks, passerines, and others[1,99,100]. Most of these species are nonpathogenic in their avian hosts. Diagnosis and treatment are as described for *P. cathemerium*.

TREMATODES

Collyriclum faba

Collyriclum faba has been reported in the skin and subcutaneous tissues of Galliformes and Passeriformes[101,102]. *Collyriclum faba* belongs to the Troglotrematid family of flukes. Specific details on the morphology and life cycle of *C. faba* are lacking. Infection is usually unapparent, though some birds may become anemic and emaciated. Diagnosis is by identifying adult flukes in the subcutaneous tissues. No effective treatment is available. Control of the intermediate hosts prevents the transmission of *C. faba*. *Collyriclum faba* is not known to infect humans.

Echinoparyphium recurvatum

Echinoparyphium recurvatum has been reported in the small intestines of chickens, turkeys, ducks, pigeons, and other birds. It belongs to the Echinostomatid family of flukes. Snails serve as first intermediate hosts, while other snails, and frogs serve as second intermediate hosts.

Chickens become infected through the ingestion of second intermediate hosts[103]. Infection may result in emaciation, anemia, and weakness. Enteritis is a common postmortem finding. Affected birds are lethargic and have diarrhea.

A diagnosis is made by identifying the eggs in the feces or the flukes within the intestines. No effective treatment is available. Control of the intermediate host prevents disease transmission. Morley and co-workers reported that parasite viability was associated with survival of the host snail[104]. Tributyltin, copper, or irgarol 1051 may be used to control snail populations. *Echinoparyphium recurvatum* has also been reported from dogs, cats, rats, and primates, including humans. However, there is no danger of direct transmission of infection from birds to humans.

Hypoderaeum conoideum

Hypoderaeum conoideum has been reported in the small intestine of chickens and other birds. It belongs to the Echinostomatid family of flukes. Specific details on the life cycle of *H. conoideum* are unknown. However, ingestion of an infected mollusk, i.e., a snail, is an essential part of the transmission cycle. Munoz-Antoli and co-workers reported that the freshwater snail, *Lymnaea peregra*, serves as the natural first intermediate host[105]. Other freshwater snails, *Physella acuta* and *Gyraulus chinensis*, can serve as second intermediate hosts. The pathologic effects and clinical signs of *H. conoideum* infection in chickens and other avian species remain unknown.

A diagnosis is made by identifying the *H. conoideum* eggs in the feces or the adults in the small intestines. No effective treatment is available. The control of the intermediate host can help to interrupt the transmission cycle. *Hypoderaeum conoideum* has not been reported in humans.

Prosthogonimus spp.

Morphology. Adult *Prosthogonimus* are 6 mm to 8 mm long and 5 mm to 6 mm wide, and have spiny cuticles (Figure 10.6). The *Prosthogonimus* eggs, which measure 26 μ to 32 μm by 10 μ to 15 μm, have an operculum on one end and a small spine on the other end.

Hosts. *Prosthogonimus* species have been found in the bursa of Fabricius and oviduct of chickens and other birds[101]. Parasite species identified include *P. macrorchis*

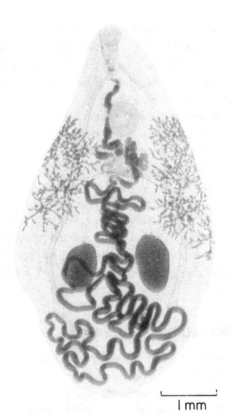

Fig. 10.6 Adult *Prosthogonimus macrorchis.* Courtesy of Marietta Voge, University of California.

(U.S.), *P. pellucidus* (Europe), *P. ovatus* (Europe, Asia, Africa), and *P. longus-morbificans* (Europe).

Life Cycle. Adult flukes shed their eggs in the feces. Two intermediate hosts, a snail and dragonfly, are needed to perpetuate the life cycle. Infection occurs via ingestion of an infected insect. Metacercariae are released in the small intestines and subsequently migrate to the cloaca. Finally, they migrate to the bursa of Fabricius or to the oviduct, where maturation occurs[106].

Pathologic Effects and Clinical Disease. Pathologic changes include inflammation of the oviduct and associated coelomitis. Leok and co-workers reported degeneration and exfoliation of the mucosal epithelium in the bursa[107]. Affected birds are inappetent and have reduced weight gains, decreased egg production, and malformed eggs[101].

Diagnosis, Treatment, and Prevention. Diagnosis is by identification of fluke eggs in the feces or flukes in the oviduct[101]. There is no effective treatment. Elimination of the intermediate hosts prevents infection.

Public Health Considerations. *Prosthogonimus* do not infect humans.

CESTODES
Cyclophyllidea
Amoebotaenia cuneata

Amoebotaenia cuneata measures 4 mm long. The anterior end is triangular in shape due to the pointed scolex. The rostellum is armed with a single row of 12 to 14 distinctive hooks that are 25 μ to 32 μ long[108]. *Amoebotaenia cuneata* has been recovered from the small intestine of chickens and other avian species[101]. Gravid proglottids passed in the feces are ingested by an earthworm intermediate host. Earthworm species that have served as intermediate hosts include the genus *Allotophora, Pheritima, Ocnerodrilus,* and *Lumbricus*[108]. *Amoebotaenia cuneata* is not pathologic. Thus, clinical disease is not observed.

Diagnosis is by identifying gravid proglottids in feces or adult worms in the intestines, where they appear as white projections among the duodenal villi. Treatment is generally not warranted. Control of the intermediate host helps prevent completion of the transmission cycle. *Amoebotaenia cuneata* does not infect humans.

Choanotaenia infundibulum

Morphology. Adult *Choanotaenia infundibulum* measure up to 23 cm long, and possess an armed rostellum bearing a single row of 16 to 22 hooks that are 25 μ to 30 μ long each. The eggs of *C. infundibulum* have elongated filaments and embryonal hooks that measure 18 μ long[108].

Hosts and Life Cycle. *Choanotaenia infundibulum* has been reported in the small intestine of chickens and other birds[101,108]. Gravid proglottids are passed in the feces and are ingested by intermediate hosts, including horseflies, houseflies, grasshoppers, termites, and beetles[108,109].

Pathologic Effects and Clinical Disease. *Choanotaenia infundibulum* is nonpathogenic unless present in high numbers. It is usually not associated with clinical disease.

Diagnosis, Treatment, and Prevention. Diagnosis is by identifying gravid proglottids in the feces or adult worms in the intestine. Dibutyltin dilaurate has been used effectively for treatment for *C. infundibulum* infections[108]. Control of the intermediate host disrupts completion of the transmission cycle.

Public Health Considerations. *Choanotaenia infundibulum* does not infect humans.

Davainea proglottina

Morphology. Adult *Davainea proglottina* (Syn. *Taenia proglottina*) measure up to 4 mm long and have no more than nine proglottids. The rostellum is armed with three to six rows of hooks[101] (Figure 10.7).

Hosts. *Davainea proglottina* has been reported in the duodenum of chickens, pigeons, and other birds[101,111].

Life Cycle. Gravid segments contain *D. proglottina* eggs, which hatch when ingested by a snail or slug. Development of the infective larval stage in the intermediate host occurs in three to four weeks. Birds become infected upon ingestion of the intermediate host. Maturation requires about two weeks. More than 1,500 cysticercoids may develop in the slug intestinal tract and can remain

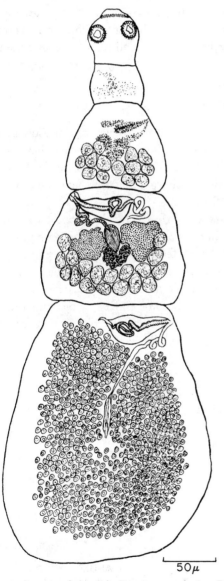

Fig. 10.7 A diagram of an adult *Davainea proglottina*. Reproduced from Lapage, G. (1962) with permission.

infective for up to 11 months[108]. *Davainea proglottina* have been documented to live as long as three years[108].

Pathologic Effects. *Davainea proglottina* is highly pathogenic. Up to 4,000 tapeworms have been reported in a single infection[111]. Hemorrhagic enteritis occurs due to the attachment of adult tapeworms on the duodenal mucosa, which results in inflammation, hemorrhage, and mucosal thickening.

Clinical Disease. Affected birds have diarrhea, lethargy, and ruffled feathers. Levine reported a 12% reduction in weight in affected birds[112].

Diagnosis, Treatment, and Prevention. Diagnosis is by identifying the gravid proglottids in the feces or the adult tapeworms in intestinal scrapings[101]. The tapeworm may be eliminated with Butynorate (dibutyltin dilaurate), which is approved for treatment of *D. proglottina*. Control of the intermediate host prevents transmission.

Public Health Considerations. *Davainea proglottina* is not zoonotic.

Fimbriaria fasciolaris

Fimbriaria fasciolaris adult worms measure 5 cm to 43 cm long by 1 mm to 5 mm wide. Adult worms have a distinctive flaring anterior neck region (pseudoscolex) and unsegmented strobila. The rostellum is armed with 10 to 12 hooks measuring 17 μ to 27 μm in length[108]. *Fimbriaria fasciolaris* has been reported in the small intestine of anseriformes and chickens[101,111]. Tapeworm cysticercoids of *F. fasciolaris* develop in a copepod crustacean (*Diaptomus* sp. or *Cyclops* sp.). Birds subsequently become infected when they drink water containing infected copepods[108]. *Fimbriaria fasciolaris* is nonpathogenic. Thus, clinical disease is not observed.

Diagnosis is by identifying the proglottids in the feces or the adults in the intestines. Treatment is generally not warranted. Reducing exposure to contaminated water containing the infected copepods prevents infection. *Fimbriaria fasciolaris* is not zoonotic.

Hymenolepis cantaniana

Hymenolepis cantaniana is 2 cm long and 1 mm wide, and bears rostellar hooks[108]. *Hymenolepis cantaniana* has been reported in the small intestine of chickens and other birds[111]. Specific details on the life cycle of *H. cantaniana* are sparse. It is known that the dung beetle serves as the intermediate host[108]. Each beetle can carry 100 or more cysticercoids. *Hymenolepis cantaniana* is considered nonpathogenic; therefore, clinical disease is not observed.

A definitive diagnosis is made by identifying the gravid proglottids in the feces or the adults in the intestines. Because *H. cantaniana* is considered nonpathogenic, treatment is not needed. Control of the intermediate host aids in the prevention of *H. cantaniana* infection. *Hymenolepis cantaniana* has not been reported in humans.

Hymenolepis carioca

Morphology. *Hymenolepis carioca* is a slender, threadlike worm measuring 3 cm to 8 cm long and 0.5 mm wide. The rostellum is unarmed, but rostellar sacs are present[108].

Hosts and Life Cycle. *Hymenolepis carioca* occurs in the intestines of the chicken and other avian species[111]. Details on the life cycle of *H. carioca* are lacking. Birds become infected by ingesting an insect intermediate host, usually a beetle (Figure 10.8)[113]. Dung beetles or ground beetles are the most common source of infection[108]. The metacestode stage develops in the insect and the adult stage develops in the chicken two to four days post-infection.

Pathologic Effects and Clinical Disease. *Hymenolepis carioca* is not usually considered pathogenic. Birds have been known to harbor several hundred worms without any pathologic lesions[108]. However, Jha and co-workers reported chronic inflammation and enteritis in birds infected with *H. carioca*[114]. Because *H. carioca* is usually nonpathogenic, clinical disease is not observed.

Diagnosis, Treatment, and Prevention. Diagnosis is by identification of the gravid proglottids in the feces or the adult tapeworm in the intestines. Butynorate (dibutyltin dilaurate) is the only approved drug for the treatment of *H. carioca* infection[108]. It can be administered at the level of 500 mg/kg of feed[115]. Control of the intermediate host (beetles) prevents disease transmission.

Public Health Considerations. *Hymenolepis carioca* has not been reported in humans.

Hymenolepis megalops

Hymenolepis megalops is a small tapeworm. Adult worms measure 3 mm to 6 mm long and bear a 1-mm to 2-mm scolex[108]. The rostellum is unarmed. *Hymenolepis megalops* has been recovered from the cloaca or bursa of Fabricius of waterfowl[108]. Gravid proglottids are passed in the feces and are ingested by an ostracod crustacean. Waterfowl subsequently become infected after eating the infected intermediate host[108]. *Hymenolepis megalops* is considered pathogenic but few details are available. Likewise, details on the clinical manifestations for *H. megalops* are scarce. As for other members of the genus, dibutyltin dilaurate would probably be effective. Control of the intermediate host prevents transmission. *Hymenolepis megalops* is not zoonotic.

Raillietina cesticillus

Morphology. Adult *R. cesticillus* can measure up to 15 cm long[108]. It has a distinctive scolex, which has a wide rostellum with 300 to 500 hammer-shaped hooks[108]. Gravid proglottids contain eggs that are 75 μ to 88 μm in diameter (Figure 10.9).

Hosts and Life Cycle. *Raillietina cesticillus* has been reported in the small intestine of chickens and other avian species[101,111,116]. Gravid proglottids are passed in the feces and ingested by an intermediate host (Figure 10.10). More than 100 species of beetles can serve as intermediate host[108]. Birds become infected by ingesting infected beetles. It takes approximately two to four weeks to complete the tapeworm life cycle.

TRANSMISSION OF HYMENOLEPIS CARIOCA

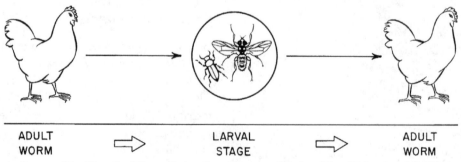

ADULT WORM   LARVAL STAGE   ADULT WORM

Fig. 10.8   A schematic diagram of the life cycle of *Hymenolepis carioca.* Courtesy of Marietta Voge, University of California.

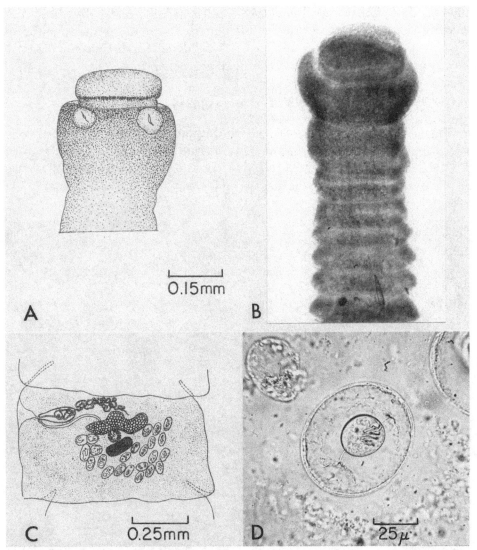

Fig. 10.9 *Raillietina cesticillus.* (A), (B) Scolex with distinctively shaped rostellum. (C) Mature proglottid. (D) Egg. (A),(C) Reproduced from Wehr, E.E. (1965) with permission. (B),(D) Courtesy of W.M. Reid, University of Georgia.

TRANSMISSION OF RAILLIETINA CESTICILLUS

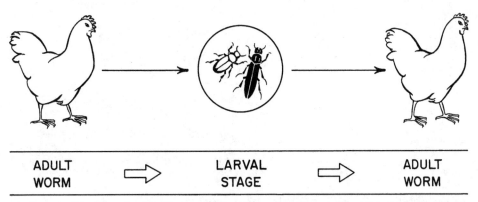

Fig. 10.10 A schematic diagram of the life cycle of *Raillietina cesticillus.* Courtesy of Marietta Voge, University of California.

Pathologic Effects and Clinical Disease. Pathologic findings include enteritis with degeneration of epithelial cells, infiltration by macrophages and lymphocytes, and proliferation of connective tissue[114]. Clinical disease is not observed in birds affected with *R. cesticillus.*

Diagnosis, Treatment, and Prevention. Diagnosis is by identification of the gravid proglottids in the feces, or the adult tapeworm in the small intestines. Butynorate (dibutyltin dilaurate) is approved for the treatment of *R. cesticillus* infection[117]. Pote and co-workers reported 100% efficacy of fenbendazole when administered in the diet at 240 ppm (104.3 mg/kg BW) for six days[118]. Control of the intermediate host prevents completion of the life cycle.

Public Health Considerations. *Raillietina cesticillus* is not zoonotic.

Raillietina echinobothrida

Morphology. Adult *Raillietina echinobothrida* worms measure up to 25 cm in length[116]. The rostellum is armed with two rows of large hooks[116]. Gravid proglottids contain eight to 12 eggs each (Figure 10.11)[119].

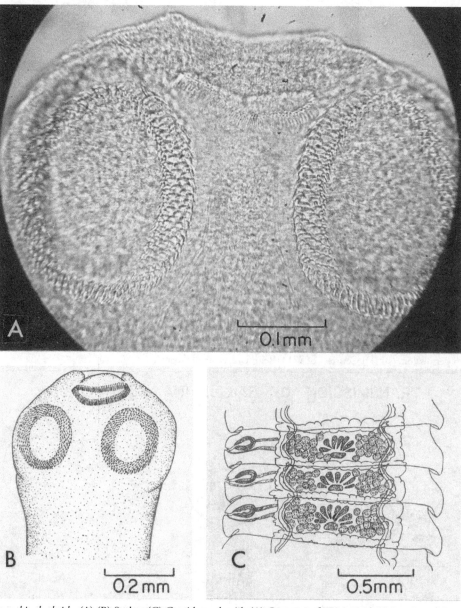

Fig. 10.11 *Raillietina echinobothrida.* (A),(B) Scolex. (C) Gravid proglottid. (A) Courtesy of W.M. Reid, University of Georgia. (B) Reproduced from Lapage, G. (1962) with permission. (C) Reproduced from Wardle, R.A. and McLeod, J.A. (1952) with permission.

Hosts. *Raillietina echinobothrida* has been reported in the small intestine of chickens, grey quails (*Coturnix coturnix*), and other birds[111,116,120].

Life Cycle. Gravid proglottids are passed in the feces and ingested by an ant, the intermediate host[111]. These eggs hatch and develop into infective larvae within the ant's body cavity[121]. The avian host becomes infected by ingesting an infected ant. It takes three weeks to complete the life cycle of *R. echinobothrida*.

Pathologic Effects and Clinical Disease. *Raillietina echinobothrida* is highly pathogenic and causes intestinal wall nodules due to worm penetration. Nodules measure 1 mm to 6 mm in diameter[122], and are visible on the serosal surface (Figure 10.12). In addition, catarrhal, hyperplastic enteritis with lymphocytic, polymorphonuclear, and eosinophilic infiltrates has been reported with *R. echinobothrida* infections[108]. Samad and co-workers reported anemia with an increase in total leukocyte counts, and a decrease in total serum protein[123]. Affected birds are weak, emaciated, and often have diarrhea[116]. Anemia has also been noted[123].

Diagnosis, Treatment, and Prevention. Diagnosis is by finding gravid proglottids in the feces, along with clinical signs and pathological lesions. Treatment with dibutyltin dilaurate is most likely effective. Ant control disrupts the transmission cycle.

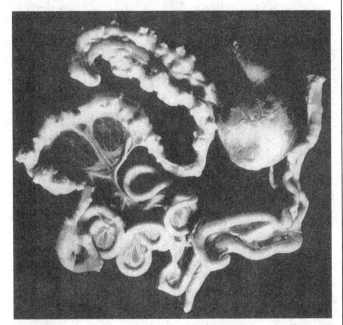

Fig. 10.12 Lesions produced by *Raillietina echinobothrida* in the chicken intestine. Reproduced from Wehr, E.E. (1965) with permission.

Public Health Considerations. *Raillietina echinobothrida* is not zoonotic.

Raillietina georgiensis

Adult *Raillietina georgiensis* measure 15 cm to 38 cm by 3.5 mm. The scolex bears two rows of 230 rostellar hooks that are 12 μm to 23 μm long and have eight to 10 circles of 8-μ to 13-μ acetabular hooks[108].

Raillietina georgiensis is found in the small intestine of turkeys. Gravid proglottids passed in the feces are ingested by a small brown ant (*Pheidole vinelandica*). The eggs hatch and infective larvae develop in the ant's body cavity. It takes approximately three weeks to complete the life cycle[108]. Severely infected birds develop enteritis. However, most birds do not show any clinical signs of disease.

Diagnosis is by identifying gravid proglottids in the feces or adults in the intestines. Dibutyltin dilaurate is probably effective against *R. georgiensis* but it is not registered for use against turkey tapeworms[108]. Control of the intermediate host prevents completion of the transmission cycle. *Raillietina georgiensis* does not infect humans.

Raillietina tetragona

Morphology. Adult *Raillietina tetragona* measure up to 25 cm long and 3 mm wide. The tapeworm is distinguished from other members of the genus by its oval suckers, which have eight to 12 rows of 3-μm to 8-μm long hooks. The rostellum is armed with 90 to 100 hooks measuring 6 μ to 8 μ long. These are arranged in either single or double row[108].

Hosts and Life Cycle. *Raillietina tetragona* has been reported in the small intestine of chickens, pigeons, and other birds[116]. The life cycle of *R. tetragona* is similar to that of *R. echinobothrida*[116]. The ant is the intermediate host[116].

Pathologic Effects and Clinical Disease. Reduced glycogen levels in the liver and intestinal mucosa have been found in birds infected with *R. tetragona*[124]. Jha and co-workers reported enteritis with epithelial cell degeneration, lymphocyte and macrophage infiltration, and connective tissue proliferation. Total white blood cells were also diminished[114,125]. Nadakal and Nair reported weight loss and decreased egg production in experimentally infected birds[124].

Diagnosis, Treatment, and Prevention. Diagnosis is by identifying proglottids in the feces or adults in the intestine. Dibutyltin dilaurate has been an effective treatment for *R. tetragona*. Oral oxfendazole was 100%

effective in chickens at 7.5 mg/kg for adult tapeworms and 10 mg/kg for immature tapeworms[126]. Likewise, praziquantel was 100% effective at 5 mg/kg, 7.5 mg/kg, or 10 mg/kg for immature tapeworms and 100% effective at 10 mg/kg for adult tapeworms in chickens[127]. In addition, Rajendran and Nadakal[128] reported that praziquantel at a dosage of 0.15 ml/kg in liquid form was also effective when given intramuscularly in the chicken. Elowni and co-workers did not find niclosamide to be effective[129]. Control of the intermediate host disrupts transmission.

Public Health Considerations. *Raillietina tetragona* does not infect humans.

NEMATODES

Superfamily Rhabditoidea

Strongyloides avium

Strongyloides avium has been reported in chickens, turkeys, geese, grouse, and quail[130,131]. Infection occurs through ingestion of the infective, free-living larvae[130]. Adult female worms inhabit the small intestine and ceca. First-stage larvae are passed in the feces. Larvae reach the infective third stage in the environment. *Strongyloides avium* is pathogenic in young birds, where it causes enteritis and a cecal wall thickening. Adult birds show no clinical signs of infection, while young birds develop bloody diarrhea[130].

Diagnosis is by identifying the larvae in the feces, using a direct smear or Baermann technique, along with clinical signs and lesions. Adult worms can also be identified in the small intestines and cecum. Tetramisole has some efficacy against *S. avium*[131]. Proper sanitation and good management are important for preventing infection with *S. avium*. Frequent removal of the feces can limit the spread of infection. *Strongyloides avium* has not been reported in humans.

Strongyloides oswaldoi

Strongyloides oswaldoi has been reported in the small intestines of chickens[132]. The life cycle is similar to that of *S. avium*. *Strongyloides oswaldoi* is pathogenic in young birds but not in adults. Enteritis and a thickened cecal wall have been reported in young birds. Adult birds have unapparent infections. Affected younger birds often have bloody diarrhea[132]. Diagnosis and prevention of *S. oswaldoi* are as described for *S. avium*.

Superfamily Heterakoidea

Ascaridia bonasae

Ascaridia bonasae has been found in the small intestine of the grouse. This species has often been mistaken for *A. galli* but it is smaller in size. Males measure 10 mm to 35 mm with 1.8-mm to 2.7-mm spicules of equal length. Females measure 30 mm to 50 mm in length[131]. The life cycle of *A. bonasae* is similar to that of *A. galli*. It is unknown whether *A. bonasae* causes pathologic changes or clinical disease. Diagnosis, treatment, and prevention are as described for *A. galli*. *Ascaridia bonasae* does not infect humans.

Ascaridia columbae

Ascaridia columbae has been reported in the small intestine, esophagus, proventriculus, gizzard, liver and coelomic cavity of pigeons and doves[131]. Geese and chukars may serve as paratenic hosts[133]. Adult male *A. columbae* measure 50 mm to 70 mm long and possess 1.2-mm to 1.9-mm spicules of equal length. Unlike other avian *Ascaridia* species, *A. columbae* males have the fourth pair of ventral papillae located adjacent to the anus. Females measure 20 mm to 95 mm[131]. The life cycle of *A. columbae* is similar to that of *A. galli*, except that the second larval stage can penetrate the intestines to reach the lung and liver, where further development does not occur[134]. *Ascaridia columbae* larvae migrate to the liver and produce granulomatous lesions with leucocytic infiltration[134]. Affected birds may develop diarrhea.

Diagnosis, treatment, and prevention are as described for *A. galli*. *Ascaridia columbae* is not zoonotic.

Ascaridia compar

Ascaridia compar is found in the small intestines of grouse, partridges, pheasants, and quail. Adult male worms measure 36 mm to 48 mm long and have 1.8-mm long spicules. Unlike other *Ascaridia* sp., *A. compar* males possess four pairs of pre-anal papillae (two pairs located near the pre-anal sucker and two pairs anterior to the anus). Adult females measure 84 mm to 96 mm long[131]. The life cycle of *A. compar* is similar to that of *A. galli*. Vassilev[135] reported that *A. compar* in partridges develops only in the lumen and does not penetrate the intestinal wall. The larvae undergo a two-stage molt which occurs at six to seven days and then at 12 to 13 days post-infection. *Ascaridia compar* eggs can remain viable for at least 493 days[135]. Pathologic changes and clinical disease caused by *A. compar* have not been described.

Diagnosis, treatment[33], and prevention are as described for *A. galli*. *Ascaridia compar* is not zoonotic.

Ascaridia dissimilis

Ascaridia dissimilis has been reported in the small intestines of turkeys. *Ascaridia dissimilis* is similar to *A. galli* in morphology. Males measure 35 mm to 65 mm in length and possess 1.3-mm to 2.2-mm long spicules that have rounded ends. Unlike other members of the genus, males have the first pair of pre-anal papillae opposite the pre-anal sucker, and the closely adjacent ventral pair of post-anal papillae directly behind the anus. Females measure 50 mm to 105 mm[131]. The life cycle of *A. dissimilis* is similar to that of *A. galli*. However, *A. dissimilis* eggs embryonate in nine to 10 days and the larvae mature in the lumen around 30 days. *Ascaridia dissimilis* eggs can survive on the turkey egg shell[136]. Mortality has been associated with heavy worm burdens of *A. dissimilis*[137,138]. A high number of turkey flocks are affected with *A. dissimilis*[139] and aberrant migration of *A. dissimilis* has resulted in white hepatic foci as a result of granuloma formation[140]. Affected birds develop diarrhea[141].

Diagnosis, treatment[142], and prevention are as described for *A. galli*. *Ascaridia dissimilis* is not zoonotic.

Ascaridia galli

Morphology. *Ascaridia galli* (Syn. *Ascaridia lineata*) (the "chicken roundworm") is a large, white worm that has three large lips[131]. Males range in size from 50 mm to 76 mm long by 490 μ to 1210 μ wide. There is a circular pre-anal sucker with a chitinous wall. The tail has narrow caudal alae and 10 pair of papillae. The first pair of ventral caudal papillae is anterior to the pre-anal sucker, while the fourth pair is separated from the other pairs (Figure 10.13). The spicules are symmetrical and narrow, and there is a slight indentation of the tail. The female worm measures 60 mm to 116 mm by 900 μ to 1,800 μ. The eggs of *A. galli* are elliptical and thick-shelled, and measure 70 μ to 80 μ by 45 μ to 50 μ[131,143] (Figure 10.14).

Hosts. *Ascaridia galli* has been reported in the small intestine of chickens, turkeys, doves, ducks, geese, and guinea fowl[131].

Life Cycle. The life cycle of *A. galli* is direct. Transmission is via ingestion of an embryonated egg, which hatches in the proventriculus or duodenum. Larvae live free in the duodenum for nine days before penetrating the mucosa[131]. They return to the lumen eight to nine days later, where they mature by 28 to 30 days post-ingestion[131]. Grasshoppers and

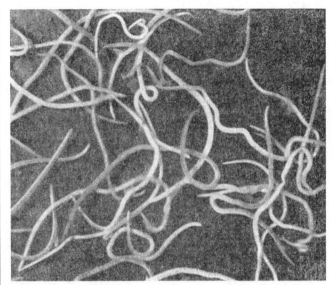

Fig. 10.13 *Ascaridia galli* from the chicken small intestine. Reproduced from Wehr, E.E. (1965) with permission.

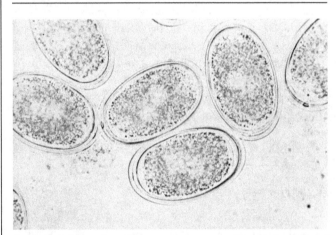

Fig. 10.14 *Ascaridia galli* eggs at 400 × magnification. Reproduced from Benbrook, E.A. and Sloss, M.W. (1961) with permission.

earthworms can ingest the infective egg and remain infective to the bird host, although no development occurs in these paratenic hosts. Adult *A. galli* pass eggs, which become infective in 10 to 12 days, in the feces. Eggs are very resistant to environmental stress, such as low temperature, and can survive for prolonged periods of time in the environment. Resistance to *A. galli* infection may involve genetic factors[144].

Pathologic Effects and Clinical Disease. Pathologic effects have been associated with severe *A. galli* infection, and include intestinal blockage, weight loss, anemia, hypoglycemia, increased urates, atrophic thymus glands, depressed growth, and death[145]. Although anemia was present, there were no effects on blood protein levels, packed cell volumes, or hemoglobin levels[146]. Total leukocyte counts were elevated[147]. Infection with *A. galli* may exacerbate other disease conditions and may facilitate transmission of avian reoviruses[131]. Worms have also been recovered from bird eggs[148]. Affected birds may develop diarrhea and weight loss.

Diagnosis. Diagnosis is by identification of *A. galli* eggs in the feces or adult worms in the small intestine, along with clinical signs and lesions.

Treatment. Effective treatments include piperazine compounds. For chickens and turkeys, piperazine can be given in the water (0.1% to 0.2%). Chickens otherwise can be given a single oral treatment of 50 to 100 mg/bird. Turkeys younger than 12 weeks should receive 100 mg/bird orally, while those older than 12 weeks should receive 100 to 400 mg/bird orally[131]. Levamisole (25 mg/kg) was more effective than thiabendazole (70 mg/kg) when given orally for four days. A water-suspensible fenbendazole at 60.6 ppm in the drinking water via automatic medicators for six hours on three consecutive days was also effective[149]. Ivermectin, 0.07 to 0.14 mg/kg per adult guinea fowl, was effective when given subcutaneously[150].

Prevention. Proper sanitation and good management practices are effective control strategies. Because the eggs do not embryonate until 10 to 12 days, proper sanitation and good management practices aid in preventing infections.

Public Health Considerations. *Ascaridia galli* has not been reported in humans.

Ascaridia numidae

Ascaridia numidae has been reported in the small intestine and cecum of guinea fowl. *Ascaridia numidae* is smaller than *A. galli*. Males measure 19 mm to 35 mm long and possess 3-mm spicules. Males also have 10 pairs of caudal papillae; two pairs are pre-anal and two pairs are adanal. Females measure 30 mm to 50 mm long[131]. The life cycle of *A. numidae* is similar to that of *A. galli* except that *A. numidae* larvae remain in the lumen for four to 14 days prior to penetration of the small intestinal mucosa[131]. The pathologic changes found in birds infected with *A. numidae* have not been fully described. Affected birds can have diarrhea. Diagnosis, treatment, and prevention are as described for *A. galli*. *Ascaridia numidae* is not of public health concern.

Heterakis dispar

Morphology. Adult male worms measure 7 mm to 18 mm long and have a pre-anal sucker that measures 109 μ to 256 μ in diameter with 390-μ to 730-μ spicules. Females measure 16 mm to 23 mm. Eggs of *H. dispar* are 59 μ to 62 μ by 39 μ to 41 μ[131].

Hosts and Life Cycle. *Heterakis dispar* has been identified in the ceca of ducks and geese[131]. Eggs pass out in the feces and become infective in approximately two weeks. Following ingestion by a suitable avian host, eggs hatch in the upper intestine, and the larvae migrate to the cecum within 24 hours. Alternatively, eggs passed in the feces may also be ingested by an earthworm. Birds ingesting earthworms carrying larval *H. dispar* also become infected[131].

Pathologic Effects and Clinical Disease. *Heterakis dispar* is nonpathogenic. Thus, clinical signs are not observed.

Diagnosis, Treatment, and Prevention. A definitive diagnosis is made by identification of the *H. dispar* eggs in the feces or adult worms in the cecum. Fenbendazole has been effective in the treatment of *H. gallinarum* in turkeys and chickens and would likely be an effective treatment for *H. dispar*. Proper sanitation and good hygiene help prevent transmission of *H. dispar*. Frequent removal of feces reduces environmental contamination.

Public Health Considerations. *Heterakis dispar* does not infect humans.

Heterakis gallinarum

Morphology. *Heterakis gallinarum* (the "cecal worm") is a white worm that has three equal-sized lips, lateral membranes that extend the length of the body, and an esophagus that has a well-developed bulb and valvular apparatus[131]. Males measure 7 mm to 13 mm long and have a straight tail, two large lateral bursal wings, a well-developed pre-anal sucker, 12 pairs of caudal papillae, and asymmetrical spicules (one measuring 0.85 mm to 2.8 mm long and the other measuring 0.37 mm to 1.1 mm long with a curved tip)[131]. Females are 10 mm to 15 mm long and have a narrow pointed tail (Figure 10.15)[151]. The eggs of *H. gallinarum* have a thick shell, are elliptical, and measure 63 μ to 75 μ by 36 μ to 50 μ[131] (Figure 10.16).

Hosts. *Heterakis gallinarum* has been found in the ceca of chickens, ducks, geese, grouse, guinea fowl, partridges, pheasants, quail, turkeys, and other birds[131].

Life Cycle. Eggs are passed in the feces and embryonate in the environment within two weeks. These infective eggs are ingested and the larvae are hatched within the small intestine and migrate to the ceca. Earthworms can also ingest eggs of *H. gallinarum* and thus serve as a source

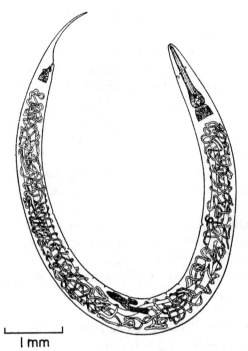

Fig. 10.15 *Heterakis gallinarum* female. Reproduced from Lapage, G. (1968) with permission.

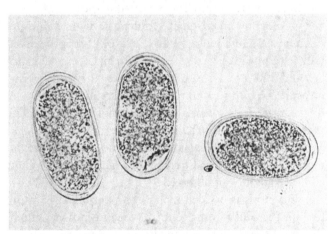

Fig. 10.16 *Heterakis gallinarum* egg at 410 × magnification. Reproduced from Benbrook, E.A. and Sloss, M.W. (1961) with permission.

of infection for birds[131]. Cecal worm ova can also serve as a carrier for the protozoan *Histomonas meleagridis*.

Pathologic Effects and Clinical Disease. Ring-necked pheasants, guinea fowl, and chickens are more susceptible to disease than are other avian species[152]. *Heterakis gallinarum* causes inflammation and thickening of the cecal wall. In the pheasant, pathologic changes include congestion, petechial hemorrhages, and thickening of the mucosa consistent with a chronic diffuse typhlitis[211].

Mucosal and submucosal cecal nodules have been reported in severe cases[153]. Hepatic granulomas have been reported in the chicken[154]. Clinical disease is uncommon in birds infected with *H. gallinarum*.

Diagnosis, Treatment, and Prevention. Diagnosis is by identifying *H. gallinarum* eggs in the feces or adults in the cecum. Fenbendazole eliminates infection with *H. gallinarum* when administered at a dose of 120 ppm in the feed for three days or 45 ppm for six days for turkeys[155], and 30 ppm for five or six days or 60 ppm for three days in chickens[156]. Pullet hens may be treated with fenbendazole (30 ppm or 60 ppm in the feed for five days)[157]. Liquid piperazine diluted to 3 ml of solution/liter drinking water to provide 30 to 50 mg of piperazine per liter has proven effective for treating infected quail[33]. Lastly, ivermectin (0.07 or 0.14 mg/kg per adult bird subcutaneous [SQ]) was effective in guinea fowl[150]. Proper sanitation and good management practices are effective control strategies. Frequent manure removal reduces worm development and further contamination of the environment.

Public Health Considerations. *Heterakis gallinarum* does not infect humans.

Heterakis isolonche

Morphology. *Heterakis isolonche* is similar in morphology to *H. gallinarum*. Males are 5.9 mm to 15 mm long; have a 70-μ to 150-μ diameter pre-anal sucker; and long, symmetrical 0.72-μ to 2.33-μ spicules. Female worms measure 9 mm to 12 mm long. Eggs of *H. isolonche* are 65 μ to 75 μ by 37 μ to 46 μ.

Hosts and Life Cycle. *Heterakis isolonche* has been recovered from the ceca of ducks, grouse, pheasants, prairie chickens, quail, and turkeys[131,158]. The life cycle of *H. isolonche* is similar to that of *H. gallinarum*.

Pathologic Effects and Clinical Disease. Severe mortality, up to 50%, has been reported in infected pheasants[131]. *Heterakis isolonche* invades the cecal mucosa and causes lymphocytic infiltration and granulation resulting in nodule formation. These nodules can coalesce to form a thickened cecal wall[131]. In pheasants and turkeys, nodules are composed of granulomata and fibrous hyperplastic tissue[158]. Pathology is not observed in the quail or grouse. Affected birds may lose weight and have diarrhea.

Diagnosis, Treatment, and Prevention. Diagnosis is by identifying *H. isolonche* eggs in the feces or adult worms in the ceca. Fenbendazole is most likely effective, since it is recommended in the treatment of *H. gallinarum* infection. Proper sanitation and good management practices are effective control strategies. Frequent manure removal reduces environmental contamination.

Public Health Considerations. *Heterakis isolonche* has not been reported in humans.

Superfamily Subuluroidea

Aulonocephalus lindquisti

Aulonocephalus lindquisti are red worms with a finely striated cuticle and a head with six 65-µ to 70-µ grooves extending from the mouth[131]. Males measure 8 mm to 10.6 mm long by 420 µ to 490 µ wide and have 1.16-mm to 1.3-mm long spicules. Females measure 10 mm to 14.8 mm long by 430 µ to 590 µ wide and have a tail that ends in a thin spike. Eggs measure 58 µ by 42 µ to 45 µ[131].

Aulonocephalus lindquisti has been reported in the cecum and large intestine of bobwhites and blue (scaled) quail[131]. Specific details on the life cycle of *A. lindquisti* are unknown. *Aulonocephalus lindquisti* is considered nonpathogenic. Clinical disease has not been observed.

Diagnosis is by identifying *A. lindquisti* eggs in the feces or the adults in the ceca. Treatment is not warranted. Proper sanitation and good management practices prevent future infections. *Aulonocephalus lindquisti* is not zoonotic.

Subulura brumpti

Morphology. *Subulura brumpti* are small nematodes whose anterior end is curved dorsally[131]. They have a hexagonal mouth with six lips that each bear a median papillae[131]. Males measure 6.9 mm to 10 mm long by 340 µ to 420 µ wide, and have a 0.98-mm to 1.1-mm long esophagus, lateral alae that extend to the middle of the esophagus, and a tail that is curved ventrally[131]. Males also have 10 pairs of caudal papillae (three pre-anal pairs, two adanal pairs, and five post-anal pairs), 1.22-mm to 1.5-mm long spicules, and a 170-µ to 220-µ wide pre-anal sucker[131]. Females measure 9 mm to 13.7 mm long by 460 µ to 560 µ wide, have a 1-mm to 1.3-mm long esophagus, and a straight and conical tail that ends in a point[131]. Eggs are thin-shelled, spherical, and 82 µ to 86 µ by 66 µ to 76 µ, and are embryonated when passed in the feces[131].

Hosts. *Subulura brumpti* has been reported in chickens, turkeys, doves, ducks, grouse, guinea fowl, partridges, pheasants, and quail[131].

Life Cycle. *Subulura brumpti* eggs are passed in the cecal droppings and are immediately infective to an intermediate host, including beetles or cockroaches. After ingestion by the intermediate host, larvae hatch in four to five hours and develop into the infective third-stage larvae within the insect body cavity. The second-stage larvae was observed eight days post-infection and the encysted infective third-stage larvae was observed 12 to 16 days post-infection[159]. This intermediate host is then ingested by a definitive avian host and a fourth-stage larva develops within two weeks. By day 18 post-infection, the final molt occurs, and adult *S. brumpti* begin to lay eggs six weeks post-infection[131,160].

Pathologic Effects and Clinical Disease. *Subulura brumpti* does not appear to be pathogenic[160]. Thus, clinical signs are typically not observed.

Diagnosis, Treatment, and Prevention. Diagnosis is by identifying eggs in the feces and adult worms in the cecum. Treatment is not warranted. Because *S. brumpti* is immediately infective to the intermediate hosts, control of the life cycle is of utmost importance to control future infections.

Public Health Considerations. *Subulura brumpti* has not been reported in humans.

Subulura strongylina

Subulura strongylina has been reported in the ceca of chickens, guinea fowl, and quail. Adult male worms measure 4.4 mm to 12 mm long, and have a V- or O-shaped curved tail, a 169-µ wide pre-anal sucker, 11 pairs of caudal papillae, and 890-µ to 1,200-µ long spicules[131]. Female worms measure 5.6 mm to 18 mm long[131]. Eggs measure 84 µ by 67 µ and are embryonated when passed in the feces[131]. The life cycle of *S. strongylina* likely resembles that of *S. brumpti*. *Subulura strongylina* is not pathogenic. There were no reportable lesions produced in the quail ceca[131]. Thus, clinical signs are not observed.

Diagnosis is by identifying *S. strongylina* eggs in the feces or the adults in the ceca. Treatment is not warranted. Because *S. strongylina* is immediately infective to the intermediate hosts, its control is of utmost importance to control future infections. *Subulura strongylina* does not infect humans.

Subulura suctoria

Subulura suctoria has been reported in the small intestine and ceca of chickens, turkeys, guinea fowl, partridges, pheasants, and quail[131]. *Subulura suctoria* is larger than *S. brumpti*. Males measure 11.8 mm to 13.8 mm long by 359 µ wide and have 1-mm to 1.5-mm long curved spicules. Female worms measure 20 mm to 33 mm long. Eggs are 51 µ to 70 µ by 45 µ to 64 µ[131]. The life cycle is similar to that of *S. brumpti*. Beetles serve as the intermediate host[131]. *Subulura suctoria* is nonpathogenic[161,162]. Thus, clinical disease had not been reported.

Diagnosis and prevention are as described for *S. brumpti*. Treatment is not needed, since *S. suctoria* is nonpathogenic. However, ivermectin given subcutaneously (0.07 mg/kg or 0.14 mg/kg) to adult guinea fowl was effective[150]. *Subulura suctoria* is not of public health concern.

Superfamily Strongyloidea

Cyathostoma bronchialis

Morphology. Adult *Cyathostoma bronchialis* are sexually dimorphic. Adult males measure 8 mm to12 mm long by 200 μ to 600 μ wide, and have long and slender spicules measuring 540 μ to 870 μ long[131]. Adult females measure 16 mm to 30 mm long by 750 μ to 1500 μ wide. Eggs are operculated and measure 68 μ to 90 μ by 43 μ to 60 μ.

Hosts. *Cyathostoma bronchialis* has been reported naturally in the larynx, trachea and bronchi, and abdominal air sacs of ducks, geese and turkeys, and experimentally in chickens[131,163].

Life Cycle. Infection can occur through direct infection with third-stage larvae, or via ingestion of an infected earthworm intermediate host. Following ingestion, third-stage larvae migrate to the lungs via the coelomic cavity and airsacs[164]. From the lungs, larvae migrate to the trachea, where they mature and copulate within two weeks of ingestion[164].

Pathologic Effect. Fernando and co-workers reported that experimentally infected geese develop bronchitis of the primary, secondary, and tertiary bronchi. There is hyperplasia of the epithelium in the primary bronchus. Generalized pneumonitis was also reported due to the aspiration of *C. bronchialis* eggs[165].

Clinical Disease. Morbidity rates of up to 80% and mortality rates of up to 20% have been reported in a flock of domestic geese[166]. Affected birds may develop respiratory difficulty and gaping.

Diagnosis, Treatment, and Prevention. Diagnosis is by identification of the eggs in the feces, observation of clinical signs, or recovery of the adults in the trachea. Thiabendazole, as recommended for *Syngamus trachea*, is effective. Proper sanitation, including frequent removal of feces, aids in preventing infection with *C. bronchialis*.

Syngamus trachea

Morphology. *Syngamus trachea* is also called the gape worm, redworm, or forked worm[131]. Adults are sexually dimorphic.

Males are 2 mm to 6 mm long by 200 μ wide, with short, slender 57-μ to 64-μ spicules. Females are 5 mm to 20 mm long by 350 μ wide (Figure 10.17). The eggs are elliptical, operculated, and measure 90 μ by 49 μ[131] (Figure 10.18). Adult worms appear bright red, and the male and female form a Y-shape as they are locked in copulation[131]. The mouth of *S. trachea* has an orbicular shape that has a hemispheric chitinous capsule containing eight sharp teeth at the base. There is a chitinous plate surrounding the mouth that is formed by six festoons. The male has an asymmetrical bursa that is obliquely truncated with short rays. The female has a conical tail with a pointed process and a vulva that is placed in the upper quadrant of the body[131].

Hosts. *Syngamus trachea* has been reported in the trachea, bronchi, and bronchioles of chickens, turkeys, geese, guinea fowl, pheasants, peafowl, quail, and some passeriforms[101,131].

Life Cycle. The life cycle of *S. trachea* may be direct or indirect. In the direct life cycle, birds become infected by ingesting embryonated eggs or infective larvae. In the indirect life cycle, birds become infected by ingesting earthworm intermediate hosts[131]. Adult females release eggs into the tracheal lumen. The eggs are carried to the oropharynx, swallowed, and are passed into the feces. Eggs of *S. trachea*

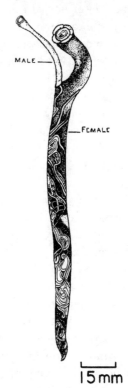

Fig. 10.17 *Syngamus trachea* male and female. Reproduced from Wehr, E.E. (1965) with permission.

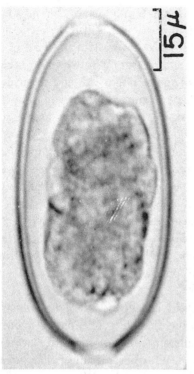

Fig. 10.18　Egg of *Syngamus trachea*. Reproduced from Soulsby, E.J.L. (1982) with permission.

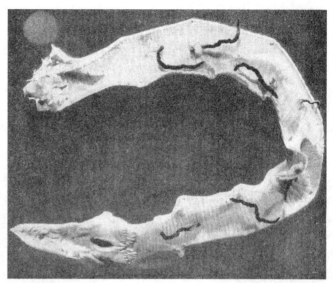

Fig. 10.19　*Syngamus trachea* adults attached to the tracheal mucosa in a chicken. Reproduced from Wehr, E.E. (1965) with permission.

embryonate and hatch in eight to 14 days, depending on environmental temperature and moisture content.

Free-living larvae may be ingested by an earthworm, slug, or snail, and live within the body cavity or encyst in its muscles, where they can remain infective for up to four years[131]. Following ingestion, infective larvae penetrate the crop or esophageal wall and migrate to the lungs. They can also enter the duodenum, penetrate the intestinal wall, and enter the lungs via the portal blood vessels[167]. In the lungs, they molt and develop into adults within two weeks after ingestion.

Pathologic Effects. *Syngamus trachea* attach to the posterior tracheal mucosa (Figure 10.19), where they cause tracheal obstruction with bloody mucus and tracheitis. As a result of localized inflammation, nodules may form at the site of attachment of male worms. The females detach and reattach so nodules are less likely to form at their attachment sites. Nodules are common in turkeys and pheasants but not in chickens and guinea fowl[131]. Hwang and co-workers reported marked heterophilia, monocytosis, eosinophilia, and lymphocytopenia, and a decreased packed cell volume in experimentally affected turkeys[168].

Clinical Disease. Young birds are more severely infected than older birds. Affected birds develop characteristic signs of respiratory difficulty, including dyspnea, asphyxia, coughing, and the characteristic open mouth with head extension ("gape").

Diagnosis. Diagnosis is by identifying the eggs in the feces along with the characteristic gape, or by identifying the adults in the trachea.

Treatment. Some have reported that thiabendazole is effective in treating birds infected with *S. trachea*[101]. However, others have reported that in chickens, thiabendazole (500 mg/kg) was least effective when compared to albendazole (15 mg/kg) or mebendazole (40 mg/kg)[169]. Levamisole (2 mg/100g body weight, given subcutaneously) has been effective for treating pheasants[33]. Fenbendazole (100 ppm in the feed for four days) also eliminated the infection in pheasants[157]. Albendazole (5 mg/kg or 10 mg/kg) given orally for three to five days was effective in turkeys[170]. For geese, flubendazole was effective when given at 30 ppm in the feed for seven days[171].

Prevention. Proper sanitation and good management practices can reduce infections. Frequent removal of feces reduces environmental contamination.

Public Health Considerations. *Syngamus trachea* does not infect humans.

Superfamily Trichostrongylidae

Amidostomum anseris

Morphology. *Amidostomum anseris* is a slender red worm in the family Trichostrongylidae, subfamily Amidostomatinae. Adults have a buccal cavity containing three pointed teeth. Males measure 10 mm to 17 mm long by 250 μ to 350 μ wide, and possess spicules 200 μ in length. Females measure 12 mm to 24 mm long by 200 μ to 400 μ wide. The thin-shelled eggs measure 85 μ to 110 μ by 50 μ to 82 μ[131].

Hosts and Life Cycle. *Amidostomum anseris* has been reported under the koilin layer of the gizzard in the duck, goose, and pigeon[131]. Eggs are passed in the feces and hatch within a few days. Infective larvae are ingested by a susceptible host bird. Adult worms are found in the gizzard about 40 days after ingestion[131].

Pathogenic Effects and Clinical Disease. In severely infected birds, gizzard linings become hemorrhagic and necrotic, and they slough. Affected birds are anorexic, emaciated, and lethargic, and may develop a staggering gait and impacted esophagus[172].

Diagnosis. A definitive diagnosis can be made by identifying the *A. anseris* eggs in the feces or the adults in the gizzard.

Treatment. Cambendazole (60 mg/kg) is effective against adult worms and larvae[173]. Pyrantel (100 mg/kg) is effective for adult worms. Mebendazole (10 mg/kg for three days) and fenbendazole have also proven effective[131,174]. Vanparijs reported that flubendazole was effective at 30 ppm in the feed for seven consecutive days in geese[171]. Cencek and co-workers reported success with ivermectin (200 μg/kg SQ) in geese[175].

Prevention. Proper sanitation and good management practices help prevent future infections.

Public Health Considerations. *Amidostomum anseris* has not been reported in humans.

Amidostomum skrjabini

Amidostomum skrjabini is smaller than *A. anseris*. Males measure 7.5 mm to 8.8 mm long by 100 μ to 130 μ wide, and have 115-μ to 125-μ spicules. Females measure 9 mm to 11 mm long by 101 μ to 120 μ wide. Eggs are 70 μ to 80 μ by 40 μ to 50 μ[131]. *Amidostomum skrjabini* (*Sclerostoma monodon*, *Strongylus acutus*, *S. monodon*, *Amidostomum monodon*, *A. chevreuxi*, *A. anatinum*, *A. fuligulae*, *A. biziurae*, *A. boschadis*, *A. orientale*, and *A. acutum*) has been reported under the gizzard koilin layer of ducks and pigeons. Chickens may be infected experimentally[131]. The life cycle of *A. skrjabini* is similar to that of *A. anseris*. The koilin layer of the gizzard often hemorrhages and sloughs. Affected birds can be anorexic and emaciated. Diagnosis, treatment, and prevention are as described for *A. anseris*. *Amidostomum skrjabini* has not been reported in humans.

Epomidiostomum uncinatum

Epomidiostomum uncinatum is in the family Trichostrongylidae, subfamily Amidostomatinae. It has been found under the gizzard koilin layer of ducks, geese, and pigeons. Chickens may be experimentally infected[131]. *Epomidiostomum uncinatum* is similar to *Amidostomum* except that its buccal capsule does not have teeth, and its anterior end bears a pair of nodules. Males measure 6.5 mm to 7.3 mm long by 150 μ wide and have spicules measuring 120 μ to 130 μ long. Females measure 10 mm to 11.5 mm long by 230 mm to 240 mm wide. Eggs measure 74 μ to 90 μ long by 45 μ to 50 μ wide[131]. *Epomidiostomum uncinatum* has been reported in ducks, geese, and pigeons. *Epomidiostomum uncinatum* eggs are passed in the feces and can become infective third-stage larvae within four days. These infective larvae are then ingested by a susceptible bird[176]. The extent to which *E. uncinatum* causes pathologic changes or clinical disease is unknown.

Diagnosis is by identifying eggs of *E. uncinatum* in feces or the adults in the gizzard. Treatment regimens used for *Amidostomum* may also be effective against *E. uncinatum*. Proper sanitation and good management practices are likely to be effective in preventing future infections. *Epomidiostomum uncinatum* has not been reported in humans.

Trichostrongylus tenuis

Morphology. *Trichostrongylus tenuis* is a slender worm in the family Trichostrongylidae. Adults have three small lips. Males measure 5.5 mm to 9 mm long by 48 μ wide, and have brown, twisted spicules. Adult female worms measure 6.5 mm to 11 mm long by 77 μ to 100 μ wide. Eggs are thin-shelled[131].

Hosts and Life Cycle. *Trichostrongylus tenuis* has been reported in the small intestine and cecum of chickens, ducks, geese, grouse, guinea fowl, pigeons, quail, and turkeys[131,177]. The life cycle of *T. tenuis* is direct. Eggs are passed in the feces and hatch in 36 to 48 hours and become infective in about two weeks. These infective larvae are then ingested by a susceptible bird host.

Pathologic Effects and Clinical Disease. Pathologic changes include mucosal congestion, inflammation, and thickening. Watson and co-workers reported plicae depression in the ceca of heavily infected grouse[178]. Affected birds lose weight, become anemic, and experience depressed egg production[177].

Diagnosis, Treatment, and Prevention. Diagnosis is by identifying the *T. tenuis* egg in the feces or the adult worm in the small intestines. *Trichostrongylus tenuis* has been effectively treated using cambendazole (30 mg/kg), citarin (40 mg/kg), flubendazole (30 ppm in the feed for seven days), mebendazole (10 mg/kg for three days), pyrantel tartrate (50 mg/kg), or thiabendazole (75 mg/kg)[131,171,173,174]. Proper sanitation and good management practices prevent infections.

Public Health Considerations. *Trichostrongylus tenuis* does not infect humans.

Superfamily Metastrongyloidea

Pelecitus spp.

Morphology. *Pelecitus* spp. belong to the family Metastrongylidae. Adult *Pelecitus* have a corkscrew-shaped body. Males measure 8 mm to 11 mm long, have three to four pairs of pre-anal papillae and one to two pairs of post-anal papillae, and possess a 75-μ to 92-μ long and a 70-μ to 81-μ long spicule. Females measure 19.5 mm long[179].

Hosts. *Pelecitus* species have been reported in subcutaneous tissues of a variety of bird species, including pigeons[180] and macaws[181]. *Pelecitus calamiformis, P. tercostatus,* and *P. quadripapillosus* have been reported in psittacines[181,182]. They are found primarily in the neck, legs, or feet. *Pelecitus major* and *P. spiralis* have been reported in passerines.

Life Cycle. *Pelecitus* filariae were observed in congested and hemorrhagic cervical connective tissue of the pigeon[180]. Adult *Pelecitus* were found in the peritracheal connective tissue and in the deep zone of the subcutaneous tissue of the neck in the pigeon[180]. Infection may be associated with chronic tenosynovitis in psittacines[183] and subcutaneous nodules on the feet of macaws[181].

Pathologic Effects and Clinical Disease. Infections are usually asymptomatic. However, lameness has been reported in some infections involving the leg[181].

Diagnosis, Treatment, and Prevention. Diagnosis is often made when adult worms are found during necropsy. There is no effective pharmaceutical treatment for *Pelecitus* infections. Surgical removal of the worms is the only effective treatment[181]. Proper sanitation and good management practices reduce re-infection. Removal of infected birds limits transmission.

Public Health Considerations. *Pelecitus* species found in avian species have not been reported in humans.

Superfamily Spiruroidea

Cheilospirura hamulosa

Morphology. *Cheilospirura hamulosa* (Syn. *Acuaria hamulosa*) has two triangular lips. Adult worms have four long longitudinal cordons which are not anastomosing or recurrent. Male worms measure 9 mm to 19 mm in length; possess a 1.6-mm to 1.8-mm long by 12-μ wide, short, curved spicule; and a 180-mm to 200-mm by 64-μ slender spicule; and have a tightly coiled tail, two caudal alae, and 10 pairs of caudal papillae[131]. Adult females measure 16 mm to 25 mm long and have a pointed tail. Eggs measure 40 μ by 27 μ[131].

Hosts. *Cheilospirura hamulosa* has been found under the koilin layer of the gizzard of chickens, grouse, guinea fowl, pheasants, quail, and turkeys[131].

Life Cycle. The life cycle of *C. hamulosa* includes a grasshopper, beetle, weevil, or sand hopper intermediate host[184]. Larvae develop in the muscles of the intermediate host and become infective to the bird host in 22 days. After ingestion, larvae mature in the bird at around 76 days[131].

Pathologic Effects and Clinical Disease. *Cheilospirura hamulosa* is generally nonpathogenic. However, heavy infestations may result in nodule formation in the gizzard. Menezes and co-workers also reported finding hemorrhages, ulcers, and mucosa and koilin thickening in both pheasants and chickens with low parasite burdens[185]. Histologically, there was evidence of chronic diffuse inflammation. Clinical signs are typically not observed in birds infected with *C. hamulosa*.

Diagnosis, Treatment, and Prevention. Diagnosis is by identifying eggs of *C. hamulosa* in the feces or the adult worms in the gizzard. Treatment is generally not warranted. Because the life cycle of *C. hamulosa* involves an intermediate host, control of the intermediate host helps prevent future infections.

Public Health Considerations. *Cheilospirura hamulosa* does not infect humans.

Cheilospirura spinosa

Morphology. *Cheilospirura spinosa* is a member of the family Acuariidae. Males measure 14 mm to 20 mm long by 183 μ to 232 μ wide, and have two different types of spicules. One type measures 660 μ to 720 μ long and the other measures 192 μ long. The male caudal alae are similar to those of *C. hammulosa*. Female worms measure 34 mm to 40 mm long by 315 μ to 348 μ wide. Eggs are 39 μ to 42 μ by 25 μ to 27 μ[131,186].

Hosts. *Cheilospirura spinosa* has been reported under the koilin layer of the gizzard in game birds, including grouse, partridges, pheasants, quail, and turkeys[131].

Life Cycle. The life cycle of *C. spinosa* is similar to that of *C. hamulosa*. Grasshoppers serve as the intermediate host. Worms reach maturity in the avian host 32 days after ingestion of the intermediate host[131, 184].

Pathologic Effects and Clinical Disease. Mild infections are usually nonpathogenic. Heavy infection results in hemorrhages of the gizzard lining. Clinical signs are generally not observed.

Diagnosis, Treatment, and Prevention. Diagnosis is by identifying eggs of *C. spinosa* in the feces or adult worms in the gizzard. Treatment is not warranted. Because *C. spinosa* requires an intermediate host, control of the intermediate host helps prevent future infections.

Public Health Considerations. *Cheilospirura spinosa* does not infect humans.

Cyrnea colini

Morphology. *Cyrnea coli* is a member of the family Habronematidae. Adult worms are slender, yellowish, and resemble *Cheilospirura hamulosa*. Adults have four lips which bear four papillae[131]. Males measure 6 mm long by 250 μ wide, and have a 58-μ deep buccal cavity, 10 pairs of pedunculated papillae, and two distinct spicules— one 2-mm long and the other 365-μ to 400-μ long. Females measure 14 mm to 18 mm long by 315 μ wide, and have a 75-μ deep buccal cavity. Eggs measure 40.5 μ by 22.5 μ[131].

Hosts. *Cyrnea colini* has been reported in the proventriculus, especially near the junction with the gizzard, in chickens, grouse, prairie chickens, quail, and turkeys[156].

Life Cycle. Eggs are passed in the feces and are ingested by the cockroach, *Blatella germanica*[131]. The *C. colini* larvae mature in the cockroach 18 days after being ingested. Mature worms can be found in the bird 41 days after ingesting the intermediate host[131].

Pathologic Effects and Clinical Disease. *Cyrnea colini* is nonpathogenic. Thus, clinical signs are not observed.

Diagnosis, Treatment, and Prevention. Diagnosis is by identifying eggs of *C. colini* in the feces or adult worms in the proventriculus. Treatment is not needed, since *C. colini* is nonpathogenic. Because the cockroach is the intermediate host, its control prevents completion of the *C. colini* life cycle.

Public Health Considerations. *Cyrnea colini* does not infect humans.

Dispharynx nasuta

Morphology. *Dispharynx nasuta* is a member of the family Acuariidae. Male worms measure 7 mm to 8.3 mm long by 230 μ to 315 μ wide, and possess four pairs of pre-anal and five pairs of post-anal papillae. Males also have a 400-μ long slender, curved spicule and a shorter, 150-μ long spicule. Females measure 9 mm to 10.2 mm long by 360 μ to 565 μ wide. Eggs are embryonated when passed in the feces[131].

Hosts. *Dispharynx nasuta* has been reported in the proventriculus, esophagus, and small intestine of chickens, grouse, guinea fowl, partridges, pheasants, pigeons, quail, turkeys, princess parrots (*Polytelis alexandrae*), mourning doves, and numerous passerines[7,131].

Life Cycle. Embryonated eggs are passed in the feces, where they are ingested by pill bugs (*Armadillidium vulgare*) or sow bugs (*Porcellio scaber*), which serve as intermediate hosts of *D. nasuta*. Within four days after ingestion, larvae escape and are found in the tissues of the intermediate host's body cavity, and they mature into infective larvae by 26 days. Upon ingestion of the intermediate host, the larvae reach sexual maturity in the avian host and begin to pass embryonated eggs by day 27 after ingestion[131].

Pathologic Effects and Clinical Disease. In heavy infections, ulceration is seen in the proventriculus, and the proventricular wall becomes thickened and macerated[131]. Worms burrow into the mucosa, and can be found under the thickened proventricular tissue[131]. Lesions consist of multifocal petechial hemorrhages, excess mucus, mononuclear infiltrates, and epithelial desquamation from passerines. Affected birds may become emaciated.

Diagnosis, Treatment, and Prevention. Diagnosis is by identifying eggs of *D. nasuta* eggs in the feces or adult worms in the proventriculus. Mebendazole has shown some efficacy against *D. nasuta*. Because an intermediate host is required for the *D. nasuta* life cycle, control of the intermediate host is necessary for the prevention of future infections.

Public Health Considerations. *Dispharynx nasuta* does not infect humans.

Echinura uncinata

Morphology. *Echinura uncinata* is similar in appearance to *Cheilospirura* and *Dispharynx*. Adult male worms measure 8 mm to 10 mm long by 300 μ to 500 μ wide, and have two dissimilar spicules (one measuring 700 μ to 900 μ long and the other measuring 350 μ long). Females measure 12 mm to 18.5 mm long by 515 μ wide, and possess a 250-μ long tail. Eggs measure 28 μ to 37μ by 17 μ to 23 μ, and are embryonated when laid in the feces[131].

Hosts. *Echinura uncinata* has been reported in the esophagus, proventriculus, gizzard, and small intestine of ducks, geese, swans, and other birds[131,187].

Life Cycle. Embryonated eggs are passed in the feces, and are ingested by water fleas (*Daphnia* spp.). Larvae become infective in 12 to 14 days. After these infected water fleas are ingested by the definitive avian host, larvae reach maturity and begin to lay eggs within five days after ingestion[131].

Pathologic Effects and Clinical Disease. Following infection, mucosal nodules develop at the sites of worm attachment. Caseated pus may be associated with these nodules[131]. The surface of the proventriculus may become covered by a thick exudate containing heterophils and mononuclear cells[187]. Affected birds become emaciated and appear lethargic. Some birds may be asymptomatic[131].

Diagnosis, Treatment, and Prevention. Diagnosis is by identifying the eggs of *E. uncinata* in the feces or adult worms in the intestines. Treatment protocols have not been developed for *E. uncinata*. Because water fleas serve as the intermediate hosts reducing exposure to them prevents future infections.

Public Health Considerations. *Echinura uncinata* does not infect humans.

Gongylonema ingluvicola

Morphology. *Gongylonema ingluvicola* bears shield-like markings over the body. The male measures 17 mm to 20 mm long by 224 μ to 250 μ wide, has a variable number of genital papillae, and has two dissimilar spicules (17 mm to 19 mm long by 7 μ to 9 μ wide with a barbed point, and 100 μ to 120 μ long by 15 μ to 20 μ wide). Females measure 32 mm to 55 mm long by 320 μ to 490 μ wide[131].

Hosts and Life Cycle. *Gongylonema ingluvicola* has been reported in the crop, esophagus, and proventriculus of chickens, partridges, pheasants, quail, and turkeys[131]. Details of the life cycle of *G. ingluvicola* are lacking, but it involves a beetle (*Copris minutus*) or cockroach as an intermediate host[131].

Pathologic Effects and Clinical Disease. Although burrows can be formed in the crop mucosa, there is minimal pathologic damage with *G. ingluvicola*. Because the

pathologic effects of *G. ingluvicola* are minimal, clinical disease is rarely reported.

Diagnosis, Treatment, and Prevention. Diagnosis is by identifying eggs of *G. ingluvicola* in the feces or adult worms in the upper gastrointestinal tract, proximal to the proventriculus. Treatment is not needed because clinical signs are rarely observed. Because the life cycle of *G. ingluvicola* involves an intermediate host, its control prevents future infections.

Public Health Considerations. *Gongylonema ingluvicola* has not been reported in humans.

Oxyspirura mansoni

Morphology. *Oxyspirura mansoni* (avian eyeworm) has a circular mouth surrounded by a chitinous ring with six lobes and papillae located in each of the clefts of this ring[131]. *Oxyspirura mansoni* also has three pairs of teeth (two subdorsal pairs and one subventral pair). Male worms are 8.2 mm to 16 mm long by 350 μ wide, and have a curved tail, six pairs of papillae (four pre-anal pairs and two post-anal pairs), and two dissimilar spicules (3 mm to 4.55 mm long and 180 μ to 240 μ long). Females measure 12 mm to 20 mm long by 270 μ to 430 μ wide. Eggs measure 50 μ to 65 μ by 45 μ, and are embryonated when passed in the feces[131].

Hosts. *Oxyspirura mansoni* has been reported in the nictitating membrane, conjunctival sacs, and nasolacrimal ducts of chickens, ducks, grouse, guinea fowl, peafowl, pigeons, quail, turkeys, and numerous free-living birds[131,188].

Life Cycle. Embryonated eggs of *O. mansoni* pass in the feces and are ingested by the cockroach intermediate host. Larvae develop in the cockroach body cavity to become infective around 50 days[131]. Larvae encyst in the adipose tissue or alimentary tract. These larvae can also remain free in the body cavity or legs of the cockroach. After the cockroach is ingested by the avian host, the infective larvae are released in the crop, migrate up the esophagus to the mouth to enter the nasolacrimal duct, and finally to the conjunctival sac and nictitating membranes of the eye. Adult worms shed embryonated eggs into the tears, where they are swallowed and passed out with the feces[131].

Pathologic Effects and Clinical Disease. Infection leads to ophthalmia and swollen nictitating membranes. Affected birds may scratch at their eyes. Moreover, the nictitating membrane is swollen and protrudes out of the corner of the eye. Eyelids can also stick together and white debris can be present under these eyelids. Severe infections can result in the loss of an eye[131].

Diagnosis, Treatment, and Prevention. Diagnosis is by identifying the eggs of *O. mansoni* in the feces or adult worms in the eye. Specific details on effective treatment regimens of *O. mansoni* are lacking. Because the cockroach is the intermediate host of *O. mansoni,* its control helps prevent future infections.

Public Health Considerations. *Oxyspirura mansoni* has not been reported in humans.

Oxyspirura petrowi

Morphology. *Oxyspirura petrowi* is a member of the family Thelaziidae. Adult worms have seven pairs of cephalic papillae (four submedian pairs and three circumoral pairs). Male worms are 6.3 mm to 8.6 mm long by 185 μ to 330 μ wide and have a 121-μ to 320-μ long slender spicule with a sharp tip. Females measure 7.7 mm to 12.3 mm long by 200 μ to 455 μ wide. Eggs measure 35 μ to 44 μ by 15 μ to 31 μ[131].

Hosts and Life Cycle. *Oxyspirura petrowi* has been reported in the nictitating membrane of grouse, pheasants, and prairie chickens[131]. The life cycle of *O. petrowi* is similar to that of *O. mansoni.*

Pathologic Effects and Clinical Disease. The pathologic effects and clinical disease caused by *O. petrowi* are similar to those of *O. mansoni.*

Diagnosis, Treatment, and Prevention. Diagnosis is by identifying the eggs of *O. petrowi* in the feces or adult worms in the eye. Specific details on effective treatment regimens for *O. petrowi* are lacking. Because the life cycle of *O. petrowi* involves the cockroach as an intermediate host, its control prevents future infections.

Public Health Considerations. *Oxyspirura mansoni* has not been reported in humans.

Tetrameres americana

Morphology. *Tetrameres americana,* the "stomach" or "globular stomach" worm has three small lips surrounding a buccal cavity. Adult worms are sexually dimorphic[131]. Males measure 5 mm to 5.5 mm long by 116 μ to 133 μ wide, and have two rows of posteriorly directed spines that extend the length of the body, cervical papillae, a long and slender tail, and spicules measuring either 100 μ long or 290 μ to 312 μ long. Females measure 3.5 mm to 4.5 mm long by 3 mm wide and are globular in shape. Females are also red in color and have four longitudinal furrows. Eggs measure 42 μ to 50 μ by 24 μ and are embryonated when passed in the feces[131].

Hosts. *Tetrameres americana* has been reported in the proventriculus of chickens, ducks, grouse, pigeons, quail, and turkeys[131].

Life Cycle. The red, globular-appearing adult female worms may be observed through the serosal surface of the proventriculus, while the males are primarily observed on the mucosal surface. Embryonated eggs are passed in the feces and later ingested by an intermediate host[184]. Intermediate hosts include grasshoppers (*Melanoplus femurrubrum* and *M. differentialis*) and a cockroach (*Blatella germanica*)[184]. Following ingestion of the intermediate host, *S. americana* larvae escape and develop to the adult stage. Adult female worms enter the gastric glands to mate and lay eggs around 45 days post-ingestion[184].

Pathologic Effects. Following infection, the walls of the proventriculus may become markedly thickened[131]. Multiple dark red nodules, 2 mm to 6 mm in diameter, may be present on the proventricular wall[189]. Adult worms within the fundic glands may result in compression of the walls and glands[190].

Clinical Disease. Affected birds may not show any clinical disease. However, heavily infected birds are anemic and emaciated[191]. Affected pigeons also develop lethargy, vomiting, weight loss, diarrhea, and pale skin[129,189,190].

Diagnosis, Treatment, and Prevention. Diagnosis is by identifying eggs in the feces or adult worms in the proventriculus. Piperazine has been used to treat *T. fissipina* and would likely be effective for *T. americana*. Because *T. americana* is immediately infective to the intermediate host, control of the intermediate host helps prevent future infections.

Public Health Considerations. *Tetrameres americana* is not infectious to humans.

Tetrameres crami

Morphology. *Tetrameres crami* is smaller than *T. americana*. Adult males measure 2.9 mm to 4.1 mm long by 70 μ to 92 μ wide. Two forms of spicule may be found in the males. One is curved and measures 136 μ to 185 μ long and the other is twisted and measures 272 μ to 350 μ long. Female worms measure 1.5 mm to 3.3 mm by 1.2 mm to 2.2 mm wide and have a 113-μ to 156-μ long tail. Eggs measure 41 μ to 57 μ by 26 μ to 34 μ and are embryonated when passed in the feces[131].

Hosts and Life Cycle. *Tetrameres crami* has been reported in the proventriculus of both free-living and domestic ducks[131]. The life cycle of *T. crami* is similar to that of *T. americana,* and involves an amphipod

(*Gammarus fasciatus* and *Hyalella knickerbock*) intermediate host[192]. *Tetrameres crami* larvae become infective to the duck 29 days after ingestion by the intermediate host. In the duck, *T. crami* matures around 33 days after ingestion of the amphipod[192].

Pathologic Effects and Clinical Disease. Pathologic changes have not been described. Heavy infections may result in emaciation.

Diagnosis, Treatment, and Prevention. Diagnosis is by identifying *T. crami* eggs in the feces or adult worms in the proventriculus. Piperazine has been used against *Tetrameres fissispina* and would likely be effective for *T. crami*. Because *T. crami* is immediately infective to the intermediate host, control of the intermediate host will help to prevent future infections.

Public Health Considerations. *Tetrameres crami* is not infectious to humans.

Tetrameres fissispina

Morphology. *Tetrameres fissispina* is similar in appearance to *T. americana*. Adult males measure 3 mm to 6 mm long by 90 μ to 200 μ wide, and have four rows of spines and spicules that measure either 280 μ to 490 μ or 82 μ to 150 μ long. Females measure 1.7 mm to 6 mm long by 1.3 mm to 5 mm wide and have a 71-μ long tail. Eggs measure 48 μ to 56 μ by 26 μ to 30 μ and are embryonated when passed in the feces[131].

Hosts and Life Cycle. *Tetrameres fissispina* has been found in the proventriculus of free-living and domestic ducks and geese, and in chickens, guinea fowl, pigeons, quail, and turkeys[131]. The life cycle of *T. fissispina* is similar to that of *T. americana,* and includes amphipods, cockroaches, earthworms, and grasshoppers as intermediate hosts[156]. *Tetrameres fissispina* larvae become infective to birds 10 days after ingestion by the intermediate host. In the bird, larvae mature in 18 days[131]. Fish may also serve as a paratenic host[156].

Pathologic Effects and Clinical Disease. Following infection, the proventriculus becomes thickened, and there is degeneration, edema, and leukocytic infiltration of the proventricular glands, as well as catarrhal enteritis[193,194]. Affected birds are emaciated.

Diagnosis, Treatment, and Prevention. Diagnosis is by identifying *T. fissispina* eggs in the feces or adult worms in the proventriculus. Piperazine is an effective treatment. Because *T. fissispina* is immediately infective to the intermediate host, its control helps prevent future infections.

Public Health Consideration. *Tetrameres fissispina* is not infectious to humans.

Tetrameres pattersoni

Morphology. *Tetrameres pattersoni* is similar in appearance to *T. americana*[131]. Females are red and are found in the proventricular glands, whereas the males are on the proventricular mucosal surface. Males measure 4.2 mm to 4.6 mm long by 140 μ to 170 μ wide, and have two rows of spines along the body and one spicule. Female worms measure 5 mm long by 2 mm to 2.3 mm wide, and have an enlarged area between the vulva and anus. Eggs are 42 μ to 46 μ by 25 μ to 30 μ and are embryonated when passed in the feces[131].

Hosts and Life Cycle. *Tetrameres pattersoni* has been reported in quail[131]. The life cycle of *T. pattersoni* is similar to that of *T. americana,* and includes intermediate hosts such as grasshoppers (*Melanoplus femurrubrum* or *Chortophaga viridifasciata*) or cockroaches (*Blatella germanica*)[195].

Pathologic Effects and Clinical Disease. Following infection, the proventricular walls may become thickened. Affected birds can be emaciated.

Diagnosis, Treatment, and Prevention. Diagnosis is by identifying *T. pattersoni* eggs in the feces or adult worms in the proventriculus. Piperazine is effective against *T. fissispina* and would likely also be effective against *T. pattersoni*. Because *T. pattersoni* is immediately infective to the intermediate host, control of the intermediate host helps prevent future infections.

Public Health Considerations. *Tetrameres pattersoni* is not infectious to humans.

Superfamily Filaroidea

Aproctella stoddardi

Morphology. *Aproctella stoddardi* is a member of the family Dipetalonematidae. *Aproctella stoddardi* is a slender worm that has a simple mouth with no defined lips[156]. Males measure 6 mm to 7.6 mm long by 60 μ to 140 μ wide, and have thick, curved spicules that measure 50 μ to 60 μ long or 73 μ to 90 μ long. Females measure 13 mm to 16.5 mm long by 71 μ to 260 μ wide. Microfilariae are present in the uteri[131].

Hosts and Life Cycle. *Aproctella stoddardi* has been reported in the coelomic cavity of doves, grouse, bobwhite quail, and turkeys[131]. Specific details on the life cycle of *A. stoddardi* are lacking. However, a biting arthropod is proposed as the intermediate host[131].

Pathologic Effects and Clinical Disease. *Aproctella stoddardi* is generally considered nonpathogenic but can be associated with a granulomatous pericarditis[131]. Clinical disease has not been reported in birds infected with *A. stoddardi*.

Diagnosis, Treatment, and Prevention. Diagnosis is by identifying adult worms in the body cavity. Treatment is not needed because *A. stoddardi* is considered to be non-pathogenic. Because a biting arthropod is proposed to be the intermediate host, control of biting insects is necessary to prevent future infections.

Public Health Considerations. *Aproctella stoddardi* has not been reported in humans.

Singhfilaria hayesi

Morphology. *Singhfilaria hayesi* is a member of the family Onchocerciidae. Adult male *S. hayesi* measure 13.6 mm long by 250 μ wide, and bear two types of spicules, an 81-μ long, tooth-shaped spicule and a 125-μ long spicule that is divided into a thick blade-like shaft and a short thin shaft. Males also bear a pair of post-anal papillae. Female worms measure 35 mm to 40 mm long by 420 μ to 500 μ wide. Microfilariae are present in the uteri[131].

Hosts and Life Cycle. *Singhfilaria hayesi* has been found in the subcutaneous tissues of the neck in quail and turkeys. Specific details on the life cycle of *S. hayesi* are lacking.

Pathologic Effects and Clinical Disease. *Singhfilaria hayesi* is nonpathogenic. Thus, clinical signs are not observed.

Diagnosis, Treatment, and Prevention. Diagnosis is by identifying adult worms in the subcutaneous tissues of the neck region. Treatment is not necessary because *S. hayesi* is nonpathogenic. Because the life cycle is unknown, specific preventive strategies have not been developed.

Public Health Considerations. *Singhfilaria hayesi* has not been reported in humans.

Superfamily Dracunculoidea

Avioserpens species

Morphology. *Avioserpens* spp. are dracunculid nematodes which cause "subcutaneous worm" or "guinea worm" infection. Female worms measure 25 cm long by 0.8 mm wide, and have a chitinous-rimmed mouth bearing two prominent lateral papillae[131].

Hosts. *Avioserpens* species have been reported in the subcutaneous tissues of the neck in waterfowl. *Avioserpens mosgovoyi*, *A. sichuanensis*, and *A. taiwana* (Syn. *Filaria*

taiwana, *Oshimaia taiwana*, *A. dentriculophasma*, and *Petroviprocta vigissi*) have been reported in ducks[131].

Life Cycle. Adult female worms release embryonated eggs that contain the first-stage larvae[131]. Larvae hatch and escape through a hole in the skin made by the adult female *A. taiwana*. They are ingested by the intermediate host, an aquatic copepod (*Mesocyclops leuckarti*, *Thermocyclops hyalinus*, and *Cyclops sternus*)[196]. Larvae penetrate the intestinal wall, enter the hemocoele, and molt three to four days after ingestion by the copepod. Larvae undergo a second molt three to four days later. Males may be found in the host mesentery 18 days after the ingestion of the copepod, while females are found in the subcutaneous tissues of the host 20 days after ingesting the copepod[131].

Pathologic Effects and Clinical Disease. Granulomas have been noted in the skin of the submandibular area and thighs[131]. Clinical disease is rarely reported in affected birds.

Diagnosis, Treatment, and Prevention. Diagnosis is by identifying adult worms at necropsy. There is no effective pharmaceutical treatment for *Avioserpens* infection. Worms may be removed surgically. Reducing exposure to the intermediate host can reduce transmission.

Public Health Considerations. *Avioserpens* species have not been reported in humans.

Superfamily Trichuroidea

Capillaria annulata

Morphology. *Capillaria annulata* is a slender worm that has a cuticular swelling at the back of its head[131]. Males measure 10 mm to 26 mm long by 52 μ to 74 μ wide and have a 1.12-mm to 1.63-mm long spicule. Females measure 25 mm to 60 mm long by 77 μ to 120 μ wide. Eggs are operculated, measure 55 μ to 65 μ by 26 μ to 28 μ and have characteristic bipolar plugs[131].

Hosts. *Capillaria annulata* has been found in the esophagus and crop of chickens, grouse, guinea fowl, partridges pheasants, quail, and turkeys[131].

Life Cycle. Eggs pass out in the feces and require 24 days or more to develop. Following ingestion by an earthworm (*Eisenia foetidus* or *Allolobophora caliginosus*)[197], larvae encyst in the body wall. Larvae become infective three to four weeks after being ingested by the earthworm[197]. When the earthworm is ingested by a suitable avian host, larvae mature and begin to release eggs three to four weeks later.

Pathologic Effects and Clinical Disease. The burrowing of *C. annulata* into the crop wall causes a local thickening, and enlargement of the mucosal glands. In heavy worm burdens, the crop mucosal surface may slough[131]. Affected birds appear emaciated, lethargic, and anemic.

Diagnosis, Treatment, and Prevention. Diagnosis is by identifying *C. annulata* eggs in the feces or adult worms in the crop or esophagus. Subcutaneous administration of methyridine (100 mg/kg) has been effective in some bird species[198]. Many of the studies evaluating effective treatments have been performed on the related species, *C. obsignata*. Mebendazole at a dosage of 120 mg/kg in the feed for 14 days was effective[199]. Proper sanitation and good management practices, along with earthworm control, help prevent future infections in the flock.

Public Health Considerations. *Capillaria annulata* has not been reported in humans.

Capillaria contorta

Morphology. *Capillaria contorta* has a slender body but does not have the dorsal cephalic cuticular swelling found on *C. annulata*. Males measure 8 mm to 17 mm long by 60 μ to 70 μ wide, have two terminal laterodorsal prominences on the tail, and a slender, transparent 800-μ long spicule covered with a sheath that has numerous fine, hairlike processes. Females measure 15 mm to 60 mm long by 140 μ to 180 μ wide[131].

Hosts and Life Cycle. *Capillaria contorta* has been reported in the oropharynx, esophagus, and crop of ducks, chickens, guinea fowl, partridges, pheasants, quail, and turkeys[131]. Eggs are passed in the feces and require approximately one month for embryonation. After ingestion by the avian definitive host, the *C. contorta* larvae mature into adults approximately one to two months after being ingested.

Pathologic Effects and Clinical Disease. The crop becomes thickened and inflamed. There can also be sloughing of the crop mucosa in severe infections. Affected birds are lethargic and emaciated.

Diagnosis, Treatment, and Prevention. Diagnosis is by identifying eggs of *C. annulata* in the feces or adult worms in the crop. Haloxon was highly effective in quail with *C. contorta* when administered at the 0.075% to 0.5% level in the feed for five to seven days[200]. Higher concentrations were toxic. Alternative treatments have been studied using *C. obsignata*. Olsen reported that levamisole (2 mg/100 g body weight) given subcutaneously or tetramisole (3 g/10 liters drinking water) has been effective for treating infected pheasants and quail[33]. Proper sanitation and good management practices help prevent future infections in the flock.

Public Health Considerations. *Capillaria contorta* has not been reported in humans.

Capillaria obsignata

Morphology. *Capillaria obsignata* (Syn. *C. dujardini*) is a fine, hair-like worm. Males measure 7 mm to 13 mm long by 49 μ to 53 μ wide, and have a 1.1-mm to 1.5-mm long spicule covered by a sheath that is spineless but has transverse folds on its surface. Females measure 10 mm to 18 mm long by 80 μ wide. Eggs measure 44 μ to 46 μ by 22 μ to 29 μ and have a reticulated pattern on the shell[163].

Hosts and Life Cycle. *Capillaria obsignata* has been reported in the small intestine and cecum of chickens, geese, guinea fowl, pigeons, quail, and turkeys[131]. *Capillaria obsignata* has a direct life cycle. Development is complete in 65 to 72 hours at 35°C or in 13 days at 20°C. The prepatent period is 20 to 21 days[201]. Pigeons remained infected for nine months[201].

Pathologic Effects and Clinical Disease. There is thickening of the small intestinal and cecal wall. Catarrhal or hemorrhagic enteritis may also be present[201]. Affected birds become emaciated and develop diarrhea[272]. There are no changes in white blood cell count or packed cell volume, but globulins and total proteins may be increased[201–203]. However, severely infected pigeons may have decreased total protein, albumen, plasma carotenoids, and liver vitamin A[204].

Diagnosis, Treatment, and Prevention. Diagnosis is by identifying eggs of *C. obsignata* in the feces or adult worms in the small intestine and cecum. Fenbendazole was 97% effective against *C. obsignata* infection in turkeys when fed at a concentration of 45 ppm for six days[155]. It was also greater than 99% efficacious in chickens[205], but was less efficacious when fed at 80 ppm for three days or 48 ppm for five days[156]. Fenbendazole added to the feed at 80 ppm for three days or 30 ppm for six days was 99% effective in eradicating *C. obsignata* from chickens[205,206]. Kirsch reported nearly 100% efficacy when fenbendazole was fed at 30 or 60 ppm for five days for pullet hens with *C. obsignata* infection[157]. Others achieved high efficacy of flubendazole when fed to broiler breeder chickens as 60 ppm for seven days[175].

Methyridine administered subcutaneously as a 5% aqueous solution delivered 25 to 45 mg methyridine per bird, and was 99% to 100% effective[198]. Effectiveness was reduced to 67% when the dose was reduced to 23 mg per bird. In contrast, piperazine citrate, phenothiazine, thiabendazole, and bephenium were inactive against

C. obsignata. Proper sanitation and good management practices help prevent future infections in the flock.

Public Health Considerations. *Capillaria obsignata* has not been reported in humans.

ARTHROPODS

Class Insecta

Order Diptera

Family Calliphoridae

The family Calliphoridae is composed of several genera which include the screwworm flies (*Cochliomyia* and *Chrysomyia*), blowflies (*Lucilia,* and *Phormia*), and bottle flies (*Calliphora* and *Phaenicia*)[207]. The primary screwworms include the New World screwworm (*Cochliomyia hominovorax*) and the Old World (*Chrysomyia bezziana*) screwworm. Primary screwworm flies cause obligate myiasis, because they lay their eggs only in fresh wounds. In contrast, secondary screwworm flies constitute the majority of calliphorids, which deposit their eggs in carion. These cause facultative myiasis[207], because larvae feed on dead tissues and only secondarily invade healthy tissues.

Morphology. Adult calliphorids measure approximately 10 mm and have a metallic blue-green body with a yellowish orange face. Eggs are 1.25 mm long[207]. Calliphorid larvae are distinguished from other flies by their characteristic posterior spiracles (Figure 10.20).

Hosts and Life Cycle. Calliphorids have been reported on the skin wounds of a variety of bird and mammalian species. For the primary screwworm flies, the eggs are deposited on fresh wounds and hatch within a day[207]. Larvae develop within one week and pupate. Adults emerge anytime from 10 days to eight weeks, depending on environmental temperature and humidity.

Pathologic Effects. Maggots produce superficial dermal myiasis but larvae will invade the deeper tissues during their development. The secondary myiasis-producing flies often follow the invasion tracts caused by the primary myiasis-producing flies.

Clinical Disease, Treatment, and Prevention. Skin wounds become necrotic and develop a fetid odor. Diagnosis is by identifying the characteristic calliphorid larvae with their posterior spiracles. Treatment is via wound flushing and removal of the maggots. Debridement of necrotic tissue also assists in wound healing.

Prevention. Treatment of open wounds and fly control helps reduce further infestations.

Public Health Considerations. Although humans can be infected by calliphorid flies, infected birds are not a hazard to humans.

Family Ceratopogonidae

Ceratopogonids are often called midges, "punkies," or "no-see-ums." They attack both birds and mammals. *Culicoides* species commonly found in poultry include *C. obsoletus, C. furens, C. sanguisuga,* and *C. crepuscularis*[208].

Morphology. Ceratopogonids are 1 mm to 4 mm long and have 15-segmented antennae. They have mouth parts well suited for blood feeding. Larvae are translucent white and measure 2 mm to 5 mm long[208].

Hosts and Life Cycle. Ceratopogonids can affect a wide variety of avian and mammalian hosts. Females require a blood meal for egg development. Eggs are laid on moist substrates and hatch within two to 10 days. Eggs are 250 μ to 500 μ long and banana-shaped[208]. Larvae develop through four instar stages before pupating. Pupae are found in the water. The life span of adults ranges from two to seven weeks.

Pathologic Effects and Clinical Disease. Ceratopogonids cause irritation to birds. More importantly, they

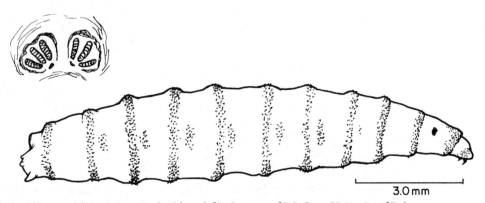

Fig. 10.20 A Calliphorid larvae with posterior spiracles (above left). Courtesy of E.P. Catts, University of Delaware.

can serve as vectors to such blood-borne pathogens as *Leucocytozoon* and *Haemoproteus*[208]. Clinical disease is often not noted, but there can be production losses. Young birds may develop anemia with heavy infestations.

Diagnosis, Treatment, and Prevention. Diagnosis is made by identifying the adults. There is no effective treatment for ceratopogonid bites. Control of biting midges is difficult because it is difficult to regulate their breeding environments. Mesh netting can reduce exposure to birds.

Public Health Considerations. Ceratopogonids can serve as vectors to human diseases.

Family Culicidae

Culicids, the mosquitoes, are blood-sucking flies which commonly feed on birds. More important, however, is their role as vectors of other pathogens. Important genera include *Anopheles, Aedes,* and *Culex.*

Morphology. Adults measure 2.5 mm to 6 mm long and have a slender abdomen and long proboscis. The morphology of the egg, larva, and pupa varies with mosquito species (Figure 10.21).

Hosts. A variety of birds and mammals serve as hosts for culicids. Common mosquitoes associated with birds include *Culex quinquefasciatus* (Southern house mosquito), *C. tarsalis* (encephalitis mosquito), *Psorophora confinnis, Aedes stimulans, A. aegypti,* and *A. vexans.*

Life Cycle. Female mosquitoes lay eggs, either individually or on rafts, on the water surface or on a moist substrate, depending on the mosquito species. Eggs hatch in one to two days and remain in the larval stage for one to two weeks and the pupal stage for two to three days. The life span of an adult is approximately one month.

Pathologic Effects and Clinical Disease. Only the female mosquito sucks blood. Its "bite" can cause pruritus and inflammation at the site of penetration. Mosquitoes can serve as mechanical and biological vectors to many pathogens, including *Plasmodium, Trypanosoma,* encephal-omyelitis viruses, and the avian pox virus. There may be pruritus and local inflammation in some affected birds.

Diagnosis, Treatment, and Prevention. Diagnosis is by identifying the adult mosquito. There is no effective treatment for mosquito bites on birds. Mosquito control,

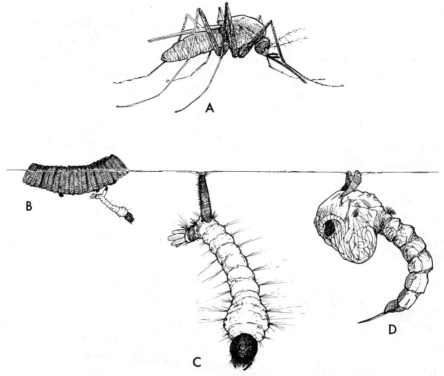

Fig. 10.21   General morphology of mosquitoes (Culicidae). (A) Adult female. (B) Eggs. (C) Larva. (D) Pupa. Courtesy of E.P. Catts, University of Delaware.

including elimination of standing water, aids in reducing mosquito populations.

Public Health Considerations. Mosquitoes can bite humans and serve as reservoirs of various zoonotic pathogens.

Family Cuterebridae
Dermatobia hominis. **Morphology.** *Dermatobia hominis* ("human botfly" or "torsalo") larvae may infest the skin of some birds. Adult *D. hominis* are 12 mm long and have a grey-metallic blue body with an orange face[207]. Larvae have a narrow anterior portion and a larger posterior portion, giving it a "bottle-shaped" appearance (Figure 10.22). Larvae are cream colored and have narrow belts of spines[207].

Hosts and Life Cycle. *Dermatobia hominis* has been reported on humans and other mammals, as well as birds. Adult female flies lay eggs near the host's nares. Eggs hatch in one to two weeks. After hatching, larvae enter through the nares or mouth and migrate through connective tissue for about a week before lodging in the subcutaneous tissue. The larva creates a small opening in the overlying skin, which it then uses as a breathing pore and also as a pore through which to excrete wastes. A subcutaneous cyst develops in two to three weeks. When the larvae is fully grown, it backs out of the opening in the skin and falls to the ground and pupates[209].

Pathologic Effects and Clinical Disease. *Dermatobia hominis* larvae produce dermal cysts[210]. Secondary bacterial infections may result in skin ulceration.

Diagnosis, Treatment, and Prevention. Diagnosis is by identifying *D. hominis* larvae in dermal cysts, which must be removed surgically. Prevention is via fly control to prevent future infections.

Public Health Considerations. *Dermatobia hominis* affects humans but infected birds are not a direct hazard to humans.

Family Hippoboscidae
Pseudolynchia canariensis. **Morphology.** Adult flies are dark brown, dorsoventrally flattened, and measure 6 mm long[208]. They have transparent wings and a short, stout beak[208] (Figure 10.23).

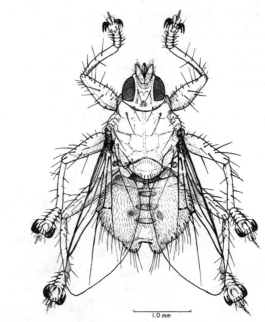

Fig. 10.23 *Pseudolynchia canariensis* adult. Courtesy of E.P. Catts, University of Delaware.

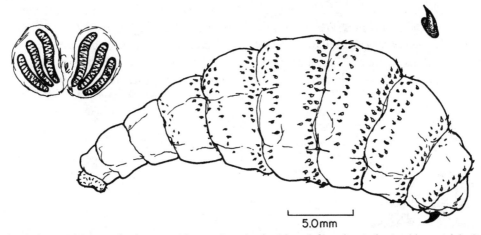

Fig. 10.22 A third-stage larvae of *Dermatobia hominis* with posterior spiracles (above left) and typical spine (above right). Courtesy of E.P. Catts, University of Delaware.

Hosts and Life Cycle. The pigeon is the host for *Pseudolynchia canariensis.* The life cycles of hippoboscids are unique in that larvae mature in the female, and pupate upon being ejected. The larvae pupate for approximately one month, and adults live for 45 days[208].

Pathologic Effects and Clinical Disease. Adult *P. canariensis* suck blood and therefore may cause anemia, especially in young birds. They also serves as a vector for blood-borne pathogens, including *Haemoproteus.* Affected birds can develop anemia and reduced egg production.

Diagnosis, Treatment, and Prevention. Diagnosis is by demonstrating *P. canariensis* on the bird. Permethrin spray (0.05%) is likely to be effective[211]. Pyrethrin dust (0.25%) has also been effective[212]. A thorough physical examination of incoming birds reduces the risk of introducing *P. canariensis* in the flock. Dusting birds with a 1% pyrethrin compound represents an effective preventive measure[213].

Public Health Considerations. Although humans are not a host of *P. canariensis,* humans can develop a hypersensitivity reaction at the site of fly feeding.

Family Muscidae

Most flies in the family Muscidae family are non-biting, coprophagus flies. Important genera include *Musca, Fannia, Muscina,* and *Stomoxys.* Of these, only flies in the genus *Stomoxys* suck blood. Common *Musca* species include *M. domestica* (the housefly), *Fannia canicularis* (the "lesser" or "little" housefly), *F. scalaris* (the "latrine" fly), and *Muscina stabulans* (the "false stable" fly). A common *Stomoxys* genus is *Stomoxys calcitrans* (the "stable" fly). Members of the family produce accidental myiasis in birds[207].

Morphology. Adults of *Musca, Fannia,* and *Muscina* are blackish gray with nonmetallic bodies. Larvae of *Musca* and *Muscina* measure 10 mm to 12 mm long and are tapered at the anterior end and truncated at the posterior end (Figure 10.24). *Fannia* larvae are flattened and have noticeable lateral processes (Figure 10.25). *Stomoxys* resemble the housefly but are slightly darker in color and

are more robust. *Stomoxys* larvae are similar to those of *Musca* and *Muscina*[207].

Hosts. *Muscidae* flies have been associated with birds and mammals. *Musca, Fannia,* and *Muscina* are associated with animal wastes[207], whereas *Stomoxys* can suck blood from a variety of birds and mammals.

Life Cycle. Muscid flies lay their eggs in decaying organic matter. *Musca, Fannia,* and *Muscina* also deposit their eggs in animal wastes, while *Stomoxys* prefer decaying vegetation[207].

Pathologic Effects and Clinical Disease. Muscid flies can cause accidental myiasis of open wounds. In addition, they serve as mechanical vectors of intestinal pathogens such as *Salmonella*[214]. *Stomoxys* flies are also bloodsuckers and can cause local inflammation at the bite location. Because they feed on animals, they can transmit blood-borne agents. Moreover, *S. calcitrans* is the intermediate host for *Hymenolepis carioca,* a chicken tapeworm. *Stomoxys* flies can cause local inflammation at the bite site.

Diagnosis, Treatment, and Prevention. Diagnosis is by identification of the larvae in the tissues. Flushing of the wounds and antibiotics are necessary to treat myiasis. Fly control is necessary to reduce fly populations. Moreover, prompt removal of animal wastes and decaying organic material reduces fly breeding sites.

Public Health Considerations. Muscid flies can affect humans by causing myiasis of open wounds or by serving as vectors for diseases. In addition, *Stomoxys* flies can cause a painful bite.

Family Sarcophagidae

The sarcophagid, or "flesh" flies, are large flies that infest a wide variety of birds and mammals. Common genera include *Sarcophaga* and *Wohlfahrtia.* Of these, *S. haemorrhoidalis* is among the most common[208].

Morphology. Sarcophagid flies are medium to large gray and black flies that measure 8 mm to 14 mm long[207].

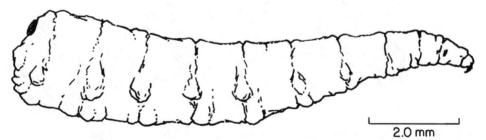

Fig. 10.24   A muscid larvae (*Musca, Muscina, Stomoxys*). Courtesy of E.P. Catts, University of Delaware.

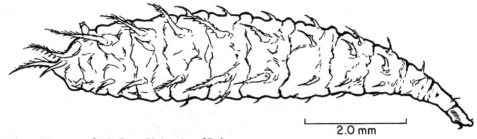

Fig. 10.25   A *Fannia* larva. Courtesy of E.P. Catts, University of Delaware.

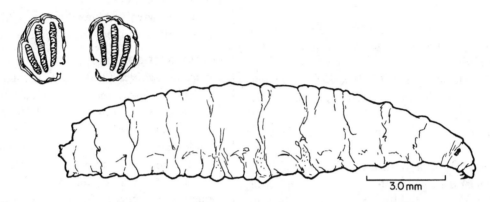

Fig. 10.26   A sarcophagid larva with posterior spiracles (above left). Courtesy of E.P. Catts, University of Delaware.

Sarcophagid fly larvae are tapered and are recognized by their posterior spiracles (Figure 10.26).

Hosts and Life Cycle. Sarcophagid flies cause myiasis in a variety of bird and mammalian hosts. Instead of laying eggs, females deposit larvae on wounds. These larvae develop in four to seven days and pupate for approximately four days. Sarcophagid flies can complete their life cycle in two weeks[207].

Pathologic Effects and Clinical Disease. Sarcophagid larvae may invade healthy tissue when there is accidental myiasis. Clinical disease is not noted unless maggots invade deeper tissues.

Diagnosis, Treatment, and Prevention. Diagnosis is by identifying larvae in the tissues. Flushing the wound to remove maggots is an important step in treating myiasis. Fly control reduces fly populations. Reduction of animal wastes and decaying organic matter eliminates fly breeding areas.

Public Health Considerations. Sarcophagid flies cause myiasis in humans. However, infected birds are not a direct hazard to humans.

Family Simulidae

Simuliids (blackflies, turkey gnats, or buffalo gnats) are short, stout, biting flies. The most important genus is *Simulium*. Common species parasitizing birds include *S. bracteatum*, *S. jenningsi*, *S. slossonae*, *S. meridionae*, *S. occidentale*, *S. croxtoni*, *S. euryadminiculum*, *S. rugglesi*, *S. slossonae*, and *S. congareenarum*.

Morphology. Adults have a small, robust body with conical antennae with seven to nine segments, an arched thorax, and wings with thickened veins.

Hosts and Life Cycle. Simuliids can affect a variety of bird and mammalian species. Blackflies lay their eggs only in running water. Following hatching, larvae develop for three to 10 weeks before pupating. Pupae are found under water, where they can remain for a few days to one week. Adults emerge in the spring, summer, or early fall, depending on the species.

Pathologic Effects and Clinical Disease. Simuliids commonly feed on poultry. More importantly, they serve as vectors for such blood-borne pathogens as *Leucocytozoon*. Affected birds can have production losses and anemia can be seen in young birds.

Diagnosis, Treatment, and Prevention. Diagnosis is by identifying the gnat. Control is difficult because simuliids develop in streams. The use of insecticides may affect free-living animals. Netting may prevent birds from being attacked.

Public Health Considerations. Simuliids readily feed upon humans, and serve as vectors for human diseases. However, there are no direct hazards from affected birds to humans.

Order Phthiraptera

Cuclotogaster heterographa

Morphology. *Cuclotogaster heterographa* (chicken head louse) is gray and measures 2 mm long[215]. The head is unusual—it is longer than it is wide—and has an anterior portion that is evenly rounded. The widest portion of the head is posterior to the five-segmented antenna[215] (Figure 10.27).

Hosts. *Cuclotogaster heterographa* is found in the feathers, especially in the head and neck region, of chickens and other birds.

Life Cycle. The life cycle of *Cuclotogaster heterographa* is completed in two to three weeks. Although they can live for several months, they can only live for five to six days in the absence of a host. Transmission occurs via direct contact.

Pathologic Effects and Clinical Disease. *Cuclotogaster heterographa* damages the feathers of affected birds. Affected birds are restless and have depressed weight gains and reduced egg production. Feathers may appear to be of poor quality and have a "moth-eaten" appearance.

Diagnosis, Treatment, and Prevention. Diagnosis is by identifying *C. heterographa* in the feathers. Treatment includes synthetic pyrethroids, organophosphorus, carbamate, or pyrethroid insecticides. If treatment is used, birds need to be treated at least twice on a seven- to 10-day interval[208]. Repeat treatment is needed to control the lice that hatch after the initial treatment, because the available chemicals do not kill the eggs[208]. A thorough physical examination helps to minimize introduction of *C. heterographa* into the flock.

Public Health Considerations. *Cuclotogaster heterographa* is not of public health significance.

Goniocotes gallinae

Goniocotes gallinae (fluff louse) is found in the feathers, especially the down feathers, of chickens. *Goniocotes gallinae* measures 1.5 mm long and has a yellow, rounded shape[215]. The head is wider than it is long and has a rounded anterior portion and an angular posterior portion. The antennae have five segments[215] (Figure 10.28).

The life cycle is unknown, though transmission is though direct contact. *Goniocotes gallinae* is generally nonpathogenic, though with heavy infestations, feathers may appear "moth-eaten." Hyperchromic anemia has been reported[196]. With heavy infestations, affected birds become

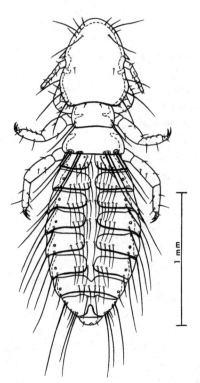

Fig. 10.27 Dorsal view of a female *Cuclotogaster heterographa*. Courtesy of R.D. Price, University of Minnesota.

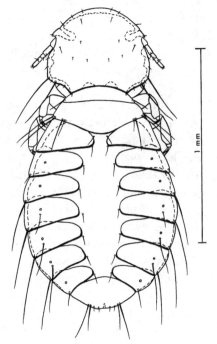

Fig. 10.28 Dorsal view of a female *Goniocotes gallinae*. Courtesy of R.D. Price, University of Minnesota.

restless and have reduced egg production and weight gain. Diagnosis is by identification of *G. gallinae*. Treatments recommended for *C. heterographa* are effective for *G. gallinae*. A thorough physical examination of the flock helps to minimize introducing *G. gallinae* into the flock. *Goniocotes gallinae* is not of public health significance.

Goniodes spp.

Morphology. The genus *Goniodes* is represented by three common species: *G. dissimilis* (brown chicken louse), *G. gigas*, and *G. numidae* (guinea feather louse). Members of the genus are the largest lice found on chickens. They are brown, and measure 3 mm long[215]. The antennae have five segments. The front portion of the head is rounded while the back is angular. The head is wider than it is long. Although similar in body shape, *Goniodes* is larger than *Goniocotes*. *Goniodes dissimilis* has four long hairs on the posterior margin of the head (Figure 10.29), while *G. gigas* has six long hairs on the posterior margin[215].

Hosts and Life Cycle. *Goniodes* species parasitize chickens and other birds[215]. *Goniodes gigas* requires one month to complete its life cycle. Females deposit up to 14 eggs, which hatch in about a week[215]. After reaching maturity, males only live up to 19 days, and females up to 24 days. The life cycles of *G. dissimilis* and *G. numidae*

remain unknown, but are most likely similar to that of *G. gigas*. Transmission is via direct contact[215].

Pathologic Effects and Clinical Disease. *Goniodes* are nonpathogenic. Thus, clinical signs are typically not observed.

Diagnosis, Treatment, and Prevention. Diagnosis is by identifying the adult louse. Treatment for *Goniodes* is similar to that recommended for *Cuclotogaster heterographa*. A thorough physical examination of incoming birds helps to minimize the risk of introducing *Goniodes* into the flock.

Public Health Considerations. *Goniodes* are host-specific and do not infest humans.

Lipeurus and closely related species

Common *Lipeurus* lice found on birds include *Lipeurus caponis* (wing louse), *L. numidae* (slender guinea louse), and *L. lawrensis*. In addition, the closely related *Oxylipeurus polytrapezius* (slender turkey louse), *O. corpelentus*, and *O. dentatus*[208,215] have also been reported in birds. *Lipeurus caponis* is a long, slender, gray louse measuring 2.5 mm long[215]. The head is longer than it is wide, and the anterior portion of the head is rounded. The antennae have five segments[215] (Figure 10.30).

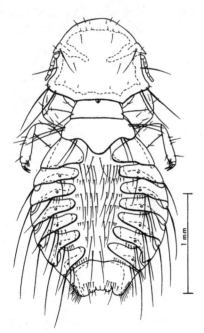

Fig. 10.29 Dorsal view of a female *Goniodes dissimilis*. Courtesy of R.D. Price, University of Minnesota.

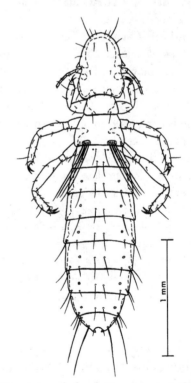

Fig. 10.30 Dorsal view of a female *Lipeurus caponis*. Courtesy of R.D. Price, University of Minnesota.

Lipeurus species have been reported in the feathers of the chicken and other birds[215]. Specific details on the life cycle of *Lipeurus* are unknown, but the complete life cycle occurs within three to five weeks[216]. *Lipeurus caponis* is primarily found on the ventral side of the primary flight, tail, or back feathers[217]. They are nonmotile and usually nonpathogenic. Other *Lipeurus* species are also relatively nonpathogenic. Therefore, clinical disease is not noted with *Lipeurus*. However, heavy infestation can result in restlessness and unthriftiness.

Diagnosis is by identifying *Lipeurus* on the bird. Treatment for *Lipeurus* is similar to that recommended for *Cuclotogaster heterographa*. An herbal extract of *Cedrus deodara*, *Azadirachta indica*, and *Embelia ribes*, when sprayed on chickens for three successive days, was effective, though mild skin irritation developed[218]. A thorough physical examination of incoming birds minimizes the risk of introducing *Lipeurus* lice species into the flock. *Lipeurus* lice species are not of public health significance.

Menacanthus stramineus

Morphology. *Menacanthus stramineus* (chicken body louse) (Syn. *Eomenacanthus stramineus*), *M. cornutus*, and *Menacanthus pallidulus* are yellow and measure 3 mm to 3.5 mm long. They have a triangular head and club-shaped antennae[208] (Figure 10.31).

Hosts and Life Cycle. *Menacanthus* spp. are found on the vent feathers of chickens, guinea fowl, and turkeys[208]. Eggs are deposited on the base of the feather shaft, especially in the vent region. Females live for about 12 days and lay up to four eggs per day[219]. Eggs hatch in four to five days[219]. The life cycle is completed in about two weeks. Transmission is via direct contact.

Pathologic Effects. *Menacanthus stramineus* is especially prevalent in the less feathered areas of the breast, thigh, and vent. There can be small blood clots near the vent region when *M. stramineus* bites through the soft quills and causes bleeding[217]. Blood loss may result in hyperchromic anemia[196].

Clinical Disease, Treatment, and Prevention. Affected birds may be restless and unthrifty. There can also be decreased production. Diagnosis is by identifying *M. stramineus* on the bird. Treatments recommended for *M. stramineus* are similar to those recommended for *Cuclotogaster heterographa*. A thorough physical examination of incoming birds minimizes the risk of introducing *M. stramineus* into the flock.

Public Health Considerations. *Menacanthus stramineus* does not infest humans.

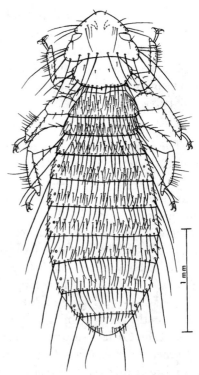

Fig. 10.31 Dorsal view of a female *Menacanthus stramineus*. Courtesy of R.D. Price, University of Minnesota.

Menopon gallinae

Menopon gallinae (shaft louse) has been recovered from the feathers of chickens, guinea fowl, and other bird species[208,215]. *Menopon gallinae* is yellow and measures 2 mm in length. It has a triangular head with club-shaped antennae[208] (Figure 10.32).

Few details are known of the life cycle of *M. gallinae*. Eggs are deposited at the base of the feathers of the breast and thighs[217]. Hyperchromic anemia has been reported in affected birds[196]. However, it is usually nonpathogenic and so clinical signs are generally not observed. Heavy infestations may cause restlessness, lowered production, and unthriftiness.

Diagnosis is made by identifying *M. gallinae* on the bird. Treatments recommended for *M. gallinae* are similar to those recommended for *Cuclotogaster heterographa*. In one study, an herbal compound of *Cedrus deodara*, *Azadirachta indica*, and *Embelia ribes* diluted 1:10 to 1:50 and sprayed for three successive days eliminated the infestation[218]. *Menopon gallinae* does not infest humans, but may serve as a reservoir for *Chlamydiophila psittaci*.

Syringophillus spp.

Syringophillus lice species have been recovered from the quill feathers of the wing and body plumage of chickens and other birds[208]. Species found include *S. hipectinatus* (quill mite)

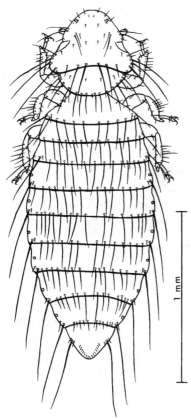

Fig. 10.32 Dorsal view of a female *Menopon gallinae*. Courtesy of R.D. Price, University of Minnesota.

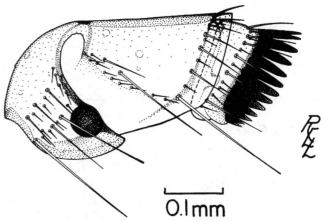

Fig. 10.33 The head of *Ceratophyllus gallinae*. Courtesy of R.E. Lewis, Iowa State University.

environment (i.e. litter). Incubation requires two to four days and there are three larval instars[208]. The third larval instar spins a cocoon in which the larva develops into an adult in about two weeks[208]. Transmission occurs by direct contact.

Pathologic Effects and Clinical Disease. *Ceratophyllus gallinae* can cause anemia. *Ceratophyllus gallinae* causes pale skin and decreased production.

Diagnosis, Treatment, and Prevention. Diagnosis is by identifying *C. gallinae* on the bird or in the environment. Treatment for *C. gallinae* is similar to that recommended for *E. gallinae*. It is important not only to treat the bird but also to focus on the sanitation and disinfection of the environment to eliminate *C. gallinae*.

Public Health Considerations. *Ceratophyllus gallinae* readily feeds on humans.

Ceratophyllus niger

Ceratophyllus niger (Western chicken flea) has been reported on the external body surface of chickens and other birds, as well as rodents and humans[208]. *Ceratophyllus niger* is similar in appearance to *C. gallinae*. Likewise, the life cycle of *C. niger* is similar to that of *C. gallinae*.

Ceratophyllus niger can cause anemia, resulting in pale skin and decreased production. Diagnosis is by identifying *C. niger* on the bird or from its environment. Treatment for *C. niger* is similar to that recommended for *E. gallinae*. It is important not only to treat the bird but also to focus on the sanitation and disinfection of the environment to eliminate *C. niger*.

Echidnophaga gallinacea

Morphology. *Echidnophaga gallinacea* (chicken flea or sticktight flea) is a small flea, measuring only up to 1.5 mm in length. The distinguishing feature of *E. gallinacea* is the

from chickens, turkeys, and golden pheasants; *S. columbae* (pigeon quill mite) from pigeons; *S. minor* from house sparrows; and *S. bipectinatus* from poultry[208]. *Syringophillus* measure 0.9 mm long by 0.15 mm wide[208]. The life cycle is completed in 38 to 41 days. Unfertilized eggs can hatch and the released larvae are male[208]. *Syringophillus* infestations can result in partial or complete loss of the feathers. Powdery debris obtained near the remaining quill stump can contain the mites, and are useful diagnostic specimens. No effective treatments have been developed for *Syringophillus* infestation. *Syringophillus* mites do not infest humans.

Order Siphonaptera

Ceratophyllus gallinae

Morphology. Adult *Ceratophyllus gallinae* (European chicken flea)[208] are brown and measure 2 mm long. Adults bear a pronotal comb but lack a genal comb (Figure 10.33).

Hosts and Life Cycle. *Ceratophyllus gallinae* has been reported in chickens and turkeys. It has also been noted on free-living birds and mammals, including humans[208]. The life cycle of *C. gallinae* is similar to that of *Ctenocephalides* sp. Adults mate while on the host and the eggs often fall into the

lack of genal and pronotal combs. The head has an angular appearance (Figure 10.34).

Hosts. *Echidnophaga gallinacea* is commonly found on unfeathered portions of the head of chickens, pheasants, pigeons, quail, and turkeys. It has also been reported on blackbirds, blue jays, hawks, owls, and sparrows[208]. Humans and numerous mammalian species can also be infested.

Life Cycle. Unlike other fleas, adults of *E. gallinacea* become sessile and remain deeply embedded in the skin[208]. One to four eggs are ejected per day into the surrounding environment. The eggs incubate for six to eight days before hatching[220]. Larvae feed on flea excrement. Larvae develop for 14 to 31 days and then spin cocoons. They remain in these cocoons for nine to 19 days[221]. Infection occurs when the host enters an infested area rather than by direct transmission, because the fleas remain attached to the host.

Pathologic Effects and Clinical Disease. *Echidnophaga gallinacea* can occur in large numbers on the unfeathered portions of the head (i.e., comb, wattles, and area surrounding the eyes). A lymphoplasmacytic reaction in the dermis with visible embedded flea mouthparts has been reported[222]. *Echidnophaga gallinacea* can result in pale skin and decreased production.

Diagnosis, Treatment, and Prevention. Diagnosis is by identifying *E. gallinacea* on the host. Pyrethroid permethrin spray (0.125% to 0.25%) on nest boxes and litter is effective[223]. Treatment with a topical pyrethrin product in a viscous base or dusting with 5% carbaryl is also effective[224]. Treatment of the bird and the environment is needed to effectively control infestations. Removal of infested litter and proper sanitation of the buildings to kill immature larvae are needed to control *E. gallinacea* infections. Removal of infected birds and reducing exposure to mammalian pests are necessary to prevent future infections.

Public Health Considerations. *Echinophaga gallinacea* can feed on humans, causing pruritus and swelling at sites of feeding. Moreover, they can also serve as vectors for *Yersinia pestis* (plague), *Rickettsia* spp. (typhus), and *Salmonella tyhpimurium*[214].

Order Hemiptera

Cimex lectularius

Morphology. Adults of the family Cimicidae (bed bugs) are dorsoventrally flattened, measure 2 mm to 5 mm long by 1.5 mm to 3 mm wide, and have three pair of legs and a pair of four-segmented antennae. Cimicids have piercing-sucking mouthparts composed of three segments, wing pads, and a hard, chitinous exoskeleton[208] (Figure 10.35). The eggs of cimicids are white and have an operculum on the anterior end.

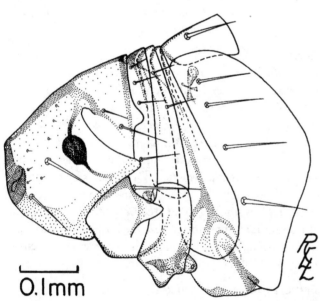

Figure. 10.34 The head of *Echidnophaga gallinacea*. Courtesy of R.E. Lewis, Iowa State University.

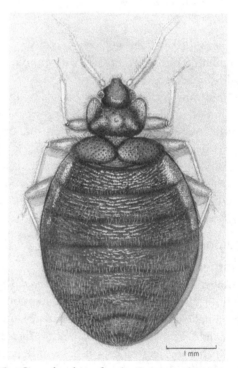

Fig. 10.35 *Cimex lectularius* female. Courtesy of M. Dorothy Cox, Loma Linda University.

Hosts and Life Cycle. *Cimex lectularius* has been reported on the external body surface of chickens and other birds, as well as on many species of mammals. Female bugs deposit eggs in crevices. Depending on the temperature, eggs can hatch in four to 20 days. Immature bugs develop through five instar stages before reaching the adult stage in one to three months[131].

Pathologic Effects and Clinical Disease. Affected birds may become anemic and may experience swelling and pruritus at the feeding sites. Affected birds may have pale combs and experience a decrease in feed consumption, weight gain, and/or egg production.

Diagnosis. Diagnosis is by identifying *C. lectularius* on the bird. Because *C. lectularius* often feeds at night, it may be necessary to examine the cracks and crevices of the animal room or housing system to detect the adults.

Treatment. Pyrethrin has been effective for eliminating those *C. lectularius* found in the bird. It is important to also treat the housing environment to effectively control *C. lectularius*.

Prevention. A thorough examination of all incoming birds minimizes the risk of introducing *C. lectularius* into the flock and environment.

Public Health Considerations. *Cimex lectularius* readily feeds on humans.

Triatoma sanguisuga

Morphology. *Triatoma sanguisuga* is a member of the family Reduviidae. These are referred to as cone-nose bugs or assassin bugs[208]. Reduviids have three pairs of legs, one pair of four-segmented antennae, and a three-segmented proboscis. Adults have two pairs of wings. The immature fourth and fifth instars have wing pods[225]. The reduviid body is shaped like a cylinder. The beak curves backward into a groove. They measure up to 25 mm long[208].

Hosts and Life Cycle. *Triatoma sanguisuga* has been reported in chickens[208]. The life cycle of *T. sanguisuga* is similar to that of the bed bugs such as *C. lectularius*. *Triatoma sanguisuga* serves as a reservoir for equine encephalomyelitis virus[208].

Pathologic Effects and Clinical Disease. *Triatoma sanguisuga* may cause anemia, but is usually nonpathogenic. Thus, clinical signs are not usually observed.

Diagnosis, Treatment, and Prevention. Diagnosis is by identifying *T. sanguisuga* on the bird or in the environment. Treatment for *T. sanguisuga* is similar to that for *C. lectularius*. It is difficult to control *T. sanguisuga* because they can fly long distances and are only found on the host

for feeding. Control is best achieved by eliminating *T. sanguisuga* in the environment.

Public Health Considerations. *Triatoma sanguisuga* readily feeds on humans and causes hypersensitivity reactions.

Class Arachnida

Ticks

Family Argasidae
Argas spp. **Morphology.** *Argas* spp. (fowl ticks) affect a wide variety of bird species. The species in birds include *A. persicus, A. sanchezi, A. radiatus, A. miniatus, A. reflexus, A. hermanni, A. neghmei, A. robertsi,* and *A. aboreus*[208]. Members of the genus are oval ticks measuring 4 mm to 11 mm long. They have a wrinkled integument with radiating disks bounded laterally by quadrangular cells (Figure 10.36).

Hosts. *Argas* parasitize birds and mammals. They have been reported on chickens, turkeys, ducks, geese, guinea fowl, pigeons, canaries, doves, hawks, magpies, owls, quail, sparrows, thrushes, vultures, and ostriches[208].

Life Cycle. *Argas persicus* has a four-month life cycle, typical of the genus[208]. Larvae feed for five to 10 days, then molt into nymphs. The nymphs have two or three instar stages, depending on the species, and then finally molt to

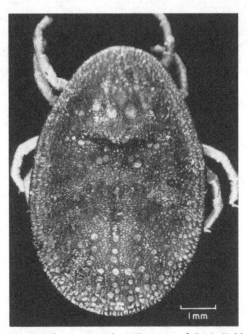

Fig. 10.36 Female *Argas sanchezi*. Courtesy of G.M. Kohls, Rocky Mountain Laboratory.

the adult stage. Feeding occurs nocturnally. It has been noted that *A. persicus* can survive for two years without feeding[208].

Pathologic Effects. Heavily infested birds become anemic. *Argas* can also serve as a vector of *Borrelia anserina,* the causative agent of avian spirochetosis[226], and *Aegyptianella pullorum,* the causative agent of aegyptianellosis[227].

Clinical Signs. Heavily infested birds appear weak, emaciated, and pale. *Argas persicus* can cause tick paralysis. The extent to which other members of the genus cause paralysis is unknown.

Diagnosis, Treatment, and Prevention. Diagnosis is by identifying the tick during nocturnal feeding. Although removal of the tick from the body of the bird is a necessary treatment, *Argas* feeds only at night, so treatment should target the bird housing to remove a majority of the tick population. To prevent future infestations, the entire housing area must be treated because the adults and nymphs feed on the host for only a short period of time.

Public Health Considerations. *Argas* may occasionally feed on humans[228]. *Argas* also can serve as a reservoir for several human pathogens.

Ornithodorus **spp.** *Ornithodorus* parasitizing birds includes *O. turicata, O. parkeri, O. talaje,* and *O. moubata* complex[229]. *Ornithodorus* ticks are similar in appearance to *Argas.* The life cycles of *Ornithodorus* ticks are similar to that of *Argas,* except that most *Ornithodorus* larvae remain attached to the host for many days, similar to that observed among the hard ticks. In addition, after the larval blood meal, *Ornithodorus* molt twice without additional feedings[229]. Heavily infected birds may become anemic and appear weak, emaciated, and pale.

Diagnosis is by identifying ticks on the host. Treatment consists of careful removal of the tick. To prevent future infestations, there must be treatment of the premises to help reduce the population. *Ornithodorus* ticks readily feed on humans and in doing so, cause local inflammatory reactions.

Family Ixodidae
Amblyomma **spp. and** *Hyalomma* **spp.** *Amblyomma* ticks are commonly found attached to the skin of birds. Common species include *Amblyomma americanum* (lone star tick), *A. maculatum, A. tuberculatum, A. variegatum,* and *A. hebraeum.* The related genus *Hyalomma* also parasitizes birds. The *Hyalomma* species reported on birds include *H. marginatum marginatum, H. marginatum rufipes, H. excavatum, H. impelatum,* and *H. truncatum*[208].

Morphology. *Amblyomma americanum* is representative of the genus, and measures 3 mm long. Engorged females can be up to 11 mm long[229] (Figure 10.37). Males have a shiny brownish red scutum, pale lateral stripes, and two U-shaped markings posteriorly. Females have similar ornamentation, except for a pale spot posteriorly.

Hosts and Life Cycle. *Amblyomma americanum* is not host-specific, and has been reported on a variety of birds and mammals[208]. *Amblyomma americanum* is a three-host tick. Females lay 2,000 to 10,000 eggs. These hatch in three to four weeks. Larvae feed, molt, and temporarily leave the host as they develop to the nymphal stage, and finally to the adult stage. The life cycle of *Hyalomma* is similar[229].

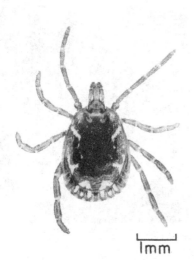 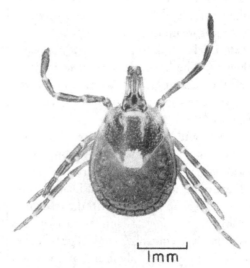

Fig. 10.37 *Amblyomma americanum.* (Left) Male. (Right) Female. Courtesy of G.M. Kohls, Rocky Mountain Laboratory.

Pathologic Effects and Clinical Disease. Heavy infestations cause anemia and result in debilitation and lethargy.

Diagnosis, Treatment, and Prevention. Diagnosis is by identifying the tick on the host. Careful removal of the entire tick, including mouthparts, is needed, along with treatment of the environmental premises. To prevent future infestations, there must be treatment of the premises because the adults and nymphs feed on the host for only a short period of time.

Public Health Considerations. *Amblyomma* and related species can serve as vectors for several human diseases so care must be taken in handling them on infected birds.

Haemaphysalis leporispalustris. *Haemaphysalis leporispalustris* (rabbit tick) can be found attached to the skin of chickens and other birds[228]. Besides *H. leporispalustris*, other *Haemaphysalis* reported on birds include *H. punctata* and *H. concinna.* All are three-host ticks. *Haemaphysalis leporispalustris* is a relatively small tick, measuring only 2.2 mm to 2.6 mm long. It has a rectangular basis capitulum (Figure 10.38). Females can measure up to 10 mm when engorged. Although the rabbit is the host, the immature larvae and nymphs can feed on chickens and other birds. Adults live for up to a year[228]. *Haemaphysalis leporispalustris* can cause anemia, lethargy, and emaciation when present in high numbers.

Diagnosis is by identifying the tick on the host. Treatment includes the physical removal of the tick from the host. The entire housing area must be treated to prevent future infestations. *Haemaphysalis leporispalustris* and related species can serve as vectors for several zoonotic diseases.

Ixodes spp. **Morphology.** *Ixodes* ticks have characteristic anal grooves that join anterior to the anus. The mouthparts are long[230]. The scutum lacks eyes, festoons, and other ornamentation (Figure 10.39). Males have seven shields that cover the ventral surface. These are absent from the female. *Ixodes* are 2 mm to 3 mm in length, but engorged females measure 7 mm to 16 mm[230].

Hosts. *Ixodes* tick species have been occasionally reported on birds. The immature forms of *I. scapularis, I. pacificus, I. ricinus, I. persulcatus,* and *I. holocyclus* have been documented on birds.

Life Cycle. *Ixodes* are three-host ticks[230]. The length of time in each life cycle stage varies with the species. Life cycles may require from seven months up to three years to complete, depending on tick species[231].

Pathologic Effects and Clinical Disease. Because *Ixodes* have long mouth parts, these can remain in the tissue after the tick has been removed. This can cause inflammation and secondary bacterial infection can occur. Heavy infestations can cause anemia. Heavy infestations can result in lethargic and debilitated animals.

Diagnosis, Treatment, and Prevention. Diagnosis is by identification of the tick on the bird. Careful removal of the tick is necessary. Because *Ixodes* have long mouthparts, removal of the entire tick must be performed to prevent inflammation and secondary bacterial infections. To prevent future infestations, there must be treatment of the

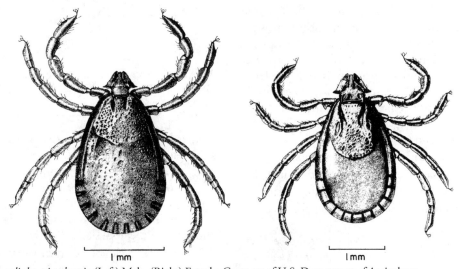

Fig. 10.38 *Haemaphysalis leporispalustris.* (Left) Male. (Right) Female. Courtesy of U.S. Department of Agriculture.

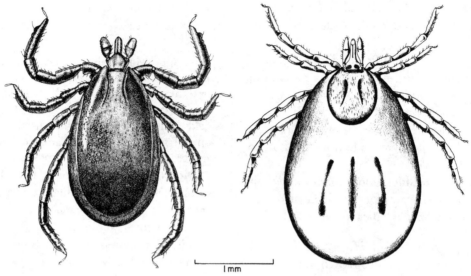

Fig. 10.39　*Ixodes scapularis.* (Left) Male. (Right) Female. Courtesy of U.S. Department of Agriculture.

premises because the adults and nymphs feed on the host for only a short period of time.

Public Health Considerations. *Ixodes* tick species can serve as a reservoir for several human diseases, so care must be taken in handling them on infected birds.

Mites

Suborder Astigmata

Cytodites nudus. *Cytodites nudus* (Syn. *Cytoleichus nudus*) (air sac mite) measures 480μ to 650 μ long by 325 μ to 500 μ wide and has short setae and a smooth dorsal integument. The legs are short and end in stalked ambulacral suckers (in the female). Males have reduced, sessile, ambulacral suckers (Figure 10.40)[232]. *Cytodites nudus* has been reported in chickens and other birds. *C. nudus* may be transmitted through aerosolization of sputum during coughing. Affected birds have increased mucus in the trachea and bronchi, pulmonary edema, emphysema, pneumonia, enteritis, and peritonitis. Granulomatous pneumonia has been reported. Affected birds cough, become weak, lose weight, and develop intermittent sneezing and head shaking[233].

Diagnosis is by identifying mites in pulmonary lesions. Ivermectin treatment has been effective in some birds. The elimination of affected birds aids in controlling this infection. *Cytodites nudus* is not of public health significance.

Knemidocoptes gallinae. *Knemidocoptes gallinae* (Syn. *Neocnemidocoptes laevis gallinae*, *Knemidocoptes laevis* var. *gallinae*)(depluming mite, depluming itch mite) has been

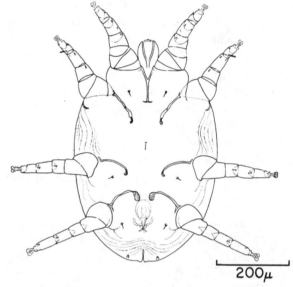

Fig. 10.40　*Cytodites nudus* male, ventral view. Reproduced from Baker, E.W., Evans, T.M., Gould, D.J., Hull, W.B. and Keegan, H.L. (1956) with permission.

reported on the skin of chickens, pigeons, and pheasants[208]. A closely related species, *N. laevis laevis,* has been reported from the pigeon. Adults measure 204 μ to 210 μ long by 144 μ to 150 μ wide[208]. Females measure 340 μ to 435 μ long and resemble *K. mutans* except that there is a transverse and unbroken dorsal striae as well as discrete tibiae and tarsi and vestigial pretarsal stalks[234] (Figure 10.41).

The life cycle of *K. gallinae* is similar to that of *K. mutans.* Mites burrow into the basal shafts of the feathers

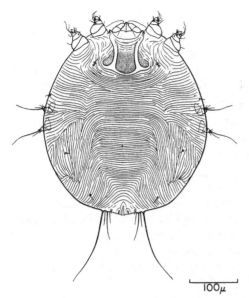

Fig. 10.41 *Knemidocoptes gallinae* female, dorsal view. Reproduced from Hirst, S. (1922) with permission.

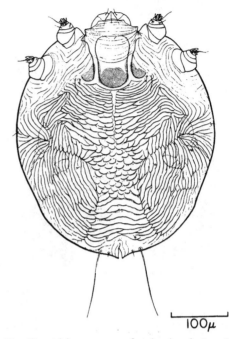

Fig. 10.42 *Knemidokoptes mutans* female, dorsal view. Reproduced from Hirst, S. (1922) with permission.

to cause pruritus[208]. Scales and small papules are produced and result in thickened and wrinkled skin. Affected birds lose feathers. The feathers of the head, neck, back, abdomen, and upper legs are most likely affected. Affected birds also lose weight, and egg production declines. Diagnosis is by identifying mites under the scales or beneath the quills. Treatment for *K. gallinae* is similar to that described for *K. mutans*. Control is via isolation of infected birds. A thorough physical examination minimizes the risk of introducing *K. gallinae* into the flock. *Knemidocoptes gallinae* is not a public health significance.

Knemidocoptes mutans. **Morphology.** *Knemidocoptes mutans* (scaly-leg mite) measures 350 μ to 450 μ long by 280 μ to 380 μ wide[234–236]. Adults are short-legged and have a striated epidermis[208] (Figure 10.42).

Hosts and Life Cycle. The natural host of *Knemidocoptes mutans* is the chicken. The life cycle of *K. mutans* is completed on the skin in 10 to 14 days. Females burrow into the epidermis and deposit eggs in the epidermal tunnel. Eggs hatch in three to eight days, and larvae migrate to the skin surface where they undergo successive molts to the adult stage[234].

Pathologic Effects and Clinical Disease. Lesions are produced on the unfeathered positions of the leg, or occasionally on the skin of the comb or wattles. Lesions include irritation, inflammation, vesicle formation, serous exudation and crust formation. As the infection worsens, there can be distortion of the legs, lameness, and loss of digits[237]. Affected birds develop proliferations and crust formation on the scales of the shank. Scales become upturned (Figure 10.43).

Diagnosis, Treatment, and Prevention. Diagnosis is by identifying mites from scrapings of lesions. Birds can be treated by dipping the legs in a warm acaricidal solution. Alternatively, birds can be treated with ivermectin[237]. Affected birds should be culled or isolated. Houses should be cleaned prior to obtaining new birds.

Public Health Considerations. *Knemidocoptes mutans* is not of public health significance.

Knemidocoptes pilae. *Knemidocoptes pilae* (scaly-face mite) causes scaly-face and scaly-leg in the parakeet. Adult males measure 200 μ to 219 μ long by 143 μ to 152 μ wide. Females measure 315 μ to 428 μ long by 252 μ to 378 μ wide. The adult and immature stages resemble *K. mutans*[234] (Figure 10.44).

The life cycle of *K. pilae* is similar to *K. mutans*. *Knemidocoptes pilae* invades feather follicles, skin folds, and the featherless epidermis of the face, foot, and cere, by direct penetration[234,238]. Mites may be seen in the deeper layers of the stratum corneum, where they cause hyperkeratosis and sloughing of the keratin[239]. Affected birds initially have whitish, yellow powdery debris over affected areas (Figure 10.45). On the face, the lesions are first noted at

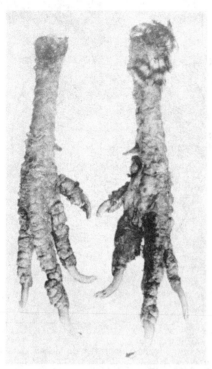

Fig. 10.43 Leg lesions caused by *Knemidocoptes mutans* in a chicken. Reproduced from Benbrook, E.A. and Sloss, M.W. (1961) with permission.

the base of the cere and the corners of the mouth. These lesions extend to cover the eyes, forehead, and cere. The beak also becomes distorted and friable[234,239].

Diagnosis is by identifying mites in the skin and scrapings from the lesions[240]. Treatment with ivermectin has been effective in some cases. The isolation and thorough examination of parakeets reduce the risk of infection to the rest of the flock. *Knemidocoptes pilae* is not of public health significance.

Laminosioptes cysticola. **Morphology.** *Laminosioptes cysticola* (fowl cyst mite, flesh mite) measures 250 μ long by 110 μ wide, and has a smooth dorsal integument with long setae (Figure 10.46). The gnathosome is reduced in size[208], and the first two pairs of legs are short and end with a claw-like tarsus. The third and fourth pairs are longer with tarsi ending with long pad-like attachments.

Hosts and Life Cycle. *Laminosioptes cysticola* has been reported in chickens, pheasants, geese, pigeons, and other birds[208]. Details of the life cycle of *L. cysticola* are lacking but females lay embryonated eggs. The entire life cycle occurs on the host.

Pathologic Effects and Clinical Disease. Affected birds develop small, yellow nodules in the subcutaneous tissues. These nodules become calcified after the death of the mite[208]. Affected birds may not show clinical signs. Carcasses may appear unpalatable for consumption. Wing droop and

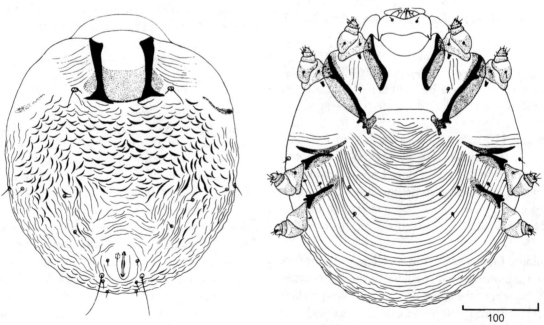

100

Fig. 10.44 *Knemidocoptes pilae* female. (Left) Dorsal view. (Right) Ventral view. Reproduced from Fain, A. and Elsen, P. (1967) with permission.

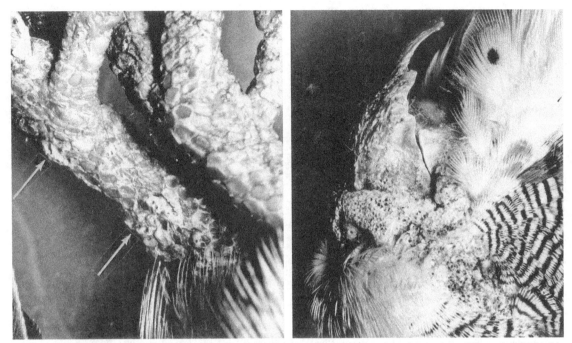

Fig. 10.45 Lesions on the face (left) and leg (right) caused by *Knemidocoptes pilae*. Reproduced from Fain, A. and Elsen, P. (1967) with permission.

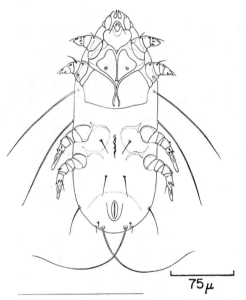

Fig. 10.46 *Laminosioptes cysticola* female, ventral view. Courtesy of Institute of Acarology.

an unsteady gait occur with heavy infestations around the region of the brachial plexus and sciatic nerves[241].

Diagnosis, Treatment, and Prevention. Microscopic examination of the skin and subcutis may reveal *L. cysticola*. In addition, a diagnosis can be made by finding a nodule and crushing it under a cover glass to confirm the presence of *L. cysticola*. Treatment regimens have not been developed. Control of *L. cysticola* is difficult. Isolation of affected birds, in conjunction with proper disinfection of facilities, is recommended.

Public Health Considerations. *Laminosioptes cysticola* is not of public health significance.

Suborder Mesostigmata
***Dermanyssus gallinae*. Morphology.** *Dermanyssus gallinae* (chicken mite, poultry red mite, red mite, roost mite, poultry mite, red roost mite) measures 700 μm by 400 μm, though engorged females can measure over 1 mm. They have characteristic ventral body plates. The sternal shield has two pairs of setae, a truncated genital plate, and an anal plate with a broad shield[232] (Figure 10.47).

Hosts. *Dermanyssus gallinae* has been reported on chickens, turkeys, pigeons, canaries, and free-living birds[208]. It can also affect rodents and humans as incidental hosts.

Life Cycle. The life cycle of *D. gallinae* can be completed within a week[208]. Eggs laid in the environment hatch in two to three days. Larvae can molt within one to two days without having taken a blood meal. Two nymphal stages occur, during which they feed and molt in one to two days to the adult stage[208]. Feeding occurs only at night.

Pathologic Effects and Clinical Disease. Heavily infested birds become anemic, the skin becomes inflamed,

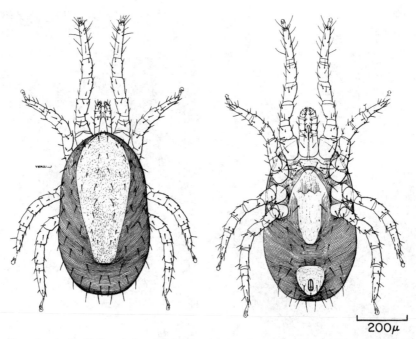

Fig. 10.47   *Dermanyssus gallinae* female. (Left) Dorsal view. (Right) Ventral view. Reproduced from Hirst, S. (1922) with permission.

and scabs form. This mite serves as a reservoir for equine encephalitis virus and other blood-borne pathogens. Heavily infested birds become pale, lethargic, and restless, and can have depressed weights and reduced egg production.

Diagnosis, Treatment, and Prevention. Diagnosis is by identifying the mite. Nocturnal examinations facilitate detection. Treatment for *D. gallinae* is similar to that described for *O. bacoti*. A thorough physical examination of incoming birds minimizes the likelihood of introducing *D. gallinae* to the flock. Because *D. gallinae* feeds on the bird only at night, environmental sanitation is important in controlling this parasite.

Public Health Consideration. *Dermanyssus gallinae* feeds on humans, and causes localized skin reaction. Because it can also serve as a reservoir of arboviruses, there should be caution when handling infected birds.

Ornithonyssus bacoti. *Ornithonyssus bacoti* commonly infests wild rodents, but also affects chickens and other birds. The biology of this mite is presented in Chapter 11, Parasites of Rats and Mice. In birds, *O. bacoti* may cause anemia. Birds become pale and lethargic, and production (meat and eggs) is decreased.

Diagnosis is by identifying mites on the bird or in the environment. Affected birds can be treated with an approved insecticide. Treatments should occur twice over a five- to

seven-day interval to ensure that the treatment will affect both adults and juvenile stages. Permethrin sprays are effective and have residual effects for up to nine weeks[211] when applied as a 0.05% concentration. The use of carbamate powder as a dusting agent is also effective[208]. Because *O. bacoti* is primarily a rodent parasite, rodent control is essential to prevent future infections. Treatment with approved pesticides in the animal facilities is the most important prevention strategy because the mite is only on the bird during feeding. *Ornithonyssus bacoti* readily feeds on humans and can inflict a painful bite. It can also harbor several human pathogens.

Ornithonyssus bursa. *Ornithonyssus bursa* (Syn. *Liponyssus bursa, Bdellonyssus bursa*) (tropical fowl mite) is found on the feathers and skin of chickens, pigeons, canaries, ducks, sparrows, mynah birds, and others. *Ornithonyssus bursa* is similar in appearance to *O. bacoti* and *O. sylviarum*[208]. Compared to *O. bacoti,* it has shorter dorsal plate setae. Compared to *O. sylviarum,* it has two pairs of setae on the posterior end of its dorsal plate (Figure 10.48). The life cycle, pathologic findings, clinical signs, diagnosis, and prevention are similar to those of *O. sylviarum*[242]. *Ornithonyssus bursa* will feed on humans and cause skin irritation.

Ornithonyssus sylviarum. **Morphology.** *Ornithonyssus sylviarum* (Syn. *Liponyssus sylviarum, Bdellonyssus sylviarum*)

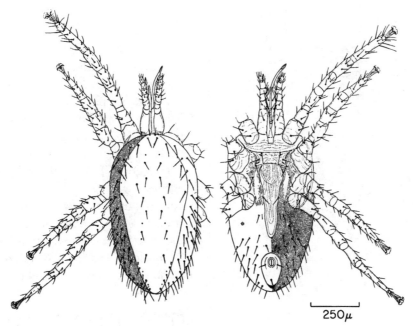

Fig. 10.48 *Ornithonyssus bursa* female. (Left) Dorsal view. (Right) Ventral view. Reproduced from Baker, E.W., Evans, T.M., Gould, D.J., Hull, W.B. and Keegan, H.L. (1956) with permission.

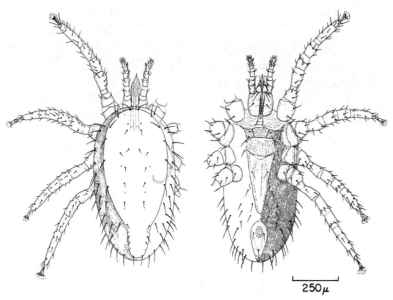

Fig. 10.49 *Ornithonyssus sylviarum* female. (Left) Dorsal view. (Right) Ventral view. Reproduced from Baker, E.W., Evans, T.M., Gould, D.J., Hull, W.B. and Keegan, H.L. (1956) with permission.

(northern fowl mite) is similar in appearance to *O. bacoti*, except that the setae on its dorsal plate are smaller than those found on the other parts of the dorsum. In *O. bacoti*, these setae are larger on the dorsal plate than on the rest of the dorsum (Figure 10.49). Moreover, to distinguish *O. sylviarum* from *O. bursa*, the tropical fowl mite, it is noted that *O. sylviarum* has a single pair of setae at the posterior dorsal plate, versus *O. bursa*, which bears two pairs of setae in this location (Figure 10.50). Adults measure 800 μ long.

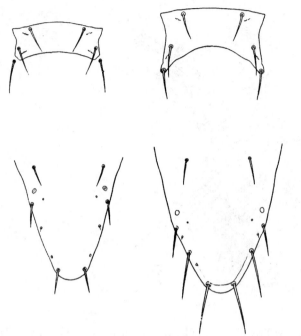

Fig. 10.50 Comparison of the distinguishing characteristics of *Ornithonyssus sylviarum* (left) and *O. bursa* (right) females. Sternal plates (top) and posterior end of the dorsal shields (bottom). Reproduced from Hirst, S. (1922) with permission.

Hosts and Life Cycle. *Ornithonyssus sylviarum* has been recovered from chickens, pigeons and other birds[243], and may also temporarily feed on rodents and humans.

The entire life cycle of *O. sylviarum* occurs on the host and can be completed in less than one week[242]. Adult mites can survive for two to three weeks in the absence of a host.

Pathologic Effects and Clinical Disease. Heavy infestations can cause anemia. Skin, especially near the vent region, can be scabby and thickened due to the mites. Affected birds have matted and discolored feathers. Birds may be restless, pale, and lethargic, and can have decreased production (weight gain or egg production).

Diagnosis, Treatment, and Prevention. Diagnosis is by identifying mites on the bird. Treatment for *O. sylviarum* is similar to that of *O. bacoti*. A thorough physical examination of incoming birds, followed by treatment of affected birds, minimizes infestation of the flock.

Public Health Considerations. *Ornithonyssus sylviarum* feeds on humans and may cause pruritus.

ACKNOWLEDGEMENTS

The authors would like to thank Irene Choi, Marisa Ames, and Peter Kobalka of the Avian Disease Investigation Laboratory, Department of Veterinary Preventive Medicine, The Ohio State University, for their technical assistance; and Dolores Fischer, Department of Veterinary Preventive Medicine at The Ohio State University, for her secretarial assistance.

TABLE 10.1 Parasites of birds—circulatory/lymphatic system.

Parasite	Geographic distribution	Hosts	Location in host	Method of infection	Pathologic effects	Zoonosis	Reference
Flagellates							
Trypanosoma avium	Worldwide	Galliformes, Anseriformes, Passeriformes	Blood	Black fly or mosquito bite	None	None known	1
Coccidia							
Atoxoplasma spp.	Worldwide	Passeriformes	Mononuclear leukocytes	Transmitted by mites	Death	Not reported	49,50
Toxoplasma gondii	Worldwide	Birds	Spleen, heart, lung, liver, brain	Ingestion of sporulated oocysts in cat feces	Tissue cysts, chorioretinitis	Common zoonosis	82
Piroplasmids and Haemosporidia							
Aegyptianella pullorum	Africa, Asia, Europe	Birds	Erythrocytes, heart	Soft tick vector	Anemia, diarrhea, pulmonary hypertension	Not reported	227
Babesia moshkovskii	Asia, Africa	Chickens, other birds	Erythrocytes	Tick vector	Unknown	Not reported	1
Haemoproteus columbae	Worldwide	Pigeons, other Columbiformes	Erythrocytes, lung, liver, spleen	Bite of pigeon ked, *Pseudolynchia canariensis*	Generally unapparent, variable anorexia, anemia, splenomegaly	Not reported	1
Haemoproteus meleagridis	Unknown	Turkeys	Erythrocytes, spleen, heart	Arthropod vector	None	Not reported	89
Haemoproteus nettionis	Unknown	Waterfowl	Erythrocytes, spleen, heart	*Culicoides* bite	None	Not reported	1
Haemoproteus meleagridis	Unknown	Columbiformes	Erythrocytes, spleen, heart	Bite of hippoboscid fly	None	Not reported	1
Haemoproteus spp.	Worldwide	Birds	Erythrocytes, spleen, heart	Arthropod vector	Variable	Not reported	44, 86–88
Leucocytozoon andrewsi	Unknown	Chickens, pheasants	Leucocytes, erythrocytes, visceral organs	*Simulium* bite	None	Not reported	94
Leucocytozoon caulleryi	Asia, North America	Chickens, guinea fowl, pheasants	Leucocytes, erythrocytes, visceral organs	*Culicoides* bite	Anemia, diarrhea, reduced production	Not reported	90,91
Leucocytozoon marchouxi	Worldwide	Columbiformes	Leucocytes, erythrocytes, visceral organs	Arthropod vector	None	Not reported	1
Leucocytozoon sabrazesi	Asia	Chickens, pheasants	Leucocytes, erythrocytes, visceral organs	Arthropod vector	Anemia, diarrhea	Not reported	93

(*Continued*)

275

TABLE 10.1 (Continued)

Parasite	Geographic distribution	Hosts	Location in host	Method of infection	Pathologic effects	Zoonosis	Reference
Leucocytozoon simondi	Unknown	Anseriformes	Leucocytes, erythrocytes, visceral organs	Simulium bite	Splenomegaly, hepatitis, anemia, leukocytosis, pneumonia	Not reported	95
Leucocytozoon smithi	Unknown	Turkeys	Leucocytes, erythrocytes, visceral organs	Simulium bite	Splenomegaly, hepatomegaly, icterus, enteritis, pneumonia	Not reported	96
Leucocytozoon spp.	Worldwide	Galliformes, other birds	Leucocytes, erythrocytes, visceral organs	Arthropod vector	Variable	Not reported	93,94
Plasmodium catberium	Unknown	Canaries, other Passeriformes	Erythrocytes, liver, skeletal muscle	Mosquito bite	Vasculitis	Not reported	97
Plasmodium circumflexum	Worldwide	Passerines, other birds	Erythrocytes, liver, lung	Mosquito bite	None	Not reported	98
Plasmodium durae	Unknown	Turkeys, other birds	Erythrocytes, liver, lung	Mosquito bite	Cardiomyopathy	Not reported	99
Plasmodium fallax	Unknown	Guinea fowl, other birds	Erythrocytes, lung, liver	Mosquito bite	Mildly pathogenic	Not reported	1
Plasmodium gallinaceum	Asia	Galliformes	Erythrocytes, lung, liver	Mosquito bite	Anemia, cerebral vasculitis, splenomegaly, high mortality	Not reported	1
Plasmodium hermani	Unknown	Turkeys, other Galliformes, Anseriformes, Passeriformes	Erythrocytes, lung, liver	Mosquito bite	Anemia, splenomegaly	Not reported	100
Plasmodium juxtanucleare	Americas, Asia	Chickens, other Galliformes	Erythrocytes, lung, liver	Mosquito bite	Anemia, splenomegaly, pericardial effusion, high mortality	Not reported	1
Plasmodium matutinum	Worldwide	Canaries, other birds	Erythrocytes, lung, liver	Unknown arthropod vector	Highly pathogenic	Not reported	1
Plasmodium relictum	Unknown	Many birds	Erythrocytes, lung, liver	Mosquito bite	Anemia, splenomegaly, hepatomegaly	Not reported	1

276

TABLE 10.2 Parasites of birds—enterohepatic system.

Parasite	Geographic distribution	Hosts	Location in host	Method of infection	Pathologic effects	Zoonosis	Reference
Flagellates							
Chilomastix gallinarum	Worldwide	Galliformes, Anseriformes	Ceca	Fecal-oral	None	Not reported	5
Cochlosoma anatis	Worldwide	Geese, turkeys	Intestines	Fecal-oral	Enteritis	Not reported	13
Cochlosoma spp.	Worldwide	Passeriformes	Intestines	Fecal-oral	Enteritis	Not reported	14,15
Giardia psittaci	Worldwide	Psitaciformes, Passeriformes, Anseriformes,	Small intestine	Fecal-oral	Enteritis	Not reported	19
Hexamita columbae	Worldwide	Pigeons	Intestines	Fecal-oral	Catarrhal enteritis	Not reported	22
Hexamita meleagridis	Worldwide	Galliformes, psittacines	Small intestine, ceca, bursa	Fecal-oral	Enteritis	Not reported	2
Hexamita spp.	Unknown	Finches, parrots	Small intestine, ceca	Fecal-oral	Unknown	Not reported	20,26
Histomonas meleagridis	Worldwide	Turkeys, pheasants, peafowl, chickens	Ceca, liver	Fecal-oral, or ingestion of organism in *Heterakis* eggs	Enteritis, hepatitis	Not reported	30
Pentatrichomonas gallinarum	Worldwide	Galliformes	Ceca, liver	Fecal-oral	None	Not reported	1
Tetratrichomonas anatis	Worldwide	Ducks	Ceca	Fecal-oral	None	Not reported	1
Tetratrichomonas anseris	Worldwide	Geese	Ceca	Fecal-oral	None	Not reported	1
Tetratrichomonas gallinarum	Worldwide	Galliformes	Ceca	Fecal-oral	None	Not reported	34
Trichomonas gallinae	Worldwide	Galliformes, Columbiformes, Passeriformes, Psitaciformes	Mouth and upper digestive tract	Ingestion of organism passed in pigeon milk or in contaminated water	Caseous nodules or ulcers	Not reported	3
Tritrichomonas eberthi	Worldwide	Chickens, turkeys, ducks	Ceca	Fecal-oral	None	Not reported	43
Amoebae							
Endolimax gregariniformis	Worldwide	Galliformes, Anseriformes, others	Ceca	Fecal-oral	None	Not reported	1
Entamoeba anatis	Worldwide	Ducks	Large intestine	Fecal-oral	None	Not reported	1
Entamoeba gallinarum	Worldwide	Galliformes, Anseriformes	Ceca	Fecal-oral	None	Not reported	1

(Continued)

277

TABLE 10.2 (*Continued*)

Parasite	Geographic distribution	Hosts	Location in host	Method of infection	Pathologic effects	Zoonosis	Reference
Coccidia							
Blastocystis spp.	Unknown	Chickens, other birds	Intestines	Ingestion of sporulated oocyst	None	Not reported	1
Cryptosporidium baileyi	Worldwide	Cockatiels, other birds	Intestine, lung, other organs	Ingestion of sporulated oocyst	Usually none	Not reported	53,57
Cryptosporidium meleagridis	Worldwide	Turkeys, other Galliformes, other birds	Intestine, lung, other organs	Ingestion of sporulated oocyst	Occasional enteritis	Reported	51,52
Cryptosporidium spp.	Worldwide	Various birds	Gastrointestinal tract, other locations	Ingestion of sporulated oocyst	Variable	Not reported	20,29,60
Eimeria acervulina	Worldwide	Chickens	Small intestine (jejunum)	Ingestion of sporulated oocyst	Occasional enteritis	Not reported	1
Eimeria adenoeides	Worldwide	Turkeys	Lower intestinal tract	Ingestion of sporulated oocyst	Severe hemorrhagic enteritis	Not reported	1
Eimeria anatis	Worldwide	Ducks	Small intestine	Ingestion of sporulated oocyst	None	Not reported	1
Eimeria battakhi	Unknown	Ducks	Intestine	Ingestion of sporulated oocyst	None	Not reported	1
Eimeria columbae	Worldwide	Pigeons	Intestine	Ingestion of sporulated oocyst	None	Not reported	1
Eimeria danailova	Unknown	Ducks	Small intestine	Ingestion of sporulated oocyst	Catarrhal and hemorrhagic enteritis	Not reported	1
Eimeria necatrix	Worldwide	Chickens	Small intestine (jejunum)	Ingestion of sporulated oocyst	Enteritis	None	1
Eimeria brunetti	Worldwide	Chickens	Small intestine (jejunum) to colon	Ingestion of sporulated oocyst	Necrotic enteritis	Not reported	1
Eimeria dispersa	Worldwide	Galliformes	Small intestine	Ingestion of sporulated oocyst	Mild enteritis	Not reported	1
Eimeria dunsingi	Unknown	Parakeets	Small intestine	Ingestion of sporulated oocyst	Enteritis	Not reported	1
Eimeria gallopavonis	Worldwide	Turkeys	Large intestine	Ingestion of sporulated oocyst	Mild enteritis	Not reported	1
Eimeria gorakhpuri	Unknown	Guinea fowl	Large intestine	Ingestion of sporulated oocyst	None	Not reported	1
Eimeria grenieri	Unknown	Guinea fowl	Intestine	Ingestion of sporulated oocyst	Mild enteritis	Not reported	1
Eimeria haematodi	Unknown	Lorikeets	Intestine	Ingestion of sporulated oocyst	Unknown	Not reported	1
Eimeria bagani	Worldwide	Chickens	Small intestine (duodenum)	Ingestion of sporulated oocyst	Mild enteritis, villus tips primarily	Not reported	1

Species	Distribution	Host	Site	Transmission	Clinical signs		Reference
Eimeria inocua	Worldwide	Turkeys	Small intestine	Ingestion of sporulated oocyst	None	Not reported	1
Eimeria kotlani	Unknown	Geese	Large intestine	Ingestion of sporulated oocyst	Hemorrhagic enteritis	Not reported	1
Eimeria labbeana	Worldwide	Pigeons, doves	Intestine	Ingestion of sporulated oocyst	Enteritis, stunting	Not reported	1
Eimeria mandali	Worldwide	Peafowl	Intestine	Ingestion of sporulated oocyst	None	Not reported	1
Eimeria maxima	Worldwide	Chickens	Small intestine (jejunum)	Ingestion of sporulated oocyst	Hemorrhagic enteritis	Not reported	1
Eimeria mayurai	Worldwide	Peafowl	Small intestine (jejunum)	Ingestion of sporulated oocyst	Enteritis	Not reported	1
Eimeria meleagridis	Worldwide	Turkeys	Small intestine (jejunum)	Ingestion of sporulated oocyst	None	Not reported	1
Eimeria meleagrimitis	Worldwide	Turkeys	Small intestine	Ingestion of sporulated oocyst	Catarrhal enteritis	Not reported	1
Eimeria mitis	Worldwide	Chickens	Small intestine	Ingestion of sporulated oocyst	Occasional enteritis	Not reported	1
Eimeria mivati	Worldwide	Chickens	Small intestine (duodenum)	Ingestion of sporulated oocyst	Enteritis, sometimes death	Not reported	1
Eimeria mulardi	Unknown	Ducks	Intestine	Ingestion of sporulated oocyst	None	Not reported	1
Eimeria nocens	Unknown	Geese	Intestine	Ingestion of sporulated oocyst	Enteritis	Not reported	1
Eimeria numidae	Worldwide	Guinea fowl	Intestine	Ingestion of sporulated oocyst	Catarrhal enteritis	Not reported	1
Eimeria pavonina	Worldwide	Peafowl	Intestine	Ingestion of sporulated oocyst	None	Not reported	1
Eimeria pavonis	Worldwide	Peafowl	Intestine	Ingestion of sporulated oocyst	None	Not reported	1
Eimeria praecox	Worldwide	Chickens	Small intestine (jejunum)	Ingestion of sporulated oocyst	None	Not reported	1
Eimeria saitamae	Unknown	Ducks	Small intestine	Ingestion of sporulated oocyst	Enteritis	Not reported	1
Eimeria schachdagica	Unknown	Ducks	Intestine	Ingestion of sporulated oocyst	None	Not reported	1
Eimeria stigmosa	Unknown	Geese	Large and small intestines	Ingestion of sporulated oocyst	None	Not reported	1
Eimeria subrotunda	Worldwide	Turkeys	Small intestine (duodenum)	Ingestion of sporulated oocyst	None	Not reported	1
Eimeria tenella	Worldwide	Chickens	Ceca	Ingestion of sporulated oocyst	Hemorrhagic to fibrinonecrotic enteritis, diarrhea, anorexia, death	Not reported	3

(Continued)

279

TABLE 10.2 (Continued)

Parasite	Geographic distribution	Hosts	Location in host	Method of infection	Pathologic effects	Zoonosis	Reference
Eimeria tropicalis	Unknown	Pigeons	Intestine	Ingestion of sporulated oocyst	Enteritis	Not reported	1
Eimeria spp.	Worldwide	Quail, pheasants, other Galliformes	Intestines	Ingestion of sporulated oocyst	Variable	Not reported	33
Isospora spp.	Worldwide	Various birds	Intestines	Ingestion of sporulated oocyst	Variable	Not reported	74–76
Tyzzeria parvula	Unknown	Geese	Small intestine	Ingestion of sporulated oocyst	None	Not reported	1
Tyzzeria perniciosa	Unknown	Ducks	Small intestine	Ingestion of sporulated oocyst	Hemorrhagic enteritis	Not reported	1
Wenyonella anatis	Unknown	Ducks	Intestine	Ingestion of sporulated oocyst	None	Not reported	1
Wenyonella columbae	Unknown	Pigeons	Small intestine	Ingestion of sporulated oocyst	None	Not reported	1
Wenyonella gallinae	Unknown	Chickens	Large intestine	Ingestion of sporulated oocyst	Hemorrhagic enteritis	Not reported	1
Trematodes							
Digenetic							
Catatropis verrucosa	Europe, North America	Chickens, other birds	Ceca, rectum	Ingestion of cercaria encysted on snail shell or vegetation	Mild typhlitis	Not reported	101
Echinoparyphium recurvatum	Worldwide	Chickens, other birds	Small intestine	Ingestion of infected mollusk (snail) or amphibian (tadpole)	Severe enteritis, anemia, emaciation	Not reported	101
Echinostoma spp.	Worldwide	Chickens, other birds	Intestines	Ingestion of infected mollusk (snail)	Variable	Not reported	101
Hypoderaeum conoideum	Worldwide	Chickens, other birds	Small intestine	Ingestion of infected mollusk (snail)	Unknown	Reported	101
Notocotylus attenuatus	Asia, Europe	Chickens, other birds	Ceca, rectum	Ingestion of cercaria encysted on snail shell or vegetation	Slight cecal erosion	Not reported	101
Notocotylus thienemanni	Europe	Chickens, other birds	Ceca	Ingestion of cercaria encysted on snail shell or vegetation	Probably slight cecal erosion	Not reported	101
Platynosomum spp.	Worldwide	Cockatoos	Liver, bile ducts	Ingestion of intermediate host	Hemorrhagic typhlitis	Not reported	101
Postharmostomum gallinum	Worldwide	Chickens, pigeons, other birds	Small intestine, ceca	Ingestion of infected snail	Hemorrhagic typhlitis	Not reported	101
Ribeiroia ondatrae	North America	Chickens, other birds	Proventriculus	Ingestion of metacercaria in fishes	None	Not reported	101

280

		Birds	Ceca, small intestine		None	Not reported	101
Zygocotyle lunata	North America	Birds	Ceca, small intestine	Ingestion of metacercaria encysted on vegetation	None	Not reported	101

Cestodes

Cyclophyllidea

Amoebotaenia cuneata	Worldwide	Chicken, other birds	Small intestine	Ingestion of intermediate host (earthworms)	Mild to unapparent infection	Not reported	108
Choanotaenia infundibulum	Worldwide	Chicken, other birds	Small intestine	Ingestion of intermediate host (flies, beetles, other insects)	Mild or unapparent except in heavy infections	Not reported	109
Cotugnia digonopora	Africa, Asia, Europe	Chicken, other birds	Intestine	Ingestion of intermediate host (ants)	Enteritis	Not reported	108
Cotugnia spp.	Unknown	Pigeons	Small intestine	Unknown	Unknown	Not reported	108
Davainea proglottina	Worldwide	Chickens, pigeons, other birds	Duodenum	Ingestion of intermediate host (snails, slugs)	Diarrhea, weight loss, ruffled plumage, enteritis	Not reported	112
Fimbriaria fasciolaris	Worldwide	Chickens, Anseriforms	Small intestine	Ingestion of intermediate host (copepods)	None	Not reported	108
Hymenolepis cantaniana	Asia, Europe, North America	Chickens	Small intestine	Ingestion of intermediate host (dung beetles)	None	Not reported	108
Hymenolepis carioca	Hawaii, North America	Chickens, other birds	Small intestine	Ingestion of intermediate host (dung beetles, stable flies, flour beetles)	May cause enteritis	Not reported	114
Hymenolepis megalops	Unknown	Waterfowl	Cloaca, bursa of Fabricius	Ingestion of intermediate host (crustaceans)	Unknown	Not reported	108
Metroliasthes lucida	Africa, Asia, North America	Turkeys, other birds	Small intestine	Ingestion of intermediate host (grasshoppers, beetles)	Unknown	Not reported	108
Raillietina cesticillus	Worldwide	Chickens, other birds	Small intestine	Ingestion of intermediate host (beetles)	Sometimes decreased growth rate, emaciation	Not reported	118
Raillietina echinobothrida	Worldwide	Chickens, quail, other birds	Small intestine	Ingestion of intermediate host (ants)	Intestinal nodules, enteritis, diarrhea, emaciation, sometimes death	Not reported	123

(Continued)

TABLE 10.2 *(Continued)*

Parasite	Geographic distribution	Hosts	Location in host	Method of infection	Pathologic effects	Zoonosis	Reference
Raillietina georgiensis	Unknown	Turkeys	Intestines	Ingestion of intermediate host (ants)	Enteritis	Not reported	108
Raillietina tetragona	Worldwide	Chickens, pigeons, other birds	Small intestine	Ingestion of intermediate host (ants)	Enteritis	Not reported	114,124
Raillietina spp.	Unknown	Psittacines	Small intestine	Unknown	Unknown	Not reported	20
Nematodes							
Rhabditoidea							
Strongyloides avium	Americas, Asia	Chickens, other birds	Small intestine, ceca	Ingestion or skin penetration of infective larva	Enteritis in young birds	Not reported	130
Strongyloides oswaldoi	South America	Chickens	Adult: intestine Larva: lungs	Ingestion or skin penetration of infective larva	Enteritis in young birds	Not reported	132
Heterakoidea							
Ascaridia bonasae	North America	Grouse	Small intestine	Ingestion of embryonated egg on soil or in insect transport host	Unknown	Not reported	131
Ascaridia columbae	Worldwide	Pigeons, doves	Small intestine, liver, lung	Ingestion of embryonated egg	Hepatitis	Not reported	131,133
Ascaridia compar	Asia, Europe, North America	Grouse, partridges, pheasants, quail	Small intestine	Ingestion of embryonated egg on soil or in insect transport host	Unknown	Not reported	135
Ascaridia dissimilis	North America	Turkeys	Small intestine	Ingestion of embryonated egg on soil or in insect transport host	Enteritis, hepatic granulomata, death	Not reported	136
Ascaridia galli	Worldwide	Chickens, turkeys, doves, ducks, geese, guinea fowl	Small intestine	Ingestion of embryonated egg on soil or in insect transport host	Anemia, enteritis, intestinal blockage, thymic atrophy, death	Not reported	131,147
Ascaridia numidae	Unknown	Guinea fowl	Small intestine, ceca	Ingestion of embryonated egg on soil or in insect transport host	Unknown	Not reported	131

Species	Geographic distribution	Host	Location	Transmission	Pathology		Reference
Heterakis beramporia	Asia	Chickens	Ceca	Ingestion of embryonated egg on soil or in earthworms	Cecal nodules	Not reported	101
Heterakis dispar	Asia	Ducks, geese	Ceca	Ingestion of embryonated egg on soil or in earthworms	None	Not reported	131
Heterakis gallinarum	Worldwide	Chickens, other birds	Ceca	Ingestion of embryonated egg on soil or in earthworms	Vector of *Histomonas meleagridis*	None	101
Heterakis isolonche	Worldwide	Pheasants, other birds	Ceca	Ingestion of embryonated egg on soil or in earthworms	Cecal nodules, typhlitis	Not reported	158
Subuluroidea							
Aulonocephalus lindquisti	Unknown	Quail	Small intestine, ceca	Unknown	None	Not reported	131
Subulura brumpti	Worldwide	Galliformes, ducks	Ceca	Ingestion of intermediate host (beetles, grasshoppers, cockroaches)	None	Not reported	131
Subulura differens	Worldwide	Galliformes	Distal small intestine	Ingestion of intermediate host (arthropods)	None	Not reported	184
Subulura minetti	India	Chickens	Ceca	Unknown	None	Not reported	184
Subulura strongylina	Americas	Chickens, guinea fowl, quail	Ceca	Ingestion of intermediate host (arthropods)	None	Not reported	131
Subulura suctoria	Former Soviet Union, South America	Galliformes	Ceca, small intestine	Ingestion of intermediate host (arthropods)	None	Not reported	131,162
Trichostrongyloidea							
Amidostomum anseris	Unknown	Ducks, geese, pigeons	Gizzard	Ingestion of larva	Gizzard hemorrhages, necrosis	Not reported	131
Amidostomum skrjabini	Unknown	Ducks, pigeons	Gizzard	Ingestion of larva	Gizzard hemorrhages, necrosis	Not reported	131
Epomidiostomum uncinatum	Unknown	Ducks, geese, pigeons	Gizzard	Ingestion of larva	Unknown	Not reported	176
Ornithostrongylus hastatus	Europe	Galliformes	Intestine	Ingestion of larva	Unknown	Not reported	101

(Continued)

TABLE 10.2 (Continued)

Parasite	Geographic distribution	Hosts	Location in host	Method of infection	Pathologic effects	Zoonosis	Reference
Ornithostrongylus quadriradiatus	Worldwide	Pigeons, other birds	Crop, proventriculus, duodenum	Ingestion of larva	Catarrhal to hemorrhagic enteritis	Not reported	101
Trichostrongylus tenuis	Worldwide	Galliformes, Anseriformes	Ceca, small intestine	Ingestion of larva	Catarrhal to hemorrhagic enteritis	Not reported	177
Spiruroidea							
Acuaria skrjabini	Worldwide	Passerines	Gizzard	Ingestion of insect intermediate host	Degeneration of mucosal glands of the gizzard	Not reported	131
Cheilospirura hamulosa	Worldwide	Galliformes	Esophagus, crop, gizzard	Ingestion of intermediate host (grasshoppers, sandhoppers, beetles, weevils)	Anemia, ulceration, nodule formation in gizzard	Not reported	131,185
Cheilospirura spinosa	Worldwide	Galliformes	Gizzard	Ingestion of intermediate host (grasshoppers)	Anemia, hemorrhages of gizzard lining	Not reported	131
Cyrnea colini	Unknown	Galliformes	Proventriculus	Ingestion of intermediate host (cockroaches)	None	Not reported	131
Dispharynx nasuta	Worldwide	Pigeons, other birds	Proventriculus	Ingestion of intermediate host (sowbugs, pillbugs)	Proventricular nodules, inflammation, hemorrhaging, and ulceration	Not reported	131,185, 186
Echinura uncinata	Unknown	Anseriformes, other birds	Esophagus, proventriculus, gizzard, small intestine	Ingestion of intermediate host (water fleas)	Anemia, hemorrhages of gizzard lining	Not reported	131,187
Gongylonema ingluvicola	Worldwide	Galliformes	Crop, esophagus, proventriculus	Ingestion of intermediate host (cockroaches)	Mild inflammation of crop	Not reported	131
Hartertia gallinarum	Africa	Chickens, other birds	Small intestine	Ingestion of intermediate host (arthropods)	Emaciation diarrhea, death	Not reported	184
Histiocephalus laticaudatus	Europe	Chickens	Gizzard	Unknown	Hemorrhagic inflammation of the gizzard, nodule formation	Not reported	101,131

Species	Distribution	Host	Location	Transmission	Pathology		References
Streptocara crassicauda	Unknown	Ducks	Crop, esophagus, proventriculus, gizzard	Ingestion of intermediate host (amphipods)	Esophagitis, pharyngitis	Not reported	101,131
Tetrameres americana	Africa, Americas	Chickens, grouse, quail, turkeys, pigeons, ducks	Proventriculus	Ingestion of intermediate host (cockroaches, grasshoppers)	Proventriculitis	Not reported	131,184
Tetrameres confusa	Asia, South America	Chickens, pigeons, other birds	Proventriculus	Ingestion of intermediate host	Proventriculitis	Not reported	131
Tetrameres crami	Africa, Americas	Ducks	Proventriculus	Ingestion of intermediate host	Emaciation	Not reported	131,192
Tetrameres fissipina	Worldwide	Ducks, geese, other birds	Proventriculus	Ingestion of intermediate host (water fleas, amphipods, grasshoppers, cockroaches, earthworms)	Proventriculitis	Not reported	131,193, 194
Tetrameres pattersoni	North America	Quail	Proventriculus	Ingestion of intermediate host (grasshoppers, cockroaches)	Proventriculitis	Not reported	131,195
Trichuroidea							
Capillaria anatis	Worldwide	Galliformes, Anseriformes	Small intestine, ceca	Unknown	Enteritis	Not reported	131
Capillaria annulata	Worldwide	Galliformes	Esophagus, crop	Ingestion of earthworm paratenic host	Thickening and necrosis of the crop glands	Not reported	101
Capillaria bursata	Worldwide	Galliformes	Small intestine	Ingestion of earthworm paratenic host	Unknown	Not reported	131
Capillaria caudinflata	Europe, North America	Galliformes, Anseriformes	Small intestine	Ingestion of earthworms	Unknown	Not reported	131
Capillaria contorta	Worldwide	Galliformes	Esophagus, crop	Ingestion of embryonated egg or earthworms	Thickening and necrosis of the crop glands	Not reported	131
Capillaria montevidensis	Uruguay	Chickens	Ceca	Unknown	None	Not reported	131
Capillaria obsignata	Worldwide	Galliformes	Small intestine, ceca	Ingestion of embryonated egg	Intestinal thickening, catarrhal or hemorrhagic enteritis	Not reported	201–204

(Continued)

TABLE 10.2 *(Continued)*

Parasite	Geographic distribution	Hosts	Location in host	Method of infection	Pathologic effects	Zoonosis	Reference
Capillaria uruguanensis	Uruguay	Chickens	Ceca, large intestine	Unknown	None	Not reported	131
Acanthocephala							
Mediorhynchus gallinarum	Asia	Chickens	Small intestine	Unknown	Unknown	Not reported	131
Polymorphus boschadis	Unknown	Ducks, swans	Intestines	Unknown	Hemorrhagic enteritis, death of young birds	Not reported	131
Polymorphus minutus	Europe, North America	Chickens, ducks, other birds	Small intestine	Ingestion of intermediate host (crustaceans, fishes)	Nodule formation in intestinal wall	Not reported	131
Prosthorhynchus formosus	North America	Chickens, Passeriformes	Small intestine	Ingestion of intermediate host (isopods)	Unknown	Not reported	131

286

TABLE 10.3 Parasites of birds—musculoskeletal system

Parasite	Geographic distribution	Hosts	Location in host	Method of infection	Pathologic effects	Zoonosis	Reference
Coccidia							
Arthrocystis galli	Unknown	Chicken	Muscles	Ingestion of sporozoites	Unknown	Not reported	1
Sarcocystis falcatula	Worldwide	Canaries, other birds; definitive host = opossum	Muscles, lungs	Ingestion of sporozoites	Pulmonary edema, pneumonitis, hepatitis	Not reported	78,79
Sarcocystis horvathi	Worldwide	Chickens; definitive hosts = dog, cat	Muscles	Ingestion of sporozoites	Benign muscle cysts	Not reported	1
Sarcocystis rileyi	Worldwide	Ducks; definitive hosts = skunk, opossum, dog, cat	Muscles	Ingestion of sporozoites	Benign muscle cysts	Not reported	1
Sarcocystis spp.	Worldwide	Psittaciformes	Muscles	Ingestion of sporozoites	None	Not reported	20

TABLE 10.4 Parasites of birds—respiratory system.

Parasite	Geographic distribution	Hosts	Location in host	Method of infection	Pathologic effects	Zoonosis	Reference
Coccidia							
Cryptosporidium spp.	Worldwide	Cockatiels	Lungs	Ingestion of sporulated oocyst	Pneumonia	Not reported	53
Sarcocystis falcatula	Worldwide	Canaries, other birds; definitive host = opossum	Muscles, lungs	Ingestion of sporozoites	Pulmonary edema, pneumonitis, hepatitis	Not reported	78,79
Trematodes							
Clinostomum attenuatum	Worldwide	Chickens, pigeons	Trachea	Ingestion of infected amphibians	Unknown	Not reported	101
Nematodes							
Strongyloidea							
Cyathostoma bronchialis	Worldwide	Ducks, geese, turkeys	Larynx, trachea, bronchi, abdominal air sacs	Ingestion of infective larva or transport host (earthworms)	Bronchitis, pneumonitis	Not reported	164,165
Syngamus trachea	Worldwide	Chickens, other Galliformes, Passeriformes	Trachea, bronchi, bronchioles	Ingestion of embryonated egg, infective larva, or transport host (earthworms, snails, slugs)	Tracheitis, tracheal nodules	Not reported	131,168
Syngamus skrjabinomorpha	Former Soviet Union	Chickens, geese	Trachea	Ingestion of embryonated egg, infective larva, or transport host (earthworms, snails, slugs)	Unknown	Not reported	110
Arachnida							
Mites							
Astigmates							
Cytodites nudus	Worldwide	Chickens, other birds	Respiratory tract	Direct contact	Pulmonary edema, pneumonia, increased tracheal and bronchial mucus	Not reported	233

288

TABLE 10.5 Parasites of birds—skin and connective tissue.

Parasite	Geographic distribution	Hosts	Location in/on host	Method of infection	Pathologic effects	Zoonosis	Reference
Trematodes							
Collyriclum faba	North America, Europe	Chickens, other birds	Skin, subcutaneous tissues	Unknown	Anemia, emaciation	Not reported	102
Philophthalmus gralli	Asia, Hawaii	Chickens, other birds	Conjunctival sac	Ingestion of cercaria encysted on snail shell or vegetation	Conjunctival congestion and erosion	Reported	108
Philophthalmus problematicus	Philippine Islands	Chickens	Conjunctival sac	Ingestion of cercaria encysted on snail shell or vegetation	Conjunctival congestion and erosion	Not reported	108
Nematodes							
Metastrongyloidea							
Eulimdana spp.	Worldwide	Pigeons	Subcutaneous tissues of the neck, shoulder, esophagus, crop	Unknown	Cellulitis, tenosynovitis	Not reported	244
Pelecitus spp.	Worldwide	Passeriformes, Anseriformes, Psittaciformes	Subcutaneous tissues of the neck, legs, feet	Unknown	Cellulitis, tenosynovitis	Not reported	182
Spiruroidea							
Ceratospira spp.	Unknown	Psittaciformes	Conjunctival sac	Ingestion of arthropod intermediate host	Unknown	Not reported	245
Oxyspirura mansoni	Worldwide	Galliformes, Columbiformes	Conjunctival sac	Ingestion of intermediate host (cockroaches)	Ophthalmia, swollen nicitiating membranes	Not reported	131
Oxyspirura petrowi	Worldwide	Galliformes	Conjunctival sac	Ingestion of intermediate host (cockroaches)	Ophthalmia, swollen nicitiating membranes	Not reported	131
Dracunculoidea							
Avioserpens spp.	Worldwide	Anseriformes	Subcutaneous tissues of the neck	Ingestion of intermediate host (copepod)	Subcutaneous granulomata	Not reported	131
Filaroidea							
Aproctella stoddardi	Unknown	Galliformes	Coelomic cavity	Unknown biting arthropod	Granulomatous pericarditis	Not reported	131
Singhfilaria hayesi	Unknown	Quail, turkeys	Subcutaneous tissues of neck region	Unknown biting arthropod	None	Not reported	131

(*Continued*)

289

TABLE 10.5 (Continued)

Parasite	Geographic distribution	Hosts	Location in/on host	Method of infection	Pathologic effects	Zoonosis	Reference
Arthropods							
Diptera (flies)							
Calliphoridae	Worldwide	Birds, mammals	Skin wounds	Eggs deposited by female fly	Dermal myiasis; fetid skin wounds	Reported	207
Ceratopogonidae (midges)	Worldwide	Birds, mammals	Skin	Direct contact	Irritation, pathogen transmission	Common	208
Culicidae (mosquitoes)	Worldwide	Birds, other terrestrial vertebrates	Skin	Direct contact	Pruritus, local inflammation, pathogen transmission	Common	208
Hippoboscidae (keds) (*Pseudolynchia canariensis*)	Worldwide	Pigeons	Skin, plumage	Direct contact	Anemia	Reported	208
Muscidae (filth flies)	Worldwide	Birds, mammals	Skin	Direct contact	Irritation, pathogen transmission, accidental myiasis	Common	207
Oestridae (bots) (*Dermatobia hominis*)	Worldwide	Birds, mammals	Subcutaneous tissues	Eggs deposited by female fly	Dermal cysts	Common ("Human botfly")	209
Sarcophagidae (flesh flies)	Worldwide	Birds, mammals	Skin wounds	Larvae deposited by female fly	Dermal myiasis; fetid skin wounds	Reported	207
Simulidae (blackflies)	Worldwide	Birds, mammals	Skin	Direct contact	Irritation, pathogen transmission	Common	208
Phthiraptera (lice)							
Anaticola anseris	Unknown	Geese	Plumage	Direct contact	Unknown	Not reported	208
Anaticola crassicornis	Unknown	Ducks	Plumage	Direct contact	Unknown	Not reported	208
Campanulotes bidentatus compare	Unknown	Pigeons	Plumage	Direct contact	Unknown	Not reported	208
Chilopistes meleagridis	Unknown	Turkeys	Plumage	Direct contact	Unknown	Not reported	208
Columbicola columbae	Unknown	Pigeons	Plumage	Direct contact	Unknown	Not reported	208
Cuclotogaster heterographa	Worldwide	Chickens	Plumage, especially of neck, head	Direct contact	Feather damage, irritation, restlessness, weight loss, retarded growth	Not reported	208
Goniocotes gallinae	Worldwide	Chickens	Plumage, especially down feathers	Direct contact	Feather damage, restlessness	Not reported	215
Goniodes spp.	Worldwide, especially in temperate climates	Chickens, other birds	Plumage	Direct contact	None	Not reported	215

Lagopoecus sinensis	China	Chickens	Plumage	Direct contact	Unknown	Not reported	208
Lipeurus spp.	Worldwide	Chickens, other birds	Plumage, especially of primary flight, tail, or back feathers	Direct contact	Restlessness	Not reported	215,216
Menacanthus cornutus	Worldwide	Chickens	Plumage	Direct contact	Irritation, unthriftiness, sometimes death	Not reported	215
Menacanthus pallidulus	Worldwide	Chickens	Plumage	Direct contact	Irritation, unthriftiness, sometimes death	Not reported	215
Menacanthus stramineus	Worldwide	Chickens, turkeys, guinea fowl, other birds	Plumage, especially near vent	Direct contact	Anemia, feather damage, restlessness	Not reported	208
Menopon gallinae	Worldwide	Chickens, guinea fowl, other birds	Plumage	Direct contact	Anemia, irritation, restlessness, unthriftiness	Serves as reservoir of *Chlamydophila psittaci*	196
Oxylipeurus dentatus	Asia, South America	Chickens	Plumage	Direct contact	Unknown	Not reported	215
Syringophilus spp.	Worldwide	Chickens, other birds	Plumage	Direct contact	Feather loss	Not reported	208
Trinoton anserinum	Unknown	Geese	Plumage	Direct contact	Unknown	Not reported	208
Trinoton querquedulae	Unknown	Ducks	Plumage	Direct contact	Unknown	Not reported	208

Siphonaptera (fleas)

Ceratophyllus gallinae	Worldwide	Chickens, turkeys, mammals	Plumage, skin	Direct contact	Anemia, irritation, local edema, dermal ulcers	Reported	208
Ceratophyllus niger	North America	Chickens, turkeys, other birds, mammals	Skin	Direct contact	Anemia	Reported	208
Echidnophaga gallinacea	Worldwide	Chickens, other birds, mammals	Skin; usually on head and other unfeathered areas	Direct contact	Lymphoplasmacytic dermatitis	Common; may transmit agents of plague, typhus; harbors *Salmonella typhimurium*	221,224

Hemiptera (bugs)

Cimex boueti	Worldwide	Chickens	Skin	Direct contact	Anemia, local swelling and pruritus	Reported	208
Cimex columbarius	Europe	Pigeons	Skin	Direct contact	Anemia, local swelling and pruritus	Reported	208,225

(Continued)

TABLE 10.5 (Continued)

Parasite	Geographic distribution	Hosts	Location in/on host	Method of infection	Pathologic effects	Zoonosis	Reference
Cimex hemipterus	Worldwide	Chickens, bats	Skin	Direct contact	Anemia, local swelling and pruritus	Common	225
Cimex lectularius	Europe	Pigeons, other birds, mammals	Skin	Direct contact	Anemia, local swelling and pruritus	Common	208
Haematosiphon inodorus	Americas	Chickens, turkeys, raptors	Skin	Direct contact	Anemia, local swelling and pruritus	Reported	101
Hesperocimex cochimiensis	Mexico	Chickens, other birds	Skin	Direct contact	Anemia, local swelling and pruritus	Reported	208
Hesperocimex coloradensis	North America	Chickens, other birds	Skin	Direct contact	Anemia, local swelling and pruritus	Reported	225
Hesperocimex sonorensis	North America	Chickens, other birds	Skin	Direct contact	Anemia, local swelling and pruritus	Reported	225
Ornithocoris pallidus	Unknown	Chickens	Skin	Direct contact	Anemia, local swelling and pruritus	Reported	208
Ornithocoris toledoi	South America	Chickens	Skin	Direct contact	Anemia, local swelling and pruritus	Common	208
Triatoma protracta	South America	Chickens, mammals	Skin	Direct contact	Variable anemia	Reported	246
Triatoma sanguisa	South America	Chickens	Skin	Direct contact	Variable anemia	Reported	246
Arachnida							
Ticks (Hard)							
Amblyomma spp.	Worldwide	Birds	Skin	Direct contact	Anemia	Common	229
Haemaphysalis leporispalustris	Worldwide	Rabbits, chickens, other birds	Skin	Direct contact	Anemia	Reported	228
Ixodes spp.	Worldwide	Birds, mammals	Skin	Direct contact	Anemia, local inflammation, secondary bacterial infection	Common	230,231
Ticks (Soft)							
Argas spp.	Worldwide	Birds	Skin	Direct contact	Anemia, pathogen transmission	Reported; serve as reservoirs of human pathogens	226,227

	Worldwide	Birds, mammals	Skin	Direct contact	Anemia	Common	228
Ornithodoros spp.	Worldwide		Skin	Direct contact	Anemia	Common	228
Mites							
Astigmates							
Dermoglyphus elongatus	Worldwide	Birds	Quill feathers	Direct contact	Feather loss	Not reported	208
Dermoglyphus minor	Worldwide	Birds	Quill feathers	Direct contact	None	Not reported	208
Epidermoptes bilobatus	Worldwide	Chickens	Skin	Direct contact	Dermatitis, feather loss	Not reported	208
Knemidokoptes gallinae	North America, Europe, Africa; probably worldwide	Chickens, pigeons, pheasants	Skin of body, head, upper legs	Direct contact	Dermatitis, pruritus, feather loss, dermal scales, papules	Not reported	208
Knemidokoptes mutans	Worldwide	Chickens	Skin, beneath epidermal scales of legs	Direct contact	Irritation, inflammation, vesicles, crusts on legs, deformity of legs, lameness	Not reported	208
Knemidokoptes pilae	Worldwide	Parakeets	Skin, usually base of beak, legs	Direct contact	Crust formation on face and legs, beak deformities	Not reported	239
Laminosioptes cysticola	Worldwide	Chickens, turkeys, pheasants, grouse, pigeons	Subcutis	Direct contact	Subcutaneous nodules	Not reported	208
Megninia spp.	Worldwide	Birds	Down feathers, contour feathers	Direct contact	Sometimes dermal irritation	Not reported	208
Pterolichus obtusus	Worldwide	Chickens	Wing feathers, tail feathers	Direct contact	Sometimes reduced vigor	Not reported	208
Rivoltasia bifurcata	Worldwide	Chickens	Skin, downy parts of quill feathers	Direct contact	Pruritus, feather damage	Not reported	208
Mesostigmates							
Haemolaelaps casalis	Worldwide	Chickens	Skin, feathers	Direct contact	None	Reported	208
Haemolaelaps glasgowi	Europe	Chickens	Skin, feathers	Direct contact	None	Reported	208
Ornithonyssus bursa	Worldwide	Chickens, other birds	Skin, feathers	Direct contact	Anemia, irritation, matted feathers	Reported	208
Ornithonyssus sylviarum	Worldwide	Chickens, pigeons, other birds, mammals	Skin, feathers	Direct contact	Anemia, matted and discolored feathers, scab formation, thickened skin, retarded growth	Reported	208
Dermanyssus gallinae	Worldwide	Chickens, other birds, mammals	Skin	Direct contact	Anemia, dermatitis, irritation, lethargy, restlessness, decreased production, pathogen transmission	Reported; serves as reservoir of human pathogens	208

(Continued)

TABLE 10.5 (Continued)

Parasite	Geographic distribution	Hosts	Location in/on host	Method of infection	Pathologic effects	Zoonosis	Reference
Prostigmates							
Eutrombicula spp.	Americas	Birds, humans	Skin	Direct contact	Abscess formation	Common ("chigger")	208
Neoschoengastia americana	Americas	Birds	Skin	Direct contact	Irritation	Not reported	208
Neotrombicula autumnalis	Americas	Birds, humans	Skin	Direct contact	Abscess formation	Common ("chigger")	208
Syringophilus bipectinatus	Worldwide	Birds	Quills of wing and body	Direct contact	Feather loss	Not reported	208

TABLE 10.6 Parasites of birds—urogenital system.

Parasite	Geographic distribution	Hosts	Location in host	Method of infection	Pathologic effects	Zoonosis	Reference
Coccidia							
Cryptosporidium spp.	Worldwide	Chickens, other birds	Ureters	Ingestion of sporulated oocyst	Ureteral hyperplasia	Not reported	55
Eimeria truncata	Unknown	Geese	Kidney	Ingestion of oocyst passed in urine	Nephritis	Not reported	1
Trematodes							
Plagiorchis arcuatus	Europe	Chickens	Oviduct	Presumably by ingestion of infected insect	Unknown	Not reported	101
Prosthogonimus macrorchis	North America	Chickens, other birds	Oviduct, bursa of Fabricius	Ingestion of second intermediate host (dragonflies)	Coelomitis, decreased production, anorexia	Not reported	101
Prosthogonimus pellucidus	Europe	Chickens, other birds	Oviduct, bursa of Fabricius	Ingestion of second intermediate host (dragonflies)	Coelomitis, decreased production, anorexia	Not reported	101
Prosthogonimus ovatus	Africa, Asia, Europe	Chickens, other birds	Oviduct, bursa of Fabricius	Ingestion of second intermediate host (dragonflies)	Coelomitis, decreased production, anorexia	Not reported	107
Prosthogonimus longus-morbificans	Europe	Chickens, other birds	Oviduct, bursa of Fabricius	Ingestion of second intermediate host (dragonflies)	Coelomitis, decreased production, anorexia	Not reported	101

REFERENCES

1. Levine, N. (1985) *Veterinary Protozoology.* Iowa State University Press, Ames, Iowa. 414 pages.

2. McDougald, L.R. (1997) Other protozoan diseases of the intestinal tract. In: Calnek, B.W. (ed.). *Diseases of Poultry,* 10th ed., Iowa State University Press, Ames, Iowa. pp. 890–899.

3. Levine, N.D. (1961) *Protozoan parasites of domestic animals and man.* Burgess, Minneapolis, Minnesota. 412 pages.

4. Kosters, J., Cubillos, A., and Ulloa, J. (1976) *Chilomastix* sp. en gansos domesticos de Chile. *Bol. Chile. Parasitol.* **31,** 84–85.

5. Davis, D.E., Schwartz, L.D., and Jordan, H.E. (1964) A case report: *Chilomastix* sp. infection in pen-raised quail. *Avian Dis.* **8,** 465–470.

6. Kosters, J., Grimm, F., Ippen, R., and Schroder, H.D. (1987) *Erkrankungen der Zootiere.* Verhandlungsbericht des 29. Internationalen Symposiums uber die Erkrankungen der Zootiere von 20. Mai bis 24. Mai 1987 in Cardiff. Akademie-Verlag, Berlin, German Democratic Republic. pages 57–60.

7. Kosters, J., Cubillos, A., Ulloa, J., and Schutze, H.R. (1979) Control of *Chilomastix* infection in domestic poultry with metronidazole. *Berliner-und-Munchener-Tierarztliche-Wochenschrift* **13,** 266–268.

8. Pecka, Z. (1991) Domestic geese (*Anser anser* L.) as a new host of *Cochlosoma anatis* Kotlán, 1923. *Folia Parasitologica.* **38,** 91–92.

9. Lindsay, D.S., Larsen, C.T., Zajac, A.M., and Pierson, F.W. (1999) Experimental *Cochlosoma anatis* infections in poultry. *Vet. Parasitol.* **81,** 21–27.

10. Travis, B. (1938) A synopsis of the flagellate genus *Cochlosoma* Kotlan, with the description of two new species. *J. Parasitol.* **24,** 343–351.

11 Tyzzer, E.E. (1929) Coccidiosis in gallinaceous birds. *Am. J. Hyg.* **10,** 269–383.

12. Filippich, L.J. and O'Donoghue, P.J. (1997) *Cochlosoma* infections in finches. *Aust. Vet. J.* **75,** 561–563.

13. Cooper, G.L., Shivaprasad, H.L., Bickford, A.A., Nordhausen, R., Munn, R.J., and Jeffrey, J.S. (1995) Enteritis in turkeys associated with an unusual flagellated protozoan (*Cochlosoma anatis*). *Avian Dis.* **39,** 183–190.

14. Bollinger, T.K., Barker, I.K., and Fernando, M.A. (1996) Effects of the intestinal flagellate, *Cochlosoma anatis,* on intestinal mucosal morphology and disaccharidase activity in Muscovy ducklings. *Int. J. Parasitol.* **26,** 533–542.

15. Bollinger, T.K. and Barker, I.K. (1996) Runting of ducklings associated with *Cochlosoma anatis* infection. *Avian Dis.* **40,** 181–185.

16. Erlandsen, S.L. and Bemrick, W.J. (1987) SEM evidence for a new species, *Giardia psittaci. J. Parasitol.* **73,** 623–629.

17. Box, E.D. (1981) Observations on *Giardia* of budgerigars. *J. Protozoology.* **28,** 491–494.

18. Dieter, R.A., Jr., Dieter, R.S., Dieter, R.A., 3rd, and Gulliver, G. (2001) Zoonotic diseases: health aspects of Canadian geese. *Int. J. Circumpolar Health.* **60,** 676–684.

19. Filippich, L.J., McDonnell, P.A., Munoz, E., and Upcroft, J.A. (1998) *Giardia* infection in budgerigars. *Aust. Vet. J.* **76,** 246–249.

20. Tsai, S.-S., Hirai, K., and Itakura, C. (1992) Histopathological survey of protozoa, helminths, and ascarids of imported and local psittacine and passerine birds in Japan. *Jap. J. Vet. Res.* **40,** 161–174.

21. Chilvers, B.L., Cowan, P.E., Waddington, D.C., Kelly, P.J., and Brown, T.J. (1998) The prevalence of infection of *Giardia* spp. and *Cryptosporidium* spp. in wild animals on farmland, southeastern North Island, New Zealand. *Int. J. Environ. Health Res.* **8,** 59–64.

22. Harper, F.D.W. (1991) *Hexamita* species present in some avian species in South Wales. *Vet. Rec.* **128,** 130.

23. Harlin, R.W. (1996) Husbandry and diseases of domestic pigeons. In: Rosskopf, W.J. and Woerpel, R.W. (eds.). *Diseases of Cage and Aviary Birds,* 3rd ed., Williams and Wilkins, Baltimore, Maryland, pages 946–947.

24. McNeil, E. and Hinshaw, W.R. (1941). *Hexamita meleagridis* sp. nov. from the turkey. *Am. J. Hyg.* **34,** 71–82.

25. Hegngi, F.N., Karunakaran, D., Opengart, K.N., Larsen, C.T., and Pierson, F.W. (1997) Case report: Hexamitiasis in turkeys raised in the Shenandoah Valley of Virginia. *Poultry Sci.* **76,** 147.

26. Wenrich, D.H. (1943) Observations on the morphology of *Histomonas* (Protozoa, Mastigophora) from pheasants and chickens. *J. Morphology* **72,** 279–303.

27. Hu, J. and McDougald, L.R. (2003) Direct lateral transmission of *Histomonas meleagridis* in turkeys. *Avian Dis.* **47,** 489–492.

28. Norton, R.A., Hoerr, F.J., Clark, F.D., and Ricke, S.C. (1999) Ascarid associated hepatic foci in turkeys. *Avian Dis.* **43,** 29–38.

29. Hegngi, F.N., Doerr, J., Cummings, T.S., et al. (1999) The effectiveness of benzimidazole derivatives for the treatment and prevention of histomonosis (Blackhead) in turkeys. *Vet. Parasitol.* **81,** 29–37.

30. McDougald, L.R. (1998) Intestinal protozoa important to poultry. *Poult. Sci.* **77,** 1156–1158.

31. McDougald, L.R. and Hu, J. (2001) Blackhead disease (*Histomonas meleagridis*) aggravated in broiler chickens by concurrent infection with cecal coccidiosis (*Eimeria tenella*). *Avian Dis.* **45,** 307–312.

32. Hu, J. and McDougald. L.R. (2004) The efficacy of some drugs with known antiprotozoal activity against *Histomonas meleagridis* in chickens. *Vet. Parasitol.* **121,** 233–238.

33. Olsen, G.H. (1993) Common infections and parasitic diseases of quail and pheasants. *Proc. Assn. Avian Veterinarians.* 146–148.

34. Pecka, Z. (1991) Study of the pathogenicity of *Tetratrichomonas gallinarum. Veterinarni-Medicina* **36,** 183–188.

35. Wenrich, D.H. (1930) Comparative morphology of *Trichomonas* flagella of man. *J. Parasitol.* **17,** 117.

36. McKeon, T., Dunsmore, J., and Raidal, S.R. (1997) *Trichomonas gallinae* in budgerigars and columbid birds in Perth, Western Australia. *Aust. Vet. J.* **75,** 652–655.

37. Erwin, K.G., Kloss, C., Lyles, J., et al. (2000) Survival of *Trichomonas gallinae* in white-winged dove carcasses. *J. Wildl. Dis.* **36,** 551–554.

38. Cover, A.J., Harmon, W.M., and Thomas, M.W. (1994) A new method for the diagnosis of *Trichomonas gallinae* infection by culture. *J. Wildl. Dis.* **30,** 457–459.

39. Inghelbrecht, S., Vermeersch, H., Ronsmans, S., Remon, J.P., DeBacker, P., and Vercruysse, J. (1996) Pharmacokinetics and anti-trichomonal efficacy of a dimetridazole tablet and water-soluble powder in homing pigeons (*Columba livia*). *J. Vet. Pharmacol. Ther.* **19,** 62–67.

40. McLoughlin, D.K. (1966) Observations on the treatment of *Trichomonas gallinae* in pigeons. *Avian Dis.* **10,** 288–290.

41. Duchatel, J.P. and Vindevogel, H. (1998) In vitro sensitivity to ronidazole of different *Trichomonas gallinae* strains isolated from pigeons. *Ann. Med. Vet.* **142,** 333–338.

42. Munoz, E., Castella, J., and Gutierrez, J.F. (1998) In vivo and in vitro sensitivity of *Trichomonas gallinae* to some nitromidazole drugs. *Vet. Parasitol.* **78,** 239–246.

43. Friedhoff, K.T., Kuhnigk, C., and Muller, I. (1991) Experimental infections in chickens with *Chilomastix gallinarum, Tetratrichomonas gallinarum,* and *Tritrichomonas eberthi. Parasitol. Res.* **77,** 329–334.

44. Dusek, R.J. and Forrester, D.J. (2002) Blood parasites of American crows (*Corvus brachyrhynchus*) and fish crows (*Corvus ossifragus*) in Florida, U.S.A. *Comp. Parasit.* **69,** 92–96.

45. Votypka, J. and Svobodova, M. (2004) *Trypanosoma avium:* Experimental transmission from black flies to canaries. *Parasitology Res.* **92**, 147–151.

46. Desser, S.S. (1977) Ultrastructural observations on the epimastigote stages of *Trypanosoma avium* in *Simulium rugglesi. Can. J. Zool.* **55**, 1359–1367.

47. Ponce Gordo, F., Martinez-Diaz, R.A., and Herrera, S. (2004) *Entamoeba struthionis* n. sp. (*Sarcomastigophora: Endamoebidae*) from ostriches (*Struthio camelus*). *Vet. Parasitol.* **119**, 327–335.

48. Crouch, C.F., Andrews, S.J., Ward, R.G., and Francis, M.J. (2003) Protective efficacy of a live attenuated anti-coccidial vaccine administered to 1-day-old chickens. *Avian Pathol.* **32**, 297–304.

49. Ball, S.J., Brown, M.A., Daszak, P., and Pittilo, R.M. (1998) Atoxoplasma (Apicomplexa: Eimeriorina: Atoxoplasmatidae) in the greenfinch (*Carduelis chloris*). *J. Parasitol.* **84**, 813–817.

50. Quiroga, M.I., Aleman, N., Vazquez, S., and Nieto, J.M. (2000) Diagnosis of atoxoplasmosis in a canary (*Serinus canarius*) by histopathologic and ultrastructural examination. *Avian Dis.* **44**, 465–469.

51. Sreter, T. and Varga, J. (2000) Cryptosporidiosis in birds—a review. *Vet. Parasitol.* **87**, 267–279.

52. Morgan, U.M., Xiao, L., Limor, J., et al. (2000) *Cryptosporidium meleagridis* in an Indian ring-necked parrot (*Psittacula krameri*). *Aust. Vet. J.* **78**, 182–183.

53. Abe, N. and Iseki, M. (2004) Identification of *Cryptosporidium* isolates from cockatiels by direct sequencing of the PCR-amplified small subunit ribosomal RNA gene. *Parasitol. Res.* **92**, 523–526.

54. Morgan, U.M., Monis, P.T., Xiao, L., et al. (2001). Molecular and phylogenetic characterisation of *Cryptosporidium* from birds. *Int. J. Parasitol.* **31**, 289–296.

55. Trampel, D.W., Pepper, T.M., and Blagburn, B.L. (2000) Urinary tract cryptosporidiosis in commercial laying hens. *Avian Dis.* **44**, 479–484.

56. Sironi, G., Rampin, T., and Burzoni, G. (1991) Cryptosporidiosis in game birds. *Vet. Rec.* **129**, 337–338.

57. Tumova, E., Skrivan, M., Marounek, M., Pavlasek, I., and Ledvinka, Z. (2002) Performance and oocyst shedding in broiler chickens orally infected with *Cryptosporidium baileyi* and *Cryptosporidium meleagridis. Avian Dis.* **46**, 203–207.

58. Abbassi, H., Wyers, M., Cabaret, J., and Naciri, M. (2000) Rapid detection and quantification of *Cryptosporidium baileyi* oocysts in feces and organs of chickens using a microscopic slide flotation method. *Parasitol. Res.* **86**, 179–187.

59. Sreter, T., Szell, Z., and Varga, I. (2002) Anticryptosporidial prophylactic efficacy of enrofloxacin and paromomycin in chickens. *J. Parasitol.* **88**, 209–211.

60. Lindsay, D.S., Blagburn, B.L., Hoerr, F.J., and Smith, P.C. (1991) Cryptosporidiosis in zoo and pet birds. *J. Protozool.* **38**, 180S–181S.

61. Vanparijs, O., Hermans, L., and Marsboom, R. (1991) Efficacy of diclazuril against *Eimeria dispersa* in turkeys. *Avian Dis.* **35**, 599–600.

62. McDougald, L.R., Fuller, A.L., Mathis, G.F., and Wang, G.T. (1990) Efficacy of maduramicin ammonium against coccidiosis in turkeys under laboratory and floor-pen conditions. *Avian Dis.* **34**, 634–638.

63. Watkins, K.L., Bafundo, K.W., and Donovan, D.J. (1990) Anticoccidial effect of monesin against *Eimeria mitis* and *Eimeria dispersa. Poult. Sci.* **69**, 1009–1011.

64. Cabel, M.C., Norton, R.A., Yazwinski, T.A., and Waldroup, P.W. (1991) Efficacy of different anticoccidialis against experimental coccidiosis in large white turkeys. *Poult. Sci.* **70**, 289–292.

65. Chandler, A.C. and Read, P.R. (1961) *Introduction to Parasitology,* 10th ed. Wiley and Sons, New York, New York, 822 pages.

66. Nakai, Y., Tsuchiya, H., and Takahashi, S. (1992) Cultivation of *Eimeria tenella* in Japanese quail embryos (*Coturnix coturnix japonica*). *J. Parasitol.* **78**, 1024–1026.

67. Tsuji, N., Kawazu, S., Ohta, M., et al. (1997) Discrimination of eight chicken *Eimeria* species using the two step polymerase chair reaction. *J. Parasitol.* **83**, 977–970.

68. Mathis, G.F., Froyman, R., and Kennedy, T. (2004) Coccidiosis control by adding toltrazuril in the drinking water for a 2-day period. *Vet. Parasitol.* **121**, 1–9.

69. Giannenas, I., Florou-Paneri, P., Papazahariadou, M., Christaki, E., Botsoglou, N.A., and Spais, A.B. (2003) Effect of dietary supplementation with oregano essential oil on performance of broilers after experimental infection with *Eimeria tenella. Arch. Tierernahr.* **57**, 99–106.

70. El-Abasy, M., Motobu, M., Na, K.J., et al. (2003) Protective effects of sugar cane extracts (SCE) on *Eimeria tenella* infection in chickens. *J. Vet. Med. Sci.* **65**, 865–871.

71. Conway, D.P., Mathis, G.F., Johnson, J., Schwartz, M., and Baldwin, C. (2001) Efficacy of diclazuril in comparison with chemical and ionophorous anticoccidials against *Eimeria* spp. in broiler chickens in floor pens. *Poult. Sci.* **80**, 426–430.

72. Allen, P.C. and Danforth, H.D. (1998) Effects of dietary supplementation with n-3 fatty acid ethyl esters on coccidiosis in chickens. *Poult. Sci.* **77**, 1631–1635.

73. Williams, P. (1998) Epidemiological aspects of the use of live anticoccidial vaccines for chickens. *Int. J. Parasitol.* **28**, 1089–1098.

74. Box, E.D. (1975) Exogenous stages of *Isospora serini* (Aragao) and *Isospora canaria* sp. n. in the canary (*Serinus canarius* Linnaeus). *J. Protozool.* **22**, 165–169.

75. Grulet, O., Landau, I., and Baccam, D. (1982) *Isospora* from domestic sparrow (*Passer domesticus*) multiple species. *Ann. Parasitol. Hum. Comp.* **57**, 209–236.

76. Olson, V.A., Gissing, G.J., Barta, J.R., and Middleton, A.L. (1998) A new *Isospora* sp. from *Carduelis tristis* (Aves: Fringillidae) from Ontario, Canada. *J. Parasitol.* **84**, 153–156.

77. Speer, C.A. and Dubey, J.P. (1999) Ultrastructure of shizonts and merozoites of *Sarcocystis falcatula* in the lungs of budgerigars (*Melopsittacus undulatus*). *J. Parasitol.* **85**, 630–637.

78. Suedmeyer, W.K., Bermudez, A.J., Barr, B.C., and Marsh, A.E. (2001) Acute pulmonary *Sarcocystis falcatula*-like infection in three Victoria crowned pigeons (*Goura victoria*) housed indoors. *J. Zoo. Wildl. Med.* **32**, 252–256.

79. Smith, J.H., Neill, P.J., Dillard, A.E. 3rd, and Box, E.D. (1990) Pathology of experimental *Sarcocystis falcatula* infections of canaries (*Serinus canarius*) and pigeons (*Columba livia*). *J. Parasitol.* **76**, 59–68.

80. Dubey, J.P., Cawthorn, R.J., Speer, C.A., and Wobeser, G.A. (2003) Redescription of the sarcocysts of *Sarcocystis rileyi* (Apicomplexa: Sarcocystidae). *J. Eukaryot. Microbiol.* **50**, 476–482.

81. Kajerova, V., Literak, I., Bartova, E., and Sedlak, K. (2003) Experimental infection of budgerigars (*Melopsittacus undulatus*) with a low virulent k21 strain of *Toxoplasma gondii. Vet. Parasitol.* **116**, 297–304.

82. Williams, S.M., Fulton, R.M., Render, J.A., Mansfield, L., and Bouldin, M. (2001) Ocular and encephalic toxoplasmosis in canaries. *Avian Dis.* **45**, 262–267.

83. Dubey, J.P., Graham, D.H., Dahl, E., et al. (2003) *Toxoplasma gondii* isolates from free-ranging chickens from the United States. *J. Parasitol.* **89**, 1060–1062.

84. Mushi, E.Z., Binta, M.G., Chabo, R.G., Mathaio, M., and Ndebele, R.T. (1999) *Haemoproteus columbae* in domestic pigeons in Sebele, Gaborone, Botswana. *Onderstepoort J. Vet. Res.* **66**, 29–32.

85. El-Metenawy, T.M. (1999) Therapeutic effects of some antihaematozoal drugs against *Haemoproteus columbae* in domestic pigeons. *Dtsch. Tierarztl. Wochenschr.* **106,** 72.

86. Blanco, G., Rodriguez-Estrella, R., Merino, S., and Bertellotti, M. (2001) Effects of spatial and host variables on hematozoa in white-crowned sparrows wintering in Baja California. *J. Wildl. Dis.* **37,** 786–790.

87. Peirce, M.A. and Bevan, B.J. (1977) Blood parasites of imported psittacine birds. *Vet. Rec.* **100,** 282–283.

88. Cardona, C.J., Ihejirika, A., and McClellan, L. (2002) *Haemoproteus lophortyx* infection in bobwhite quail. *Avian Dis.* **46,** 249–255.

89. Atkinson, C.T., Forrester, D.J., and Greiner, E.C. (1988) Pathogenicity of *Haemoproteus meleagridis* (Haemosporina: Haemoproteidae) in experimentally infected domestic turkeys. *J. Parasitol.* **74,** 228–239.

90. Nakamura, K., Mitarai, Y., Tanimura, N., et al. (1997) Pathogenesis of reduced egg production and soft-shelled eggs in laying hens associated with *Leucocytozoon caulleryi* infection. *J. Parasitol.* **83,** 375–327.

91. Isobe, T., Yoshihara, S., and Shimura, K. (1993) Resistance of chicks against reinfection with *Leucocytozoon caulleryi. Avian Dis.* **37,** 27–30.

92. Ito, A. and Gotanda, T. (2004) Field efficacy of recombinant R7 vaccine against chicken leucocytozoonosis. *J. Vet. Med. Sci.* **66,** 483–487.

93. Bennett, G.F., Earle, R.A., Peirce, M.A., Huchzermeyer, F.W., and Squires-Parsons, D. (1991) Avian leucocytozoidae the leucocytozoids of the *Phasianidae* sensu lato. *J. Natural History* **25,** 1407–1428.

94. Fallis, A.M., Jacobson, R.L., and Raybould, J.N. (1973) Haematozoa in domestic chickens and guinea fowl in Tanzania and transmission of *Leucocytozoon neavei* and *Leucocytozoon schoutedeni. J. Protozool.* **20,** 438–442.

95. Shutler, D., Ankney, C., Davison, C., and Mullie, A. (1999) Effects of the blood parasite *Leucocytozoon simondi* on growth rates of anatid ducklings. *Can. J. Zool.* **77,** 1573–1578.

96. Steele, E.J. and Noblet, G.P. (2001) Gametogenesis, fertilization and ookinete differentiation of *Leucocytozoon smithi. J. Eukaryot. Microbiol.* **48,** 118–125.

97. Carmona, M., Finol, H.J., Marquez, A., and Noya, O. (1996) Skeletal muscle ultrastructural pathology in *Serinus canarius* infected with *Plasmodium cathemerium. J. Submicro. Cytol. Pathol.* **28,** 87–91.

98. Meyer, C.L. and Bennett, G.F. (1976) Observations on the sporogony of *Plasmodium circumflexum* Kikuth and *Plasmodium polare* Manwell in New Brunswick. *Can. J. Zool.* **54,** 133–141.

99. Huchzermeyer, F.W. (1988) Avian pulmonary hypertension syndrome. IV. Increased right ventricular mass in turkeys experimentally infected with *Plasmodium durae. Onderstepoort J. Vet. Res.* **55,** 107–108.

100. Forrester, D.J., Nayar, J.K., and Young, M.D. (1987) Natural infection of *Plasmodium hermani* in the Northern Bobwhite, *Colinus virginianus,* in Florida. *J. Parasit.* **73,** 865–866.

101. Soulsby, E.J.L. (1982) *Helminths, Arthropods and Protozoa of Domesticated Animals,* 7th ed., Lea and Febiger, Philadelphia, 809 pages.

102. Byrd, E.E. (1970) The brown thrasher, *Toxostoma rufum* (L.), as a host for *Collyriclum faba* (Bremser). *J. Parasitology* **56,** 195–196.

103. McCarthy, A.M. (1999) The influence of second intermediate host species on the infectivity of metacercarial cysts of *Echinoparyphium recurvatum. J. Helminthol.* **73,** 143–145.

104. Morley, N.J., Leung, K.M., Morritt, D., and Crane, M. (2004) Toxicity of anti-fouling biocides to encysted metacercariae of *Echinoparyphium recurvatum* (Digenea: Echinostomatidae) and their snail hosts. *Chemosphere* **56,** 353–358.

105. Munoz-Antoli, C., Toledo, R., and Esteban, J.G. (2000) The life cycle and transmission dynamics of the larval stages of *Hypoderaeum conoideum. J. Helminthol.* **74,** 165–172.

106. Macy, R.W. (1934) *Prosthogonimus macrorchis* n. sp., the common oviduct fluke of domestic fowls in the Northern United States. *Trans. Am. Microscop. Soc.* **53,** 30–34.

107. Leok, C.S., Inoue, I., Sato, T., Haritani, M., Tanimura, N., and Okada, K. (2002) Morphology of the oviduct fluke, *Prosthognonimus ovatus,* isolated from Indonesian native chickens and histopathological observation of the infected chickens. *J. Vet. Med. Sci.* **64,** 1129–1131.

108. McDougald, L.R. (2003) Cestodes and trematodes. In: Saif, Y.M., Barnes, H.J., Glisson, J.R., Fadly, A.M., McDougald, L.R., and Swayne, D.E. (eds.). *Diseases of Poultry,* 11th ed., Iowa State University Press, Ames, Iowa, 961–971.

109. Ponnudurai, G., Harikrishnan, T., and Anna, T. (2003) Incidence of cysticercoids of poultry tapeworm *Choanotaenia infundibulum* in *Musca domestica* in Namakkal, Tamil Nadu. *Ind. J. Poult. Sci.* **38,** 308–310.

110. Lapage, G. (1962) *Veterinary Helminthology and Entomology,* 5th ed., Bailliere, Tindall, and Cox, London, England, 600 pages.

111. Reid, W.M. (1962) Chicken and turkey tapeworms. *Georgia Agr. Exp. Sta. Univ. Georgia* 71 pages.

112. Levine, P.P. (1938) The effect of infection with *Davainea proglottina* on the weights of growing chickens. *J. Parasitol.* **24,** 550–551.

113. Horsfall, M.W. (1938) Meal beetles as intermediate hosts of poultry tapeworms. *Poultry Sci.* **17,** 8–11.

114. Jha, A.N., Sahai, B.N., Jha, G.J., Prasad, G., Singh, S.P., and Sahay, M.N. (1981) The histopathology and histochemistry of the intestine in common poultry cestodiasis with a note on the incidence of parasites in Patna Bihar India. *Indian J. Anim. Sci.* **51,** 655–660.

115. Edgar, S.A. (1956) The removal of chicken tapeworms by di-n-butyltin dilaurate. *Poult. Sci.* **35,** 64–73.

116. Wehr, E.E. (1965) Cestodes of poultry. In: Biester, H.E. and Schwarte, L.H. (eds.) *Diseases of Poultry,* 5th ed. Iowa State University Press, Ames, Iowa, 1006–1034.

117. Kerr, K.B. (1952) Butynorate, an effective and safe substance for the removal of *R. cesticillus* from chickens. *Poult. Sci.* **31,** 328–336.

118. Pote, L.M., Couvillion, C.E., Keirs, R.W., et al. (1992) Dose-filtration to confirm the level of fenbendazole for control of *Raillietina cesticillus* in broiler chickens. *Avian Dis.* **36,** 722–724.

119. Wardle, R.A. and McLeod, J.A. (1952) *The Zoology of Tapeworms.* University of Minnesota Press, Minneapolis, Minnesota, 780 pages.

120. Otify, Y.Z. (1989) Tapeworms of quails (*Coturnix coturnix*) in Egypt. *J. Egypt. Soc. Parasitol.* **19,** 81–84.

121. Olsen, O.W. (1967) *Animal Parasites: Their Biology and Life Cycles.* 2nd ed. Burgess, Minneapolis, Minnesota, 431 pages.

122. Nadakal, A.M., Mohandas, K., John, K.O., and Muraleedharan, K. (1973) Contribution to the biology of the fowl cestode *Raillietina echinobothrida* with a note on its pathogenicity. *Trans. Am. Microsc. Soc.* **92,** 273–276.

123. Samad, M.A., Alam, M.M,, and Bari, A.S. (1986) Effect of *Raillietina echinobothrida* infection on blood values and intestinal tissues of domestic fowls of Bangladesh. *Vet. Parasitol.* **21,** 279–284.

124. Nadakal, A.M. and Nair, K.V. (1979) Studies on the metabolic disturbances caused by *Raillietina tetragona* (Cestoda) infection in domestic fowl. *Indian J. Exp. Biol.* **17,** 310–311.

125. Vijayakumaran Nair, K. and Nadakal, A.M. (1981) Haematological changes in domestic fowl experimentally infected with the cestode *Raillietina tetragona* (Molin, 1858) *Vet. Parasitol.* **8,** 49–58.

126. Nurelhuda, I.E., Elowni, E.E., and Hassan, T. (1989) Anticestodal action of oxfendazole on *Raillietina tetragona* in experimentally infected chickens. *Br. Vet. J.* **145,** 458–461.

127. Nurelhuda, I.E., Elowni, E.E., and Hassan, T. (1989) Anthelmintic activity of praziquantel on *Raillietina tetragona* in chickens. *Parasitol. Res.* **75**, 655–656.

128. Rajendran, M. and Nadakal, A.M. (1988) The efficacy of praziquantel (Droncit R) against *Raillietina tetragona* (Molin, 1958) in the domestic fowl. *Vet. Parasitol.* **26**, 253–260.

129. Elowni, E.E., Nurelhuda, I.E.M., and Hassan, T. (1989) The effect of niclosamide on *Raillietina tetragona*. *Vet. Res. Communications.* **13**, 451–453.

130. Cram, E.B. (1930) New host records for *Strongyloides avium*. *J. Parasitol.* **17**, 55–56.

131. Norton, R.A. and Ruff, M.D. (2003) Nematodes and acanthocephalans. In: Saif, Y.M., Barnes, H.J., Glisson, J.R., Fadly, A.M., McDougald, L.R., and Swayne, D.E. (eds.). *Diseases of Poultry.* 11th ed. Iowa State University Press, Ames, Iowa, 931–961.

132. Travassos, L.P. (1932) Nota sobre *Strongyloides*. *Ann. Acad. Brasil. Sci.* **4**, 39–40.

133. Vassilev, I. (1993) On the ecology of *Ascaridia columbae* (Gmelin, 1790). *Helminthologia* (Bratislava) **30**, 135–138.

134. Wehr, E.E. and Hwang, J.C. (1964) The life cycle and morphology of *Ascaridia columbae* (Gmelin, 1790) Travassos 1913. (Nematoda: Ascarididae) in the domestic pigeon (*Columba livia domestica*). *J. Parasitol.* **50**, 131–137.

135. Vassilev, I. (1987) The development of *Ascaridia compar* Schrank 1790 in the host. *Khelmintologiya* **23**, 30–35.

136. Seaton, E.M., Monahan, C.M., and Morishita, T.Y. (2001) Presence and recovery of *Ascaridia dissimilis* ova on the external shell surface of turkey eggs. *Avian Dis.* **45**, 500–503.

137. Hemsley, R.V. (1971) Fourth stage *Ascaridia* spp. larvae associated with high mortality in turkeys. *Can. Vet. J.* **12**, 147–149.

138. Norton, R.A., Hopkins, B.A., Skeeles, J.K., Beasley, J.N., and Kreeger, J.M. (1992) High mortality of domestic turkeys associated with *Ascaridia dissimilis*. *Avian Dis.* **36**, 469–473.

139. Norton, R.A., Bayyari, B.A., Skeeles, J.K., Huff, W.E., and Beasley, J.N. (1994) A survey of two commercial turkey farms experiencing high levels of liver foci. *Avian Dis.* **38**, 887–894.

140. Norton, R.A., Clark, F.D., and Beasley, J.N. (1999) An outbreak of histomoniasis in turkeys infected with a moderate level of *Ascaridia dissimilis* but no *Heterakis gallinarum*. *Avian Dis.* **43**, 342–348.

141. Willoughby, D.H., Bickford, A.A., Charlton, B.R., Cooper, G.L., and Linares, J.A. (1995) *Ascaridia dissimilis* larval migration associated with enteritis and low market weights in meat turkeys. *Avian Dis.* **39**, 837–843.

142. Yazwinski, T.A., Rosenstein, M., Schwartz, R.D., Wilson, K., and Johnson, Z. (1993) The use of fenbendazole in the treatment of commercial turkeys infected with *Ascaridia dissimilis*. *Avian Path.* **22**, 177–181.

143. Benbrook, E.A. and Sloss, M.W. (1961) *Veterinary Clinical Parasitology*, 3rd edition, Iowa State University Press, Ames, Iowa, 206 pages.

144. Schou, T., Permin, A., Roepstorff, A., Sorensen, P., and Kjaer, J. (2003) Comparative genetic resistance to *Ascaridia galli* infections of 4 different commercial layer-lines. *Brit. Poult. Sci.* **44**, 182–185.

145. Reid, W.M. and Carmon, J.L. (1958) Effects of numbers of *Ascaridia galli* in depressing weight gains in chicks. *J. Parasitol.* **44**, 183–186.

146. Ikeme, M.M. (1971) Observations on the pathogenicity and pathology of *Ascaridia galli*. *Parasitology* **63**, 169–179.

147. Arunachalam, K., Manomohan, C.B., Vargheese, C., and George, C. (2003) Haematological changes in broiler chickens experimentally infected with *Ascardia galli*. *Indian J. Poult. Sci.* **38**, 27–31.

148. Ebako, G.M., Seaton, E.M., Morishita, T.Y., Monahan, C.M., and Bremer, C. (2002) *Ascaridia galli* in hen's egg from a flock with low fecal ova count. *J. Anim. Vet. Adv.* **1**, 193–194.

149. Sander, J.E. and Schwartz, R.D. (1994) Evaluation of three water-suspensible formulations of fenbendazole against *Ascaridia galli* infection in broiler chickens. *Avian Dis.* **38**, 350–353.

150. Okaeme, A.N. and Agbontale, J. (1989) Ivermectin in the treatment of helminthiasis in caged raised adult guinea-fowl (*Numida meleagris galeata* Pallas). *Rev. Elev. Med. Vet. Pays. Trop.* **42**, 227–230.

151. Lapage, G. (1968) *Veterinary Parasitology*, 2nd revised edition, Thomas, Springfield, Illinois, 1182 pages.

152. Lund, E.E. and Chute, A.M. (1972) Reciprocal responses of eight species of galliform birds and three parasites: *Heterakis gallinarum, Histomonas meleagridis,* and *Parahistomonas wenrichi*. *J. Parasitol.* **58**, 940–945.

153. Kaushik, R.K. and Deorani, V.P.S. (1969) Studies on tissue responses in primary and subsequent infections with *Heterakis gallinae* in chickens and on the process of formation of caecal nodules. *J. Helminthol.* **43**, 69–78.

154. Riddell, C. and Gajadhar, A. (1988) Cecal and hepatic granulomas in chickens associated with *Heterakis gallinarum* infection. *Avian Dis.* **32**, 836–838.

155. Norton, R.A., Yazwinski, T.A., and Johnson, Z. (1991) Research note: Use of fenbendazole for the treatment of turkeys with experimentally induced nematode infections. *Poult. Sci.* **70**, 1835–1837.

156. Yazwinski, T.A., Andrews, P., Holtzen, H., Presson, B., Wood, N., and Johnson, Z. (1986) Dose-titration of fenbendazole in the treatment of poultry nematodiasis. *Avian Dis.* **30**, 716–718.

157. Kirsch, R. (1984) Treatment of nematodiasis in poultry and game birds with fenbendazole. *Avian Dis.* **28**, 311–318.

158. Griner, L.A., Migaki, G., Penner, L.R., and McKee, A.E. Jr. (1977) Heterakidosis and nodular granulomas caused by *Heterakis isolonche* in the ceca of gallinaceous birds. *Vet. Pathol.* **14**, 582–590.

159. Karunamoorthy, G., Chellappa, D.J., and Anandan, R. (1994) The life history of *Subulura brumpti* in the beetle *Alphitobius diaperinus*. *Indian Vet. J.* **71**, 12–15.

160. Cuckler, A.C. and Alicata, J.E. (1944) The life history of *Subulura brumpti*, a cecal nematode of poultry in Hawaii. *Trans. Am. Microbiol. Soc.* **63**, 345–357.

161. Barus, V. (1970) Studies on the nematode *Subulura sactoria*. *Folia Parasitol.* (Prague) **17**, 191–199.

162. Barus, V. and Blazek, K. (1970) Studies on the nematode *Subulura sactoria*. III. Development in the definitive host. *Folia Parasitol.* (Prague) **17**, 141–151.

163. Zieris, H. and Betke, P. (1991) Cyathostoma bronchialis (Muhling 1884), Ordnung Strongylida, Family Syngamidae bei Mandarinenten (*Aix galericulata*) als Todesursache. *Monatschefte fur Vet.* **46**, 146–149.

164. Fernando, M.A., Hoover, I.J., and Ogungbade, S.G. (1973) The migration and development of *Cyathostoma bronchialis* in geese. *J. Parasitol.* **59**, 759–764.

165. Fernando, M.A., Stockdale, P.H.G., and Ogungbade, S.G. (1973) Pathogenesis of the lesions caused by *Cyathostoma bronchialis* in the respiratory tract of geese. *J. Parasitol.* **59**, 980–986.

166. Griffiths, H.J., Leary, R.M., and Fenstermacher, R. (1954) A new record for gapeworm (*Cyathostoma bronchialis*) infections of domestic geese in North America. *Am. J. Vet. Res.* **15**, 298–299.

167. Fernando, M.A., Stockdale, P.H.G., and Remmler, C. (1971) The route of migration development and pathogenesis of *Syngamus trachea* (Montagu, 1811) Chapin, 1925, in pheasants. *J. Parasitol.* **57**, 107–116.

168. Hwang, J.C. (1964) Hemogram of turkey poults experimentally infected with *Syngamus trachea*. *Avian Dis.* **8,** 380–390.

169. Devada, K. and Sathianesan, V. (1989) Comparative anthelmintic efficacy of mebendazole thiabendazole, and albendazole against *Syngamus trachea* infection in chicken. *Kerala J. Vet. Sci.* **20,** 59–64.

170. Istvan, V., Gyorgy, B., Zoltan, S., and Csaba, B. (1998) Efficacy of albendazole against *Syngamus trachea* in experimentally infected turkeys. *Magyar Allatorvosok Lapja.* **120,** 336–338.

171. Vanparijs, O. (1983) Anthelmentic activity of flubendazole in naturally infected geese and the economic importance of deworming. *Avian Dis.* **28,** 526–529.

172. MacNeill, A.C. (1970) *Amidostomum anseris* infection in wild swans and goldeneye ducks. *Can. Vet. J.* **11,** 164–166.

173. Enigk, K. and Dey-Hazra, A. (1971) Zur Behandlung de häufigsten nematodeninfektionen des hausgeflügels. *Dtsch. Tieraerztl. Wochenschr.* **78,** 178–181.

174. Enigk, K., Dey-Hazra, A., and Batke, J. (1973) Zur Wirksamkeit Von Mebendazol Bei Helminthosen Von Huhn und Gaus. *Avian Pathol.* **2,** 67–74.

175. Cencek, T., Ziomko, I., Kuczynska, E., and Tomczyk, G. (1992) *Amidostomum anseris* in geese efficacy of antihelminth drugs. *Medycyna Weterynaryjna* **48,** 421–423.

176. Leiby, P.D. and Olsen, O.W. (1965) Life history studies on Nematodes of the genera *Amidostomum* (Strongloidea) and *Epomidiostomum* (*Trichostrongyloidea*) occurring in the gizzards of waterfowl. *Proc. Helminthol. Soc. Wash.* **32,** 32–49.

177. Shaw, J.L. and Moss, R. (1990) Effect of the caecal nematode *Trichostrongylus tenuis* on egg-laying by captive red grouse. *Res. Vet. Sci.* **48,** 59–63.

178. Watson, H., Lee, D.L., and Hudson, P.J. (1987) The effect of *Trichostrongylus tenuis* on the caecal mucosa of young, old and anthelmintic-treated wild red grouse, *Lagopus lagopus scoticus. Parasitology* **94,** 405–411.

179. Rutherford, D.M. (1974) *Pelecitus,* a peritracheal nematode in the pigeon. *New Zealand Vet. J.* **22,** 147.

180. Pizarro, M., Villegas, P., Rodriguez, A., and Rowland, G.N. (1994) Filariasis (*Pelecitus* sp.) in the cervical subcutaneous tissue of a pigeon with trichomoniasis. *Avian Dis.* **38,** 385–389.

181. Allen, J.L., Kollias, G.V., Greiner, E.C., and Boyce, W. (1985) Subcutaneous filariasis (*Pelecitus* sp.) in a yellow-collared macaw (*Ara auricollis*). *Avian Dis.* **29,** 891–894.

182. Oniki, Y., Kinsella, J.M., and Willis, E.O. (2002) *Pelecitus helicinus* Railliet and Henry, 1910 (Filarioidea, Dirofilariinae) and other nematode parasites of Brazilian birds. *Mem. Inst. Oswaldo Cruz* **97,** 597–598.

183. Bartlett, C.M. and Anderson, R.C. (1987) Additional comments on species of *Pelecitus* (Nematoda: Filarioidea) from birds. *Can. J. Zool.* **65,** 2813–2814.

184. Cram, E.B. (1931) Developmental stages of some nematodes of the Spiruroidea parasite in poultry and game birds. *U.S. Dept. Agric. Tech. Bull. No. 227,* 1–27.

185. Menezes, R.C., Tortelly, R., Gomes, D.C., and Pinto, R.M. (2003) Pathology and frequency of *Cheilospirura hamulosa* (Nematoda, Acuarioidea) in Galliformes hosts from backyard flocks. *Avian Pathol.* **32,** 151–156.

186. Gomes, D.C., Menezes, R.C., Vicente, J.J., Lanfredi, R.M., and Pinto, R.M. (2004) New morphological data on *Cheilospirura hamulosa* (Nematoda, Acuarioidea) by means of bright-field and scanning electron microscopy. *Parasitol. Res.* **92,** 225–231.

187. Griffiths, G.L., Hopkins, D., Wroth, R.H., and Gaynor, W. (1985) *Echinura uncinata* infestation in mute swan cygnets (*Cygnus olor*). *Aust. Vet. J.* **62,** 132.

188. Schwabe, C.W. (1951) Studies on *Oxyspirura mansoni:* the tropical eyeworm of poultry II. Life history. *Pac. Sci.* **5,** 18–35.

189. Hubbard, G.B. and Kelm, S.W. (1984) Diagnostic exercise. *Lab. Animal Sci.* **34,** 441–442.

190. Flatt, R.E. and Nelson, L.R. (1969) *Tetrameres americana* in laboratory pigeons (*Columba livia*). *Lab. Anim. Care* **19,** 853–856.

191. Fatunmbi, O.O. and Adene, D.F. (1979) Occurrence and pathogenicity of tetrameriasis in guinea fowl and chickens in Nigeria. *Vet. Rec.* **105,** 330.

192. Swales, W.E. (1933) *Tetrameres* crami sp. Nov., a nematode parasitizing the proventriculus of a domestic duck in Canada. *Can. J. Res.* **8,** 334–336.

193. Tsvetaeva, N.P. (1960) Pathomorphological changes in the proventriculus of the ducks by experimental tetrameriasis. *Helminthologia* **2,** 143–150.

194. Endo, M. and Inoue, I. (1989) Observations on tetrameriasis in race pigeons (*Columba livia* var. *domestica*). *Bull. Coll. Agric. Vet. Med. Nihoir Univ.* **46,** 83–88.

195. Cram, E.B. (1933) Observations on the life history of *Tetrameres pattersoni. J. Parasitol.* **10,** 97–98.

196. Prelezov, P., Gundasheva, D., and Groseva, N. (2002) Haematological changes in chickens, experimentally infected with biting lice (Phthiraptera-Insecta). *Bulgarian J. Vet. Med.* **5,** 29–37.

197. Wehr, E.E. (1936) Earthworms as transmitters of *Capillaria annulata,* the crop worm of chickens. *North Am. Vet.* **17,** 18–20.

198. Wehr, E.E., Colglazier, M.L., Burtner, R.H., and Wiest, L.M. Jr. (1967) Methyridine, an effective anthelmintic for intestinal threatworm, *Capillaria obsignata,* in pigeons. *Avian Dis.* **11,** 322–326.

199. Pavlovic, I., Rosic, G., Bajic, V., Lazarov, D., and Misic, Z. (1996) Effect of mebendazole in treatment of helminthoses of game birds and pigeons maintained in controlled conditions. *Veterinarski Glasnik* **50,** 779–784.

200. Colglazier, M.L., Wehr, E.E., Burtner, R.H., and Wiest, L.M. Jr. (1967) Haloxon as an anthelmintic against the cropworm *Capilaria contorta* in quail. *Avian Dis.* **11,** 257–260.

201. Wakelin, D. (1965) Experimental studies on the biology of *Capillaria obsignata,* Madson, 1945, a nematode parasite of the domestic fowl. *J. Helminthol.* **39,** 399–412.

202. Levine, P.P. (1938) Infection of the chicken with *Capillaria columbae* (RUD). *J. Parasitol.* **24,** 45–52.

203. Berghen, P. (1966) Serum protein changes in *Capillaria obsignata* infections. *Exp. Parasitol.* **19,** 34–41.

204. Chubb, L.G., Freeman, B.M., and Wakelin, D. (1964) The effect of *Capillaria obsignata,* Madsen, 1945, on the vitamin A and ascorbic acid metabolism in the domestic fowl. *Res. Vet. Sci.* **5,** 154–160.

205. Taylor, S.M., Kenny, J., Houston, A., and Hewitt, S.A. (1993) Efficacy, pharmacokinetics and effects on egg-laying and hatchability of two dose rates of in-feed fenbendazole for the treatment of *Capillaria* species infections in chickens. *Vet. Rec.* **133,** 519–521.

206. Pote, L.M. and Yazwinski, T.A. (1985) Efficacy of fenbendazole in chickens. *Arkansas Farm Res.* **34,** 2.

207. James, M.T. 1947. The flies that cause myiasis in man. *U.S. Dept. Agr., Misc. Publ. 631.* 175 pp.

208. Arends, J.J. (2003) External Parasites and Poultry Pests. In: Diseases of Poultry. Saif, Y.M., Barnes, H.J., Glisson, J.R., Fadly, A.M., McDougald, L.R., and Swayne, D.E. (eds.). Iowa State Press, Ames, Iowa, pages 905–927.

209. Banegas, A.D. and Mourier, H. (1967) Laboratory observations on the life history and habits of *Dermatobia hominis* (Diptera: Cuterebridae): I. Mating behavior. *Ann. Entomol. Soc. Am.* **60**, 878–881.

210. Guimaraes, J.H. and Papavero, N. (1966) A tentative annotated bibliography of *Dermatobia hominis* (Diptera, Cuterebridae). *Arquiv. Zool.* **14**, 223–294.

211. Arthur, F.H. and Axtell, R.C. (1982) Comparisons of permethrin formulations and application methods for northern fowl mite control on caged laying hens. *Poult. Sci.* **61**, 879–884.

212. Owiny, J.R. and French, E.D. (2000) Ectoparasites in a pigeon colony. *Comp. Med.* **50**, 229–230.

213. Bishopp, F.C. (1929) The pigeon fly—an important pest of pigeons in the United States. *J. Econ. Entomol.* **22**, 974–980.

214. Yunker, C.E. (1964) Infections of laboratory animals potentially dangerous to man: Ectoparasites and other arthropods, with emphasis on mites. *Lab. Anim. Care* **14**, 455–465.

215. Emerson, K.C. (1956) Mallophaga (chewing lice) occurring on the domestic chicken. *J. Kansas Entomol. Soc.* **29**, 63–79.

216. Wilson, F.H. (1939) The life-cycle and bionomics of *Lipeurus caponis* (Linn.). *Ann. Entomol. Soc. Am.* **32**, 318–320.

217. Roberts, I.H. and Smith, C.L. (1956) Poultry lice. In: *Yearbook of Agriculture.* U.S. Dept. Agr., Washington, D.C., pages 490–493.

218. Das, S.S., Bhatia, B.B., and Kumar, A. (1993) Efficacy of Pestoban-D against common poultry lice. *Indian J. Vet. Res.* **2**, 25–26.

219. Stockdale, H.J. and Raun, E.S. (1965) Biology of the chicken body louse, *Menacanthus stramineus. Ann. Entomol. Soc. Am.* **58**, 802–805.

220. Parman, D.C. (1923) Biological notes on the hen flea, *Echidnophaga gallinacea. J. Agr. Res.* **23**, 1007–1009.

221. Suter, P. (1965) Life cycle of *Echidnophaga gallinacea. Proc. 12th Intern. Congr. Entomol., London* **1964**, 830–831.

222. Gustafson, C.R., Bickford, A.A., Cooper, G.L., and Charlton, B.R. (1997) Sticktight fleas associated with fowl pox in a backyard chicken flock in California. *Avian Dis.* **41**, 1006–1009.

223. Titchener, R.N. (1983) The use of permethrin to control an outbreak of hen fleas (*Ceratophyllus gallinae*). *Poult. Sci.* **62**, 608–611.

224. Cooper, J.E. and Mellau, L.S.B. (1992) Sticktight fleas (*Echidnophaga gallinacea*) on birds. *Vet. Rec.* **130**, 108.

225. Usinger, R.L. (1966) *Monograph of Cimicidae.* Entomological Society of America, College Park, Maryland. 585 pages.

226. Da Massa, A.J. and Adler, H.E. (1979) Avian spirochetosis: natural transmission by *Argas (Persicargas) sanchezi* (Ixodoidea: Argasidae) and existence of different serologic and immunologic types of *Borrelia anserina* in the United States. *Am. J. Vet. Res.* **40**, 154–157.

227. Gothe, R. (1992) *Aegyptianella*: an appraisal of species, systematics, avian hosts, distribution, and developmental biology in vertebrates and vectors and epidemiology. *Adv. Dis. Vector Res.* **9**, 67–100.

228. Bishopp, F.C. and Trembley, H.L. (1945) Distribution and hosts of certain North American ticks. *J. Parasitol.* **31**, 1–54.

229. Cooley, R.A. and Kohls, G.M. (1944) The genus Amblyomma (Ixodidae) in the United States. *J. Parasitol.* **30**, 77–111.

230. Cooley, R.A. and Kohls, G.M. (1945) The genus *Ixodes* in North America. *National Institutes of Health Bulletin 184* U.S. Public Health Serv., 246 pages.

231. Arthur, D.R. and Snow, K.R. (1968) *Ixodes pacificus.* Cooley and Kohls, 1943: Its life history and occurrence. *Parasitology* **58**, 893–906.

232. Baker, E.W., Evans, T.M., Gould, D.J., Hull, W.B. and Keegan, H.L. (1956) *A Manual of Parasitic Mites of Medical or Economic Importance.* Tech. Publ. Natl. Pest Control Assoc., Inc. New York, 170 pages.

233. Ayroud, M. and Dies, K.H. (1992) *Cytodites nudus*-induced granulomatous pneumonia in chickens. *Can. Vet. J.* **33**, 754–755.

234. Fain, A. and Elsen, P. (1967) Les acariens de la famille Knemidokoptidae producteurs de gale chez les oiseaux (Sarcoptiformes). *Acta. Zool. Pathol. Antverpiensia* **45**, 3–142.

235. Hirst, S. (1922) Mites injurious to domestic animals. British Museum of Natural History Econ. Ser. 13, 107 pages.

236. Nevin, F.R. (1935) Anatomy of *Cnemidocoptes mutans* (R. and L.), the scaly-leg mite of poultry. *Ann. Entomol. Soc. Am.* **28**, 338–367.

237. Morishita, T.Y., Johnson, G., Johnson, G., Thilsted, J., Promsopone, B., and Newcomer, C. (2005) Digit necrosis associated with scaly-leg mite infestation. *J. Avian Med. Surg.* **19**, 230–233.

238. Blackmore, D.K. (1963) Some observations on Cnemidocoptes pilae, together with its effect on the budgerigar (*Melopsittacus undulatus*). *Vet. Rec.* **75**, 592–595.

239. Yunker, C.E. and Ishak, K.G. (1957) Histopathological observations on the sequence of infection in knemidokoptic mange of budgerigars (*Melopsittacus undulatus*). *J. Parasitol.* **43**, 664–672.

240. Beck, W. (2000) Scaly face mite infection by *Knemidocoptes pilae* (Acaridida: Knemidocoptes) in a budgerigar—Biology of *Knemidocoptes pilae*, pathogenesis, clinical features, diagnosis and treatment. *Kleintierpraxis* **45**, 453–457.

241. Smith, K.E., Quist, C.F., and Crum, J.M. (1997) Clinical illness in a wild turkey with *Laminosioptes cysticola* infestation of the viscera and peripheral nerves. *Avian Dis.* **41**, 484–489.

242. Sikes, R.K. and Chamberlain, R.W. (1954) Laboratory observations on three species of bird mites. *J. Parasitol.* **40**, 691–697.

243. Cameron, D. (1938) The northern fowl mite (*Liponyssus sylviarum* C. and F., 1877). *Can. J. Res.* **16**, 230–254.

244. Eslami, A. (1987) Filariosis in a pigeon caused by *Eulimdana clava* (Wedl, 1856) Founikoff, 1934. *J. Vet. Facul. Univ. Tehran* **42**, 1–4.

245. Theodoropoulos, G. and Greve, J.H. (1985) Observations on the morphology of the eyeworm, *Ceratospira inglisi* (Nematoda: Thelaziidae) from a Moluccan cockatoo. *Proc. Helm. Soc. Wash.* **52**, 132–133.

246. Ryckman, R.E. (1962) Bisystematics and hosts of the *Triatoma protracta* complex in North America (Hemiptera: Reduviidae) (Rodentia: Cricetidae). *Univ. Calif. (Berkeley) Publ. Entomol.* **27**, 93–240.

CHAPTER

11

Parasites of Rats and Mice

David G. Baker, DVM, MS, PhD, DACLAM

INTRODUCTION

For most of the 20th century, and continuing into the 21st century, laboratory rats and mice have been the animals of choice for much of biomedical research because they serve as models for the study of numerous human medical conditions and physiological processes. It therefore should come as no surprise that laboratory animal rodent pathogens,

including parasites, have been well-studied and characterized. Laboratory rats and mice commonly were found to be affected by a plethora of both internal and external parasites in the early days of biomedical research[1,2].

Tremendous improvements in sanitation, nutrition, housing systems, environmental control, disease surveillance and treatment, and animal quality have resulted in a marked reduction in parasite prevalence and incidence. In addition, laboratory animal veterinarians, technicians, and researchers have gained greater understanding of the effects of natural parasitic diseases on research results[3]. This knowledge has driven efforts to exclude natural parasitic diseases from the animal colony. In modern facilities, it is uncommon to find laboratory rats and mice parasitized with more than a very narrow spectrum of pathogens[4].

Despite tremendous improvements in laboratory animal science, laboratory rats and mice are sometimes found to be naturally harboring parasites thought to have disappeared. For example, the recent finding of *Demodex musculi* in immune-deficient transgenic mice[5] illustrates the need to remain vigilant about parasites, even those not reported for many years. Prior to the report of Hill and colleagues, this parasite had not been reported in laboratory mice for nearly a century[6].

Information in this chapter is organized phylogenetically. It should be appreciated that phylogenetic classification schemes vary. While this chapter primarily covers the parasitic diseases of laboratory rats and mice, the exhaustive coverage of the first edition is retained, serving as a reference for parasitic diseases of wild-caught rats and mice, including those of rat and mouse species less frequently used in research.

PROTOZOA

Phylum Sarcomastigophora

Class Mastigophora (flagellates)

Several flagellates are known to occur in rats and mice. Although most are considered to be nonpathogenic, some are distinctly pathogenic and others are of unknown pathogenicity. All are rare. Natural infection of the hemoflagellates, for instance, requires the presence of suitable arthropod vectors, which should not be present in well-managed production or research facilities.

Hemoflagellates

Trypanosoma conorhini *Trypanosoma conorhini* is a nonpathogenic flagellate found in wild Norway and black rats, and in its insect vector, a reduviid bug, *Triatoma rubrofasciata*. It is found in Asia and parts of South America. Natural infection has not been reported in laboratory animals but could possibly occur in specimens obtained from their natural habitat or in facilities infested with the insect vector. The laboratory mouse (*Mus musculus*), rat (*Rattus norvegicus*), Mongolian gerbil (*Meriones unguiculatus*), guinea pig (*Cavia porcellus*), and rabbit (*Oryctolagus cuniculus*) have been infected experimentally[7]. Asian monkeys have been found infected with *T. conorhini* and may be the original hosts of this parasite. The trypomastigote form is 27 μ to 54 μ long, including a free flagellum. The body has a long, pointed posterior end and a prominent undulating membrane. The kinetoplast is of medium size, lies some distance from the posterior end, and has a pot-shaped structure anterior to it.

Trypanosoma lewisi Morphology. *Trypanosoma lewisi* measures 25 μ to 36 μ in length and has a long, slender body which tapers to a point at the posterior end. There is a medium-sized non-terminal kinetoplast, a well-defined undulating membrane, and a free anterior flagellum (Figure 11.1)[8]. Recently, a longer form, measuring 35 μ to 39 μ, has been identified in *Rattus norvegicus* in India[9].

Hosts. *Trypanosoma lewisi* has been reported in wild Norway rats (*R. norvegicus*) and black rats (*R. rattus*) in Egypt and Brazil[10,11]. Laboratory rats may become infected from wild rats when the flea intermediate host is present in the animal facility. There is a single report of natural infection with *T. lewisi* in *Gerbilus pyramidous*[12]. *Trypanosoma*

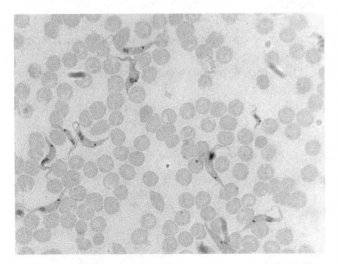

Fig. 11.1 *Trypanosoma lewisi* trypomastigotes in a rat blood smear. Romanowski stain. 1000×. Reproduced from Baker, D.G. (2005) with permission.

lewisi is not naturally found in mice, due to antibody-dependent, cell-mediated immunity[13]. *T. lewisi* has been experimentally and only transiently transmitted to laboratory mice, Mongolian gerbils, and guinea pigs[14].

Life Cycle. The northern rat flea (*Nosopsyllus fusciatus*), and possibly the oriental rat flea (*Xenopsylla cheopis*), serve as natural arthropod hosts and vectors of *T. lewisi*. Fleas are infected while taking a blood meal. The ingested trypomastigote form penetrates the gastric epithelial cells of the flea and produces long, free transitional forms by multiple fission. The epithelial cells are destroyed through several intracellular multiplications, and the transitional forms pass to the rectum. Here the epimastigote form develops, attaches to the wall of the rectum, and multiplies for the life of the flea. About five days after infection, some epimastigote stages transform into metacyclic (infectious) trypomastigotes, which cannot reproduce in the flea. These pass out in the feces. *Trypanosoma lewisi* is a stercorarian trypanosome; that is, transmission is via the contaminated feces of infected arthropod hosts. Rats become infected by the ingestion of fleas or moist flea feces, but are not infected by the bite of the flea. The trypanosomes appear in the rat blood five to seven days after infection, multiply for about a week, and disappear. The rat louse *Polyplax spinulosa* may also serve as a mechanical vector[15].

Pathologic Effects. *Trypanosoma lewisi* infection is usually nonpathogenic. A spontaneous arthritis may develop in naturally infected four- to five-week-old rats[16], and is characterized by erythema and edema of the distal extremities. The rear paws are most frequently involved and the tibiotarsal joint most severely affected. Histologically, joint lesions are characterized by purulent arthritis, with inflammation of the adjacent subcutaneous and muscular tissues. Exudates from affected joints contain trypomastigotes. Experimental infection has resulted in anemia when rats were concurrently immunosuppressed with corticosteroids[17].

Disease may also develop in experimentally infected rats following irradiation, splenectomy, and adrenalectomy. *Trypanosoma lewisi* may be associated with a wide range of physiologic changes in the rat host. Many of these may go unrecognized. Possible physiologic changes include immunoregulation[18], lipopolysaccharide hyperreactivity[19], autoimmune hemolytic anemia with splenomegaly and glomerulonephritis[20], increased susceptibility to other pathogens such as *Toxoplasma gondii*[21] and *Salmonella typhimurium*[22], decreased total iron binding capacity[23], and altered liver enzyme activities[24]. Immune mechanisms responsible for eliminating *T. lewisi* are likely similar to those responsible for clearing the biologically similar *T. musculi* in mice. The interested reader is referred to that section for a discussion of those mechanisms.

Clinical Disease. *Trypanosoma lewisi* rarely causes clinical symptoms, even in heavily infected rats. Those infected early in gestation may abort[25]. Lincicome and co-workers[26] showed that infected rats gain up to 31% more weight than uninfected controls. Parasite-induced increases in weight gain were more pronounced in younger rats than in adults. The mechanism underlying this observation remains unknown, but may involve thiamine production[27].

Diagnosis. Preliminary diagnosis of infection is by demonstrating trypanosomes in blood smears. Historically, inoculation of suspected blood into uninfected young rats has been used to confirm infection. More recently however, polymerase chain reaction (PCR) assays have been developed as an alternative to animal inoculations[28].

Treatment. Rats may be cleared of *T. lewisi* infection by daily treatment with 54 mg/kg rifampicin for 30 days[29]. However, it may be more practical to simply eliminate the affected animals from the colony.

Prevention. Infection with *T. lewisi* is unlikely to occur in a modern animal facility. Infection is prevented by excluding fleas, lice, and wild rodents. Occasionally, wild rats may be used in research, and should be treated for arthropod infestation upon arrival in quarantine.

Public Health Considerations. Human infections with *T. lewisi*-like trypanosomes have been reported in a malnourished child[30] and in adults[31]. In all cases, the patients recovered spontaneously.

Trypanosoma musculi **Morphology.** *Trypanosoma musculi* (Syn. *T. duttoni*) is morphologically indistinguishable from *T. lewisi*.

Hosts. This usually nonpathogenic species occurs in wild mice throughout the world[27]. Laboratory mouse strains differ in their susceptibility to infection, as well as in the character of the induced immune response. Mice of the C3H/He/J, CBA/J, and A/J strains are most susceptible, while BALB/c, DBA/2, and C57Bl/6 and related strains, are less susceptible[32,33]. Likewise, different species of wild mice differ in susceptibility to infection, while hybrids are equally susceptible to infection[34]. Wild strains of *T. musculi* may differ in their host effects, when compared to the Partinico II (laboratory) strain[35]. *Trypanosoma musculi* is not usually transmitted to rats.

Life Cycle. As another stercorarian trypanosome, the life cycle of *T. musculi* is similar to that of *T. lewisi*. Its vector is the northern rat flea, *Nosopsyllus fasciatus*.

Pathologic Effects. The development of *T. musculi* as a model of human trypanosomiasis has resulted in the publication of a large volume of information on murine trypanosomiasis. *Trypanosoma musculi* is generally considered nonpathogenic, though distinct histologic changes are observable during the period of parasitemia. These include splenic, lymph node, renal glomerula, and hepatic hyperplasia, as well as transient thymic involution[36]. These changes occur because parasites establish primarily in the liver, and less so in the spleen, lungs, and kidneys, following infection[37]. Anemia may also be present[36]. Infection with *T. musculi* elevates host serum total protein, hepatic enzymes, creatinine, and gamma globulin[38].

Control of the infection is through both non-immunological (reproduction-inhibiting) and immunological factors[32,37]. Both CD4+ T-lymphocytes and B-lymphocytes are important components of acquired immunity[39]. Infection renders mice more sensitive to the systemic effects of lipopolysaccharide[19]. Aged mice, and those exposed to stressors, such as malnutrition, cold temperatures, pregnancy, or concurrent helminth infection, may develop more severe disease. They may also develop pronounced or prolonged parasitemia following infection[19,39]. Likewise, athymic mice develop chronic infection and elevated parasitemia[40]. Following recovery from acute infection, *T. musculi* may reside in a distinct, latent form in the renal vasculature for the life of the mouse, thereby serving to maintain immunity through chronic immune stimulation[41].

Clinical Disease. Clinical signs are not observed. Similar to infection of rats with *T. lewisi*, infected mice reportedly gain more weight than do uninfected controls[42,43].

Diagnosis, Treatment, and Prevention. These aspects are similar to those described for *T. lewisi*.

Public Health Considerations. There are no reports of humans being infected with *T. musculi*.

Enteric flagellates

Several enteric flagellates occur in mice and rats, including the trichomonads, retortamonads, oxymonads, and diplomonads. It is likely that many of those with direct life cycles remain common in laboratory mice and rats[44]. However, relatively few studies have documented their occurrence.

The trichomonads belong to the order Trichomonadida, characterized by three to five anterior flagella and a recurrent flagellum, which is either free or associated with a cell body, forming an undulating membrane[45]. *Tritrichomonas* has three anterior flagella and no pelta (a crescent-shaped, silver-stained structure anterior to the axostyle). The other genera all have a pelta. *Trichomitus* has three, *Trichomonas* and *Tetratrichomonas* have four, and *Pentatrichomonas* has five anterior flagella. Other genera of importance include *Trichomitus* and *Hexamastix*.

The retortamonads belong to the order Retortamonadida. These are small flagellates with two to four flagella, one of which is turned backward and associated with a cytostome. Trophozoite and cyst stages are known. Genera of interest include *Retortamonas* and *Chilomastix*.

The oxymonads belong to the order Oxymonadida. The principal genus of interest in laboratory rats and mice is *Monocercomonoides*. Members of this genus are small, oval to pyriform flagellates with two pairs of flagella, an anterior nucleus, and a slender axostyle.

The diplomonads belong to the order Diplomonadida. They are small, unicellular, bilaterally symmetrical flagellates. They have four flagella associated with each of two anteriorly located nuclei. One flagellum on each side is directed backward and in some cases is associated with a ventral cytostome. Genera of importance include *Giardia*, *Octomitus*, and *Spironucleus*.

Chilomastix bettencourti **Morphology.** Trophozoites of this typically nonpathogenic flagellate measure 8.3 μ to 20.9 μ (mean 13.3 μ) by 6.6 μ to 8.4 μ (mean 7.4 μ). They are pyriform, with an anterior nucleus; a large cytostomal groove near the anterior end; three anterior flagella; a fourth, short flagellum which undulates within the cytostomal groove; and a cytoplasmic fibril along the anterior end and sides of the cytostomal groove (Figure 11.2)[46]. The cysts are usually lemon-shaped and contain one nucleus and the organelles of the trophozoite[47].

Hosts. *Chilomastix bettencourti* occurs in the cecum of the mouse, Norway rat, black rat, and hamster (*Mesocricetus auratus*)[27]. It is structurally identical to *C. mesnili* of primates. Its prevalence in laboratory rats and mice is unknown. It is probably common in conventional colonies[44,48].

Life Cycle. Like other trichomonads, *C. bettencourti* has a direct life cycle. Infection occurs following ingestion of infective cysts passed in the feces.

Pathologic Effects and Clinical Disease. *Chilomastix bettencourti* is considered nonpathogenic. Infection has not been reported to be associated with clinical disease.

Diagnosis. Infection with trichomonads is confirmed following identification of motile trophozoites in direct

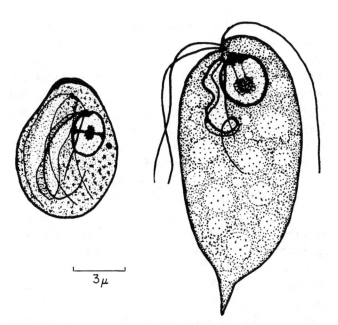

Fig. 11.2 *Chilomastix bettencourti.* (Left) Cyst. (Right) Trophozoite. Reproduced from Wenrich, D.H. (1930) with permission.

wet mounts. Species differentiation requires collection of fecal samples into special fixatives, followed by staining of fixed smears. The type of fixative influences the quality of diagnostic preparation, with a mixture of ethanol, methanol, isopropanol, and formaldehyde or polyvinyl alcohol, producing the least parasite distortion[49]. Fixed slides may be stained with trichrome stain. Staining of prepared slides with Calcofluor white M2R has proven suitable for detecting the cysts of *C. mesnili*[50], and may also be suitable for detecting *C. bettencourti*.

Treatment and Prevention. Because *C. bettencourti* is not considered pathogenic, treatment is not generally attempted.

Public Health Considerations. *Chilomastix bettencourti* is not considered a human health hazard.

Giardia muris **Morphology.** *Giardia muris* (Syn. *Lamblia intestinalis*, *Megastoma entericum*) is a member of the order Diplomonadida and family Hexamitidae. Trophozoites are pyriform with a broadly rounded anterior end, a ventral adhesive disc, eight flagella emerging at different locations, two slender axostyles, and a pair of darkly staining median bodies. The latter are small and rounded, and are characteristic of the genus. Trophozoites measure 7 μ to 13 μ long by 5 μ to 10 μ wide[51] (Figure 11.3).

Hosts. *Giardia muris* has been found in the anterior small intestine of the mouse, rat, hamster, and other wild rodents[52,53,54]. Historically, *G. muris* was common in laboratory rodent colonies[55]. The current prevalence is unknown but presumed to be low. Inbred mouse strains differ in their susceptibility and response to infection. For example, experimentally infected A/J, C3H/He, and C3H/HeJ mice have a shorter prepatent period and become chronically infected compared to BALB/c or DBA/2 mice, which rapidly eliminate their infections[56,57]. Immune-deficient mice are naturally more prone to prolonged infections than are immune-competent mice[57].

Life Cycle. The life cycle of *G. muris* is direct. Trophozoites attach to enterocytes by the ventral sucking disc, and feed through absorbing nutrients. Reproduction is by longitudinal binary fission, which may rapidly increase trophozoite numbers[58]. As trophozoites pass down the intestinal tract, they go through a process of encystation to become environmentally resistant cysts. These represent the typical infective stage, although trophozoites may also survive ingestion to establish infection in a susceptible host[59]. Binary fission may also occur within the cyst stage, resulting in two daughter trophozoites which are released following ingestion by a suitable host. While some authors have reported no gender effect on cyst excretion in experimentally infected mice[60], others have reported that cyst excretion is greater in males[61].

Pathologic Effects. Infection with *G. muris* is generally considered nonpathogenic. Architectural changes,

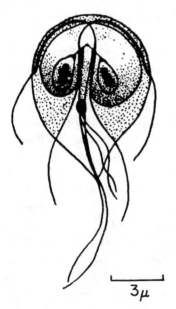

Fig. 11.3 *Giardia muris* trophozoite. Reproduced from Lavier, G. (1924) with permission.

however, are observed in chronic infections including increased numbers of intraepithelial lymphocytes, an increased rate of villus cell turnover, a reduction in villus height, and chronic enteritis[62]. There is also a pronounced deficiency in intestinal disaccharidases that corresponds to the time of maximum trophozoite numbers[63]. Overwhelming infection may result in enteric vascular compromise and systemic dissemination of trophozoites[64].

Clinical Disease. Experimental infection of weanling mice with *G. muris* results in decreased food intake and retarded growth[65].

Diagnosis. Diagnosis is made by identifying trophozoites or cysts in fecal wet mounts. A small amount of iodine may be added to stain internal structures such as the axostyle and median body. Trichrome staining of polyvinyl alcohol-fixed intestinal or fecal contents facilitates diagnosis. Fecal cyst excretion is not a reliable indicator of intestinal parasite burden[66].

Treatment. There are no effective antiprotozoal treatments for eliminating *G. muris*. Metronidazole eliminated the infection in 58.3% of naturally infected mice in one study, and was more efficacious than tinidazole, secnidazole, and furazolidone[67].

Prevention. Most reputable commercial producers of laboratory rodents have currently eliminated *G. muris* from their animal colonies. Therefore, animals should only be purchased from such sources. Rigid sanitation is an important component of prevention. Cysts of *G. muris* are inactivated by ultraviolet light[68] and chlorine-based disinfectants[69].

Public Health Considerations. *G. muris* is not considered a public health concern.

Giardia simoni *Giardia simoni* occurs in the anterior small intestine of the rat, hamster, and various wild rodents throughout the world. It does not infect *Mus musculus*. The trophozoites are of the *G. duodenalis*-type and measure 11 μ to 19 μ long by 5 μ to 11 μ wide, with a "claw-shaped" median body typical of the morphologic type[51] (Figure 11.4). While considerably less is known of the host-parasite relationship of this flagellate, versus *G. muris*, it is probably similar to that of *G. muris*.

Hexamastix muris *Hexamastix muris* (Syn. *Octomitus muris*, *Syndyomita muris*) is a trichomonad belonging to the order Trichomonadida and family Monocercomonadidae. The monocercomonads differ from other members of the order in that they lack an undulating membrane and a costa. *Hexamastix muris* has an anterior nucleus and cytostome, a conspicuous axostyle, a prominent parabasal

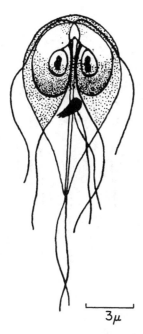

Fig. 11.4 *Giardia simoni* trophozoite. Reproduced from Lavier, G. (1924) with permission.

body, five anterior flagella, and a trailing flagellum. Trophozoites measure 5 μ to 12 μ long. It occurs in the cecum of the rat, hamster, and other rodents throughout the world. Its prevalence is unknown but the organism is likely common. While considered nonpathogenic, infection with *H. muris* has been shown to increase intraepithelial lymphocyte numbers and increase villus cell production rates in rats[62].

Monocercomonoides sp. *Monocercomonoides* sp. belongs to the order Oxymonadida. Members of the genus lack a cytostome, but possess an anterior nucleus, two pairs of anterior flagella, a pelta, an axostyle which is usually filamentous, and one to four strand-like funises. The funis is a costa-like structure which extends backward just beneath the body surface. Trophozoites measure 5 μ to 15 μ long. *Monocercomonoides* sp. has been reported in the cecum of the rat and hamster in North America[70]. Its prevalence is unknown. *Monocercomonoides* sp. is considered nonpathogenic.

Octomitus pulcher Octomitus pulcher (Syn. *O. intestinalis, Hexamita pulcher*) is a member of the order Diplomonadida and family Hexamitidae. It occurs in the cecum of the mouse, rat, hamster, ground squirrel, and other wild rodents throughout the world[27]. Trophozoites are 6 μ to 10 μ long and 3 μ to 7 μ wide (Figure 11.5). Trophozoites are bilaterally symmetrical with a pyriform

body, two anterior nuclei, six anterior flagella, and two posterior flagella[45]. There are two axostyles which originate at the anterior end; these come together and fuse as they pass posteriorly, emerging from the body as a single central rod. In one study, *O. pulcher* was identified in 7.8% of laboratory mice[44]. *Octomitus pulcher* is not known to be pathogenic.

Pentatrichomonas hominis This nonpathogenic flagellate occurs in the cecum and colon of mice, rats, hamsters, dogs, cats, cattle, and primates, including humans[71]. Trophozoites measure 7 μ to 12 μ long and have five anterior flagella, an undulating membrane, and an axostyle that is more slender than that of *T. muris*[72]. The prevalence of *P. hominis* in laboratory colonies is unknown.

Retortamonas sp. *Retortamonas* sp. belongs to the order Retortamonadida and family Retortamonadidae. Members of the order produce true cysts, which represent the infective stage. The cysts are pyriform or ovoid. Trophozoites are pyriform or fusiform and are drawn out posteriorly, with an anterior nucleus; a large anterior cytostome; an anterior flagellum; a posteriorly directed trailing flagellum which emerges from the cytostomal groove; and a cytostomal fibril around the anterior end and sides of the cytostome (Figure 11.6). *Retortamonas* sp. are considered non-pathogenic and have been reported in

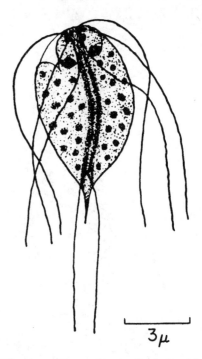

Fig. 11.5 *Octomitus pulcher* trophozoite. Reproduced from Wenrich, D.H. (1930) with permission.

the cecum of wild Norway rats in the eastern United States[73]. The prevalence in laboratory colonies is unknown.

Spironucleus muris **Morphology.** *Spironucleus muris* (formerly *Hexamita muris*) belongs to the order Diplomonadida and family Hexamitidae. Trophozoites are pyriform and rotationally symmetrical. There are two sets of anterior flagella, one set on each side of the trophozoite. For each set, three flagella are free, while a fourth passes through the body to emerge as a trailing posterior flagellum. There are also two separate axostyles[74]. Trophozoites measure 7 μ to 9 μ long and 2 μ to 3 μ wide (Figure 11.7). Cysts are ellipsoid and measure 7.5 μ to 13 μ by 4.5 μ to 6 μ[75]. Two nuclei can be observed in fresh cysts containing one organism. In those cysts where fission has occurred, four nuclei are visible within two daughter trophozoites (Figure 11.8).

Hosts. *Spironucleus muris* infects the mouse, rat, hamster, and various wild rodents throughout the world[77]. Host-specific strains have been identified[78]. Historically, *S. muris* was commonly found in laboratory colonies of rats and mice[55]. Current prevalence is unknown but probably still high. Inbred mouse strains differing in major histocompatibility type also differ in magnitude and course of infection. For example, 129/J mice experimentally infected with *S. muris* shed significantly fewer cysts than BALB/c, ByJ, C3H/HeJ, and DBA/1J mice[76].

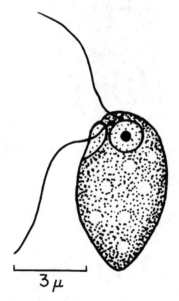

Fig. 11.6 *Retortamonas* sp. trophozoite. Courtesy of N.D. Levine, University of Illinois.

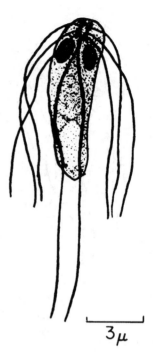

Fig. 11.7 *Spironucleus muris* trophozoite. Reproduced from Wenrich, D.H. (1930) with permission.

Life Cycle. The life cycle is direct. Following ingestion of infectious cysts, excystation occurs, releasing trophozoites which colonize the crypts of Lieberkuhn, primarily in the posterior small intestine and cecum. Multiplication of trophozoites is by longitudinal binary fission. Infectious cysts are passed in the feces. The minimum infective dose for a mouse is one cyst[79]. Cysts lose infectivity as contaminated feces desiccate[74].

Pathologic Effects. Immune-deficient animals, such as athymic (*nu/nu*) or irradiated rats and mice, develop severe chronic enteritis and weight loss following infection with *S. muris*. The intestinal mucosa is reddened, and the lumen filled with fluid and gas. Intestinal crypts are hyperplastic and may be distended with trophozoites. Microvilli and villi may be shortened, and enterocyte turnover is increased[80]. There is an increased number of intraepithelial lymphocytes from three weeks onward corresponding to the start of elimination of the infection[81] (Figure 11.9). Infection with *S. muris* may alter immune reactivity in mice[82] but not in rats[83].

Clinical Disease. Infection with *S. muris* is usually asymptomatic in immune-competent mice and rats. Weanling and immune-compromised hosts may develop acute diarrhea, weight loss, rough hair coat, lethargy, abdominal distension, and hunched posture, and they may

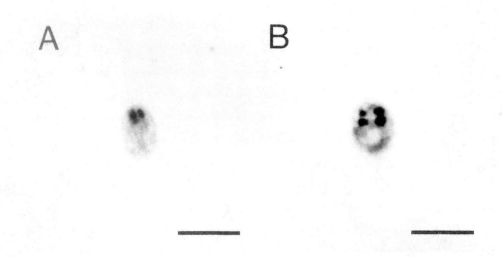

Fig. 11.8 Cysts of *Spironucleus muris* from a preserved mouse fecal smear. Both cysts have undergone internal division. (A) Two nuclei are in focus and a third is in partial focus. (B) All four nuclei are seen. Bar = 5μ. Trichrome stain, 3400 ×. Reproduced from Baker, D.G., Malineni, S., and Taylor, H.W. (1998) with permission.

occasionally die[81]. Older animals may develop more chronic disease, characterized by weight loss and listlessness; diarrhea is uncommon and death is rare.

Diagnosis. Infection is diagnosed by histologic examination of intestinal sections stained with periodic acid-Schiff or silver stains, or by light microscopic examination of intestinal content or fecal wet mounts. Phase-contrast microscopy facilitates examination of wet mounts by allowing one to distinguish cysts of *S. muris* from yeasts.

Treatment. There is no entirely effective treatment for eliminating *S. muris* infection, though some have reported cessation of clinical signs following administration of dimetridazole (3 g/5L drinking water for 14 days) or metronidazole at various dosages[81,84]. Because the flagellate is generally considered nonpathogenic, eradication is rarely considered necessary.

Prevention. It is difficult to find mice or rats free of *S. muris*. If *S. muris*-free rodents are needed, breeders should be asked to specifically test for the organism. Upon arrival, *S. muris*-free rats and mice should be isolated from infected animals.

Public Health Considerations. *Spironucleus muris* is not considered a public health concern.

Tetratrichomonas microti This nonpathogenic flagellate (Syn. *Trichomonas microti*) occurs in the cecum of the mouse, rat, hamster, vole, and other rodents in North America, and has been experimentally transmitted from the hamster to the rat[70]. Trophozoites are 4 μ to 9 μ long and have four free anterior flagella and an undulating membrane about the length of the cell body[85]. Little is known of the biology or pathogenesis of *T. microti* (Figure 11.10)

Trichomitus wenyoni *Trichomitus wenyoni* (formerly *Trichomonas wenyoni*) is a parasite in the subfamily Trichomonadinae. Trophozoites measure 4 μ to 16 μ by 2.5 μ to 6 μ and have three anterior flagella and a recurrent flagellum adhering to the undulating membrane, which runs the length of the cell body[86] (Figure 11.10). It has been found in the Norway rat, house mouse, and hamster. It also occurs in the rhesus monkey and baboon. Little is known of its biology. Its prevalence in rodent colonies is unknown.

Tritrichomonas minuta *Tritrichomonas minuta* belongs to the family Trichomonadidae, subfamily Tritrichomonadinae. It occurs in the cecum and colon of the mouse, rat, and hamster[27]. Relatively little is known of the biology and pathogenesis of *T. minuta*. It is assumed to be similar to *T.*

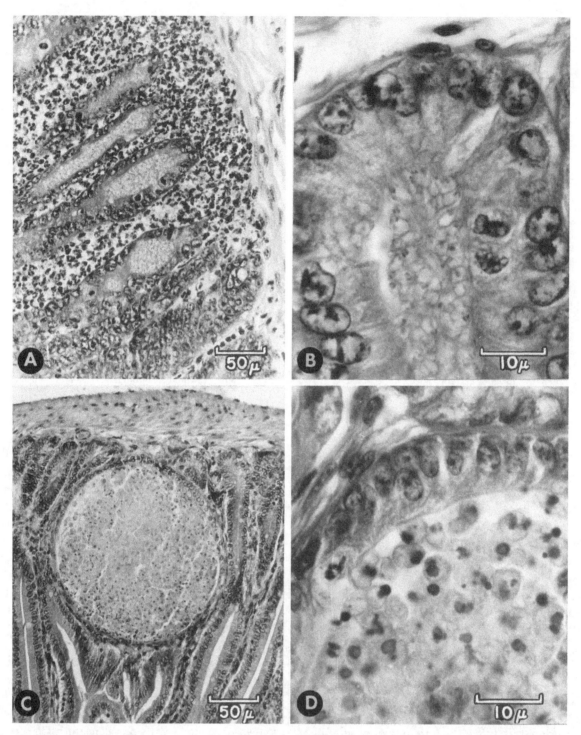

Fig. 11.9 *Spironucleosis* in the duodenum of a mouse. (A) Acute infection. Note cellular infiltration and organisms in crypts. (B) Higher magnification of organisms in crypt. (C) Chronic infection. Note pseudocyst in intestinal wall. (D) Higher magnification of portion of pseudocyst. Courtesy of A. Meshorer, Weizmann Institute of Science.

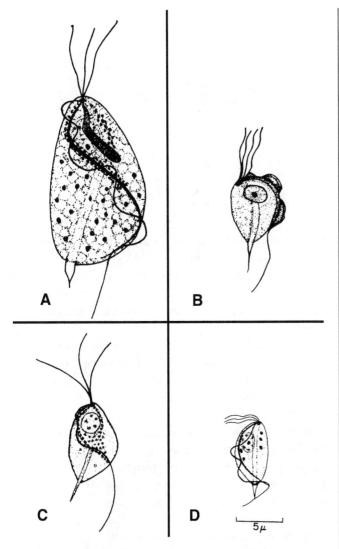

Fig. 11.10 Trichomonad trophozoites infecting rats and mice. (A) *Tritrichomonas muris*. (B) *Tetratrichomonas microti*. (C) *Trichomitus wenyoni*. (D) *Tritrichomonas minuta*. Reproduced from Wenrich, D.H. (1930) and Wenrich, D.H. and Saxe, L.H. (1950) with permission.

muris, and is differentiated from that parasite by its much smaller size. Trophozoites measure only 4 μ to 9 μ long by 2 μ to 5 μ wide[73] (Figure 11.10). Its prevalence in conventional rodent colonies is unknown.

Tritrichomonas muris **Morphology.** *Tritrichomonas muris* belongs to the family Trichomonadidae, subfamily Tritrichomonadinae. Trophozoites measure 16 μ to 26 μ by 10 μ to 14 μ[27] (Figure 11.10). It has an anterior vesicular nucleus. Anterior to this is a blepharoplast from which arise the three anterior flagella, a posterior flagellum, a fibrillar costa, a stiff rod-like axostyle, and a parabasal body and filament[45].

Hosts. This non-pathogenic flagellate is common in the cecum, colon, and small intestine of wild and laboratory mice, rats, golden and Armenian hamsters, Mongolian gerbils, and other rodents[44,48,87,88]. Cross infection between the mouse, rat, and hamster has been accomplished experimentally[70,89]. Because *T. muris* is not considered a pathogen, few laboratories test for it, and it is typically not reported in surveys of laboratory rat and mouse pathogens[4]. Therefore, though previously common[55], the current prevalence of infection of laboratory rats and mice with *T. muris* is unknown.

Life Cycle. Historically, it has been asserted that no cysts are formed, and transmission is by ingestion of trophozoites passed in the feces. More recently, "pseudocyst" and intermediate forms were identified in fecal smears from golden and Armenian hamsters[89]. There is incomplete agreement concerning existence of a true cyst form[90]. The pseudocyst was determined to represent the infective stage. Pseudocysts had internalization of the three anterior flagella and the undulating membrane with its recurrent flagellum[87]. The minimal infectious dose of pseudocysts for athymic mice was determined to be 5, with a prepatent period of 10 days[79]. Reproduction is by simple binary fission[91].

Pathologic Effects and Clinical Disease. *Tritrichomonas muris* is considered nonpathogenic. No clinical signs have been associated with infection.

Diagnosis. Trichomonad infections are diagnosed by examination of fresh fecal wet smears of large intestinal contents. Motile trophozoites are readily identified, and often occur in large numbers. Definitive diagnosis to the species level is by trichrome staining of fixed smears or by electron microscopy and examination of morphologic features[45].

Treatment. Because *T. muris* is considered nonpathogenic, treatment is usually not attempted. However, there may be cases in which it is deemed desirable to eliminate the parasite from the colony. Roach and co-workers[88] reported the successful elimination of *T. muris* from a mouse colony by using a 1% sucrose solution containing 2.5 mg/ml metronidazole or tinidazole in the drinking water. Removal of neonatal mice from infected to uninfected dams, similar to the procedure described to eliminate *Helicobacter hepaticus*[92], effectively eliminates *T. muris* from rats (D. Baker, unpublished observation). Caesarean-section, followed by fostering pups onto uninfected dams (rederivation), is also useful for eliminating the parasite from the colony. It is likely that embryo transfer would likewise be effective.

Prevention. Laboratory animal veterinarians, in consultation with investigators, should determine whether it is desired to exclude *T. muris* from the animal facility. If it is determined that *T. muris* should be excluded, animals should be purchased only from sources certifying them free of this parasite, or rederived upon arrival.

Public Health Considerations. *Tritrichomonas muris* is not a public health concern.

Class Sarcodina (amoebae)

Endolimax ratti

Endolimax ratti may be synonymous with *E. nana,* a morphologically identical amoeba known to inhabit the cecum and colon of a wide range of vertebrate host species, including humans and other primates[27]. *Endolimax ratti* is considered nonpathogenic in rats. Trophozoites measure 6 µ to 15 µ in diameter. Cysts are oval and measure 5 µ to 14 µ long and contain up to four nuclei when mature. The current prevalence of *E. ratti* in laboratory rats is unknown.

Entamoeba muris

This nonpathogenic species is common in the cecum—and less commonly, is found in the colon—of wild mice and rats[93]. Even up to recent times, *E. muris* was also common in laboratory colonies[48]. The current prevalence in laboratory rodents is unknown. Trophozoites measure 25 µ to 30 µ in diameter, while cysts measure 9 µ to 23 µ in diameter and contain eight nuclei when mature[94,95] (Figure 11.11). Transmission is by the fecal-oral route.

Phylum Apicomplexa

Class Coccidia

The coccidia belong to the order Eucoccidiorida, in which there are several families of rodent parasites. Those found in laboratory mice and rats are generally considered nonpathogenic and rare. Very little information is available concerning current prevalence rates of these parasites.

Cryptosporidium muris

Morphology. *Cryptosporidium* sp. belongs to the family Cryptosporidiidae. Mice may be infected by two species of *Cryptosporidium: C. muris* and *C. parvum.* Oocysts of *C. muris* measure 5.3 µ by 7.9 µ[96]. No sporocyst of either *C. muris* or *C. parvum* has been identified. Instead, the sporulated oocyst contains four naked sporozoites.

Hosts. *Cryptosporidium muris* or *C. muris*-like coccidia have been reported from a wide range of mammalian hosts. Recent morphologic and phylogenetic analyses have

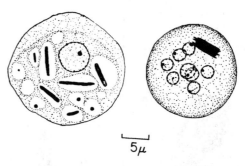

Fig. 11.11 *Entamoeba muris.* (Left) Trophozoite. (Right) Cyst. Reproduced from Hoare, C.A. (1959) with permission.

demonstrated that *C. muris* is not a uniform species, and that the isolates primarily infecting rodents probably constitute a different species from that infecting cattle and other large mammals[97,98]. *Cryptosporidium muris* has been found in wild mice and rats throughout the world[99,100]. Reports from laboratory colonies are rare[96].

Life Cycle. Infection occurs through ingestion of oocysts in contaminated feed and water. Sporozoites are released in the stomach and infect the glandular gastric epithelium. Like other members of the genus, *C. muris* is an intracellular, extracytoplasmic parasite. The parasite inhabits a parasitophorous vacuole just under the host cell membrane. *Cryptosporidium muris* undergoes multiple rounds of schizogony before undergoing sexual reproduction and final production of oocysts. The oocysts sporulate and become infective prior to passing out in the host feces. Some of these oocysts are thin-walled and rupture *in situ,* resulting in repeated autoinfection which intensifies the infection. The prepatent period is about 10 days.

Pathologic Effects. Gastric glands of naturally infected mice become filled with numerous free or embedded parasites. The glands contain degenerated and atrophied epithelial cells, but there is no evidence of inflammation[96]. Other investigators have reported that infected mice develop gastric mastocytosis, which peaks on days 20 to 30 post-inoculation[101]. Experimentally infected nude mice develop dilated, hypertrophied gastric glands which are filled with numerous parasites[102]. Resistance to disease caused by *C. muris* is age-related, and develops quickly after weaning. Susceptibility has also been linked to differences in major histocompatibility complex genes. These differences are correlated with differences in patterns of interleukin-4 secretion[103].

Clinical Disease. Clinical signs typically are not observed in healthy, conventional mice and rats[104].

Diagnosis, Treatment, and Prevention. Infection may be diagnosed by direct observation of oocysts in fecal flotation preparations or through the use of commercial tests based on the indirect fluorescent antibody test. There is currently no effective treatment for cryptosporidiosis in mice. Infected colonies should be rederived or eliminated. Mice and rats should be purchased from reputable sources and wild rodents excluded from the facility.

Public Health Considerations. *Cryptosporidium muris* is not known to infect humans.

Cryptosporidium parvum

Morphology. Oocysts of *C. parvum* are smaller than those of *C. muris,* are ovoid to spherical, and measure 4 μ to 5 μ by 3 μ (Figure 11.12).

Hosts. *Cryptosporidium parvum* infects most if not all mammalian species, including rodents and humans[105]. Neonatal and immunodeficient hosts are far more susceptible to infection and disease than are immunologically competent hosts[106].

Life Cycle. The life cycle of *C. parvum* is similar to that of *C. muris.* However, while *C. muris* infects the gastric glands, *C. parvum* infects the microvillous region of the small intestine, principally the ileum.

Pathologic Effects. Immunocompetent adult rodents develop patent infections but these are mild and the animals suffer few ill effects from infection, and then recover quickly[105].

Clinical Disease. Immunocompetent hosts show no clinical signs of infection. In contrast, in experimentally infected neonatal, severe combined immunodeficient (SCID), and other immunodeficient or immunosuppressed

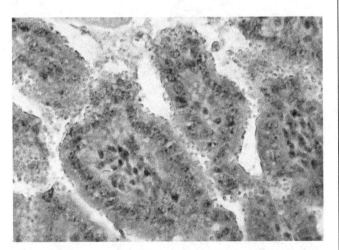

Fig. 11.12 *Cryptosporidium parvum* in mouse ileum. Courtesy of Dr. C. Sterling, University of Arizona.

mice or rats, a severe and eventually fatal chronic infection occurs, characterized by diarrhea, dehydration, and depression, with infection in the ileum, cecum, and colon[107].

Diagnosis. Infection may be diagnosed by direct observation of oocysts in fecal flotation preparations, acid-fast staining of oocysts in fecal smears, or commercial tests based on the indirect fluorescent antibody test.

Treatment and Prevention. Currently there are no effective treatments for cryptosporidial infection. Mice and rats should be purchased from reputable sources, and wild rodents excluded from the facility. Potentially infected, immunocompromised people should not handle laboratory mice or rats.

Public Health Considerations. *Cryptosporidium parvum* is a zoonosis, and can cause severe disease in immunocompromised people. All personnel working with rodents shedding this parasite should use personal protective equipment and adhere to rigid standard operating procedures for hygiene and personal protection. People who are known to have or are suspected of having an immunodeficiency should not work with rodents infected with *C. parvum.*

Eimeria falciformis

Morphology. The oocyst is oval or spherical, with a smooth, colorless wall[108,109] (Figure 11.13). It measures 14 μ to 26 μ by 11 μ to 24 μ. Oocyst size increases midway through the patent period[110].

Hosts. *Eimeria falciformis* occurs primarily within epithelial cell crypts of the large intestine of the mouse[111]. It is rare in laboratory colonies. In contrast, *E. falciformis* undergoes schizogony in experimentally infected laboratory rats but does not complete its life cycle[112].

Life Cycle. The life cycle is similar to that of *E. nieschulzi.* The prepatent period is four to seven days and the patent period is three to four days[113].

Pathologic Effects. Among immune competent strains of mice, C3H/He and CBA/H are highly susceptible; C57BL/10 mice are moderately so; and BALB/c mice are relatively resistant to infection than older mice[114]. All strains are highly resistant to challenge infection[115]. Nude mice are highly susceptible to increased oocyst shedding and mortality, and lack resistance to re-infection[115]. Infection of mice with large numbers of *E. falciformis* has been associated with catarrhal enteritis, hemorrhages, and epithelial sloughing. Mortality is higher in younger mice[114]. Infection confers resistance to challenge[116,117]. Infection with *E. falciformis* may non-specifically augment cellular immunity and thereby alter other host-pathogen relationships[118,119].

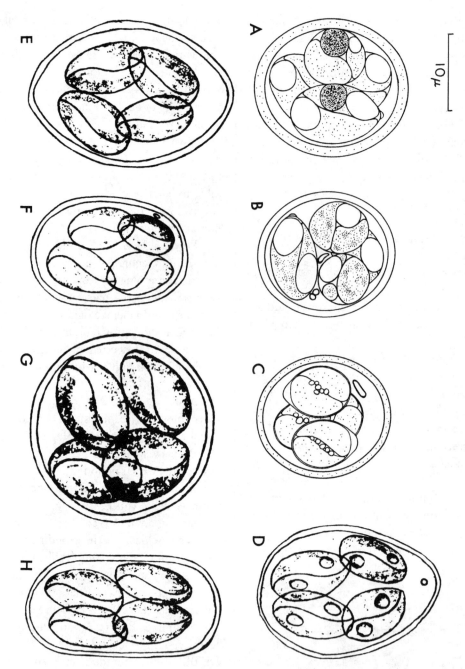

Fig. 11.13 *Eimeria* of the mouse (sporulated oocysts). (A) *E. falciformis.* (B) *E. ferrisi.* (C) *E. hansonorum.* (D) *E. hindlei.* (E) *E. keilini.* (F) *E. krijgsmanni.* (G) *E. musculi.* (H) *E. schueffneri.* (A), (B), (C) reproduced from Levine, N.D. and Ivens, V. (1965) with permission; (D), (E), (F), (G), (H) reproduced from Yakimoff, W.L. and Gousseff, W.F. (1938) with permission.

Clinical Disease. Mild infections are asymptomatic. Heavy infections may result in anorexia, diarrhea, and occasionally, death. Severity of clinical signs is a function of the size of the inoculum and is linked to the major histocompatibility complex, and therefore differs among mouse strains[114].

Diagnosis, Treatment, and Prevention. Diagnosis is based on identification of oocysts in the feces. Treatment recommendations are lacking. Infected colonies should be rederived or eliminated. Control is based on exclusion of wild mice, sound quarantine and sanitation procedures, and purchase of parasite-free animals from reputable sources.

Public Health Considerations. *Eimeria falciformis* is not a public health concern.

Eimeria miyairii

This coccidium occurs in the small intestine of the wild Norway rat, and possibly the black rat, throughout the world. It is not uncommon[77]. There are no recent reports of its occurrence in laboratory colonies. The oocyst is spherical to semispherical, with a thick, rough, yellow-brown, radially striated wall[120,121] (Figure 11.14). It measures 17 μ to 29 μ by 16 μ to 26 μ (mean 24 μ by 22 μ)[122]. Nothing is known of its pathogenicity in rats.

Eimeria nieschulzi

Morphology. *Eimeria nieschulzi* (Syn. *Eimeria halli*) is another coccidian parasite in the family Eimeriidae. The oocyst of *E. nieschulzi* is ellipsoidal to ovoid, is tapered at both ends, and has a smooth, colorless-to-yellow wall (Figure 11.14). Oocysts measure 16 μ to 26 μ by 13 μ to 21 μ. Sporocysts are elongate ovoid. Sporozoites are 10 μ to 12 μ long and contain a central nucleus[122].

Hosts. *Eimeria nieschulzi* is common in wild Norway and black rats[77], but is uncommon in laboratory colonies. Mice are not susceptible to infection with *E. nieschulzi*[123].

Life Cycle. Oocysts containing a single cell, or sporont, are passed in the feces. In the presence of oxygen, sporulation occurs after about three days. Four sporocysts are formed, each containing two sporozoites. The rat is infected by ingestion of sporulated oocysts. Sporozoites escape from the oocysts and enter the intestinal epithelium to undergo four generations of schizogony, during which schizonts form. Each of these contains several merozoites. Fourth-generation merozoites enter epithelial cells and form microgametocytes and macrogametes. The microgametocytes produce a large number of flagellated microgametes by multiple fission. The macrogametes enlarge and, after fertilization by a microgamete, form a wall and become oocysts[124] (Figure 11.15). These oocysts enter the intestinal lumen from the epithelial cells and pass out in the feces. The prepatent period is seven days[122].

Pathologic Effects. The pathogenesis of *E. nieschulzi* is similar to that described for other coccidial infections, and consists primarily of damage and atrophy to the intestinal villi, decreased intestinal disaccharidase activities[125], and alterations in transport of nutrients across the intestinal wall[126]. Infection induces accumulation of mucosal mast cells and release of rat mucosal mast cell protease in immune-competent rats, but not in immune-deficient rats[127]. Infection with *E. nieschulzi* may also elevate circulating neutrophil counts[128] and may interfere with immunologic responses induced by other pathogens[129,130].

Clinical Disease. Reports of naturally acquired disease caused by *E. nieschulzi* are rare. Natural clinical disease has been reported in young rats. In one report, rats developed severe diarrhea, weakness, emaciation, and occasionally, death[131]. Similar, though somewhat less severe, signs have been reported following experimental infection[132]. Typical of coccidial infections, the severity of the disease depends on the size of the infecting dose of oocysts and the immune status and exposure history of the host. Animals which recover are relatively immune to challenge due to high levels of IgG and IgA antibodies[132].

Diagnosis. Tentative diagnosis is based on the presence of oocysts in the feces, but accurate identification is sometimes difficult and may require careful examination of oocysts

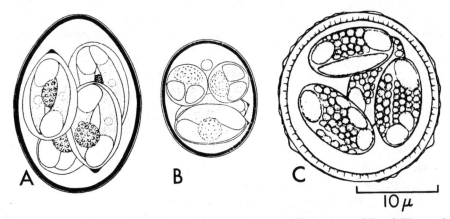

Fig. 11.14 *Eimeria* of the rat (sporulated oocysts). (A) *E. nieschulzi.* (B) *E. separata.* (C) *E. miyairii.* (A) and (B) reproduced from Becker, E.R., Hall, P.R., Hager, A. (1932) with permission; (C) reproduced from Matubayasi, H. (1938) with permission.

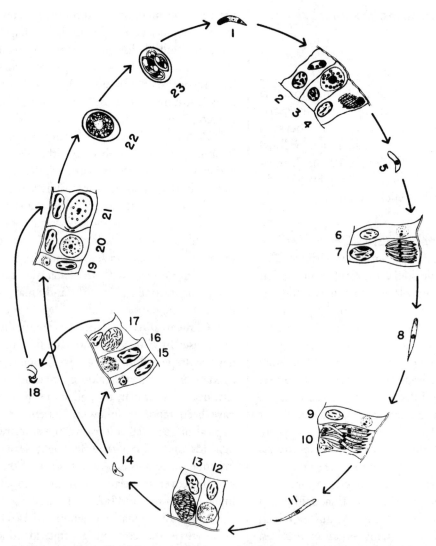

Fig. 11.15   Life cycle of *Eimeria nieschulzi.* (1) Sporozoite. (2) Sporozoite after entering host intestinal cell. (3) First-generation schizont in host cell (merozoites shown in cross section; note refractile globule). (4) First-generation merozoites in host cell. (5) First-generation merozoite. (6) Second-generation schizont in host cell. (7) Second-generation merozoites in host cell. (8) Second-generation merozoite. (9) Third-generation schizont in host cell. (10) Third-generation merozoites in host cell. (11) Third-generation merozoite. (12) Fourth-generation schizont in host cell. (13) Fourth-generation merozoites in host cell. (14) Fourth-generation merozoite. (15) Young microgametocyte in host cell. (16) Older microgametocyte in host cell. (17) Mature microgametocyte in host cell (surface view). (18) Microgamete. (19) Young macrogamete in host cell. (20) Developing macrogamete in host cell (note plastic granules inside macrogamete). (21) Young oocyst (zygote) in host cell. (22) Unsporulated oocyst in feces. (23) Sporulated oocyst in feces. Reproduced from Levine, N.D. (1957) with permission.

and schizonts for distinct morphologic features[133]. Oocysts may be shed in the absence of disease. A diagnosis of clinical disease can be made only at necropsy by finding lesions containing coccidia in association with signs of disease.

Treatment. Infection with *E. nieschulzi* is self-limiting both in the individual and the colony. There are several coccidiostatic drugs, but none have been specifically efficacious against *E. nieschulzi* in the rat. Rederivation through

caesarean section or embryo transfer eliminates the infection. Ideally, infected colonies should be culled.

Prevention. Prevention depends on exclusion of wild rats, purchase of rats only from reputable sources, effective quarantine and testing, and strict attention to facility sanitation.

Public Health Considerations. *Eimeria nieschulzi* is not transmissible to humans.

Eimeria pragensis

Eimeria pragensis is quite similar to *E. falciformis* and was for many years considered a subspecies of *E. falciformis*[134]. Oocysts measure 21.2 μ by 18.3 μ[135]. Mice are the only known hosts of *E. pragensis*. It is uncommon in wild mice[77]. The prevalence in laboratory colonies is unknown. Patency occurs on day seven to day eight and the patent period is four to 16 days[113]. Heavy infection may result in pathologic changes that sequentially include large intestinal cryptal and absorptive epithelial cell destruction, submucosal edema, neutrophil infiltration, mucosal necrosis, crypt hyperplasia, and finally, granulomatous colitis. Infection is followed by lymphoid hyperplasia in the lymph nodes and spleen. Clinical signs are evident in heavy infection, and may include depression, anorexia, weight loss, diarrhea or dysentery, dehydration, and death[136]. Immune-deficient mice are unable to clear the infection[137].

Eimeria separata

Morphology. The oocyst of *E. separata* is ellipsoidal with a smooth, colorless, or pale yellow wall (Figure 11.14). The oocysts of a small number of coccidia are known to increase in size during specific portions of the patent period. Early in the patent period, oocysts of *E. separata* measure 9.9 μ to 14.3 μ by 8.8 μ to 12.1 μ (mean = 11.7 μ by 10.1 μ). Oocyst size increases late in the patent period, reaching maximum dimensions of 14.3 μ to 17.6 μ by 13.2 μ to 15.4 μ (mean = 16.3 μ by 14.2 μ)[138].

Hosts. *Eimeria separata* is common in the cecum and colon of wild rats throughout the world[77]. It is likely rare in laboratory colonies, but current prevalence data is lacking. Experimental transmission of *E. separata* to certain strains of *M. musculus* has been reported[135,139], but *E. separata* does not naturally infect mice.

Life Cycle. The life cycle is similar to that of *E. nieschulzi*[122].

Pathologic Effects. Infection of rats with even large numbers of sporulated oocysts is not considered pathogenic[140]. Infection induces early accumulation of intraepithelial lymphocytes and strong immunity[141], increases cecum and colon weights[132], and results in alterations in intestinal ion transport[142] and in local elevations in inflammatory cytokines[143]. Other host-parasite interactions are also altered[144].

Clinical Disease. Clinical signs, other than poor weight gain, are generally not observed in rats infected with even large numbers of *E. separata*[139].

Diagnosis, Treatment, and Prevention. Diagnosis is based on finding characteristic oocysts in the feces. Treatment recommendations are as described for *E. nieschulzi*. Infected colonies should be rederived or culled. Prevention of infection is based on exclusion of wild rats from the research colony, adequate quarantine and testing, and purchase of parasite-free rats from reputable sources.

Public Health Considerations. *Eimeria separata* is not considered a public health concern.

Eimeria spp.

Several other species of *Eimeria* infect the mouse (Figure 11.13). These include *E. arasinaensis*, *E. ferrisi*, *E. hansonorum*, *E. hindlei*, *E. keilini*, *E. krijgsmanni*, *E. musculi*, *E. musculoidei*, *E. paragachaica*, *E. papillata*, *E. schueffneri*, and *E. vermiformis*. Like *E. separata*, *E. contorta* normally infects rats, but will also complete its life cycle in mice[135,145]. Very little is known concerning the prevalence, pathogenicity, clinical signs, or control of these species. All are rare or not reported in laboratory mice.

Frenkelia spp.

Morphology. *Frenkelia* spp. are coccidian parasites in the family Sarcocystidae and are biologically similar to *Sarcocystis* spp.[160] Tissue cysts of *Frenkelia sp.* were first reported in the brain of laboratory-reared Fischer 344 rats[161]. The cysts are thin-walled and multilobulated, with many compartments outlined by fine interlacing septae. Each compartment contains numerous crescent-shaped, periodic acid-Shiff (PAS)-positive bradyzoites (Figure 11.16)[162].

Hosts. *Frenkelia* spp. occur in many species of rodents, including rats, voles (*Microtus agrestis*), chinchillas (*Chinchilla laniger*), meadow mice (*Microtus modestus*), muskrats, lemmings (*Lemmus lemmus*), red-backed mice (*Clethrionomys glareolus*), and others. Raptorial birds serve as the definitive hosts. Whereas infections in raptorial birds are routinely diagnosed, infection in a laboratory rodent, a rat, has only been reported once[161].

Life Cycle. The life cycles of *Frenkelia* spp. are typical of the family, and involve predator-prey relationships. The definitive hosts of *Frenkelia* spp. are raptorial birds in the families Falconiformes and Strigiformes. These include the hawks, eagles, vultures, and owls. Intermediate hosts, including rats and mice, become infected by ingesting sporocysts or sporulated oocysts shed in the feces of definitive hosts. Only asexual reproduction occurs in the rodent intermediate host.

Pathologic Effects and Clinical Disease. Following infection, merozoite formation (merogony) occurs in the rodent liver. Merogony may result in hepatic necrosis, and perivascular cellular infiltration in several organs. Brady-zoite tissue cysts are found in the brain and cervical spinal cord, typically with no local reaction[161]. However, cyst growth may occasionally cause pressure necrosis, followed by inflammatory changes characterized by granulomatous encephalitis with giant cell formation, perivascular and meningeal infiltrates, and gliosis. Infections with *Frenkelia* spp. are asymptomatic.

Diagnosis. Diagnosis of *Frenkelia* spp. infection, if it occurs at all, will likely be as an incidental finding of histopathology.

Treatment. There are no published guidelines concerning treatment of *Frenkelia* spp. in laboratory rodents. Infected colonies should be culled and the source of infection determined.

Prevention. Since *Frenkelia* spp. have obligate two-host life cycles, infection of laboratory rodents is extremely unlikely. Raptorial birds should not be housed near laboratory rodents, and rodent feed and bedding stocks should be

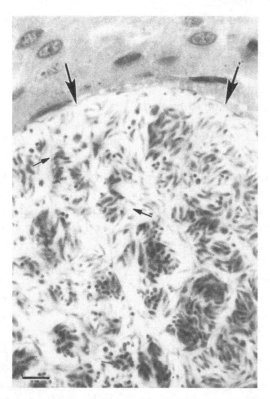

Fig. 11.16 *Frenkelia microti* cysts in the brain of a vole. High magnification of numerous lobulated cysts reveals smooth, thin cyst wall (arrows). Hemotoxylin and eosin stain. Bar = 10 μm. Courtesy of J.P. Dubey, United States Department of Agriculture. Reproduced from Dubey, J.P. and Odening, K. (2001) with permission.

protected from contamination with raptor feces, including that introduced by filth-bearing insect transport hosts.

Public Health Considerations. *Frenkelia* spp. are not considered public health hazards.

Hammondia hammondi

Morphology. *Hammondia hammondi* is a coccidian parasite in the family Sarcocystidae. Oocysts shed in cat feces measure 10.6 μ by 11.4 μ[163]. Bradyzoite cysts form primarily in skeletal and cardiac muscle in the rodent intermediate host.

Hosts. The definitive host of *H. hammondi* is the cat. Intermediate hosts include rats, mice, deer mice (*Peromyscus* sp.), multimammate rats, hamsters, and several other mammalian species. *Hammondia hammondi* is not infective to humans. The prevalence of *H. hammondi* in cats is very low[164]. The prevalence of *H. hammondi* in wild rodents is unknown, but reports of natural infection are rare[165]. Spontaneous hammondiosis has not been reported in laboratory rodents.

Life Cycle. The life cycle of *H. hammondi* is similar to that of *T. gondii,* except that there is no extraintestinal phase of the life cycle in the cat, the intermediate hosts become infected only by ingestion of oocysts, and cats become infected only by ingesting intermediate hosts[166].

Pathologic Effects. *Hammondia hammondi* is not pathogenic in rodents. Elongated intracellular bradyzoite cysts form primarily in skeletal and cardiac muscle, yet are incidental.

Clinical Disease. *Hammondia hammondi* is not thought to cause clinical disease in rodents. However, most studies of intermediate hosts have focused on mice. Similar studies are needed using rats.

Diagnosis. Diagnosis of *H. hammondi* infection is similar to that of *T. gondii.* Infection with *H. hammondi* may give cross-reacting positive results to *T. gondii* serology unless monoclonal antibodies are used[167]. The two infections can also be distinguished via bioassay in mice. Sporulated oocysts are infective to mice, but bradyzoites and tachyzoites of *H. hammondi* are not. In contrast, both *T. gondii* bradyzoites and tachyzoites are infective to mice[166]. Also, *H. hammondi* tissue cysts are more frequent in striated muscle than in the brains of mice used for bioassay, while the opposite is true for *T. gondii.* This feature alone, however, is inadequate for differentiating the two infections[167].

Treatment. There is no effective treatment for *H. hammondi* infection in rodents. Affected colonies should be culled.

Prevention. Natural infection of laboratory rodents with *H. hammondi* is unlikely to occur so long as feed and bedding stocks are protected from contamination with cat feces.

Public Health Considerations. *Hammondia hammondi* is not considered a human health hazard.

Hepatozoon muris

Morphology. *Hepatozoon muris* (Syn. *Hepatozoon perniciosum, Leucocytozoon muris, Leucocytozoon ratti, Leucocytogregarina innoxia*) is a coccidian parasite belonging to the family Haemogregarinidae. These are heteroxenous (two-host) parasites of the circulatory system of vertebrate hosts and the digestive tract of invertebrate hosts. Schizonts, which are found in the liver, are 10 μ to 30 μ in diameter[168] (Figure 11.17). Gamonts, which occur in the lymphocytes, appear in stained blood smears as elongated oval or reniform bodies, 8 μ to 12 μ by 3 μ to 6 μ, with a light blue, non-granular cytoplasm and a pink central nucleus. The cytoplasm of the lymphocyte around the parasite is unstained. Free forms of the parasite, which occur in the blood, are slender and curved or straight, and are often pointed at one end.

Hosts. *Hepatozoon muris* occurs only in rats of the genus *Rattus. Hepatozoon muris* has been found in wild rats throughout the world[169], though the current prevalence is unknown. Infection of laboratory-raised rats is presumed to be rare.

Life Cycle. The rat becomes infected by ingesting the invertebrate host, the spiny rat mite, *Laelaps echidninus.* Sporozoites are released in the intestine, enter the hepatic portal system, and are transported to the liver. Schizogony takes place in the hepatic parenchymal cells. Merozoites enter the lymphocytes in the circulating blood and become gamonts. The gamonts are ingested by the mite; fertilization and sporogony occur in the arthropod host (Figure 11.18)[170].

Pathologic Effects. *Hepatozoon muris* is generally considered nonpathogenic in rats. Following natural infection, parasite burdens increase gradually over the course of a few months. The infection induces profound leukocytosis and monocytosis, and may also cause splenomegaly, hepatic degeneration, and anemia. Grossly, affected rats are pale, the liver and spleen are enlarged, and the lungs may have minute surface hemorrhages. Other organs may show degenerative changes[171].

Clinical Disease. Mild parasite burdens are asymptomatic. In contrast, heavily infected rats develop anorexia, lethargy, emaciation, terminal diarrhea, and death. A mortality of 50% has been reported in rats experimentally

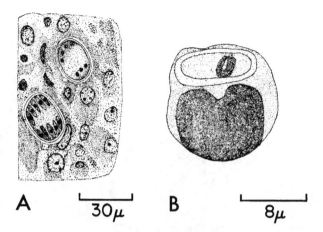

Fig. 11.17 *Hepatozoon muris* in the rat. (A) Schizonts in liver tissue. (B) Gamont in lymphocyte. Reproduced from Wenrich, D.H. (1949) with permission.

infected by the parasite. Growing rats are more susceptible to overwhelming infection than are mature rats[171].

Diagnosis. Diagnosis is based on recognition of the parasite in blood smears and tissue sections in association with signs and lesions. Gametocytes may be demonstrated within leukocytes on stained blood smears, while merozoites may be observed in liver sections.

Treatment. No effective drugs are known. Eradication of mites prevents transmission of the parasite. Affected colonies should be eliminated. Macintire and co-workers report on the treatment of dogs infected with *H. americanum.* Treatment with anticoccidial agents ameliorated clinical disease, but did not eliminate tissue stages[172]. Likewise, Krampitz and Haberkorn administered toltrazuril subcutaneously or in the drinking water or feed of bank voles (*Clethrionomys glareolus*) infected with *H. erhardovae.* Clinical recovery occurred following nearly all routes and dosages, but infection was not reproducibly eliminated with any of the regimens[173]. It is unlikely that antiprotozoal treatment would be preferred to rederivation and elimination of infected laboratory rats.

Prevention. This parasite should not occur in laboratory-reared rats in well-managed animal facilities because the mite intermediate host should not be available. Rats should be purchased from reputable sources.

Public Health Considerations. *Hepatozoon muris* is not known to occur in humans.

Hepatozoon musculi

Hepatozoon musculi has not been reported from laboratory mice since early in the last century[174]. It differs from *H. muris*

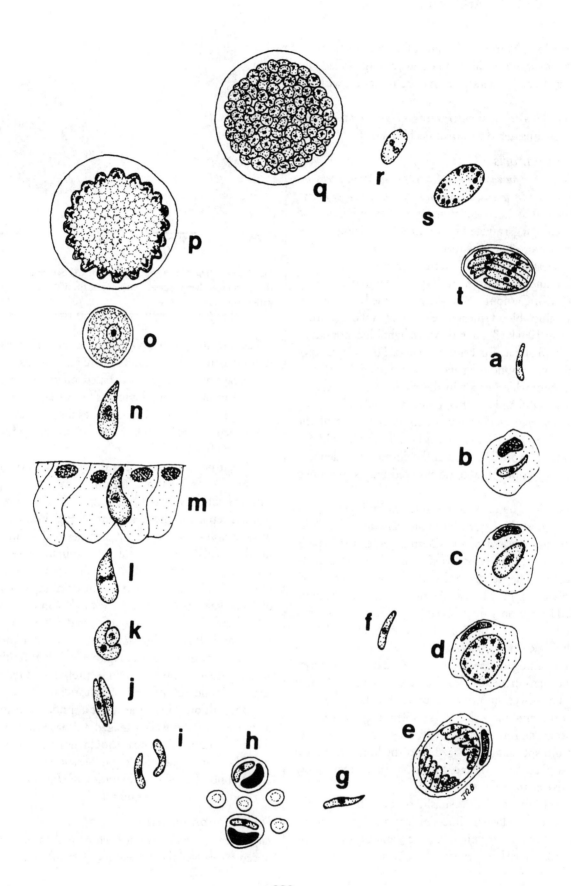

Fig. 11.18 *Hepatozoon muris.* Life cycle: a. sporozoite; b-f. merogony; g. invasion of blood cells by gamonts; i. gamonts free in blood meal of mite; j, k. syzygy and maturation of gametes; l-n. syngamy and migration of zygote (ookinete) to extraintestinal tissues; o. young oocyst; p, q. formation of numerous sporoblasts; r. single sporoblast; s, t. maturation of sporoblasts containing 12–24 sporozoites. Reproduced from Lee, J.J., Leedale, G.F., and Bradbury, P. (2000) with permission.

in that schizogony takes place only in the bone marrow. The prevalence in wild populations of mice is unknown.

Isospora ratti

Isospora ratti belongs to the family Eimeriidae. This parasite was found in the intestinal contents of a wild Norway rat several years ago but has not been reported since[108]. Little is known of the biology of this parasite. Oocysts are subspherical, smooth, and measure 22 μ to 24 μ by 20 μ to 21 μ (Figure 11.19).

Klossiella muris

Morphology. *Klossiella muris* is a one-host parasite in the family Klossiellidae, and is the type species for the genus. The sporocyst is the antemortem diagnostic stage, has a thin wall, measures 16 μ by 13 μ, and contains 30 to 35 banana-shaped sporozoites[174,175].

Hosts. *Klossiella muris* infects mice and rats[176,177]. Historically, prevalence was high in laboratory colonies but low in wild populations. Current prevalence in wild and laboratory rodents is unknown.

Life Cycle. The mouse is infected by ingesting sporulated sporocysts. Sporozoites are released and distributed hematogenously to the endothelial cells of the renal glomeruli, where schizogony occurs (Figure 11.20). Merozoites enter the epithelial cells of the convoluted tubules of the kidney, where they form gamonts which become macrogametes and microgametes. After fertilization, the zygote or sporont grows and divides by budding to form 12 to 16 sporoblasts, each of which becomes a sporocyst. The sporocysts rupture the host cell and pass out of the body in the urine[175].

Pathologic Effects. *Klossiella muris* is generally considered nonpathogenic, but may result in interstitial nephritis[178]. Kidneys may be enlarged, and pale areas and small gray necrotic foci are seen on the surface[179]. Microscopically, organisms occur in the tubular epithelial cells, glomerular endothelium, and convoluted tubule lumens. The parasites are most common in the cortex, where they cause little inflammation, although destruction of tubular epithelium has been reported. Foci of interstitial cellular

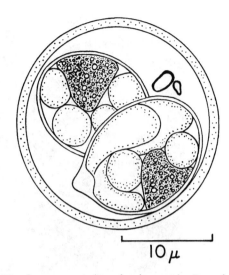

Fig. 11.19 *Isospora ratti* (sporulated oocyst). Reproduced from Levine, N.D. and Ivens, V. (1965) with permission.

infiltration are seen, but not in association with the organisms[175]. Interstitial pneumonia, pulmonary congestion, and splenomegaly are additional lesions which may be observed in animals infected with *K. muris*[178].

Clinical Disease. No clinical signs have been reported in mice or rats experimentally infected with *K. muris*. Some mice naturally infected with *K. muris* become emaciated[178]. Infected mice have impaired metabolic capability under cold conditions[180].

Diagnosis. Diagnosis, when it occurs at all, will most likely be made on gross and microscopic examination of renal architecture and on recognition of the organisms in tissue sections[178]. The presence of perivascular, follicular, lymphocytic infiltration in the outer zone of the medulla is said to be of diagnostic significance[181]. Giemsa staining of impression smears reveals the sporogonic stages of the parasite[177]. The extent of colony involvement can be determined by examination of urine for sporocysts.

Treatment. Currently there is no treatment for *K. muris* infection. Van Pelt and Dieterich treated a colony of infected mice with various therapies, including nitrofurantoin or sulfonamides added to the drinking water, but none of these treatment regimens eradicated the parasite[178]. Infected colonies should be eliminated or rederived.

Prevention. Given the paucity of reports of this parasite in laboratory mice and rats, it is assumed that infection is rare. Exclusion of wild rodents and other good management practices are important in maintaining a *Klossiella*-free colony.

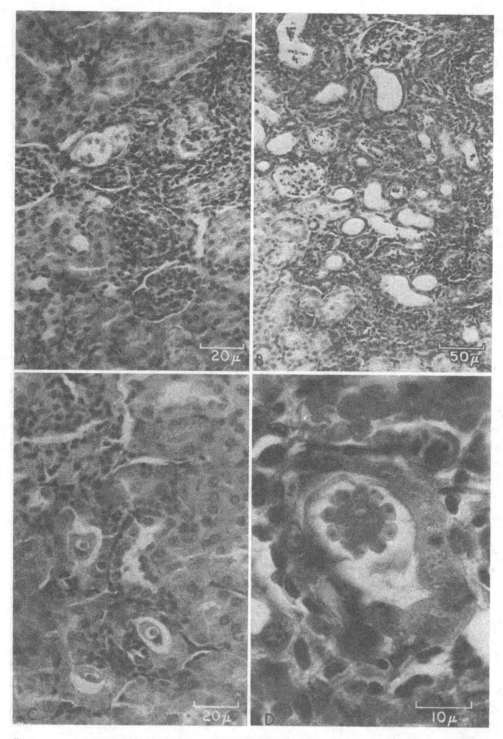

Fig. 11.20 *Klossiella muris* in mouse kidney. (A) Schizogony. (B), (C) Early stage of sporogony. (D) Late stage of sporogony. Courtesy of N. Meshorer, Weizmann Institute of Science.

Public Health Considerations. *Klossiella muris* is not considered a risk to human health.

Sarcocystis muris

Morphology. *Sarcocystis muris* is a member of the family Sarcocystidae. Sporocysts, released in the feces of infected cats, measure 8.5 μ by 10.3 μ[182].

Hosts. Mice serve as the intermediate host for *S. muris*. Infection of wild mice has been reported in many parts of the world[183]. Host genotype influences susceptibility to infection, with hybrid mice being more susceptible[184]. Many years ago *S. muris* was common in laboratory rodent colonies, but is now extremely uncommon[185]. Rats are not susceptible to infection with *S. muris*.

Life Cycle. In the mouse intermediate host, the life cycle begins when the mouse ingests sporocysts containing infectious sporozoites. These are released in the intestinal tract. Following hematogenous dissemination, bradyzoite cysts develop primarily in the diaphragm and tongue, and to a lesser extent, the myocardium. This occurs within four weeks of infection (Figure 11.21)[186]. Cysts are infective to cats, in which the sexual phase of the life cycle occurs[183]. Rodents may also serve as the definitive host, becoming infected through cannibalism.

Pathologic Effects. *Sarcocystis muris* is known to cause architectural changes in infected muscle fibers and in uninfected fibers elsewhere in the infected rodent host[187]. Heavy infection results in myositis and muscle necrosis[185]. Cellular and architectural changes resulting in splenomegaly, attributable to white pulp hyperplasia, have also been noted in mice infected with *S. muris*. There is also a progressive accumulation of splenic B-cells. These changes are associated with suppression of cellular aspects of immunity[188].

Clinical Disease. *Sarcocystis muris* does not generally cause clinical disease in the rodent intermediate host. Heavy infections have resulted in hemorrhaging and abortion[185].

Diagnosis. Diagnosis of *S. muris* is most likely to occur during routine histopathologic examination of laboratory mice. *S. muris* must be differentiated from other cyst-forming coccidia, including *Toxoplasma gondii*, *Isospora felis*, and *Hammondia hammondi*. These all form bradyzoite cysts which are < 1 mm in diameter, while the cysts of *S. muris* are larger[185]. Diagnosis is aided by examining cyst morphology on PAS-stained tissues.

Treatment. Rommel and co-workers have reported the successful elimination of *S. muris* infection using combination therapy consisting of sulfaquinoxaline plus

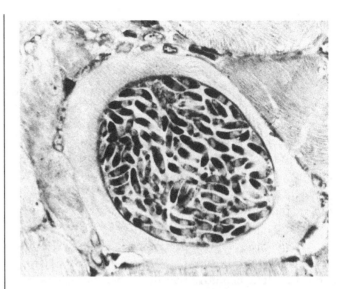

Fig. 11.21 Cross section of a *Sarcocystis muris* sarcocyst in a mouse myocyte. Giemsa stain, 750 ×. Reproduced from Dubey, J.P. (1991) with permission.

pyrimethamine[189]. Ideally however, infected colonies should be eliminated.

Prevention. Caretakers who own cats should be instructed to practice strict personal hygiene to prevent introduction of *S. muris* into the mouse colony. Feral cats should not be allowed near feed and bedding storage areas, because sporocysts released from infected cats may remain infective for at least 20 days under suitable conditions. Cockroaches have been shown to serve as vectors for *S. muris* during this time[190].

Public Health Considerations. *Sarcocystis muris* is not considered a public health hazard.

Sarcocystis spp. in the mouse

Mice may also be infected with *Sarcocystis dispersa*, *S. scotti*, and *S. sebeki*. The definitive hosts of each of these are various species of owls[27]. Rodent feed and bedding stocks should be protected from contamination from owl feces. Mice may also become infected with *Sarcocystis* spp., described below for the rat.

Sarcocystis spp. in the rat

Morphology. Several *Sarcocystis* spp. have been reported from wild rats. These include *S. cymruensis*, *S. dirumpens*, *S. murinotechis*, *S. singaporensis*, *S. sulawesiensis*, *S. villivillosi*, and *S. zamani*[191,192,193]. The elongated cysts (or Miescher's tubes) of *Sarcocystis* spp. occur in cardiac and skeletal muscle tissues throughout the body, or in vascular endothelium, depending on parasite species. Cysts are bounded by a parasitophorous vacuole membrane. Zoites liberated from cysts are crescent shaped, and differ by species in length and width.

Hosts. In the wild, *Sarcocystis* spp. use a range of intermediate hosts, including *Rattus* sp., multimammate rats, house mice, gerbils, Siberian dwarf hamsters (*Phodopus sungorus*), and bandicoot rats (*Bandicota indica*). Many years ago, *Sarcocystis* spp. infections were common in laboratory rodents[194]. Nowadays, laboratory rats are rarely infected. Definitive hosts include snakes and cats. The prevalence of natural infection in wild snakes is high, while cats are uncommonly infected.

Life Cycle. Typical of the family, the life cycles of *Sarcocystis* spp. involve predator-prey relationships. The definitive hosts of *S. singaporensis, S. villivillosi,* and *S. zamani* are snakes. The definitive host of *S. cymruensis* is the cat, while the definitive hosts of *S. sulawesiensis, S. dirumpens,* and *S. murinotechis* are not known. Predators become infected while consuming rodents infected with tissue cysts. Rats become infected by ingestion of sporocysts shed in predator feces.

Pathologic Effects. Of the species found in rats, *S. singaporensis* is the most pathogenic, so much so that *S. singaporensis* has been proposed as a means of wild rat population control. While many rats develop fatal protozoal pneumonia, surviving rats mount a rapid and specific immune response[195].

Clinical Disease. Infections with most *Sarcocystis* spp. are asymptomatic. However, *S. singaporensis* causes terminal anorexia, labored breathing, and death[196].

Diagnosis. Diagnosis of sarcocystosis is based on the demonstration of the characteristic tissue cysts in histologic sections. The cyst wall may be smooth or bear projections. Cyst wall morphology is a key feature used to differentiate parasite species. Serologic tests have also been developed but are not likely to be practical due to the low prevalence of infection in laboratory rats.

Treatment. There are currently no effective therapies for sarcocystosis in rats. In mice, *S. muris* infection can be eliminated by combined treatment with sulfaquinoxaline plus pyrimethamine[189]. It is not known whether this combination will also clear rats of *Sarcocystis* spp.

Prevention. Infection of laboratory rats is extremely unlikely when snakes and cats are not housed near laboratory rodents, and rodent feed and bedding stocks are protected from contamination with snake and cat feces. Caretakers should practice adequate hygiene to prevent spread of contamination from house cats and pet snakes.

Public Health Considerations. The *Sarcocystis* spp. of rats are not public health risks.

Toxoplasma gondii

Morphology. *Toxoplasma gondii* is a common coccidian parasite belonging to the family Sarcocystidae. In the rodent host, bradyzoite cysts are most numerous in the brain, and are often up to 50 μ in diameter (Figure 11.22).

Hosts. The definitive host of *T. gondii* is the cat. Intermediate hosts include virtually all warm-blooded animals, including rats and mice. Globally, rodents, including rats and mice, have frequently been found naturally infected with *T. gondii*[197,198].

Life Cycle. Cats become infected through ingestion of infected intermediate hosts or by ingestion of sporulated oocysts excreted from another cat. Following infection, asexual, and later, sexual, development occurs in the feline intestinal tract. Ultimately, unsporulated oocysts are released into the environment. Oocysts can survive for long periods under moderate conditions of temperature and humidity. As a result, oocysts may contaminate feed or bedding intended for use in the laboratory environment.

Laboratory rodents become infected following ingestion of feed or bedding contaminated with oocysts. Following ingestion of sporulated oocysts, sporozoites penetrate and multiply within the lamina propria of the small intestine. Thereafter, parasites disseminate and form bradyzoite cysts in brain, lung, heart, muscle, liver, spleen, kidneys, uterus, intestine, lymph nodes, and other organs[199]. Tissue cysts are formed inside the cell as the host develops both cellular and humoral immunity. Tissue cysts may persist for many months, years, or the life of the host. Once established in a rodent colony, offspring may also become infected through transplacental transmission[197].

Pathologic Effects. *Toxoplasma gondii* is an intracellular parasite capable of affecting all organs, with particular affinity for the central nervous system and tissues of the mononuclear phagocytic system. Severe infection, or infection with virulent strains of *T. gondii*, may compromise hematopoietic function and result in death due to dissemination to extraintestinal organs[200]. Rats that survive longer may die of encephalitis or the compromise of other vital organs. In mild infections, there may be no obvious pathologic effects. Tissue cysts do not ordinarily provoke inflammatory host responses. However, ruptured cysts elicit lymphocytic inflammation.

Clinical Disease. Rats are among the most resistant hosts to *T. gondii* infection, and rarely show clinical signs.

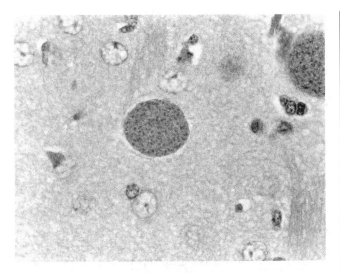

Fig. 11.22 *Toxoplasma gondii.* A well-developed tissue cyst in the brain of a rat 29 days after infection. Hematoxylin and eosin, 650 ×. Original photograph courtesy of Dr. J.P. Dubey, United States Department of Agriculture. Reproduced from Baker, D.G. (2005) with permission.

However, the clinical outcome of infection is highly dependent on parasite strain, stage inoculated, and route of inoculation. Infection of *T. gondii* in newborn or young rats often results in fatal pneumonia[201]. Older rats inoculated with few parasites become chronically infected but rarely show clinical signs of infection. Rats administered with large numbers of sporulated oocysts may experience fatal infection[202]. Beyond these, *T. gondii* alters cognitive function in the rat, such that the rat's innate aversion to cats is diminished, thereby facilitating predation and completion of the life cycle[203]. This would only be an issue in the laboratory setting if infected rats were used in behavioral studies.

Diagnosis. Spontaneous toxoplasmosis in laboratory rodents is rare. Diagnosis of *T. gondii* infection is based on the demonstration of parasites in tissue sections or stained cell preparations, serologic tests (a commercial modified agglutination test kit is available), bioassays of suspect material in mice, or PCR assays[197,204].

Treatment. There are no effective treatments for *T. gondii* infection in rats. Infected rats should be culled, because they are likely unfit for most research applications. Valuable stocks or strains may be rederived free of *T. gondii* by embryo transfer.

Prevention. Rodent feed and bedding must be protected from contamination with cat feces. Careful management practices must be instated if cats and laboratory mice are housed in the same facility. An adequate vermin control program should be in place, because cockroaches may serve as mechanical vectors of *T. gondii* through ingestion of oocyst-containing cat feces. Rodents become infected when they consume contaminated cockroaches[190]. Caretakers should be encouraged to practice strict personal hygiene after handling their personal cats at home to prevent entry of *T. gondii* into the animal facility.

Public Health Considerations. *Toxoplasma gondii* represents a potentially serious risk to human health. The most common sources of human infection include consumption of undercooked pork and lamb, and less commonly, ingestion of sporulated oocysts in cat feces. Human fetuses and immune-compromised people are at increased risk of potentially life-threatening illness with *T. gondii*. The risk to human health is much lower when handling *T. gondii*-infected rodents, because oocysts are not shed in the feces of intermediate hosts. Research personnel handling experimentally infected rodents must exercise caution to avoid needle sticks.

Class Piroplasmidia

Babesia microti

Morphology. *Babesia microti* (Syn. *Babesia rodhaini*) is a piroplasmid in the family Babesiidae. This is a small species of *Babesia*. Intraerythrocytic forms appear singly as round, ovoid, elongate, or amoeboid trophozoites; in pairs as pyriform merozoites; or in tetrads as cross-shaped structures each composed of four merozoites (Figure 11.23)[27].

Hosts. *Babesia microti* infects several species of rodents, including rats and mice. Humans may also become infected. Infection of wild rodents is common, whereas infection of laboratory rodents is extremely rare.

Life Cycle. The life cycle is indirect. Erythrocytic forms are ingested by ticks (*Ixodes* sp.) during the consumption of a blood meal. Sexual reproduction likely occurs within the tick. The parasite is transmitted transstadially, but not transovarially as in other *Babesia* sp. Another rodent is infected during a subsequent blood meal taken by an infected tick. Trophozoites are injected during the blood meal. These enter erythrocytes and multiple by schizogony.

Pathologic Effects. Hemoglobinuria and death sometimes occur in experimentally infected rats[205]. Degenerative changes occur in the convoluted tubules of the kidneys, and large amounts of hematin are deposited in the kidneys and liver. Natural infections are generally considered nonpathogenic. Cellular immunity is critical for the clearance of *B. microti* in mice[206].

Clinical Disease. Natural infection with *B. microti* is not associated with clinical disease in immunologically competent hosts. Experimentally infected aged mice experience increased mortality when compared to younger animals[207].

Diagnosis, Treatment, and Prevention. Diagnosis is based on identifying parasites in erythrocytes on thin blood smears. There are currently no effective therapies recommended for treatment of babesiosis in rodents. Infected colonies should be eliminated. Ticks and wild rodents should be excluded from the laboratory animal facility. Wild rodents brought into the facility should be treated for tick infestations while in quarantine, and tested for babesiosis.

Public Health Considerations. *Babesia microti* is a known zoonotic agent. Splenectomized persons are at heightened risk of developing clinical babesiosis.

Babesia rodhaini

Morphology. *Babesia rodhaini* measures 2 μ to 4 μ long and 2 μ to 3 μ wide. Multiplication stages include four trophozoites, each measuring 2 μ by 1 μ, which are arranged in a cruciform pattern. Trophozoites ingest host cell cytoplasm by phagotrophy as do *Plasmodium*. Hemoglobin is digested more completely and there is no formation of hemozoin, a parasite metabolite released during schizogony[208].

Hosts. *Babesia rodhaini* naturally infects erythrocytes of the tree rat (*Thamnomys surdaster*)[209]. Mice, Norway

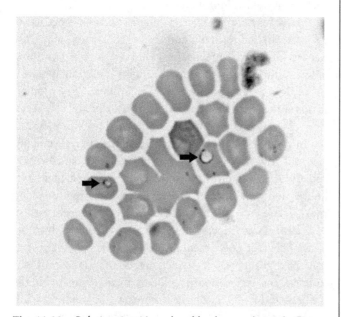

Fig. 11.23 *Babesia microti* in rodent blood smear (arrows). Giemsa stain, 1000 ×. Specimen courtesy of Sam Telford III, Tufts University.

rats, cotton rats (*Sigmodon hispidus*), and hamsters have been experimentally infected, but natural infection has not been reported in laboratory rodents. Subpatent infections have been established experimentally by inoculation of splenectomized primates, including guenon (vervet) monkeys (*Cercopithecus pygerythrus*), Guinea baboons (*Papio papio*), and chimpanzees (*Pan troglodytes*), as well as in an intact, black-capped capuchin monkey (*Cebus apella*)[210]. Experimental infection in rodents is commonly used as an animal model of human babesiosis.

Life Cycle. The life cycle is similar to that of *B. microti*. The life cycle is indirect, with sexual reproduction occurring within the tick intermediate hosts.

Pathologic Effects. Experimentally infected mice develop anti-erythrocyte and anti-parasite IgG antibodies[211], leading to severe hemolytic anemia, hyperplasia of cells involved in the mononuclear phagocytic system, focal liver necrosis, nephritis, and hematuria[209]. The incubation period is three to 10 days, and the infection reaches a peak in six to 13 days[212]. Similar changes occur in experimentally infected rats[213].

Clinical Disease. Clinical signs are not typically observed until severe pathologic changes have occurred. Then, experimentally infected mice become pale and die[209].

Diagnosis. Diagnosis is based on identification of the parasite in erythrocytes.

Treatment. While partial elimination of *B. rodhaini* has been achieved using clindamycin and tetracycline, there are currently no effective therapies recommended for treatment of babesiosis in rodents[214].

Prevention. Ticks should be excluded from the laboratory animal facility. Wild rodents brought into the facility should be treated for tick infestations while in quarantine.

Public Health Considerations. *Babesia rodhaini* is not considered infectious for humans. However, because *B. rodhaini* has been reported in non-human primates, splenectomized and immune-compromised people should exercise caution when working around infected animals.

Class Haemosporidia

Plasmodium inopinatum

Plasmodium inopinatum belongs to the family Plasmodiidae. It was reported from a wild rat in Belgium many years ago, but has not been reported since. Experimental infections may be established in mice, rats, hamsters, tree rats (*Thamnomys surdaster*), and fat mice (*Steatomys*)[215].

Plasmodium spp.

Several species of *Plasmodium* are maintained in laboratory rodents for malarial research. In each case, the natural host is a murine rodent. Three of the most common are discussed here.

Plasmodium berghei occurs naturally in the tree rat in central Africa[216]. It is transmissible to the Norway rat, mouse, hamster, and various wild rodents, but not to the guinea pig or rabbit. Severe malaria is produced in the mouse and in pregnant rats. Non-pregnant rats experience a milder form of disease[217]. In addition, *P. berghei* has been associated with other conditions, including paralysis[218] and alteration of chemical receptors in the rat brain[219].

Plasmodium chabaudi was obtained from a tree rat in central Africa[220]. It can be easily transmitted to the mouse, in which it causes severe, fatal malaria[221]. Rats are more difficult to infect and are therefore rarely used as a host species.

Plasmodium vinckei was obtained from a mosquito in central Africa[222]. Several subspecies have been described. *Plasmodium vinckei* develops in certain African rats (*Thamnomys, Aethomys*) and the mouse and causes a severe type of malaria in the latter species. It is not transmissible to the Norway rat.

Phylum Microsporidia

Encephalitozoon cuniculi

Morphology. The biology of *Encephalitozoon cuniculi* is presented in detail in Chapter 15, Parasites of Rabbits. As noted in that chapter, analysis of small subunit RNA has resulted in the reclassification of this pathogen to the fungi[146]. Spores are oval, and measure about 1.5 µ by 2.5 µ, with a thick, resistant spore wall. The spore contains a nucleus near one end and a polar tube forming five to six coils at the other end.

Hosts. *Encephalitozoon cuniculi* exists in at least three strains and infects several species of mammals, including rats, mice, and humans[147]. The extent to which strains are cross-infective and/or represent distinct species is unknown. Though never common in laboratory rodent colonies, *E. cuniculi* is now considered rare[148]. However, the current actual prevalence of *E. cuniculi* in rat and mouse colonies is unknown. Infection remains common in wild rodent populations[149,150].

Life Cycle. The life cycle of *E. cuniculi* is presented in Chapter 15, Parasites of Rabbits. Briefly, transmission is through the ingestion of spores excreted in the urine.

Spores usually form clusters in the brain, kidney, liver, macrophages, and less commonly, peritoneal exudates, heart muscle, pancreas, spleen, and other organs.

Pathologic Effects and Clinical Disease. In rodents, infection with *E. cuniculi* has been primarily associated with lesions in the brain, kidneys, and to a lesser extent, liver (Figure 11.24). In one study, granulomatous encephalitis caused by *E. cuniculi* was found throughout the brain in 21% of 365 adult laboratory rats[151]. The granulomas (glial nodules) consisted of collections of activated glial cells surrounded by lymphocytes. Perivascular spread of sporoblasts was observed in the brain, without an associated inflammatory response. The pathogen was also found in interstitial infiltrates in rat kidneys[151]. Other investigators have found granulomas in sections of cervical spinal cord[152]. Immunity to *E. cuniculi* is dependent on both CD4+ and CD8+ T cells[153], and may be suppressed by *E. cuniculi* itself in some strains of mice[154].

Historically, *E. cuniculi* was a frequent contaminant in cell cultures. Several years ago, Petri reported the infection in 25% of tumor cells of a transplantable ascites sarcoma[155]. The infected tumor cells became less pathogenic than usual and did not give rise to solid tumors after subcutaneous inoculation of rats. Rats and mice infected with *E. cuniculi* typically show no clinical signs.

Diagnosis. Exudates from suspected animals should be air-dried, fixed with methanol, stained, and examined for spores. Normally, only a small portion of peritoneal mononuclear cells are infected. Spores can be demonstrated using special stains. For example, *E. cuniculi* stains positively with Giemsa, Goodpasture's carbol fuchsin, iron hematoxylin, and gram stains, while *Toxoplasma gondii* does not. Conversely, *T. gondii* stains well with hematoxylin and eosin, whereas *E. cuniculi* stains poorly. Serologic assays have been developed for colony surveillance, though these have found greatest utility in monitoring rabbit colonies. Polymerase chain reaction assays[156], single-strand conformation polymorphism analysis[157], and other newer diagnostic modalities will likely assume greater diagnostic roles in the future.

Treatment. Novel synthetic polyamines have been shown to be effective in the treatment of experimentally infected mice[158]. Fenbendazole has been used successfully for eliminating *E. cuniculi* in rabbits[159]. However, infected rodent colonies should be culled.

Prevention. Because of improvements in husbandry standards, infection of laboratory rodent colonies is rare. Careful management practices should be instituted when

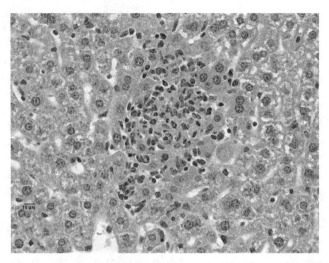

Fig. 11.24 *Encephalitozoon cuniculi.* Granuloma in the liver of a mouse contains a cluster of small (1 × 1.5μ) ovoid, Gram-positive microsporidia spores. Bar = 10 μ. Courtesy of E. Didier, Tulane University Medical School.

housing rodents and potentially infected rabbits in the same animal facility.

Public Health Considerations. *Encephalitozoon cuniculi* may cause severe disease in immunocompromised people. Therefore, such people should exercise caution when working with potentially infected laboratory animals.

CESTODES

Nearly all cestode life cycles require multiple hosts. Improvements in laboratory animal husbandry practices typically preclude exposure to infectious stages in the research environment. However, cestode infections are not uncommon in wild rodents, and breakdown in management practices may expose laboratory animals to infection. In addition to those described, rodents may occasionally serve as intermediate hosts for *Taenia pisiformis* and *Echinococcus multilocularis.*

Cataenotaenia pusilla

Cataenotaenia pusilla is a tapeworm in the family Cataenotaenidae. It has been reported in wild and laboratory house mice and laboratory hamsters, and from wild rats[77,223]. It is likely that other closely related rodents are also susceptible to infection. Adults are 30 mm to 160 mm long. The scolex bears four suckers but lacks a rostellum. Gravid proglottids are longer than wide, and are released in the feces. The eggs measure 22 μ to 28 μ by 12 μ to 15 μ. Intermediate hosts of *C. pusilla* are grain or storage mites, including *Glycophagus domesticus* and *Tyroglyphus farinae*[223]. Adult worms inhabit the small intestine of the rodent definitive host, where they appear to cause no pathological effects. The genus includes at least seven other species, all of which have been found in rodents.

Hymenolepis diminuta

Morphology. *Hymenolepis diminuta* is known as the "rat tapeworm." The adult worm measures 20 mm to 60 mm in length and 3 mm to 4 mm in width. *Hymenolepis diminuta* has a pear-shaped scolex bearing four deep suckers. Its scolex is similar to that of *Rodentolepis nana* and *R. microstoma,* except that *H. diminuta* bears no hooks (is unarmed). Mature proglottids are much wider than long, measuring 20 mm to 60 mm in length and 3 mm to 4 mm in width (Figure 11.25). Gravid segments break away from the strobila and are passed in the feces. The egg is almost spherical, measures 62 μ to 88 μ by 52 μ to 81 μ, and contains an embryo which possesses three pairs of small hooks (Figure 11.26). Unlike *R. nana,* the embryo of *H. diminuta* lacks polar filaments. The eggs of *H. diminuta* are more resistant to the environment than those of *R. nana,* and can survive in the feces for up to six months.

Hosts. *Hymenolepis diminuta* occurs in the upper small intestine of mice, rats, other rodents, and primates, including humans. It is common in wild rodents[77] but rare in laboratory populations. Rat strains differ in susceptibility to infection. In one study, inbred rats of the TM and DA strains developed 60% and 30% fewer total adult worms, respectively, versus F344/N, JAR-2, LOU/M, and outbred Wistar rats[224].

Life Cycle. The life cycle of *H. diminuta* requires an insect intermediate host. This is usually a mealworm beetle (*Tenebrio molitor*), flour beetle (*Tribolium confusum*), moth, or flea (*Nosopsyllus fasciatus*). Eggs are ingested by intermediate hosts, hatch, and develop into cysticercoid larvae. Infection of the definitive host is by ingestion of the infected arthropod. The larva is liberated from the cysticercoid, and the scolex evaginates and attaches itself to the intestinal mucosa. Adult worms are found in 19 to 21 days. Unlike *R. nana,* the cysticercoid of *H. diminuta* cannot develop within the definitive host.

Pathologic Effects. Light infections with *H. diminuta* are nonpathogenic[225]. The number of worms present in the intestinal tract is somewhat self-limiting, through the

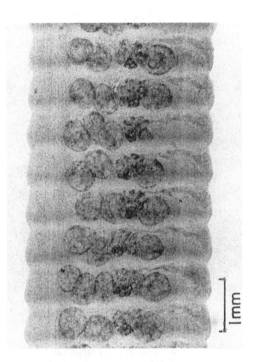

Fig. 11.25 *Hymenolepis diminuta,* mature proglottids. Courtesy of Marietta Voge, University of California.

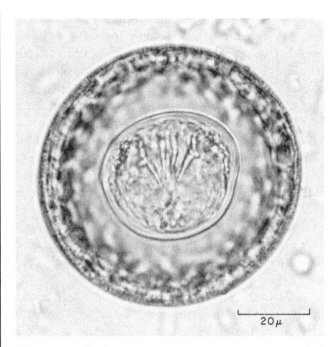

Fig. 11.26 *Hymenolepis diminuta,* embryonated egg. Courtesy of Marietta Voge, University of California.

development of a strong but short-lived immune resistance to further infection[226]. Heavy infection may cause acute catarrhal enteritis or chronic enterocolitis with lymphoid hyperplasia[227]. However, even mild infections may alter host physiology, including increased intestinal permeability[228].

Clinical Disease. Infection with *H. diminuta* is generally asymptomatic. Because the life cycle includes an obligatory intermediate host, and worm populations are density-dependent, heavy worm burdens are rare.

Diagnosis, Treatment, and Prevention. Diagnosis is based on finding eggs or proglottids in the feces, or adult worms in the small intestine. Little information is available concerning treatment of mice infected with *H. diminuta* using modern anthelmintics. Treatments recommended for *R. nana* will likely also be effective against *H. diminuta*. However, infected colonies should be culled, because infection may alter host physiology. Prevention of infection depends on procurement of animals from reputable dealers, as well as exclusion of wild rodents and potential arthropod vectors from animal facilities.

Public Health Considerations. Though less common than infection with *R. nana,* infection of humans with *H. diminuta* does occur. However, human infection requires ingestion of infected arthropod intermediate hosts.

Rodentolepis nana

Morphology. *Rodentolepis nana* (Syn. *Hymenolepis nana, Hymenolepis fraterna, Vampirolepis nana*), is also known as the "dwarf tapeworm" of mice. It is a member of the class Eucestoda and family Hymenolepididae. *Rodentolepis nana* is a slender worm, usually about 25 mm to 40 mm long and less than 1 mm wide[229]. Worm length is affected by the host's immune status and the temperature at which the host is housed[230]. The scolex bears four unarmed suckers, and the rostellum is armed with a single ring of 20 to 27 small hooklets (Figure 11.27). Mature proglottids are wider than long and trapezoidal (Figure 11.28). The egg is oval and measures 44 µ to 62 µ by 30 to 55 µ (Figure 11.29). The embryo is spherical and thin-walled with a knob at each pole, from which six fine filaments emerge. The onchosphere (hexacanth embryo) possesses three pairs of small hooks.

Hosts. *Rodentolepis nana* occurs in the small intestines of rodents, particularly mice and hamsters[231], though infections in other rodents have also been reported[232]. Parasite strains are not universally cross-infective between rodent species[233]. Rats may also become infected. Some investigators consider the rat to be an unnatural host[234], though in one survey, wild rats, but not wild mice, were found naturally infected with *R. nana*[77].

Historically, many primates, including humans, have been considered to be susceptible to rodent strains of *R. nana*. In fact, in some parts of the world, human infections are quite common[235]. However, recent studies have suggested that rodent and human isolates of *R. nana* may be different and not cross-infective[236]. Laboratory strains of mice differ in the speed of onset of immune response to *R. nana*. Mice of the C57 strain respond more rapidly, while C3H mice are delayed responders[237].

Historically, the prevalence or *R. nana* in laboratory rodents was high[238]. This is no longer the case. However, mice or other rodents purchased from pet stores may still be found to be infected[239], and animal workers who own these pets risk introducing the parasite into the laboratory animal population unless strict attention is paid to personal hygiene.

Life Cycle. The dwarf tapeworm is the only cestode known to be transmitted directly, because eggs passed in the feces of the definitive host are infective to another definitive host. The eggs hatch in the small intestine, and the embryos penetrate the intestinal villi and become cysticercoid larvae in four to five days within the villus

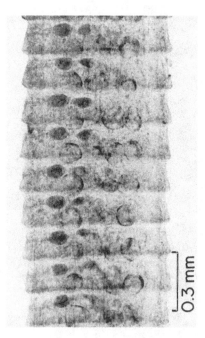

Fig. 11.28 *Rodentolepis nana,* mature proglottids. Courtesy of Marietta Voge, University of California.

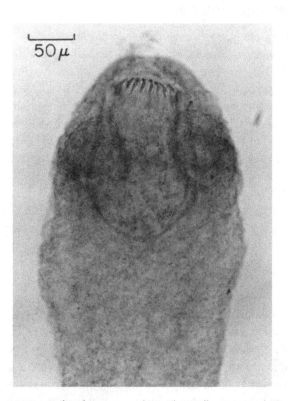

Fig. 11.27 *Rodentolepis nana* scolex with rostellum retracted. Courtesy of Marietta Voge, University of California.

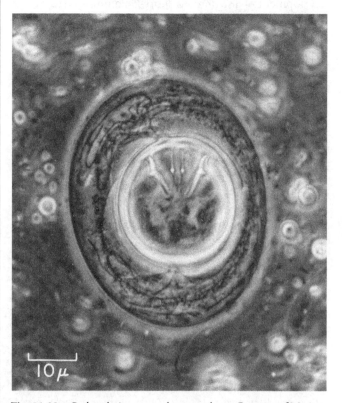

Fig. 11.29 *Rodentolepis nana,* embryonated egg. Courtesy of Marietta Voge, University of California.

mucosa. The larvae then reenter the intestinal lumen, attach to the mucosa, and develop into mature worms in 10 to 11 days. Thus the life cycle, in direct transmission, is completed in 14 to 16 days[229].

Indirect transmission also occurs. Infective larvae develop in grain beetles (*T. molitor* and *T. obscurus*), flour beetles (*Tribolium confusum*), and fleas (*Pulex irritans, Ctenocephalides canis,* and *Xenopsylla cheopis*), and the definitive host becomes infected by ingestion of the infected insect[240]. The egg hatches in the insect gut and the onchosphere penetrates the hemocoele and develops into a cysticercoid larva. The length of the indirect life cycle is variable because the time required for larval development in the insect varies with the environmental temperature.

A further variation in the life cycle is autoinfection, or the immediate hatching of eggs within the intestine of the same host in which they were produced[241]. The embryos develop into mature adults without leaving the original host.

Rodentolepis nana is also unusual in that the life span of the adult in the intestine is usually limited to a few weeks. Successful establishment of re-infection depends on the nature of the previous infection. When direct transmission occurs, the host tissue is invaded and a degree of immunity develops. However, when transmission is indirect, the initial infection is acquired by ingesting fully developed larvae in insects, the tissue phase is omitted, and immunity does not develop[242]. Autoinfection does not usually occur in hosts initially infected by direct transmission because of immunity produced during the tissue phase of the original infection.

Pathologic Effects. The effects of this parasite depend on the number of worms present. Heavy infection causes severe catarrhal enteritis[227]. Chronic infections were reported to produce abscesses and focal granulomatous lymphadenitis of mesenteric lymph nodes[243]. Serum albumin levels decline for the first 20 days post-infection in rats experimentally infected with *R. nana*. This is accompanied by increased γ-globulin levels, indicating a developing immune response. Thereafter, albumin levels return toward normal, coincident with worm expulsion[244]. Other physiologic changes include: decreased serum concentrations of glucose and total proteins, increased serum lipid concentration[245], and decreases in intestinal tissue protein and lipid[246]. There is also increased histamine or a histamine-like compound in the intestine of *R. nana*-infected rats[247], and increased intestinal eosinophilia[248].

Clinical Disease. Heavy infection causes retarded growth, weight loss, and intestinal obstruction in the mouse[229]. Clinical signs may not be observed in less severe cases.

Diagnosis. Diagnosis is based on the identification of the eggs in the feces or the adult worms in the intestine at necropsy (Figure 11.30). Adults of *R. nana* may be distinguished from those of *H. diminuta* by overall size, and because the scolex of *R. nana* bears hooks, while the scolex of *H. diminuta* does not.

Treatment. Infection may be eliminated with a single oral dose of praziquantel, administered at a dosage of 35 mg/kg to mice, or 10 mg/kg to rats[249]. Also in rats, infection can be eliminated with four consecutive days of nitroscanate added to the feed at a rate providing 50 mg/kg of the drug[250]. However, infected animals should be rederived or eliminated.

Prevention. Because infection with this parasite can be spread in many ways, control is difficult once the infection is established within the facility. Sanitation and insect control are essential. Because of the high prevalence of infection in wild rodents, these animals should not be allowed to enter the animal facility or contaminate feed or bedding stores.

Public Health Considerations. In spite of reports suggesting that human and rodent isolates of *R. nana* are different and not cross-infective, animal care personnel should exercise caution when working with infected rodents. Contaminated feed and bedding should be incinerated.

Rodentolepis microstoma

Morphology. *Rodentolepis microstoma* (Syn. *Hymenolepis microstoma, Vampirolepis microstoma*) is a member of the class Eucestoda and family Hymenolepididae. It is known as the "bile duct" tapeworm of mice. *Rodentolepis microstoma* is a small, slender, white worm. Adults are 80 mm to 350 mm in length, and 2 mm in width. The size of the adult worm is influenced by a number of factors, including sex hormones of the male mouse host. Orchiectomy reduces the size of adult worms, while ovariectomy has no effect[251]. Like *R. nana*, *R. microstoma* has an armed rostellum. The rostellum bears 23 to 28 small hooklets. The round eggs measure 80 μ to 90 μ in diameter[252] and contain polar filaments[253].

Hosts. The mouse is the primary host of *R. microstoma*. Infection is common in wild mice[253]. Mouse strains differ in their ability to mount an effective immune response to *R. microstoma*; AKR are mice that are more resistant to secondary infection than C3HeB/FeJ mice[254].

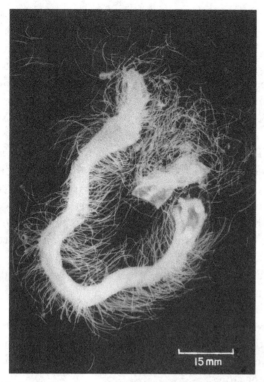

Fig. 11.30 *Rodentolepis nana,* adults in small intestine of mouse. Reproduced from Heyneman, D. (1961) with permission.

Cotton rats and the Syrian hamsters have also been infected experimentally[255]. The latter developed clinical signs of cestodiasis[252]. Recently, *R. microstoma* was found in humans in Western Australia[235]. The rat is not a natural host, and is not susceptible to experimental infection. In fact, some investigators have been unable to infect rats even experimentally[252,256].

Life Cycle. After ingestion of the infected flour beetle intermediate host, oncospheres are found in the first 20 cm of the mouse small intestine distal to the pylorus. By four days post-infection, worms are migrating to the bile duct, where they mature, and attain their full size by 25 days post-infection. The prepatent period is 14 days[252], after which worms are rarely found in the gut[257]. Autoinfection as reported for *R. nana* does not occur[252]. Recently, it has been reported that a "tailless" form of *R. microstoma* may develop cysticercoids in the intestine of some strains of immunodeficient mice[258]. This finding suggests that the direct life cycle may have originated from the indirect life cycle. This is supported by the time required for development of the fully matured cysticercoids in mice, which is longer in mice than in beetles.

Pathologic Effects. Even mild infections are associated with localized biliary inflammation and mucosal erosion[259]. Experimental infection results in pronounced intestinal mastocytosis[260], hepatitis and biliary ductule hyperplasia[255], increased rates of hepatic fatty acid and cholesterol synthesis, decreased testicular fatty acid synthesis and weights, increased metabolic rate[261], and other physiologic changes[262]. Hepatic damage was reduced when mice were housed at higher environmental temperatures[45].

Clinical Disease. Clinical signs are not typically observed in mice infected with *R. microstoma.*

Diagnosis. Diagnosis is made by finding the adult worm in the bile duct. *Rodentolepis microstoma* may be further differentiated from *R. nana* by the larger size of the eggs in the former.

Treatment. Little information is available on treatment of mice infected with *R. microstoma.* It is likely that treatments effective against *R. nana* will also be effective against *R. microstoma.* However, infected mice should be culled or rederived.

Prevention. Natural infection of laboratory mice with *R. microstoma* has not been reported recently. Exclusion of wild mice and beetle intermediate hosts should prevent establishment of this parasite in the modern laboratory animal facility.

Public Health Considerations. As noted above, *R. microstoma* has been reported in humans[235]. However, it is unlikely that animal workers will become infected with this parasite while working in the animal facility.

Rodentolepis straminea

Rodentolepis straminea is morphologically similar to *R. microstoma.* The two species are most easily differentiated from each other, and from *R. nana,* by careful examination of the eggs and scolex. The round eggs of *R. microstoma* measure 80 µ to 90 µ in diameter, while the slightly more oval eggs of *R. straminea* measure 35 µ to 48 µ by 44 µ to 57 µ. Also, eggs of *R. microstoma* have five to six polar filaments and those of *R. nana* have three to five, and they are absent in eggs of *R. straminea.* The scolex of *R. microstoma* bears 23 to 29 rostellar hooks, while that of *R. straminea* bears 22 to 36 hooks[253].

Rodentolepis straminea has been reported in wild rodents in many parts of the world. The life cycle of *R. straminea* is similar to that of *R. microstoma,* with the exception of differences in the range of definitive hosts.

The preferred definitive hosts of *R. straminea* include *M. auratus, M. musculus,* and *Apodemus* spp.

Taenia taeniaformis

Morphology. *Taenia taeniaformis* (Syn. *Hydatigera taeniaformis*) is a cyclophyllidean tapeworm. Adult tapeworms are found in domestic and exotic cats, while the metacestode stage of *T. taeniaformis* (strobilocercus larval stage formerly named *Cysticercus fasciolaris*) is found in the rodent intermediate host. Cysts reach a diameter of up to 10 mm and contain a strobilocercus, which measures 60 mm to 100 mm in length[264].

Hosts. *Taenia taeniaformis* is the most common tapeworm species found in cats. Suitable rodent intermediate hosts include house mice, Norway rats, Syrian hamsters, Persian gerbils (*Meriones persicus*), voles, and Eastern gray squirrels (*Sciurus carolinensis*). Infection is uncommon in wild rats and mice[77]. Rabbits may also occasionally serve as intermediate hosts[263]. However, strain differences, based on infectivity and restriction endonuclease patterns, exist among rodent isolates of *T. taeniaformis*[265].

Life Cycle. Following ingestion of an infectious egg, the larva migrates through the intestinal wall of the rodent and develops to a strobilocercus in the liver. Approximately two months are required for the strobilocercus to mature and become infective to the cat definitive host[266].

Pathologic Effects and Clinical Disease. Larvae migrate to the liver. Here they establish migration tracts that become surrounded by a thick zone of inflammation, but are not considered to have significant deleterious effects[264]. Infections in the rodent intermediate host are asymptomatic[264].

Diagnosis, Treatment, and Prevention. Diagnosis is typically made at necropsy, by identifying the strobilocercus in the liver. Mebendazole has been used to kill strobilocerci in mice[267]. However, infections in the rodent intermediate host typically are discovered at necropsy, and so are not treated. Infected colonies should be eliminated. Laboratory rodent feed and bedding stocks should be protected from contamination with cat feces.

Public Health Considerations. Adults of *T. taeniaformis* have been recovered from the intestines of humans. It is not known how these people became infected, but it is likely that they consumed the infective strobilocercus from a rabbit or rodent host. Unless animal workers engage in such behavior, it is extremely unlikely that they will become infected with this parasite. Therefore, *T. taeniaformis* is not considered to be a public health hazard.

NEMATODES

Improvements in laboratory animal husbandry and medicine have resulted in a significant decline in the prevalence of nematode parasite infections of laboratory rats and mice. Still, breaks in sanitation procedures, importation of wild rodents, or procurement of rodents from infected sources may permit the introduction of nematode parasites into the laboratory animal colony.

Superfamily Rhabditoidea

Strongyloides ratti

Morphology. The threadworm, *Strongyloides ratti*, is a member of the superfamily Rhabditoidea. The main importance of this parasite has been as an experimental model in developmental biology and parasitology. Only the adult female worm is known to be parasitic. The adult worm is small, measuring only 2.1 mm to 3.1 mm (mean 2.37 mm)[269].

Hosts. *Strongyloides ratti* is common in the intestines of wild Norway rats and black rats throughout the world[270,271], though some of these reports may actually be of *S. venezuelensis,* a similar species. *Strongyloides ratti* has not been reported from modern laboratory animal facilities. Mice are also susceptible to infection, but are not considered to be a natural host[272].

Life Cycle. Like other members of the genus, the life cycle of *S. ratti* includes both parasitic (homogonic) and free-living (heterogonic) phases (Figure 11.31). Eggs typically hatch before being passed in the feces of the infected host. Under appropriate environmental conditions, homogonic development results in the generation of third-stage infective larvae. These enter a suitable host through the hair follicles to the sebaceous glands[268]. Larvae rapidly disseminate via the bloodstream before entering the lungs. Larvae molt in the lungs before ascending the trachea and being swallowed. Worms mature within four days post inoculation, and colonize from the pylorus to a distance of roughly 45 cm into the small intestine.

Peak populations are found within the first 15 cm of the small intestine[273]. The prepatent period is five days[268]. Trans-mammary transmission also occurs and may be the most common means of infection in suckling rats[274]. In contrast, heterogonic development results in the generation of larvae, which mature in the environment to male and female adult worms and then mate. Eggs produced from these matings develop into third-stage infective larvae. While other *Strongyloides* sp. may undergo multiple generations of heterogonic development, *S. ratti* undergoes only one generation of heterogonic development[273]. As immunity develops or worm burdens increase, worms redistribute from the small intestine to the large intestine[275]. Typically, adult worms are expelled from the intestine starting 14 to 18 days after infection, with the development of an immune response[276,277].

Pathologic Effects. Infection with *S. ratti* is not associated with alterations in intestinal function in immunocompetent rats[278], and causes minimal damage in the lungs[279]. Larvae that invade skin elicit dermatitis at the site of penetration. The severity of the reaction is similar in rats that experience primary versus challenge infection[280].

Clinical Disease. Infection with *S. ratti* is not associated with clinical disease of the intestinal tract[278]. Skin-penetrating larvae may cause local dermatitis[280].

Diagnosis, Treatment, and Prevention. Infection with *S. ratti* may be diagnosed by finding the characteristic larvae

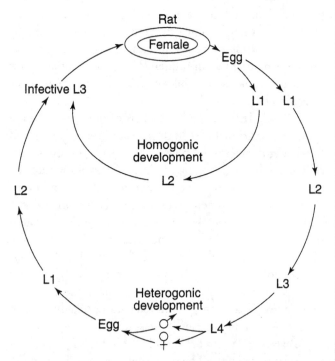

Fig. 11.31 The life cycle of *Strongyloides ratti* has both parasitic and free-living phases. The progeny of the parasitic female phase can develop by two different routes, termed heterogonic and homogonic. (L) Larval stage. Reproduced from Viney, M.E. (1999) with permission.

on fecal examination. Infection with *S. ratti* may be eliminated using benzimidazole anthelmintics such as albendazole[281] and thiabendazole[282]. Infection with *S. ratti* has not been diagnosed in a laboratory animal colony in recent times.

Public Health Considerations. *Strongyloides ratti* is not considered to be a public health hazard.

Strongyloides venezuelensis

Morphology. *Strongyloides venezuelensis* superficially resembles *S. ratti*. The two can be differentiated by a number of morphologic features[269]. The two most useful features include spiral-shaped ovaries in *S. venezuelensis* adult female worms and eggs which develop to early cleavage stages when passed in host feces. In contrast, the ovaries of *S. ratti* adult female worms are straight, and most larvae have hatched when passed in the host feces. Adult female *S. venezuelensis* are 2 mm to 3.2 mm long[269,283].

Hosts. *Strongyloides venezuelensis* is common in the intestine of wild rats[284]. Other reported hosts include the cotton rat[285], Mongolian gerbil[286], Syrian golden hamster[287], and laboratory mouse[288]. Mice are much more susceptible to infection with *S. venezuelensis* than with *S. ratti*, and thereby serve as a useful model for human strongyloidiasis[289]. However, inbred mouse strains differ in susceptibility. For example, 129/SvJ mice are naturally less susceptible than C57BL/6 mice, possibly due to higher intestinal concentrations of chondroitin sulphate, which prevents worm establishment[288]. *Strongyloides venezuelensis* should not occur in modern laboratory animal facilities.

Life Cycle. The life cycle of *S. venezuelensis* is generally similar to that of *S. ratti*. Infecting larvae penetrate compromised skin, migrate through the subcutaneous tissues and the muscle, and arrive in the lungs, probably hematogenously. Larvae leave the lung via the trachea, then pass through the esophagus and stomach, and reach the small intestine[290]. Transmammary passage also occurs, and may partially explain why *S. venezuelensis* infection occurs primarily in suckling rats[291]. Testosterone appears to increase susceptibility to infection in rats[292].

Pathologic Effects. Pathologic effects are similar to those induced by *S. ratti*. Experimental infection with large numbers of parasites results in dermatitis, hemorrhagic and eosinophilic pneumonia, and other pulmonary changes indicative of a type-1 hypersensitivity response[293]. Intestinal mucosal mast cells are important in causing the expulsion of *S. venezuelensis*[294].

Clinical Disease. Clinical disease has only been reported in rats experimentally inoculated with large numbers of infective larvae[295]. In those cases, clinical signs, including death, were associated with pulmonary migration of larvae. Pulmonary function studies also indicate that airways are hyperresponsive[293].

Diagnosis, Treatment, and Prevention. Infection with *S. venezuelensis* may be diagnosed by finding the characteristic embryonated or blastular eggs on fecal examination. Infection with *S. venezuelensis* may be eliminated using single injections of levamisole (26 mg/kg) or ivermectin (0.2 to 0.5 mg/kg)[296]. Oral preparations of ivermectin (0.2 mg/kg) also are highly effective against both larval and adult forms[297]. Infection with *S. venezuelensis* has not been diagnosed in a laboratory animal colony.

Public Health Considerations. *Strongyloides venezuelensis* is not considered to be a public health hazard.

Superfamily Heterakoidea

Heterakis spumosa

Morphology. *Heterakis spumosa* is a member of the superfamily Heterakoidea and family Heterakidae. Members of this superfamily resemble members of the superfamily Ascaridoidea. Adult worms have three small lips and a cylindrical esophagus that swells posteriorly, ending in a distinct bulb. The male is 6.4 mm to 9.9 mm long by 0.20 mm to 0.26 mm in diameter, with a distinct spicule. The female is 7 mm to 13 mm by 0.68 mm to 0.74 mm. The egg has a thick, mammillated shell and measures 55 μ to 60 μ by 40 μ to 50 μ[298].

Hosts. This parasite is common in wild Norway and black rats, and in a range of other wild rodents throughout the world, including wild field mice (*Apodemus* spp.), moles (*Mogera* spp.), and others[54,299,300]. Experimental infections in laboratory mice are frequently established to study host-parasite relationships[301]. *Heterakis spumosa* has not been reported from laboratory animal colonies for many years.

Life Cycle. The life cycle is direct. Eggs passed in the feces embryonate in about two weeks. When ingested they hatch in the stomach, and the larvae migrate to the cecum and colon, where they mature in about 26 to 47 days[298]. High circulating testosterone levels in sexually mature and intact male mice profoundly affect the host-parasite relationship. Testosterone effects include an extended period of parasite egg release, increased number of eggs released, shortened prepatent period, accelerated development and growth of worms so that young adult worms may be observed in the colon by 21 days post-infection, and increased worm survival within the host[302].

Pathologic Effects and Clinical Disease. *Heterakis spumosa* is generally regarded as nonpathogenic. Clinical signs have not been reported.

Diagnosis. Diagnosis is based on the identification of eggs in the feces or of adult worms in the large intestine.

Treatment. There is scant literature on treatment of *Heterakis spumosa*-infected rodents. In one study, subcutaneous injection of 50 or 100 mg/kg into experimentally infected rats resulted in complete elimination of the infection[303]. Other investigators have reported that a combination of febantel (25 mg/kg) and pyrantel (2.5 mg/kg), administered orally, acted synergistically to clear the infection, while either drug alone was ineffective[301].

Prevention. Sanitation, vermin control, and procurement of animals from reputable sources prevent entry of *H. spumosa* into the modern animal facility.

Public Health Considerations. *Heterakis spumosa* has not been reported to infect humans.

Superfamily Oxyuroidea

Aspiculuris tetraptera

Morphology. *Aspiculuris tetraptera* is morphologically similar to *Syphacia obvelata*[304]. The males are 2 mm to 4 mm long and 120 μ to 190 μ wide, with a short conical tail that is 117 μ to 169 μ long. Both spicule and gubernaculum are absent. The females are 3 mm to 4 mm long and 215 μ to 275 μ wide, with a conical tail that is 445 μ to 605 μ long. The eggs are symmetrically ellipsoidal and 70 μ to 98 μ long by 29 μ to 50 μ wide (Figure 11.32).

Aspiculuris tetraptera and *S. obvelata* may be differentiated on the basis of shape of the esophageal bulb, size of cervical alae, position of the vulva in the female, size and presence or absence of a spicule or gubernaculum in the male, and size and shape of the egg[304]. Mixed infections with *S. obvelata* are common[305]. *Aspiculuris tetraptera* may also be differentiated from other members of the genus, though this is not considered practical[306].

Hosts. *Aspiculuris tetraptera* remains common in laboratory mice[4]. Other rodents are also susceptible to infection, though generally less so. These include members of the genera *Apodemus*, *Clethrionomys*, *Cricetus*, *Mastomys* (*Praomys*), *Meriones*, *Microtus*, *Peromyscus*, *Rattus*, and others[48,307–309].

Life Cycle. The life cycle of *A. tetraptera* is direct. Unembryonated eggs are passed in the feces. Unlike in *S. obvelata* and *S. muris*, eggs are not cemented to the perianal skin. Eggs embryonate in the environment, and are infective in five to eight days at 27°C[310]. The eggs are resistant to dessication and many disinfectants, but are sensitive to high temperatures. Infection is by ingestion of infective eggs. Larvae hatch and develop in the posterior colon and then migrate anteriorly and develop to maturity in the proximal colon. They remain in the lumen of the intestine and do not invade the mucosa. The prepatent period is 23 days.

Pathologic Effects and Clinical Disease. *Aspiculuris tetraptera* is generally regarded to have no clinical significance.

No clinical signs are observed in mice infected with *A. tetraptera*.

Diagnosis, Treatment, and Prevention. Diagnosis is by finding the eggs in fecal floatation preparations or adult worms in the cecum and colon. *Aspiculuris tetraptera* may be eliminated from animal colonies by feeding fenbendazole-medicated feed, as described for the *Syphacia* spp[311]. The longer embryonation time (versus *Syphacia* spp.) facilitates eradication. Other investigators have eliminated *A. tetraptera* using 1% ivermectin (2 mg/kg) applied by

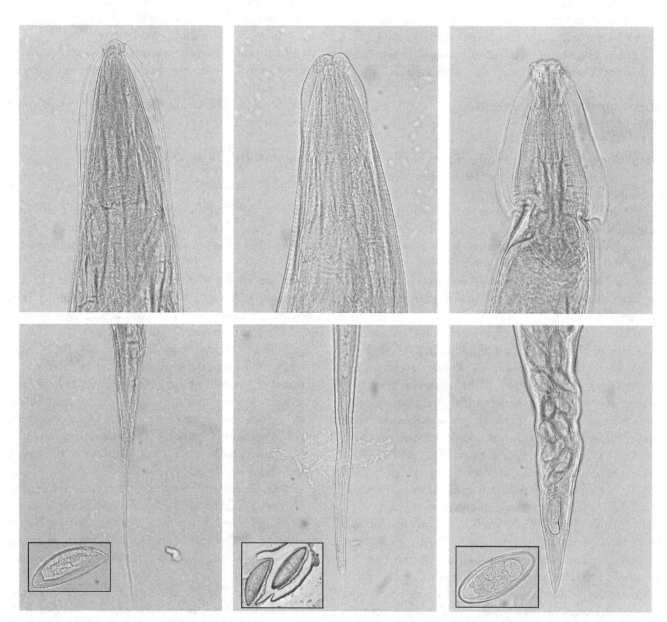

Fig. 11.32 Heads, tails, and eggs of the adult female pinworms *Syphacia muris* (left), *Syphacia obvelata* (middle), and *Aspiculuris tetraptera* (right). Heads and tails photographed at 250 ×. Eggs photographed at 400 ×. Reproduced from Baker, D.G. (2005) with permission.

micropipette between the scapulae. Two treatments were administered ten days apart[312]. Guidelines for preventing entry of *S. obvelata* and *S. muris* (see below) also should prevent infections with *A. tetraptera*.

Public Health Considerations. *Aspiculuris tetraptera* is not considered a public health hazard.

Syphacia muris

Morphology. *Syphacia muris* is the common pinworm of rats. The adult worm has a rounded anterior region and a tapered posterior region that ends in a sharply pointed tail (Figure 11.32). Typical of the superfamily, the mouth is surrounded by three distinct lips. The male is 1,200 μ to 1,300 μ long and 100 μ wide. The anterior mamelon is near the middle of the body. The tail of the adult male is bent ventrally. The male worm has a single, long, prominent spicule and a gubernaculum. The female is 2,800 μ to 4,000 μ long, with the vulva in the anterior quarter of the body. The egg is vermiform, slightly flattened on one side, and measures 72 μ to 82 μ long by 25 μ to 36 μ wide (Figure 11.32). *Syphacia muris* closely resembles *S. obvelata*. The two can be differentiated using morphologic features described for *S. obvelata*.

Hosts. *Syphacia muris* primarily infects rats, including non-domestic species such as the Malaysian wood rat (*Rattus tiomanicus*)[313]. Other susceptible hosts include laboratory mice, gerbils, and the Syrian hamster[314,315]. Infections in laboratory colonies remain common[4].

Life Cycle. The life cycle of *S. muris* is similar to that of *S. obvelata*. Adult worms inhabit the cecum and colon. Eggs are deposited by the female on the perianal area of the host or in the colon. Unlike *S. obvelata*, female *S. muris* demonstrate periodicity in egg laying, preferentially depositing eggs in the afternoon[316]. Eggs embryonate within hours of release into the environment. Infection of the rat occurs by ingestion of embryonated eggs from the perianal area or the cage environment[317]. Larvae migrate to the large intestine and mature. The prepatent period is seven to eight days[318]. Eggs may remain infective in the laboratory environment for at least four weeks[319].

Pathologic Effects. Like other pinworm infections of rodents, *S. muris* is generally considered to be nonpathogenic. While overt lesions are not observed, infection with *S. muris* is known to alter host physiology. For example, rats infected with *S. muris* have impaired intestinal electrolyte transport[320] and decreased weight gain[321].

Clinical Disease. Other than decreased weight gain, clinical signs have not been observed in rats infected with *Syphacia muris*.

Diagnosis. Infection with *S. muris* is diagnosed by finding adult worms in the large intestine. The cecum is removed, and opened in a petri dish containing a small amount of warm water or saline. Within minutes the worms migrate away from the fecal mass and into the liquid, where they may be observed by using a dissecting scope or magnifying glass. Antemortem diagnosis is accomplished by finding eggs on clear tape applied to the perianal region. Tape tests are best performed in the afternoon, because perianal egg counts are higher during this time than in the morning[304,316].

Treatment. Pinworms can be surprisingly difficult to eliminate from the animal facility. While several treatment strategies have been reported[322], the most efficacious and cost-effective means is providing feed that contains fenbendazole (150 mg/kg of feed), given for at least two weeks[322]. Fenbendazole not only has larvacidal and adulticidal efficacy, but is also ovicidal[323,324]. While most clinicians advocate simultaneous disinfection of all surfaces within the animal room, others have found using medicated feed to be adequate to eliminate the infection[325].

Prevention. Guidelines for preventing entry of *S. muris* into the animal facility are similar to those for *S. obvelata*. Incoming animals should be treated with fenbendazole-medicated feed and tape-tests examined prior to shipment and arrival[325]. Re-occurrence of infection appears to be more common when personnel other than professional animal caretakers are responsible for colony husbandry and facility sanitation[326]. Control depends on colony surveillance and strict attention to cleaning protocols that remove and disinfect potentially contaminated fomites.

Public Health Considerations. *Syphacia muris* is not a public health hazard.

Syphacia obvelata

Morphology. Adult male *S. obvelata* are 1,100 μ to 1,500 μ long and 120 μ to 140 μ wide, with a long tail bearing a distinct spicule and gubernaculum. The mouth is surrounded by three simple lips but lacks a buccal capsule. The anterior end bears small cervical alae while the tail is bent ventrally. Three cuticular projections (mamelons) are present on the ventral surface. Adult female worms are 3,400 μ to 5,800 μ long and 240 μ to 400 μ wide (Figure 11.32). The eggs are thin-shelled, unembryonated, crescent shaped, and flattened on one side. Eggs measure 111 μ to 153 μ long by 33 μ to 55 μ wide (Figure 11.32).

Hosts. *Syphacia obvelata*, the common mouse pinworm, is one of the most common parasites of laboratory mice. Many laboratory mouse colonies were infected until recently[55]. Advances in husbandry, and facility design and attention to pathogen detection and control have greatly reduced the prevalence of infection, though it remains high[4,305]. Laboratory rats are also susceptible to infection with *S. obvelata*[327]. Other susceptible species include hamsters, gerbils, voles, mastomys (*Praomys coucha*), Algerian mice (*M. spretus*), and primates, including humans[48,327–329].

Life Cycle. Larvae and adult worms inhabit the cecum and colon. The life cycle of *S. obvelata* is direct. Eggs are deposited on the perianal region, where they embryonate within hours. Infection is by ingestion of infective eggs from the perineum, or ingestion of contaminated food or water. Some have suggested that retrofection may also occur, but this has not been supported by controlled studies[330]. The prepatent period is 11 to 15 days[304]. Few controlled studies have been done on egg survival. In one study, eggs were viable on cellophane tape at room temperature for only 42 hours, and up to 14 days at 1°C to 4°C[331]. In contrast, eggs of the closely related rat pinworm, *S. muris,* may remain infective for at least four weeks under laboratory conditions[319].

Pathologic Effects. No specific enteric lesions have been attributed to light infections with *S. obvelata*. In contrast, very heavy parasite loads may lead to catarrhal enteritis, hepatic granulomas, and perianal irritation. In spite of their seemingly innocuous nature, infection with *S. obvelata* can alter host physiology, thereby confounding research results[3].

Clinical Disease. Typically, clinical disease is not observed in rodents infected with *S. obvelata*. While infections are usually subclinical, rectal prolapse, intussusception, fecal impaction, poor weight gain, and rough hair coat have been reported in heavily infected rodents, although generally without adequate exclusion of other pathogens[332].

Diagnosis. Diagnosis is based on demonstration of eggs in the feces or on the perianal region, or of adult worms in the cecum and colon at necropsy. Dependability of the different diagnostic methods varies widely. In one study, demonstration of adult worms in the intestine was the most dependable method (80.8% positive), demonstration of the eggs in the perianal region by clear cellophane tape the next most dependable (67.1% positive), and demonstration of eggs in fecal smears the least dependable (3.2% positive)[333]. Similar findings have been reported by others[312]. The age of the host at the time of examination is also important. In a study using the perianal

examination method, the positive rate at three weeks of age was 30% and at four weeks of age was 100%[333]. Thereafter, the infection rate diminished with age to 80% at five weeks and only 15% at seven weeks. Other studies have confirmed the observation that infection rates are maximal at four to five weeks of age[304].

Syphacia obvelata can be differentiated from other common pinworms of mice and rats (Figure 11.32). *Syphacia obvelata* is differentiated from *S. muris* on the basis of egg size, adult length, position of excretory pore in both sexes, position of the vulva in the female, tail length, and position of the anterior and middle mamelons in the male[304]. It is differentiated from *A. tetraptera* by the size and shape of the egg, shape of the esophageal bulb, size of cervical alae, position of the vulva in the female, and size and presence of a spicule and gubernaculum in the male[333]. Mixed infections with *A. tetraptera* are common[305].

Treatment. Eradication of pinworm infection is complicated by the potential survival of eggs in the environment, and the ease of movement of eggs throughout the facility. The most effective method of eradication involves feeding fenbendazole-medicated feed, similar to that used to eliminate *S. muris* from rats[325]. Several alternative treatment approaches have been described. While some of these approaches may be equally successful, they are generally labor intensive[322]. Eradication efforts are facilitated by strict adherence to sanitation protocols, including thorough detergent washing of all surfaces and objects associated with the animal room.

Prevention. Prevention of infection is complicated by the continued high prevalence of this parasite in laboratory rodent colonies, and the potentially long survival times of infectious eggs. Incoming animals should be treated with fenbendazole-medicated feed and tape-tests examined prior to shipment and arrival[325]. Filter top cages greatly reduce cage-to-cage (aerosol) transmission of *S. obvelata*[334].

Public Health Considerations. Human infections with *S. obvelata* are uncommon. Personnel working with infected rodents should always practice excellent personal hygiene.

Superfamily Trichostrongyloidea

Heligmosomoides polygyrus

Morphology. *Heligmosomoides polygyrus,* formerly known as *Nematospiroides dubius,* is a trichostrongylid nematode.

Adult female worms are approximately 9 mm to 12 mm long and are tightly coiled into a spiral. Adult male worms are smaller, and measure 4 mm to 6 mm long. The ellipsoidal, thin-walled eggs measure 70 μ to 84 μ by 37 μ to 53 μ[335].

Hosts. *Heligmosomoides polygyrus* is widely distributed among wild rodents in North America and Europe. Recently, its main importance has been as an experimental model in parasite immunology and screening of anthelmintics. In that regard, wild and laboratory strains differ somewhat in their duration of infection; infections with laboratory strains are relatively short-lived[336]. Among mouse strains, C3H mice are more susceptible to chronic experimental infection, whereas NIH and BALB/c mice acquire resistance and expel the worms[337]. Natural laboratory infections are rare.

Life Cycle. The life cycle of *H. polygyrus* is typical of the family. Eggs passed in the feces hatch in the environment. Larvae became infective in about four to five days[338]. Following ingestion by a suitable host, larvae travel to the small intestine and mature to the adult stage. The prepatent period is nine to 12 days[339].

Pathologic Effects and Clinical Disease. Natural infections have been considered to be nonpathogenic. Experimental infections alter growth trajectories and morphology of neonatal mice[340], alter the hemogram in an iron-responsive manner, and induce splenomegaly[338]. A strong Th2-associated immune response rapidly induces an immediate hypersensitivity reaction that results in clearing of the parasite[341]. In mouse strains such as the FVB, the immune response may be accompanied by pathological changes in the intestinal mucosa, including granuloma, decreased villus-to-crypt ratio, increased mesenteric lymph node, goblet and Paneth cell hyperplasia, and splenic reactivity[342]. Natural infections are not associated with clinical signs of disease.

Diagnosis. Infections with *H. polygyrus* may be diagnosed by finding the characteristic eggs in fecal floatation or by finding adult worms during necropsy.

Treatment. Infections with adult worms may be eliminated by treating mice with ivermectin (10 mg/kg SQ), but higher dosages (20 mg/kg) may be required to eliminate arrested larvae[343]. Treatment of transgenic or inbred mice with ivermectin should be attempted cautiously, because toxicity has been reported in some strains of mice[344]. Preferably, infected colonies should be eliminated.

Prevention. Given the low incidence of *H. polygyrus* infection in laboratory mice, the risk of infection is low.

However, mice should only be procured from reputable sources.

Public Health Considerations. *Heligmosomoides polygyrus* is not considered a public health hazard.

Nippostrongylus brasiliensis

Morphology. *Nippostrongylus brasiliensis* (Syn. *Nippostrongylus muris, Heligmosomum muris*) is a trichostrongylid nematode in the superfamily Trichostrongyloidea. Adult worms are slender; the female is 2.5 mm to 6.2 mm long and the male 2.1 mm to 4.5 mm long. The egg is ellipsoidal and thin-shelled and measures 52 μ to 63 μ by 28 μ to 35 μ (Figure 11.33)[345].

Hosts. *Nippostrongylus brasiliensis* is common in the Norway rat throughout the world. It also occurs naturally, but much less frequently, in the black rat and rarely in the mouse. Experimental hosts in which the parasite will attain sexual maturity include the mouse, hamster, Mongolian gerbil, rabbit, chinchilla, and to a lesser extent, the cotton rat. Rat strains differ in their permissiveness to infection, with albino rats being the most permissive[345]. The parasite does not occur naturally in laboratory rodents, and its primary importance is as a model of immunology, host-parasite interactions, and anthelmintic testing.

Life Cycle. The life cycle is direct, and similar to that of *H. polygyrus.* Eggs passed in the feces hatch within 24 hours and develop into infective larvae in another three to four days. Infection is normally by larval penetration of the skin. The larvae migrate through the lungs and then, by way of the trachea, esophagus, and stomach, to the small intestine. Eggs are passed in the feces after six days, and adults live from a few weeks to several months, though longer-lived infections may occur with laboratory-adapted strains of *N. brasilienis*[346].

Pathologic Effects and Clinical Disease. Light infections cause inflammation in the skin, lungs, and intestine, which subsides after a few days[345]. Small intestinal epithelial cells are flattened and villi are shortened and fused[347]. Severe infections cause verminous pneumonia. Clinical signs are not evident in light infections. Heavy infections result in hunched posture, rough hair coat, lethargy, respiratory distress, and death.

Diagnosis, Treatment, and Prevention. Diagnosis depends on identification of the eggs in feces or adult worms in the intestine. Animals infected with *N. brasiliensis* should be culled. If that is not possible, avermectins, benzimidazoles, and other anthelmintics useful for eradicating trichostrongylid nematodes should also be effective

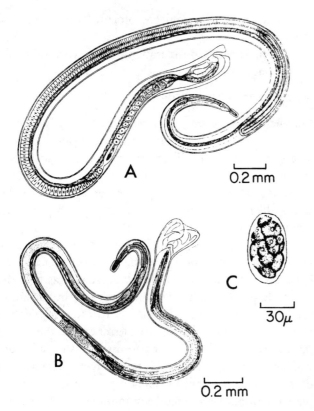

Fig. 11.33 *Nippostrongylus brasiliensis.* (A) Female. (B) Male. (C) Egg. Courtesy of W. Taliaferro, Argonne National Laboratory.

in eliminating *N. brasiliensis,* though few controlled studies have been reported. Prevention is through sanitation, exclusion of wild rodents, and purchase of parasite-free animals from reputable vendors.

Public Health Considerations. *Nippostrongylus brasiliensis* is not considered to be a public health hazard.

Superfamily Metastrongyloidea

Angiostrongylus cantonensis

Morphology. *Angiostrongylus cantonensis* (Syn. *Parastrongylus cantonensis*) is the rat lungworm. Adult worms are filariform (Figure 11.34). Male worms are 12 mm to 18 mm long, while female worms are 20 mm to 25 mm long[348].

Hosts. *Angiostrongylus cantonensis* infects rats of the genus *Rattus,* and a wide range of other rodents in many parts of the world[349]. While infections are more common in Asia, wild rats living near major harbors elsewhere in the world are also commonly infected[350]. Infections have not been reported in laboratory rats, but could occur where

wild rats have access to laboratory rodent facilities. Mice are frequently used as an experimental model of infection. Susceptible non-rodent species include primates[348], fruit bats[351], horses, dogs, opossums (*Didelphis virginiana*)[350], and others. Adult worms develop in these abnormal hosts, but infection is typically, though not always, restricted to the brain.

Life Cycle. The life cycle is indirect. Adults live in the pulmonary artery of the rat definitive host. Eggs released into the circulation lodge in small pulmonary vessels, embryonate, and hatch. Larvae are coughed up, swallowed, and expelled in the feces. Obligate intermediate hosts include terrestrial, aquatic, and amphibious snails, as well as slugs[352]. Development to the infective third-stage larva occurs in about 17 days. Several animals may serve as paratenic hosts, including freshwater shrimp, crabs, planarians, frogs, toads, and snail-eating lizards. Following ingestion by a rat, larvae migrate to the brain and remain in the neural parenchyma for up to two weeks. From there, larvae migrate to the subarachnoid space and then migrate via the venous system to the pulmonary artery, where they develop to the adult stage. The prepatent period is 37 to 45 days[353].

Pathologic Effects and Clinical Disease. Pathologic effects in the rat are generally limited to the central nervous system and the lungs, and are associated with reactions to migrating larvae. Light infections are typically asymptomatic. Heavy infections result in clinical signs associated

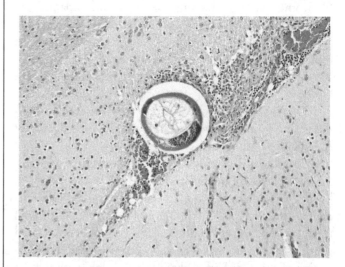

Fig. 11.34 *Angiostrongylus cantonensis* in a squirrel monkey. Cross section of a larva surrounded by eosinophilic and granulomatous inflammation with focal hemorrhage in the leptomeninges. Courtesy of Dae Young Kim, University of Missouri-Columbia.

with central nervous system disease. These may include weight loss, paralysis, blindness, and death[354,355].

Diagnosis, Treatment, and Prevention. Antemortem diagnosis depends on identifying larvae in the feces. Several anthelmintics have been effective in eliminating larval stages of *A. cantonensis*. These include albendazole[356], mebendazole[357], and levamisole[358]. Adult worms are more difficult to eliminate[358,359]. This infection should not occur in conventional rats, due to the lack of available intermediate hosts.

Public Health Considerations. *Angiostrongylus cantonensis* represents a significant indirect zoonotic threat as a cause of eosinophilic meningitis of humans, a serious and sometimes fatal condition[360]. However, human infections require the consumption of raw or undercooked snails or paratenic hosts.

Angiostrongylus costaricensis

Morphology. Adult worms are filariform, with the body tapering toward both ends (Figure 11.35). The tail is ventrally curved in both sexes. Males are 17 mm to 22 mm long and females are 28 mm to 42 mm long[362].

Hosts. *Angiostrongylus costaricensis* occurs in wild rodents in Central and South America. The principal definitive host is the cotton rat. Other suitable hosts include the black rat (*R. rattus*), rice rat (*Oryzomys palustris*), and others[361]. Patent infections have occurred in accidental hosts such as New World monkeys, raccoons, and dogs[363,364]. The epidemiologic significance of the dog as a reservoir host is unknown.

Life Cycle. The life cycle of *A. costaricensis* is similar to that of *A. cantonensis,* except that adult worms are in the subserosal arteries of the cecum and the cranial mesenteric arteries. Eggs lodge in the capillary plexus of the lamina propria. First-stage larvae penetrate into the intestinal lumen and pass out of the body with the feces[361]. The prepatent period is 24 days[360]. Intermediate hosts include slugs (*Vaginulus plebeius* and others) and terrestrial snails (*Bradybaena similaris*)[365]. Infective third-stage larvae are released in mucoid secretions of the intermediate host. In humans, development culminates with the production of eggs that hatch and release larvae. These, however, are trapped inside granulomata in the intestinal wall and are not released into the feces[364]. The role of paratenic hosts for *A. costaricensis* is less well known than for *A. cantonensis.*

Pathologic Effects and Clinical Disease. In mild infections, adult worms are found in the subserosal arteries of the cecum and in the ileocecocolic branch of the cranial mesenteric artery. As the worm burden increases, worms are also found higher in the main trunk of the cranial mesenteric artery, as well as in the jejunal branch[361]. Changes in the cecum vary from slight perivascular edema and discoloration around affected vessels to an enlarged, thin-walled cecum containing inspissated feces. Histopathologic changes include focal to diffuse subserosal edema, atrophy of the mesenteric fat, and enlargement of the ileocecocolic lymph nodes. Worm eggs and larvae may be found in the lymph nodes and on the serosal surface or in all layers of the cecal mucosa. Inflammatory cell infiltration around eggs and larvae are absent or minimal[361]. Similar parasite stages induce Th-1 mediated granuloma formation in abnormal hosts, including mice and humans[366]. Clinical disease has not been reported in rats.

Diagnosis, Treatment, and Prevention. Diagnosis is by identifying first-stage larvae in the feces, adult worms in the cranial mesenteric artery, and typical eggs and larvae in cecal mucosa. No information is available concerning treatment of rodents infected with *A. costaricensis*. Anthelmintic treatment of infected humans has not been effective. This parasite has not been reported in laboratory colonies, and the obligate intermediate hosts are not available for consumption in the animal facility. Therefore, no specific preventive measures are warranted.

Public Health Considerations. Like *A. cantonensis, A. costaricensis* represents an indirect threat to human health.

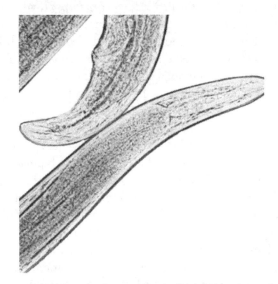

Fig. 11.35 *Angiostrongylus costaricensis.* (Right) Anterior and (left) posterior ends of adult females. 125 ×. Reproduced from Tesh, R.B., Ackerman, L.J., Dietz, W.H., and Williams, J.A. (1973) with permission.

Inadvertent ingestion of infectious larvae of *A. costaricensis* in snail and slug mucoid secretions on vegetables or in the intermediate hosts themselves leads to the development of eosinophilic granulomata in the mesenteric arteries of humans, sometimes with fatal consequences[367].

Angiostrongylus spp.

Other *Angiostrongylus* spp. have been reported in rodents. These include *A. dujardini,* which occurs in the pulmonary arteries and right ventricle of the wood mouse (*Apodemus sylvaticus*) and *Clethrionomys glareolus*[368]. *Angiostrongylus mackerrasae* occurs in rats[369]. *Angiostrongylus (Rodentocaulus) ondatrae* occurs in the muskrat, and *A. schmidti* is found in the pulmonary arteries of the rice rat[370].

Superfamily Filaroidea

Litomosoides carinii

Litomosoides carinii is a filarial nematode commonly found in wild cotton rats and in *Holochilus brasiliensis nanus,* a small semi-aquatic South American rodent[371]. Infection can be experimentally transmitted to laboratory mice and rats, multimammate rats, and Mongolian gerbils[372,373]. *Litomosoides carinii* has been used a model of human filariasis.

Superfamily Trichuroidea

Calodium hepaticum

Morphology. Adult male *Calodium hepaticum* (Syn. *Capillaria hepatica, Hepaticola hepatica*) measure 17 mm to 32 mm in length by 40 μ to 80 μ in width. Females reach 100 mm in length and 200 μ in width. Both sexes have a short, anterior, muscular esophagus attached to a long, glandular portion. The male has a lightly cuticularized terminal spicule up to 500 μ long, a protrusible spicule sheath that forms a funnel-shaped dilatation, and a blunt tail with a pair of subventral lobes. The vulva of the female lies posterior to the end of the esophagus. Eggs have bipolar plugs and are 48 μ to 62 μ long and 29 μ to 37 μ wide[374] (Figure 11.36). Eggs are similar to those of other trichurids, but differ in that their shell contains many small perforations and appears striated by rod-like structures.

Hosts. *Calodium hepaticum* occurs in the liver of a wide range of hosts throughout the world. It is common in wild rodents, especially in wild rats[375,376], and occurs occasionally in other wild mammals, including simian primates, and rarely in the woodchuck (*Marmota monax*), rabbit, dog, cat, other domestic animals, and humans. Several rodent species

may be infected in the wild, or experimentally in the laboratory. However, *C. hepaticum* has not been reported in commercially produced or laboratory-reared mice or rats.

Life Cycle. Eggs are deposited in the liver tissue, but are not released until either the tissue is eaten by another host and eggs are liberated and passed in the feces, or until the first host dies and the liver decomposes. Eggs embryonate in four to six weeks after exposure to air. Infection occurs only when embryonated eggs are ingested. They hatch in the intestine, and infective larvae penetrate the intestinal mucosa and pass via the portal system to the liver, where they develop to maturity in about 30 days. Male worms disappear from the liver around 33 days post-infection, leaving only female worms packed with eggs[377].

Pathologic Effects and Clinical Disease. The liver surface of infected animals contains white or yellow patches or nodules. Histologically, these are seen to contain the nematode and numerous eggs[378]. These large clusters of eggs cause localized liver damage and scarring[378]. Despite hepatic pathology, infection with *C. hepaticum* does not appear to affect the general health of rodents.

Diagnosis, Treatment, and Prevention. Diagnosis is based on demonstration of the parasite and the typical eggs in histologic sections of liver. Infected laboratory rodents should be culled from the colony or rederived parasite-free. Because of the unusual life cycle of this parasite, natural transmission in the laboratory is unlikely. Entry, death, and cannibalism of wild rodents could result in small numbers of cases within the animal facility.

Public Health Considerations. This parasite is pathogenic for humans, in which parasite eggs cause granulomatous lesions in the liver[379]. However, cases of human infection are rare, and generally occur in children one to five years of age. Transmission to animal facility staff is unlikely and special precautions should not be necessary.

Capillaria spp.

Several species of capillarids occur in the gastrointestinal or urinary tracts of mice and/or rats. *C. annulosa* infects the small intestine of rats; *C. bacielata* infects the esophagus of rats and mice; *Capillaria gastrica* infects the stomach of rats, mice, and voles; and *C. intestinalis* and *C. tavernae* infect the intestine of rats. Species in the urinary bladder of rats include *C. papillosa* and *C. prashadi*[272].

Trichuris arvicolae

Trichuris arvicolae is a whipworm of bank voles, field voles (*Microtus agrestis*), and common voles (*M. arvalis*).

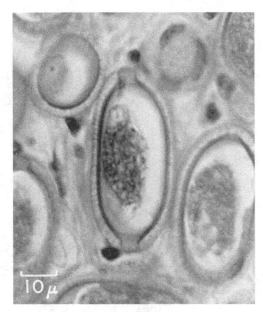

Fig. 11.36 *Calodium hepaticum* eggs in tissue section. Courtesy of E.F. Staffeldt, Argonne National Laboratory.

Trichuris arvicolae is biologically and morphologically similar to *T. muris,* and can be reliably differentiated from the latter species by morphologic comparison of egg size and vaginal length and by endonuclease restriction mapping[380]. Eggs of *T. arvicolae* are 67 μ to 79 μ long and 31 μ to 43 μ wide[381]. Males of the two species are nearly identical, though subtle differences in spicule morphology exist[381].

Trichuris muris

Morphology. *Trichuris muris* is morphologically similar to *T. arvicolae,* and can be reliably differentiated from the latter by morphologic comparison of egg size and vaginal length. Eggs are 62 μ to 68 μ long and 28 μ to 32 μ wide[381]. Males of the two species are nearly identical, though subtle differences in spicule morphology exist[381]. The two species can also be differentiated by endonuclease restriction mapping[380].

Hosts. *Trichuris muris* has been identified from 18 genera of rodents from the following families: Arvicolidae, Bathyergidae, Cricetidae, Echimyidae, Hystrichidae, Muridae, and Sciuridae[381]. Infection is common in wild rats[77] but uncommon in wild mice[382].

Life Cycle. The life cycle of *T. muris* is direct. Adult worms are intra-epithelial in the cecum and colon, where worms excavate intra-epithelial tunnels[383]. The tunnel is a syncytium of enterocyte origin and is induced by secretion of digestive enzymes from the region of the worm head. The worm appears to feed upon the syncytial protoplasm[384]. Eggs are passed in the feces and embryonate in the environment within two months[385]. Eggs hatch following ingestion, releasing infectious first-stage larvae[385]. Larvae establish in the cecal and colonic mucosa and molt through larval stages to the adult stage. In most mouse strains, the development of immunity to *T. muris* results in expulsion of adult worms ("self-cure") and resistance to reinfection. In this regard, *T. muris* serves as a model of intestinal nematode infection[386].

Pathologic Effects and Clinical Disease. Infection with *T. muris* results in minimal intestinal pathology. Infection with *T. muris* is not reported to cause clinical disease.

Diagnosis, Treatment, and Prevention. Diagnosis is made by histologic identification of the parasite in the host intestinal tract and by identifying characteristic trichurid parasite eggs in the feces. Infections may be eliminated with oxantel (25 mg/kg once) or with mebendazole (50 mg/kg orally for two treatments given on consecutive days)[387]. Natural infections of laboratory animals have not been reported. Regardless, entry of wild rodents could result in this species entering the laboratory animal colony.

Public Health Considerations. *Trichuris muris* is not known to infect humans and therefore is not considered a public health threat.

Trichuris spp.

Several other *Trichuris* spp. have been recovered from rodents. From North America, these include *T. dipodomys, T. fossor, T. madisonensis, T. neotomae, T. opaca,* and *T. peromysci.* From Africa, these include *T. carlieri, T. contorta, T. gerbillis, T. gundii, T. parvispicularis,* and *T. vondwei. Trichuris petrowi* occurs in the Asian part of Russia[381]. Relatively little is known of these species.

Trichosomoides crassicauda

Morphology. *Trichosomoides crassicauda* is a hairlike worm in the superfamily Trichuroidea. It is known as the "bladder threadworm". The female worm is about 10 mm long and 200 μ in diameter. Its small size makes it difficult to see without the aid of a dissecting microscope. The male is much smaller than the female, and measures only 1.5 mm to 3.5 mm in length, and is a permanent hyperparasite harbored within the reproductive tract of the female (Figure 11.37)[388]. Eggs are embryonated when passed, oval, brown with a thick shell and bipolar plugs, and measure 60 μ to 70 μ by 30 μ to 35 μ (Figure 11.38).

Hosts. *Trichosomoides crassicauda* is a common urinary tract parasite of wild rats[77], and was reported recently in a pet rat[389]. It should be noted that the source of that infection may actually have been a laboratory animal facility, though this seems unlikely[389]. Many years ago *T. crassicauda* was regularly found in laboratory rats; however, this is no longer the case.

Life Cycle. Adult female worms occur free in the urinary bladder or live in the wall of the urinary bladder and occasionally the upper ureter and renal pelvis (Figure 11.39). Embryonated eggs are passed in the urine. These can survive in the environment at room temperature for up to 52 days[390]. Infection is by ingestion of embryonated eggs. The primary means of transmission is from adult rats to offspring prior to weaning[391]. Eggs hatch in the stomach, and larvae penetrate the stomach wall and within a few hours are carried by the blood to the lungs and other parts of the body. Most larvae die; only those that reach the kidneys or urinary bladder survive[392]. The complete life cycle requires eight to nine weeks, with the prepatent period as short as 55 days. Typically however, eggs are not usually present in the urine of rats infected as neonates until eight to 12 weeks of age[391]. Infection is more common in male rats than in females[393].

Pathologic Effects. *Trichosomoides crassicauda* is mildly pathogenic. Embedded female worms cause the formation of white masses measuring about 3 mm by 0.8 mm. Histologic examination of these lesions reveals epithelial hyperplasia with a noticeable lack of inflammation, suggesting that the relatively avascular hyperplastic epithelium may represent an immunologically protected site[394], though serologic responses have been detected[395]. Worms are seen lying on, or embedded in, the mucosa (Figure 11.40). Other lesions include nephritis, pulmonary granuloma formation, and eosinophilia[396].

Clinical Disease. Natural infection with *T. crassicauda* usually is unapparent. Urinary calculi and bladder tumors have been associated with *T. crassicauda* infection, but a causal relationship has not been established[397].

Diagnosis. Diagnosis of the infection is by demonstration of the parasite in the urinary bladder or in histologic sections of the bladder wall, or by demonstration of the characteristic eggs in the urine. Antemortem urine examination may be facilitated by filtering collected urine through a prefilter[391]. Given the rarity of infection, however, urine is not commonly examined. Therefore, diagnosis most often depends on examination of the urinary bladder at necropsy. Other, more labor-intensive methods

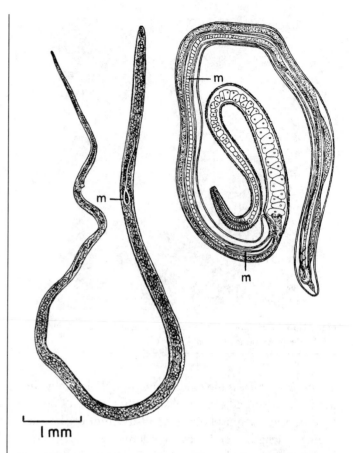

Fig. 11.37 *Trichosomoides crassicauda.* (Left) Mature female with male (m) as a permanent hyperparasite in uterus. (Right) Immature female with male in vagina. Reproduced from Yorke, W. and Maplestone, P.A. (1926) with permission.

include cryostat sections of the urinary bladder stained with acridine orange and viewed under a fluorescence microscope, as well as stabilization of the bladder surface prior to examination using scanning electron microscopy[398].

Treatment and Prevention. Ivermectin (3 mg/kg of a 0.4% w/v solution) administered orally has been shown to be effective for eliminating the infection[399]. Prevention depends on procurement of high-quality animals from reputable sources, and exclusion of wild rats and those associated with the pet trade.

Public Health Considerations. *Trichosomoides crassicauda* is not considered a public health hazard because it does not infect humans.

ACANTHOCEPHALA

Acanthocephala have always been extremely rare in laboratory rodents, even before modern improvements in

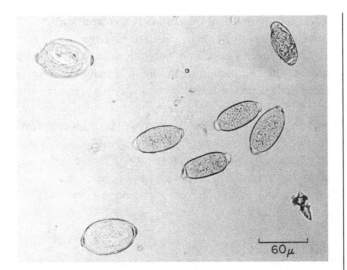

Fig. 11.38 *Trichosomoides crassicauda* eggs. Reproduced from Habermann, R.T. and Williams, F.P. Jr. (1958) with permission.

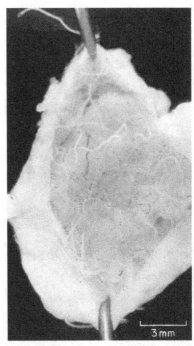

Fig. 11.39 *Trichosomoides crassicauda* females in the bladder of a rat. Courtesy of J.M. Tufts, Ralston Purina Company.

laboratory animal husbandry. However, breaks in vermin control may permit the introduction of acanthocephalan parasites into the laboratory animal colony.

Moniliformis moniliformis

Morphology. *Moniliformis moniliformis* (Syn. *Moniliformis dubius*) has a thick, rounded, annulated body (Figure 11.41). Males are 6 cm to 8 cm long, and females 10 cm to 32 cm long. The proboscis is club-shaped or cylindrical and armed with several rows of distinctive crescentic hooks. The egg is 90 μ to 125 μ by 50 μ to 62 μ and embryonated when passed in the feces (Figure 11.42)[400].

Hosts. *Moniliformis moniliformis* occurs in wild Norway and black rats, and in other rodents throughout the world. It is most common in tropical and subtropical regions, especially where the cockroach intermediate host is plentiful. It is less common in temperate regions. Entry into modern animal facilities is extremely unlikely.

Life Cycle. The adult worm inhabits the intestinal tract of the rodent host. Eggs pass out of the body in the feces. These are ingested by a suitable arthropod intermediate host and hatch in the gut as larvae (acanthors), which penetrate the gut wall, develop into immature acanthellas, and then become infective acanthellas or cystacanths in the hemocoel of the intermediate host[401]. The cystacanth is released when the infected intermediate host is ingested by a rodent. The acanthella escapes from the cyst, attaches to the gut wall, and grows into an adult worm in the anterior small intestine. Suitable intermediate hosts include several species of cockroaches[402], including the American cockroach (*Periplaneta americana*), in addition to various beetles. Development from egg to infective acanthella in the intermediate host requires approximately seven weeks, while development of infective acanthella to adult worms in the definitive host requires 31 to 38 days[403]. Female worms each release about 5,500 eggs per day, or about 600,000 eggs over the course of a 106-day patent period[404].

Pathologic Effects. The adult worms localize to a small portion of the rodent small intestine. Infections produce mild thickening of the gut mucosa, with inflammation of the lamina propria, goblet and Paneth cell hypertrophy, and copious production of sulphomucins and sialomucins. Necrosis and penetration of the intestinal wall, with secondary peritonitis, may occur with heavy infections[405,406]. Experimental infection alters stress hormone levels in rats[407].

Clinical Disease. Clinical signs of infection are uncommon, but can include systemic disease secondary to penetration of the intestinal wall.

Diagnosis, Treatment, and Prevention. Diagnosis is based on the identification of either the eggs in the feces or adult worms in the intestine at necropsy. There is no documented treatment for *M. moniliformis* in rats. Human

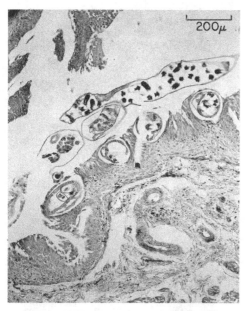

Fig. 11.40 *Trichosomoides crassicauda* in the lumen and mucosa of the urinary bladder of a rat. Reproduced from Habermann, R.T. and Williams, F.P. Jr. (1958) with permission.

infections have been treated with pyrantel pamoate[408]. Infected colonies should be culled or rederived and vermin control measures instituted. Sanitation and insect control prevent the completion of the life cycle and the entry of the parasite into the research colony. Proper cleaning after an outbreak is essential, because the embryonated egg may remain infectious for cockroaches for years under optimal environmental conditions[409].

Public Health Considerations. Human infections have been reported[408]. Humans can become infected only by ingestion of an infected invertebrate host, usually a cockroach.

ARTHROPODS

Improvements in animal facility design, construction, and operation have contributed to a great reduction in the number of free-living facultative, as well as obligate external, parasites. These improvements directly benefit laboratory animal health, interrupt the life cycles of parasites with arthropods as intermediate hosts, and reduce exposure of animal facility personnel to arthropod pests. Occasionally, however, structural problems in the facility, breaks in sanitation procedures, or other lapses in standard operating procedures may permit entry of arthropod parasites.

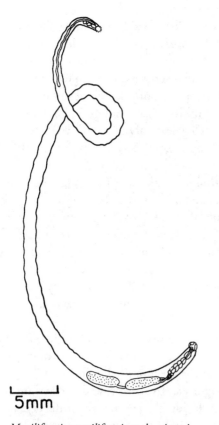

Fig. 11.41 *Moniliformis moniliformis* male. Anterior end at top. Reproduced from Olsen, O.W. (1967) with permission.

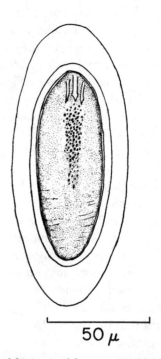

Fig. 11.42 *Moniliformis moniliformis* egg. Reproduced from Moore, D.V. (1946) with permission.

Class Insecta

Several insects commonly parasitize wild rats and mice. Lapses in facility sanitation procedures; loss of the structural integrity of the facility; and entry of incoming rodents (wild or domestic), other animals, or personnel may allow insects to enter even the modern laboratory animal facility.

Order Diptera (flies)

Although many flies (Diptera) cause disease in vertebrate animals, few are important pathogens for laboratory rats and mice. Parasitism caused by larval flies is highly varied and characteristically temporary. Continued parasitism of laboratory rodents requires repeated contacts or invasions from outside the laboratory.

Cuterebra sp.

Morphology. *Cuterebra* sp. are also known as rodent botflies. Adults superficially resemble bumblebees. They are large, robust, hairy flies with uniformly dark wings and are 15 mm to 30 mm long. Many species have conspicuous white markings that contrast with an overall black or blueblack coloration. Eggs are yellow and 1 mm long; the firststage infective larva is minute and spindle-shaped. The second-stage larva is 5 mm to 20 mm long, and the third larval stage is 30 mm long (Figure 11.43).

Hosts. The genus *Cuterebra* contains more than 40 species, all of which occur in the Western Hemisphere. Most species show a high degree of specificity to both host and site of larval development on the host. Wild rodents, lagomorphs, and primates native to the Western Hemisphere are the natural hosts. Other rodents, including laboratory rats and mice, domestic animals, and humans may serve as accidental hosts. Only partial larval development may occur in some accidental hosts[410].

Common North American species include *C. angustifrons, C. approximata, C. austeni, C. fontinella, C. grisea, C. latifrons, C. neomexicana, C. polita,* and *C. tenebrosa,* which affect deer mice, wood rats, and related wild rodents; *C. emasculator,* which affects squirrels; and *C. cuniculi, C. horripilum, C. jellisoni, C. lepivora, C. princeps,* and *C. ruficrus,* which affect the cottontail rabbit and hares[411–414]. Infestation is common in rodents obtained from their natural habitats.

Life Cycle. *Cuterebra* adults are not parasitic. Gravid females often enter buildings through ground-level openings and deposit their eggs either singly or in broken rows near a host, but not on the host itself. The eggs hatch in one to two weeks under temperate conditions, about 25°C. Infective larvae generally enter the host through the nares and mouth[415]. The larvae apparently migrate through connective tissue and, after about one week, appear in the subcutaneous tissue. A small opening in the host's skin is produced at the posterior end of the larva for breathing and excretion. The larva molts and grows rapidly in the next two to three weeks, which induces a large subcutaneous cyst (warble) to develop. When fully grown, the third-stage larva enlarges the warble pore, backs out of the cyst, drops to the bedding, cage floor, or ground, and pupates. The total period of larval development lasts three to five weeks[415]. Pupal development takes up to four to six months if it is interrupted by winter diapause. Adult flies will not mate in a building, so continuing laboratory infestation is not likely. The incidence of cuterebriasis is greatest during the summer and fall in temperate regions.

Pathologic Effects. *Cuterebra* larvae produce subcutaneous cysts in affected hosts. There are usually one to three larvae per host[416]. They produce little lasting pathology in native hosts. Chronic inflammation occurs around the cyst, but healing is usually rapid once the larva emerges[417]. Secondary infection is uncommon. Anemia, reduced hemoglobin, leukocytosis, and splenomegaly have been observed[416,417]. The pathologic effects are more severe in non-native hosts such as the laboratory rat, mouse, and others[410]. Extensive inflammation, secondary infection, and protracted healing of cysts are common, and larval migration and development tend to be erratic[410].

Clinical Disease. Clinical signs of disease are generally associated with warble formation, accompanying inflammation, and secondary bacterial infection. Death of the host sometimes occurs about one week after infective larvae reach the site of warble development, or when the mature larvae emerges[410].

Diagnosis. Diagnosis is based on recovery of characteristic larvae from dermal cysts. Generally, there is only one larva per cyst. Accurate species identification cannot be made from larval or egg morphology.

Treatment. Rodent botfly infection is treated by surgically removing larvae from the dermal cysts, flushing the cyst cavity with antiseptic solution, and applying antibiotic ointment.

Prevention. Preventing entry of rodent botflies into the animal facility is achieved by insect-proofing animal buildings. In temperate areas, hosts obtained from their natural habitat should be examined carefully for evidence of external parasites and treated appropriately.

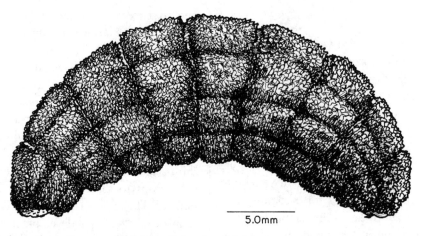

Fig. 11.43 *Cuterebra,* third-stage larva. Courtesy of E.P. Catts, University of Delaware.

Public Health Considerations. *Cuterebra* infection has been reported in humans[418], but is uncommon. Infected laboratory animals are not a direct hazard to personnel.

Oestromyia leporina

Morphology. Adults of *Oestromyia leporina,* also known as the Old World rodent botfly, have an overall blue-black appearance, with an orange and yellow head. Larvae are 12 mm to 15 mm long and plump, and have bands of pale, flattened spines on all segments (Figure 11.44).

Hosts. Larvae of *O. leporina* are common dermal, cyst-producing parasites of voles, rabbits, and the muskrat in Europe, and have been reported in Asian pikas (*Ochotona* sp.)[419,420].

Life Cycle. The life cycle is similar to that of *Cuterebra* except that gravid females oviposit directly on their hosts and larvae penetrate intact skin[421]. In Europe, the adult flight season and egg-laying occur in late summer. The pupa phase can last up to 10 months[421].

Pathologic Effects. Larvae occur singly in cutaneous cysts, with usually only one larva per host. There is little inflammation, and the cyst heals within about three weeks after the mature larva has emerged[422].

Clinical Disease. Clinical signs are generally limited to the cutaneous cyst. Other signs may occur if cyst development occurs in an aberrant location.

Diagnosis, Treatment, and Prevention. Diagnosis is based on demonstration of the parasite in cutaneous cysts. Treatment is as described for *Cuterebra.* As described for *Cuterebra,* entry of rodent botflies into the animal facility is prevented by insect-proofing animal buildings. Because females oviposit directly on hosts, screening is an effective method of prevention. In endemic areas, hosts obtained from their natural habitat should be examined carefully for evidence of external parasites at the time of entry into the facility.

Public Health Considerations. There are no reports of infestation of humans with *O. leporina.*

Order Phthiraptera (lice)

Hoplopleura spp.

Morphology. *Hoplopleura acanthopus, H. captiosa,* and *H. pacifica* are sucking lice of wild rats and mice. *Hoplopleura* sp. (Figure 11.45) are slender lice, 1 mm to 2 mm long, and have seven to eight lateral abdominal plates. Each plate is large and rectangular. The abdomen also has numerous ventral plates, and each abdominal segment usually bears two to three dorsal plates. The eggs are oval, about 0.5 mm long, and are attached to hairs by the female with a drop of cement[423]. The three nymphal stages have a characteristic heart-shaped abdomen but usually lack spiracles[424,425].

Hosts. *Hoplopleura acanthopus* is found on meadow voles, red-backed mice (*Clethrionomys rutilus*), deer mice, European field mice (*M. minutus*), lemming mice (*Synaptomys* sp.), and pine mice (*Pitymys* sp.) throughout the world and is occasionally found on the house mouse[426,427]. Infestation of laboratory mice has not been reported recently. *Hoplopleura captiosa* infests the house mouse. It occurs globally[425,428]. *Hoplopleura pacifica,* or the tropical rat louse, is a parasite of black rats, Norway rats, and other wild rats throughout the world[429,430].

Life Cycle. The life cycle is poorly understood, but is probably similar to *Polyplax* sp., with transmission by direct contact.

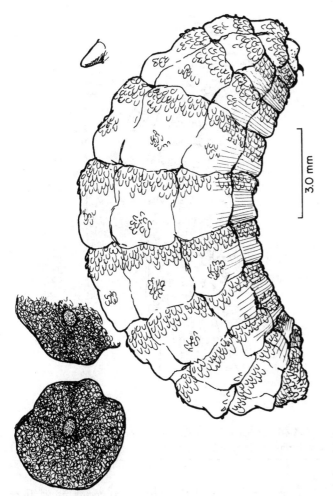

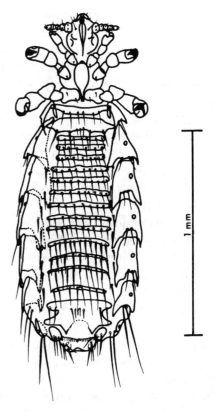

Fig. 11.45 *Hoplopleura acanthopus* female, ventral view. Courtesy of K.C. Kim, Pennsylvania State University.

Fig. 11.44 *Oestromyia leporina* larva (insets). Posterior spiracles (left) and typical spine (right). Courtesy of E.P. Catts, University of Delaware.

Pathologic Effects and Clinical Disease. The pathologic effects of *Hoplopleura* are similar to those described for *Polyplax*. *Hoplopleura acanthopus* transmits *Brucella brucei,* a common pathogen of small field rodents[431]. Clinical signs are likely as described for *Polyplax*.

Diagnosis, Treatment, and Prevention. Diagnosis, treatment, and prevention are as described for *Polyplax*.

Public Health Considerations. These lice are of no known direct public health importance, but can transmit murine typhus and other human pathogens[430].

Polyplax serrata

Morphology. *Polyplax serrata* is the common mouse louse. Adult females are slender and about 1.5 mm long. Males are thicker and shorter (1 mm) (Figure 11.46). Adults of both sexes may be seen without magnification. The head resembles *P. spinulosa*. The ventral thoracic plate is nearly triangular (versus pentagonal for *P. spinulosa*). The abdomen has seven lateral plates on each side and seven to 13 dorsal plates. The first lateral plate is divided. The setae of the fourth lateral plate are unequal in length; the dorsal one is much longer than the ventral one (versus equal lengths for *P. spinulosa*). Eggs are elongated, have a cone-like operculum with a row of pores along the cone, and are attached near the base of hair shafts.

Hosts. *Polyplax serrata* has been reported from wild and laboratory mice[2,432]. Infestation with *P. serrata* was not detected in a recent survey of more than 14,000 mice submitted to a commercial diagnostic laboratory[4].

Life Cycle. The life cycle is similar to that of *P. spinulosa*[433]. Eggs hatch in five to six days. After hatching, first-stage nymphs may be found widely distributed over the body surface. More mature stages of nymphs, as well as the adults, generally favor the anterior dorsum of the host[433]. Nymphal stages may be identified by setal arrangements[433], and develop to the adult stage in seven days. The average minimum life cycle is 13 days[433]. Louse populations are constrained by the development of a host immune response and by host grooming behavior[434,435]. Transmission from host to host is by direct contact. Female mice use olfactory cues to discriminate between *P. serrata*-infected and -uninfected male mice in an oxytocin-dependant manner, and exhibit a preference for the odor of uninfected males[436].

Pathologic Effects. Because this is a blood-sucking louse, heavy infestation with *P. serrata* may cause anemia and debilitation. Histopathologic findings are compatible with Type-I hypersensitivity[437]. These changes are largely immune mediated, involve both immediate and delayed responses, and restrict louse populations[435,438]. Arthropod-borne infections transmitted by *P. serrata* are known to include *Eperythrozoon coccoides* and *Francisella tularensis*[439].

Clinical Disease. Heavy infestations with *P. serrata* cause erythema, pruritus, self-trauma, loss of condition, and occasionally, death[437].

Diagnosis. Diagnosis is by direct examination of the pelage of dead or anesthetized mice under a bright light and dissecting microscope. The pelage should be examined under low power, focusing on the epidermal surface. The hair over the dorsum, nuchal crest area of the skull, dorsal neck region, and area between the scapulae generally yield the most parasites. The hair in these areas should be parted and examined for moving or stationary lice and for viable or hatched egg cases. An alternate method for detecting lice involves placing the euthanized mouse on a sheet of black paper surrounded by clear adhesive tape, sticky side up. After an overnight wait, discard the carcass and examine the paper under a dissecting microscope for lice and other arthropod parasites.

Treatment. *Polyplax serrata* may be eliminated through rederivation or chemical treatment. Rederivation procedures are labor intensive, may put valuable stock at risk, and may slow or halt research efforts, but are highly effective. Historically, chemical treatments have been applied as dusts, insecticidal powders, or dips. These are labor intensive and often not 100% effective. Among chemical treatments available, the pyrethroids, such as permethrin, are effective and generally safe. Pyrethroids may be applied as dips or sprays. They should be applied twice, 14 days apart[440]. Pyrethroids may be fatal to mice if overdosed[441]. The insecticide fipronil effectively eliminates lice when applied twice, 10 days apart, to the mouse's entire body[440]. However, fipronil has been reported to increase plasma progesterone, decrease plasma estrogen levels, and lengthen the estrous cycle of female Wistar rats[442]. Ivermectin administered at 200 to 400 μg/kg is also effective in controlling lice on mice[440].

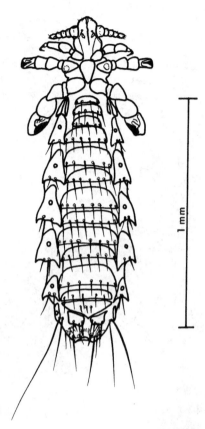

Fig. 11.46 *Polyplax serrata* female, ventral view. Courtesy of K.C. Kim, Pennsylvania State University.

It should be noted that the avermectins may affect host physiology and/or cause toxicity in a number of inbred or genetically modified mouse strains[443]. For example, ivermectin has anticonvulsant properties[444], is neurotoxic in P-glycoprotein deficient CF-1 mice[445], and causes neurologic signs and occasional death in C57BL mouse pups[344]. Ivermectin also alters sensitive behaviors in some mouse strains, including exploration of a novel open field, the acoustic startle reflex, and the prepulse inhibition of the acoustic startle reflex, a measure of sensory gating[446].

Prevention. Mice should only be obtained from sources shown to have stock free of ectoparasites. Wild mice should be excluded from the animal facility.

Public Health Considerations. *Polyplax serrata* is not considered to be a direct public health hazard. However, like *P. spinulosa*, *P. serrata* could potentially serve as a vector for some blood-borne human pathogens.

Polyplax spinulosa

Morphology. *Polyplax spinulosa* is known as the spined rat louse. It is most commonly found in the fur of the midbody, shoulders, and neck. It is slender, yellow-brown, and 0.6 mm to 1.5 mm long. The head is rounded, lacks eyes, and bears two five-segmented antennae. There is also a long hair on the posterior angle of the head. The third segment of the male antenna bears a pointed apophysis. The ventral thoracic plate is pentagonal. The abdomen has seven lateral plates on each side and seven to 13 dorsal plates. The first lateral plate is divided. The setae of the fourth lateral plate are almost the same length. The eggs are elongated and have a cone-like operculum with a row of pores along the cone.

Hosts. *Polyplax spinulosa* (the "spined rat louse") is the common louse of both laboratory and wild rats. Susceptible rat species include both *R. norvegicus* and *R. rattus*[77,447]. Several species of closely related murine rodents, including mice, voles, and other species of wild rats, can be infested[448,449]. *Polyplax spinulosa* may also infest guinea pigs[450]. As a group, however, lice tend to be more host-specific than many other external parasites. Infestation of laboratory rats has become rare with improvements in husbandry and veterinary standards.

Life Cycle. Eggs are laid and fastened to the hair near the skin. Eggs hatch in five to six days. Nymphs emerge from the operculum and undergo three molts to the adult stage. The three nymphal stages resemble adults but are paler and lack reproductive organs. The entire life cycle takes place on the host and is completed in 26 days. Adults survive 28 to 35 days. Transmission between animals is by direct contact.

Pathologic Effects. *Polyplax spinulosa* is a blood-sucking louse; heavy infestation may result in dermatitis and anemia. Rats may be concurrently infested with mites that may contribute to skin pathology. This louse serves as a vector of *Brucella brucei*, *Borrelia duttoni*, *Mycoplasma haemomuris* (formerly *Haemobartonella muris*), *Rickettsia typhi*, and *Trypanosoma lewisi*.

Clinical Disease. Rat genetic background has been shown to affect the degree and duration of pediculosis[451]. Infested animals may develop an unthrifty appearance, constant scratching and irritation, restlessness, and debilitation. Eventually, infestation may induce partial immunity through exposure to a louse midgut epithelial protein, resulting in decreased louse burdens[451].

Diagnosis. Diagnosis is achieved by finding and identifying adult lice, nymphs, or eggs on the fur.

Treatment. Several insecticides have been used successfully to treat pediculosis. Effective formulations have included dusts, sprays, and dips. Although lice do not usually leave the host, treatments should be applied both to the animals and to their bedding. Virtually all insecticides formulated for treatment of pediculosis in veterinary species should be effective in eradicating *P. spinulosa*. Ivermectin administered by subcutaneous injection at a dosage of 600 µg/kg is also effective[452].

Prevention. Entry of *P. spinulosa* into the animal colony can be prevented by purchasing parasite-free rats, using effective quarantine procedures, and excluding vermin. Insecticide treatment and sanitation are effective control measures if infestation occurs.

Public Health Considerations. *Polyplax spinulosa* is not considered to be a direct public health risk. However, as an arthropod vector of human blood-borne pathogens, caution is warranted when working with infested wild rats or with laboratory rats infested from wild populations of lice.

Order Siphonaptera (fleas)

Fleas should not be found in modern, well-managed animal facilities. However, they may gain access to the facility through vectors such as animal caretakers, incoming laboratory animals, or wild rodents; or they may enter on fomites such as contaminated feed or bedding bags. While most species of flea have host preferences, they are not strictly host-specific. The following section will focus on fleas which preferentially infest rodents.

Leptopsylla segnis

Morphology. *Leptopsylla segnis,* also known as the "mouse flea", is small, (1 mm to 2 mm long) and is distinguished from other fleas by a pair of spiniform bristles on each side of the frons and four blunt teeth in the genal comb (Figure 11.47).

Hosts. *Leptopsylla segnis* is a common parasite of house mice throughout the world. It also occurs frequently on Norway rats, black rats, European field mice, and wild guinea pigs (*Cavia aperea*)[447,450,453]. *Leptopsylla segnis* has been found on a high percentage of wild rodents in Europe and in urban areas of the United States[454].

Life Cycle. The life cycle is similar to *Ctenocephalides* of dogs and cats, except that the larval stages of *L. segnis* are usually limited to the nest or burrow of the rodent host, where flea eggs accumulate. Eggs hatch, releasing larvae that grow and molt through three larval stages. Larvae feed on adult flea feces. The third larval stage spins a cocoon and metamorphoses (pupates) into adult fleas. Adults emerge from the cocoons in three to four weeks. Adult fleas repeatedly pierce the skin and feed on the blood of their hosts[263]. Flea populations are generally highest in the spring[450] and increase with rats' age and body size[447]. Adult female fleas live an average of about 23 days, and as long as 51 days, whereas adult males live an average of about 19 days, and as long as 37 days[455]. Female fleas may lay more than 400 eggs during their lifetime[456].

Pathologic Effects and Clinical Disease. The pathologic effects of this flea on its natural host are unknown. Clinical signs have not been reported for rodents. Moderate to severe infestations could be expected to affect growth rates and overall body condition, and could lead to death.

Diagnosis, Treatment, and Prevention. Diagnosis is made by identifying the flea on the host. Presumably, preparations typically useful for eliminating infestations with *Ctenocephalides* sp. on dogs and cats would also be useful for eliminating this parasite from rodent colonies. The environment of the animal room should also be thoroughly sanitized to eliminate eggs and the source of the infestation identified and eliminated. Flea infestation is prevented through proper storage and inspection of feed and bedding bags, exclusion of wild rodents, procurement of research animals from approved sources, effective quarantine procedures, and personal hygiene of facility personnel.

Public Health Considerations. This flea is an intermediate host for the tapeworms *Hymenolepis diminuta* and *Rodentolepis nana*. *Leptopsylla segnis* is also capable of transmitting the agent of typhus (*Rickettsia*)[457], and possibly also the virus that causes hemorrhagic fever with renal syndrome. The latter, however, is only likely to be transmitted mechanically without propagation in the flea host[458].

Nosopsyllus fasciatus

Morphology. *Nosopsyllus fasciatus,* the Northern rat flea, is 1.5 mm to 2.5 mm long and is a rich amber color. It is distinguished from other fleas by the absence of a genal comb, by the presence of a pronotal comb, and by the number of teeth in the pronotal comb (Figure 11.48).

Hosts. *Nosopsyllus fasciatus* occurs on various species of wild rats and mice throughout the world, including the Norway rat, black rat, and house mouse. It is the flea that is most frequently found on wild rats in Europe, and it is common on wild rodents from urban areas in the United States[454]. Although it has not been reported from rodents raised in the laboratory setting, it could be introduced on rats and mice obtained from their natural environment or through entry of wild rodents into the animal facility[77]. Rarely, *N. fasciatus* is recovered from hamsters and from non-rodent hosts, including cats and dogs[459].

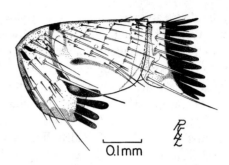

Fig. 11.47   *Leptopsylla segnis.* Courtesy of R.E. Lewis, Iowa State University.

Life Cycle. The life cycle is similar to that of *Ctenocephalides* except that the larval stages are usually limited to the nest or burrow. Adults are most plentiful during the cooler months of the year.

Pathologic Effects and Clinical Disease. Little is known of the pathologic effects and clinical disease caused by *N. fasciatus*. It is likely that these aspects are similar to those found in other flea infestations. *Nosopsyllus fasciatus* is a vector of *Trypanosoma lewisi* and *T. duttoni,* and is an intermediate host for the tapeworms *Hymenolepis diminuta* and *Rodentolepis nana*.

Diagnosis, Treatment, and Prevention. Diagnosis is made by identifying the parasite on the host. Treatment regimens effective for eliminating *Ctenocephalides* sp. from dogs and cats should also effectively eliminate *N. fasciatus* from rodents. Procurement of parasite-free animals from reputable sources, exclusion of wild rodents, as well as inspection, isolation, and routine treatment of all newly acquired wild rodents captured in their native environment prevent entry of this parasite into the animal facility.

Public Health Considerations. Because this flea is an intermediate host for the tapeworms *H. diminuta* and *R. nana,* it is a potential hazard for animal workers. It is also an important vector for the agents of plague (*Yersinia pestis*) and typhus (*Rickettsia*). The bite of this flea is irritating to humans and causes a reaction similar to that caused by the bites of the *Xenopsylla cheopis* and *Ctenocephalides* sp.

Xenopsylla cheopis

Morphology. *Xenopsylla cheopis,* also known as the "Oriental" or "Indian" rat flea, is similar in size to *Ctenocephalides felis* and *C. canis* of dogs and cats, but is light amber in color and lacks both genal and pronotal combs. The head is smoothly rounded anteriorly[440] (Figure 11.49).

Hosts. *Xenopsylla cheopis* occurs on the Norway rat and black rat[447]. Other rodent hosts include the house mouse, ground squirrel, common vole (*M. arvalis*), and others; non-rodent hosts include cottontail rabbits[440]. Although the origin of *X. cheopis* was probably North Africa or India, it is not found throughout the world. It occurs commonly on wild rodents in urban areas in the United States, particularly in the Midwest and port cities. It has been reported in one laboratory mouse colony[460].

Life Cycle. The life cycle is similar to that of *Leptopsylla segnis*. Adults may survive to up to 100 days if a host is available, and up to 38 days without a blood meal if environmental humidity levels are high[440].

Pathologic Effects and Clinical Disease. The pathologic effects of *X. cheopis* on its natural host have not been reported. In addition to a number of human pathogens, *X. cheopis* may also transmit *Hepatozoon erhardovae* to murine rodents[461]. Clinical signs have not been reported for rodents.

Diagnosis. Diagnosis is made by identifying the parasite on the host. While similar in appearance to the human flea, *Pulex irritans*, *X. cheopis* can be distinguished by a vertical rod on the mesothorax, which is absent in *P. irritans*[263]. The latter also does not typically infest rodents.

Treatment and Prevention. Treatment of infested animals would be as described for dogs and cats infested with *Ctenocephalides* sp. Prevention of flea infestation is as described for *L. segnis*.

Public Health Considerations. This flea is an intermediate host for the tapeworms *Hymenolepis diminuta* and *Rodentolepis nana*. Therefore, it is a potential hazard for animal facility personnel. *Xenopsyllus cheopis* transmits *Yersinia pestis,* the cause of plague, and *Rickettsia typhi,* the cause of endemic typhus[462]. The bite of this flea is extremely irritating to humans and produces a reaction similar to that caused by the bite of the dog or cat flea.

Other fleas

Several other species of fleas have been recovered from rats and mice. Most of these reports are from wild rodents. Important aspects of the biology and control of these parasites are similar to those described for *L. segnis, N. fasciatus,* and *X. cheopis*. Fleas that have been recovered from rats and mice include *N. londiniensis, Echidnophaga gallinacea* ("sticktight" flea), *X. ramesis, P. irritans* (human flea), *C. felis* (cat flea), *C. canis* (dog flea), and others[447,453]. Other fleas may be found on rats or mice, but may simply represent transfers from preferred rodent or non-rodent hosts. These fleas include *Orchopeas sexdentatus, Atyphloceras multidentatus, Hoplopsyllus anomalus, Diamanus montanus,* and others[454].

Order Hemiptera (bugs)

True bugs are rarely found in laboratory animal settings; however, they are frequently found on wild rodents. Besides being directly parasitic, some bugs serve as vectors of rodent and human diseases. The family Reduviidae is comprised of some 20 subfamilies. All members of the family are predacious except the Triatominae, which are all parasitic, primarily on endothermal vertebrates. In addition, most triatomes serve as vectors of human and animal diseases, which makes them among the most biomedically important of the bugs. The genera *Paratriotoma, Rhodnius,* and *Triatoma* are the most likely to affect laboratory species. In contrast, *Cimex* sp. (the bedbugs) do not serve as vectors of any infectious diseases, but may potentially be found on laboratory rodents.

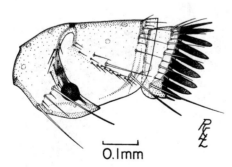

Fig. 11.48 *Nosopsyllus fasciatus.* Courtesy of R.E. Lewis, Iowa State University.

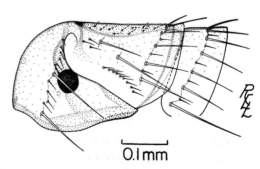

Fig. 11.49 *Xenopsylla cheopis.* Courtesy of R.E. Lewis, Iowa State University.

Cimex lectularis

Cimex lectularis, the human bedbug, is a small, roughly 4-mm to 5-mm long, blood sucking bug. Bedbugs leave the protection of hiding places to feed nocturnally on humans and other animals, including rats and mice[460]. Bedbugs may live longer than a year without a blood meal, so elimination of bedbugs requires the use of pesticides.

Panstrongylus, Paratriatoma, Rhodnius, Triatoma

Morphology. These are also known as "kissing" bugs, "assassin" bugs, or "cone-nosed" bugs. They are obligate blood-feeding ectoparasites. These bugs have three pairs of legs, one pair of four-segmented antennae, a three-segmented proboscis, and two compound eyes[463]. In addition, adults have two simple eyes or ocelli and two pairs of wings. The immature stages do not have functional wings, but the fourth and fifth instar nymphs have wing pads. Eggs are smooth or rough. *Rhodnius prolixus* (Figure 11.50) is typical of these bugs.

Hosts. The usual reservoir host for *Triatoma* and *Paratriatoma* is a pack or wood rat. However, the rock squirrel (*Citellus variegatus*) and armadillo (*D. novemcinctus*) sometimes serve as reservoir host. The usual reservoir hosts for *Rhodnius* are domestic animals and humans[464]. The reservoir hosts for *Panstrongylus* include armadillos (Dasypodidae)[465] and the South American opossum (*Didelphis marsupialis*)[466]. Kissing bugs will feed on wild and laboratory mice and rats[467]. The many species of kissing bugs are found throughout most of the tropical and temperate regions of the Western Hemisphere.

Life Cycle. Kissing bugs are usually not a problem in laboratory settings. These bugs pass through five immature instars to the adult. They usually feed for 10 to 20 minutes and then quickly return to dark, secluded areas in cracks and crevices. Immature stages require at least one blood meal and usually feed two or three times as advanced instars before molting to the next stage. The adults live for more than a year and feed at least once per week, facilitating transmission of blood-borne agents. Females require more blood than do males. Eggs are laid singly and are dropped or glued to the surface at random, depending on the species. The time required for kissing bugs to develop is highly variable, and depends on the temperature, nutrition, and species. Typically, development requires four to eight months under optimum conditions[467].

Pathologic Effects and Clinical Disease. Pathologic changes are rarely reported following examination of rodents infested with kissing bugs. Infestation with kissing bugs does not typically lead to clinical signs.

Diagnosis. Diagnosis is made by finding the parasite on the host or in cracks and crevices in animal buildings.

Treatment. Kissing bugs are not easily killed, and they have developed resistance to a number of residual insecticides. They are relatively strong flyers and can travel long distances. They are seldom found on the host, and therefore control within animal facilities should be directed toward their resting or hiding places. Residual insecticides should be applied as either sprays, dusts, or fumigants to those surfaces where bugs are most likely to crawl upon entering the facility or to places where they hide between feedings[468].

Prevention. Kissing bugs can be prevented from entering the facility by ensuring the structural integrity of the building, properly maintaining door jams, and visually inspecting feed and bedding bags prior to transporting them into the facility.

Public Health Considerations. *Trypanosoma cruzi* (the cause of Chagas' disease), and possibly also hepatitis B virus, may be transmitted by kissing bugs[469]. Repeated bites from these bugs sometimes cause hypersensitivity reactions in humans[470].

Class Arachnida (mites/ticks)

Demodex musculi

Morphology. *Demodex musculi* is a prostigmatid mite in the family Demodicidae. *Demodex musculi* is a very small mite with a characteristic "cigar-shaped" body.

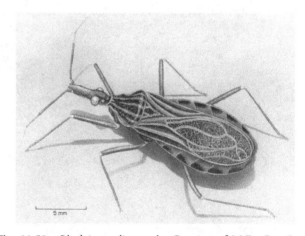

Fig. 11.50 *Rhodnius prolixus* male. Courtesy of M.D. Cox, Loma Linda University.

The elongated abdomen is striated on its dorsal and ventral surfaces. Adult males are about 130 μ in length, while adult females are about 150 μ in length[6]. Adult *D. musculi* are shorter than other *Demodex* sp. that may infest mice[5]. Nymphal and adult stages have four pairs of short, stout legs on the thorax. Setae are absent[440].

Hosts. *Demodex musculi* is considered to be very host-specific, and has only rarely been reported to infest mice. The host range of this parasite is unknown. Until recently[5], *D. musculi* had not been reported in mice for nearly a century[6]. It is possible, however, that the parasite was not identified and reported simply because it was overlooked. In addition to *D. musculi,* at least four other *Demodex* sp. have been reported from various species of mice[471-474]. Of these, only *D. flagellurus* has been recovered from laboratory mice.

Life Cycle. Virtually nothing is known of the life cycle of *D. musculi.* It is likely similar to that of *D. canis,* which infests dogs.

Pathologic Effects and Clinical Disease. Infestations are generally nonpathogenic in immunologically competent mice infested with *D. musculi.* Recently, *D. musculi* was reported in a colony of transgenic mice[5]. Mouse strains represented in that study included B6,CBA-TgN(CD3E)26Cpt (CD3E) mice, which lack mature T-lymphocytes and natural killer cells; B6,SENCARB-TgN(pk5prad1)7111Sprd (*Prad* 1) mice, which are considered to be immunologically competent, but they over express human cyclin D1 and have severe thymic hyperplasia; and double-Tg F1 offspring from these two lines. In addition, *D. musculi* from these mice was experimentally transmitted to SCID and nu/nu (CD-1) mice. *Demodex musculi* was not recovered from immunologically normal sentinel mice in the same room, nor from other strains housed elsewhere in the facility[5]. None of the infested mice developed clinical signs or dermatitis.

Because *D. musculi* is rarely diagnosed, little is known of its pathologic potential. Likewise, minimal tissue reaction has been observed in the tissues of mice infested with other *Demodex* sp.[474] Infestations with *D. musculi* are asymptomatic.

Diagnosis. Mites may be found by examining hairs plucked from the dorsum of the back or from deep skin scrapings collected from the same location, or by histology. Scrapings must be deep enough to include hair follicles. Diagnosis of *D. musculi* should prompt consideration of an underlying immunodeficiency.

Treatment. Little is known about effective treatment strategies for *D. musculi.* Treatments that successfully eliminate *Demodex* sp. from other host species also should eliminate *D. musculi.* Immune-compromised rodents may pose special challenges.

Prevention. The prevalence of *D. musculi* is unknown, but is probably low. The lack of prevalence data complicates formulating recommendations for prevention.

Public Health Considerations. *Demodex musculi* is not considered a public health hazard, because human infestations have not been reported.

Laelaps echidninus

Morphology. *Laelaps echidninus* is known as the "spiny rat mite." *Laelaps echidninus* is occasionally referred to as *Echinolaelaps echidninus.* However, *Echinolaelaps* is a subgenus of *Laelaps* and organisms are not typically referred to by subgenus[475]. Adults of *L. echidninus* are non-burrowing, long-legged, and globular in shape (Figure 11.51). The ventral plates are characteristic. The sternal plate is semi-rectangular, slightly longer than wide, and bears three pairs of setae. The epigynial plate is elongate and flask-shaped, has four pairs of setae, and is concave on its posterior margin. The anterior margin of the anal plate is convex, fitting closely within the concavity of the epigynial plate. All body setae are long and stout, and the first three pairs of coxae bear short, thick ventral spurs. The females are about 1.1 mm long with heavily sclerotized, reddish brown shields. The males are 0.88 mm long[475].

Hosts. *Laelaps echidninus* is common on wild rats[77]. Other natural hosts include the cotton rat and other wild rodents. Laboratory rats and mice are also susceptible, and though rare, infestation of laboratory rodents still occurs.

Life Cycle. Female mites are viviparous. Within five to 17 days of reaching the adult stage, females produce live, hexapod larvae, sometimes by parthenogenesis. Larvae do not feed, but molt into first-stage nymphs in 10 to 13 hours. These feed and molt into second-stage nymphs in three to 11 days. These also feed and molt into adults in three to nine days. Therefore, the entire life cycle requires at least 16 days[476]. Females can live two to three months if fed, but survive only a week without food. The mites live in the bedding and come out at night to feed on abraded skin and body fluids. Although they sometimes suck blood, they can also feed on a variety of other substances, including lacrimal secretions and serous exudate from a living host[477]. They sometimes ingest their own larvae. Under laboratory conditions, they have never been seen to break the intact skin of their host.

Pathologic Effects. Although *L. echidninus* is a blood-sucking arthropod, it is generally considered nonpathogenic. *Laelaps echidninus* serves as the natural vector of the hemogregarine protozoan *Hepatozoon muris*[171]. Experimentally, *Laelaps* sp. also harbor *Francisella tularensis,* the cause of tularemia[478].

Clinical Disease. Natural infestation with *L. echidninus* has not been associated with clinical signs. Experimentally infected suckling mice have been shown to develop footpad lesions[477].

Diagnosis, Treatment, and Prevention. Diagnosis is based on recognition of the mite on a host or in the bedding or cage crevices. There are no guidelines for treatment of *L. echidninus.* Treatments described for other mite infestations would likely be successful. Because *L. echidninus* spends much of its life off the host, control programs should address treatment of the immediate host environment, as discussed for treatment of *O. bacoti.* Prevention is best achieved by excluding wild rodents, maintaining high standards of facility cleanliness, and purchasing animals from reputable vendors.

Public Health Considerations. This parasite is not considered a public health hazard.

Liponyssoides sanguineus

Morphology. *Liponyssoides sanguineus* (Syn. *Allodermanyssus sanguineus*), the "house mouse mite," superficially resembles *O. bacoti* and *Dermanyssus gallinae.* These three mites are readily distinguishable with careful examination[479]. The female has elongate, whiplike chelicerae resembling those of *D. gallinae* (Figure 11.52)[480]. *Liponyssoides sanguineus* has two dorsal shields, an elongate anterior one and a reduced posterior one, and three pairs of setae on the sternal plate. Unengorged females are 650 μ to 750 μ long, and sometimes distend to more than 1 mm after feeding.

Hosts. *Liponyssoides sanguineus* is a blood-sucking mite that occurs on the house mouse, Mongolian gerbil, Egyptian gerbil (*M. libycus*), wild Norway rat, other wild rodents, and humans. It has been found globally. There is only one report of laboratory animal infestation[481].

Life Cycle. The female ingests blood intermittently and oviposits after each feeding[482]. Eggs hatch in four to five days, and the larvae molt in three days without feeding. Both the first and second nymphal stages feed only once; the former molts after four to five days and the latter after six to 19 days. The complete cycle requires 17 to 23 days, and the female can survive up to 51 days without feeding. *Liponyssoides sanguineus* is nidicolous, occurring on the host only when feeding. At other times it dwells in cracks and crevices in close proximity to the host.

Pathologic Effects and Clinical Disease. The effects of *L. sanguineus* on rodent hosts are unknown. In one

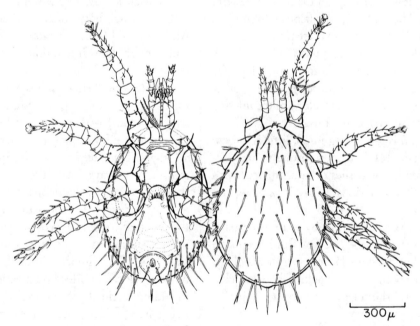

Fig. 11.51 *Laelaps echidninus* female. (Left) Ventral view. (Right) Dorsal view. Reproduced from Strandtmann, R.W. and Mitchell, C.J. (1963) with permission.

report, Levine and Lage reported no clinical signs in infested mice or gerbils[481].

Diagnosis, Treatment, and Prevention. Diagnosis is based on recognition of the mite on a host or on bedding, cages, or racks; under wall moldings; or in ducts, vents, or chutes. Control and prevention strategies have not been adequately investigated, but are likely similar to those described for *O. bacoti*.

Public Health Considerations. The bite of this mite causes dermatitis in humans, similar to that described for *O. bacoti*. Another important zoonotic consideration is the capability of *L. sanguineus* to serve as a vector for *Rickettsia akari,* the cause of rickettsialpox in humans[483].

Myobia musculi

Morphology. *Myobia musculi* is the fur mite of mice. It is a non-burrowing mite in the family Myobiidae. This mite is small, unsclerotized, elongate, and has transverse integumental striae (Figure 11.53)[484]. The male and female differ only in size, setation, and genitalia. The gnathosoma is small, with minute, simple palpi and small, stylet-like chelicerae. The first pair of legs is short, compressed, and highly adapted for hair clasping. The other three pairs are less modified; true claws are absent, but each tarsus ends in a large, claw-like structure, the empodium or empodial claw. The mite is approximately twice as long as

it is wide, and the lateral margins of the posterior body (idiosoma) form bulges between each pair of legs. Females are approximately 400 µ to 500 µ long, and males are 285 µ to 320 µ long. The anus is dorsal. Genitalia consist of a posterior opening on the female dorsum, and an elongate, dorsal, internal penis (aedeagus) in the male. The adult dorsum bears a series of large, slightly expanded, fluted setae.

Eggs are oval and about 200 µ to 250 µ long, resemble miniature louse eggs (nits), and are attached to the bases of hairs at their lower poles[485]. The first larval stage has three pairs of legs. The first pair is used for clasping hair and the second and third pairs are for walking. The larval mouthparts appear as a slender, whip like proboscis. The second larva is larger, and possesses a large, claw-like empodium on the third tarsi and limb buds of the developing fourth legs. Nymphs are larger than the larvae and possess three pairs of walking legs and an anterior pair of hair-clasping legs. In the first nymphal stage, the fourth pair of legs is rudimentary while in the second nymphal stage this pair is well developed and possesses setae and clawlike empodia. Nymphs also have extended mouthparts.

Hosts. *Myobia musculi* infests wild and laboratory mice, and to a lesser extent, rats and closely related rodents throughout the world[77]. Though once common, infestations in mouse colonies are now uncommon. In a large

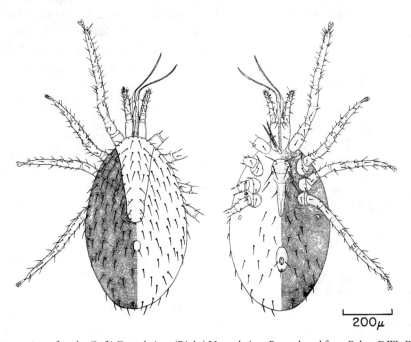

Fig. 11.52 *Liponyssoides sanguineus* female. (Left) Dorsal view. (Right) Ventral view. Reproduced from Baker, E.W., Evans, T.M., Gould, D.J., Hull, W.B., and Keegan, H.L. (1956) with permission.

survey recently conducted at a commercial diagnostic laboratory, infestation was detected in only 0.12% of mice submitted[4].

Life Cycle. Eggs hatch in about seven to eight days[486]. The larval period lasts 10 days, with eight-legged nymphal forms appearing on the 11th day post-hatching. Adults may be observed as early as the 15th day, and are capable of laying eggs within 24 hours[486]. Therefore, the complete life cycle requires about 23 days. All motile stages feed on extracellular tissue fluids. Transmission is by direct transfer of female mites. Neonatal mice become infested as early as the seventh to eighth day of life, shortly after the appearance of the hair coat. New infestations are characterized by an initial increase in mite populations, followed by a decrease coinciding with the development of host immunity[487]. Mite populations generally equilibrate by around eight to 10 weeks. At this point, the host cannot eradicate the parasite, but parasitic populations cannot significantly expand. The equilibrium population level may be carried for long periods of time, even years. Cyclic fluctuations of 20 to 25 days in the equilibrium population level may represent waves of egg hatches[486].

Pathologic Effects. The degree of pathogenicity to mice varies among mouse strains. Nude and other hairless mice are not susceptible. Strains derived from C57BL/6 or NC/Jic mice are genetically predisposed to more severe

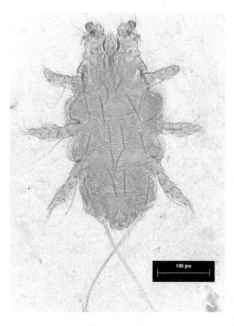

Fig. 11.53 *Myobia musculi* adult female, dorsal view. Reproduced from Baker, D.G. (in press) with permission.

forms of disease[488,489]. Gross skin changes vary from unapparent to mild dermatitis to more severe lesions that include ulceration and pyoderma. Lesions are most common on the head, neck, shoulders, and flank[490]. There appears to be no direct relationship between mite numbers and severity of lesions[491]. In uncomplicated chronic infestations, the epithelium is mildly hyperkeratotic and there is an increase in the presence of chronic inflammatory cells underlying the epithelium, with an increased rate of epithelial cell mitosis[492]. More severe lesions include ulceration and pyoderma[491]. Histologic as well as clinical characteristics support an immediate hypersensitivity component[489].

Other pathologic changes have been associated with acariasis. These include localized lymphadenopathy, variable splenic hypertrophy, epicarditis, pleural thickening, secondary amyloidosis, hypergammaglobulinemia, hypoalbuminemia, and decreased mean hemoglobin concentration[493].

Clinical Disease. Clinical signs associated with *M. musculi* infestation are variable[494], and increase in severity as mice age[490]. Light infestations typically cause no obvious signs and are usually unapparent. However, mouse strains differ in susceptibility and severity of clinical signs. Clinical signs range from mild alopecia and reddening of the skin to extreme pruritus with self-excoriation and deep ulceration[489]. Alopecia begins in the flank area and may become generalized. Deep ulcerations may be complicated by secondary infection[490]. Systemic effects may include decreased life span[492], decreased body weight[490], development of an IgE antibody response[489], and decreased reproductive indices[491].

Diagnosis. The following method of diagnosing *M. musculi* infestations has been described as being very effective[312]: A 5.5-cm by 10-cm strip of transparent shipping tape is applied to the back of a euthanized mouse. The tape is left in place for at least six hours and then examined by light microscopy. A less reliable method is direct examination of the pelage of dead or anesthetized mice under a bright light and dissecting microscope. The hair over the dorsum, nuchal crest area of the skull, cervical dorsum, and area between the scapulae generally yield the greatest number of parasites. If this method is chosen, the hair in these areas should be parted and examined for moving or stationary mites[485].

Treatment. Many compounds have been used in attempts to eradicate mite infestations. Currently used acaricides are at least as effective as older treatments, and are less toxic to the host. One commonly used treatment strategy involves 1% ivermectin diluted 1:100 with a mixture of propylene glycol and water (1:1)[495]. Other investigators[489], including the present author, have found that simply diluting the ivermectin in distilled water and spraying or misting it over the mice also works well. Using this formulation, three weekly treatments apparently did not completely eradicate mites, but did result in negative ectoparasite examinations for up to 18 weeks after the last treatment[495].

Other investigators have used a micropipette to deliver 1% ivermectin (2 mg/kg) once between the scapulae of mice[312]. Ivermectin (200 μg/kg body weight) administered twice subcutaneously one week apart eliminated mites for up to 35 days, which was the duration of the study. One injection of ivermectin reduced, but did not eliminate, the infestation[496]. Other investigators have reported that a single injection of a higher dose (300 μg/kg) will eradicate the infestation[497]. However, follow-up examinations were only performed for a few weeks. In one report, ivermectin administered in drinking water at 10 μg/ml, 25 μg/ml, or 50 μg/ml for four consecutive days successfully eliminated infestation with *M. musculi* and *Myocoptes musculinus*[498]. However, in another report, administration of ivermectin in the drinking water (32 mg/L) for three 10-day periods, separated by a 7-day rest period, did not result in complete elimination of mites until nine weeks after the last treatment[499]. Ivermectin must be used with caution in mice due to potential toxicity in transgenic or young mice.

Permethrins have also been used to control mite infestations. Useful preparations include dips or dusts; the latter is applied to the bedding or to the mice[500]. Chlorpyrifos (Dursban®) has been shown to be effective when six grams of the compound were applied to bedding during twice weekly cage changing for three weeks[501]. Mite infestations were eradicated and no clinical signs of toxicity were observed. However, in some mice, brain acetylcholinesterase levels declined but then returned to normal following completion of the treatment regimen[501]. It should be noted that if an acaricide is ineffective on *in ovo* forms, and lacks residual activity, a second application should take place sometime after day eight, when all eggs will have hatched, but before day 16, when new adults may have laid new eggs[486].

Few acaricidal treatments are 100% effective. Survival of even a few mites constitutes a potential source for reinfestation of the colony. To facilitate eradication, it is also important to thoroughly clean and disinfect all elements of rodent caging, including filter tops. Mite infestation is often a recurring problem, with complete resolution seemingly unattainable. Final eradication may require rederivation of the colony.

Prevention. Because mites may alter host physiology, and infestations may be difficult to eradicate, prevention is preferred over treatment. Mite infestation may be prevented by only procuring mice from reputable sources, carefully examining preshipment health records, examining or treating mice during quarantine, and excluding wild rodents from the animal facility.

Public Health Considerations. *Myobia musculi* is not considered a human health hazard.

Myocoptes musculinus

Morphology. *Myocoptes musculinus* is a non-burrowing mite in the family Myocoptidae. The female is white, oval, and approximately 300 μ to 380 μ long by 130 μ wide (Figure 11.54)[502]. The body is striated; the dorsal striae are scale-like and the ventral ones appear as minute denticles. The genital opening is triangular but, when closed, appears as a transverse slit between the fourth pair of legs. The anus is posterior and ventral, and associated with a pair of long terminal setae. The chelicerae are large and chelate. The first and second legs have six free segments and terminate in short stalks bearing ambulacral suckers. The third and fourth pairs of legs have six segments, but ambulacral suckers are absent. The legs are modified for clasping hairs; they are enlarged and strongly chitinized. The male is smaller (about 160 μ to 210 μ by 135 μ), less striated, and more heavily sclerotized than the female. Anterior to the third pair of legs, it resembles the female, but the posterior portion differs. The aedeagus is located in a deltoid genital opening, the anus is accompanied by a small pair of suckers, and the idiosoma is posteriorly bilobate. The fourth pair of legs is greatly enlarged and has five free segments, none of which are modified for hair-clasping.

Hosts. *Myocoptes musculinus* infests wild and laboratory mice[77]. Infestations were common prior to recent improvements in laboratory animal husbandry. However, in a large survey recently conducted at a commercial diagnostic laboratory, infestation was detected in only 0.10% of mice submitted[4]. A single report of *M. musculinus* infestation of guinea pigs has been described[503].

Life Cycle. The stages of the life cycle include egg, larva, two nymphal stages, and adult. The eggs average

0.20 mm by 0.045 mm in size and hatch within five days. *Myocoptes* eggs are usually attached to the distal part of the hair shaft, in contrast to *Myobia* sp. eggs, which are attached closer to the base of the shaft[502]. All stages occur in the pelage and a complete cycle requires about 14 days. In monospecific infestations, *M. musculinus* occupies the face, head, neck, inguinal region, and base of the tail[504]. If *M. musculi* is also present, *M. musculinus* exhibits some predilection for the skin of the inguinal areas, abdominal ventrum, and back. In heavy mixed infestations, there is some tendency for *M. musculinus* to crowd out populations of *M. musculi*[485]. *Myocoptes musculinus* is considered a more ambulatory species than *M. musculi,* and tends to spread out over greater areas of the body. Transmission requires close, direct contact. Infestation of neonates may occur within four to five days, when hair first appears, with mites attaching to the vibrissae of the young[504]. All life stages of *M. musculinus* migrate to new hosts.

Pathologic Effects. Pathologic changes are often not observed in the skin of mice infested with *M. musculinus.* However, reaction to mite infestation is strain-dependent. Hairless mice are not susceptible. Some conventional, inbred strains such as the C57Bl/6, and less commonly, the BALB/c, develop pruritic dermatopathology typically associated with allergic-type hypersensitivity. Lesions include ulcerative dermatitis, erythema, lymphadenopathy, lymphocytopenia, granulocytosis, and extensive mast cell infiltration of the affected skin and local lymph nodes. These changes are accompanied by greatly elevated serum IgE[505]. Similar changes occur in the skin of NC mice, an atopy-prone inbred strain[506].

Clinical Disease. *Myocoptes musculinus* is considered a surface dweller that feeds on superficial epidermal layers[504]. Clinical signs of infestation are usually absent or unnoticed. When present they may include alopecia, and erythema, pruritus, traumatic dermatitis, dulling of the coat, and wasting also occur[505]. In the guinea pig, *M. musculinus* causes suppurative mange[503].

Diagnosis. Infestations may be reliably diagnosed by using the dorsal tape test as described for *M. musculi,* or by direct examination of the pelage of dead or anesthetized mice under a bright light and dissecting microscope as described for *Polyplax serrata.* The hair over the inguinal areas, abdominal ventrum, and dorsum generally yield the greatest number of parasites. The hair in these areas should be parted and examined for moving or stationary mites.

Myocoptes musculinus must be distinguished from other non-burrowing murine mites, including *M. musculi, Radfordia affinis,* and *Trichoecius romboutsi.* The first two species are readily separated from *M. musculinus* in that only their first pair of legs is modified for clasping hairs.

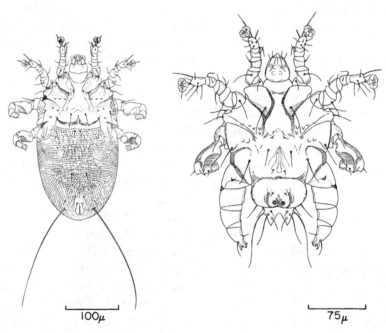

Fig. 11.54 *Myocoptes musculinus.* (Left) Female, ventral view. (Right) Male, ventral view. Reproduced from Baker, E.W., Evans, T.M., Gould, D.J., Hull, W.B., and Keegan, H.L. (1956) with permission.

Myocoptes musculinus is larger than *T. romboutsi,* the female has a broader body, and the male has two long and two short terminal setae, rather than four long terminal setae[507].

Treatment and Prevention. Treatment and prevention recommendations are as described for *M. musculi.*

Public Health Considerations. *Myocoptes musculinus* does not infest humans.

Notoedres muris

Morphology. *Notoedres muris* (Syn. *Notoedres alepis*) is the "mange ear mite of rats." The adult female measures 400 μ by 350 μ long (Figure 11.55). Adult female *Notoedres* sp. may be differentiated from mites of the genus *Sarcoptes.* The anus of adult female *N. muris* is located dorsally, and the adult female *N. muris* lacks heavy dorsal spines, cones, and triangular scales[440]. Also, the middorsal integumental striations are not scale-like, paragenital setae are absent, and the perianal setae are relatively small[508,509]. In contrast, the adult male and immature forms of *N. muris* closely resemble *S. scabiei. Notoedres muris* also resembles *Trixacarus diversus*[510]. The two can be differentiated because *N. muris* lacks a shield and triangular scales on the dorsum, while both are possessed by *T. diversus.*

Hosts. Rats are the natural hosts of *N. muris*[77]. Infestation has also been reported in a variety of wild rodents, including the European hamster (*Cricetus cricetus*), marsh rat (*Holochilus brasiliensis*), and California vole (*M. californicus*)[511–513]. While infestation remains common in wild rats, the mite is rarely observed in laboratory populations.

Life Cycle. Eggs are laid in burrows in the stratum corneum and hatch in four or five days[514]. Pre-adult stages (larva and nymphs) live an average of 14.5 days. The entire life cycle requires 19 to 21 days. Fertilization is thought to occur in the burrows. Transmission is by direct contact.

Pathologic Effects. Following infestation, mites are usually restricted to the stratum corneum, but occasionally they penetrate this layer, giving rise to a more severe skin reaction and serum exudation[514]. Epidermal cells in affected areas proliferate and gradually cornify[508]. Encapsulation of the mite by fibrous tissue does not occur. Localized inflammation, characterized by an increase in neutrophils and lymphocytes, is sometimes so intense as to obscure the dermal fibrous tissues beneath the lesion.

Clinical Disease. Notoedric mange of the rat affects the pinnae, nose, tail, and sometimes the external genitalia and limbs, causing a pruritic and papular, crusting dermatitis[515]. Typical lesions on the pinnae are papilloma-like horny excrescences with yellowish crusts (Figure 11.56).

Those on the nose are also wart-like and horny, but caudal and dermal lesions are erythematous and vesicular or papular.

Diagnosis. Differential diagnosis includes allergic and autoimmune causes, mycotic infections, and self-inflicted trauma. Although the presence of mites and eggs in skin scrapings is diagnostic for mange, care must be taken to differentiate notoedric mange of rats from mange caused by *T. diversus*[516].

Treatment. Beco and co-workers[517] treated *Notoedres*-infested hamsters with ivermectin (400 μg/kg) by subcutaneous injection for eight weekly treatments. At the end of the treatment period, skin scrapings were negative in only 60% of hamsters treated. Therefore, use of ivermectin for the elimination of *N. muris*-infested rats and other rodents should be accompanied by thorough post-treatment examinations. In this regard, burrowing mites may be more difficult to eliminate than non-burrowing mites, possibly requiring repeated treatments at weekly intervals until the infestation is cleared. It is also important to thoroughly clean and disinfect rodent caging to prevent reinfestation. In fact, some investigators have suggested that bedding changes alone may facilitate eradication of *Notoedres* sp. from rodent colonies[518]. A single topical treatment with selamectin (6 to 12 mg/kg) successfully eliminated *N. cati* in a group of 17 cats[519].

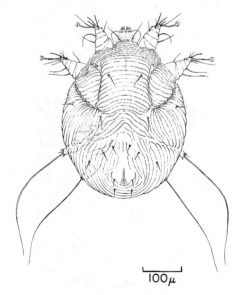

Fig. 11.55 *Notoedres muris* female, dorsal view. Reproduced from Baker, E.W., Evans, T.M., Gould, D.J., Hull, W.B., and Keegan, H.L. (1956) with permission.

Prevention. Animals should only be procured from reputable sources, and should undergo a period of quarantine, ideally including treatment with acaricides. Wild rodents should be excluded from the animal facility.

Public Health Considerations. *Notoedres muris* is not known to infest humans and is therefore not considered a public health concern.

Notoedres spp.

Other *Notoedres* spp. known to infest murid rodents include *N. musculi,* a parasite of the house mouse in Europe, *N. oudemansi,* a parasite of black rats and hedgehogs (*Erinaceus albiventris*) in Africa, *N. pseudomuris* from Ryukyu mice (*M. caroli*) in Taiwan, *N. jamesoni* from bandicoot rats (*Bandicota bengalensis*) in India, *N. paucipilis* from the creek rat (*Pelomys fallax*) in Africa, and *N. douglasi,* a parasite from grey squirrels in California[440,520]. Relatively little is known of the biology of these parasites.

Ornithonyssus bacoti

Morphology. *Ornithonyssus bacoti* (Syn. *Bdellonyssus bacoti, Liponyssus bacoti*) is known as the "tropical rat mite." It is a bloodsucking mesostigmatid mite. The female is white or tan and 750 μ long. When engorged with blood it is dark red or black, and more than 1 mm in length. Body plates are well developed and include an elongate, narrow dorsal shield that does not cover the entire dorsum (Figure 11.57), a rectangular sternal plate with three pairs of setae, an elongate, fingerlike epigynial plate, and an anal plate (Figure 11.58). The setae on the dorsal plate are as long as the other dorsal setae. The chelicerae are well developed, chelate, protrusible, and equal

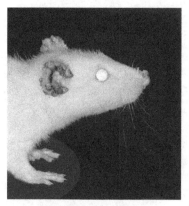

Fig. 11.56 Notoedric mange in a rat. Reproduced from Flynn, R.J. (1960) with permission. Courtesy of J.K. Glaser, Argonne National Laboratory.

in diameter throughout. The male is smaller and possesses chelicerae modified for copulation. A fingerlike spermatodactyl, for the transfer of sperm, is on the movable chela. A single holoventral plate covers the entire intercoxal area and is usually fused with the anal shield[229].

Hosts. *Ornithonyssus bacoti* infests a wide range of mammalian and avian hosts. Natural hosts of *O. bacoti* include several species of rats, mice, hamsters, gerbils, voles, and other wild rodents[447,521-526]. Nonrodent hosts include cats, dogs, chickens and other birds, opossums, humans, and the lesser white-toothed shrew[522,526-528]. *Ornithonyssus bacoti* occurs on wild hosts throughout the world. Laboratory outbreaks involving research animals, as well as facility personnel, have been reported[529,530].

Life Cycle. Adult mites suck blood. The adult female survives about 70 days, deposits up to 100 eggs in the bedding or in crevices, and feeds every two to three days during this period. Larvae hatch in one to four days and molt within one day without feeding. The first nymphal stage sucks blood and generally molts five to 14 days after feeding. It can survive for a month without food. The second nymphal stage is sluggish, does not feed, and molts in one to two days. Adults copulate 24 hours after emerging, and the life cycle can be completed in 13 days. *Ornithonyssus bacoti* is an obligate, intermittent blood feeder. All stages live in close proximity to the host, but usually only nymphs and adults occur on the host[531]. When not on the host, mites retreat to hiding areas such as cage bedding, filter tops, cage racks, etc.

Pathologic Effects. This mite ingests blood and causes debility and anemia[532]. *Ornithonyssus bacoti* can transmit several other pathogens, including the agents of murine typhus (*R. typhi*), rickettsialpox (*R. akari*), Q fever (*Coxiella burnetii*), Lyme disease (*Borrelia burgdorferi*), hemorrhagic fever with renal syndrome, and plague (*Y. pestis*)[533-535]. However, *O. bacoti* is probably not an important natural vector of any of these pathogens. It is, however, a common vector of *L. carinii* and closely related filarial nematode species which infect cotton rats and other wild rodents[524,536].

Clinical Disease. Clinical signs are generally limited to decreased reproduction in affected mouse colonies, though severe infestation may lead to death[532].

Diagnosis. Infestation of an animal colony with *O. bacoti* is easily diagnosed. Engorged mites are readily seen on bedding, cages, filter tops, and racks, but typically not on the animals. Identification is based on morphologic characteristics.

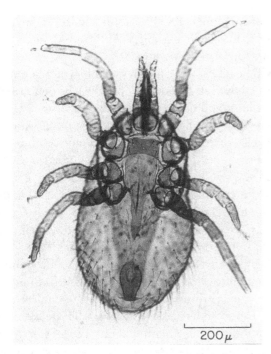

Fig. 11.57 *Ornithonyssus bacoti* female, ventral view. Courtesy of C. Taylor, Rocky Mountain Laboratory, U.S. Public Health Service.

Treatment. Many compounds have been used in attempts to eradicate mite infestations, including *O. bacoti*. These are more fully discussed in the section describing treatment of *M. musculi* infestation. Unlike most of the other non-burrowing mites, however, direct application of chemicals to the animals may not be necessary, because the parasite is only on the host when feeding. Malathion (1%) has been effectively used to eradicate *O. bacoti* from rodent colonies[537]. Chlorpyrifos (Dursban®) has likewise been used to eliminate *M. musculi* and would likely eliminate *O. bacoti* as well[501]. It is likely that other, newer, safer acaricides such as pyrmethrins[500], which can also be applied to the caging, would also be effective. Ivermectin applied topically, by injection, or in the drinking water, as described for treatment of *M. musculi,* would likely also be effective, but these routes of administration have not been tested against *O. bacoti*.

Prevention. Infestation with mites can be prevented by maintaining a high degree of sanitation, procuring animals from uninfested sources, and excluding wild rodents from the facility.

Public Health Considerations. This mite readily feeds on humans, causing a condition known as tropical rat mite dermatitis[526]. Humans are most often attacked in the absence of its preferred hosts. *Ornithonyssus bacoti* can

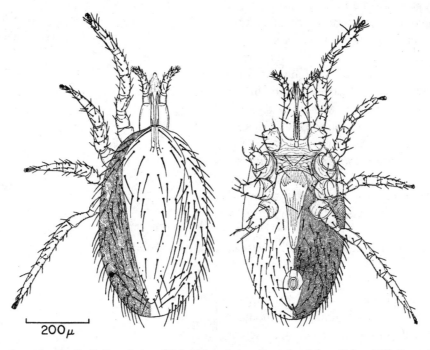

Fig. 11.58 *Ornithonyssus bacoti* female. (Left) Dorsal view. (Right) Ventral view. Reproduced from Baker, E.W., Evans, T.M., Gould, D.J., Hull, W.B., and Keegan, H.L. (1956) with permission.

harbor certain pathogens following their ingestion in a blood meal, as previously described. These pathogens include *R. typhi, R. acari, C. burnetti, F. tularensis,* Eastern equine encephalitis virus, hemorrhagic fever with renal syndrome virus, *B. burgdorferi,* and *Y. pestis*[533–535]. Therefore, animals infested with this mite should be handled with caution.

Psorergates simplex

Morphology. *Psorergates simplex* is also known as the "follicle mite of mice." It is a minute, rounded mite which ranges in length from approximately 90 µ to 150 µ long (Figure 11.59)[538]. Adults and nymphs have four pairs of legs. These are radially arranged, each with five telescoping segments; the larva has three pairs of legs. The mite can be distinguished from other similarly sized mites by the presence of a medially directed spine on the ventral surface of each femur. Each tarsus terminates in a pair of simple claws and a pad-like empodium. The palpal segments are undifferentiated and coalesced. Chelicerae are minute, protrusible, stylet-like and enclosed in a small, conical rostrum. The anus is ventral with a tubercle on each side. The female has a pair of long, whip-like setae on each tubercle; the male has a single seta on each side[440] and a dorsal penis.

Hosts. Mice are the natural hosts of *P. simplex.* Infestation of wild mice appears to be relatively uncommon. Though once commonplace, infestation of laboratory mice is now extremely rare. In a large survey recently conducted at a commercial diagnostic laboratory, infestation was not detected in more than 14,000 mice submitted[4]. It appears that mouse strain may influence susceptibility to infestation. In one study, Swiss stock were infested, while those of C3H, BALB/c, DBA, A, and C57 strains were not[507].

Life Cycle. The life cycle of *P. simplex* is incompletely known. All stages are found in a single follicle or lesion (Figure 11.60). Colonization of a follicle apparently results from the entrance of a gravid female. Transmission is by direct contact.

Pathologic Effects. Infestation of mice with *P. simplex* is characterized by formation of skin nodules or "pouches" (Figure 11.61)[540]. These are small (up to 2 mm), distended, whitish, cyst-like dermal structures that contain mites and cellular debris. Histologically, the nodules resemble comedones and consist of invaginated sacs of squamous epithelium filled with mites, mite products, and keratinaceous debris. Skin nodules are thought to form as a

result of epidermal growth to accommodate internal pressure of space-occupying mites. All life cycle stages of the mite are found in the nodules[539].

Clinical Disease. Clinical signs are typically restricted to formation of skin nodules. These may be unapparent in the live host, and only noticed upon inversion of the skin at necropsy. Typically, skin nodules form in the skin of the legs, back, trunk, abdomen, shoulders, and head, but may occur anywhere[540]. Nodules tend to be larger in the loose skin of the trunk, and smaller where the skin is tighter, such as the face and legs. A second, auricular clinical manifestation occurs rarely. This form develops slowly, and may have a severe, mange-like appearance, with thick, yellow crusting of one or both surfaces of the pinna[541].

Diagnosis. *Psorergates simplex* can be diagnosed by examination of the inverted subcuticular surface of the pelt for the characteristic cyst-like nodules. Nodule contents may be expressed by pressure of a scalpel blade or by scraping and the contents mounted under a cover slip in water, glycerine, or 10% potassium hydroxide for microscopic examination. Care must be taken to distinguish between psorergatic and notoedric ear mange. Definitive diagnosis is made by identification of the mite.

Treatment. Little information is available on modern treatments for psorergatic mange of rodents. A single

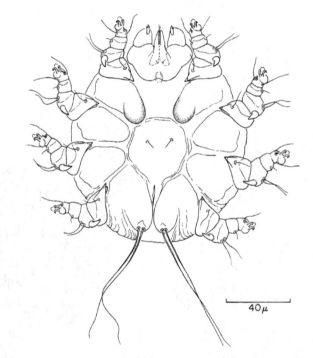

Fig. 11.59 *Psorergates simplex* female, ventral view. Courtesy of A.D. Smith, Rocky Mountain Laboratory, U.S. Public Health Service.

treatment with ivermectin, administered by subcutaneous injection of 200 µg/kg, has been reported to be effective in clearing *P. ovis*-infested sheep[542] and stumptailed macaques infested with *Psorergates* sp.[543]. It is likely that ivermectin would also be effective against *P. simplex*.

Prevention. *Psorergates simplex* is rare in modern rodent facilities. Infestation may be prevented by procuring mice only from uninfested sources; including quarantine, treatment, and sentinel surveillance in the pathogen control program; and excluding wild rodents from the animal facility.

Public Health Considerations. *Psorergates simplex* is not known to infest humans.

Radfordia affinis

Morphology. *Radfordia affinis* (Syn. *Myobia affinis*) is another mouse fur mite. It is a nonburrowing, pelage-inhabiting mite in the family Myobiidae. *Radfordia affinis* is morphologically similar to *M. musculi* (Figure 11.62)[544]. The two can be differentiated by scrutiny of the tarsal terminus of the second pair of legs. *Radfordia affinis* has two tarsal claws of unequal length, while *M. musculi* has a single empodial claw. *Radfordia affinis* may be differentiated from *R. ensifera* of rats, again by comparing of the tarsal claws of the second pair of legs. The claws are paired and unequal in length in *R. affinis* and paired and equal in length in *R. ensifera*[545]. Relatively little is known of the life cycle of *R. affinis*. It is assumed that the life cycle is similar to that of *M. musculi*.

Hosts. The house mouse is the natural host of *R. affinis*. Infestations of both laboratory and wild mice have been reported[546,547]. Historically, infestation of laboratory mice was common in many parts of the world. However, in a large survey recently conducted at a commercial diagnostic laboratory, infestation was detected in only 0.01% of mice submitted[4].

Life Cycle. The life cycle of *R. affinis* is similar to that of *M. musculi*.

Pathologic Effects and Clinical Disease. Relatively little is known of the pathologic effects or clinical disease caused by *R. affinis*. It is likely that lesion development and clinical signs are similar to those described for *M. musculi*.

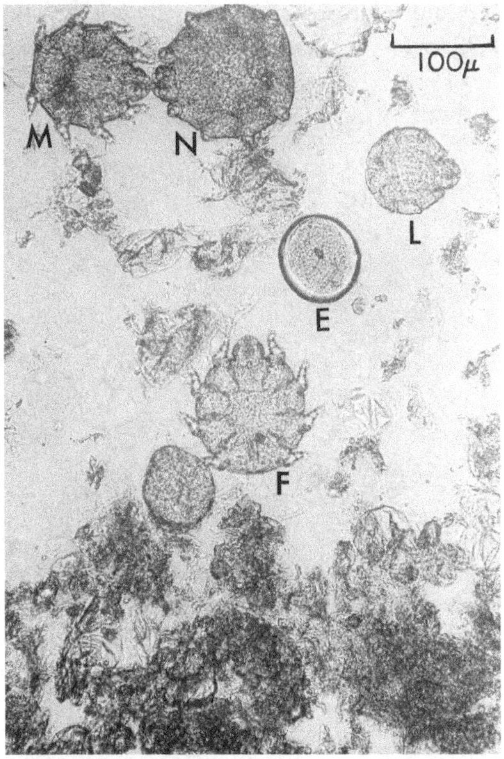

Fig. 11.60 *Psorergates simplex* egg (E), female (F), larva (L), male (M), and nymph (N). Reproduced from Flynn, R.J. and Jaroslow, B.N. (1956) with permission.

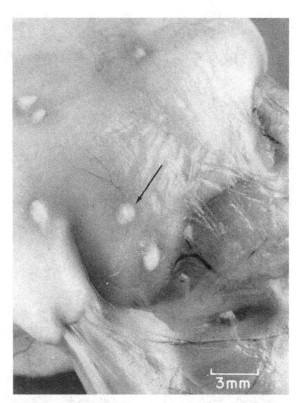

Fig. 11.61 Nodules in skin (visceral surface) of a mouse caused by *Psorergates simplex*. Reproduced from Flynn, R.J. and Jaroslow, B.N. (1956) with permission.

Diagnosis, Treatment, and Prevention. Practices effective for *M. musculi* should also be effective for *R. affinis*.

Public Health Considerations. *Radfordia affinis* does not infest humans.

Radfordia ensifera

Morphology. *Radfordia ensifera* (Syn. *Myobia ensifera*, *Myobia ratti*) is the rat fur mite. It is morphologically and biologically similar to *S. affinis* of mice. The two can be distinguished by comparing the tarsal claws of the second pair of legs. The claws are paired and unequal in length in *R. affinis* and paired and equal in length in *R. ensifera* (Figure 11.63)[545].

Hosts. *Radfordia ensifera* was once common in laboratory rat colonies. In a large survey recently conducted at a commercial diagnostic laboratory, infestation was detected in only 0.02% of rats submitted[4]. Infestation of wild rats remains common[447].

Life Cycle. The life cycle of *R. ensifera* is likely similar to that of *M. musculi* of mice.

Pathologic Effects and Clinical Disease. Relatively little is known of the pathobiology or clinical symptoms of *R. ensifera*. One report described clinical disease, including pruritus, alopecia, and self-excoriation in rats infested with *R. ensifera*, similar to that described for *M. musculi*[548]. It is likely that as for other mite infestations, debilitation, overcrowding, and poor husbandry may exacerbate disease.

Diagnosis. *Radfordia ensifera* infestations may be reliably diagnosed using the dorsal tape test as described for *M. musculi*[312].

Treatment and Prevention. It is likely that treatment and prevention strategies useful for eliminating and preventing *M. musculi* infestations will also be successful against *R. ensifera*. In one report, microdot delivery of 1% ivermectin (2 mg/kg body weight) to the dorsal skin, given three times at approximately two week intervals, eliminated *R. ensifera* from a colony of Long Evans rats[549].

Public Health Considerations. *Radfordia ensifera* is not known to infest humans.

Trichoecius romboutsi

Morphology. *Trichoecius romboutsi* (Syn. *Myocoptes romboutsi*) is a non-burrowing mite in the family Myocoptidae[550]. *Trichoecius romboutsi* is smaller than *M. musculinus*;

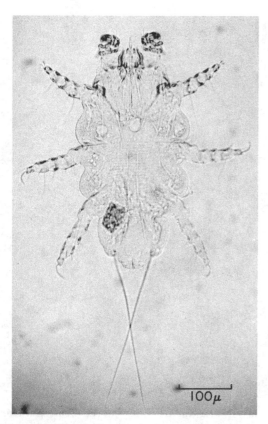

Fig. 11.62 *Radfordia affinis* female. Reproduced from Flynn, R.J. (1963) with permission.

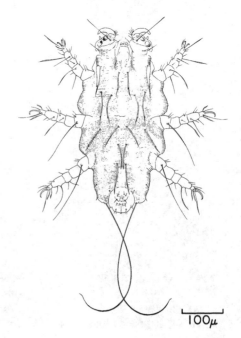

Fig. 11.63 *Radfordia ensifera* female, dorsal view. Reproduced from Baker, E.W., Evans, T.M., Gould, D.J., Hull, W.B., and Keegan, H.L. (1956) with permission.

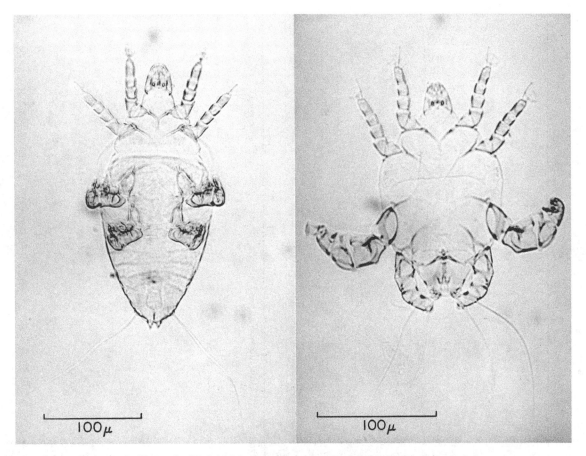

Fig. 11.64 *Trichoecius romboutsi*. (Left) Female. (Right) Male. Reproduced from Flynn, R.J. (1963) with permission.

the female is about 200 μ to 280 μ and the male about 160 μ to 190 μ long (Figure 11.64)[550]. The female is narrower than *M. musculinus* and the male has four long, rather than two long and two short, terminal setae.

Hosts. *Trichoecius romboutsi* has been reported from mice in the United States and Europe[550]. The mite was found in a survey of commercial mouse breeders in the United States in 1955[507]. However, in a similar survey 10 years later, the mite was not observed[551]. Its prevalence in laboratory colonies is now considered rare. In a large survey recently conducted at a commercial diagnostic laboratory, infestation was not detected in more than 14,000 mice submitted[4]. However, *T. romboutsi* closely resembles *M. musculinus,* and failure to identify it may account for the lack of reports of its occurrence.

Life Cycle. Relatively little is known of the life cycle of *T. romboutsi*. It is probably similar to that of *M. musculinus*. Life cycle stages include the egg, larva, two nymphal stages, and adults[550].

Pathologic Effects and Clinical Disease. Relatively little is known of the pathologic effects and clinical disease associated with *T. romboutsi*. However, it is likely that these are similar to the condition caused by *M. musculinus*.

Diagnosis, Treatment, and Prevention. These aspects of infestation with *T. romboutsi* are likely similar to *M. musculinus,* and therefore as described for *M. musculi*.

Public Health Considerations. *Trichoecius romboutsi* is not considered a public health hazard, because infestation of humans with this parasite has not been reported.

Trixacarus diversus

Trixacarus diversus (Syn. *Sarcoptes anacanthos*) is a sarcoptid mite that closely resembles *N. muris*[516]. Natural hosts include rats, mice, and hamsters. Infested rats may develop

TABLE 11.1 Parasites of rats and mice—circulatory/lymphatic system.

Parasite	Geographic distribution	Hosts	Location in host	Method of infection	Pathologic effects	Zoonosis	Reference
Flagellates							
Trypanosoma conorhini	Asia, South America	Rats, Asian monkeys	Blood	Passed in feces of reduviid bug	None	Not reported	7
Trypanosoma cruzi	Americas	Rodents and other mammals	Blood, myocardium	Passed in feces of reduviid bug	Myocarditis, anemia, splenomegaly, lymphadenitis	Trypanosomiasis ("Chaga's disease")	552
Trypanosoma lewisi	Worldwide	Rats	Blood	Passed in flea feces	Usually none; may cause arthritis of distal extremities	Reported in children and immune-suppressed adults	10
Trypanosoma musculi	Worldwide	Mice	Blood	Passed in flea feces	Usually none	Not reported	36
Leishmania donovani	Asia, Africa	Rodents and other mammals	Phagocytic cells, visceral organs	Sand fly bite; skin contamination with crushed flies or fly feces	Splenomegaly, hepatomegaly, lymphadenopathy	Visceral leishmaniosis ("kala-azar")	27
Leishmania tropica	Asia, Mediterranean Basin	Wild rodents (also found in dogs, cats, man)	Phagocytic cells, skin, mucous membranes	Sand fly bite; skin contamination with crushed flies or fly feces	Cutaneous ulcers	Cutaneous leishmaniasis	27
Coccidia							
Hepatozoon muris	Worldwide	Rat	Lymphocytes, liver	Ingestion of mite vector, *Laelaps echidninus*	May cause splenomegaly, hepatitis, anemia	Not reported	27
Hepatozoon musculi	Great Britain	Mice	Lymphocytes, bone marrow	Unknown	Unknown	Not reported	27
Piroplasmids and Haemosporidia							
Babesia microti	Worldwide	Rats, other rodents, dogs	Erythrocytes	Tick transmission	Renal degeneration, hemoglobinuria, sometimes death	Reported	27
Babesia rodhaini	Worldwide	Tree rats (*Thamnomys surdaster*)	Erythrocytes	Tick transmission	Hemolytic anemia, mononuclear phagocytic system hyperplasia, hepatitis	Not reported	209
Plasmodium berghei	Africa	Tree rats	Erythrocytes	Mosquito transmission	Malaria in mouse and pregnant rat	Not reported	217
Plasmodium chabaudi	Africa	Tree rats	Erythrocytes	Mosquito transmission	Malaria in mouse	Not reported	220
Plasmodium inopinatum	Europe	Wild rats	Erythrocytes	Mosquito transmission	Malaria	Not reported	215
Plasmodium vinckei	Africa	Tree rats	Erythrocytes	Mosquito transmission	Malaria in mouse	Not reported	222

Nematodes

Metastrongyloidea

Angiostrongylus (Parastrongylus) cantonensis	Asia, North America, Pacific Islands	Wild rats and other rodents; bats, horses, dogs, opossums, others	Pulmonary artery, brain	Ingestion of mollusk intermediate host, or paratenic host	Pulmonary and central nervous system reactions to migrating larvae	Reported (Eosinophilic meningitis)	350
Angiostrongylus costaricensis	Central and South America	Cotton rats, rats, others	Cranial mesenteric artery, subserosal arteries of the cecum	Ingestion of intermediate host	Arteritis	Reported (Intestinal eosinophilic granulomata)	361
Angiostrongylus spp.	Worldwide	Wild rodents	Pulmonary artery	Ingestion of intermediate host	Pulmonary reactions to migrating larvae	Possible, depending on species	229, 368–370

TABLE 11.2   Parasites of Rats and Mice—Enterohepatic System.

Parasite	Geographic distribution	Hosts	Location in host	Method of infection	Pathologic effects	Zoonosis	Reference
Flagellates							
Chilomastix bettencourti	Worldwide	Mice, rats, hamsters	Cecum	Ingestion of cysts	None	None	47
Enteromonas hominis	Worldwide	Rats, hamsters, rabbits, primates	Cecum	Ingestion of organism passed in feces	None	Reported	27
Giardia muris	Worldwide	Mice, rats, hamsters, other rodents	Anterior small intestine	Ingestion of cysts passed in feces	Enteritis, villus changes	Not reported	66
Giardia simoni	Worldwide	Rats, hamsters	Anterior small intestine	Ingestion of cysts passed in feces	Associated with jejunal tympanites in rats	Not reported	27
Hexamastix muris	Worldwide	Rats, hamsters, other rodents	Cecum	Ingestion of organism passed in feces	Villus changes	Not reported	27, 62
Monocercomonoides sp.	North America	Rats, hamsters	Cecum	Ingestion of organism passed in feces	None	Not reported	27, 70
Octomitus pulcher	Worldwide	Mice, rats, hamsters, squirrels, other rodents	Cecum	Ingestion of organism passed in feces	None	Not reported	27
Pentatrichomonas hominis	Worldwide	Mice, rats, hamsters, dogs, cats, cattle, primates	Cecum, colon	Ingestion of organism passed in feces	None	Reported	71, 72
Retortamonas sp.	North America	Rats	Cecum	Ingestion of cysts passed in feces	None	Not reported	27, 73
Spironucleus muris	Worldwide	Rats, mice, hamsters, other rodents	Small intestine, cecum	Ingestion of cysts passed in feces	Enteritis in immune-deficient mice	Not reported	81
Tetratrichomonas microti	North America	Mice, rats, hamsters, voles, other rodents	Cecum	Ingestion of organism passed in feces	None	Not reported	85
Trichomitus wenyoni	North America	Mice, rats, hamsters, rhesus monkeys, baboons	Cecum, colon	Ingestion of organism passed in feces	None	Not reported	86
Tritrichomonas muris	Worldwide	Rats, Mice, other rodents	Cecum, colon, small intestine	Ingestion of "pseudocyst"	None	Not reported	45, 89
Tritrichomonas minuta	North America, Europe	Mice, rats, hamsters	Cecum, colon	Ingestion of organism passed in feces	None	Not reported	27
Amoebae							
Endolimax ratti	Worldwide	Rats	Cecum, colon	Ingestion of cysts passed in feces	None	Not reported	27
Entamoeba muris	Worldwide	Mice, rat, hamster	Cecum, colon	Ingestion of cysts passed in feces	None	Not reported	93
Coccidia							
Cryptosporidium muris	North America	Mice, rats	Stomach	Ingestion of sporulated oocyst in feces	Gastric mastocytosis	Not reported	96, 102, 104
Cryptosporidium parvum	North America	Mice, most other mammals	Small intestine	Ingestion of sporulated oocyst in feces	Enteritis in immune-deficient mammals	Common	105

Eimeria falciformis	Worldwide	Mice	Large intestine	Ingestion of sporulated oocyst in feces	Catarrhal enteritis, death	Not reported	110
Eimeria miyairii	Worldwide	Rats	Small intestine	Ingestion of sporulated oocyst in feces	None	Not reported	122
Eimeria nieschulzi	Worldwide	Rats	Small intestine	Ingestion of sporulated oocyst in feces	Enteritis, villus changes, diarrhea, death	Not reported	133
Eimeria separata	Worldwide	Rats	Cecum, colon	Ingestion of sporulated oocyst in feces	Mild enteritis	Not reported	27
Eimeria spp.	Worldwide	Mice	Intestine	Ingestion of sporulated oocyst in feces	None	Not reported	27, 108, 134
Isospora ratti	North America	Rats	Intestine	Presumably by ingestion of sporulated oocyst in feces	Unknown	Not reported	108
Trematodes							
Ascocotyle (Phagicola) sp.	Worldwide	Rats	Small intestine	Ingestion of metacercaria encysted in fish	Unknown	Reported	556
Echinostoma spp.	Worldwide	Rats, other rodents, birds (species dependent)	Small intestine, cecum, rectum	Ingestion of mollusk intermediate host	Enteritis (species dependent)	Reported	557
Plagiorchis spp.	Worldwide	Mice, rats, hamsters	Intestine	Ingestion of infected snail intermediate host	Unknown	Common	558
Postharmostomum helicis	North America	Deer mice, other rodents	Cecum	Ingestion of infected snail intermediate host	Typhlitis	Not reported	559
Stellantchasmus falcatus	Asia	Rats, mice, dogs, cats, man	Small intestine	Ingestion of metacercaria encysted in fish	Unknown	Reported	560
Cestodes							
Cyclophyllidea							
Cataenotaenia pusilla	Africa, Europe	Mice, rats, hamsters	Intestine	Ingestion of arthropod intermediate host	None	Not reported	223
Hymenolepis citelli	North America	Ground squirrels, mice, rats, kangaroo rats	Intestine	Ingestion of arthropod intermediate host	Unknown	Not reported	561
Hymenolepis diminuta	Worldwide	Rats, mice, other rodents, primates	Small intestine	Ingestion of arthropod intermediate host	Catarrhal enteritis	Reported	224
Raillietina celebensis	Worldwide	Wild rats, man	Intestine	Unknown	Unknown	Reported	562
Rodentolepis (Hymenolepis) microstoma	Worldwide	Mice, cotton rats, hamsters	Duodenum, biliary system, liver	Ingestion of arthropod intermediate host	Biliary inflammation, mucosal erosion	Reported	252
Rodentolepis (Hymenolepis) nana	Worldwide	Mice, rats, hamsters, other rodents	Intestine	Direct transmission or ingestion of arthropod intermediate host	Catarrhal enteritis, abscesses, focal granulomatous lymphadenitis, retarded growth, weight loss, death	Probably not susceptible to rodent strains	233, 236

(Continued)

TABLE 11.2 (*Continued*)

Parasite	Geographic distribution	Hosts	Location in host	Method of infection	Pathologic effects	Zoonosis	Reference
Larval							
Echinococcus granulosis	Worldwide	Rodents, many domesticated mammals, primates, man	Liver, lungs, brain, peritoneal cavity	Ingestion of eggs passed in canine feces	Unapparent unless hydatid interferes with local tissues	Common "Hydatid disease"	563
Echinococcus multilocularis	Worldwide	Deer mice, voles, hamsters, lemmings, other rodents, man	Liver	Ingestion of eggs passed in canine feces	Liver cysts, death	Common "Hydatid disease"	564
Taenia taeniaeformis	Worldwide	Mice, rats, hamsters, gerbils, voles, other wild rodents	Liver	Ingestion of embryonated egg passed in cat feces	Strobilocercus in liver; may cause hepatic sarcoma	Reported	264
Adult							
Cataenotaenia pusilla	Worldwide	Mice, rats	Small intestine	Ingestion of intermediate host (grain mite)	None	Not reported	223
Nematodes							
Rhabditoidea							
Strongyloides ratti	Worldwide	Rats	Adult: duodenum, jejunum; Larva: lungs	Ingestion or skin/mucosal penetration	Dermatitis	Not reported	268, 269, 273
Strongyloides sigmodontis	Americas	Cotton rats	Adult: intestine; Larva: lungs	Ingestion or skin/mucosal penetration	None	Not reported	565, 566
Strongyloides venezuelensis	Worldwide	Rats, mice, cotton rats, gerbils, hamsters	Adult: duodenum, jejunum; Larva: lungs	Ingestion or skin/mucosal penetration, transmammary	Dermatitis, pneumonia	Not reported	291, 295
Heterakoidea							
Heterakis spumosa	Worldwide	Rats, mice, moles, other rodents	Cecum, colon	Ingestion of embryonated egg	None	Not reported	298
Oxyuroidea							
Aspiculuris tetraptera	Worldwide	Mice, other rodents	Cecum, colon	Ingestion of embryonated egg	Usually none	Not reported	304
Syphacia muris	Worldwide	Rats, mice, gerbils, hamsters	Cecum, colon	Ingestion of embryonated egg; retrofection	Weight loss, impaired intestinal electrolyte transport	Not reported	318, 322
Syphacia obvelata	Worldwide	Mice, rats, hamsters, voles, other rodents, primates	Cecum, colon	Ingestion of embryonated egg; retrofection	Catarrhal enteritis, hepatic granulomas, perianal irritation	Rare	327, 330

374

	Geographic distribution	Host	Site in host	Mode of infection	Pathology	Prevalence	Reference
Trichostrongyloidea							
Heligmonoides murina	Africa	Mice	Small intestine	Ingestion of larva	None	Not reported	308
Heligmosomoides polygyrus	Europe, North America	Rodents	Small intestine	Ingestion of larva	None in immunologically normal hosts	Not reported	339
Longistriata spp.	North America	Rats, mice	Small intestine	Ingestion of larva or skin penetration	None	Not reported	308, 567
Nippostrongylus brasiliensis	Worldwide	Rat, mice	Small intestine	Larval penetration of skin	Dermatitis, pneumonitis, enteritis	Not reported	345
Orientostrongylus ezoensis	Asia	Rats	Small intestine	Ingestion of larva	None	Not reported	568
Trichostrongylus sigmodontis	North America	Cotton rats, rice rats	Small intestine	Ingestion of larva	None	Not reported	569
Spiruroidea							
Gongylonema musculi	Europe	Mice	Esophagus, stomach	Ingestion of intermediate host (insects)	None	Not reported	308
Gongylonema neoplasticum	Worldwide	Rodents, lagomorphs	Esophagus, stomach	Ingestion of intermediate host (cockroaches, mealworms, fleas)	Gastric ulcers	Not reported	570
Mastophorus spp.	Worldwide	Rodents	Stomach	Ingestion of intermediate host (cockroaches)	None	Not reported	571
Physaloptera spp.	Americas, Europe	Rodents	Stomach	Ingestion of intermediate host (insects)	Gastroenteritis	Not reported	308, 572
Rictularia spp.	Worldwide	Mice, rats, squirrels	Small intestine	Ingestion of intermediate host (arthropods)	None	Rare	308, 573
Trichuroidea							
Trichuris arvicolae	Worldwide	Voles	Cecum, colon	Ingestion of embryonated egg	None	Not reported	381
Trichuris muris	Worldwide	Rats, mice, other rodents	Cecum, colon	Ingestion of embryonated egg	None	Not reported	381
Calodium hepaticum (*Capillaria hepatica*)	Worldwide	Rodents, many other mammals	Liver	Ingestion of embryonated egg	Hepatitis	Reported	379, 574
Capillaria spp.	Worldwide	Mice, rats, other rodents	Esophagus, intestine, small intestine, stomach (species dependent)	Ingestion of embryonated egg or ingestion of earthworm (species dependent)	None	Not reported	229, 298
Trichinella spiralis	Worldwide	Rats, mice, many other mammals	Adult: intestinal mucosa; Larva: skeletal muscle, various organs	Ingestion of encysted larva	Enteritis	Common	575

(Continued)

TABLE 11.2 *(Continued)*

Parasite	Geographic distribution	Hosts	Location in host	Method of infection	Pathologic effects	Zoonosis	Reference
Acanthocephala							
Moniliformis clarki	North America	Wild rodents, primates	Small intestine	Ingestion of intermediate host	Enteritis	Not reported	576
Moniliformis dubius	Africa, Asia, Europe	Wild rodents	Small intestine	Ingestion of intermediate host	Enteritis	Reported	577
Moniliformis moniliformis	Worldwide	Rodents, dogs, apes	Small intestine	Ingestion of intermediate host	Enteritis, peritonitis	Reported	578

TABLE 11.3 Parasites of Rats and Mice—Musculoskeletal System.

Parasite	Geographic distribution	Hosts	Location in host	Method of infection	Pathologic effects	Zoonosis	Reference
Coccidia							
Sarcocystis muris	Worldwide	Mice (cats = definitive host)	Striated and smooth muscle	Ingestion of sporulated sporocysts; cannibalism	Cysts in muscle, myositis, splenomegaly	Not reported	185
Sarcocystis dispersa, S. scotti, S. sebeki	Worldwide	Mice (owls = definitive host)	Striated and smooth muscle	Ingestion of sporulated sporocysts; or through cannibalism	Cysts in muscle	Not reported	27
Sarcocystis cymruensis	Worldwide	Wild rats and other rodents (cat = definitive host)	Cardiac and skeletal muscle	Ingestion of sporulated sporocysts; or through cannibalism	Cysts in muscle	Not reported	191
Sarcocystis singaporensis, S. villivillosi, S. zamani	Asia	Wild rats and other rodents (snakes = definitive host)	Muscle	Ingestion of sporulated sporocysts; or through cannibalism	Cysts in muscle; protozoal pneumonia (*S. singaporensis*)	Not reported	27, 192
Sarcocystis sulawesiensis, S. dirumpens, S. murinotechis	Asia	Wild rats and other rodents (definitive host unknown)	Muscle	Ingestion of sporulated sporocysts; or through cannibalism	Cysts in muscle	Not reported	27, 193, 196

TABLE 11.4 Parasites of Rats and Mice—Skin and Connective Tissues.

Parasite	Geographic distribution	Hosts	Location in host	Method of infection	Pathologic effects	Zoonosis	Reference
Coccidia							
Besnoitia spp.	Americas	Wild rodents	Connective tissues, serosal membranes	Ingestion of sporulated oocyst	Acute, fatal or chronic disease	Not reported	580, 581
Cestodes							
Larval							
Diphyllobothrium (Spirometra) erinacei	Worldwide	Wild rodents	Subcutis and muscle	Ingestion of first intermediate host (crustaceans)	Cysts in subcutis and muscle	Reported ("Sparganosis")	582
Mesocestoides corti	Americas	Wild rodents, dogs, cats, other mammals	Peritoneal cavity, liver, other organs	Ingestion of first intermediate host (oribatid mites)	Cysts in liver, other abdominal organs; occasionally debilitation; sometimes ascites, death	Reported	583
Mesocestoides lineatus	Africa, Asia, Europe	Wild rodents, dogs, cats, other mammals	Peritoneal cavity, pleural cavity	Ingestion of first intermediate host	Cysts in abdominal organs; occasionally debilitation; sometimes ascites, death	Reported	584
Taenia taeniaformis	Worldwide	Wild rodents, lagomorphs	Liver	Ingestion of eggs passed by definitive host (cats)	Generally none	Not reported	585
Spirometra mansonoides	Americas	Deer mice, hamsters, voles, man	Connective tissue	Ingestion of first intermediate host (crustaceans)	Cysts in connective tissue, alteration of growth rate	Reported ("Sparganosis")	229
Nematodes							
Rhabditoidea							
Pelodera strongyloides	Worldwide	Wild rodents, other domestic mammals, man	Skin lesions	Wound contamination with larva	Dermatitis	Reported	586
Metastrongyloidea							
Aelurostrongylus abstrusus	Worldwide	Wild rodents serve as paratenic hosts; definitive hosts are cats	Abdominal cavity	Ingestion of mollusk (snail, slug) intermediate hosts	Larval cysts in omentum	Not reported	229
Filaroidea							
Litomosoides carinii	Americas	Cotton rats, gerbils, rats, mice, other rodents	Adult: thoracic, pericardial, peritoneal cavities Microfilaria: blood	Infected mites	Eosinophillic inflammation	Not Reported	587, 588

378

Arthropods

Phthiraptera (lice)

	Distribution	Hosts	Location	Transmission	Pathology	Significance	Reference
Hoplopleura spp.	Worldwide	Mice, deer mice, cotton rats, voles, other rodents	Pelage	Direct contact	Pruritus, anemia; *H. acanthopus* transmits *Brucella brucei*	Potential vector of human pathogens	229, 426, 427
Polyplax borealis	Europe	Red-backed mice, tree voles (*Phenacomys*)	Pelage	Direct contact	Irritation	Not reported	589
Polyplax serrata	Worldwide	Mice, European field mice	Anterior dorsal pelage	Direct contact	Pruritus, anemia, debilitation, death; vector of rodent pathogens	Potential vector of human pathogens	437, 440
Polyplax spinulosa	Worldwide	Rats, mice, voles, wild rats, guinea pigs	Anterior dorsal pelage	Direct contact	Pruritus, anemia, debilitation, death; vector of rodent pathogens	Potential vector of human pathogens	440

Siphonaptera (fleas)

	Distribution	Hosts	Location	Transmission	Pathology	Significance	Reference
Leptopsylla segnis	Worldwide	Mice, rats, European field mice, Guinea pigs	Pelage	Direct contact	Unknown pathology; intermediate host for *Hymenolepis diminuta*, *Rodentolepis nana*	Potential vector of human pathogens	440
Nosopsyllus fasciatus	Worldwide	Rats, mice, other rodents, man	Pelage	Direct contact	Unknown pathology; intermediate host for *Hymenolepis diminuta*, *Rodentolepis nana*; vector of rodent pathogens	Potential vector of human pathogens	440
Nosopsyllus londiniensis	Worldwide	Mice, rats	Pelage	Direct contact	Unknown	Not reported	590
Xenopsylla cheopis	Worldwide	Rats, mice, squirrels, voles, guinea pigs, rabbits, man, other mammals	Pelage	Direct contact	None; Intermediate host for *Hymenolepis diminuta*, *Rodentolepis nana*; vector of rodent pathogens	Common; vector of human pathogens	440

(Continued)

TABLE 11.4 (Continued)

Parasite	Geographic distribution	Hosts	Location in host	Method of infection	Pathologic effects	Zoonosis	Reference
Hemiptera (bugs)							
Cimex spp.	Africa	Small domestic mammals, bats, birds, man	Skin	Direct contact	Anemia, annoyance	Common; may be vector of Hepatitis B	591
Dipetalogaster maximus	Mexico (Baja California)	Wood rats	Skin	Direct contact	Anemia	Common; vector of *Trypanosoma cruzi*	592
Panstrongylus megistus	South America	Wild rodents, armadillos, South American opossums, man	Skin	Direct contact	Anemia; vector of *Trypanosoma cruzi*	Common; vector of *T. cruzi*	593
Paratriatoma hirsuta	North America	Wood rats, rock squirrels, armadillos	Skin	Direct contact	Anemia	Reported	594, 595
Rhodnius prolixus	Americas	Domestic animals, man	Skin	Direct contact	Anemia; vector of *T. cruzi, T. rangeli*	Common; vector of *T. cruzi*	464
Triatoma spp.	Americas	Domestic animals, wood rats, armadillos, man	Skin	Direct contact	Anemia; vector of *Trypanosoma cruzi, T. rangeli, T. conorhini*	Common; vector of human trypanosomes	594, 596
Arachnida							
Mites							
Astigmates							
Myocoptes musculinus	Worldwide	Mice, guinea pigs	Skin, pelage	Direct contact	Dermatitis, self-inflicted trauma alopecia	Not reported	485
Notoedres spp.	Worldwide	Wild rodents	Skin	Direct contact	Unknown	Not reported	440, 509, 520
Notoedres muris	Worldwide	Rats, other rodents	Skin, usually of ears	Direct contact	Dermatitis	Not reported	515
Trichoecius romboutsi	Europe, North America	Mice	Skin, pelage	Direct contact	Dermatitis	Not reported	550
Trichoecius muris	Europe	Rats	Skin, pelage	Direct contact	Dermatitis	Not reported	550
Trixacarus diversus	Europe	Rats, mice, hamsters	Skin	Direct contact	Scabby dermatitis, alopecia	Unknown	516
Mesostigmates							
Eulaelaps stabularis	Asia, Europe, North America	Rats, mice, other rodents, other small mammals, man	Skin, pelage	Direct contact	None	Reported; vector of *Francisella tularensis*	480, 597
Haemogamasus pontiger	Worldwide	Rats, mice, other rodents, man	Skin, pelage	Direct contact	None	Reported	480

Species	Geographic distribution	Host	Site	Transmission	Pathology	Zoonosis	References
Haemolaelaps spp.	Worldwide	Rats, mice, other small mammals, birds, man	Skin, pelage, plumage	Direct contact	None	Reported	475, 480
Hirstionyssus butantanensis	South America	mice	Skin, pelage	Direct contact	None	Not reported	598
Laelaps echidninus	Worldwide	Rats, cotton rats, other rodents	Skin, pelage	Direct contact	Vector of *Hepatozoon muris*	Reported; potential vector of *F. tularensis*	475
Laelaps nuttalli	Worldwide	Rats, mice, other rodents	Skin, pelage	Direct contact	None	Not reported	599
Liponyssoides sanguineus	Worldwide	Mice, rats, gerbils, other rodents, man	Skin	Direct contact	Unknown	Reported; vector of *Rickettsia akari*	481
Ornithonyssus bacoti	Worldwide	Rats, mice, hamsters, gerbils, voles, man, other mammals	Skin	Direct contact	Anemia, death; vector of rodent pathogens	Reported; vector of human pathogens	527, 528
Prostigmates							
Demodex musculi	Unknown	Mice	Skin	Direct contact	None in immunologically competent mice	Not reported	471–474
Demodex ratti	Unknown	Rats	Skin	Direct contact	Unknown	Not reported	600
Myobia musculi	Worldwide	Mice, rats, guinea pigs	Skin, pelage	Direct contact	Dermatitis, alopecia, pruritus, self-inflicted dermal trauma	Not reported	485–487, 491
Psorergates simplex	Worldwide	Mice	Hair follicles	Direct contact	Caseous nodules in skin, dermal cysts, dermatitis of ears	Not reported	440, 539
Psorergates oettlei	Africa	Multimammate mice	Skin	Direct contact	Scabby dermatitis, alopecia	Not reported	509
Radfordia affinis	Worldwide	Mice	Skin, pelage	Direct contact	Dermatitis, alopecia, pruritus	Not reported	440, 546
Radfordia ensifera	Worldwide	Rats	Skin, pelage	Direct contact	Self-inflicted dermal trauma	Not reported	440
Trombicula (Neotrombicula) autumnalis	Europe	Rats, mice, man, other mammals	Skin	Direct contact	None	Common ("chigger")	440
Pentastomids							
Porocephalus crotali	Americas	Cotton rats, deer mice	Serosal surfaces	Ingestion of eggs passed by definitive host (pit vipers)	Cysts in viscera, mesentery, abdominal wall, thoracic wall	Not reported	601, 602

TABLE 11.5 Parasites of Rats and Mice—Nervous, Respiratory, and Urogenital Systems.

Parasite	Geographic distribution	Hosts	Location in host	Method of infection	Pathologic effects	Zoonosis	Reference
Coccidia							
Klossiella muris	Worldwide	Mice, rats	Kidneys	Ingestion of sporocysts passed in urine	Interstitial nephritis, interstitial pneumonia, splenomegaly	Not reported	175
Nematodes							
Trichuroidea							
Capillaria papillosa	Europe	Rats	Urinary bladder	Ingestion of egg	None known	Not reported	453
Capillaria polonica	Europe	Rats	Urinary bladder	Ingestion of egg	None known	Not reported	453
Capillaria (Pearsonema) plica	Worldwide	Rats (also dogs, cats, foxes)	Urinary bladder, kidneys	Ingestion of earthworm	Usually none	Not reported	374
Trichosomoides crassicauda	Worldwide	Rats	Urinary bladder, kidneys, ureters	Ingestion of embryonated egg	Masses in bladder wall, urinary calculi, nephritis, pulmonary granulomata, eosinophilia	Not reported	389, 392
Trichosomoides nasalis	Africa, Asia, Europe	Wild rats, grass rats, golden hamsters	Nasal mucosa	Ingestion of embryonated egg	Rhinosinusitis	Not reported	454
Spirurida							
Thelazia callipaeda	Asia, Europe, North America	Rats (also found in rabbits, dogs, monkeys, man)	Eyes (lacrimal system, conjunctiva)	Transmitted from fly intermediate host during feeding on ocular secretions	Scleral congestion, lacrimation, keratoconjunctivitis, photophobia	Reported	455

severe clinical disease culminating in death[516]. The parasite is rarely identified, even from wild rodents. Therefore, relatively little is known of its biology, treatment, or control. It is likely that in these areas it closely resembles *N. muris*.

REFERENCES

1. Sparrow, S. (1976) The microbiological and parasitological status of laboratory animals from accredited breeders in the United Kingdom. *Lab. Anim.* **10**, 365–373.

2. Nakagawa, M., Saito, M., Suzuki, E., Nakayama, K., Matsubara, J., and Muto, T. (1984) Ten years-long survey on pathogen status of mouse and rat breeding colonies. *Jikken Dobutsu* **33**:115–120.

3. Baker, D.G. (2004) *Natural Pathogens of Laboratory Animals: Their Effects on Research.* American Society for Microbiology Press, Washington, D.C.

4. Livingston, R.S. and Riley, L.K. (2003) Diagnostic testing of mouse and rat colonies for infectious agents. *Lab. Anim.* **32**, 44–51.

5. Hill, L.R., Kille, P.S., Weiss, D.A., Craig, T.M., and Coghlan, L.G. (1999) *Demodex musculi* in the skin of transgenic mice. *Contemp. Top. Lab. An. Sci.* **38**, 13–18.

6. Hirst, S. (1917) Remarks on certain species of the genus *Demodex*, Owen (the *Demodex*) of man, the horse, dog, rat, and mouse. *Ann. Mag. Nat. Hist.* **20**, 233–235.

7. Cross, J.H., Hsu, M.Y., and Hung, C.K. (1983) Studies on trypanosomes in the Taiwan monkey. *Southeast Asian J. Trop. Med. Public Health* **14**, 536–542.

8. Baker, D.G. (2005) Parasitic Diseases. In: Suckow, M. (ed) *The Laboratory Rat*, 2nd ed., Elsevier Inc.

9. Saxena, V.K. and Miyata, A. (1993) An unusual morphological type of *Trypanosoma (Herpetosoma) lewisi* (Kent, 1880) detected in the blood of *Rattus norvegicus* in India. *J. Commun. Dis.* **25**, 15–17.

10. Allam, K.A., El Bassioni, S.O., and Nour El-Hoda, A.M. (2002) Some field and laboratory studies on *Rattus rattus* subspecies and *Rattus norvegicus* in two Egyptian governorates of different ecological characters. *J. Egypt. Soc. Parasitol.* **32**, 805–812.

11. Linardi, P.M. and Botelho, J.R. (2002) Prevalence of *Trypanosoma lewisi* in *Rattus norvegicus* from Belo Horizonte, State of Minas Gerais, Brazil. *Mem. Inst. Oswaldo Cruz* **97**, 411–414.

12. Sakla, A.A. and Monib, M.E.M. (1984). Redescription of the life cycle of *Trypanosoma (Herpetosoma) lewisi* from upper Egyptian rats. *J. Egypt. Soc. Parasitol.* **14**, 367–376.

13. Albright, J.W. and Albright, J.F. (1981) Differences in resistance to *Trypanosoma musculi* infection among strains of inbred mice. *Infect. Immun.* **33**, 364–371.

14. Smith, O. (1972) Survival and growth pattern of *Trypanosoma lewisi* in two heterologous hosts: albino mouse and guinea-pig. *Acta Zool. Pathol. Antverp.* **55**, 3–18.

15. Khachoian, V.I. and Arakelian, L.A. (1978). Case of the transmission of the rat trypanosome by lice. *Parazitologiia* **12**, 451–453.

16. Fujiwara, K. and Suzuki, Y. (1967) Spontaneous arthritis in laboratory rats associated with trypanosomal infection. *Bull. Exp. Animals* **16**, 103–105.

17. Sherman, I.W. and Ruble, J.A. (1967) Virulent *Trypanosoma lewisi* infections in cortisone-treated rats. *J. Parasitol.* **55**, 258–262.

18. Ndarathi, C.M. (1992). Cellular responses to culture-derived soluble exoantigens of *Trypanosoma lewisi*. *Parasitol. Res.* **78**, 324–328.

19. Ferrante, A., Carter, R.F., Ferluga, J., and Allison, A.C. (1984) Lipopolysaccharide hyperreactivity of animals infected with *Trypanosoma lewisi* or *Trypanosoma musculi*. *Infect. Immun.* **46**, 501–506.

20. Thoongsuwan, S. and Cox, H.W. (1978) Anemia, splenomegaly, and glomerulonephritis associated with autoantibody in *Trypanosoma lewisi* infections. *J. Parasitol.* **64**, 669–673.

21. Catarinella Arrea, G., Chinchilla Carmona, M., Guerrero Bermudez, O.M., and Abrahams, E. (1998). Effect of *Trypanosoma lewisi* (Kinetoplastida: Trypanosomatidae) on the infection of white rats with *Toxoplasma gondii* (Eucoccidia: Sarcocystidae) oocysts. *Rev. Biol. Trop.* **46**, 1121–1123.

22. Nielsen, K., Sheppard, J., Holmes, W., and Tizard, I. (1978). Increased susceptibility of *Trypanosoma lewisi* infected, or decomplemented rats to *Salmonella typhimurium*. *Experimentia* **34**, 118–119.

23. Lee, C.M., George, Y.G., and Aboko-Cole, G. (1977) Iron metabolism in *Trypanosoma lewisi* infection: serum iron and serum iron-binding capacity. *Z. Parasitenkd.* **53**, 1–6.

24. Lee, C.M. and Boone, L.Y. (1983) Rat liver glucose-6–phosphate dehydrogenase isozymes: influence of infection with *Trypanosoma*. *Comp. Biochem. Physiol. B* **75**, 505–508.

25. Shaw, G.L. and Quadagno, D. (1975) *Trypanosoma lewisi* and *T. cruzi*: effect of infection on gestation in the rat. *Exp. Parasitol.* **37**, 211–217.

26. Lincicome, D.R., Rossan, R.N., and Jones, W.C. (1963) Growth of rats infected with *Trypanosoma lewisi*. *Exp. Parasitol.* **14**, 54–65.

27. Levine, N.D. (1985) *Veterinary Protozoology*. Iowa State University Press, Ames. 414 pages.

28. Desquesnes, M., Ravel, S., and Cuny, G. (2002) PCR identification of *Trypanosoma lewisi*, a common parasite of laboratory rats. *Kinetoplastid Biol. Dis.* **1**, 2.

29. el-Ridi, A.M., Hamdy, E.I., Nasr, N.T., Gerges, Z.I., and Sobhy, M.M. (1985) Effect of some antibiotics and chemotherapeutics on *Trypanosoma lewisi* infection in albino rats. *J. Egypt. Soc. Parasitol.* **15**, 119–123.

30. Johnson, P.D. (1933) A case of infection by *Trypanosoma lewisi* in a child. *Trans. R. Soc. Trop. Med. Hyg.* **26**, 467–468.

31. Shrivastava, K.K. and Shrivastava, G.P. (1974) Two cases of *Trypanosoma (Herpetosoma)* species infection of man in India. *Trans. R. Soc. Trop. Med. Hyg.* **68**, 143–144.

32. Albright, J.W., Pierantoni, M., and Albright, J.F. (1990) Immune and nonimmune regulation of the population of *Trypanosoma musculi* in infected host mice. *Infect. Immun.* **58**, 1757–1762.

33. Magluilo, P., Viens, P., and Forget, A. (1983) Immunosuppression during *Trypanosoma musculi* infection in inbred strains of mice. *J. Clin. Lab. Immunol.* **10**, 151–154.

34. Derothe, J.M., Loubes, C., Perriat-Sanguinet, M., Orth, A., and Moulia, C. (1999) Experimental trypanosomiasis of natural hybrids between house mouse and subspecies. *Int. J. Parasitol.* **29**, 1011–1016.

35. Chiejina, S.N., Street, J., Wakelin, D., and Behnke, J.M. (1993) Response of inbred mice to infection with a new isolate of *Trypanosoma musculi*. *Parasitology* **107**, 233–236.

36. Hirokawa, K., Eishi, Y., Albright, J.W., and Albright, J.F. (1981) Histopathological and immunocytochemical studies of *Trypanosoma musculi* infection in mice. *Infect. Immun.* **34**, 1008–1017.

37. Albright, J.W., Jiang, D., and Albright, J.F. (1997) Innate control of the early course of infection in mice inoculated with *Trypanosoma musculi*. *Cell. Immunol.* **176**, 146–152.

38. Moon, A.P., Williams, J.S., and Witherspoon, C. (1968) Serum biochemical changes in mice infected with *Trypanosoma rhodesiense* and *Trypanosoma duttoni*. *Exp. Parasitol.* **22**, 112–121.

39. Utsuyama, M., Albright, J.W., Holmes, K.L., Hirokawa, K., and Albright, J.F. (1994) Changes in the subsets of CD4$^+$ T cells in *Trypanosoma musculi* infection: delay of immunological cure in young mice and the weak ability of aged mice to control the infection. *Int. Immunol.* **6**, 1107–1115.

40. Rank, R.G., Roberts, D.W., and Weidanz, W.P. (1977) Chronic infection with *Trypanosoma musculi* in congenitally athymic nude mice. *Infect. Immun.* **16**, 715–716.

41. Monroy, F.P. and Dusanic, D.G. (2000) The kidney form of *Trypanosoma musculi:* A distinct stage in the life cycle? *Parasitol. Today* **16**, 107–110.

42. Lincicome, D.R. and Shepperson, J. (1963) Increased rate of growth of mice infected with *Trypanosoma duttoni. J. Parasitol.* **49**, 31–34.

43. Humphrey, P.A., Ashraf, M., and Lee, C.M. (1997) Growth of trypanosomes in vivo, host body weight gains, and food consumption in zinc-deficient mice. *J. Natl. Med. Assoc.* **89**, 48–56.

44. Jalili, N.A., Demes, P., and Holkova, R. (1989) The occurrence of protozoa in the intestinal microflora of laboratory mice. *Bratisl. Lek. Listy.* **90**, 42–44.

45. Lee, J.J., Leedale, G.F., and Bradbury, P (eds.) (2000) *The Illustrated Guide to the Protozoa.* 2nd ed. Society of Protozoologists, Allen Press Inc. Lawrence, Kansas, 1432 pages.

46. Wenrich, D.H. (1930) Intestinal flagellates of rats. In: Hegner, R. and Andrews, J. (eds.) *Problems and methods of research in protozoology.* Macmillan, New York, 124–142.

47. Abraham, R. (1961) A new protozoon of the genus *Chilomastix. Z. F. Parasitenkunde* **21**, 159–163.

48. Higgins-Opitz, S.B., Dettman, C.D., Dingle, C.E., Anderson, C.B., and Becker, P.J. (1990) Intestinal parasites of conventionally maintained BALB/c mice and *Mastomys coucha* and the effects of a concomitant schistosome infection. *Lab. Anim.* **24**, 246–252.

49. Jensen, B., Kepley, W., Guarner, J., et al. (2000) Comparison of polyvinyl alcohol fixative with three less hazardous fixatives for detection and identification of intestinal parasites. *J. Clin. Microbiol.* **38**, 1592–1598.

50. Kawamoto, F., Mizuno, S., Fujioka, H., et al. (1987) Simple and rapid staining for detection of *Entamoeba* cysts and other protozoans with fluorochromes. *Jpn. J. Med. Sci. Biol.* **40**, 35–46.

51. Feely, D.E., Erlandsen, S.L., and Chase, D.G. (1984) Structure of the trophozoite and cyst. In: Erlandsen, S.L. and Meyer, E.A. (eds.) *Giardia and Giardiasis.* Plenum Press, New York, 3–31.

52. Lavier, G. (1924) Deux espèces de *Giardia* du rat d'égout parisien (*Epimys norvegicus*). *Ann. Parasitol.* **2**, 161–168.

53. Sogayar, M.I., and Yoshida, E.L. (1995) *Giardia* survey in live-trapped small domestic and wild animals in four regions in the southwest region of the state of Sao Paulo, Brazil. *Mem. Inst. Oswaldo Cruz* **90**, 675–678.

54. Ito, M. and Itagaki, T. (2003) Survey on wild rodents for endoparasites in Iwate Prefecture, Japan. *J. Vet. Med. Sci.* **65**, 1151–1153.

55. Casebolt, D.B., Lindsey, J.R., and Cassell, G.H. (1988) Prevalence rates of infectious agents among commercial breeding populations of rats and mice. *Lab. An. Sci.* **38**, 327–329.

56. Belosevic, M., Faubert, G.M., Skamene, E., and MacLean, J.D. (1984) Susceptibility and resistance of inbred mice to *Giardia muris. Infect. Immun.* **44**, 282–286.

57. Roberts-Thomson, I.C. (1993) Genetic studies of human and murine giardiasis. *Clin. Infect. Dis.* **16**, S98–104.

58. de Carneri, I., Trane, F., and Mandelli, V. (1977) *Giardia muris:* oral infection with one trophozoite and generation time in mice. *Trans. R. Soc. Trop. Med. Hyg.* **71**, 438.

59. de Carneri, I., and Trane, F. (1977) Oral infection of mice with trophozoites of *Giardia muris. Am. J. Trop. Med. Hyg.* **26**, 566–567.

60. Heyworth, M.F. (1988) Time-course of *Giardia muris* infection in male and female immunocompetent mice. *J. Parasitol.* **74**, 491–493.

61. Daniels, C.W. and Belosevic, M. (1995) Comparison of the course of infection with *Giardia muris* in male and female mice. *Int. J. Parasitol.* **25**, 131–135.

62. MacDonald, T.T. and Fergusen, A. (1978) Small intestinal epithelial cell kinetics and protozoal infection in mice. *Gastroenterology* **74**, 496–500.

63. Scott, K.G., Logan, M.R., Klammer, G.M., Teoh, D.A., and Buret, A.G. (2000) Jejunal brush border microvillous alterations in *Giardia muris*-infected mice: role of T lymphocytes and interleukin-6. *Infect. Immun.* **68**, 3412–3418.

64. el-Shewy, K.A. and Eid, R.A. (2003) Intravascular detection of *Giardia* trophozoites in naturally infected mice. An electron microscopic study. *Parasite* **10**, 169–174.

65. Buret, A., Gall, D.G., and Olson, M.E. (1990) Effects of murine giardiasis on growth, intestinal morphology, and disaccharidase activity. *J. Parasitol.* **76**, 403–409.

66. Olveda, R.K., Andrews, J.S. Jr., and Hewlett, E.L. (1982) Murine giardiasis: localization of trophozoites and small bowel histopathology during the course of infection. *Am. J. Trop. Med. Hyg.* **31**, 60–66.

67. Cruz, C.C., Ferrari, L., and Sogayar, R. (1997) A therapeutic trial in *Giardia muris* infection in the mouse with metronidazole, tinidazole, secnidazole, and furazolidone. *Rev. Soc. Bras. Med. Trop.* **30**, 223–228.

68. Hayes, S.L., Rice, E.W., Ware, M.W., and Schaefer, F.W. 3rd. (2003) Low pressure ultraviolet studies for inactivation of *Giardia muris* cysts. *J. Appl. Microbiol.* **94**, 54–59.

69. Leahy, J.G., Rubin, A.J., and Sproul, O.J. (1987) Inactivation of *Giardia muris* cysts by free chlorine. *Appl. Environ. Microbiol.* **53**, 1448–1453.

70. Saxe, L.H. (1954) Transfaunation studies on the host specificity of the enteric protozoa of rodents. *J. Protozool.* **1**, 220–230.

71. Fukushima, T., Mochizuki, K., Yamazaki, H., et al. (1990) *Pentatrichomonas hominis* from beagle dogs—detection method, characteristics and route of infection. *Jikken Dobutsu* **39**, 187–192.

72. Wenrich, D.H. (1924) Trichomonad flagellates in the caecum of rats and mice. *Anat. Record* **29**, 118.

73. Andrews, J. and White, H.F. (1936) An epidemiological study of protozoa parasitic in wild rats in Baltimore, with special reference to *Endamoeba histolytica. Am. J. Hyg.* **24**, 184–206.

74. Brugerolle, G., Kunst[[yacute]][[rcaron]], I., Senaud, J., and Friedhoff, K.T. (1980) Fine structure of trophozoites and cysts of the pathogenic diplomonad *Spironucleus muris. Z. Parasitenkd.* **62**, 47–61. *Parasitol.* **82**, 951–956.

75. Kunstyr, I. (1977) Infectious form of *Spironucleus* (*Hexamita*) *muris:* banded cysts. *Lab. Anim.* **11**, 185–188.

76. Baker, D.G., Malineni, S., and Taylor, H.W. (1998) Experimental infection of inbred mouse strains with *Spironucleus muris. Vet. Parasitol.* **77**, 305–310.

77. Owen, D. (1976) Some parasites and other organisms of wild rodents in the vicinity of an SPF unit. *Lab. Anim.* **10**, 271–278.

78. Kunstýř, I., Poppinga, G., and Friedhoff, K.T. (1993) Host specificity of cloned *Spironucleus* sp. originating from the European hamster. *Lab. Anim.* **27**, 77–80.

79. Stachan, R. and Kunstýr, I. (1983) Minimal infectious doses and prepatent periods in *Giardia muris, Spironucleus muris* and *Tritrichomonas muris. Zentralbl. Bakteriol. Mikrobiol. Hyg. (A)* **256**, 249–256.

80. Kunstýř, I., Ammerpohl, E., and Meyer, B. (1977) Experimental spironucleosis (hexamitiasis) in the nude mouse as a model for immunologic and pharmacologic studies. *Lab. Anim. Sci.* **27**.

81. Whitehouse, A., France, M.P., Pope, S.E., Lloyd, J.E., and Ratchliffe, R.C. (1993) *Spironucleus muris* in laboratory mice. *Aust. Vet. J.* **70**, 193.

82. Brett, S.J. (1983) Immunodepression in *Giardia muris* and *Spironucleus muris* infections in mice. *Parasitology* **87**, 507–515.

83. Mullink, J.W., Ruitenberg, E.J., and Kruizinga, W. (1980) Lack of effect of *Spironucleus* (*Hexamita*) *muris* on the immune response to tetanus toxoid in the rat. *Lab. Anim.* **14**, 127–128.

84. Shibuya, M., Yanabe, M., Osugi, N., and Tanaka, T. (1993) A trial designed to obtain a specific pathogen free Syrian hamster colony by administration of chemicals. *Jikken Dobutsu* **41**, 379–381.

85. Wenrich, D.H. and Saxe, L.H. (1950) *Trichomonas microti*, n. sp. (Protozoa: Mastigophora). *J. Parasitol.* **36**, 261–269.

86. Wenrich, D.H. and Nie, D. (1949) The morphology of *Trichomonas wenyoni* (Protozoa, Mastigophora). *J. Morphol.* **85**, 519–531.

87. Mattern, C.F. and Daniel, W.A. (1980) *Tritrichomonas muris* in the hamster: pseudocysts and the infection of newborn. *J. Protozool.* **27**, 435–439.

88. Roach, P.D., Wallis, P.M., and Olson, M.E. (1988) The use of metronidazole, tinidazole and dimetridazole in eliminating trichomonads from laboratory mice. *Lab. Anim.* **22**, 361–364.

89. Lipman, N.S., Lampen, N., and Nguyen, H.T. (1999) Identification of pseudocysts of *Tritrichomonas muris* in Armenian hamsters and their transmission to mice. *Lab. Anim. Sci.* **49**, 313–315.

90. Chinchilla, M., Portilla, E., Guerrero, O.M., and Marin, R. (1987) The presence of cysts in *Tritrichomonas muris*. *Rev. Biol. Trop.* **35**, 21–24.

91. Levine, N.D. (1961) *Protozoan parasites of domestic animals and of man*. Burgess, Minneapolis, Minnesota. 412 pages.

92. Singletary, K.B., Kloster, C.A., and Baker, D.G. (2003) Optimal age at fostering for derivation of *Helicobacter hepaticus*-free mice. *Comp. Med.* **53**, 33–38.

93. Lin, T.-M. (1971) Colonization and encystation of *Entamoeba muris* in the rat and the mouse. *J. Parasitol.* **57**, 375–382.

94. Neal, R.A. (1950) An experimental study of *Entamoeba muris* (Grassi, 1879); its morphology, affinities and host-parasite relationship. *Parasitology* **40**, 343–365.

95. Hoare, C.A. (1959) Amoebic infections in animals. *Vet. Rev. Annotations* **5**, 91–102.

96. Ozkul, I.A. and Aydin, Y. (1994) Natural *Cryptosporidium muris* infection in the stomach in laboratory mice. *Vet. Parasitol.* **55**, 129–132.

97. Lindsay, D.S., Upton, S.J., Owens, D.S., Morgan, U.M., Mead, J.R., and Blagburn, B.L. (2000) *Cryptosporidium andersoni* n. sp. (Apicomplexa: Cryptosporidae) from cattle, *Bos taurus*. *J. Eukaryot. Microbiol.* **47**, 91–95.

98. Morgan, U.M., Xiao, L., Monis, P., et al. (2000) Molecular and phylogenetic analysis of *Cryptosporidium muris* from various hosts. *Parasitology* **120**, 457–464.

99. Chalmers, R.M., Sturdee, A.P., Bull, S.A., Miller, A., and Wright, S.E. (1997) The prevalence of *Cryptosporidium parvum* and *C. muris* in *Mus domesticus*, *Apodemus sylvaticus* and *Clethrionomys glareolus* in an agricultural system. *Parasitol. Res.* **83**, 478–482.

100. Abd el-Wahed, M.M., Salem, G.H., and el-Assaly, T.M. (1999) The role of wild rats as a reservoir of some internal parasites in Qalyobia governorate. *J. Egypt. Soc. Parasitol.* **29**, 495–503.

101. Rhee, J.K., Surl, C.G., and Kim, H.C. (1997) Effects of *Cryptosporidium muris* (strain MCR) infection on gastric mucosal mast cells in mice. *Korean J. Parasitol.* **35**, 245–249.

102. Taylor, M.A., Marshall, R.N., Green, J.A., and Catchpole, J. (1999) The pathogenesis of experimental infections of *Cryptosporidium muris* (strain RN 66) in outbred nude mice. *Vet. Parasitol.* **86**, 41–48.

103. Davami, M.H., Bancroft, G.J., and McDonald, V. (1997) *Cryptosporidium* infection in major histocompatibility complex congenic strains of mice: variation in susceptibility and the role of T-cell cytokine responses. *Parasitol. Res.* **83**, 257–263.

104. Aydin, Y. and Ozkul, I.A. (1996) Infectivity of *Cryptosporidium muris* directly isolated from the murine stomach for various laboratory animals. *Vet. Parasitol.* **66**, 257–262.

105. Current, W.L. and Garcia, L.S. (1991) Cryptosporidiosis. *Clin. Microbiol. Rev.* **4**, 325–358.

106. Enriquez, F.J. and Sterling, C.R. (1991) *Cryptosporidium* infections in inbred strains of mice. *J. Protozool.* **38**, 100S–102S.

107. McDonald, V., Deer, R., Uni, S., Iseki, M., and Bancroft, G.J. (1992) Immune responses to *Cryptosporidium muris* and *Cryptosporidium parvum* in adult immunocompetent or immunocompromised (nude and SCID) mice. *Infect. Immun.* **60**, 3325–3331.

108. Levine, N.D. and Ivens, V. (1965) The coccidian parasites (Protozoa: Sporozoa) of rodents. *Illinois Biol. Monograph 33*. University of Illinois Press, Urbana, Illinois. 365 pages.

109. Yakimoff, W.L. and Gousseff, W.F. (1938) The coccidia of mice (*Mus musculus*). *Parasitology* **30**, 1–3.

110. Cordero del Campillo, M. (1959) Estudios sobre *Eimeria falciformis* (Einer, 1870) parasito del raton: I. Observaciones sobre el periodo prepatente, esporulación, morfologia de los ooquistes y estudio biométrico de los mismos, producción de ooquistes y patogenicidad. *Rev. Iberica Parasitol.* **19**, 351–368.

111. Schito, M.L., Barta, J.R., and Chobotar, B. (1996) Comparison of four murine *Eimeria* species in immunocompetent and immunodeficient mice. *J. Parasitol.* **82**, 255–262.

112. Mayberry, L.F. and Marquardt, W.C. (1973) Transmission of *Eimeria separata* from the normal host, *Rattus*, to the mouse, *Mus musculus*. *J. Parasitol.* **59**, 198–199.

113. Shehu, K. and Nowell, F. (1998) Cross-reactions between *Eimeria falciformis* and *Eimeria pragensis* in mice induced by trickle infections. *Parasitology* **117**, 457–465.

114. Mahrt, J.L. and Shi, Y.F. (1988) Murine major histocompatibility complex and immune response to *Eimeria falciformis*. *Infect. Immun.* **56**, 270–271.

115. Stockdale, P.G., Stockdale, M.J., Rickard, M.D., and Mitchell, G.F. (1985) Mouse strain variation and effects of oocyst dose in infection of mice with *Eimeria falciformis*, a coccidian parasite of the large intestine. *Int. J. Parasitol.* **15**, 447–452.

116. Nash, P.V. and Speer, C.A. (1988) B-lymphocyte responses in the large intestine and mesenteric lymph nodes of mice infected with *Eimeria falciformis*. *J. Parasitol.* **74**, 144–152.

117. Stiff, M.I. and Vasilakos, J.P. (1990) Effect of in vivo T-cell depletion on the effector T-cell function of immunity to *Eimeria falciformis*. *Infect. Immun.* **58**, 1496–1499.

118. Lantier, F., Yvore, P., Marly, J., Pardon, P., and Kerboeuf, D. (1981) Coccidia parasitism increases resistance of mice to subcutaneous inoculation with *Salmonella abortus ovis*. *Ann. Rech. Vet.* **12**, 169–172.

119. Misael Chinchilla, C., Olga Marta Guerrero, B., and Roberto Marin, R. (1986) Effect of *Eimeria falciformis* on the development of toxoplasmosis in mice. *Rev. Biol. Trop.* **34**, 1–6.

120. Becker, E.R., Hall, P.R., Hager, A. (1932) Quantitative, biometric and host-parasite studies on *Eimeria miyairii* and *Eimeria separata* in rats. *Iowa State Coll. J. Sci.* **6**, 299–316.

121. Matubayasi, H. (1938) Studies on parasitic protozoa in Japan: IV. Coccidia parasitic in wild rats (*Epimys rattus alexandrinus* and *E. norvegicus*). *Annot. Zool. Japon.* 17, 144–163.

122. Roudabush, R.L. (1937) The endogenous phases of the life cycles of *Eimeria nieschulzi, Eimeria separata,* and *Eimeria miyairii* coccidian parasites of the rat. *Iowa St. Coll. J. Sci.* 11, 135–163.

123. Marquardt, W.C. (1966) Attempted transmission of the rat coccidium *Eimeria nieschulzi* to mice. *J. Parasitol.* 52, 691–694.

124. Levine, N.D. (1957) Protozoan parasites of laboratory animals. *Proc. Animal Care Panel* 7, 98–126.

125. Mayberry, L.F., Bristol, J.R., Cajas, O., and Tellez, G. (1986) Small intestinal sucrase activity during experimental infections with *Nippostrongylus brasiliensis* and/or *Eimeria nieschulzi* in rats. *Z. Parasitenkd.* 72, 561–564.

126. Heading, C.E., Ball, S.J., and Meade, H.M. (1985) Intestinal absorption studies with glycyl-proline, glycine and ethanol in rats infected with *Eimeria nieschulzi*. *Life Sci.* 37, 395–402.

127. Huntley, J.F., Newlands, G.F., Miller, H.R., McLauchlan, M., Rose, M.E., and Hesketh, P. (1985) Systemic release of mucosal mast cell protease during infection with the intestinal protozoal parasite, *Eimeria nieschulzi*. Studies in normal and nude rats. *Parasite Immunol.* 7, 489–501.

128. McQuiston, T.E. and Schurr, K.M. (1978) The effect of *Eimeria nieschulzi* on leukocyte levels in the rat. *J. Protozool.* 25, 374–377.

129. Upton, S.J., Mayberry, L.F., Bristol, J.R., Favela, S.H., and Sambrano, G.R. (1987) Suppression of peripheral eosinophilia by the coccidian *Eimeria nieschulzi* (Apicomplexa: Eimeriidae) in experimentally infected mice. *J. Parasitol.* 73, 300–308.

130. Bristol, J.R., Upton, S.J., Mayberry, L.F., and Rael, E.D. (1989) Suppression of phytohemagglutinin induced splenocyte proliferation during concurrent infection with *Eimeria nieschulzi* and *Nippostrongylus brasiliensis*. *Experientia* 45, 762–763.

131. Pérard, C. (1926) Sur la coccidiose du rat. *Acad. Vet. France Bull.* 102, 120–124.

132. Smith, N.C., Ovington, K.S., Deplazes, P., and Eckert, J. (1995) Cytokine and immunoglobulin subclass responses of rats to infection with *Eimeria nieschulzi*. *Parasitology* 111, 51–57.

133. Colley, F.C. (1968) Fine structure of schizonts and merozoites of *Eimeria nieschulzi*. *J. Protozool.* 15, 374–382.

134. Cerna, Z. and Senaud, J. (1969) *Eimeria pragensis* sp. n., a new coccidian parasite from the intestine of mice (*Mus musculus*). *Folia Parasitologica (Praha)* 16, 171–175.

135. Mesfin, G.M. and Bellamy, J.E. (1978) The life cycle of *Eimeria falciformis* var. *pragensis* (Sporozoa: Coccidia) in the mouse, *Mus musculus*. *J. Parasitol.* 64, 696–705.

136. Mesfin, G.M., Bellamy, J.E., and Stockdale, P.H. (1978) The pathological changes caused by *Eimeria falciformis* var *pragensis* in mice. *Can. J. Comp. Med.* 42, 496–510.

137. Mesfin, G.M. and Bellamy, J.E. (1979) Thymic dependence of immunity to *Eimeria falciformis* var. *pragensis* in mice. *Infect. Immun.* 23, 460–464.

138. Duszynski, D.W. (1971) Increase in size of *Eimeria separata* oocysts during patency. *J. Parasitol.* 57, 948–952.

139. Levine, N.D. and Ivens, V. (1988) Cross-transmission of *Eimeria* spp. (Protozoa, Apicomplexa) of rodents—a review. *J. Protozool.* 35, 434–437.

140. Marquardt, W.C., Pafume, B.A., and Bush, D. (1987) Immunity to *Eimeria separata* (Apicomplexa: Eimeriina): Expose-and-challenge studies in rats. *J. Parasitol.* 73, 342–344.

141. Shi, M.Q., Huther, S., Burkhardt, E., and Zahner, H. (2000) Immunity in rats against *Eimeria separata:* oocyst excretion, effects on endogenous stages and local tissue response after primary and challenge infections. *Parasitol. Res.* 86, 891–898.

142. Cirak, V.Y., Kowalik, S., Burger, H.J., Zahner, H., and Clauss, W. (2004) Effects of *Eimeria separata* infections on Na+ and Cl- transport in the rat large intestine. *Parasitol. Res.* 92, 490–495.

143. Shi, M.Q., Hirzmann, J., Dafa(alla, T.H., and Zahner, H. (2001) In vivo expression profiles of cytokine and iNOS mRNAs in rats infected with *Eimeria separata*. *Vet. Parasitol.* 97, 131–140.

144. Mayberry, L.F., Bristol, J.R., and Villalobos, V.M. (1985) Intergeneric interactions between *Eimeria separata* (Apicomplexa) and *Nippostrongylus brasiliensis* (Nematoda) in the rat. *Experientia* 41, 689–690.

145. Duszynski, D.W. (1972) Host and parasite interactions during single and concurrent infections with *Eimeria nieschulzi* and *E. separata* in the rat. *J. Protozool.* 19, 82–88.

146. Didier, E.S., Stovall, M.E., Green, L.C., Brindley, P.J., Sestak, K., and Didier, P.J. (2004) Epidemiology of microsporidiosis: sources and modes of transmission. *Vet. Parasitol.* 126, 145–166.

147. Didier, E.S., Vossbrinck, C.R., Baker, M.D., Rogers, L.B., Bertucci, D.C., and Shadduck, J.A. (1995) Identification and characterization of three *Encephalitozoon cuniculi* strains. *Parasitology* 111, 411–421.

148. Gannon, J. (1980) A survey of *Encephalitozoon cuniculi* in laboratory animal colonies in the United Kingdom. *Lab. Anim.* 14, 91–94.

149. Muller-Doblies, U.U., Herzog, K., Tanner, I., Mathis, A., and Deplazes, P. (2002) First isolation and characterization of *Encephalitozoon cuniculi* from a free-ranging rat (*Rattus norvegicus*). *Vet. Parasitol.* 107, 279–285.

150. Halanova, M., Cislakova, L., Valencakova, A., Balent, P., Adam, J., and Travnicek, M. (2003) Serological screening of occurrence of antibodies to *Encephalitozoon cuniculi* in humans and animals in Eastern Slovakia. *Ann. Agric. Environ. Med.* 10, 117–120.

151. Attwood, H.D. and Sutton, R.D. (1965) *Encephalitozoon* granuloma in rats. *J. Pathol. Bacteriol.* 89, 735–738.

152. Didier, E.S., Bertucci, D.C., Green, L.C., Stovall, M.E., and Didier, P.J. (2001) *Encephalitozoon cuniculi* infection in mice with the chronic granulomatous disease (CGD) disorder. *J. Eukaryot. Microbiol.* 79S–80S.

153. Braunfuchsova, P., Salat, J., and Kopecky, J. (2002) Comparison of the significance of CD4+ and CD8+ T lymphocytes in the protection of mice against *Encephalitozoon cuniculi* infection. *J. Parasitol.* 88, 797–799.

154. Valencakova, A., Halanova, M., Balent, P., et al. (2004) Immune response in mice infected by *Encephalitozoon cuniculi* and suppressed by dexamethasone. *Acta Vet. Hung.* 52, 61–69.

155. Petri, M. (1966) The occurrence of *Nosema cuniculi* (*Encephalitozoon cuniculi*) in the cells of transplantable, malignant ascites tumours and its effect upon tumour and host. *Acta Pathol. Microbiol. Scand.* 66, 13–30.

156. Kock, N.P., Petersen, H., Fenner, T., et al. (1997) Species-specific identification of microsporidia in stool and intestinal biopsy specimens by the polymerase chain reaction. *Eur. J. Clin. Microbiol. Infect. Dis.* 16, 369–376.

157. Fedorko, D.P., Nelson, N.A., Didier, E.S., Bertucci, D., Delgado, R.M., and Hruszkewycz, A.M. (2001) Speciation of human microspordia by polymerase chain reaction single-strand conformation polymorphism. *Am. J. Trop. Med. Hyg.* 65, 397–401.

158. Bacchi, C.J., Weiss, L.M., Lane, S., et al. (2002) Novel synthetic polyamines are effective in the treatment of experimental

microsporidiosis, an opportunistic AIDS-associated infection. *Antimicrob. Agents Chemother.* **46**, 55–61.

159. Suter, C., Muller-Doblies, U.U., Hatt, J.M., and Deplazes, P. (2001) Prevention and treatment of *Encephalitozoon cuniculi* infection in rabbits with fenbendazole. *Vet. Rec.* **148**, 478–480.

160. Mugridge, N.B., Morrision, D.A., Johnson, A.M., et al. (1999) Phylogenetic relationships of the genus *Frenkelia:* a review of its history and new knowledge gained from comparison of large subunit ribosomal ribonucleic acid gene sequences. *Int. J. Parasitol.* **29**, 957–972.

161. Hayden, D.W., King, N.W., and Murthy, A.S.K. (1976) Spontaneous *Frenkelia* infection in a laboratory-reared rat. *Vet. Pathol.* **13**, 337–342.

162. Dubey, J.P. and Odening, K. (2001) Toxoplasmosis and related infections. Samuel, B., Pybur, M., and Kocan, A.M. (eds.) In: *Parasitic Diseases of Wild Mammals.* Iowa State University Press, Ames, Iowa. 478–519.

163. Dubey, J.P. and Sreekumar, C. (2003) Redescription of *Hammondia hammondi* and its differentiation from *Toxoplasma gondii. Int. J. Parasitol.* **33**, 1437–1453.

164. Christie, E., Dubey, J.P. and Pappas, P.W. (1977) Prevalence of *Hammondia hammondi* in the feces of cats in Ohio. *J. Parasitol.* **63**, 929–931.

165. Mason, R.W. (1978) The detection of *Hammondia hammondi* in Australia and the identification of a free-living intermediate host. *Z. Parasitenkd.* **57**, 101–106.

166. Frenkel, J.K. and Dubey, J.P. (1975) *Hammondia hammondi* gen. nov., sp. nov., from domestic cats, a new coccidian related to *Toxoplasma* and *Sarcocystis. Z. Parasitenkd.* **46**, 3–12.

167. Riahi, H., Leboutet, M.J., Labrousse, F., Boutielle, B., and Darde, M.L. (2000) Monoclonal antibodies to *Hammondia hammondi* allowing immunological differentiation from *Toxoplasma gondii.* **86**, 1362–1366.

168. Wenrich, D.H. (1949) Protozoan parasites of the rat. In: Farris E.J. and Griffith, J.Q. (eds.). *The Rat in Laboratory Investigation.* J.B. Lippincott, Philadelphia, Pennsylvania. 486–501.

169. Price, E.W. and Chitwood, B.G. (1931) Incidence of internal parasites in wild rats in Washington, D.C. *J. Parasitol.* **18**, 55.

170. Evans, W.S., Novak, M., and Basilevsky, A. (1985) Effects of environmental temperature, sex, and infection with Hymenolepis microstoma on the liver and bile duct weights of mice. *J. Parasitol.* **71**, 106–109.

171. Miller, W.W. (1908) *Hepatozoon perniciosum* (n.g., n.s.); a hemogregarine pathogenic for white rats; with a description of the sexual cycle in the intermediate host, a mite (*Laelaps echidninus*). *Bull. U.S. Hyg. Lab.* **46**, 7–51.

172. Macintire, D.K., Vincent-Johnson, N.A., Kane, C.W., Lindsay, D.S., Blagburn, B.L., and Dillon, A.R. (2001) Treatment of dogs with *Hepatozoon americanum:* 53 cases. *J. Am. Vet. Med. Assoc.* **218**, 77–82.

173. Krampitz, H.E. and Haberkorn, A. (1988) Experimental treatment of *Hepatozoon* infections with the anticoccidial agent toltrazuril. *Zentralbl. Veterinarmed. B.* **35**, 131–137.

174. Porter, A. (1908) *Leucocytozoön musculi,* sp. n., a parasitic protozoön from the blood of white mice. *Proc. Zool. Soc. London* Part III, 703–716.

175. Taylor, J.L., Wagner, J.E., Kusewitt, D.F., and Mann, P.C. (1979) *Klossiella* parasites of animals: A literature review. *Vet. Parasitol.* **5**, 137–144.

176. Hartig, F. and Hebold, G. (1970) *Klossiella* parasitism in the kidneys of albino rats. *Exp. Pathol.* **4**, 367–377.

177. Wilson, V.C.L.C. and Edrissian, G.H. (1974) Proceedings: An infection of *Klossiella muris* Smith and Johnson, 1902, in a wild *Mus musculus* from Iran. *Trans. R. Soc. Trop. Med. Hyg.* **68**, 8.

178. Van Pelt, R.W. and Dieterich, R.A. (1985) Renal infection associated with *Klossiella muris:* A different perspective. *Vet. Med.* **80**, 66–68.

179. Yang, Y.H., and Grice, H.C. (1964) *Klossiella muris* parasitism in laboratory mice. *Can. J. Comp. Med. Vet. Sci.* **28**, 63–66.

180. Rosenmann, M. and Morrison, P.R. (1975) Impairment of metabolic capability in feral house mice by *Klossiella muris* infection. *Lab. Anim. Sci.* **25**, 62–64.

181. Otto, H. (1957) Befunde an mäusenieren bei coccidiose (*Klossiella muris*). *Frankf. Z. Pathol.* **68**, 41–48.

182. Ruiz, A. and Frenkel, J.K. (1976) Recognition of cyclic transmission of *Sarcocystis muris* by cats. *J. Infect. Dis.* **133**, 409–418.

183. Rifaat, M.A., Salem, S.A., Khalil, H.M., Azab, M.E., Baki, M.A., and Gaffar, F.M. (1976) The epidemiology of *Sarcocystis muris* in rodents from Egypt. *J. Egypt. Public Health Assoc.* **51**, 321–329.

184. Derothe, J.M., Le Brun, N., Loubes, C., Perriat-Sanguinet, M., and Moulia, C. (2001) Susceptibility of natural hybrids between house mouse subspecies to *Sarcocystis muris. Int. J. Parasitol.* **31**, 15–19.

185. Tillmann, T., Kamino, K., and Mohr, U. (1999) *Sarcocystis muris*—a rare case in laboratory mice. *Lab. Anim.* **33**, 390–392.

186. Dubey, J.P. (1991) Sarcocystosis of the skeletal and cardiac muscle, mouse. In: Mohr, U., Jones, T.C., and Hunt, R.D. (eds.) *Cardiovascular and Musculoskeletal Systems. Monographs on Pathology of Laboratory Animals.* Sponsored by the International Life Sciences Institute. Springer-Verlag. 165–169.

187. Radchenko, A.I. and Beier, T.V. (2001) Effect of developing *Sarcocystis muris* tissue cysts on ultrastructural change of murine muscle fibers. *Tsitologiia* **43**, 708–713.

188. Gill, H.S., Charleston, W.A., and Moriarty, K.M. (1988) Cellular changes in the spleens of mice infected with *Sarcocystis muris. Immunol. Cell. Biol.* **66**, 337–343.

189. Rommel, M., Schwerdtfeger, A. and Blewaska, S. (1981) The *Sarcocystis muris*-infection as a model for research on the chemotherapy of acute sarcocystosis of domestic animals. *Zentralbl. Bakteriol. Microbiol. Hyg. A.* **250**, 268–276.

190. Smith, D.D. and Frenkel, J.K. (1978) Cockroaches as vectors of *Sarcocystis muris* and of other coccidia in the laboratory. *J. Parasitol.* **64**, 315–319.

191. Ashford, R.W. (1978) *Sarcocystis cymruensis* n. sp., a parasite of rats *Rattus norvegicus* and cats *Felis catus. Ann. Trop. Med. Parasitol.* **72**, 37–43.

192. Jakel, T., Khoprasert, Y., Sorger, I., et al. (1997) Sarcosporidiasis in rodents from Thailand. *J. Wildl. Dis.* **33**, 860–867.

193. Hafner, U. and Frank, W. (1986) Morphological studies on the muscle cysts of *Sarcocystis dirumpens* (Hoare 1933) in several host species revealing endopolygeny in metrocytes. *Z. Parasitenkd.* **72**, 453–461.

194. Twort, J.M. and Twort, C.C. (1932) Disease in relation to carcinogenic agents among 60,000 experimental mice. *J. Pathol. Bacteriol.* **35**, 219–242.

195. Jakel, T., Scharpfenecker, M., Jitrawang, P., et al. (2001) Reduction of transmission stages concomitant with increased host immune responses to hypervirulent *Sarcocystis singaporensis,* and natural selection for intermediate virulence. *Int. J. Parasitol.* **31**, 1639–1647.

196. Jakel, T., Burgstaller, H., and Frank, W. (1996) *Sarcocystis singaporensis:* studies on host specificity, pathogenicity, and potential use as a biocontrol agent of wild rats. *J. Parasitol.* **82**, 280–287.

197. Dubey, J.P. and Frenkel, J.K. (1998) Toxoplasmosis of rats: a review, with considerations of their value as an animal model and their possible role in epidemiology. *Vet. Parasitol.* **77**, 1–32.

198. Dubey, J.P. (1990) *Toxoplasma gondii* infections in wildlife. *J.A.V.M.A.* **196**, 274–276.

199. Dubey, J.P. (1997) Distribution of tissue cysts in organs of rats fed *Toxoplasma gondii* oocysts. *J. Parasitol.* **83**, 755–757.

200. Petakov, M., Stojanovic, N., Jovcic, G., Bugarski, D., Todorovic, V., and Djurkovic-Djakovic, O. (2002) Hematopoiesis during acute *Toxoplasma gondii* infection in mice. *Haematologia* **32**, 439–455.

201. Lewis, W.P. and Markell, E.K. (1958) Acquisition of immunity to toxoplasmosis by the newborn rat. *Exp. Parasitol.* **7**, 463–467.

202. Dubey, J.P. (1996) Pathogenicity and infectivity of *Toxoplasma gondii* oocysts for rats. *J. Parasitol.* **82**, 951–956.

203. Berdoy, M., Webster, J.P., and Macdonald, D.W. (2000) Fatal attraction in rats infected with Toxoplasma gondii. *Proc. R. Soc. Lond. B Biol. Sci.* **267**, 1591–1594.

204. Hafid, J., Flori, P., Raberin, H., and Tran Manh Sung, R. (2001) Comparison of PCR, capture ELISA and immunoblotting for detection of *Toxoplasma gondii* in infected mice. *J. Med. Microbiol.* **50**, 1100–1104.

205. Sureau, P. and Capponi, M. (1955) Note sur un piroplasmide de *Rattus norvegicus* observe dans la region du centre Viet-Nam. *Bull. Soc. Pathol. Exotique* **48**, 823–828.

206. Clawson, M.L., Paciorkowski, N., Rajan, T.V., et al. (2002) Cellular immunity, but not gamma interferon, is essential for resolution of *Babesia microti* infection in BALB/c mice. *Infect. Immun.* **70**, 5304–5306.

207. Habicht, G.S., Benach, J.L., Leichtling, K.D., Gocinski, B.L., and Coleman, J.L. (1983) The effect of age on the infection and immunoresponsiveness of mice to *Babesia microti. Mech. Ageing Dev.* **23**, 357–369.

208. Rudzinska, M.A. and Trager, A. (1962) Intracellular phagotrophy in *Babesia rodhaini* as revealed by electron microscopy. *J. Protozool.* **9**, 279–288.

209. Paget, G.E., Alcock, S.J., and Ryley, J.F. (1962) The pathology of *Babesia rodhaini* infections in mice. *J. Pathol. Bacteriol.* **84**, 218–220.

210. Hawking, F. (1973) Infectivity of *Plasmodium berghei* and of *Babesia rodhaini* to various primates. *Am. J. Trop. Med. Hyg.* **22**, 163–167.

211. Matsuda, H., Hasegawa, K., and Kozaki, S. (1987) Development of anti-erythrocyte antibodies in mice infected with *Babesia rodhaini. Zentralbl. Bakteriol. Mikrobiol. Hyg. (A)* **266**, 543–551.

212. Rodhain, J. (1950) Sur la pluralité des espèces de *Babesia* des rongeurs: Àpropos de la spécificité de *Babesia rodhaini* van den Berghe et al. *Ann Inst. Pasteur* **79**, 777–785.

213. Schroeder, W.F., Cox, H.W., and Ristic, M. (1966) Anaemia, parasitaemia, erythrophagocytosis, and haemagglutinins in *Babesia rodhaini* infection. *Ann. Trop. Med. Parasitol.* **60**, 31–38.

214. Wijaya, A., Wulansari, R., Ano, H., Inokuma, H., and Makimura, S. (2000) Therapeutic effect of clindamycin and tetracyline on *Babesia rodhaini* infection in mouse model. *J. Vet. Med. Sci.* **62**, 835–839.

215. Resseler, R. (1956) Un nouveau plasmodium de rat en Belgique: *Plasmodium inopinatum* n.sp. *Ann. Soc. Belg. Med. Trop.* **36**, 259–263.

216. Vincke, I.H. and Lips, M. (1948) Un nouveau *Plasmodium* d'un rongeur sauvage du Congo, *Plasmodium berghei* n.sp. *Ann. Soc. Belge. Med. Trop.* **28**, 97–104.

217. Desowitz, R.S. (1999) *Plasmodium berghei* in the white rat: severe malaria of pregnancy does not occur in the progeny of mothers infected during gestation. *Ann. Trop. Med. Parasitol.* **93**, 415–417.

218. Mercado, T.I. (1965) Paralysis associated with *Plasmodium berghei* malaria in the rat. *J. Infect. Dis.* **115**, 465–472.

219. Kokwaro, G., Edwards, G., Roberts, P., Ward, S., Winstanley, P., and Watkins, W. (1997) Infection with *Plasmodium berghei* alters benzodiazepine receptor in rat brain. *Arch. Med. Res.* **28**, 425–427.

220. Landau, I. (1965) Description de *Plasmodium chabaudi* n. sp., parasite de rongeurs africains. *Compt. Rend. Acad. Sci.* **260**, 3758–3761.

221. Ott, K.J. and Stauber, L.A. (1967) *Eperythrozoon coccoides:* Influence on course of infection of *Plasmodium chabaudi* in mouse. Science **155**, 1546–1548.

222. Rodhain, J.(1952) *Plasmodium vinckei* n.sp., un deuxième plasmodium parasite de rongeurs sauvages au Katanga. *Ann. Soc. Belge. Med. Trop.* **32**, 275–279.

223. Owen, D. (1976) Cestodes in laboratory mice: Isolation of *Cataenotaenia pusilla. Lab. Anim.* **10**, 59–64.

224. Ishih, A., Nishimura, M., and Sano, M. (1992) Differential establishment and survival of *Hymenolepis diminuta* in syngeneic and outbred rat strains. *J. Helminthol.* **66**, 132–136.

225. Insler, G.D. and Roberts, L.S. (1976) *Hymenolepis diminuta:* lack of pathogenicity in the healthy rat host. *Exp. Parasitol.* **39**, 351–357.

226. Andreassen, J. and Hopkins, C.A. (1980) Immunologically mediated rejection of *Hymenolepis diminuta* by its normal host, the rat. *J. Parasitol.* **66**, 898–903.

227. Habermann, R.T. and Williams, F.P. Jr. (1958) The identification and control of helminths in laboratory animals. *J. Natl. Cancer Inst.* **29**, 979–1009.

228. Zimmerman, N.P., Bass, P., and Oaks, J.A. (2001) Modulation of caudal intestinal permeability in the rat during infection by the tapeworm *Hymenolepis diminuta. J. Parasitol.* **87**, 1260–1263.

229. Soulsby, E.J.L. (1982) *Helminths, Arthropods and Protozoa of Domesticated Animals,* 7th ed., Lea and Febiger, Philadelphia, Pennsylvania, 809 pages.

230. Novak, M., Koschinsky, M., Smith, T., and Evans, W.S. (1986) Growth and development of *Hymenolepis nana* in mice maintained at different environmental temperatures. *Int. J. Parasitol.* **16**, 13–17.

231. Katiyar, J.C., Gupta, S., and Sen, A.B. (1983) Susceptibility, chemotherapeutic reaction and immunological response of rat and mouse to *Hymenolepis nana*—a comparative study. *Indian J. Exp. Biol.* **21**, 371–374.

232. Gruber, H.E., Johnson, T.L., Kinsella, J.M., Greiner, E.C., and Gordon, B.E. (2001) Tapeworm identification in the fat sand rat (*Psammomys obesus obesus*). *Contemp. Top. Lab. Anim. Sci.* **40**, 22–24.

233. Ito, A. and Kamiyama, T. (1984) *Hymenolepis nana:* worm recovery from congenitally athymic nude and phenotypically normal rats and mice. *Exp. Parasitol.* **58**, 132–137.

234. Ito, A., and Kamiyama, T. (1987) Cortisone-sensitive, innate resistance to *Hymenolepis nana* infection in congenitally athymic nude rats. *J. Helminthol.* **61**, 124–128.

235. Macnish, M.G., Ryan, U.M., Behnke, J.M., and Thompson, R.C. (2003) Detection of the rodent tapeworm *Rodentolepis* (= *Hymenolepis*) *microstoma* in humans. A new zoonosis? *Int. J. Parasitol.* **33**, 1079–1085.

236. Macnish, M.G., Morgan, U.M., Behnke, J.M., and Thompson, R.C. (2002) Failure to infect laboratory rodent hosts with human isolates of *Rodentolepis* (= *Hymenolepis*) *nana. J. Helminthol.* **76**, 37–43.

237. Conchedda, M., Gabriele, F., Bortoletti, G., and Palmas, C. (1995) Onset of resistance to light *Hymenolepis nana* infection in mice of different strains. *Parasitologia* **37**, 53–58.

238. Simmons, M.L., Williams, H.E., and Wright, E.B. (1964) Parasite screening and therapeutic value of organic phosphates in inbred mice. *Lab. Animal Care* **14**, 326.

239. Pinto, R.M., Goncalves, L., Gomes, D.C., and Noronha, D. (2001) Helminth fauna of the golden hamster *Mesocricetus auratus* in Brazil. *Contemp. Top. Lab. Anim. Sci.* **40**, 21–26.

240. Voge, M. and Heyneman, D. (1957) Development of *Hymenolepis nana* and *Hymenolepis diminuta* (Cestoda: Hymenolepididae) in the intermediate host *Tribolium confusum*. *Univ. Calif (Berkeley) Publ. Zool.* **59**, 549–580.

241. Heyneman, D. (1961) Studies on helminth immunity: III. Experimental verification of autoinfection from cysticercoids of *Hymenolepis nana* in the white mouse. *J. Infect. Diseases* **109**, 10–18.

242. Heyneman, D. (1962) Studies on helminth immunity: I. Comparison between lumenal and tissue phases of infection in the white mouse by *Hymenolepis nana* (Cestoda: Hymenolepididae). *Am. J. Trop. Med. Hyg.* **2**, 46–63.

243. Simmons, M.L., Richter, C.B., Franklin, J.A., and Tennant, R.W. (1967) Prevention of infectious diseases in experimental mice. *Proc. Soc. Exp. Biol. Med.* **126**, 830–837.

244. Katiyar, J.C., Tangri, A.N., Ghatak, S., and Sen, A.B. (1973) Serum protein pattern of rats during infection with *Hymenolepis nana*. *Indian J. Exp. Biol.* **11**, 188–190.

245. Sidky, H.A., Seoudi, O.A., and Gaffar, S.A. (1982) Effect of *Hymenolepis nana* on blood serum glucose, total proteins, and total lipids of infected mice. *J. Egypt. Soc. Parasitol.* **12**, 187–190.

246. Sanad, M.M. (1991) Effect of *Hymenolepis nana* on the protein and lipid in the intestinal mucosal cells of mice. *J. Egypt. Soc. Parasitol.* **21**, 75–80.

247. Katiyar, J.C. and Sen, A.B. (1970) Occurrence of histamine in the intestine of rats harboring cysticercoids of *Hymenolepis nana*. *Indian J. Exp. Biol.* **8**, 191–193.

248. Niwa, A. and Miyazato, T. (1996) Enhancement of intestinal eosinophilia during *Hymenolepis nana* infection in mice. *J. Helminthol.* **70**, 33–41.

249. Gupta, S., Katiyar, J.C., Sen, A.B., et al. (1980) Anticestode activity of 3,5 dibromo-2′-chlorosalicylanilide-4′-isothiocyanate—a preliminary report. *J. Helminthol.* **54**, 271–273.

250. Gonenc, B. and Sarimehmetoglu, H.O. (2001) Continuous feed medication with nitroscanate for the removal of *Hymenolepis nana* in naturally infected mice and rats. *Dtsch. Tierarztl. Wochenschr.* **108**, 434–436.

251. Novak, M., Collins, M., and Evans, W.S. (1980) The growth of *Hymenolepis microstoma* in intact and gonadectomized mice. *Z. Parasitenkd.* **61**, 243–247.

252. Dvorak, J.A., Jones, A.W., and Kuhlman, H.H. (1961) Studies on the biology of *Hymenolepis microstoma* (Dujardin, 1845). *J. Parasitol.* **47**, 833–838.

253. Casanova, J.C., Santalla, F., Durand, P., Vaucher, C., Feliu, C., and Renaud, F. (2001) Morphological and genetic differentiation of *Rodentolepis straminea* (Goeze, 1752) and *Rodentolepis microstoma* (Dujardin, 1845) (Hymenolepididae). *Parasitol. Res.* **87**, 439–444.

254. Murray, P.D., Foster, W.B., and Passmore, H.C. (1984) *Hymenolepis microstoma*: mouse strain differences in resistance to a challenge infection. *Exp. Parasitol.* **58**, 325–332.

255. Litchford, R.G. (1963) Observations on *Hymenolepis microstoma* in three laboratory hosts: *Mesocricetus auratus*, *Mus musculus*, and *Rattus norvegicus*. *J. Parasitol.* **49**, 403–410.

256. Goodall, R.I. (1972) The growth of *Hymenolepis microstoma* in the laboratory rat. *Parasitology* **65**, 137–142.

257. De Rycke, P.H. (1966) Development of the cestode *Hymenolepis microstoma* in *Mus musculus*. *Z. Parasitenkd.* **27**, 350–354.

258. Andreassen, J., Ito, A., Ito, M., Nakao, M., Nakaya, K. 2004. *Hymenolepis microstoma*: direct life cycle in immunodeficient mice. *Journal of Helminthology* **77**, 1–5.

259. Pappas, P.W. and Mayer, L.P. (1976) The effect of transplanted *Hymenolepis microstoma*, the mouse bile duct tapeworm, on CF-1 mice. *J. Parasitol.* **62**, 329–332.

260. Novak, M. and Nombrado, S. (1988) Mast cell responses to *Hymenolepis microstoma* infection in mice. *J. Parasitol.* **74**, 81–88.

261. Mayer, L.P. and Pappas, P.W. (1976) *Hymenolepis microstoma*: Effect of the mouse bile duct tapeworm on the metabolic rate of CF-1 mice. *Exp. Parasitol.* **40**, 48–51.

262. Rath, E.A. and Walkey, M. (1987) Fatty acid and cholesterol synthesis in mice infected with the tapeworm *Hymenolepis microstoma*. *Parasitology* **95**, 79–92.

263. Bowman, D.D. and Lynn, R.C. (1999) *Georgis' Parasitology for Veterinarians*. 7th ed. Elsevier Health Sciences, Philadelphia, Pennsylvania, 414 pages.

264. Jithendran, K.P. and Somvanshi, R. (1998) Experimental infection of mice with *Taenia taeniaformis* eggs from cats—course of infection and pathological studies. *Indian J. Exp. Biol.* **36**, 523–525.

265. Azuma, H., Okamoto, M., Oku, Y., and Kamiya, M. (1995) Intraspecific variation of *Taenia taeniaformis* as determined by various criteria. *Parasitol. Res.* **81**, 103–108.

266. Singh, B.B. and Rao, B.V. (1965) Some biological studies on *Taenia taeniaformis*. *Ind. J. Helminthol.* **18**, 151–160.

267. Verheyen, A., Vanparijs, O., Borgers, M., and Thienpont, D. (1978) Scanning electron microscopic observations of *Cysticercus fasciolaris* (= *Taenia taeniaformis*) after treatment of mice with mebendazole. *J. Parasitol.* **64**, 411–425.

268. Abadie, S.H. (1963) The life cycle of *Strongyloides ratti*. *J. Parasitol.* **49**, 241–248.

269. Little, M.D. (1966) Comparative morphology of six species of *Strongyloides* (Nematoda) and redefinition of the genus. *J. Parasitol.* **52**, 69–84.

270. Fisher, M.C. and Viney, M.E. (1998) The population genetic structure of the facultatively sexual parasitic nematode *Strongyloides ratti* in wild rats. *Proc. R. Soc. Lond. B. Biol. Sci.* **265**, 703–709.

271. Fedorko, J.M. (1999) *Schistosoma japonicum* in the black rat, *Rattus rattus mindanensis*, from Leyte, Philippines in relation to *Oncomelania* snail colonies with reference to other endoparasites. *Southeast Asian J. Trop. Med. Public Health* **30**, 343–349.

272. Dawkins, H.J., Thomason, H.J., and Grove, D.I. (1982) The occurrence of *Strongyloides ratti* in the tissues of mice after percutaneous infection. *J. Helminthol.* **56**, 45–50.

273. Viney, M.E. (1999) Exploiting the life cycle of *Strongyloides ratti*. *Parasitol. Today* **15**, 231–235.

274. Kawanabe, M., Nojima, H., and Uchikawa, R. (1988) Transmammary transmission of *Strongyloides ratti*. *Parasitol. Res.* **75**, 50–56.

275. Uchikawa, R., Nojima, H., and Sato, A. (1989) The effects of single and repeated inoculations of various larval doses on *Strongyloides ratti* burden and distribution in rats. *J. Parasitol.* **75**, 577–584.

276. Moqbel, R. and Denham, D.A. (1977) *Strongyloides ratti*: 1. Parasitological observations on primary and secondary infections in the small intestine of rats. *J. Helminthol.* **51**, 301–308.

277. Olson, C.E. and Schiller, E.L. (1978) *Strongyloides ratti* infections in rats. I. Immunopathology. *Am. J. Trop. Med. Hyg.* **27**, 521–526.

278. Weesner, R.E., Kolinjivadi, J., Giannella, R.A., Huitger-O'Connor, T., and Genta, R.M. (1988) Effect of *Strongyloides ratti* on small bowel function in normal and immunosuppressed host rats. *Dig. Dis. Sci.* **33**, 1316–1321.

279. Genta, R.M. and Ward, P.A. (1980) The histopathology of experimental strongyloidiasis. *Am. J. Pathol.* **99**, 207–220.

280. McHugh, T.D., Jenkins, T., and McLaren, D.J. (1989) *Strongyloides ratti:* studies of cutaneous reactions elicited in naive and sensitized rats and of changes in surface antigenicity of skin-penetrating larvae. *Parasitology* **98**, 95–103.

281. Grove, D.I., Lumsden, J., and Northern, C. (1988) Efficacy of albendazole against *Strongyloides ratti* and *S. stercoralis* in vitro, in mice, and in normal and immunosuppressed dogs. *J. Antimicrob. Chemother.* **21**, 75–84.

282. Mojon, M., Saura, C., Roojee, N., and Tran Manh Sung, R. (1987) Albendazole and thiabendazole in murine strongyloidiasis. *J. Antimicrob. Chemother.* **19**, 79–85.

283. Wertheim, G. (1970) Growth and development of *Strongyloides venezuelensis* Brumpt, 1934 in the albino rat. *Parasitology* **61**, 381–388.

284. Taira, N., Hirooka, M., and Saeki, H. (1994) Isolation of *Strongyloides venezuelensis* from *Rattus norvegicus* in Kagoshima Prefecture. *J. Vet. Med. Sci.* **56**, 255–258.

285. Attamimi, F., Noviana, D., Muktiandini, A., et al. (2002) Enhanced protection against the migratory phase, but defective protection against the intestinal phase of *Strongyloides venezuelensis* infection in cotton rats, *Sigmodon hispidus. J. Vet. Med. Sci.* **64**, 1031–1035.

286. Baek, B.K., Whang, I.S., Islam, M.K., Kim, B.S., and Kakoma, I. (2002) Persistent infection with *Strongyloides venezuelensis* in the Mongolian gerbil (*Meriones unguiculatus*). *Korean J. Parasitol.* **40**, 181–186.

287. Shi, B.B., Ishikawa, N., Itoh, H., et al. (1995) Goblet cell hyperplasia induced by *Strongyloides venezuelensis*—infection in Syrian golden hamster, *Mesocricetus auratus. Int. J. Parasitol.* **25**, 399–402.

288. Nakamura-Uchiyama, F., Nagao, T., Obara, A., Ishiwata, K., and Nawa, Y. (2001) Natural resistance of 129/SvJ mice to *Strongyloides venezuelensis* infection. *Parasite Immunol.* **23**, 659–663.

289. Sato, Y. and Toma, H. (1990) *Strongyloides venezuelensis* infections in mice. *Int. J. Parasitol.* **20**, 57–62.

290. Takamure, A. (1995) Migration route of *Strongyloides venezuelensis* in rodents. *Int. J. Parasitol.* **25**, 907–911.

291. Carter, K.C. and Wilson, P.A. (1989) The course of infection in rats given small primary doses of *Strongyloides ratti* and *S. venezuelensis. J. Helminthol.* **63**, 107–114.

292. Rivero, J.C., Inoue, Y., Murakami, N., and Horii, Y. (2002) Age- and sex-related changes in susceptibility of Wistar rats to *Strongyloides venezuelensis* infection. *J. Vet. Med. Sci.* **64**, 519–521.

293. Negrao-Correa, D., Silveira, M.R., Borges, C.M., Souza, D.G., and Teixeira, M.M. (2003) Changes in pulmonary function and parasite burden in rats infected with *Strongyloides venezuelensis* concomitant with induction of allergic airway inflammation. *Infect. Immun.* **71**, 2607–2614.

294. Khan, A.I., Horii, Y., Tiuria, R., Sato, Y., and Nawa, Y. (1993) Mucosal mast cells and expulsive mechanisms of mice against *Strongyloides venezuelensis. Int. J. Parasitol.* **23**, 551–555.

295. Taira, N., Nakamura, Y., Almeida, M.A., and Saeki, H. (1995) Massive experimental infection with *Strongyloides venezuelensis* in rats and absence of sudden death. *J. Vet. Med. Sci.* **57**, 855–858.

296. Campos, R., Pinto, P.L., Amato Neto, V., et al. (1989) Treatment of experimental infection by *Strongyloides venezuelensis* in rats, with the use of injectable ivermectin and levamisole. *Rev. Inst. Med. Trop. Sao Paulo* **31**, 48–52.

297. Amato Neto, V., Carignani, F.L., Matsubara, L., and Braz, L.M. (1997) The treatment of rats experimentally infected with *Strongyloides venezuelensis* by orally administered ivermectin. *Rev. Soc. Bras. Med. Trop.* **30**, 481–484.

298. Smith, P.E. (1953) Life history and host-parasite relations of *Heterakis spumosa*, a nematode parasite in the colon of the rat. *Am. J. Hyg.* **57**, 194–221.

299. Smith, P.E. (1953) Host specificity of *Heterakis spumosa* Schneider, 1866 (Nematoda: Heterakidae). *Proc. Helminthol. Soc. Wash. D.C.* **20**, 19–21.

300. Yokohata, Y., Abe, H., Jiang, Y.P., and Kamiya, M. (1989) Gastrointestinal helminth fauna of Japanese moles, *Mogera* spp. *Jpn. J. Vet. Res.* **37**, 1–13.

301. Mehlhorn, H., and Harder, A. (1997) Effects of the synergistic action of febantel and pyrantel on the nematode *Heterakis spumosa:* a light and transmission electron microscopy study. *Parasitol. Res.* **83**, 419–434.

302. Harder, A., Wunderlich, F., and Marinovski, P. (1992) Effects of testosterone on *Heterakis supumosa* infections in mice. *Parasitology* **105**, 335–342.

303. Kirsch, R. (1975) The effectiveness of fenbendazole against adults and immature stages of *Nematospiroides dubius* and *Heterakis spumosa. Zentralbl. Veterinarmed B.* **22**, 441–447.

304. Tafts, L.F. (1976) Pinworm infections in laboratory rodents: a review. *Lab. Anim.* **10**, 1–13.

305. Bazzano, T., Restel, T.I., Pinto, R.M., and Gomes, D.C. (2002) Patterns of infection with the nematodes *Syphacia obvelata* and *Aspiculuris tetraptera* in conventionally maintained laboratory mice. *Mem. Inst. Oswaldo Cruz* **97**, 847–853.

306. Baker, D.G. (2004) Letter to the Editor. *Contemp. Top. Lab. Anim. Sci.* **43**, 7.

307. Mathies, A.W. Jr. (1959) Certain aspects of the host-parasite relationship of *Aspiculuris tetraptera*, a mouse pinworm. I. Host specificity and age resistance. *Exp. Parasitol.* **8**, 31–38.

308. Yamaguti, S. (1961) The nematodes of vertebrates, vol. 3 part 1. In: *Systema Helminthum.* Interscience Publishers, Inc., New York, p. 544.

309. Pinto, R.M., Gomes, D.C., and Noronha, D. (2003) Evaluation of coninfection with pinworms (*Aspiculuris tetraptera, Dentostomella translucida*, and *Syphacia obvelata*) in gerbils and mice. *Contemp. Top. Lab. Anim. Sci.* **42**, 46–48.

310. Chan, K.-F. (1955) The distribution of larval stages of *Aspiculuris tetraptera* in the intestine of mice. *J. Parasitol.* **41**, 529–532.

311. Boivin, G.P., Ormsby, I., and Hall, J.E. (1996) Eradication of *Aspiculuris tetraptera*, using fenbendazole-medicated food. *Contemp. Top. Lab. Anim. Sci.* **35**, 69–70.

312. West, W.L., Schofield, J.C., and Bennett, B.T. (1992) Efficacy of the "micro-dot" technique for administering topical 1% ivermectin for the control of pinworms and fur mites in mice. *Contemp. Top. Lab. Anim. Sci.* **31**, 7–10.

313. Krishnasamy, M., Singh, K.I., Ambu, S., and Ramachandran, P. (1980) Seasonal prevalence of the helminth fauna of the wood rat *Rattus tiomanicus* (Miller) in West Malaysia. *Folia Parasitol. (Praha)* **27**, 231–235.

314. Hussey, K.L. (1957) *Syphacia muris* vs. *S. obvelata* in laboratory rats and mice. *J. Parasitol.* **43**, 555–559.

315. Ross, C.R., Wagner, J.E., Wightman, S.R., and Dill, S.E. (1980) Experimental transmission of *Syphacia muris* among rats, mice, hamsters and gerbils. *Lab. Anim. Sci.* **30**, 35–37.

316. van der Gulden, W.J. (1967) Diurnal rhythm in egg production by *Syphacia muris. Exp. Parasitol.* **21**, 344–347.

317. Stahl, W.B. (1963) Studies on the life cycle of *Syphacia muris*, the rat pinworm. *Keio J. Med.* **12**, 55–60.

318. Lewis, J.W., and D'Silva, J. (1986) The life-cycle of *Syphacia muris* Yamaguti (Nematoda: Oxyuroidea) in the laboratory rat. *J. Helminthol.* **60**, 39–46.

319. Dix, J., Astill, J., and Whelan, G. (2004) Assessment of methods of destruction of *Syphacia muris* eggs. *Lab. Anim.* **38**, 11–16.

320. Lübcke, R., Hutcheson, F.A.R., and Barbezat, G.O. (1992) Impaired intestinal electrolyte transport in rats infested with the common parasite *Syphacia muris*. *Dig. Dis. Sci.* **37**, 60–64.

321. Wagner, M. (1988) The effect of infection with the pinworm (*Syphacia muris*) on rat growth. *Lab. Anim. Sci.* **38**, 476–478.

322. Pritchett, K.R. and Johnston, N.A. (2002) A review of treatments for the eradication of pinworm infections from laboratory rodent colonies. *Contemp. Top. Lab. Anim. Sci.* **41**, 36–46.

323. Kirsch, R. (1978) *In vitro* and *in vivo* studies on the ovicidal activity of fenbendazole. *Res. Vet. Sci.* **25**, 263–265.

324. Lacey, E., Brady, R.L., Prichard, R.K., and Watson, T.R. (1987) Comparison of inhibition of polymerisation of mammalian tubulin and helminth ovicidal activity by benzimidazole carbamates. *Vet. Parasitol.* **23**, 105–119.

325. Huerkamp, M.J., Benjamin, K.A., Zitzow, L.A., et al. (2000) Fenbendazole treatment without environmental decontamination eradicates *Syphacia muris* from rats in a large, complex research institution. *Contemp. Top. Lab. Anim. Sci.* **39**, 9–12.

326. Huerkamp, M.J., Benjamin, K.A., Webb, S.K., and Pullium, J.K. (2004) Long-term results of dietary fenbendazole to eradicate *Syphacia muris* from rat colonies. *Contemp. Top. Lab. Anim. Sci.* **43**, 35–36.

327. Kellogg, H.S. and Wagner, J.E. (1982) Experimental transmission of *Syphacia obvelata* among mice, rats, hamsters, and gerbils. *Lab. An. Sci.* **32**, 500–501.

328. Lewis, J.W. (1968) Studies on the helminth parasites of voles and shrews from Wales. *J. Zool.* **154**, 313–331.

329. Behnke, J.M., Barnard, C., Hurst, J.L., McGregor, P.K., Gilbert, F., and Lewis, J.W. (1993) The prevalence and intensity of infection with helminth parasites in *Mus spretus* from the Setubal Peninsula of Portugal. *J. Helminthol.* **67**, 115–122.

330. Chan, K.-F. (1952) Life cycle studies on the nematode *Syphacia obvelata*. *Am. J. Hyg.* **56**, 14–21.

331. Grice, R.L. and Prociv, P. (1993) *In vitro* embryonation of *Syphacia obvelata* eggs. *Int. J. Parasitol.* **23**, 257–260.

332. Harwell, J.F. and Boyd, D.D. (1968) Naturally occurring oxyuriasis in mice. *J.A.V.M.A.* **153**, 950–953.

333. Sasa, M., Tanaka, H., Fukui, M., and Takata, A. (1962) Internal parasites of laboratory animals. In: Harris, R.J.C (ed.) *The problems of Laboratory Animal Disease.* Academic Press, New York, 195–214.

334. Wescott, R.B., Malczewski, A., and Van Hoosier, G.L. (1976) The influence of filter top caging on the transmission of pinworm infections in mice. *Lab. Anim. Sci.* **26**, 742–745.

335. Owen, D.G. (1992) *Parasites of Laboratory Animals.* Laboratory Animal Handbook No. 12. Royal Society of Medicine Services Limited, London, 170 pages.

336. Quinnell, R.J., Behnke, J.M., and Keymer, A.E. (1991) Host specificity of and cross-infectivity between two strains of *Heligmosomoides polygyrus*. *Parasitology* **102**, 419–427.

337. Behnke, J.M. and Wakelin, D. (1977) *Nematospiroides dubius*: stimulation of acquired immunity in inbred strains of mice. *J. Helminthol.* **51**, 167–176.

338. Baker, N.F. (1955) The pathogenesis of trichostrongyloid parasites: some effects of Nematospiroides dubius on the erythrocyte patterns and spleens of mice. *Exp. Parasitol.* **4**, 526–541.

339. Fahmy, M.A.M. (1956) An investigation on the life cycle of *Nematospiroides dubius* (Nematoda: Heligomosomoidea) with special reference to the free-living stages. *Z. F. Parasitenkunde* **17**, 394–399.

340. Kristan, D.M. (2002) Maternal and direct effects of the intestinal nematode *Heligmosomoides polygyrus* on offspring growth and susceptibility to infection. *J. Exp. Biol.* **205**, 3967–77.

341. Svetic, A., Madden, K.B., Zhou, X.D., et al. (1993) A primary intestinal helminthic infection rapidly induces a gut-associated elevation of the Th2–associated cytokines and IL-3. *J. Immunol.* **150**, 3434–3441.

342. Cywinska, A., Czuminska, K., and Schollenberger, A. (2004) Granulomatous inflammation during *Heligmosomoides polygyrus* primary infections in FVB mice. *J. Helminthol.* **78**, 17–24.

343. Wahid, F.N., Behnke, J.M., and Conway, D.J. (1989) Factors affecting the efficacy of ivermectin against *Heligmosomoides polygyrus* (*Nematospiroides dubius*) in mice. *Vet. Parasitol.* **32**, 325–340.

344. Skopets, S., Wilson, R.P., Griffith, J.W., and Lang, C.M. (1996) Ivermectin toxicity in young mice. *Lab. An. Sci.* **46**, 111–112.

345. Haley, A.J. (1962) Biology of the rat nematode *Nippostrongylus brasiliensis* (Travassos, 1914): II. Preparasitic stages and development in the laboratory rat. *J. Parasitol.* **48**, 13–23.

346. Dineen, J.K., Ogilvie, B.M., Kelly, J.D. (1973) Expulsion of *Nippostrongylus brasiliensis* from the intestine of rats. Collaboration between humoral and cellular components of the immune response. *Immunology* **24**, 467–475.

347. Cheema, K.J. and Scofield, A.M. (1975) Scanning electron microscopy of the intestines of rats infected with *Nippostrongylus brasiliensis*. *Int. J. Parasitol.* **12**, 199–205.

348. Ko, R.C. (1978) Occurrence of *Angiostrongylus cantonensis* in the heart of a spider monkey. *J. Helminthol.* **52**, 229.

349. Wallace, G.D. and Rosen, L. (1961) Studies on eosinophilic meningitis. I. Observations on the geographic distribution of *Angiostrongylus cantonensis* in the Pacific area and its prevalence in wild rats. *Am. J. Epidemiol.* **81**, 52–62.

350. Kim, D.Y., Stewart, T.B., Bauer, R.W., and Mitchell, M. (2002) *Parastrongylus* (= *Angiostrongylus*) *cantonensis* now endemic in Louisiana wildlife. *J. Parasitol.* **88**, 1024–1026.

351. Reddacliff, L.A., Bellamy, T.A., and Hartley, W.J. (1999) *Angiostrongylus cantonensis* infection in grey-headed fruit bats (*Pteropus poliocephalus*). *Aust. Vet. J.* **77**, 466–468.

352. Rachford, F.W. (1975) Potential intermediate and paratenic hosts for *Angiostrongylus cantonensis*. *J. Parasitol.* **61**, 1117–1119.

353. Platt, T.R. and Harris, G.S. (1985) An examination of the prepatent period and the absence of a crowding effect in *Angiostrongylus cantonensis* in laboratory rats. *J. Trop. Med. Hyg.* **88**, 323–326.

354. Limaye, L.S., Bhopale, M.K., Renapurkar, D.M., and Sharma, K.D. (1983) The distribution of *Angiostrongylus cantonensis* (Chen) in the central nervous system of laboratory rats. *Folia Parasitol.* **30**, 281–284.

355. Ishii, A.I. (1987) Pathogenic factors in the later pulmonary phase of *Angiostrongylus cantonensis*-infected rats. *Parasitol. Res.* **73**, 458–465.

356. Hwang, K.P. and Chen, E.R. (1988) Larvicidal effect of albendazole against *Angiostrongylus cantonensis* in mice. *Am. J. Trop. Med. Hyg.* **39**, 191–195.

357. Lämmler, G. and Weidner, E. (1975) The larvicidal activity of anthelmintics against *Angiostrongylus cantonensis*. *Berl. Münch. Tierärztl. Wochenschr.* **88**, 152–156.

358. Hwang, K.P. and Chen, E.R. (1994) Anthelmintic effect of levamisole against *Angiostrongylus cantonensis* in mice. *Gaoxiong Yi Xue Ke Xue Za Zhi* **10**, 536–542.

359. Maki, J. and Kanda, S. (1992) Higher sensitivity of the developing larvae of *Angiostrongylus cantonensis* than the adult worms to flubendazole and mebendazole. *Kitasato Arch. Exp. Med.* **65**, 131–136.

360. Alto, W. (2001) Human infections with *Angiostrongylus cantonensis*. *Pac. Health Dialog.* **8**, 176–182.

361. Tesh, R.B., Ackerman, L.J., Dietz, W.H., and Williams, J.A. (1973) *Angiostrongylus costaricensis* in Panama. Prevalence and pathologic findings in wild rodents infected with the parasite. *Am. J. Trop. Med. Hyg.* **22**, 348–356.

362. Morera, P. (1973) Life history and redescription of *Angiostrongylus costaricensis* Morera and Céspedes, 1971. *Am. J. Trop. Med. Hyg.* **22**, 613–621.

363. Mojon, M. (1994) Human angiostrongyliasis caused by *Angiostrongylus costaricensis*. *Bull. Acad. Natl. Med.* **178**, 625–631.

364. Rodriguez, R., Agostini, A.A., Porto, S.M., et al. (2002). Dogs may be a reservoir host for *Angiostrongylus costaricensis*. *Rev. Inst. Med. Trop. Sao Paulo* **44**, 55–56.

365. Rambo, P.R., Agostini, A.A., and Graeff-Teixeira, C. (1997) Abdominal angiostrongylosis in southern Brazil—prevalence and parasitic burden in mollusc intermediate hosts from eighteen endemic foci. *Mem. Inst. Oswaldo Cruz* **92**, 9–14.

366. Ishih, A., Baba, S., Nagata, T., and Terada, M. (2003) Intestinal granuloma formation in normal and SCID BALB/c mice infected with *Angiostrongylus costaricensis*. *Parasitol. Res.* **89**, 150–153.

367. Morera, P. and Cespedes, R. (2002) *Angiostrongylus costaricensis* n.sp. (Nematoda: Metastrongyloidea), a new lungworm occurring in man in Costa Rica. *Rev. Biol. Trop.* **50**, 783–796.

368. Alvarez, F., Iglesias, R., Bos, J., Rey, J., and San Martin-Duran, M.L. (1991) Lung and heart nematodes in some Spanish mammals. *Wiad. Parazytol.* **37**, 481–490.

369. Bhaibulaya, M. (1975) Comparative studies on the life history of *Angiostrongylus mackerrasae* Bhaibulaya, 1968 and *Angiostrongylus cantonensis* (Chen, 1935). *Int. J. Parasitol.* **5**, 7–20.

370. Kinsella, J.M. (1971) Angiostrongylus schmidti sp.n. (Nematoda: Metastrongyloidea) from the rice rat, Oryzomys palustris, in Florida, with a key to the species of Angiostrongylus Kamensky, 1905. *J. Parasitol.* **57**, 494–497.

371. Holanda, J.C., Vicente, J.J., Brazil, R.P., and Bastos Ode, C. (1985) Natural infection of *Holochilus brasiliensis nanus* Thomas, 1897 (Rodentia, Cricetidae) by *Litomosoides carinii*. *Mem. Inst. Oswaldo Cruz* **80**, 121.

372. Thompson, P.E., Boche, L., and Blair, L.S. (1968) Effects of amodiaquine against *Litomosoides carinii* in gerbils and cotton rats. *J. Parasitol.* **54**, 834–837.

373. Takahashi, N., Maeda, R., and Shibuya, T. (1996) Electron microscopic observation of eosinophils migrated to the thoracic cavity of *Litomosoides carinii*-infected mice. *Int. Arch. Allergy Immunol.* **111** Suppl 1, 51–54.

374. Olsen, O.W. (1967) *Animal Parasites: Their biology and life cycles.* 2nd ed. Burgess, Minneapolis Minnesota, 431 pages.

375. Seong, J.K., Huh, S., Lee, J.S., and Oh, Y.S. (1995) Helminths in *Rattus norvegicus* captured in Chunchon, Korea. *Korean J. Parasitol.* **33**, 235–237.

376. Ceruti, R., Sonzogni, O., Origgi, F., et al. (2001) *Capillaria hepatica* infection in wild brown rats (*Rattus norvegicus*) from the urban area of Milan, Italy. *J. Vet. Med. B Infect. Dis. Vet. Public Health* **48**, 235–240.

377. Lee, C.W. (1964) The experimental studies on *Capillaria hepatica*. *Kisaengchunghak Chapchi.* **2**, 63–80.

378. Oliveira, L., de Souza, M.M., and Adrade, Z.A. (2004) *Capillaria hepatica*-induced hepatic fibrosis in rats: paradoxical effect of repeated infections. *Rev. Soc. Bras. Med. Trop.* **37**, 123–127.

379. Govil, H. and Desai, M. (1996) *Capillaria hepatica* parasitism. *Indian J. Pediatr.* **63**, 698–700.

380. Cutillas, C., Oliveros, R., de Rojas, M., and Guevara, D.C. (2002) Determination of *Trichuris muris* from murid hosts and *T. arvicolae* (Nematoda) from arvicolid rodents by amplification and sequentiation of the ITS1–5.8S-ITS2 segment of the ribosomal DNA. *Parasitol. Res.* **88**, 574–582.

381. Feliu, C., Spakulova, M., Casanova, J.C., et al. (2000) Genetic and morphological heterogeneity in small rodent whipworms in southwestern Europe: characterization of *Trichuris muris* and description of *Trichuris arvicolae* n.sp. (Nematoda: Trichuridae). *J. Parasitol.* **86**, 442–449.

382. Behnke, J.M. and Wakelin, D. (1973) The survival of *Trichuris muris* in wild populations of its natural hosts. *Parasitology* **67**, 157–164.

383. Panesar, T.S. and Croll, N.A. (1980) The location of parasites within their hosts: site selection by *Trichuris muris* in the laboratory mouse. *Int. J. Parasitol.* **10**, 261–273.

384. Lee, T.D.G. and Wright, K.A. (1978) The morphology of the attachment and probable feeding site of the nematode *Trichuris muris* (Schrank, 1788) Hall, 1916. *Can. J. Zool.* **56**, 1899–1905.

385. Wakelin, D. (1969) The development of the early larval stages of *Trichuris muris* in the albino laboratory mouse. *J. Helminthol.* **43**, 427–436.

386. Else, K.J. and deSchoolmeester, M.L. (2003) Immunity to *Trichuris muris* in the laboratory mouse. *J. Helminthol.* **77**, 95–98.

387. Rajasekariah, G.R., Deb, B.N., Jones, M.P., Dhage, K.R., and Bose, S. (1991) Response of pre-adult and adult stages of *Trichuris muris* to common anthelmintics in mice. *Int. J. Parasitol.* **21**, 697–702.

388. Yorke, W. and Maplestone, P.A. (1926) *The nematode parasites of vertebrates.* Blakiston, Philadelphia, Pennsylvania, 536 pages.

389. Bowman, M.R., Pare, J.A., and Pinckney, R.D. (2004) *Trichosomoides crassicauda* infection in a pet hooded rat. *Vet. Rec.* **154**, 374–375.

390. Wahl, D.V. and Chapman, W.H. (1967) The application of data on the survival of eggs of *Trichosomoides crassicauda* (Bellingham) to the control of this bladder parasite in laboratory rat colonies. *Lab. Anim. Care* **17**, 386–390.

391. Weisbroth, S.H. and Scher, S. (1971) *Trichosomoides crassicauda* infection of a commercial rat breeding colony. I. Observations on the life cycle and propagation. *Lab. Anim. Sci.* **21**, 54–61.

392. Thomas, L.J. (1924) Studies on the life history of *Trichosomoides crassicauda* (Bellingham). *J. Parasitol.* **10**, 105–136.

393. Bone, J.F. and Harr, J.R. (1967) *Trichosomoides crassicauda* infection in laboratory rats. *Lab. Anim. Care* **17**, 321–326.

394. Antonakopoulos, G.N., Turton, J., Whitfield, P., and Newman, J. (1991) Host-parasite interface of the urinary bladder-inhabiting nematode *Trichosomoides crassicauda*: changes induced in the urothelium of infected rats. *Int. J. Parasitol.* **21**, 187–193.

395. Smith, V.S. (1946) Are vesicle calculi associated with *Trichosomoides crassicauda*, the common bladder nematode of rats? *J. Parasitol.* **32**, 142–149.

396. Zubaidy, A.J. and Majeed, S.K. (1981) Pathology of the nematode *Trichosomoides crassicauda* in the urinary bladder of laboratory rats. *Lab. Anim.* **15**, 381–384.

397. Chapman, W.H. (1964) The incidence of a nematode *Trichosomoides crassicauda* in the urinary bladder of laboratory rats. Treatment with nitrofurantoin and preliminary report of their influence on urinary calculi and experimental bladder tumors. *Invest. Urol.* **2**, 52–57.

398. Cornish, J., Vanderwee, M.A., Findon, G., and Miller, T.E. (1988) Reliable diagnosis of *Trichosomoides crassicauda* in the urinary bladder of the rat. *Lab. Anim.* **22**, 162–165.

399. Summa, M.E., Ebisui, L., Osaka, J.T., and de Tolosa, E.M. (1992) Efficacy of oral ivermectin against *Trichosomoides crassicauda* in naturally infected laboratory rats. *Lab. Anim. Sci.* **42**, 620–622.

400. Moore, D.V. (1946) Studies on the life history and development of *Moniliformis dubius* Meyer, 1933. *J. Parasitol.* **32**, 257–271.

401. King, D. and Robinson, E.S. (1967) Aspects of the development of *Moniliformis dubius. J. Parasitol.* **53**, 142–149.

402. Moore, J. and Crompton, D.W. (1993) A quantitative study of the susceptibility of cockroach species to *Moniliformis moniliformis* (Acanthocephala). *Parasitology* **107**, 63–69.

403. Chariyahpongpun, P., Sripalwit, P., and Wongsawad, C. (2000) Reinvestigated life history of *Moniliformis dubius* Meyer, 1933 in Chiang Mai, Thailand. *Southeast Asian J. Trop. Med. Public Health* **31**, 65–68.

404. Crompton, D.W.T., Arnold, S., and Barnard, D. (1972) The patent period and production of eggs of *Moniliformis dubius* (Acanthocephala) in the small intestine of male rats. *Int. J. Parasitol.* **2**, 319–326.

405. Varute, A.T. and Patil, V.A. (1971) Histopathology of alimentary tract of rats infected by *Moniliformis dubius* (Acanthocephala). I. Histological alterations and changes in nuclei and mucopolysaccharide distribution. *Indian J. Exp. Biol.* **9**, 195–199.

406. Singhvi, A. and Crompton, D.W. (1975) Increase in size of the small intestine of rats infected with *Moniliformis* (Acanthocephala). *Int. J. Parasitol.* **12**, 173–178.

407. Sures, B., Scheef, G., Klar, B., Kloas, W., and Taraschewski, H. (2002) Interaction between cadmium exposure and infection with the intestinal parasite *Moniliformis moniliformis* (Acanthocephala) on the stress hormone levels in rats. *Environ. Pollut.* **119**, 333–340.

408. Counselman, K., Field, C., Lea, G., Nickol, B., and Neafie, R. (1989) *Moniliformis moniliformis* from a child in Florida. *Am. J. Trop. Med. Hyg.* **41**, 88–90.

409. Arnold, S.E. and Crompton, D.W. (1987) Survival of shelled acanthors of *Moniliformis moniliformis* (Acanthocephala) under laboratory conditions. *J. Helminthol.* **61**, 306–310.

410. Catts, E.P. (1965) Host-parasite interrelationships in rodent bot fly infections. *Trans. 30th North Am. Wildlife Nat. Resources Conf. Washington., D.C.* **30**, 184–186.

411. Cogley, T.P. (1991) Warble development by the rodent bot *Cuterebra fontinella* (Diptera: Cuterebridae) in the deer mouse. *Vet. Parasitol.* **38**, 275–288.

412. Lepitzki, D.A., Woolf, A., and Bunn, B.M. (1992) Parasites of cottontail rabbits of southern Illinois. *J. Parasitol.* **78**, 1080–1083.

413. Gummer, D.L., Forbes, M.R., Bender, D.J., and Barclay, R.M. (1997) Botfly (Diptera: Oestridae) parasitism of Ord's kangaroo rats (*Dipodomys ordii*) at Suffield National Wildlife Area, Alberta, Canada. *J. Parasitol.* **83**, 601–604.

414. Wilson, W.D., Hnida, J.A., and Duszynski, D.W. (1997) Parasites of mammals on the Sevilleta National Wildlife Refuge, Socorro, New Mexico: *Cuterebra austeni* and *C. neomexicana* (Diptera: Oestridae) from *Neotoma* and *Peromyscus* (Rodentia: Muridae), 1991–1994. *J. Med. Entomol.* **34**, 359–367.

415. Catts, E.P. (1967) Biology of a California rodent botfly *Cuterebra latifrons* Coquillett (Diptera: Cuterebridae). *J. Med. Entomol.* **4**, 87–101.

416. Dunaway, P.B., Payne, J.A., Lewis, L.L., and Story, J.D. (1967) Incidence and effects of *Cuterebra* in *Peromyscus. J. Mammal.* **48**, 38–51.

417. Payne, J.A. and Cosgrove, G.E. (1966) Tissue changes following *Cuterebra* infestation in rodents. *Am. Midland Naturalist* **75**, 205–213.

418. Baird, J.K., Baird, C.R., and Sabrosky, C.W. (1989) North American cuterebrid myiasis. Report of seventeen new infections of human beings and review of the disease. *J. Am. Acad. Dermatol.* **21**, 763–772.

419. Schumann, H., Schuster, R., and Lange, J. (1985) The warble fly *Oestromyia leporina* (Diptera, Hypodermatidae) as a parasite of the wild rabbit (*Oryctolagus cuniculus*). *Angew. Parasitol.* **26**, 51–52.

420. Volf, P., Lukes, J., and Srp, V. (1990) Study on the population of the warble fly, *Oestromyia leporina* (Pallas, 1778) (Diptera: Hypodermatidae) in Bohemia. *Folia Parasitol. (Praha)* **37**, 187–190.

421. Rietschel, G. and Baumann, E. (1975) The biology of the warble-fly *Oestromyia leporina* Pallas 1778 (Diptera, Hypodermatidae), a parasite of the field-mouse *Microtus arvalis* Pall. *Z. Parasitenkd.* **46**, 141–152.

422. Rietschel, G. (1979) Histological reactions of the host induced by the larvae of the warble-fly *Oestromyia leporina* Pallas (Diptera, Hypodermatidae). *Z. Parasitenkd.* **60**, 277–289.

423. Ferris, G.F. (1951) The sucking lice. *Pacific Coast Entomol. Soc. Mem.* **1**, 1–320.

424. Cook, E.F. and Beer, J.R. (1959) The immature stages of the genus *Hoplopleura* (Anoplura: Hoplopleuridae) in North America, with description of two new species. *J. Parasitol.* **45**, 405–416.

425. Kim, K.C. (1966) A new species of *Hoplopleura* from Thailand, with notes and description of nymphal stages of *Hoplopleura captiosa* Johnson (Anoplura). *Parasitology* **56**, 603–612.

426. Durden, L.A. (1992) Parasitic arthropods of sympatric meadow voles and white-footed mice at Fort Detrick, Maryland. *J. Med. Entomol.* **29**, 761–766.

427. Kollars, T.M. Jr., Durden, L.A., and Oliver, J.H. Jr. (1997) Fleas and lice parasitizing mammals in Missouri. *J. Vector Ecol.* **22**, 125–132.

428. Durden, L.A., Kollars, T.M. Jr., Patton, S., and Gerhardt, R.R. (1997) Sucking lice (Anoplura) of mammals of Tennessee. *J. Vector Ecol.* **22**, 71–76.

429. Gomez, M.S. (1989) Presence in Barcelona of *Hoplopleura pacifica* (Anoplura, Hoplopleuridae) a parasite of *Rattus norvegicus. Ann. Parasitol. Hum. Comp.* **64**, 516–517.

430. Durden, L.A. and Page, B.F. (1991) Ectoparasites of commensal rodents in Sulawesi Utara, Indonesia, with notes on species of medical importance. *Med. Vet. Entomol.* **5**, 1–7.

431. Parnas, J., Zwolski, W., and Burdzy, K. (1960) Infection of lice *Polyplax spinulosa* and *Hoplopleura acanthopus* with *Brucella brucei. Wiad Parazytol.* **6**, 441–445.

432. Sosnina, E.F., Nazarova, I.V., and Sadekova, L.K. (1981) Lice (Anoplura) of small mammals in the Volga-Kama Preserve. *Parazitologiia* **15**, 157–162.

433. Murray, M.D. (1961) The ecology of the louse *Polyplax serrata* (Burm.) on the mouse, *Mus musculus* L. *Aust. J. Zool.* **9**, 1–13.

434. Clifford, C.M., Bell, J.F., Moore, J., and Raymond, G. (1967) Effects of limb disability on lousiness in mice. IV. Evidence of genetic factors in susceptibility to *Polyplax serrata. Exp. Parasitol.* **20**, 56–67.

435. Ratzlaff, R.E. and Wikel, S.K. (1990) Murine immune responses and immunization against *Polyplax serrata* (Anoplura: Polyplacidae). *J. Med. Entomol.* **27**, 1002–1007.

436. Kavaliers, M., Colwell, D.D., Choleris, E., et al. (2003) Impaired discrimination of and aversion to parasitized male odors by female oxytocin knockout mice. *Genes Brain Behav.* **2**, 220–230.

437. Nelson, W.A., Clifford, C.M., Bell, J.F., and Hestekin, B. (1972) *Polyplax serrata*: Histopathology of the skin of louse infested mice. *Exp. Parasitol.* **31**, 194–202.

438. Bell, J.F., Stewart, S.J., and Nelson, W.A. (1982) Transplant of acquired resistance to *Polyplax serrata* (Phthiraptera: Hoplopleuridae) in skin allografts to athymic mice. *J. Med. Entomol.* **19**, 164–168.

439. Berkenkamp, S.D. and Wescott, R.B. (1988) Arthropod transmission of *Eperythrozoon coccoides* in mice. *Lab. An. Sci.* **38**, 398–401.

440. Wall, R. and Shearer, D. (2001) *Veterinary Ectoparasites: Biology, Pathology, and Control.* Blackwell Science Ltd., London, 262 pages.

441. Constantin, M.L. (1972) Effects of insecticides on acariasis in mice. *Lab. Anim.* **6**, 279–286.

442. Ohi, M., Dalsenter, P.R., Andrade, A.J.M., and Nascimento, A.J. (2004) Reproductive adverse effects of fipronil in Wistar rats. *Toxicol. Lett.* **146**, 121–127.

443. Toth, L.A., Oberbeck, C., Straign, C.M., Frazier, S., and Rehg, J.E. (2000) Toxicity evaluation of prophylactic treatments for mites and pinworms in mice. *Contemp. Topics Lab. Anim. Sci.* **39**, 18–21.

444. Dawson, G.R., Wafford, K.A., Smith, A., et al. (2000) Anticonvulsant and adverse effects of avermectin analogs in mice are mediated through the γ-aminobutyric acid (A) receptor. *J. Pharmacol. Exp. Ther.* **295**, 1051–1060.

445. Lankas, G.R., Cartwright, M.E., and Umbenhauer, D. (1997) P-glycoprotein deficiency in a subpopulation of CF-1 mice enhances avermectin-induced neurotoxicity. *Toxicol. Appl. Pharmacol.* **143**, 357–365.

446. Davis, J.A., Paylor, R., McDonald, M.P., et al. (1999) Behavioral effects of ivermectin in mice. *Lab. Anim. Sci.* **49**, 288–296.

447. Soliman, S., Marzouk, A.S., Main, A.J., and Montasser, A.A. (2001) Effect of sex, size, and age of commensal rat hosts on the infestation parameters of their ectoparasites in a rural area of Egypt. *J. Parasitol.* **87**, 1308–1316.

448. Ugbomoiko, U.S. and Obiamiwe, B.A. (1991) Distribution and incidence of ectoparasites on small mammals in a rainforest belt of southern Nigeria. *Angew Parasitol.* **32**, 143–148.

449. el Kady, G.A., Makled, K.M., Morsy, T.A., and Morsy, Z.S. (1998) Rodents, their seasonal activity, ecto- and blood-parasites in Saint Catherine area, South Sinai Governorate, Egypt. *J. Egypt. Soc. Parasitol.* **28**, 815–826.

450. Dittmar, K. (2002) Arthropod and helminth parasites of the wild guinea pig, *Cavia aperea*, from the Andes and the cordillera in Peru, South America. *J. Parasitol.* **88**, 409–411.

451. Volf, P. (1991) *Polyplax spinulosa* infestation and antibody response in various strains of laboratory rats. *Folia Parasitol.* **38**, 355–362.

452. Uhlir, J. and Volf, P. (1992) Ivermectin: its effect on the immune system of rabbits and rats infested with ectoparasites. *Vet. Immunol. Immunopathol.* **34**, 325–336.

453. Bakr, M.E., Morsy, T.A., Nassef, N.E., and El Meligi, M.A. (1996) Flea ectoparasites of commensal rodents in Shebin El Kom, Menoufia Governorate, Egypt. *J. Egypt. Soc. Parasitol.* **26**, 39–52.

454. Schwan, T.G., Thompson, D., and Nelson, B.C. (1985) Fleas on roof rats in six areas of Los Angeles County, California: their potential role in the transmission of plague and murine typhus to humans. *Am. J. Trop. Med. Hyg.* **34**, 372–379.

455. Vashchenok, V.S. (2000) The longevity of *Leptopsylla segnis* fleas (Siphonaptera: Leptopsyllidae). *Parazitologiia* **34**, 280–287.

456. Vashchenok, V.S. (2001) Aging and changes in fecundity of the flea *Leptopsylla segnis* (Siphonaptera: Leptopsyllidae). *Parazitologiia* **35**, 460–463.

457. Dobson, M.E., Azad, A.F., Dasch, G.A., Webb, L., and Olson, J.G. (1989) Detection of murine typhus infected fleas with an enzyme-linked immunosorbent assay. *Am. J. Trop. Med. Hyg.* **40**, 521–528.

458. Dong, B. (1991) Experimental studies on the transmission of hemorrhagic fever with renal syndrome virus by gamasidea and fleas. *Zhonghua Yi Xue Za Zhi* **71**, 502–504.

459. Visser, M., Rehbein, S., and Wiedemann, C. (2001) Species of flea (Siphonaptera) infesting pets and hedgehogs in Germany. *J. Vet. Med. B Infect. Dis. Vet. Public Health* **48**, 197–202.

460. Yunker, C.E. (1964) Infections of laboratory animals potentially dangerous to man: Ectoparasites and other arthropods, with emphasis on mites. *Lab. Anim. Care* **14**, 455–465.

461. Gobel, E. and Krampitz, H.E. (1982) Histological studies of the gamogony and sporogony of *Hepatozoon erhardovae* in experimentally infected rat fleas (*Xenopsylla cheopis*). *Z. Parasitenkd.* **67**, 261–271.

462. Azad, A.F. and Traub, R. (1989) Experimental transmission of murine typhus by *Xenopsylla cheopis* flea bites. *Med. Vet. Entomol.* **3**, 429–433.

463. Ryckman, R.E. (1962) Biosystematics and hosts of the *Triatoma protracta* complex in North America (Hemiptera: Reduviidae) (Rodentia: Cricetidae). *Univ. Calif. (Berkeley) Publ. Entomol.* **48**, 93–240.

464. Christensen, H.A. and de Vasquez, A.M. (1981) Host feeding profiles of *Rhodnius pallescens* (Hemiptera: Reduviidae) in rural villages of Central Panama. *Am. J. Trop. Med. Hyg.* **30**, 278–283.

465. Dias-Lima, A.G., Menezes, D., Sherlock, I., and Noireau, F. (2003) Wild habitat and related fauna of *Panstrongylus lutzi* (Reduviidae, Triatominae). *J. Med. Entomol.* **40**, 989–990.

466. Grisard, E.C., Carvalho-Pinto, C.J., Scholz, A.F., Toma, H.K., Schlemper, B.R. Jr., and Steindel, M. (2000) *Trypanosoma cruzi* infection in *Didelphis marsupialis* in Santa Catarina and Arvoredo Islands, southern Brazil. *Mem. Inst. Oswaldo Cruz* **95**, 795–800.

467. Braga, M.V., Pinto, Z.T., and Lima, M.M. (1998) Life cycle and reproductive patterns of *Triatoma rubrofasciata* (De Geer, 1773) (Hemiptera: Reduviidae), under laboratory conditions. *Mem. Inst. Oswaldo Cruz* **93**, 539–542.

468. Pinto Dias, J.C. and Zerba, E.N. (2001) The use of insecticide fumigant canister to protect an insectarium and its residual effect against triatomine bugs, in laboratory conditions. *Rev. Soc. Bras. Med. Trop.* **34**, 507–510.

469. Silverman, A.L., Qu, L.H., Blow, J., Zitron, I.M., Gordon, S.C., and Walker, E.D. (2001) Assessment of hepatitis B virus DNA and hepatitis C virus RNA in the common bedbug (*Cimex lectularius* L.) and kissing bug (*Rhodnius prolixus*). *Am. J. Gastroenterol.* **96**, 2194–2198.

470. Vetter, R. (2001) Kissing bugs (*Triatoma*) and the skin. *Dermatol. Online J.* **7**, 6.

471. Nutting, W.B., Satterfield, L.C., and Cosgrove, G.E. (1973) *Demodex* sp. infesting tongue, esophagus, and oral cavity of *Onychomys leucogaster*, the grasshopper mouse. *J. Parasitol.* **59**, 893–896.

472. Lukoschus, F.S. and Jongman, R.H. (1974) *Demodex lacrimalis* spec. nov. (Demodicidae: Trombidiformes) from the meibomian glands of the European wood mouse, *Apodemus sylvaticus. Acarilogica* **16**, 274–281.

473. Bukva, V. (1985) *Demodex flagellurus* sp. n. (Acari: Demodicidae) from the preputial and clitoral glands of the house mouse, *Mus musculus. Folia Parasitol.* **32**, 73–81.

474. Bukva, V. (1994) *Demodex agrarii* sp. n. (Acari: Demodecidae) from cerumen and the sebaceous glands in the ears of the striped field mouse, *Apodemus agrarius* (Rodentia). *Folia Parasitol.* **41**, 305–311.

475. Strandtmann, R.W. and Mitchell, C.J. (1963) The laelaptine mites of the *Echinolaelaps* complex from the Southwest Pacific area (Acarina: Mesostigmata). *Pac. Insects* **5**, 541–576.

476. Owen, B.L. (1956) Life history of the spiny rat mite under artificial conditions. *J. Econ. Ent.* **49**, 702–703.

477. Furman, D.P. (1959) Feeding habits of symbiotic mesostigmatid mites of mammals in relation to pathogen-vector potentials. *Am. J. Trop. Med. Hyg.* **8**, 5–12.

478. Zuevskii, A.P. (1976) Role of gamasids in the epizootiology of tularemia. *Parazitologiia* **10**, 531–535.

479. Goddard, J. (2003) Mites. In: *Physician's Guide to Arthropods of Medical Importance*. Boca Raton, Florida, CRC Press, 229–247.

480. Baker, E.W., Evans, T.M., Gould, D.J., Hull, W.B., and Keegan, H.L. (1956) A manual of parasitic mites of medical or economic importance. *Tech. Publ. Natl. Pest Control Assoc., Inc.*, New York. 170 pages.

481. Levine, J.F. and Lage, A.L. (1984) House mouse mites infesting laboratory rodents. *Lab. Anim. Sci.* **34**, 393–394.

482. Nichols, E., Rindge, M.E., and Russell, G.G. (1953) The relationship of the habits of the house mouse and the mouse mite (*Allodermanyssus sanguineus*) to the spread of rickettsialpox. *Ann. Internal Med.* **39**, 92–102.

483. Boyd, A.S. (1997) Rickettsialpox. *Dermatol. Clin.* **15**, 313–318.

484. Baker, D.G. (In Press) Mouse Ectoparasites. In: Fox, J.G., Barthold, S.W., Davisson, M., Newcomer, C.E., Quimby, F.W., and Smith, A.L. (eds). *The Mouse in Biomedical Research,* 2nd ed. Academic Press, New York, NY.

485. Gambles, M.R. (1952) *Myocoptes musculinus* (Koch) and *Myobia musculi* (Schrank), two species of mite commonly parasitising the laboratory mouse. *Brit. Vet. J.* **108**, 194–203.

486. Friedman, S. and Weisbroth, S.H. (1977) The parasitic ecology of the rodent mite *Myobia musculi*. IV. Life cycle. *Lab. Anim. Sci.* **27**, 34–37.

487. Friedman, S. and Weisbroth, S.H. (1975) The parasitic ecology of the rodent mite *Myobia musculi*. II. Genetic factors. *Lab. Anim. Sci.* **25**, 440–445.

488. Dawson, D.V., Whitmore, S.P., and Bresnahan, J.F. (1986) Genetic control of susceptibility to mite-associated ulcerative dermatitis. *Lab. Anim. Sci.* **36**, 262–267.

489. Iijima, O.T., Takeda, H., Komatsu, Y., Matsumiya, T., and Takahashi, H. (2000) Atopic dermatitis in NC/Jic mice associated with *Myobia musculi* infestation. *Comp. Med.* **50**, 225–228.

490. Galton, M. (1963) Myobic mange in the mouse leading to skin ulceration and amyloidosis. *Am. J. Pathol.* **43**, 855–865.

491. Weisbroth, S.H., Friedman, S., and Sher, S. (1976) The parasitic ecology of the rodent mite, *Myobia musculi*. III. Lesions in certain host strains. *Lab. Anim. Sci.* **26**, 725–735.

492. Whitely, H.J. and Horton, D.L. (1962) The effect of *Myobia musculi* on the epidermis and hair regrowth cycle in the aging CBA mouse. *J. Pathol.* **83**, 509–514.

493. Csiza, C.K. and McMartin, D.N. (1976) Apparent acaridal dermatitis in a C57Bl/6 Nya mouse colony. *Lab. Anim. Sci.* **26**, 781–787.

494. Cook, R. (1953) Murine mange: The control of *Myocoptes musculinus* and *Myobia musculi* infestations. *Br. Vet. J.* **109**, 113–116.

495. Baumans, V., Havenaar, R., and Van Herck, H. (1988) The use of repeated treatment with Ivomec and Neguvon spray in the control of murine fur mites and oxyurid worms. *Lab. Anim.* **22**, 246–249.

496. Wing, S.R., Courtney, C.H., and Young, M.D. (1985) Effect of ivermectin on murine mites. *J. Am. Vet. Med. Assoc.* **187**, 1191–1192.

497. Vachon, P. and Aubry, L. (1996) The use of ivermectin for the treatment of mites, *Myobia musculi* and *Myocoptes musculinus* in a colony of transgenic mice. *Can. Vet. J.* **37**, 231–232.

498. Papini, R. and Marconcini, A. (1991) Treatment with ivermectin in drinking water against *Myobia musculi* and *Myocoptes musculinus* mange in naturally infected laboratory mice. *Angew. Parasitol.* **32**, 11–13.

499. Conole, J., Wilkinson, M.J., and McKellar, Q.A. (2003) Some observations on the pharmacological properties of ivermectin during treatment of a mite infestation in mice. *Contemp. Top. Lab. Anim. Sci.* **42**, 42–45.

500. Bean-Knudsen, D.E., Wagner, J.E., and Hall, R.D. (1986) Evaluation of the control of *Myobia musculi* infestations on laboratory mice with permethrin. *Lab. Anim. Sci.* **36**, 268–270.

501. Pence, B.C., Demick, D.S., Richard, B.C., and Buddingh, F. (1991) The efficacy and safety of chlorpyrifos (Dursban) for control of *Myobia musculi* infestation in mice. *Lab. Anim. Sci.* **41**, 139–142.

502. Watson, D.P. (1960) On the adult and immature stages of *Myocoptes musculinus* (Kock) with notes on its biology and classification. *Acarologia* **2**, 335–344.

503. Sengbusch, H.G. (1960) Control of *Myocoptes musculinus* on guinea pigs. *J. Econ. Entomol.* **53**, 168.

504. Watson, D.P. (1961) The effect of the mite *Myocoptes musculinus* (C.L. Koch, 1840) on the skin of the white laboratory mouse and its control. *Parasitology* **51**, 373–378.

505. Jungmann, P., Freitas, A., Bandeira, A., et al. (1996) Murine acariasis: II. Immunological dysfunction and evidence for chronic activation of Th-2 lymphocytes. *Scand. J. Immunol.* **43**, 604–612.

506. Morita, E., Kaneko, S., Hiragun, T., et al. (1999) Fur mites induce dermatitis associated with IgE hyperproduction in an inbred strain of mice, NC/Kuj. *J. Dermatol. Sci.* **19**, 37–43.

507. Flynn, R.J. (1955) Ectoparasites in mice. *Proc. Animal Care Panel* **6**, 75–91.

508. Watson, D.P. (1962) On the immature and adult stages of *Notoedres alepis* (Railliet and Lucet, 1893) and its effect on the skin of the rat. *Acarologia* **4**, 64–77.

509. Fain, A. (1965) Notes sur le genre *Notoedres* Railliet, 1893 (Sarcoptidae: Sarcoptiformes). *Acarologia* **7**, 321–342.

510. Guilhon, J. (1946) Un nouvel acarien parasite du rat blanc. *Compt. Rend. Acad. Sci.* **223**, 108–109.

511. Lidicker, W.Z. (1973) Regulation of numbers in an island population of the California vole, a problem in community dynamics. *Ecol. Monogr.* **43**, 271–302.

512. Principato, M., Piergili Fioretti, D., Moretti, A., and Polidori, G.A. (1986) Initial observation in Italy of episodes of mange caused by *Notoedres muris* (Megnin, 1877) in *Cricetus cricetus*. *Ann. Ist. Super. Sanita.* **22**, 337–339.

513. Klompen, J.S. and Nachman, M.W. (1990) Occurrence and treatment of the mange mite *Notoedres muris* in marsh rats from South America. *J. Wildl. Dis.* **26**, 135–136.

514. Gordon, R.M., Unsworth, K., and Seaton, D.R. (1943) The development and transmission of scabies as studied in rodent infections. *Ann. Trop. Med. Parasitol.* **37**, 174–194.

515. Flynn, R.J. (1960) *Notoedres muris* infestation of rats. *Proc. Animal Care Panel* **10**, 69–70.

516. Lavoipierre, M.J. (1960) Acaralogical notes. II. Some remarks on *Trixacarus diversus* Sellnick, 1944 (*Sarcoptes anacanthos* Guilhon, 1946) and on 3 recently described species of *Sarcoptes* in monkeys and bats. *Ann. Parasitol. Hum. Comp.* **35**, 166–170.

517. Beco, L., Petite, A., and Olivry T. (2001) Comparison of subcutaneous ivermectin and oral moxidectin for the treatment of notoedric acariasis in hamsters. *Vet. Rec.* **149**, 324–327.

518. Telford, S.R. III. (1998) Focal epidemic of sarcoptid (Acarina: Sarcoptidae) mite infestation in an insular population of white-footed mice. *J. Med. Entomol.* **35**, 538–542.

519. Itoh, N., Muraoka, N., Aoki, M., and Itagaki, T. (2004) Treatment of *Notoedres cati* infestation in cats with selamectin. *Vet. Rec.* **154**, 409.

520. Lavoipierre, M.J. (1968) Notes on mange mites of the genus *Notoedres* (Acarina: Sarcoptidae) from mammals of eastern Asia, with a description of four new species. *J. Med. Ent.* **5**, 313–319.

521. Swindle, M.M., Hulebak, K.L., and Yarbrough, B.A. (1985) Haematology and pathology of captive southern grasshopper mice (*Onychomys torridus*). *Lab. Anim.* 19, 195–199.

522. Durden, L.A., Klompen, J.S., and Keirans, J.E. (1993) Parasitic arthropods of sympatric opossums, cotton rats, and cotton mice from Merritt Island, Florida. *J. Parasitol.* 79, 283–286.

523. el Kady, G.A., Shoukry, A., Ragheb, D.A., el Said, A.M., Habib, A.M., and Morsy, T.A. (1995) Mites (acari) infesting commensal rats in Suez Canal zone, Egypt. *J. Egypt. Soc. Parasitol.* 25, 417–425.

524. Notarnicola, J., Bain, O., and Navone, G.T. (2000) Two new species of *Litomosoides* (Nematoda: Filarioidea) in Sigmodontines (Rodentia: Muridae) from Rio de La Plata marshland, Argentina. *J. Parasitol.* 86, 1318–1325.

525. Morsy, T.A., El Bahrawy, A.F., and El Dakhil, M.A. (2001) Ecto- and blood parasites affecting *Meriones rex* trapped in Najran, Saudi Arabia. *J. Egypt. Soc. Parasitol.* 31, 399–405.

526. Creel, N.B., Crowe, M.A., and Mullen, G.R. (2003) Pet hamsters as a source of rat mite dermatitis. *Cutis* 71, 457–461.

527. Fox, M.T., Baker, S.A., Farquhar, R., and Eve, E. (2004) First record of *Ornithonyssus bacoti* from a domestic pet in the United Kingdom. *Vet. Rec.* 154, 437–438.

528. Pizzi, R., Meredith, A., Thoday, K.L., and Walker, A. (2004) *Ornithonyssus bacoti* infestation on pets in the UK. *Vet. Rec.* 154, 576.

529. Fox, J.G. (1982) Outbreak of tropical rat mite dermatitis in laboratory personnel. *Arch. Dermatol.* 118, 676–678.

530. French, A.W. (1987) Elimination of *Ornithonyssus bacoti* in a colony of aging mice. *Lab. An. Sci.* 37, 670–672.

531. Skaliy, P. and Hayes, W.J. Jr. (1949) The biology of *Liponyssus bacoti* (Hirst, 1913) (Acarina, Liponyssidae). *Am. J. Trop. Med.* 29, 759–772.

532. Harris, J.M. and Stockton, J.J. (1960) Eradication of the tropical rat mite *Ornithonyssus bacoti* (Hirst, 1913) from a colony of mice. *Am. J. Vet. Res.* 21, 316–318.

533. Nelzina, E.N., Chernova, N.I., Vorona, I.M., and Pylenko, M.S. (1965) On the role of the rat mite *Ornithonyssus bacoti* (S. Hirst, 1913) (Parasitiformes: Gamasides) in natural foci of plague. *Med. Parazitol.* 34, 357–358.

534. Zhuge, H., Meng, Y., Wu, J., Zhu, Z., Liang, W., and Yao, P. (1998) Studies on the experimental transmission of *Rattus*-borne Hantavirus by *Ornithonyssus bacoti*. *Zhongguo Ji Sheng Chong Xue Yu Ji Sheng Chong Bing Za Zhi.* 16, 445–448.

535. Lopatina, Iu.V., Vasileva, I.S., Gutova, V.P., et al. (1999) An experimental study of the capacity of the rat mite *Ornithonyssus bacoti* (Hirst, 1913) to ingest, maintain and transmit *Borrelia*. *Med. Parazitol.* 2, 26–30.

536. Renz, A. and Wenk, A. (1981) Intracellular development of the cotton-rat filaria *Litoomosoides carinii* in the vector mite *Ornithonyssus bacoti*. *Trans. R. Soc. Trop. Med. Hyg.* 75, 166–168.

537. Ram, S.M., Satija, K.C., and Kaushik, R.K. (1986) *Ornithonyssus bacoti* infestation in laboratory personnel and veterinary students. *Int. J. Zoonoses* 13, 138–140.

538. Tyrrell, J.B. (1883) On the occurrence in Canada of two species of parasitic mites. *Proc. Can. Inst.* 1, 332–342.

539. Flynn, R.J. and Jaroslow, B.N. (1956) Nidification of a mite (*Psorergates simplex*, Tyrrell. 1883: Myobiidae) in the skin of mice. *J. Parasitol.* 42, 49–52.

540. Flynn, R.J. (1959) Follicular acariasis of mice caused by *Psorergates simplex* successfully treated with aramite. *Am. J. Vet. Res.* 20, 198–200.

541. Cook, R. (1956) Murine ear mange: The control of *Psorergates simplex* infestation. *Br. Vet. J.* 112, 22–25.

542. Soll, M.D. and Carmichael, I.H. (1988) Efficacy of injectable ivermectin against the itch mite (*Psorergates ovis*) of sheep. *Parasitol. Res.* 75, 81–82.

543. Bowman, T.A. and Griffith, J.W. (1987) Comparison of treatments for *Psorergates* mites in stumptailed macaques (*Macaca arctoides*). *Lab. An. Sci.* 37, 100–102.

544. Flynn, R.J. (1963) The diagnosis of some forms of ectoparasitism of mice. *Proc. Animal Care Panel* 13, 111–125.

545. Ewing, H.E. (1938) North American mites of the subfamily Myobiinae, new subfamily (Arachnida). *Proc. Entomol. Soc. Wash.* 40, 180–197.

546. Seamer, J. and Chesterman, F.C. (1967) A survey of disease in laboratory animals. *Lab. Anim.* 1, 117–139.

547. Bochkov, A., Arbobi, M., and Malikov, V. (2000) Notes on mites of the family Myobiidae (Acari: Prostigmata) parasitising rodents (Mammalia: Rodentia) in Iran. *Folia Parasit.* 47, 73–77.

548. Skidmore, L.V. (1934) Acariasis of the white rat (*Rattus norvegicus* form *albinus*). *Can. Entomologist* 66, 110–115.

549. Kondo, S., Taylor, A., and Chun, S. (1998) Elimination of an infestation of rat fur mites (*Radfordia ensifera*) from a colony of Long Evans rats, using the micro-dot technique for topical administration of 1% ivermectin. *Contemp. Top. Lab. Anim. Sci.* 37, 58–61.

550. Fain, A., Munting, A.J., and Lukoschus, F. (1970) Myocoptidae parasites of rodents in Holland and Belgium (Acarina: Sarcoptiformes). *Acta. Zool. Pathol. Antverp.* 50, 67–172.

551. Flynn, R.J., Brennan, P.C., and Fritz, T.E. (1965) Pathogen status of commercially produced mice. *Lab. Anim. Care* 15, 440–447.

552. Devera, R., Fernandes, O., and Coura, J.R. (2003) Should *Trypanosoma cruzi* be called "*cruzi*" complex? a review of the parasite diversity and the potential of selecting population after in vitro culturing and mice infection. *Mem. Inst. Oswaldo Cruz.* 98, 1–12.

553. Levine, N.D. (1968) *Nematode parasites of domestic animals and of man.* Burgess, Minneapolis, Minnesota, 600 pages.

554. Diagne, M., Diouf, M., Lochouarn, L., and Bain, O. (2000) *Trichosomoides nasalis* Biocca and Aurizi, 1961 and *T. spratti* n. sp. (Nematoda: Trichinelloidea), from the nasal cavity of murids. *Parasite* 7, 215–220.

555. Otranto, D., Lia, R.P., Buono, V., Traversa, D., and Giangaspero, A. (2004) Biology of *Thelazia callipaeda* (Spirurida, Thelaziidae) eyeworms in naturally infected definitive hosts. *Parasitology* 129, 627–633.

556. Scholz, T. (1999) Taxonomic study of *Ascocotyle* (*Phagicola*) *longa* Ransom, 1920 (Digenea: Heterophyidae) and related taxa. *Syst. Parasitol.* 43, 147–158.

557. Huffman, J.E. and Fried, B. (1990) *Echinostoma* and echinostomiasis. *Adv. Parasitol.* 29, 215–269.

558. Ricci, M. (1995) Contribution to a revision of the genus Plagiorchis (Trematoda: Digenea: Plagiorchiidae). *Parasitologia* 37, 25–28.

559. Ulmer, M.J. (1951) *Postharmostomum helicis* (Leidy, 1847) Robinson 1949 (Trematoda), its life history and revision of the subfamily Brachylaeminae. Part I. *Trans Am. Microscop. Soc.* 70, 189–238.

560. Wongsawad, C., Chariyahpongpun, P., and Namue, C. (1998) Experimental host of *Stellantchasmus falcatus*. *Southeast Asian J. Trop. Med. Public Health* 29, 406–409.

561. Alghali, S.T. (1986) *Hymenolepis citelli* and *H. diminuta*: worm burdens in homologous and heterologous infections in rats. *Exp. Parasitol.* 62, 14–23.

562. Baer, J.G. and Sandars, D.F. (1956) The first record of *Raillietina* (*Raillietina*) *celebensis* (Janicki, 1902), (Cestoda) in man from Australia, with a critical survey of previous cases. *J. Helminthol.* 30, 173–182.

563. Colle, I., Van Vlierberghe, H., Brenard, R., et al. (2002) Biliary complications of large *Echinococcus granulosus* cysts: report of 2 cases and review of the literature. *Acta. Clin. Belg.* **57**, 349–354.

564. Tornieporth, N.G. and Disko, R. (1994) Alveolar hydatid disease (*Echinococcus multilocularis*)—review and update. *Prog. Clin. Parasitol.* **4**, 55–76.

565. Rodriguez, B., Gonzales, R., and Chinchilla, M. (2000) Parasitic helminths from *Sigmodon hispidus* (Rodentia: Cricetidae) from seasonal and evergreen habitats in Costa Rica. *Rev. Biol. Trop.* **48**, 121–123.

566. Elangbam, C.S., Qualls, C.W. Jr., Lochmiller, R.L., and Boggs, J.F. (1990) Strongyloidiasis in cotton rats (*Sigmodon hispidus*) from central Oklahoma. *J. Wildl. Dis.* **26**, 398–402.

567. Ow Yang, C.K., Durette-Desset, M.C., and Ohbayashi, M. (1983) Nematode parasites of rodents in Malaysia. II. Trichostrongyloidea. *Ann. Parasitol. Hum. Comp.* **58**, 467–492.

568. Yokota, M., Hashimoto, M., Matsui, T. et al. (1991) A nematode, *Orientostrongylus ezoensis,* from brown rats in Sekai, Osaka Prefecture. *J. Vet. Med. Sci.* **53**, 159–160.

569. Thatcher, V.E. and Scott, J.A. (1962) The life cycle of *Trichostrongylus sigmodontis* Baylis, 1945, and the susceptibility of various laboratory animals to this nematode. *J. Parasitol.* **48**, 558–561.

570. Hitchcock, C.R. and Bell, E.T. (1952) Studies on the nematode parasite, *Gongylonema neoplasticum* (*Spiroptera neoplasticum*), and avitaminosis A in the forestomach of rats: comparison with Fibiger's results. *J. Natl. Cancer Inst.* **12**, 1345–1387.

571. Rojas Mdel, C. and Digiani, M.C. (2003) First record of *Mastophorus muris* (Gmelin, 1790) (Nematoda: Spiruroidea) from a wild host in South America. *Parasite* **10**, 375–378.

572. Mafra, A.C. and Lanfredi, R.M. (1998) Revaluation of *Physaloptera bispiculata* (Nematoda: Spiruroidea) by light and scanning electron microscopy. *J. Parasitol.* **84**, 582–588.

573. Kenney, M., Eveland, L.K., Yermakov, V., and Kassouny, D.Y. (1975) A case of *Rictularia* infection of man in New York. *Am. J. Trop. Med. Hyg.* **24**, 596–599.

574. Redrobe, S.P. and Patterson-Kane, J.C. (2005) *Calodium hepaticum* (syn. *Capillaria hepatica*) in captive rodents in a zoological garden. *J. Comp. Pathol.* **133**, 73–76.

575. Pozio, E. and Zarlenga, D.S. (2005) Recent advances on the taxonomy, systematics and epidemiology of *Trichinella. Int. J. Parasitol.* **35**, 1191–1204.

576. Crook, J.R. and Grundmann, A.W. (1964) The life history and larval development of *Moniliformis clarki* (Ward, 1917). *J. Parasitol.* **50**, 689–93.

577. Crompton, D.W. (1972) The growth of *Moniliformis dubius* (Acanthocephala) in the intestine of male rats. *J. Exp. Biol.* **56**, 19–29.

578. Reyda, F.B. and Nickol, B.B. (2001) A comparison of biological performances among a laboratory-isolated population and two wild populations of *Moniliformis moniliformis.* **87**, 330–338.

579. Ernst, J.V., Chobotar, B., Oakes, E.C., and Hammond, D.M. (1968) *Besnoitia jellisoni* (Sporozoa: Toxoplasmae) in rodents from Utah and California. *J. Parasitol.* **54**, 545–49.

580. Frenkel, J.K. (1977) *Besnoitia wallacei* of cats and rodents: with a reclassification of other cyst-forming isosporoid coccidia. *J. Parasitol.* **63**, 611–628.

581. Rommel, M. (1978) Comparative review of the developmental biology of the genera *Sarcocystis, Frenkelia, Isospora, Cystoisospora, Hammondia, Toxoplasma* and *Besnoitia. Z. Parasitenkd.* **57**, 269–283.

582. Yamane, Y. (1968) On the fine structure of *Diphyllobothrium erinacei* with special reference to the tegument. *Yonago Acta Med.* **12**, 169–181.

583. Riley, S.L. and Chernin, J. (1994) The effect of the tetrathyridia of *Mesocestoides corti* on the livers and peripheral blood of three different strains of mice. *Parasitology* **109**, 291–297.

584. Conn, D.B. (1988) Fine structure of the tegument of *Mesocestoides lineatus* tetrathyridia (Cestoda: Cyclophyllidea). *Int. J. Parasitol.* **18**, 133–135.

585. Jithendran, K.P. and Somvanshi, R. (1998) Experimental infection of mice with *Taenia taeniaformis* eggs from cats—course of infection and pathological studies. *Indian J. Exp. Biol.* **36**, 523–525.

586. Cliff, G.M. and Anderson, R.C. (1980) Development of *Pelodera strongyloides* (Schneider, 1860) Schneider, 1866 (Nematoda: Rhabditoidea) in culture. *J. Helminthol.* **54**, 135–146.

587. Scott, J.A., MacDonald, E.M., and Terman, B. (1951) A description of the stages in the life cycle of the filarial worm *Litomosomoides carinii. J. Parasitol.* **37**, 425–432.

588. Mohan, R.N. (1973) Letter: Pathological changes in white rats infected with *Litosomoides carinii. Trans. R. Soc. Trop. Med. Hyg.* **67**, 883–884.

589. Scanlon, J.E. and Johnson, P.T. (1957) On some microtine-infesting *Polyplax* (Anoplura). *Proc. Entomol. Soc. Wash. D.C.* **59**, 279–283.

590. Lewis, R.E. (1967) Contributions to a taxonomic revision of the genus *Nosopsyllus* Jordan, 1933 (Siphonaptera: Ceratophyllidae): I. African species. *J. Med. Entomol.* **4**, 123–142.

591. Newberry, K. (1990) The tropical bedbug *Cimex hemipterus* near the southernmost extent of its range. *Trans. R. Soc. Trop. Med. Hyg.* **84**, 745–747.

592. Jimenez, M.L., Llinas, J., and Palacios, C. (2003) Infection rates in *Dipetalogaster maximus* (Reduviidae: Triatominae) by Trypanosoma cruzi in the Cape Region, Baja California Sur, Mexico. *J. Med. Entomol.* **40**, 18–21.

593. Minter, D.M., Minter-Goedbloed, E., Marsden, P.D., Miles, M.A., and Boreham, P.F. (1973) The host selection pattern and infection rates of *Panstrongylus megistus* in an area of eastern Brazil. *Trans. R. Soc. Trop. Med. Hyg.* **67**, 291.

594. Usinger, R.L. (1944) The Triatominae of North and Central America and the West Indies and their public health significance. *U.S. Public Health Service Bull.* **288**. 83 pages.

595. Ryckman, R.E. (1971) The genus *Paratriatoma* in western North America. *J. Med. Entomol.* **30**, 87–97.

596. Usinger, R.L. (1966) *Monograph of Cimicidae.* Entomological Society of America, College Park, Maryland. 585 pages.

597. Uchikawa, K. and Rack, G. (1979) *Eulaelaps stabularis* (Koch, 1839) and *Eulaelaps oudemansi* Turk, 1945 (Mesostigmata: Haemogamasidae). *Acarologia* **20**, 163–172.

598. Herrin, C.S. (1974) The taxonomic status of *Hirstionyssus butantanensis* (Fonseca, 1932) (Acari: Mesostigmata). *J. Med. Entomol.* **11**, 341–346.

599. Tipton, V.J. (1960) The genus *Laelaps,* with a review of the Laelaptinae and a new subfamily Alphalaelaptinae (Acarina: Laelaptidae). *Univ. Calif. (Berkeley) Publ. Entomol.* **16**, 233–356.

600. Bukva, V. (1995) *Demodex* species (Acari: Demodecidae) parasitizing the brown rat, *Rattus norvegicus* (Rodentia): redescriptions of *Demodex ratti* and description of *D. norvegicus* sp. n. and *D. ratticola* sp. n. *Folia Parasitol. (Praha)* **42**, 149–160.

601. Esslinger, J.H. (1962) Morphology of the egg and larva of *Porocephalus crotali* (Pentastomida). *J. Parasitol.* **48**, 457–462.

602. Buckle, A.C., Riley, J., and Hill, G.F. (1997) The in vitro development of the pentastomid *Porocephalus crotali* from the infective instar to the adult stage. *Parasitology* **115**, 503–512.

CHAPTER

12

Parasites of Hamsters

F. Claire Hankenson, DVM, MS, DACLAM; and Gerald L. Van Hoosier, JR., DVM, DACLAM

INTRODUCTION

Laboratory hamsters continue to be used in many disciplines of biomedical research, including toxicology, carcinogenesis, behavioral analyses, and parasitology. These animal models, particularly Syrian or golden (*Mesocricetus auratus*) and Chinese (*Cricetulus griseus*) hamsters, are readily available through vendors in both the United States

and Europe. It is generally accepted that rodent pathogens may not only be hazardous for animals (and humans) but can severely influence the results of animal experiments. Therefore, microbiological standardization of laboratory animals is of crucial importance[1].

PROTOZOA

In hamster species, numerous protozoal species may be present, but they are thought to be of low to no clinical significance[2]. Naturally occurring protozoal infections have been found in both normal and diseased hamsters[3].

Phylum Sarcomastigophora

Giardia muris

Morphology. *Giardia muris* in hamsters is morphologically indistinguishable from similar organisms found in mice[4].

Hosts. Syrian hamster[4,5]. Results of transmission studies demonstrate that *G. muris* and *Tritrichomonas muris* from hamsters readily establish infection in naïve mice. These findings support the practice of keeping these species separate until microbiologic examinations are conducted[4].

Life Cycle. *Giardia muris* colonizes the ileum. Trophozoites reside in the small intestine. Encystation occurs in the course of passage out of the intestinal tract. *G. muris* is transmissible to mice via infected bedding material. The minimal infectious dose is estimated as five to 20 viable cysts[6]. The prepatent period is estimated to be eight days.

Clinical Disease and Pathologic Effects. Typically, *G. muris* causes no clinical disease or pathologic changes in hamsters. However, an association has been found between *G. muris* and metaplastic gastric sites in Syrian hamsters co-infected with *Helicobacter* species[7].

Diagnosis, Treatment, and Prevention. Diagnosis is as described for giardiasis of rats and mice. *Giardia muris* is more difficult to eradicate from hamsters than from mice. Treatment with metronidazole therapy at 80 mg/day failed to clear infection in hamsters, while a 5 mg/day regimen has been used successfully in mice[8]. Intragastric dosing with metronidazole or its benzoyl ester form (benzoyl-metronidazole) may not be practical for large numbers of hamsters.

Public Health Considerations. *Giardia muris* is not considered zoonotic.

Spironucleus muris

Morphology. The morphology of *S. muris* is discussed in Chapter 11, Parasites of Rats and Mice.

Hosts. Among hamsters, natural or experimental hosts of *S. muris* include the Syrian hamster[5] and the European hamster (*Cricetulus cricetus*)[9].

Life Cycle. The agent has been identified in the ceca of the Syrian hamster[5]. *S. muris* established from a hamster was found to be infectious to mice, but not to rats[10]. In addition, rat *S. muris* could not be used to infect hamsters, which suggests strain heterogeneity within *S. muris*. In general, the genetic background of the host influences infection, while the sex of the host does not. The prepatent period is estimated to be five days; the minimal infectious dose is estimated as one viable cyst[6].

Pathologic Effects. *Spironucleus* has been reported as an incidental finding or as a commensal[5,11]. Infection may impact host immune response and protozoa may penetrate lamina propria of the intestinal tract, leading to desquamation of the epithelial layer, edema, inflammation, and cell death[10]. Proliferative ileitis and acute enteritis have been reported[11].

Clinical Disease. No overt signs have been reported despite the pathologic changes in the intestinal tract.

Diagnosis, Treatment, Prevention, and Public Health Considerations. These aspects are as discussed for rats and mice.

Tritrichomonas muris

Morphology. *Trichomonas cricetus* and *T. criceti* in the Syrian hamster are now believed to be synonymous with *T. muris*[12]. The pear- to lemon- or boat-shaped trophozoites measure 4 μ to 16 μ by 2.5 μ to 5 μ with an undulating

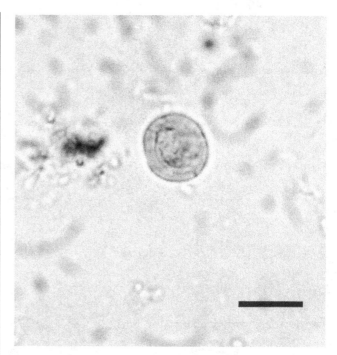

Fig. 12.1   Round refractile body (*Tritrichomonas muris* pseudocyst) detected in the feces from an Armenian hamster. Reproduced from Lipman, N.S., Lampen, N., and Nguyen, H.T. (1999) with permission.

membrane and three flagella[13]. Trophozoites can internalize their flagella to form pseudocysts[14], which appear as round to oval refractile bodies, 10 μm to 12 μm in diameter (Figure 12.1).

Hosts. Natural hosts of *T. muris* include the Armenian hamster (*Cricetulus migratorius*)[14] and Syrian hamster[4]. *T. wenyoni, T. minuta,* and forms resembling *T. microti* have also been recorded in the Syrian hamster[5].

Life Cycle. The life cycle is as described in mice. Transfaunation studies suggest that *T. muris* isolates are cross-infective between mice and hamsters[4]. *T. muris* serves as a useful biomarker of contamination in protozoa-free rodent colonies because of its low minimal infective dose[14].

Pathologic Effects and Clinical Disease. *T. muris* is not believed to be pathogenic in hamsters. Neither alterations in mucosal integrity nor presence of submucosal inflammatory infiltrates have been observed[14]. No detectable signs of gastrointestinal tract disease have been reported in hamsters.

Diagnosis. Diagnosis is accomplished by fecal flotation, using a sodium nitrate solution (specific gravity = 1.2). Pseudocysts may be identified in fecal pellets suspended in saline and treated with Lugol's iodine or trichrome stain.

Histologically, numerous trophozoites and pseudocysts of *T. muris* may be observed in tissue sections and contents of the cecum and colon of hamsters.

Treatment and Prevention. *T. muris* may be successfully eradicated from the intestinal tract using a regimen of 80 mg of metronidazole administered intragastrically for six days[4]. Hamsters should be evaluated while in quarantine, prior to admission into the animal colony, particularly if known to be of conventional health status.

Public Health Considerations. None.

Phylum Microsporidia

Encephalitozoon cuniculi

Encephalitozoon cuniculi, an obligate intracellular microsporidian, has recently been reclassified as a fungus. *E. cuniculi* has been reported from hamsters under natural and experimental conditions[15,16]. There is little information concerning the life cycle, morphologic features, diagnosis, and treatment of this pathogen in hamsters. The reader is directed to Chapter 11, Parasites of Rats and Mice for information on encephalitozoonosis in rodents.

CESTODES

Rodentolepis nana

Morphology. The morphology of *Rodentolepis* (formerly *Hymenolepis*) *nana* is described in Chapter 11, Parasites of Rats and Mice.

Hosts. *R. nana* has been found in the small intestine of *Mesocricetus auratus*[17-23]. Mice, rats, nonhuman primates, and humans are additional susceptible hosts. In addition to *R. nana*, hamsters are susceptible to infection with *R. citelli*, *R. microstoma*, *R. peromysci*, and *Hymenolepis diminuta*[18].

Life Cycle. The life cycle of *R. nana* is similar to its life cycle in mice.

Pathologic Effects and Clinical Disease. Catarrhal enteritis, chronic enteritis, abscesses of mesenteric lymph nodes, and hyperplasia of Peyer's patches have been observed in infected hamsters[18]. Heavy infestations may cause diarrhea and a pot-bellied appearance in young hamsters[19]. Clinical signs may include constipation due to worms in the small intestine[20]. Heavy infestation may cause impaction and death.

Diagnosis, Treatment, and Prevention. Diagnosis is by finding eggs in feces or finding adults in the gastrointestinal tract of the host at postmortem examination[23].

Recommended treatments include praziquantel or thiabendazole[2]. Other reports describe niclosamide as a safe and effective treatment[22]. Preventive and control measures are similar to those described for mice, and include isolation and quarantine of newly acquired animals, effective insect and wild-rodent control, and regular sanitation of cages and ancillary equipment[23].

Public Health Considerations. This pathogen can cause zoonotic disease; therefore, personnel[23] and pet owners should receive instruction in appropriate hygienic practices.

NEMATODES

Syphacia criceti

Morphology. Adult *Syphacia criceti* are slender worms (Figure 12.2). The esophagus is bulbed, and the male possesses a single spicule. Adult males are approximately 1,500 µ in length and approximately 94 µ in width. Adult females are approximately 3,500 µ in length and 210 µ in width. Eggs are approximately 116 µ by 46 µ in size[17].

Hosts and Life Cycle. The Syrian hamster is the natural host of *S. criceti*[17]. The life cycle is direct, and is similar to other members of the genus. Adult worms are found in the small intestine.

Pathologic Effects and Clinical Disease. *Syphacia criceti* is not considered pathogenic, and clinical signs are not observed following natural infection.

Treatment and Prevention. Ivermectin, piperazine, and thiabendazole are reported to be effective against *S. criceti*[2]. Prevention strategies are similar to those established for other members of the genus.

Public Health Considerations. *S. criceti* is not infective to humans.

Syphacia mesocriceti

Morphology. Adult *Syphacia mesocriceti* are small, thick worms (Figure 12.3). Like *S. criceti,* the esophagus is bulbed and the adult male possesses a single spicule. Adult males are approximately 1300 µ in length and approximately 85 µ in width. Adult females are approximately 4500 µ in length and 167 µ in width. Eggs are approximately 135 µ by 45 µ in size[17].

Hosts and Life Cycle. The Syrian hamster is the natural host of *S. mesocriceti*[17]. The life cycle is direct, and similar to those of others members of the genus. Adult worms are observed in the small intestine.

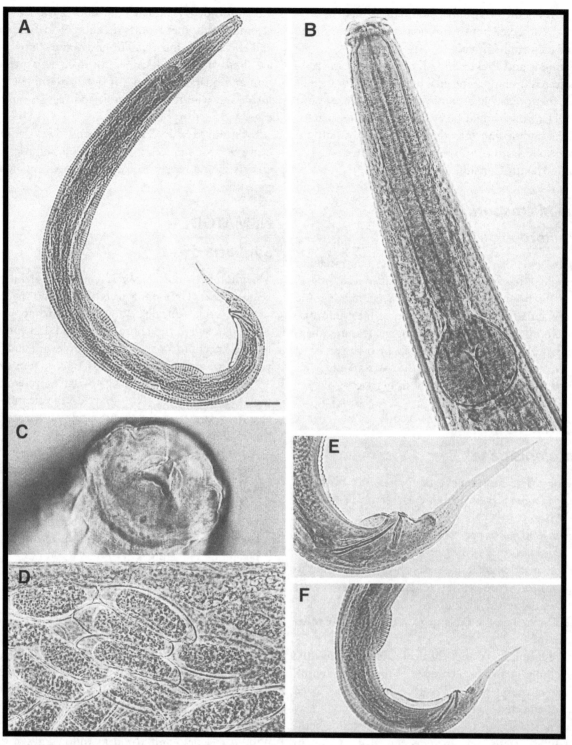

Fig. 12.2 *Syphacia criceti.* (A) Male, whole body, lateral view. Bar = 0.08 mm. (B) Anterior portion of male, lateral view. Bar = 0.02 mm. (C) Head of female, *"en face"* view. Bar = 0.01 mm. (D) Eggs *"in utero."* Bar = 0.03 mm. (E) Posterior extremity of male, lateral view. Bar = 0.02 mm. (F) Posterior portion of male, lateral view. Bar = 0.07 mm. Bar of Figure A, common to Figures B–F. Reproduced from Pinto, R.M., Goncalves, L., Gomes, D.C., and Noronha, D. (2001) with permission.

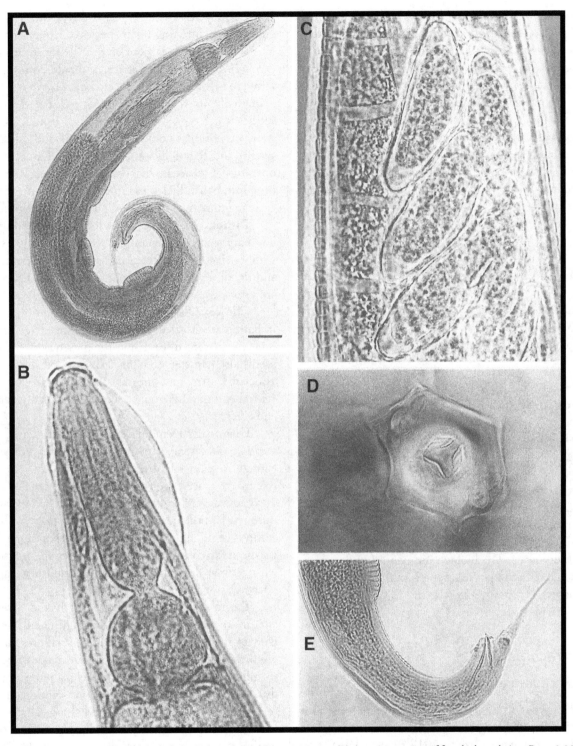

Fig. 12.3 *Syphacia mesocriceti.* (A) Male, whole body, lateral view. Bar = 0.10 mm. (B) Anterior portion of female, lateral view. Bar = 0.03 mm. (C) Eggs "*in utero.*" Bar = 0.02 mm. (D) Head of female, "*en face*" view. Bar = 0.01 mm. (E) Posterior portion of male, lateral view. Bar = 0.02 mm. Bar of Figure A, common to Figures B–E. Reproduced from Pinto, R.M., Goncalves, L., Gomes, D.C., and Noronha, D. (2001) with permission.

Pathologic Effects and Clinical Disease. Hamsters infected with *S. mesocriceti* do not appear to suffer pathologic effects, nor are any clinical signs evident.

Diagnosis. Oxyurid eggs are rare in the feces of hosts, and anal swab devices may fail to detect the larvae. Postmortem identification of worms or eggs harvested from the intestinal tract is often required.

Treatment and Prevention. No information is available concerning these aspects of control. It can be assumed that treatment and prevention strategies used to manage other rodent pinworm infections would also be successful against *S. mesocriceti*.

Other pinworm infections

In addition to those discussed above, hamsters are also susceptible to infection with other rodent pinworms. These include *Dentostomella translucida* from the Mongolian gerbil (*Meriones unguiculatus*)[24]; *Syphacia obvelata,* the mouse pinworm[21,25,26]; and *Syphacia muris,* the rat pinworm[26].

ARTHROPODS

Class Insecta

Nosopsyllus fasciatus

Hamsters are potentially susceptible to infestation by several species of flea; many of these have been reported[27]. The rat flea, *Nosopsyllus fasciatus,* may be of particular concern within the animal facility, as an intermediate host for *Rodentolepis nana*[28]. The biology and control of flea infestation is as discussed in other chapters of this text, particularly, Chapter 11, Parasites of Rats and Mice, and Chapter 10, Parasites of Birds.

Class Arachnida

Demodex aurati and D. criceti

Morphology. Adult *Demodex criceti* range in size from 87.4 μ to 103.4 μ in length and 17μ to 33.6 μ wide, while adult *D. aurati* range in size from 183.1 μ to 191.9 μ in length and 16.8 μ to 25 μ wide[29].

Hosts. The Syrian hamster is the natural host for these *Demodex* species[29,30]. The Djungarian (*Phodopus sungorus*) and Roborovski (*Phodopus roborovskii*) hamsters are also susceptible[32]. Mites are more frequently observed on male hosts than females[20,32,33].

Life Cycle. The life cycle is direct, and is similar to *Demodex* sp. infesting other species of laboratory animals. The entire life cycle is spent on host[31]. Transmission occurs through direct contact between animals. Mites are transferred to offspring at time of suckling. *D. criceti* is found in epidermal pits that rarely extend into the dermis. This species is not typically found within hair follicles. In contrast, *D. aurati* is commonly found in the pilosebacious system and hair follicles[20]. Eggs are laid singly near the openings of sebaceous glands; upon hatching, larvae penetrate into hair follicles and develop into nymphs. The life cycle requires approximately 24 days for each species.

Pathologic Effects. While these mites are normally of low pathogenicity, demodicosis is occasionally associated with dermatitis in affected hamsters. The abdominal skin and dorsum are most commonly affected[32]. Fewer lesions are seen with *D. criceti* than with *D. aurati*.

Clinical Disease. Pruritus is an uncommon finding in hamsters with demodicosis[30]. Advanced age, malnutrition, concurrent disease, and the presence of tumors may predispose hamsters to clinical disease[32,33]. Though rarely associated with signs, one may observe dorsal alopecia with ventral excoriations, roughened hair coat, scaly dermatitis, and edema[34].

Diagnosis. Demodicosis may be diagnosed using a standard skin scrape method. The scrape must be deep enough to cause slight erythema to the skin. The scraped material is placed on a slide with a few drops of warmed 10% potassium hydroxide, cover-slipped, allowed to sit 10 minutes, and then examined microscopically[34]. Histologic sections of skin and hair follicles may assist in the identification of acariasis. Presence of *Demodex* sp. in association with lesions does not necessarily establish a cause and effect relationship[23].

Treatment. Effective treatments include ivermectin and amitraz. Ivermectin can be administered (0.3 mg/kg daily by mouth) for 24 days. Treatment failures may occur, requiring retreatment[32]. Affected hamsters can be bathed in mild soap (e.g. selenium sulfide shampoo) and towel dried prior to treating with a dilute solution of amitraz (e.g. 0.013%). The solution is applied topically with a cotton ball and allowed to dry naturally. Hamsters should not be dipped[20]. Three to six topical treatments 14 days apart are recommended[20]. Subsequent miticidal treatment with coumaphos may be necessary to completely cure lesions[30].

Prevention. Hamster colonies should be maintained in a generally healthy condition, with strict adherence to sanitation protocols. Clinically affected animals should be eliminated.

Public Health Considerations. *Demodex aurati* and *D. criceti* are not zoonotic.

Demodex cricetuli

Morphology. *Demodex cricetuli* was previously incorrectly identified in Armenian hamsters as *D. aurati,* which it closely resembles[29]. Adult males are approximately 173 µ in length, with a rectangular gnathosoma. Adult females are roughly 192 µ in length. Leg structure, size, and spacing along the podosoma are similar to the male. Eggs are spindle-shaped, non-operculate, and 110 µ long by 32 µ wide. Detailed descriptions are available for all forms of the parasite, including the egg, larva, protonymph, nymph, and adult[35].

Hosts and Life Cycle. The Armenian hamster is the natural host of *D. cricetuli.* The life cycle is similar to those of other members of the species. Mites occupy hair follicles, particularly on the dorsum of the face and back. Mites reside in the cavity of the follicles. A single follicle can harbor several mites.

Pathologic Effects. Infestation with *D. cricetuli* may result in destruction of hair shafts, hyperkeratosis, parakeratosis, and lengthening of rete pegs[33]. Additional lesions include hyperemia of skin and mild serum exudation on the skin surface.

Clinical Disease. Clinical signs include pruritus, scaling dermatitis, and complete or partial alopecia of the cervical, shoulder, and mandibular regions[33].

Diagnosis, Treatment, and Prevention. Diagnosis is by deep skin scrapings as described for other members of the genus[35]. Treatment is with topical ivermectin (0.3mg/kg for 10 days). Animals are considered to be cured if skin lesions have resolved, and the results of microscopic examination of skin scrapings have remained negative for three months[32]. Methods for preventing infestation are as described for other members of the genus.

Public Health Considerations. *Demodex cricetuli* is not zoonotic.

Demodex sinocricetuli

Morphology. *Demodex sinocricetuli* has been described for all of its life stages[36]. This mite is most similar to *D. aurati,* yet the following distinguishes *D. sinocricetuli:* the length of adult males and females are similar in size and shorter, the nymph body length is shorter, and immature forms do not have ventral scutes[36]. Adult males are approximately 120 µ ± 8.5 µ in length and adult females are approximately 138.9 µ ± 11.8 µ in length[36].

Hosts and Life Cycle. The striped hamster (*Cricetulus barabensis*) is the natural host for *D. sinocricetuli.* The life cycle is similar to that of other members of the genus.

Pathologic Effects and Clinical Disease. *Demodex sinocricetuli* may occasionally cause dermatitis and localized mange[36,37].

Diagnosis, Treatment, and Prevention. Diagnosis is as reported for other members of the genus. Little information is available regarding treatment of *D. sinocricetuli.* It is assumed that ivermectin, as previously described, is effective. Methods for preventing infestation are as described for other members of the genus.

Public Health Considerations. *Demodex sinocricetuli* is not zoonotic.

Haemogamosus pontiger

Haemogamosus pontiger is similar to mites in the genera *Dermanyssus* and *Ornithonyssus. H. pontiger* has been identified in the bedding of pet hamsters. Treatment includes a change of bedding materials and the addition of 5% carbaryl (Sevin™) dust to the bedding for one week[38].

Notoedres sp.

Rarely, hamsters may become infested with *Notoedres* sp. (Figure 12.4)[39,40]. Skin lesions may become severe, and are observed on the ear pinnae, face, genitalia, tail, and limbs (Figure 12.5)[40]. Clinical signs include severe pruritus, erythema, crusts, and hyperpigmentation. Treatment with ivermectin has been successful in many, but not all, cases[40]. Infestation of hamsters with *Notoedres* sp. is similar to that described for *Notoedres* sp. infestations of mice. Additional

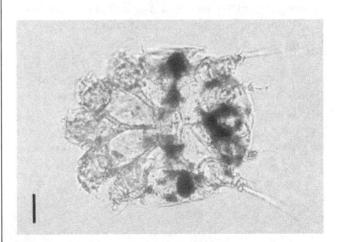

Fig. 12.4 *Notoedres* mite, characterized by a dorsal anus. Skin scraping; chloral lactophenol. Bar = 0.025 mm. Reproduced from Beco, L., Petite, A., and Olivry, T. (2001) with permission.

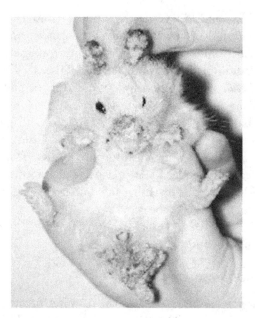

Fig. 12.5 Hamster with lesions of *Notoedres* infestation on its face and feet. Severe crusting can be observed on the muzzle, ears, and extremities. Reproduced from Beco, L., Petite, A., and Olivry, T. (2001) with permission.

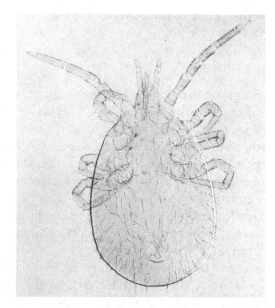

Fig. 12.6 Adult female *Ornithonyssus bacoti*. Reproduced from Fox, M.T., Baker, A.S., Farquhar, R., and Eve, E. (2004) with permission.

information concerning the biology and treatment of *Notoedres* infestation can be found in Chapter 11, Parasites of Rats and Mice.

Ornithonyssus bacoti

Though typically a parasite of rats, *Ornithonyssus bacoti* may also infest hamsters (Figure 12.6)[41,42], in which it may act as an intermediate host for *Litomosoides carinii,* a filarial nematode parasite. Typically, no clinical signs are observed. Ivermectin may be used to eliminate the infestation[42]. The reader is directed to Chapter 11, Parasites of Rats and Mice, for additional information concerning this parasite.

Radfordia sp.

Radfordia cricetulphila and *R. cricetulus* have been described in the Chinese hamster[43]. Little is known of the biology or pathogenicity of these mites. It is likely that the conditions they cause are similar to those caused by other members of the genus. The reader is directed to Chapter 11, Parasites of Rats and Mice, for information concerning *Radfordia* sp.

Spleorodens clethrionomys

Spleorodens (*Paraspeleognathopsis*) *clethrionomys* is a prostigmatid mite found in the nasal passages of the Syrian hamster[44]. The mite has also been found in the nasal passages of bank voles (*Clethrionomys glareolus*) and field voles (*Microtus agrestis*) in Europe[44]. The adult female mite is 300 μ to 360 μ (mean = 336 μ) and 114 μ to 198 μ (mean = 135 μ) wide[44]. Adult mites are milky white in color and oval in shape, with their greatest width at the humoral region behind the second coxa. The dorsal surface of the mite bears a shield with thick and heavy lines. There are four pairs of legs. In the larval mite, the tarsus of the third pair of legs bears a characteristic claw. The preferred site is on the mucosa in the posterior parts of the nasal cavities.

Pathogenic effects are unknown. Likewise, clinical signs have not been reported. Infestation with *S. clethrionomys* is an incidental finding at necropsy. Nothing is known of treatment and prevention strategies. *Spleorodens clethrionomys* is not known to inhabit the nasal passages of humans.

TABLE 12.1 Parasites of Hamsters—Enterohepatic and Respiratory Systems.

Parasite	Geographic Distribution	Hosts	Location in Host	Method of Infection	Pathologic Effects	Zoonosis	Reference
Flagellates							
Caviomonas mobilis	North America	Guinea pigs, hamsters	Cecum	Ingestion of organism passed in feces	None	Not reported	45
Chilomastix sp.	Worldwide	Mice, rats, hamsters	Cecum	Ingestion of cysts passed in feces	None	None	46
Enteromonas hominis	Worldwide	Primates, hamsters, rats, rabbits	Cecum	Ingestion of organism passed in feces	None	Reported	47
Giardia muris	Worldwide	Mice, rats, hamsters, other rodents	Anterior small intestine	Ingestion of cysts passed in feces	Enteritis, villus changes	Not reported	48
Giardia simoni	Worldwide	Rats, hamsters	Anterior small intestine	Ingestion of cysts passed in feces	None in hamsters	Not reported	47
Hexamastix muris	Worldwide	Rats, hamsters, other rodents	Cecum	Ingestion of organism passed in feces	Villus changes	Not reported	47
Monocercomonoides sp.	North America	Rats, hamsters	Cecum	Ingestion of organism passed in feces	None	Not reported	47
Octomitus pulcher	Worldwide	Mouse, rat, hamster, squirrel, other rodents	Cecum	Ingestion of organism passed in feces	None	Not reported	47
Pentatrichomonas hominis	Worldwide	Primates, mice, rats, hamsters, dogs, cats, cattle, primates	Cecum, colon	Ingestion of organism passed in feces	None	Reported	49, 50
Spironucleus muris	Worldwide	Rats, mice, hamsters, other rodents	Small intestine, cecum	Ingestion of cysts passed in feces	None in hamsters	Not reported	9
Tetratrichomonas microti	North America	Voles, hamsters, mice, rats, other rodents	Cecum	Ingestion of organism passed in feces	None	Not reported	13
Trichomitus wenyoni	North America	Mice, rats, hamsters, rhesus monkeys, baboons	Cecum, colon	Ingestion of organism passed in feces	None	Not reported	51
Tritrichomonas criceti	North America	Hamsters	Cecum, colon	Ingestion of organism passed in feces	None	Not reported	52
Tritrichomonas minuta	North America, Europe	Mice, rats, hamsters	Cecum, colon	Ingestion of organism passed in feces	None	Not reported	47
Tritrichomonas muris	Worldwide	Rats, mice, hamsters, other rodents	Cecum, colon, small intestine	Ingestion of "pseudocyst"	None	Not reported	14

(Continued)

407

TABLE 12.1 (*Continued*)

Parasite	Geographic Distribution	Hosts	Location in Host	Method of Infection	Pathologic Effects	Zoonosis	Reference
Amoebae							
Entamoeba muris	Worldwide	Mice, rats, hamsters	Cecum, colon	Ingestion of cysts passed in feces	None	Not reported	53
Cestodes							
Cyclophyllidea							
Hymenolepis diminuta	Worldwide	Rats, mice, hamsters, other rodents, primates	Small intestine	Ingestion of arthropod intermediate host	Catarrhal enteritis	Reported	54
Rodentolepis citelli	North America	Ground squirrels, hamsters, mice, rats, kangaroo rats	Intestine	Ingestion of arthropod intermediate host	Unknown	Not reported	55
Rodentolepis nana	Worldwide	Mice, rats, hamsters, other rodents	Intestine	Direct transmission or ingestion of arthropod intermediate host	Catarrhal enteritis, abscesses, focal granulomatous lymphadenitis, retarded growth, weight loss, death	Probably not susceptible to rodent strains	17
Rodentolepis microstoma	Worldwide	Mice, cotton rats, hamsters	Duodenum, biliary system, liver	Ingestion of arthropod intermediate host	Biliary inflammation, mucosal erosion	Reported	56
Rodentolepis peromysci	Worldwide	Deer mice (*Peromyscus*), hamsters, other rodents	Small intestine	Ingestion of arthropod intermediate host	Unknown	Not reported	57
Nematodes							
Oxyuroidea							
Syphacia criceti	Worldwide	Hamsters	Small intestine	Ingestion of embryonated egg	None	Not reported	17
Syphacia mesocriceti	Worldwide	Hamsters	Small intestine	Ingestion of embryonated egg	None	Not reported	17
Syphacia muris	Worldwide	Rats, mice, gerbils, hamsters	Cecum, colon	Ingestion of embryonated egg; retrofection	Weight loss, impaired intestinal electrolyte transport	Not reported	58
Syphacia obvelata	Worldwide	Mice, rats, hamsters, voles, other rodents, primates	Cecum, colon	Ingestion of embryonated egg; retrofection	Catarrhal enteritis, hepatic granulomas, perianal irritation	Rare	59

408

	Geographic distribution	Hosts	Location	Transmission	Disease		Reference
Trichostrongyloidea							
Heligmosomum juvenum	Asia	Hamsters	Small intestine	Ingestion of larva	Unknown	Not reported	60
Spirurida							
Gongylonema neoplasticum	Worldwide	Rodents, lagomorphs	Esophagus, stomach	Ingestion of intermediate host (cockroaches, mealworms, fleas)	Gastric ulcers	Not reported	61
Mastophorus sp.	Worldwide	Spiny mice (*Acomys*), voles (*Microtus*), hamsters, other rodents	Stomach	Ingestion of intermediate host (cockroaches)	Unknown	Not reported	62
Trichuroidea							
Trichosomoides nasalis	Africa, Asia, Europe	Wild rats, grass rats, golden hamsters	Nasal mucosa	Ingestion of embryonated egg	Rhinosinusitis	Not reported	63
Arachnida							
Mites							
Prostigmatids							
Spleorodens clethrionomys	Europe	Voles, hamsters	Nasal mucosa	Direct contact	Unknown	Not reported	44

409

TABLE 12.2 Parasites of Hamsters—Skin and Connective Tissue.

Parasite	Geographic Distribution	Hosts	Location in Host	Method of Infection	Pathologic Effects	Zoonosis	Reference
Arachnida							
Mites							
Astigmates							
Notoedres sp.	Europe, North America	Hamsters	Skin, usually of ears	Direct contact	Dermatitis	Not reported	39
Mesostigmates							
Haemogamasus pontiger	Worldwide	Rats, mice, hamsters, other rodents, humans	Skin, pelage	Direct contact	None	Reported	64
Ornithonyssus bacoti	Worldwide	Rats, mice, hamsters, gerbils, voles, humans, other mammals	Skin	Direct contact	Anemia, death; vector of rodent pathogens	Reported; vector of human pathogens	65
Prostigmates							
Demodex aurati	Worldwide	Hamsters	Pilosebacious system, hair follicles	Direct contact	Dermatitis, hyperpigmentation, alopecia	Not reported	29, 66
Demodex criceti	Worldwide	Hamsters	Epidermal pits	Direct contact	Dermatitis, alopecia	Not reported	29, 31, 66
Demodex cricetuli	Worldwide	Armenian hamsters (*Cricetulus migratorius*)	Hair follicles	Direct contact	Alopecia, hyperkeratosis, hyperemia	Not reported	35
Demodex sinocricetuli	Asia	Striped hamsters (*Cricetulus barabensis*)	Pilosebacious system, hair follicles	Direct contact	Dermatitis	Not reported	36
Radfordia cricetuliphila	Europe	Striped hamsters (*Cricetulus barabensis*)	Skin	Direct contact	Unknown	Not reported	67

REFERENCES

1. Implications of infectious agents on results of animal experiments. Report of the Working Group on Hygiene of the Gesellschaft fur Versuchstierkunde—Society for Laboratory Animal Science (GV-SOLAS) (1999) *Lab. Anim.* **33, Suppl 1,** S39–87.

2. Hrapkiewicz, H., Medina, L., and Holmes., D.D. (1998) Hamsters. In: *Clinical Laboratory Animal Medicine: An Introduction.* 2nd ed. Ames: Iowa State Press, 73–92.

3. Battles, A.H. (1985) The biology, care and diseases of the Syrian hamster. *Compend. Cont. Educ. Pract. Vet.* **7,** 815–825.

4. Taylor, D.M., Farquhar, C.F., and Neal, D.L. (1993) Studies on the eradication of intestinal protozoa of Syrian hamsters in quarantine and their transfaunation to mice. *Lab. Anim. Sci.* **43,** 359–360.

5. Griffiths, H.J. (1971) Some common parasites of small laboratory animals. *Lab. Anim.* **5,** 123–135.

6. Stachan, R. and Kunstyr, I. (1983) Minimal infectious doses and prepatent periods in *Giardia muris, Spironucleus muris* and *Tritrichomonas muris. Zentralbl. Bakteriol. Mikrobiol. Hyg. [A]* **256,** 249–256.

7. Patterson, M.M., Schrenzel, M.D., Feng, Y., and Fox, J.G. (2000) Gastritis and intestinal metaplasia in Syrian hamsters infected with *Helicobacter aurati* and two other microaerobes. *Vet. Pathol.* **37,** 589–596.

8. Underdown, B.J., Roberts-Thomson, I.C., Anders, R.F., and Mitchell, G.F. (1981) Giardiasis in mice: studies on the characteristics of chronic infection in C3H/He mice. *J. Immunol.* **126,** 669–672.

9. Kunstyr, I., Poppinga, G., and Friedhoff, K.T. (1993) Host specificity of cloned *Spironucleus* sp. originating from the European hamster. *Lab. Anim.* **27,** 77–80.

10. Schagemann, G., Bohnet, W., Kunstyr, I., and Friedhoff, K.T. (1990) Host specificity of cloned *Spironucleus muris* in laboratory rodents. *Lab. Anim.* **24,** 234–239.

11. Wagner, J.E., Doyle, R.E., Ronald, N.C., Garrison, R.G., and Schmitz, J.A. (1974) Hexamitiasis in laboratory mice, hamsters, and rats. *Lab. Anim. Sci.* **24,** 349–354.

12. Daniel, W.A., Mattern, C.F., and Honigberg, B.M. (1971) Fine structure of the mastigont system in *Tritrichomonas muris* (Grassi). *J. Protozool.* **18,** 575–586.

13. Wenrich, D.H. and Saxe, L.H. (1950) *Trichomonas microti,* n. sp. (protozoa, Mastigophora). *J. Parasitol.* **36,** 261–269.

14. Lipman, N.S., Lampen, N., and Nguyen, H.T. (1999) Identification of pseudocysts of *Tritrichomonas muris* in Armenian hamsters and their transmission to mice. *Lab. Anim. Sci.* **49,** 313–315.

15. Chalupsky, J., Vavra, J., and Bedrnik, P. (1979) Encephalitozoonosis in laboratory animals—a serological survey. *Folia Parasitol (Praha)* **26,** 1–8.

16. Pakes, S.P., Shadduck, J.A., and Cali, A. (1975) Fine structure of *Encephalitozoon cuniculi* from rabbits, mice and hamsters. *J. Protozool.* **22,** 481–488.

17. Pinto, R.M., Goncalves, L., Gomes, D.C., and Noronha, D. (2001) Helminth fauna of the golden hamster *Mesocricetus auratus* in Brazil. *Contemp. Top. Lab. Anim. Sci.* **40,** 21–26.

18. Wagner, J.E. (1987) Parasitic Diseases. In: Van Hoosier Jr., G.L. and McPherson, C.W. (eds.) *Laboratory Hamsters.* Academic Press, Inc., San Diego, California, 135–156.

19. Owen, D.C. (1992) *Parasites of Laboratory Animals.* Royal Society of Medicine Services Limited, London.

20. Harkness, J.E. and Wagner, J.E. (1995) *The Biology and Medicine of Rabbits and Rodents.* 4th ed. Williams and Wilkins, Media, Pennsylvania.

21. Unay, E.S. and Davis, B.J. (1980) Treatment of *Syphacia obvelata* in the Syrian hamster (*Mesocricetus auratus*) with piperazine citrate. *Am. J. Vet. Res.* **41,** 1899–1900.

22. Ronald, N.C. and Wagner, J.E. (1975) Treatment of *Hymenolepis nana* in hamsters with Yomesan (niclosamide). *Lab. Anim. Sci.* **25,** 219–220.

23. Hankenson, F.C. and Van Hoosier Jr., G.L. (2002) Biology and Diseases of Hamsters. In: Fox, J.G., Anderson, L.C., Loew, F.M., Quimby, F.W. (eds.). *Laboratory Animal Medicine.* 2nd ed. Academic Press, San Diego, California, 167–202.

24. Greve, J.H. (1985) *Dentostomella translucida,* a nematode from the golden hamster. *Lab. Anim. Sci.* **35,** 497–498.

25. Taylor, D.M. (1992) Eradication of pinworms (*Syphacia obvelata*) from Syrian hamsters in quarantine. *Lab. Anim. Sci.* **42,** 413–414.

26. Ross, C.R., Wagner, J.E., Wightman, S.R., and Dill, S.E. (1980) Experimental transmission of *Syphacia muris* among rats, mice, hamsters and gerbils. *Lab. Anim. Sci.* **30,** 35–37.

27. Visser, M., Rehbein, S., and Wiedemann, C. (2001) Species of flea (Siphonaptera) infesting pets and hedgehogs in Germany. *J. Vet. Med. B Infect. Dis. Vet. Public Health* **48,** 197–202.

28. Vogue, M. and Hyneman, D. (1957) Development of *Hymenolepis nana* and *Hymenolepis diminuta* (Cestoda Hymenolepidae) in the intermediate host *Tribolium confusum. Univ. Calif. Publ. Zool.,* **59,** 549–580.

29. Nutting, W.B. (1961) *Demodex aurati* sp.nov. and *D. criceti,* ectoparasites of the golden hamster (*Mesocricetus auratus*). *Parasitology* **51,** 515–522.

30. Hasegawa, T. (1995) A case report of the management of demodicosis in the golden hamster. *J. Vet. Med. Sci.* **57,** 337–338.

31. Nutting, W.B. and Rauch, H. (1958) *Demodex criceti* n. sp. (Acarina: Demodicidae) with notes on its biology. *J. Parasitol.* **44,** 328–333.

32. Tani, K., Iwanaga, T., Sonoda, K., Hayashiya, S., Hayashiya, M., and Taura, Y. (2001) Ivermectin treatment of demodicosis in 56 hamsters. *J. Vet. Med. Sci.* **63,** 1245–1247.

33. Skavlen, P. and Peterson, M.E. (1989) Skin Lesions in Hamsters. *Lab. Anim.* **18,** 17–18.

34. Estes, P.C., Richter, C.B., and Franklin, J.A. (1971) Demodectic mange in the golden hamster. *Lab. Anim. Sci.* **21,** 825–828.

35. Hurley, R.J. and Desch, C.E. Jr. (1994) *Demodex cricetuli:* new species of hair follicle mite (Acari: Demodecidae) from the Armenian hamster, *Cricetulus migratorius* (Rodentia: Cricetidae). *J. Med. Entomol.* **31,** 529–533.

36. Desch, C.E. Jr. and Hurley, R.J. (1997) *Demodex sinocricetuli:* new species of hair follicle mite (Acari: Demodecidae) from the Chinese form of the striped hamster, *Cricetulus barabensis* (Rodentia: Muridae). *J. Med. Entomol.* **34,** 317–320.

37. Benjamin, S.A. and Brooks, A.L. (1977) Spontaneous lesions in Chinese hamsters. *Vet. Pathol.* **14,** 449–462.

38. http://www.vin.com (2005) In: Veterinary Information Network.

39. Baies, A., Suteu, I., and Klemm, W. (1968) *Notoedres* scabies of the golden hamster. *Z. Versuchstierkd.* **10,** 251–257.

40. Beco, L., Petite, A., and Olivry, T. (2001) Comparison of subcutaneous ivermectin and oral moxidectin for the treatment of notoedric acariasis in hamsters. *Vet. Rec.* **149,** 324–327.

41. Creel, N.B., Crowe, M.A., and Mullen, G.R. (2003) Pet hamsters as a source of rat mite dermatitis. *Cutis* **71,** 457–461.

42. Fox, M.T., Baker, A.S., Farquhar, R., and Eve, E. (2004) First record of *Ornithonyssus bacoti* from a domestic pet in the United Kingdom. *Vet. Rec.* **154,** 437–438.

43. Bochkov, A.V. (1999) A new species of myobiid mite *Radfordia cricetuliphila* sp. n. (Acari: Myobiidae) from the striped hamster *Cricetulus*

barabensis (Rodentia: Cricetidae) from Buryatia. *Parazitologiia* **33,** 358–363.

44. Bornstein, S. and Iwarsson, K. (1980) Nasal mites in a colony of Syrian hamsters (*Mesocricetus auratus*). *Lab. Anim.* **14,** 31–33.

45. Brugerolle, G. and Regnault, J.P. (2001) Ultrastructure of the enteromonad flagellate *Caviomonas mobilis. Parasitol. Res.* **87,** 662–665.

46. Abraham, R. (1961) A new protozoon of the genus *Chilomastix. Z. F. Parasitenkunde* **21,** 159–163.

47. Levine, N.D. (1985) *Veterinary Protozoology.* Ames: Iowa State University Press, 414 pages.

48. Kunstyr, I., Schoeneberg, U., and Friedhoff, K.T. (1992) Host specificity of *Giardia muris* isolates from mouse and golden hamster. *Parasitol. Res.* 78, 621–622.

49. Fukushima, T., Mochizuki, K., Yamazaki, H., et al. (1990) *Pentatrichomonas hominis* from beagle dogs—detection method, characteristics and route of infection. *Jikken Dobutsu* **39,** 187–192.

50. Wenrich, D.H. (1924) Trichomonad flagellates in the caecum of rats and mice. *Anat. Record* **29,** 118.

51. Wenrich, D.H. and Nie, D. (1949) The morphology of *Trichomonas wenyoni* (Protozoa, Mastigophora). *J. Morphol.* **85,** 519–531.

52. Wantland, W.W. (1956) Trichomonads in the golden hamster. *Trans. Illinois State Acad. Sci.* **48,** 197–201.

53. Lin, T.-M. (1971) Colonization and encystation of *Entamoeba muris* in the rat and the mouse. *J. Parasitol.* **57,** 375–382.

54. Turton, J.A. (1971) Distribution and growth of *Hymenolepis diminuta* in the rat, hamster, and mouse. *Z. Parasitenkd,* **37,** 315–329.

55. Alghali, S.T. (1986) *Hymenolepis citelli* and *H. diminuta:* worm burdens in homologous and heterologous infections in rats. *Exp. Parasitol.* **62,** 14–23.

56. Dvorak, J.A., Jones, A.W., and Kuhlman, H.H. (1961) Studies on the biology of *Hymenolepis microstoma* (Dujardin, 1845). *J. Parasitol.* **47,** 833–838.

57. Stallard, H.E. and Arai, H.P. (1978) The growth and development of *Hymenolepis peromysci* Tinkle, 1972 (Cestoda: Cyclophyllidea). *Can J. Zool.* **56,** 90–93.

58. Lewis, J.W., and D'Silva, J. (1986) The life-cycle of *Syphacia muris* Yamaguti (Nematoda: Oxyuroidea) in the laboratory rat. *J. Helminthol.* **60,** 39–46.

59. Kellogg, H.S. and Wagner, J.E. (1982) Experimental transmission of *Syphacia obvelata* among mice, rats, hamsters, and gerbils. *Lab. An. Sci.* **32,** 500–501.

60. Yamaguti, S. (1961) The nematodes of vertebrates, vol. 3 part 1. In: *Systema Helminthum,* Interscience Publishers, Inc., New York: 544.

61. Hitchcock, C.R. and Bell, E.T. (1952) Studies on the nematode parasite, *Gongylonema neoplasticum* (*Spiroptera neoplasticum*), and avitaminosis A in the forestomach of rats: comparison with Fibiger's results. *J. Natl. Cancer Inst.* **12,** 1345–1387.

62. Rojas Mdel, C. and Digiani, M.C. (2003) First record of *Mastophorus muris* (Gmelin, 1790) (Nematoda: Spiruroidea) from a wild host in South America. *Parasite* **10,** 375–378.

63. Diagne, M., Diouf, M., Lochouarn, L., and Bain, O. (2000) *Trichosomoides nasalis* Biocca and Aurizi, 1961 and *T. spratti* n. sp. (Nematoda: Trichinelloidea), from the nasal cavity of murids. *Parasite* **7,** 215–220.

64. Baker, E.W., Evans, T.M., Gould, D.J., Hull, W.B., and Keegan, H.L. (1956) *A manual of parasitic mites of medical or economic importance. Tech. Publ. Natl. Pest Control Assoc., Inc.,* New York. 170 pages.

65. Creel, N.B., Crowe, M.A., and Mullen, G.R. (2003) Pet hamsters as a source of rat mite dermatitis. *Cutis* **71,** 457–461.

66. Flatt, R.E. and Kerber, W.T. (1968) Demodectic mite infestation in golden hamsters. *Lab. Animal Digest* **4,** 6–7.

67. Bochkov, A.V. (1999) A new species of myobiid mite *Radfordia cricetuliphila* sp. n. (Acari: Myobiidae) from the striped hamster *Cricetulus barabensis* (Rodentia: Cricetidae) from Buryatia. *Parazitologiia* **33,** 358–363.

Parasites of Gerbils

James D. Wilkerson, JD, DVM, DACLAM; and Diana M. Palila Berger, DVM, MS

INTRODUCTION

This chapter focuses on rodents of the genus *Meriones*, with primary emphasis on the Mongolian gerbil, *Meriones unguiculatus*. This is the species most often encountered in the laboratory setting or pet trade. Other members of the genus occasionally encountered include *M. persicus*, *M. rex*, *M. meridianus*, *M. crassus*, and *M. sacramenti*. In nature, gerbils inhabit arid regions from China to the Middle East and Russia[1].

Mongolian gerbils are generally healthy creatures with few viral or bacterial infections[2]. Likewise, gerbils serve as natural hosts for only a small number of host-specific parasites[3]. In the animal facility, most internal and external parasites found in or on gerbils have been acquired from other

rodent species. For that reason, parasites primarily associated with other host species are covered elsewhere in the text.

When evaluating treatment options for gerbils, the practitioner often must extrapolate from experience gained in treating parasitisms of other rodent species. Physiologic differences between species, in functions such as water consumption, must be considered when extrapolating treatments from one host species to another. For most drugs, the safety of treatments in gerbils has not been verified, so the practitioner should proceed deliberately but with caution. Initial treatment trials on small numbers of animals are warranted prior to treating the general population.

PROTOZOA

Gerbils are uncommon hosts of protozoan parasites. The enteric flagellates *Tritrichomonas caviae* and *Giardia* sp. have occasionally been found in gerbils[3–5]. Regarding the latter, gerbils are considered highly susceptible to infection with human forms of *Giardia* sp.[2] Gerbils may also become infected with *Entamoeba* sp.[3] Relatively little is known of the biology of these protozoa in gerbils. Additional studies are necessary to determine whether gerbils are susceptible to experimental infection with additional species of protozoa common to other laboratory rodents.

CESTODES

Hymenolepis diminuta

There is a single report of natural infection of a gerbil with *Hymenolepis diminuta*, the rat tapeworm[3]. The reader is directed to Chapter 11, Parasites of Rats and Mice, for a more complete description of the biology and clinical aspects of *H. diminuta*.

Rodentolepis nana

Morphology. A complete description of the morphology of *Rodentolepis nana* (Syn. *Hymenolepis nana*) is presented in Chapter 11, Parasites of Rats and Mice. A natural outbreak of *R. nana,* commonly called the "dwarf" tapeworm, has been reported in pet gerbils[6]. In this report, worms recovered from naturally infected gerbils were 10 mm to 45 mm long and bore a scolex, suckers, and hooked rostellum[6].

Hosts and Life Cycle. *Rodentolepis nana* has been reported in mice, rats, humans, hamsters, and gerbils. The life cycle of *R. nana* is discussed in Chapter 11, Parasites of Rats and Mice. Briefly, the life cycle is unique among cestodes in that it may be direct or indirect. Arthropods serve as intermediate hosts in the indirect life cycle. However, ingestion of eggs can lead to direct infection. Patency is reached in 20 to 30 days[6].

Pathologic Effects. Natural infection of gerbils with *R. nana* results in small intestinal distension. Microscopic lesions include enteritis of the small intestinal lamina propria, possibly in response to larvae.

Clinical Disease. While death was the presenting sign in the single naturally occurring outbreak, it could not be proven that *R. nana* was a direct cause of the mortality[6].

Diagnosis, Treatment, and Prevention. Diagnosis is as described for mice. Because of its zoonotic potential, treatment of pet gerbils infected with *R. nana* has not been recommended[6]. There are no published guidelines for treating gerbils infected with *R. nana.* The reader is directed to Chapter 11, Parasites of Rats and Mice for information concerning elimination of *R. nana* in other rodent species. Due to zoonotic potential the reader must consider whether the best course of action is removal of the infected gerbils and their euthanasia.

Public Health Considerations. It remains uncertain whether gerbil and human isolates of *R. nana* are cross-infective. Until this uncertainty is resolved, animal workers should use personal protection when handling infected animals or contaminated waste. Contaminated feed and bedding should be incinerated.

NEMATODES

Aspiculuris tetraptera

The mouse (*Mus musculus*) is the natural host for *Aspiculuris tetraptera*. The susceptibility of gerbils to infection with *A. tetraptera* is considered low[7]. Gerbils infected with *A. tetraptera* develop neither lesions nor clinical disease. Other aspects of the biology and treatment of *A. tetraptera* are covered in Chapter 11, Parasites of Rats and Mice.

Dentostomella translucida

Morphology. *Dentostomella translucida* is in the superfamily Oxyuroidea, family Heteroxynematidae, and subfamily Heteroxynematinae[8,9]. *Dentostomella translucida* has a cylindrical, elongated body, with cervical inflations of the cuticle. The cuticle is thick, transparent, and transversely striated. Two lateral longitudinal ridges extend the full length of the body[8,9]. *D. translucida* is a relatively large nematode. As originally described from the great gerbil, *Rhombomys opimus* Lichtenstein, females are 21.8 mm to 40.4 mm long and males are 14.2 mm to 18.3 mm long[10]. Specimens collected from Mongolian gerbils are typically smaller, with females ranging from 9.6 mm to 31 mm long and 0.38 mm to 1 mm wide, while males are 6.1 mm to 13.1 mm long and 0.37 mm to 0.53 mm wide (Figure 13.1)[8,11].

In both sexes, the mouth is without lips and there are five unequal teeth per esophageal sector. Females have a long, evenly proportioned body ending in a conical to bluntly rounded tail. The vulva is a transverse slit located cranial to the midbody. It opens into a thick walled, cranially directed vagina vera. This continues as a vagina uterina until it turns caudally as an unpaired uterine tube. The uterine tube remains narrow caudal to the vulva, but then widens into a common egg chamber, which divides into two uteri. The uteri are confined to the caudal half of the body. The anus is located near the caudal end of the

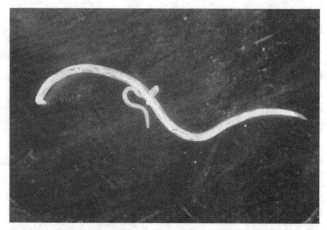

Fig. 13.1 Female (larger) and male *Dentostomella translucida* engaged in copulation. From work associated with Berger, D.M. (1991) with permission.

body. In males, a swelling of the cuticle cranial to the cloaca forms a fleshy bursa (approximately 0.5 mm to 0.73 mm in length), which ends before the tip of the tail. Males have a single, weakly sclerotized spicule that is rounded on lateral view and bifid in ventral view. There are four pairs of caudal papillae[8].

The eggs of *D. translucida* are asymmetrically oval, flattened on one side, with one end more fusiform, and measure 115 μ to 140 μ by 30 μ to 60 μ. The asymmetry is only evident on lateral view[9,11,12]. In dorsoventral view the egg of *D. translucida* could be confused with that of some other pinworms (e.g., *Aspiculuris tetraptera*). The surface layer of the eggshell is relatively thick and contains pits or bumps. Ultrastructural studies using scanning electron microscopy have shown that *D. translucida* eggs have an operculum that is located near one pole on the curved side of the egg[9]. This is the second species of the genus *Dentostomella* for which an operculum has been described. This structure was not visible by either transmission electron microscopy or light microscopy[9]. A rupture of the external layer of the shell (resulting in a bulging out of internal layers of the eggshell) or a distinct suture line was seen in the same area when eggs incubated in potassium dichromate were examined by light microscopy (Figure 13.2)[12]. These were located near the more fusiform pole on the curved side of the egg the same location from which larvae hatched *in vitro*. Splitting of the external layer in this area did not affect the development of the larvae, and the eggshell never ruptured in other areas[12].

Hosts. *Dentostomella translucida* is the common pinworm of gerbils. It has been reported from the great gerbil

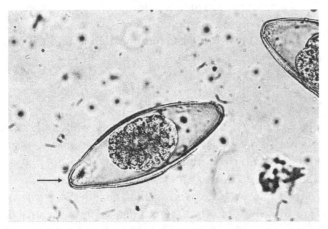

Fig. 13.2 Jagged suture line (arrow) at fusiform end of egg. Dark debris obscures a portion of the suture line toward the interior of the egg, 400×. Reproduced from Berger, D.M. (1991) with permission.

(*Rhombomys opimus* Lichtenstein) in Middle Asia (Kazakhstan, Turkmenia, Uzbekistan, and Tadzhikistan)[10,13–15], the rough-legged jerboa (*Dipus sagitta* Pallas), the midday gerbil (*Meriones meridianus* Pallas)[13], and the wild rodent (*Mastomys fumatus* Peters) in Yemen[16]. The first record of *D. translucida* from the Mongolian gerbil involved laboratory animals from three commercial sources[11]. *Dentostomella translucida* apparently has not been reported from the Mongolian gerbil under natural conditions. For example, none of the 193 animals examined in the Buriat Autonomous Soviet Socialist Republic were found to be infected[17]. *D. translucida* has been reported from laboratory-reared golden hamsters (*Mesocricetus auratus*)[18].

Attempts to transmit *D. translucida* to laboratory mice via embryonated eggs suspended in moist food and to prairie voles (*Pitymys ochrogaster* Wagner) and lemmings (*Dicrostonyx groenlandicus* Traill) via dosing with embryonated eggs have not resulted in infections[7,12].

Life Cycle. The life cycle is direct. Adult and juvenile *Dentostomella* are found in the small intestine, preferentially in the anterior third, with fewer found in the middle, and lowest counts in the posterior third[11,12]. This is an unusual location for pinworms of laboratory rodents. In other species this parasite has been found in additional organs. It has been reported to occur in the stomach of golden hamsters[18] and in the stomach, small intestine, and large intestine of great gerbils[10,14].

Typically, fewer than 10 worms are found in a single gerbil[11,12,19]. However, pregnancy and lactation may allow for increased worm burdens. In one study, a pregnant and a lactating gerbil each were infected with 40 *D. translucida*, whereas the number of worms in other females ranged from zero to 12[12]. The prepatent period is 23 to 29 days[11,12,19]. Egg laying is intermittent, but large numbers of eggs are typically found when fecal samples are positive[11,18,20].

In vitro embryonation studies have been performed in liquid mediums (tap water, water containing enzymes, or 0.5% to 1% potassium dichromate) at 37°C or room temperature (20°C to 23°C)[9,12,19]. Aside from some differences in rate of development attributable in part to differences of temperature, the descriptions of the sequence of development of the embryos were similar among the studies. In one study, after five days of incubation at room temperature, <10% of eggs underwent embryonation, whereas 90% did so with 10 days incubation[19]. In another study, only eight days of incubation at room temperature were required for embryonation, and for animals to become infected[12]. In the latter study, the gross development and behavior of larvae were studied during four separate incubation trials. At laying, the eggs contained a grainy appearing embryo that consisted of an aggregation of cells situated in the center of the egg (Figure 13.3). When incubated at 20°C to 23°C, a short, thick larva (82 μ by 27 μ) with markedly blunt ends developed in two to three days. Between days seven and eight of *in vitro* incubation, the caudal end of the larvae emerged first, and some were seen encased in a molted cuticle (Figure 13.4). Hatching *in vivo* occurs soon after ingestion of embryonated eggs[19].

Pathologic Effects and Clinical Disease. In one study, infection with *D. translucida* was not accompanied by

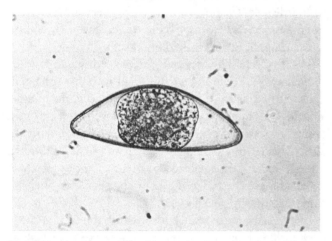

Fig. 13.3 Appearance of embryo at the time of removal of the egg from the uterus (lateral view), 400×. From work associated with Berger, D.M. (1991) with permission.

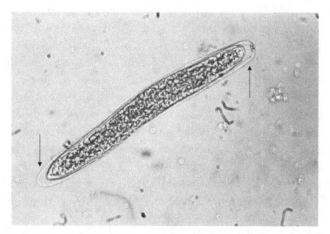

Fig. 13.4 Ensheathed (arrows), fully emerged larva, 400×. From work associated with Berger, D.M. (1991) with permission.

histologic lesions in the intestines of infected gerbils[11]. Others have reported finding eosinophils, lymphocytes, and plasma cells in the lamina propria, with thickening of the villus tips[19]. In a third study, eosinophils were seen in the nonglandular stomach as well as the small intestine; however, the level of eosinophilia did not correlate with the presence of nematodes or their numbers[12]. No evidence of either intralaminar migration or larval migration in other abdominal organs has been seen[12,19]. *Dentostomella translucida* does not cause clinical signs even in heavily parasitized gerbils[11,12].

Diagnosis. *D. translucida* may be diagnosed by fecal flotation. Due to the relatively desiccated nature of gerbil feces, fecal pellets should be soaked prior to performing flotations[11]. Presoaking fecal pellets to soften them, followed by mashing them in flotation solution, improves recovery. Detection of infection in fecal specimens in which pellets are simply rinsed or agitated in flotation solution is unlikely[12]. Although ova have been occasionally detected by cellophane-tape impressions of the perineum, this is presumed to be due to incidental contamination[11]. Post-mortem diagnosis is made by examining the small intestine for the presence of adult or larval nematodes.

Treatment. Fenbendazole-medicated feed (150 ppm) is an effective, reliable, and practical treatment for eradicating *D. translucida* from gerbils[21]. Provision of mebendazole by oral gavage (2.2 mg in 1 ml tap water, daily for five days) is also reported to be an effective, though more labor intensive, treatment[19]. Ineffective treatments include: topical misting with ivermectin (1 mg/ml solution), ivermectin-medicated drinking water (0.005 mg/ml water), and piperazine citrate-medicated drinking water (4 mg/ml deionized water)[21].

Prevention. Changing cages more than once per week may prevent re-infection[12,19].

Public Health Considerations. This parasite is not known to infect humans[22].

Syphacia muris

The rat is the natural host of *S. muris*. Gerbils and other rodents are occasional hosts[2,23]. No gerbil-specific *S. muris* strains are known. Gerbils are considered transitory hosts, who clear infections as they mature[24]. Infection with *S. muris* is not associated with pathologic effects or clinical signs in gerbils. However, gerbils may serve as a source of *S. muris* for other susceptible species[23]. Other aspects of the biology and treatment of *S. muris* are covered in Chapter 11, Parasites of Rats and Mice.

Syphacia obvelata

The natural host of *Syphacia obvelata* is the mouse. Gerbils and many other rodents may serve as occasional hosts[7,11,25]. Neither pathologic nor clinical signs have been reported in gerbils. Infected gerbils may transmit *S. obvelata* to mice or other susceptible rodent species[25]. Infection of gerbils with *S. obvelata* is transient, because as gerbils mature, their infections frequently are lost[25]. Other aspects of the biology and treatment of *S. obvelata* are covered in Chapter 11, Parasites of Rats and Mice.

ARTHROPODS

Class Insecta

Nosopsyllus laeviceps kuzenkovi

Nosopsyllus laeviceps kuzenkovi, sometimes called the gerbil flea, is a blood-sucking flea. It has been found on gerbils in Asia[26,27]. Relatively little is known of the biology of this flea, or of strategies for its elimination. It is important to correctly identify the species of all fleas found on gerbils, because *N. l. kuzenkovi* may serve as a vector for *Yersinia pestis,* the causative agent of plague[26,27].

Class Arachnida

Demodex merioni

Morphology. *Demodex merioni* (Syn. *D. meriones*) has only been reported twice[28,29]. In one report, only the body shape was described. Some individuals had a short opisthosoma, resembling that of *D. criceti,* while others had a long tapered opisthosoma, resembling that of *D. aurati*[29]. It is possible that *D. merioni* is synonymous with either D. *criceti* or *D. aurati.*

Hosts. *Demodex* are considered to be highly host-specific[30]. However, if the mites described as *D. merioni* are actually *D. criceti* or *D. aurati,* cross-species infestation may occur between hamsters and gerbils. Further studies are required to address this issue.

Life Cycle. The life cycle of *D. merioni* is presumed to be similar to those of other members of the genus.

Pathologic Effects and Clinical Disease. In one reported clinical case, a debilitated four-year-old male gerbil developed alopecia, scaliness, hyperemia, and multifocal ulcerations at the base of the tail, and to a lesser extent on the rear legs[29]. Mites were recovered from these areas. Focal ulceration, bacterial colonization, and hyperkeratosis were identified in histologic sections. In other species, presence of *Demodex* in lesions does not necessarily mean that the parasite is the cause of the lesion. Advanced age or other causes of debilitation are believed to be necessary for marked clinical signs to manifest[29,30]. It is presumed that this is also true for gerbils.

Diagnosis. Microscopic examination of deep skin scrapings reveals mites. The likelihood of detection may be increased by application of heat to the excised skin, because heat causes *D. criceti* and *D. aurati* to come to the surface of the skin, and possibly to climb hair shafts[30].

Treatment and Prevention. Therapies specific to gerbils infested with *Demodex* sp. have not been described. Those used in other species presumably would be effective, but caution should be observed in initial trials to verify safety and efficacy[30]. Provision of supportive therapy to improve general health status, clipping fur over lesions, and bathing in acaricidal dips has been suggested[24].

Public Health Considerations. *D. merioni* is not considered a human pathogen.

Liponyssoides sanguineus

Liponyssoides sanguineus is a sucking mite of mice, rats, and the spiny mouse (*Acomys sp.*)[31]. The reader is directed to Chapter 11, Parasites of Rats and Mice for a complete discussion of this parasite. In a single report, this parasite was found on two Mongolian gerbils and on a group of Egyptian gerbils (*Meriones libycus*)[32]. No clinical signs were observed[31]. *Liponyssoides sanguineus* is a vector of *Rickettsia akari,* the organism that causes Rickettsial pox in humans[31].

Tyrophagus castellani

Tyrophagus castellani is a forage or food mite that was observed during blood collection in one study group of gerbils[3]. Little is known of its biology. It is not considered a pathogen.

TABLE 13.1 Parasites of Gerbils.

Parasite	Geographic distribution	Hosts	Location in host	Method of infection	Pathologic effects	Zoonosis	Reference
Flagellates							
Entamoeba sp.	Worldwide	Gerbils	Intestine	Ingestion of cyst in feces	None	Not reported	3
Giardia sp.	Worldwide	Gerbils, other rodents	Small intestine	Ingestion of cyst in feces	None	Not reported	5
Tritrichomonas caviae	Worldwide	Guinea pigs, gerbils	Cecum, colon	Ingestion of organism passed in feces	None	Not reported	3
Cestodes							
Hymenolepis diminuta	Worldwide	Rats, mice, gerbils, other rodents, primates	Small intestine	Ingestion of arthropod intermediate host	Catarrhal enteritis	Reported	3, 32
Rodentolepis (Hymenolepis) nana	Worldwide	Mice, rats, gerbils, other rodents	Intestine	Direct transmission or ingestion of arthropod intermediate host	Catarrhal enteritis, abscesses, focal granulomatous lymphadenitis, retarded growth, weight loss, death	Unknown susceptibility to gerbil strains	6
Nematodes							
Aspiculuris tetraptera	Worldwide	Mice, gerbils, other rodents	Cecum, colon	Ingestion of embryonated egg	Usually none	Not reported	7
Dentostomella translucida	Worldwide	Gerbils	Small intestine	Ingestion of embryonated egg	Localized eosinophilia	Not reported	8, 9
Syphacia muris	Worldwide	Rats, mice, gerbils, hamsters	Cecum, colon	Ingestion of embryonated egg, retrofection	Weight loss, impaired intestinal electrolyte transport	Not reported	23
Syphacia obvelata	Worldwide	Mice, rats, hamsters, voles, gerbils, other rodents, primates	Cecum, colon	Ingestion of embryonated egg, retrofection	Catarrhal enteritis, hepatic granulomas, perianal irritation	Rare	7, 25
Arthropods							
Insecta							
Nosopsyllus laeviceps kuzenkovi	Worldwide	Gerbils	Skin	Direct contact	Unknown	Not reported, known vector of *Yersinia pestis*	26
Arachnida							
Mites							
Mesostigmatids							
Liponyssoides sanguineus	Worldwide	Mice, rats, gerbils, other rodents, humans	Skin	Direct contact	Unknown	Reported, vector of *Rickettsia akari*	31

Prostigmatids					
Demodex sp.	North America	Mongolian gerbils	Skin	Direct contact	Alopecia, scabby dermatitis	Not reported	28
Nonparasitic					
Tyrophagus castellani	Worldwide	Mammals	Periocular	Direct contact	Possible allergic dermatitis	Not reported	3

419

REFERENCES

1. Nowak, R.M. (1999) *Walker's Mammals of the World.* 6th ed., The Johns Hopkins University Press. Baltimore, Maryland, 1344–1346, 1455–1459.

2. Percy, D.H. and Barthold, S.W. (2001) *Pathology of Laboratory Rodents and Rabbits.* 2nd ed., Iowa State University Press. Ames, Iowa, 198, 203–204.

3. Vincent, A.L., Porter, D.D., and Ash, L.R. (1975) Spontaneous lesions and parasites of the Mongolian gerbil, *Meriones unguiculatus. Lab. Anim. Sci.* **25,** 711–722.

4. Foreyt, W. J. (2001) *Veterinary Parasitology Reference Manual.* 5th ed., Iowa State University Press. Ames, Iowa, 172.

5. Samuel, W.M., Pybus, M.J., and Koea, A.A. (2001) *Parasitic Diseases of Wild Mammals.* 2nd ed., Iowa State University Press. Ames, Iowa, 405.

6. Lussier, G. and Loew, F.M. (1970) Natural *Hymenolepis nana* infection in Mongolian gerbils (*Meriones unguiculatus*). *Can. Vet. J.* **11,** 105–107.

7. Pinto, R.M., Gomes, D.C., and Noronha, D. (2003) Evaluation of coinfection with pinworms (*Aspiculuris tetraptera, Dentostomella translucida,* and *Syphacia obvelata*) in gerbils and mice. *Cont. Top. Lab. Anim. Sci.* **42,** 46–48.

8. Pilitt, P.A. and Wightman, S.R. (1979) A redescription of *Dentostomella translucida* Schulz and Krepkorgorskaja, 1932 (Nematoda: Heteroxynematidae) parasite of domestic Mongolian gerbils, *Meriones unguiculatus* Milne-Edwards. *Proc. Helminthol. Soc. Wash.* **46,** 36–42.

9. Yi, J.K. and Heckman, R.A. (1988) Morphological characteristics of *Dentostomella translucida,* a nematode (Oxyuroidea) found in Mongolian gerbils. *Great Basin Naturalist* **48,** 206–215.

10. Schulz, R.E. and Krepkogorskaja, T.A. (1932) *Dentostomella translucida* n. gen., n. sp. (Nematoda, Oxyurinae) aus einem Nagetier (*Rhombomys opimus* Licht). *Zoologischer Anzeiger.* **97,** 330–334.

11. Wightman, S.R., Pilitt, P.A., Wagner, J.E. (1978) *Dentostomella translucida* in the Mongolian Gerbil (*Meriones unguiculatus*). *Lab. Anim. Sci.* **28,** 290–296.

12. Berger, D.M. (1991) Biological Characteristics and Cycle of *Dentostomella translucida* Schulz and Krepkogorskaja, 1932, in the Mongolian gerbil, *Meriones unguiculatus* (Milne-Edwards). *Masters of Science.* University of Washington, Seattle.

13. Danzan, G. (1978) Materialy po faune nematod zaitseobraznykh i gryzunov Mongol'skoi narodnoi respubliki. In *Namatody i Akantosefaly.* Trudy Gel'mintologicheskoi Laboratorii, Akademiia Nauk SSSR, Moskva. **28,** 9–16.

14. Shleikher, E.I. and Samsonova, A.V. (1953) K gel'mintofaune bol'shoi peshchanki Uzbekistana. Raboty po gel'mintologii k 75-letiiu Akademika K. I. Skriabina. (otv. red. A.M. Petrov). Akademiia Nauk SSSR, Moskva, 770–773.

15. Ryzhikov, K.M., Gvozdez, E.V., Tokobaev, M.M. et al. (1979) Opredelitel' gel'mintov gryzunov fauny SSSR: Nematody i Akantotsefaly. Nauka, Moskva. [otv. red. K.M. Ryzhikov]. 277 pages.

16. Chitwood, M.B. (1963) *Dentostomella grundmanni* n. sp. (Nematoda: Oxyuridae) from *Eutamias quadrivittatus* (Say, 1823). *Proc. Helminthol. Soc. Wash.* **30,** 70–72.

17. Machulskii, S.N. (1958) Gel'mintofauna gryzunov Buriatskoi ASSR. Raboty po Gel'mintologii k 80-letiiu Akademika K. I. Skriabina. [N.P. Shikhobalova. otv. red.]. Akademiia Nauk SSSR. 219–224.

18. Greve, J.H. (1985) *Dentostomella translucida,* a Nematode from the Golden Hamster. *Lab. Anim. Sci.* **35,** 497–498.

19. Smith, G.D. and Snider III, T.G. (1988) Experimental Infection and Treatment of *Dentostomella translucida* in the Mongolian Gerbil. *Lab. Anim. Sci.* **38,** 339–340.

20. Hendrix, C.M. 1998. *Diagnostic Veterinary Parasitology.* 2nd ed. Mosby, Inc. St. Louis, Missouri, 157– 159.

21. Wilkerson, J.D., Brooks, D., Derby, M., and Griffey, S. (2001) Comparison of practical treatment methods to eradicate pinworm (*Dentostomella translucida*) infections from Mongolian gerbils (*Meriones unguiculatus*). *Contemp. Top. Lab. Anim. Sci.* **40,** 31–36.

22. Colville, J. (1991) *Diagnostic Parasitology for Veterinary Technicians.* American Veterinary Publications, Inc. Goleta, California, 212–217.

23. Ross, C.R., Wagner, J.E., Wightman, S.R., and Dill, S.E. (1980) Experimental transmission of *Syphacia muris* among rats, mice, hamsters and gerbils. *Lab Anim. Sci.* **30,** 35–37.

24. Wagner, J.E. and Farrar, P.L. (1987) Husbandry and Medicine of Small Rodents, Gerbils. In Harkness, J.E. (ed.) *The Veterinary Clinics of North America, Small Animal Practice, Exotic Animal Medicine,* Vol. 17. No.5. W.B. Saunders Company. Philadelphia, Pennsylvania, 1074–1082.

25. Kellogg, H.S. and Wagner, J.E. (1982) Experimental transmission of *Syphacia obvelata* among mice, rats, hamsters and gerbils. *Lab. Anim. Sci.* **32,** 500–501.

26. Jun, L., Shang-Jun, L., Amin, O.M., and Yumei, Z. (1993) Blood-feeding of the gerbil flea *Nosopsyllus laeviceps kuzenkovi* (Yagubyants), vector of plague in inner Mongolia, China. *Med. Vet. Entomol.* **7,** 54– 58.

27. Amin, O.M., Jun, L., Shangjun, L., Yumei, Z., and Lianzhl, S. (1993) Development and longevity of *Nosopsyllus laeviceps Kuzenkovi* (Siphonaptera) from inner Mongolia under laboratory conditions. *J. Parasitol.* **79,** 193–197.

28. Reynolds, S.L. and Gainer, J.H. (1968) Dermatitis of Mongolian gerbils *(Meriones unguiculatus)* caused by *Demodex* sp. 19th An. Mtg. AALAS, Las Vegas, N.V. Abstract #150.

29. Schwarzbrott, S.S., Wagner, J.E., and Frisk, C. S. (1974) Demodicosis in the Mongolian Gerbil (*Meriones unguiculatus*): A Case Report. *Lab. Anim. Sci.* **24,** 666–668.

30. Wagner, J.E. (1987) Parasitic Diseases, In Van Hoosier Jr., G.L. and McPherson, C.L. (eds.) *Laboratory Hamsters.* Academic Press, Inc., Orlando, Florida, 135–156.

31. Levine, J.F. and Lage, A.L. (1984) House Mouse Mites Infesting Laboratory Rodents. *Lab. Anim. Sci.* **34,** 393–394.

32. Johnson, S.S. and Conder, G.A. (1996) Infectivity of *Hymenolepis diminuta* for the jird, *Meriones unguiculatus,* and utility of this model for anthelmintic studies. *J. Parasitol.* **82,** 492–495.

CHAPTER

14

Parasites of Guinea Pigs

Lora R. Ballweber, MS, DVM, DEVPC; and John E. Harkness, DVM, MS, MEd, DACLAM

INTRODUCTION

Guinea pigs continue to serve as useful models of many human diseases and conditions. They are susceptible to experimental infection or infestation with a variety of parasites naturally found in or on other animals; therefore they are frequently used as models of parasitic infections and infestations, including those caused by protozoa, helminths, and arthropods. These experimental infections and infestations are not discussed in this chapter, but the interested reader is referred to the biomedical literature for additional information.

PROTOZOA

Numerous protozoans have been described in guinea pigs; large intestinal flagellates and ciliates are the most numerous. These rarely cause disease, and are commonly considered part of the normal intestinal fauna. Other protozoans, for which the guinea pig serves as a natural or accidental host, may cause disease and can interfere with experimental studies.

Phylum Sarcomastigophora

Class Mastigophora

Intestinal flagellates of guinea pigs have direct life cycles and typically inhabit the lumen of the cecum and colon, where they feed on bacteria, undigested plant material, starch, and soluble nutrients[1]. In general, intestinal flagellates are considered nonpathogenic. However, no quantitative studies have been performed on the relationship between cecal fauna and host physiology.

Identification of most cecal flagellates is difficult without proper training and correct handling of specimens. Examination of fecal smears is the most common technique used for detecting motile organisms. For rapidly moving organisms, agents such as methylcellulose will increase water viscosity, thus slowing the organisms for better viewing[2]. Fresh smears can also be fixed in appropriate fixative (e.g., Schaudinn's fixative, Bouin's fixative) and stained with iron hematoxylin and protargol silver protein. Fresh smears, smears mixed with methylcellulose or nickel sulfate, and smears fixed in the vapors of 3% osmium tetroxide should be examined using phase contrast or differential interference microscopy. Because proper identification depends, in part, on the siderophilic or argyrophilic structures, good preparations of both kinds of stains are critical[1,2].

Because cecal flagellates may be part of the normal gut fauna of guinea pigs, treatment to reduce or eliminate these organisms is of questionable value. Transmission can be reduced by adhering to strict hygiene for those species that develop cysts. The route of transmission is unclear for those that do not form cysts. However, guinea pigs removed from their mothers within 15 minutes of birth are free of flagellates[3], indicating some maternal contact or contact with fecal matter may be important in transmission.

Transfaunation experiments seem to indicate that guinea pig flagellates do not readily infect other common laboratory animals such as rats, mice, or golden hamsters. However, natural infections of at least one species of guinea pig flagellate (*Caviomonas mobilis*) in golden hamsters have been reported. In addition, guinea pigs became infected after oral administration of *Octomitus marmotae* from a ground hog (*Marmota monax*) and *Tetratrichomonas microti* from a mouse[3]. Neither of these species has been reported from naturally infected guinea pigs, and it is unknown whether guinea pigs harboring their normal cecal fauna would become infected. Although it appears unlikely that healthy guinea pigs would easily become infected with flagellates from other hosts, it seems prudent to maintain separate housing of host species to ensure that cross-transmission does not occur. Human infections with intestinal flagellates of guinea pigs have not been reported.

Caviomonas mobilis

Caviomonas mobilis (Figure 14.1) is a small flagellate that lives in the cecum of the guinea pig. Trophozoites are ovoid to elongate in shape with the anterior end more rounded than the posterior end and measuring 2.2 μ to 6.6 μ long by 2 μ to 3.3 μ wide (average: 4.2 μ long by 2.9 μ wide). The single vesicular nucleus, which does not contain a nucleolus, is located in the anterior extremity. A single flagellum, two to three times the body length, originates near the nucleus. The peristyle arises near the nucleus, extends posteriad along the body surface, and terminates at the posterior end of the body. There are no cytostomes, contractile elements, mitochondria, or Golgi body, and the endoplasmic reticulum is reduced. Feeding is by pinocytosis and phagocytosis[4,5]. Cysts have not been reported. *Caviomonas mobilis* has been reported from 11% (6/56) of asymptomatic guinea pigs in the United States[4]. Although experimental oral administration of trophozoites did not result in infections of

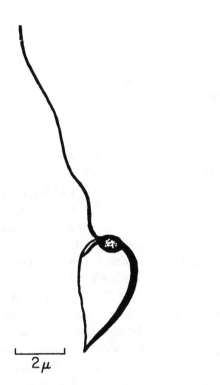

Fig. 14.1 *Caviomonas mobilis.* Reproduced from Nie, D. (1950) with permission.

golden hamsters[3], natural infections with *C. mobilis* in this host have been reported[6].

Chilomastix intestinalis

Species of the genus *Chilomastix* are piriform, with a rounded anterior end and tapered posterior end. The nucleus is round, with a large, ventral cytostome situated adjacent to it. Four basal bodies are present at the anterior pole of the cytostome from which the three anterior flagella and one cytostomal flagellum arise. Cysts are formed[7]. *Chilomastix intestinalis* trophozoites (Figure 14.2) measure 8.8 μ to 28 μ long by 6.6 μ to 11 μ wide (average: 19.4 μ long by 8.1 μ wide). The cytostome is in the shape of a "figure 8." A tongue-like process is present on the right cytostomal lip. The nucleus is located one-half to two-thirds its diameter below the anterior end of the body. The cytoplasm contains vacuoles of varying sizes. Cysts are ellipsoidal or lemon-shaped, measuring 9 μ to 11 μ long by 6.6 μ to 9.9 μ wide[7].

Chilomastix intestinalis was detected in 45% (25/56) of guinea pigs examined in the United States[7] and has been reported in guinea pigs from Africa, Asia, and South America[1,8]. Rats and golden hamsters are not susceptible to infection with *C. intestinalis*[3].

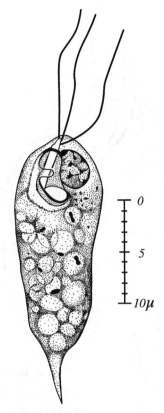

Fig. 14.2 *Chilomastix intestinalis.* Reproduced from Nie, D. (1948) with permission.

Chilomastix wenrichi

Chilomastix wenrichi trophozoites are smaller than those of *C. intestinalis,* and measure 7.5 μ to 12 μ long by 4 μ to 5 μ wide (average: 10.1 μ long by 4.3 μ wide). The cytostome lacks a tongue-like process, the nucleus is located more anteriorly than for *C. intestinalis,* and the cyst formed is smaller than that of *C. intestinalis*[4,7].

Chilomastix wenrichi has only been reported from guinea pigs in the United States, where it was detected in 12% (7/59) of asymptomatic guinea pigs examined[7]. As with *C. intestinalis*, rats are not susceptible[3].

Chilomitus caviae

Chilomitus caviae (Figure 14.3) is ellipsoidal in shape, with a convex dorsal surface and straight or concave ventral surface. Trophozoites measure 6 μ to 14 μ long by 3.1 μ to 4.6 μ wide (average: 11.2 μ long by 4.4 μ wide). Immediately below the blepharoplast is an ovoid nucleus without a nucleolus. A ring-shaped parabasal body is present, located on the left ventral side of the nucleus. The parabasal body may be equal to or exceed the nucleus in size. Three anterior free flagella and one recurrent flagellum, all of which

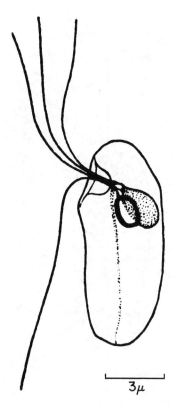

Fig. 14.3 *Chilomitus caviae.* Reproduced Nie, D. (1950) with permission.

are slightly longer than the body and of about equal length, arise from the blepharoplasts located at the base of the antero-ventral funnel. The flagella remain adherent to each other throughout their course in the funnel, but separate after reaching the exterior. A very delicate, rudimentary axostyle is present. Siderophilic bodies are present within the cytoplasm. No pelta is present and cysts do not occur[4].

Chilomitus caviae has been found in the cecum and colon of guinea pigs in the Americas, Europe, and India[9]. In one report, *C. caviae* was found in 24% (20/84) of guinea pigs examined[4]. *Chilomitus caviae* does not infect rats[3].

Chilomitus conexus

Chilomitus conexus measures 3.8 μ to 6.6 μ long by 1.3 μ to 1.8 μ wide (average: 5.2 μ long by 1.7 μ wide). The tunnel-shaped depression is located about one-third of the body length from the anterior end, with a slight outward protrusion and variable depth. Immediately below the blepharoplast is a densely staining nucleus. A small, round to ring-shaped parabasal body is located lateral to the nucleus. A well developed axostyle, originating from the

blepharoplast, extends to the posterior end but does not protrude. Intracytoplasmic, siderophilic bodies are also present[4]. *Chilomitus conexus* inhabits the cecum and colon, and was found in 1.2% (1/84) of guinea pigs examined[4]. *Chilomitus conexus* does not infect rats nor golden hamsters[3].

Enteromonas caviae

Enteromonas caviae (Syn. *Enteromonas fonsecai*) (Figure 14.4) trophozoites are piriform in shape and measure 3 μ to 5.5 μ long by 2.3 μ to 4.4 μ wide (average: 4 μ long by 3 μ wide). The vesicular nucleus is located in the anterior portion of the body and may or may not contain a nucleolus. Two blepharoplasts, which give rise to four flagella (three anterior and one recurrent), and a funis are present. The three anterior flagella are unequal in length, and the recurrent flagellum is slightly longer than the body. Reproduction is by binary fission. Cysts are formed[4]. *Enteromonas caviae* has only been reported from guinea pigs in the United States and Europe[1,4]. In one study, 7% (6/84) of guinea pigs were infected[4]. Rats are not susceptible to infection with *E. caviae*[3].

Giardia duodenalis

Morphology. *Giardia duodenalis* (Syn. *Giardia caviae*, *G. intestinalis*, *G. lamblia*) isolates recovered from guinea pigs were formerly named *G. caviae* when *Giardia* spp. were named according to the host from which they were

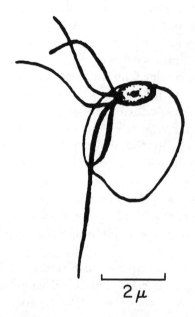

Fig. 14.4 *Enteromonas caviae.* Reproduced from Nie, D. (1950) with permission.

recovered. This parasite is bilaterally symmetrical and dorso-ventrally flattened with a pear-shaped body. A concave ventral sucking disc occupies almost the entire anterior portion of the body. Two anterior vesicular nuclei with nucleoli, two axostyles, four pairs of flagella, and a pair of median bodies are present. The trophozoites measure 8 μ to 14 μ long by 5.6 μ to 10.1 μ wide (average: 10.7 μ long by 7.2 μ wide)[10]. Cyst measurements have not been reported.

Hosts and Life Cycle. *Giardia duodenalis* has been found in guinea pigs in most regions of the world[1,11,12]. Although the life cycle has not been specifically described for this parasite in the guinea pig, in other mammals, *G. duodenalis* is transmitted by the fecal-oral route and through ingestion of feed and/or water contaminated with cysts. Cysts form within the intestinal tract and are passed with the feces. Within each cyst are two trophozoites, which leave the cyst after ingestion, attach to the brush border of the intestinal tract, and multiply through binary fission[13]. Trophozoites can also be passed with the feces, particularly during acute infections. This can also result in transmission of the parasite if ingested shortly after excretion. However, cysts are more resistant to external environmental conditions and are the stage most often responsible for continued transmission. The prepatent period is reported to be five to 16 days[13].

Pathologic Effects and Clinical Disease. Trophozoites colonize the anterior small intestine, primarily the duodenum. Overt disease in guinea pigs has only been reported on one occasion, during quarantine of a group of 15 animals[12]. Diarrhea was not evident, but some animals became weak and moribund, and one died. Animals housed in the same cage were euthanized and necropsied. Histologically, mild inflammatory lesions were present in the duodenum and jejunum, and villar height was decreased. Cystic enlargement of the duodenal crypts was also present. Numerous *Giardia* sp trophozoites were detected in the duodenal contents.

Diagnosis. Diagnosis is by microscopic examination of direct fecal smears for trophozoites and cysts. Smears should be prepared in normal saline within minutes of fecal collection. Lugol's iodine may be added to help visualize structures; however, motility will be lost because iodine kills trophozoites. Centrifugal or simple fecal flotation can also be used to detect cysts. Zinc sulfate is the recommended flotation medium. Saturated sugar also works well, although the appearance of the cysts will differ from those found with zinc sulfate flotation. The cyst wall remains intact but the organism will retract into a half-moon shape inside the cyst when saturated sugar is used as the floatation medium.

Numerous test kits using immunofluorescent antibodies are commercially available for the detection of cysts in feces. Although there are no reports using these tests in guinea pigs, they have been used in the detection of *Giardia* spp. in a wide variety of vertebrates[13,14]. However, because *Giardia* spp. are shed intermittently in the feces, it is possible that any of these methods may fail to detect infection. Therefore, multiple tests are recommended before declaring an animal to be negative for *Giardia* cysts[13]. Direct saline smear of scrapings of the duodenum can also be used to detect trophozoites at necropsy.

Treatment and Prevention. Metronidazole (20 to 40 mg/kg every 12 hours per os), and fenbendazole (20 mg/kg every 24 hours for 5 days) have been recommended for treatment of infections in guinea pigs[15]. Infections can be prevented through the use of proper sanitation. Cysts tend to survive best under cool, wet conditions, so keeping areas dry is important. Cysts are susceptible to a variety of disinfectants including quaternary ammonium compounds, Lysol (2% to 5%), Sterinol (1%), or sodium hypochlorite (1%)[15,16]. Cleaning cages with hot water at temperatures achieved by most cage washers also destroys cysts.

Public Health Considerations. Currently, it is unknown whether the genotype of *G. duodenalis* found in guinea pigs can infect humans. However, the greatest zoonotic risk is considered to be from isolates found in genotype Assemblage A, the assemblage to which *G. duodenalis* from guinea pigs belongs[17].

Hexamastix caviae

Species of the genus *Hexamastix* are generally piriform in shape, although considerable variation may occur. A pelta, blepharoplast, and parabasal body are present. The axostyle is well developed and protrudes beyond the posterior end of the body. The number of anterior flagella is variable (two to five) and may be related to degree of maturity[4]. One recurrent flagellum is also present. Reproduction is by binary fission. No cysts are formed[4,18].

Hexamastix caviae trophozoites (Figure 14.5) measure 3.8 μ to 10 μ long (which includes the protruding axostyle) by 3.3 μ to 4.7 μ wide (average: 6.5 μ long by 4 μ wide). The anterior flagella vary in length; they are approximately equal to or longer than the length of the body. The recurrent flagellum is longer than the anterior flagella. An angular nucleus containing a nucleolus is immediately posterior to the blepharoplast. *H. caviae* moves in a rapid,

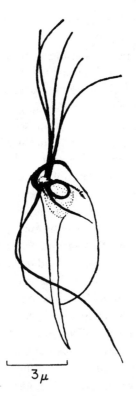

Fig. 14.5 *Hexamastix caviae.* Reproduced from Nie, D. (1950) with permission.

erratic fashion in fresh preparations. The anterior flagella are usually united and beat back and forth, whip-like. The pellicle is not rigid, accounting for the variablity in shape[4]. In one study, *H. caviae* was detected in 11% (9/84) of guinea pigs examined[4]. Rats orally administered this parasite failed to develop infection[3].

Hexamastix robustus

Hexamastix robustus is larger than *H. caviae*. It measures 6.6 μ to 13.5 μm long, including the protruding axostyle, by 3.5 μ to 7.5 μ wide (average: 10.2 μ by 5.2 μ wide). The nucleus is rounded to elongate-oval in shape, and the parabasal body is indistinct[4]. *Hexamastix robustus* was found in 14% (12/84) of guinea pigs examined[4], but, like *H. caviae,* is not infective for rats[3].

Leishmania enriettii

Morphology. Amastigotes of *Leishmania enriettii* are usually ellipsoidal in shape and larger than other leishmanial species, measuring 3 μ to 7 μ long by 2 μ to 3 μ wide (average: 5.2 μ long by 2.5 μ wide). The nucleus, kinetoplast, and rudimentary flagellum are visible in stained smears. Cultured promastigotes measure 8 μ to 10 μ long by 3 μ to

4 μ wide and the flagellum measures 10 μ to 14 μ in length.

Hosts. Natural infection with *L. enriettii* is restricted to guinea pigs[19]. Attempted experimental transmission to mice, wild guinea pigs (*Cavia aperea*), dogs, rhesus monkeys, and humans have been unsuccessful, although a small skin lesion with a few amastigotes was produced in one of eight hamsters. It is possible that the failure to produce visible skin lesions in the wild guinea pig does not equate with susceptibility to infection because there are species of *Leishmania* that produce significant lesions in laboratory animals but are benign in the natural, wild hosts[20]. While *L. enriettii* was originally isolated from spontaneously infected laboratory guinea pigs, all other records of natural infections involve farmed guinea pigs.

Life Cycle. Little is known of the life cycle of *L. enriettii.* Members of the genus have indirect life cycles and all known vectors are phlebotomine sandflies. The natural vector for *L. enriettii* is unknown. The sandflies *Phlebotomus gomezi* and *Lutzomyia monticola* have been experimentally infected[21,22]. However, transmission of *L. enriettii* did not occur when organisms from the sandflies were inoculated into the skin of an uninfected guinea pig.

Pathologic Effects and Clinical Disease. Within one to two weeks of inoculation, *L. enriettii* causes the development of a cutaneous nodule at the site of entry. The nodule enlarges and the overlying skin becomes keratotic. Parasites may disseminate hematogenously to other parts of the body, so that organisms may be found in regional lymph nodes shortly after infection. In naive guinea pigs, lesions in the acute stage are characterized by a central ulcer surrounded by a zone of heavily parasitized macrophages. Extensive necrosis of parasite-laden macrophages occurs at four to five weeks. Cutaneous ulcers are common on the feet, ears, nose, and genitalia. Ulcers occur by four weeks and reach maximum size (approximately 2 cm diameter and 4 mm thick) within six to seven weeks. Intact macrophages are not present in the ulcerated core of the lesion, but numerous extracellular parasites are present. Peripheral to the lesions at four weeks are plasma cells, lymphocytes, and multinucleated giant cells. By seven weeks, the giant cells are absent and fibroblasts are present, indicating resolution of the lesion, which can be complete by 10 weeks[23].

Infection with *L. enriettii* is characterized by a delayed-type hypersensitivity response. The reaction appears early in infection, peaks at midpoint, and remains detectable for a considerable period of time after recovery. The response accompanies the appearance of sensitized lymphocytes that respond *in vitro* to leishmanial antigens, producing lymphokines which, in turn, activate macrophages. These activated macrophages are then responsible for destruction of the organisms[24].

Diagnosis and Treatment. Detection of *L. enrietii* is by identification of amastigotes on histological examination of lesions. Culture of organisms in a number of defined media may also be used[19,20]. Treatment of natural infections has rarely been reported and success has been sporadic[19].

Public Health Considerations. There is no evidence that *L. enrietti* can infect humans. This fact, coupled with the ease in which it can be experimentally transmitted and the large numbers of easily identifiable amastigotes produced in the skin lesions of guinea pigs, made this parasite-host system a popular model for studies on cutaneous leishmaniasis.

Monocercomonas caviae

Species of *Monocercomonas* are piriform to ellipsoidal in shape with a rounded anterior end. A pelta, parabasal body, blepharoplast, axostyle, and nucleus with no nucleolus are present. Three anterior flagella and one recurrent flagellum are present, equal to or 1.5 times the length of the body. There are no cysts formed[4]. *Monocercomonas caviae* (Syn. *Monas caviae, Heteromita caviae, Trichomastix caviae, Eutrichomastix aguti*) (Figure 14.6) trophozoites measure 4.4 μ to 8.5 μ long by 2.2 μ to 4.3 μ wide (average: 6 μ long by 3.1 μ wide). The axostyle protrudes from the body approximately 1 μm, with the protrusion ending in a sharp point. In fresh preparations, *M. caviae* moves in an erratic, rapid fashion similar to other flagellates. Some variability in body shape occurs; however, the pellicle is somewhat rigid, thereby minimizing variability[4]. *Monocercomonas caviae* has been detected in guinea pigs in the United States, Europe, and Brazil[1,4,25]. In one study, 35% (29/84) of guinea pigs were infected[4]. Rats are not susceptible to infection with *M. caviae*[3].

Monocercomonas minuta

Monocercomonas minuta is smaller than either *M. caviae* or *M. pistillum*, measuring 2.6 μ to 6.0 μ long by 2 μ to 2.7 μ wide (average: 4.2 μ long by 2.3 μ wide). The indistinct axostyle does not protrude from the body. *Monocercomonas minuta* was detected in 11% (9/84) of guinea pigs examined in the United States[4]. Rats are not susceptible to infection[3].

Monocercomonas pistillum

Monocercomonas pistillum is morphologically and biologically similar to *M. caviae*, though slightly smaller in size,

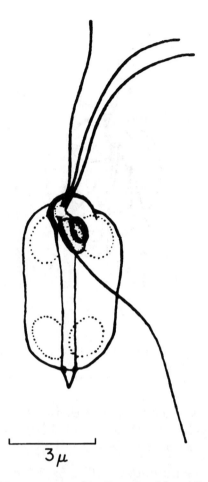

Fig. 14.6 *Monocercomonas caviae.* Reproduced from Nie, D. (1950) with permission.

measuring 4 μ to 6.5 μ long by 3 μ to 3.6 μ wide (average: 5.4 μ long by 3.3 μ wide). The axostyle does not end in a point as it does in *M. caviae* but in a squarely terminated stump[4]. *Monocercomonas pistillum* was detected in 5% (4/84) of guinea pigs examined in the United States[4]. Rats are not susceptible to infection[3].

Monocercomonoides caviae

Species of the genus *Monocercomonoides* have an anterior nucleus, two pairs of flagella, a pelta, blepharoplasts, and an axostyle. One to four strandlike, argyrophilic funises extend backward just beneath the body surface. There is neither a cytostome nor a parabasal body. Cysts are not formed[4]. *Monocercomonoides caviae* (Syn. *Monocercomonas caviae; M. hassalli*) trophozoites (Figure 14.7) are ovoid to subspherical, and measure 4 μ to 8 μ long by 2.7 μ to 6.6 μ wide. The nucleus, with central nucleolus, is located at the anterior end. Three funises are present[4]. *Monocercomonoides caviae* has been detected in guinea pigs from

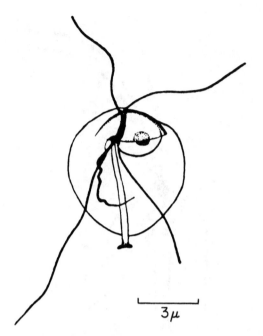

Fig. 14.7 *Monocercomonoides caviae.* Reproduced from Nie, D. (1950) with permission.

Brazil and Czechoslovakia[1] as well as in 46% (39/84) of guinea pigs from the United States[4]. Rats are not susceptible to infection with *M. caviae*[3].

Monocercomonoides exilis

Monocercomonoides exilis trophozoites are piriform to rounded in shape. It is the smallest species of the genus in guinea pigs, measuring 3.5 μ to 8.8 μ long by 2.5 μ to 5.5 μ wide (average: 5.5 μ long by 3.5 μ wide). The nucleus, with a rounded, central nucleolus, is not located as far anteriorly as in other members of the genus. A single funis, associated with the recurrent flagellum, is present[4]. *Monocercomonoides exilis* has been found in guinea pigs in the United States[4].

Monocercomonoides quadrifunilis

Monocercomonoides quadrifunilis trophozoites are piriform in shape, although other forms occur. This parasite measures 3.5 μ to 13.2 μ long by 3.3 μ to 11 μ wide. The nucleus, with a crescent-shaped, marginal nucleolus, is located at the anterior end. Four funises are present and are closely adherent to the flagella[4]. *Monocercomonoides quadrifunilis* has been found in guinea pigs in the United States.

Monocercomonoides wenrichi

Monocercomonoides wenrichi is biologically similar to *M. caviae*. Trophozoites are ovoid to globular in shape, and

measure 3.3 μ to 11.5 μ long by 3 μ to 8.4 μ wide (average: 6.6 μ long by 5.2 μ wide). The nucleus is anterior, with a marginal nucleolus. A single funis is closely adhered to the posterior flagellum[4].

Proteromonas brevifilia

Proteromonas brevifilia trophozoites (Figure 14.8) are spindle-shaped and measure 4.5 μ to 9 μ long by 1.6 μ to 4.4 μ wide (average: 6.8 μ long by 3.2 μ wide). The trophozoite contains two blepharoplasts, which give rise to two flagella, one anterior and one trailing. The nucleus, which does not contain a nucleolus, is located in the middle portion of the anterior half of the body. A paranuclear body is immediately adjacent to the nucleus and is approximately its equal in size. No cyst stage is formed[4]. This nonpathogenic species is known only from the guinea pig. It has been detected in 3% (2/70) of guinea pigs in France and 5% (3/56) of guinea pigs in the United States. It has also been detected in guinea pigs in Czechoslovakia[1].

Retortamonas caviae

Retortamonas caviae (Syn. *Embadomonas caviae*) trophozoites are piriform or fusiform, and measure 4 μ to 7 μ long by 2.4 μ to 3.2 μ wide (average: 5.5 μ long by 2.8 μ wide)[26]. The nucleus is located at the anterior end of the body and may or may not contain a nucleolus. The cytostome is immediately behind the nucleus. Two blepharoplasts are present, which give rise to two flagella, one anterior and one recurrent, both of which are usually shorter than the body. Food vacuoles may be present within the cytoplasm. Cysts occur, and contain one or two nuclei, flagella, and cytostomal fibrils. Cysts measure 3.4 μ to 5.2 μ long by 3.3 μ to 3.6 μ wide (average: 4.2 μ long by 3.5 μ wide)[26]. *Retortamonas caviae* has been found in guinea pigs in Asia and Europe[1], and in two surveys, was detected in 27% (14/52) and 9.5% (8/84) of guinea pigs from the United States[4,26]. Rats are not susceptible to infection with *R. caviae*[3].

Tritrichomonas caviae

Tritrichomonas caviae (Syn. *Trichomonas caviae*, *T. flagelliphora*) is one of the largest intestinal flagellates of the guinea pig. *Tritrichomonas caviae* is ovoid, piriform, or kidney shaped, and measures 10 μ to 22 μ long by 6 μ to 11 μ wide. At the anterior end is a large blepharoplast complex from which arise three flagella, which are usually shorter than the body. A recurrent flagellum is present and forms the edge (marginal filament) of the undulating membrane and trails beyond it. A costa and ribbon-like parabasal body are present. The cylindrical, rod-shaped axostyle comes to a

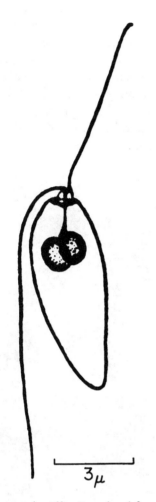

Fig. 14.8 *Proteromonas brevifilia.* Reproduced from Nie, D. (1950) with permission.

point a short distance after protruding from the posterior end of the body. A chromatic ring with two to three turns surrounds the axostyle where it emerges from the body. A structure reported initially to be the pelta has since been determined to be an extension of the axostylar capitulum[27]. Dorsal to the axostyle is the 5-μm by 3 μm, oval to ellipsoid nucleus, which contains a nucleolus. Numerous granules and vacuoles fill the cytoplasm[4]. There is no cyst stage.

Tritrichomonas caviae is cosmopolitan in distribution, having been detected in guinea pigs from Asia, Europe, and North and South America[1]. Wenrich[25] cultured *T. caviae* from 8% (1/13) of guinea pigs, while Faust[28] found it in 32% (13/41) of guinea pigs examined. This parasite has also been detected in all of a group of eight Mongolian gerbils (*Meriones unguiculatus*)[29]. *Tritrichomonas caviae* is not infectious to rats (*Rattus norvegicus*) or golden hamsters (*Mesocricetus auratus*)[3]. *Tritrichomonas caviae* is found

primarily in the cecum, but has also been detected in the duodenum, jejunum, and lower ileum[9]. Rarely, *T. caviae* has been associated with tissue invasion and ulceration of the cecum and colon[1]. However, infection has not resulted in clinical signs.

A smaller (8-μ to 13-μ long by 4.5-μ to 6.5-μ wide) trichomonad was described from material collected from a single guinea pig[4]. Although morphologically distinct from *T. caviae,* the species was not named and the author considered the guinea pig to be an accidental host.

Reclassified organisms

Colpodella edax *Colpodella edax* (Syn. *Spiromonas angusta*) has only been reported once from guinea pigs[28]. Recent evidence indicates this species, as with other members of the genus, is a predatory, non-endoparasitic flagellate[30,31]. Consequently, the parasitic nature of *C. edax* in guinea pigs is questionable.

Oikomonas termo. *Oikomonas termo* has been detected in the feces of guinea pigs in the former Soviet Union as well as in France[1]. However, like other members of the genus, this species is a free-living protozoan commonly found in water[32]. Consequently, *O. termo* is considered to be *coprozoic* rather than parasitic[33].

Selenomonas ruminantium. *Selenomonas ruminantium* (Syn. *Ancyromonas ruminantium, Selemonastix ruminantium, Selenomonas palpitans*) has been found in the ceca of guinea pigs[1,9,28] as well as the ceca of pigs and the rumen of goats, sheep, and other herbivorous mammals[34,35]. These organisms are not protozoans; rather, they are anaerobic, Gram-negative, motile bacteria with flagella attached to the concave side of the cell[36,37].

Sphaeromonas communis. *Sphaeromonas communis* has been reported from guinea pig feces[1] as well as rumen fluid of a variety of hosts and is considered a part of the normal ruminant gut flora[38]. Studies have shown that this organism, however, is a fungus rather than a protozoan[38].

Class Sarcodina

Endolimax caviae

Trophozoites of *E. caviae* measure 4.8 μ to 6.7 μ long by 5.2 μ to 7.8 μ wide (average: 5.5 μ long by 6.6 μ wide). The nucleus is spherical, measuring 1.2 μ to 2 μ in diameter. No cysts have been observed[4,28, 39]. *Endolimax caviae* has only been reported in the cecum of guinea pigs. Wenrich[25] found it in 8% (1/13) and Nie[4] found it in 18% (15/84) of guinea pigs in the United States. It has also been found in Asia[1]. Cross-transmission attempts to rats have been unsuccessful[3]. Smears of intestinal contents or feces made in normal saline can be used to detect live amoebae. Use of either phase contrast or differential interference contrast microscopy aids in visualizing the trophozoites. Staining with Lugol's iodine also helps; however, this will kill the organism. Zinc sulfate flotation may also be used to concentrate cysts. Positive identification should be made from stained smears[1].

Entamoeba caviae

Entamoeba caviae (Syn. *Entamoeba cobayae*) trophozoites measure 10.5 μ to 20 μ in diameter (average: 14.4 μ). The ectoplasm is not clearly differentiated from the endoplasm. The nucleus is ringlike, measuring 2.8 μ to 5 μ in diameter[4]. Cysts are rarely formed, and measure 11 μ to 17 μ in diameter (average: 14 μ) with eight nuclei when mature[28,40]. *Entamoeba caviae* was found in the ceca of 14% (12/84) of guinea pigs examined in the United States[4], while others found it in 46% (6/13) of animals examined in Germany[41]. *Entamoeba caviae* has also been reported from guinea pigs in France, England, and Venezuela[1,28]. Attempts to infect rats experimentally have not been successful[3,40]. *Entamoeba caviae* can be detected with the same techniques used for *Endolimax caviae*.

Phylum Apicomplexa

Class Coccidia

Cryptosporidium wrairi

Morphology. Oocysts of *C. wrairi* measure 4.8 μ to 5.6 μ long by 4 μ to 5 μ wide (average: 5.4 μ long by 4.6 μ wide)[42]. Oocysts contain four sporozoites when passed.

Hosts. Thirteen species of *Cryptosporidium* are currently recognized, including *C. wrairi*[43]. Occasionally considered to be a variant of *C. parvum*, recent evidence indicates *C. wrairi* is a separate species[44,45]. The species name was derived as an acronym for the Walter Reed Army Institute of Research[46]. Although experimental infections with *C. wrairi* have been established in some laboratory mice, lambs, and calves, natural infections only occur in the guinea pig[42,43,47]. Rat snakes (*Elaphe obsoleta*) appear to be refractory to infection with *C. wrairi*[48].

Life Cycle. The life cycle is essentially as described for other directly transmitted apicomplexan parasites[15,46]. Infections in guinea pigs 16 weeks and older may last for as little as one week, while infections in younger animals can last longer[46,49].

Pathologic Effects. Lesions tend to be most prominent in the small intestine (Figure 14.9). Acute infections are characterized by erosions, inflammation, hyperemia and edema of the lamina propria, and hyperplasia of crypt epithelium. Chronic infections are characterized by villous atrophy and bridging, metaplasia of the mucosal epithelium, and lymphocyte infiltration of the lamina propria[49-51]. Emaciation is a common finding at necropsy[51].

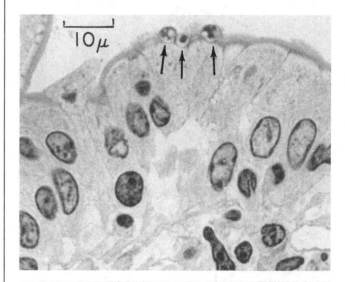

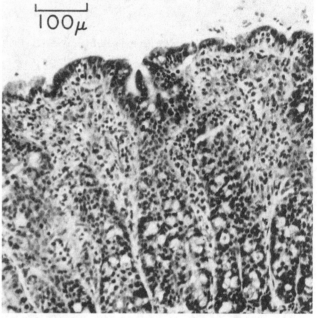

Fig. 14.9 *Cryptosporidium* sp. in a guinea pig. (Top) Organism (arrows) embedded in the striated border of the ileum. (Bottom) Ileal mucosa. Note infiltration of inflammatory cells. Reproduced from Jervis, H.R., Merrill, T.G., and Sprinz, H. (1966) with permission.

Clinical Disease. Clinical signs may be lacking in guinea pigs infected with *C. wrairi*[46,50]. Clinical signs are more common in juvenile animals versus adults[51]. The most common clinical signs include weight loss or failure to gain weight. Guinea pigs may appear potbellied and have a rough, greasy hair coat. Diarrhea is uncommon[50]; it is found in approximately one-third of clinically affected animals[51]. Morbidity and mortality range from 0% to 50%[49–51].

Diagnosis. Diagnosis is based on finding characteristic oocysts in the feces, generally using acid-fast stain, direct smears, or fecal flotation techniques. Immunofluorescence and molecular techniques, although not validated for diagnosing cryptosporidiosis in guinea pigs, have been used to detect species of *Cryptosporidium* in other animals[52,53]. Post-mortem diagnosis is based on finding the organisms in the brush border epithelium of the small intestine.

Treatment and Prevention. Treatment of cryptosporidial infections in animals has met with only limited success. Therefore, the best management tool is hygiene. Cryptosporidial oocysts are resistant to most commercial disinfectants. Chlorine and related compounds can render oocysts noninfectious, although their usefulness is limited by the long exposure times or high concentrations (e.g., 80 mg/l free chlorine for two hours) required. Oocysts are killed by heating above 65°C for at least five minutes[54].

Public Health Considerations. Although several other species of *Cryptosporidium*, including *C. parvum* of ruminants, *C. felis* of cats, *C. meleagridis* of birds, *C. canis* of dogs, and *C. hominis* of primates, have been identified in humans, *C. wrairi* has not[43]. It is likely that humans are not susceptible to infection with *C. wrairi*. However, people at risk for opportunistic infections should exercise caution when working with infected guinea pigs.

Eimeria caviae

Morphology. *Eimeria caviae* is the only member of the genus found in guinea pigs. Oocysts are ellipsoidal to subspherical, with a smooth, brownish wall and no micropyle, and they measure 17.6 μ to 24.2 μ long by 12.1 μ to 19.8 μ wide (average: 19.3 μ long by 16.5 μ wide)[55]. An oocyst residuum is present but a polar granule is absent. Oocysts are unsporulated when passed in the feces. Sporulation occurs in five to 11 days at 18°C to 22°C, although shorter sporulation times have also been reported[15,56,57]. Each oocyst contains four sporocysts measuring 11 μ to 13 μm long by 6 μ to 7 μm wide[57] (Figure 14.10)[58]. Each sporocyst contains two sporozoites.

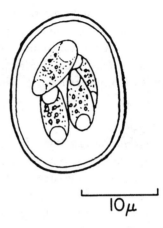

Fig. 14.10 *Eimeria caviae* of the guinea pig (sporulated oocyst). Reproduced from Ryšavý, B. (1954) with permission.

Hosts. *Eimeria caviae* has been reported from domestic and wild guinea pigs throughout the world[1,56,57,59]. At one time prevalence rates as high as 100% in laboratory colonies were recorded; however, improved management has greatly reduced the prevalence of this parasite.

Life Cycle. The life cycle of *E. caviae* is typical of the genus, and is described in Chapter 2, Biology of the Protozoa. The prepatent period is 11 to 12 days and the patent period is approximately seven days[55,60,61].

Pathologic Effects. In severe infections, necropsy findings include hyperemia, edema, petechial hemorrhages in the colonic mucosa, and white or yellow plaques in the colon and, depending on severity, the cecum. Intestinal contents may be watery or contain formed feces and blood may or may not be present. Microscopically, developmental stages are present in intact epithelial cells and free in the lumen. Epithelial sloughing may occur. Dilated cystic crypts of Lieberkühn may be present[55,60,62].

Clinical Disease. Clinical signs are generally not present unless the infection is severe. As with other enteric coccidial infections, diarrhea is among the first clinical signs observed. Anorexia and rough hair coat are usually present as well. These clinical signs usually start about 11 days post-infection and abate within a week. However, in severe cases, death may result[55,60,62].

Diagnosis, Treatment, and Prevention. Diagnosis is by identification of oocysts in fecal flotations. Identification of organisms in mucosal scrapings or histologic sections taken at necropsy can also be performed. Sulfadimethoxine (25 to 50 mg/kg every 24 hours for 10 to 14 days) and sulfamethazine have been used successfully to control infections[15,60]. Infections can be reduced through proper sanitation, reducing stress, and providing proper nutrition. *Eimeria*-free guinea pig colonies have been established by placing caesarian-derived offspring into strictly controlled housing conditions[63].

Public Health Considerations. *Eimeria caviae* does not infect humans.

Klossiella cobayae

Morphology. *Klossiella cobayae* (Syn. *Klossia caviae*) lives in the kidney of the host. First-generation schizonts measure 2 μ to 7 μ in diameter, while later generation schizonts may be larger. Sexual reproduction results in the production of zygotes. As these mature to become sporonts, they grow to 30 μ to 40 μ in diameter.

Hosts. *Klossiella cobayae* was first discovered in the kidneys of guinea pigs in Nigeria, in which the prevalence was 20% (4/20)[64]. In early studies, Pearce[65] reported 20% (12/60) and Jackson[66] reported 27% (12/44) of guinea pigs in the United States infected. Since then, *K. cobayae* has been reported from domestic guinea pigs in England, Italy, Romania (60.5% of 976 animals), Poland, and Germany (29% of 108), and in wild guinea pigs in Brazil[1,64,67]. The current prevalence of infection in laboratory guinea pigs is unknown.

Life Cycle. Infection of an animal is initiated upon ingestion of sporulated sporocysts from the environment. Sporozoites excyst in the gut lumen and enter the capillary or lymphatic system where they are transported throughout the body. They then invade capillary endothelial cells, particularly those lining the capillaries of the kidney glomerulus, and undergo schizogony.

Schizonts cause the host cell to bulge into the lumen of the capillary. Mature schizonts contain eight to 12 merozoites, each measuring 2 μ by 1 μ. The schizont and host cell ruptures, releasing merozoites, which enter epithelial cells lining the proximal convoluted tubule. Each merozoite undergoes another round of asexual development, producing large schizonts that nearly fill the lumen of the tubule, each containing approximately 100 early gametocytes. The schizont and host cell again rupture, releasing the gametocytes which enter the epithelium of the loop of Henle. Fertilization occurs and the resulting zygote undergoes sporogony. Sporonts produce 30 or more sporoblasts, each of which develops into a sporocyst. Thirty or more infective sporozoites develop within each sporocyst. The sporocysts are released into the urine when the host cell ruptures[1,64].

Pathologic Effects. Microscopic lesions associated with infection include lymphocytic and histiocytic interstitial and perivascular infiltration, as well as an increase of interstitial fibroblasts[65,67]. Gross lesions typically are not apparent, although heavily infected kidneys may have an irregular surface[65].

Clinical Disease. Clinical signs of infection are rare. Therefore, *K. cobayae* is generally considered nonpathogenic. However, necrosis of the epithelial lining of the kidney tubules, kidney dysfunction, and death of guinea pigs have been reported[68]. Therefore, pathogenic effects are considered to be important even when infection levels are low[67,68].

Diagnosis. Microscopic examination of tissue sections for the typical stages of the parasite is the only reliable method of diagnosis. Occasionally, schizogonous stages have been reported in other tissues, including endothelial cells of the lung and spleen. However, these stages somewhat resembled those of *T. gondii* and *E. cuniculi*. Because sporocysts are passed with the urine, these stages should be demonstrable through standard sedimentation procedures. However, sporocysts are not often observed in urine[1].

Treatment and Prevention. Treatments for eradicating *K. cobayae* from infected guinea pigs have not been described, partly because of the lack of reliable antemortem diagnostic techniques. Sulfonamides or other anticoccidials represent effective treatments. However, strict attention to sanitation procedures remains the cornerstone of control and prevention.

Sarcocystis caviae

Morphology. There is no description of the tissue cysts because of the early confusions with *T. gondii*. Also, *S. caviae* is a relatively rare parasite in laboratory guinea pigs.

Hosts. *Sarcocystis caviae* has only been reported from guinea pigs. The prevalence and distribution of this parasite is unknown, in part because earlier reports likely confused this parasite with *T. gondii*[1,69].

Life Cycle. All species of *Sarcocystis* have an indirect life cycle with an herbivore/omnivore intermediate host and carnivore/omnivore definitive host. Sporulated oocysts are produced by the definitive host and are passed with the feces. Intermediate hosts become infected by ingesting the infective sporocysts. Asexual development occurs within the intermediate host, resulting in sarcocysts containing numerous bradyzoites. The definitive host then becomes infected by ingesting intermediate host tissue containing the mature sarcocysts. Sarcocysts are found within tissues of the guinea pig; however, the definitive host for *S. caviae* is unknown[1].

Pathologic Effects and Clinical Disease. Pathologic changes associated with infections of *S. caviae* have not been adequately described. This parasite is not known to cause clinical disease in infected guinea pigs.

Diagnosis and Prevention. Diagnosis is by detection of sarcocysts at necropsy. Because of the morphological similarities among tissue cysts of various cyst-forming coccidian parasites, ultrastructural details of cysts or the use of immunohistochemical staining of sections with specific monoclonal antibodies may be needed to differentiate these parasites.

Treatment and Prevention. Because *S. caviae* appears to be a rare parasite, treatment strategies have not been described. Control is based on preventing fecal contamination of food and bedding materials by possible definitive hosts.

Toxoplasma gondii

Morphology. A description of the morphology of *T. gondii* oocysts is presented in Chapter 18, Parasites of Cats. In the guinea pig, intracellular cysts are ellipsoidal in cardiac and skeletal muscle and spherical in the brain, eye, and other organs. They may reach 100 µ in size and contain several hundred bradyzoites. Bradyzoites are crescent-shaped, pointed on one end and rounded on the other, and measure 4 µ to 8 µ long by 2 µ to 4 µ wide[1].

Hosts. *Toxoplasma gondii* is cosmopolitan in distribution, infecting an extraordinarily wide range of mammalian and avian intermediate hosts. Spontaneous infections have been reported in guinea pigs from the Americas and Europe[1,69,70].

Life Cycle. The life cycle of *T. gondii* is discussed in Chapter 18, Parasites of Cats. Briefly, oocysts are released in cat feces. Sporulation occurs in as little as 24 hours, producing sporulated oocysts that are infective to mammalian and avian hosts. Following ingestion of sporulated oocysts, infectious sporozoites are released and disseminate via the circulatory system to several organs in the body, including the liver, lungs, central nervous system, striated muscle, and others[13]. Bradyzoite cysts form in these locations. Cysts can remain viable for as long as five years in the guinea pig, awaiting ingestion by the definitive host[71].

Pathologic Effects and Clinical Disease. Fatal hepatitis, pneumonia, encephalitis, and abortion have been reported in guinea pigs[70,72]. Clinical signs of infection are generally not present. However, severe infection can result in clinical signs indicative of the organ system affected[1,70,72].

Diagnosis. Diagnosis is based on serologic detection of antibodies against *T. gondii*. Cysts can be detected on histologic examination of affected organs, particularly the brain, striated muscle, and liver. Inoculation of tissue homogenates from suspect animals into mice or hamsters with subsequent identification of the organism in tissue sections has also been reported, but is labor-intensive[15].

Treatment and Prevention. Sulphadiazine and pyrimethamine are used widely for suppressive treatment of toxoplasmosis in the acute stage of clinically apparent infection[73]. However, these have little effect on subclinical infections, and treatment is unlikely to eliminate the tissue cysts. The use of commercially prepared food should eliminate a potential source of oocysts. Oocysts are resistant to many disinfectants but may be killed through exposure to heat (60°C). If the parasite has been introduced, transplacental transmission can be avoided by breeding only seronegative animals[1].

Public Health Considerations. Although *T. gondii* is a zoonotic parasite of great concern to human health, the guinea pig is unlikely to be a source of infection for personnel in the laboratory setting.

Phylum Ciliophora

Balantidium caviae

Morphology. The trophozoite of *B. caviae* is ovoid to ellipsoid in shape, and measures 55 µ to 155 µ long by 45 µ to 72.5 µ wide (average: 92 µ long by 65 µ wide). With the exception of the peristomal field, the entire surface is covered with fine cilia arranged in parallel longitudinal rows. The macronucleus is small, thick, and ovoid to ellipsoidal in shape (compared with *B. coli,* in which the macronucleus is dumbbell-shaped). The micronucleus is smaller than the macronucleus and usually is found adjacent to it. Cysts are formed and measure 40 µ to 45 µ in diameter (average: 45 µ in diameter). The cyst wall is thick and may be yellow-brown in color[4].

Hosts. *Balantidium caviae* (Figure 14.11) is found in the lumen of the cecum and colon of guinea pigs throughout the world[1,4,28,62]. Little information is available on current prevalence rates. Historically, infection was common[28]. Mice, rats, and hamsters appear to be refractory to infection with *B. caviae*.

Life Cycle. The life cycle is direct, with ingestion of cysts the probable means of transmission.

Pathologic Effects and Clinical Disease. Ordinarily, *B. caviae* is nonpathogenic and appears unable to invade

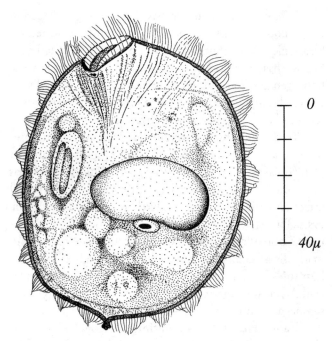

Fig. 14.11 *Balantidium caviae.* Reproduced from Nie, D. (1950) with permission.

intact mucosa. Thus, clinical signs are typically not observed. However, if the mucosal barrier is compromised, *B. caviae* may become a secondary invader[74], resulting in enteritis.

Diagnosis. *Balantidium caviae* can be detected on histologic sections of the cecum or colon[1,62]. Caution must be exercised, however, in interpreting the presence of organisms within the intestinal walls. These organisms can penetrate the host tissue post-mortem; therefore, the length of time between death and examination should be considered. Organisms can also be detected by examining fresh smears of cecal or colonic contents[1].

Treatment and Prevention. Because infections with *B. caviae* tend to be unapparent, no chemotherapy has been described. Compounds in the tetracycline group are most commonly used to treat *B. coli* infections in humans[75]. Control of this ciliate is centered on the maintenance of proper hygiene.

Cyathodinium spp.

Up to 10 species of *Cyathodinium* have been described from wild and captive guinea pigs. However, it is likely that only four of these are valid species[1,4]. Members of the genus have a pyriform-shaped trophont with cilia and tentacles ("endosprits") that are reduced to a series of short protuberances on the left side of the anterior ciliated cavity.

Cyathodinium chagasi trophonts measure 53.7 μm long by 21.9 μm wide. The ventral cavity occupies only the anterior one-fourth of the body[1].

Cyathodinium conicum is the largest species, measuring 50 μ to 80 μ long by 20 μ to 30 μ wide (average: 65 μ long by 25 μ wide). As for *C. chagasi*, the ventral cavity occupies only one-fourth of the body length[1].

Cyathodinium cunhai trophonts measure 10.2 μ to 35.5 μ long by 8 μ to 22 μ wide (average: 19 μ long by 14 μ wide). The cavity is unciliated, and occupies the anterior one-third of the organism. Eleven rows of somatic cilia are present with nine arranged around the cavity and the remaining encircling the organism. There are nine to 13 tentacles. The macronucleus and micronucleus resemble those of *C. piriforme*[4,76].

Cyathodinium piriforme (Figure 14.12)[77] trophonts measure 10 μ to 35.5 μ long by 8.8 μ to 24.4 μ wide (average: 29.2 μ long by 20.3 μ wide). Nine rows of somatic cilia are arranged around the ventral cavity, which occupies the anterior two-thirds of the body. Two rows completely encircle the organism. The other seven originate on the left lip and terminate along the inside of the right wall of the cavity. There are 9 to 14 tentacles. A round macronucleus and smaller micronucleus are located in the middle portion of the body. Cysts have been reported only rarely[4,76].

The cyathodiniids are common endosymbionts of the cecum and colon of guinea pigs. Reported historical

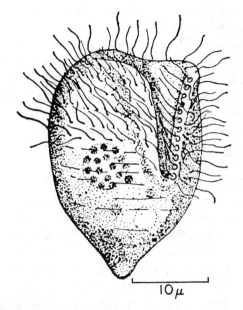

Fig. 14.12 *Cyathodinium piriforme* trophozoite. Reproduced from Kudo, R.R. (1966) with permission.

prevalences range between 4% and 78% with a worldwide geographic range[78,79]. They are easily detected in fresh smears examined with phase contrast or differential interference contrast microscopy. The organisms can also be detected in stained smears[1,2]. Infections of *C. piriforme* can be established in rats and hamsters, and *C. cunhai* can be established in rats following oral administration of organisms[3].

Enterophrya elongata

Trophonts of *Enterophrya elongata* measure 30 µ to 52 µ long by 5 µ to 14 µ wide (average: 38.8 µm long by 8.1 µ wide). The anterior end is spatulate and the posterior end is rounded or tapering. Somatic cilia cover the whole body with the anterior region, which is more densely ciliated than the posterior region. The vestibular opening is small, and located at the anterior extremity of the body. The short vestibulum is densely ciliated. The cytoproct is located at the posterior end of the body. The macronucleus is an elongated ellipse. The spherical micronucleus is near the macronucleus. There is a single contractile vacuole, which varies in location[1].

Enterophrya elongata was originally described from the cecum of wild guinea pigs in Brazil. Additional reports of *E. elongata* are sparse and it is unknown whether the species infects domestic guinea pigs[1]. It has also been found in the capybara (*Hydrochoerus hydrochaeris*), a closely related histricomorph rodent from Bolivia[80].

Kopperia intestinale

Kopperia intestinale (Syn. *Malacosoma intestinale*) is a cecal ciliate of guinea pigs. The trophont is egg-shaped, and measures 30 µ to 50 µ long by 17 µ to 30 µ wide (average: 40 µ long by 25 µ wide) with the widest part near the anterior end. Longitudinal rows of cilia (6 µ to 10 µ long) cover the entire body. The spherical to ovoid macronucleus is located anteriorly, and measures 6 µ to 10 µ in length. A micronucleus is situated near the macronucleus[1,4].

Protocaviella acuminate

Protocaviella acuminate is a relatively large, cecal ciliate. Trophonts measure 30 µ to 40 µ long by 12 µ to 15 µ wide. It has a rigid body whose anterior end is broader than the posterior end and slightly flattened laterally. The dorsal side is convex and the ventral side is concave. Dense longitudinal rows of short somatic cilia are present. A row of long cilia are present on the right lip of the ventral cavity. The spheroid macronucleus measures 5 µ to 6 µ long and

is situated near the anterior end of the body. The spherical micronucleus is posterior to the macronucleus. Reports of this organism are rare[1].

Phylum Microspora

Encephalitozoon cuniculi

Encephalitozoon cuniculi (Syn. *Nosema cuniculi*) is an obligate intracellular pathogen with both eukaryote and prokaryote characteristics. Originally considered to be a primitive protozoan, recent molecular biological studies have resulted in its reclassification as a fungus[81]. *Encephalitozoon cuniculi* infects a wide range of mammals, including guinea pigs[82–84]. Infection occurs through ingestion, inhalation, or transplacental transmission of infectious spores[15,83]. Most infections are subclinical and gross and histologic evidence of infection is usually lacking. In guinea pigs, lesions that have been reported include interstitial nephritis with tubular necrosis and fibrosis, and multifocal granulomatous encephalitis[84,85]. Treatment regimens have not been developed for guinea pigs. However, albendazole and fenbendazole have been used successfully in infected rabbits, and may be useful in guinea pigs should treatment be considered[86]. *Encephalitozoon cuniculi* is zoonotic. Three strains (I-III) have been identified. Strains I and III have been found in humans[87]. It is unknown which strain or strains naturally infect guinea pigs.

TREMATODES

Fasciola spp.

Naturally occurring trematode infections in laboratory guinea pigs are rarely encountered. When they do occur, it is usually the result of dietary supplementation with forage containing the infective metacercariae. Two species of trematodes may be found in laboratory guinea pigs, *Fasciola hepatica* and *F. gigantica*.

Morphology. Mature flukes are dorsally-ventrally flattened and leaf-shaped, measuring up to 30 mm long for *F. hepatica* and 75 mm long for *F. gigantica*. However, those recovered from guinea pigs tend to be somewhat smaller[88,89]. The eggs are oval, operculate, and yellow in color. Those of *F. hepatica* measure 130 µ to 150 µ long by 65 µ to 90 µ wide[13] and those of *F. gigantica* are slightly larger, though this species rarely reaches patency in the guinea pig[92].

Hosts. *Fasciola hepatica* and *F. gigantica* infect a wide variety of herbivorous hosts, including cattle, goats, sheep, llamas, and buffalo throughout the world. Natural infections in guinea pigs have been reported in South America, primarily in wild guinea pigs and those raised for food. Prevalences in those endemic areas range from 15% to 53%[90,91]. Infections in laboratory colonies have been reported only rarely[89].

Life Cycle. Both *F. hepatica* and *F. gigantica* have similar life cycles. These are discussed in Chapter 20, Parasites of Sheep and Goats. Briefly, the life cycles are indirect, and require a snail intermediate host. Ingested metacercariae excyst in the duodenum, and migrate through the intestinal wall, the peritoneal cavity, and the liver parenchyma. Juvenile flukes feed and develop before burrowing into the bile ducts where they mature. The prepatent period differs between the two species; it is approximately eight to 12 weeks for *F. hepatica* and 12 to 16 weeks for *F. gigantica*. Apparently *F. gigantica* in guinea pigs rarely reaches patency[92].

Pathologic Effects and Clinical Signs. Typically, natural infections of *F. hepatica* in wild guinea pigs tend to be limited to a maximum of two adult flukes[91]. Neither pathologic changes nor clinical signs associated with these infections have been documented. In experimental infections, pathologic changes and death appear to be associated with secondary bacterial infections. As few as 25 metacercariae can result in 80% to 100% mortality in guinea pigs[93].

Pathologic changes reported in natural infections with *F. gigantica* are a result of aberrant migration and cyst formation of the trematode. Posterior paresis has been reported, resulting in fatalities in a guinea pig breeding colony. *Fasicola gigantica* were present in cysts in the pelvic and peritoneal cavities, or were embedded in muscle of the lumbar vertebra. Flukes were also found in the renal pelvises and femurotibial joints, and within the thoracic cavity. Extensive tissue destruction, liver damage, and hemorrhage were present, and characteristic coffee-brown fluid was present in the cysts[89]. Histological features vary according to the age of infection and include congestion and hemorrhage around the portal vessels, central veins and sinusoids; fibronecrotic tracks; inflammation; and granuloma formation[92,94,95].

Diagnosis, Treatment, and Prevention. Diagnosis and treatment are not usually necessary in laboratory colonies in which animals are fed only commercial food. If necessary, fecal sedimentation procedures used in ruminants can be used for detecting eggs in the feces of guinea pigs. Albendazole and clorsulon are used to treat liver fluke

infections in ruminants[13] and might also be suitable for guinea pigs. Preventing infections in laboratory colonies is achieved by feeding only commercially-prepared guinea pig diet. If supplementation with greens is desired, foods grown in fluke-endemic areas should not be used.

NEMATODES

Superfamily Rhabditoidea

Pelodera strongyloides

Pelodera strongyloides is a free-living nematode that normally inhabits damp soil and decaying vegetation[96] but occasionally invades the skin or orbits of the eyes of a variety of mammals. A single case report attributes dermatitis in a guinea pig to infection with this nematode[97]. Infections are usually associated with poor environmental conditions and management. Therefore, infections may be avoided by proper husbandry and good sanitation.

Superfamily Ascaridoidea

Baylisascaris procyonis

Morphology. Adult *Baylisascaris procyonis* are tan in color and quite large, with males and females reaching lengths of 9 cm to 11 cm and 20 cm to 22 cm, respectively. Males possess pericloacal roughened areas. The eggs are ellipsoid and brown in color with a thick shell, and contain a large single-celled embryo. Eggs measure 63 μ to 88 μ long by 50 μ to 70 μ wide[98].

Hosts. *Baylisascaris procyonis* is the ascarid roundworm of raccoons and the most commonly recognized cause of clinical larva migrans affecting a wide range of wild and domestic animals, including guinea pigs. Originally endemic to North America, the parasite has become established in other areas of the world[98,99]. The guinea pig serves as one of many mammalian paratenic hosts for *B. procyonis*.

Life Cycle. Adult nematodes reside in the lumen of the small intestine of raccoons. Eggs are passed in the feces and require 11 to 14 days for the second-stage larvae to develop within, thereby becoming infective. Paratenic hosts become infected when ingesting embryonated eggs from the environment. After hatching, larvae penetrate the small intestine and migrate through the liver to the lungs. From there, they are disseminated throughout the body via the circulatory system. Larvae become encapsulated where they remain until ingested by a raccoon[98].

Pathologic Effects. Infections in paratenic hosts are asymptomatic so long as migrating larvae do not enter the brain or the eye. Larvae migrating in the brain, however, produce traumatic damage and inflammation[98]. While gross lesions are often absent in affected guinea pigs, histologic findings in the brain include multifocal eosinophilic granulomatous inflammation, multifocal neutrophilic infiltration, perivascular lymphoid cuffing, and malacia. The degree of damage is related to the number of larvae present[100,101].

Clinical Disease. In guinea pigs with cerebral larval migrans, clinical signs have included lethargy, torticollis, ataxia, recumbency with inability to rise, and opisthotonos[100,101].

Diagnosis. Diagnosis is by finding histopathologic lesions compatible with this infection and by identifying the larvae in cross section. While routine histopathology often fails to detect the larvae, especially when few are present, if found on sections, larvae usually measure 57 μ to 70 μm in diameter and have prominent, single lateral alae. There is a large, centrally located intestine with an open lumen that is laterally compressed in the mid- to posterior regions. There are usually six to nine low columnar cells within the intestine, each with a thin microvillous border. The intestine is flanked by prominent, lateral chords containing the lateral excretory columns[98].

Treatment. No treatment regimens have been described for guinea pigs. While benzimidazoles and diethylcarbamazine may be of some use, cerebral larval migrans is usually not evident until extensive damage has occurred, and anthelmintic treatment at this stage is usually ineffective[98].

Prevention. Prevention of fecal contamination of feed or bedding prevents infection. Eggs of *B. procyonis* are resistant to most chemical disinfectants commonly used in animal facilities and can remain viable for extended periods of time in dry materials such as straw and bedding. Eggs, however, are heat-sensitive. Thus, autoclaving cages and burning contaminated bedding are effective means of decontamination[98].

Public Health Considerations. *Baylisascaris procyonis* is a cause of cerebral and ocular larval migrans in humans. However, as with guinea pigs, humans become infected by ingesting eggs[98]. Because the parasite does not mature in paratenic hosts, guinea pigs are not a source of infection for humans. However, if guinea pigs do become infected, the source should be found and eliminated as quickly as possible to minimize potential human exposure.

Superfamily Heterakoidea

Paraspidodera uncinata

Morphology. Adult male worms measure 11 mm to 22 mm long and have a pre-anal sucker, two spicules of approximately equal length (470 μ to 700 μ), and a gubernaculum (136 μ to 158 μ long). Adult female worms measure 16 mm to 28 mm long. Eggs are ellipsoidal and unembryonated when passed. Different authors report a range of egg size, with some reporting 43 μ long by 31 μ wide, and others reporting 60 μ to 73 μ long by 47 μ to 53 μ wide[102–104].

Hosts. *Paraspidodera uncinata* occurs in the cecum of wild and domestic guinea pigs throughout the world. The parasite has also been reported from the agouti (*Agouti paca*) and tuco-tocos (*Ctenymys* spp.) in South America. Historically, prevalence of infection in laboratory colonies varied from 10% to 75%, while prevalence in pet store animals has been reported to be 45% and in wild animals the prevalence has been reported to be 37%[91,103–106].

Life Cycle. The life cycle has not been described in detail. Eggs produced by the females are passed in the feces and become infective in five to nine days when held at 22°C to 24°C. Infections can be established experimentally in guinea pigs by oral administration of embryonated eggs; therefore, it has been assumed that transmission is via this source. The prepatent period is 37 to 66 days and the patent period is 12 to 39 days[104,107].

Pathologic Effects and Clinical Disease. Pathologic changes within the cecum of guinea pigs infected with *P. uncinata* have not been reported and this parasite has generally been considered to be nonpathogenic. However, infections have been associated with increased eosinophils in bronchoalveolar lavage in clinically healthy animals[108].

Diagnosis, Treatment and Prevention. Diagnosis is by finding characteristic eggs in the feces or nematodes in the cecum at necropsy. Few treatment protocols have been described. Levamisole (25 mg/kg) and mebendazole (50 mg/kg) administered orally, have been shown to be effective, but piperazine has not[109,110]. Adequate sanitation is essential for preventing infection in laboratory colonies.

ARTHROPODS

Class Insecta

Order Diptera (flies)

Facultative myiasis-producing flies generally lay eggs in carrion or feces. However, flies are also attracted by suppurative wounds; necrotic areas; and skin soiled with urine, feces, or vomitus[13]. Fatal myiasis, involving at least three species of fly (*Lucilia sericata, Calliphora vicina, C. vomitoria*), has been reported in guinea pigs[111,112]. Oviposition by flies was associated with bacterial inflammation in the areas of the rectum and vulva.

Order Phthiraptera (lice)

Gyropus ovalis, Gliricola porcelli, and Trimenopon hispidum

Louse infestations have frequently been reported from laboratory guinea pigs throughout the world[106,113–117]. Species infesting guinea pigs include *Gyropus ovalis, Gliricola porcelli,* and *Trimenopon hispidum*. Historically, *G. porcelli* has been the most common, followed by *G. ovalis* with *T. hispidum* the least commonly encountered species[117,118]. Current prevalences of these lice are unknown, but are thought to be low due to improved husbandry practices in laboratory animal facilities. Life cycles for these species have not been completely described. However, life cycle stages for biting lice include the egg (or

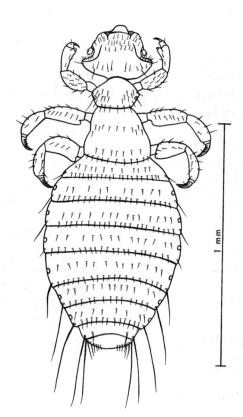

Fig. 14.13 *Gyropis ovalis* female, dorsal view. Courtesy of R.D. Price, University of Minnesota.

"nit"), three nymphal stages, and adult males and females. Transmission is primarily by direct contact[13,118].

Mature *G. ovalis* measure 1 mm to 1.2 mm long, with a maximum width of 0.5 mm (Figure 14.13). The head is triangular in shape. The maxillary palps have four easily discernable segments. There are six pairs of abdominal spiracles located ventrolaterally within poorly defined spiracular plates[118]. Mature *G. porcelli* measure 1 mm to 1.5 mm long and 0.44 mm wide (Figure 14.14). The head is slightly longer than it is wide. The maxillary palps have two easily discernable segments. There are five pairs of abdominal spiracles located ventrally within distinct spiracular plates[118]. Mature *T. hispidum* measure 1.25 mm long and 0.5 mm wide. The head is broadly triangular in shape. The antennae lie in grooves alongside the head, and appear club-shaped. The legs are stout with two tarsal claws. The abdomen is composed of five segments[118]. Louse infestations in guinea pigs may be asymptomatic, or may cause pruritus, roughened hair coat, or alopecia[116,118]. Diagnosis is by observing lice and nits on the pelage, either grossly or with the aid of a hand-held magnifying lens. Treatment regimens include ivermectin, and carbamate- or pyrethrin-based powders[15,115–118].

Class Arachnida

Mites

Suborder Astigmata

Chirodiscoides caviae *Chirodiscoides caviae* (Syn. *Camplyochirus caviiae, Indochirus utkalensis*) (Figure 14.15)[119] is the fur mite of guinea pigs. Both male and female mites are elongate. Males measure 350 μ to 376 μ long and females measure 502 μ to 528 μ long. The anterior portion is triangular, the sternal shield is striated, and all legs are modified for hair clasping with legs I and II more modified than legs III and IV[118,120].

Chirodiscoides caviae is cosmopolitan in distribution and historically was common in guinea pigs[113,114,118,120]. Improvements in laboratory animal husbandry have rendered them less common. These mites may be found attached to hairs anywhere on the body, but are more common in the posterior back region and lateral sides of the posterior quarters[118,120].

The life cycle of *C. caviae* has not been described. However, life cycle stages for mites include the egg, larva (six legs), nymph (eight legs), and adult males and females. Eggs measure 254 μ long by 69 μ wide. Transmission is primarily by direct contact[15,120]. Light infestations may be present for extended periods of time with no clinical

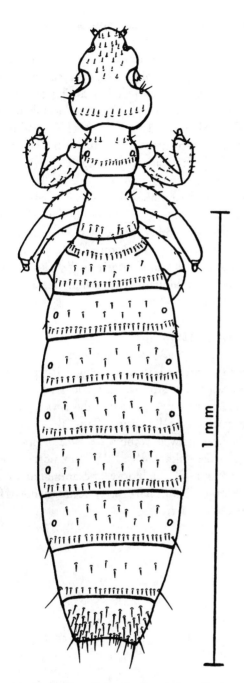

Fig. 14.14 *Gliricola porcelli* female, dorsal view. Courtesy of R.D. Price, University of Minnesota.

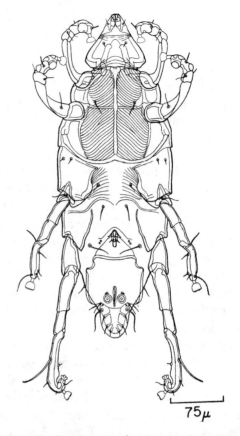

Fig. 14.15 *Chirodiscoides caviae* female, ventral view. Reproduced from Hirst, S. (1922) with permission.

evidence of disease. Pruritus, alopecia, increased grooming behavior leading to self-trauma, and ulcerative dermatitis have been reported[116,120]. Diluted ivermectin applied as a spray has been used to successfully control *C. caviae*, whereas ivermectin administered subcutaneously failed to reduce the number of mites in heavily infested guinea pigs[130,134]. Selamectin (12 mg/kg) administered twice at two-week intervals has also been successful against *C. caviae* infestations[116].

***Trixacarus caviae* Morphology.** *Trixacarus caviae* is a sarcoptiform mite of guinea pigs. Females measure 160 µ to 230 µ long and 120 µ to 180 µ wide. Males measure 120 µ to 150 µ long and 85 µ to 100 µ wide[121]. *Trixacarus caviae* is distinguished from *S. scabiei* by the position of the anus (terminal in *S. scabiei* versus dorsal in female *T. caviae*) and the form of the dorsal setae (some setae transformed into stout dorsal spines in *S. scabiei* versus all dorsal setae simple in *T. caviae*). *Trixacarus caviae* can be distinguished from *N. cati* by the dorsal scales (few, rounded scales surrounding anus in *N. cati* versus many pointed scale in *T. caviae*)[122–124].

Hosts. Prior to 1972, reports of mange in guinea pigs were attributed to either *Sarcoptes scabiei* or *Notoedres cati*[118]. However, Fain and co-workers[122] described a new species of mite associated with mange in guinea pigs. Since that time, *T. caviae* has been documented on guinea pigs worldwide[118,123,125,131,136,137,138]. It is likely that earlier cases of mange attributed to *S. scabiei* or *N. cati* were actually caused by *T. caviae,* though guinea pigs are also susceptible to infestation with *S. scabiei* and *N. cati.*

Life Cycle. The life cycle stages include eggs, larvae, two nymphal stages, and adults. All stages are generally present on the infested animal. Transmission occurs through direct contact. Larvae and nymphs are primarily responsible for establishing new infestations[121,122].

Pathologic Effects. Adult mites are found in epidermal tunnels in the skin, while larvae and nymphs are found primarily on the surface. Histologic lesions include acanthosis, hyperkeratosis, and exfoliative dermatitis. Accumulations of lymphocytes, monocytes, and eosinophils may be present. Hematologic changes may include monocytosis, neutrophilia, eosinophilia and basophilia[123,124,126,127].

Clinical Disease. *Trixacarus caviae* is the most common cause of pruritus in pet and laboratory guinea pigs. Pruritus is associated with excessive rubbing, biting, or scratching. The skin becomes thickened and alopecic. Secondary bacterial infections may also occur. Lesions tend to occur on the neck, shoulders, dorsal trunk, and ventral abdomen, although in severe cases, all parts of the body may be affected[123,125–129]. Occasionally, seizures and abnormal behaviors have been reported in *T. caviae*-infested guinea pigs[123,129,130]. The cause for this is considered to be a generalized pruritus-induced hyperesthesia[129,130].

Diagnosis, Treatment, and Prevention. Diagnosis is based on clinical signs and upon finding characteristic mites in skin scrapings. Care must be taken to distinguish *T. caviae* from *S. scabiei* and *N. cati.* Some infestations may be eliminated with ivermectin using one of the following regimens: 0.2 mg/kg orally or subcutaneously, repeated in seven to 10 days as needed; 0.4 mg/kg orally, repeated weekly for four weeks; or 0.5 mg/kg subcutaneously, repeated once in seven days[15,133–135]. The use of fipronil on the animal or to treat the environment has also been suggested[125,128]. For accompanying behavioral "fits," diazepam can be used initially at 1 to 2 mg/kg intramuscularly, and may be followed by other antiseizure medications such as primidone (25 mg/kg orally twice per day). Animals housed together should be treated for the parasite at the same time or re-infestation is likely to occur.

Public Health Considerations. *Trixacarus caviae* can transiently infest humans. Infestations result in papular urticaria and pruritus[132].

Suborder Prostigmata

Demodex caviae *Demodex caviae* is a relatively short species of *Demodex,* measuring 138 μ to 165 μ long and 65 μ to 69 μ wide. The stubby legs are located close together on the anterior portion of the body. Few reports of this parasite exist in the literature. Thus, the host and geographic ranges, as well as the prevalence of infestation on guinea pigs, are unknown[116,118,139]. Antemortem diagnosis is by skin scrapings, skin biopsy, or examination of the hair shafts. Amitraz baths have been recommended for the treatment of *D. caviae*[139].

TABLE 14.1 Parasites of Guinea Pigs—Enterohepatic System.

Parasite	Geographic distribution	Hosts	Location in host	Method of infection	Pathologic effects	Zoonosis	Reference
Flagellates							
Caviomonas mobilis	United States	Guinea pigs	Cecum	Ingestion of organism passed in feces	None	Not reported	4
Chilomastix spp.	Worldwide	Guinea pigs	Cecum	Ingestion of organism passed in feces	None	Not reported	4, 7
Chilomitus caviae	Worldwide	Guinea pigs	Cecum, colon	Ingestion of organism passed in feces	None	Not reported	4
Enteromonas cavia	Europe, United States	Guinea pigs	Cecum	Ingestion of organism passed in feces	None	Not reported	4
Giardia duodenalis	Worldwide	Guinea pigs, possibly other mammals	Anterior small intestine	Ingestion of organism passed in feces	None	Unknown whether humans are susceptible to guinea pig strain	12, 17
Hexamastix spp.	Worldwide	Guinea pigs	Cecum	Ingestion of organism passed in feces	None	Not reported	4
Monocercomonas spp.	Americas, Europe	Guinea pigs	Cecum	Ingestion of organism passed in feces	None	Not reported	4
Monocercomonoides spp.	Americas, Europe	Guinea pigs	Cecum	Ingestion of organism passed in feces	None	Not reported	4
Proteromonas brevifilia	Europe, United States	Guinea pigs	Cecum	Ingestion of organism passed in feces	None	Not reported	4
Retortamonas caviae	Worldwide	Guinea pigs	Cecum	Ingestion of organism passed in feces	None	Not reported	4, 26
Tritrichomonas caviae	Worldwide	Guinea pigs, gerbils	Cecum, colon, small intestine	Ingestion of organism passed in feces	Rare cecal and colonic ulceration	Not reported	1, 4, 27
Amoebae							
Endolimax caviae	Asia, United States	Guinea pigs	Cecum	Ingestion of cysts passed in feces	None	Not reported	1, 4, 39
Entamoeba caviae	Americas, Europe	Guinea pigs	Cecum	Ingestion of cysts passed in feces	None	Not reported	4, 41
Coccidia							
Cryptosporidium wrairi	United States	Guinea pigs	Small intestine	Presumably by ingestion of oocyst passed in feces	Slight enteritis	Not reported	49
Eimeria caviae	Worldwide	Guinea pigs, wild guinea pigs (*Cavia aperea*)	Large intestine	Ingestion of oocyst passed in feces	Sometimes hemorrhagic enteritis	Not reported	1, 55–57, 61

(Continued)

441

TABLE 14.1 (Continued)

Parasite	Geographic distribution	Hosts	Location in host	Method of infection	Pathologic effects	Zoonosis	Reference
Ciliates							
Balantidium caviae	Worldwide	Guinea pigs	Cecum, colon	Ingestion of cysts passed in feces	Secondary enteritis	Not reported	28, 62
Cyathodinium spp.	Worldwide	Guinea pigs	Cecum, colon	Ingestion of trophozoites (or cysts?) passed in feces	None	Not reported	1, 4
Enterophyra elongata	Brazil	Wild guinea pigs	Cecum	Presumed ingestion of trophozoites or cysts passed in feces	None	Not reported	1, 80
Kopperia intestinale	Unknown	Guinea pigs	Cecum	Presumed ingestion of trophozoites or cysts passed in feces	None	Not reported	1, 4
Protocaviella acuminate	Unknown	Guinea pigs	Cecum	Presumed ingestion of trophozoites or cysts passed in feces	None	Not reported	1
Trematodes							
Fasciola spp.	Worldwide	Guinea pigs, other herbivorous mammals, humans	Liver, abdominal cavity	Ingestion of metacercaria encysted on vegetation	Usually none; cysts may cause local lesions (F. gigantica)	Reported	89, 90, 93
Pseudoquinqueserialis caviae	South America	Wild guinea pigs	Intestine	Presumed ingestion of metacercaria	None	Not reported	142
Taxorchis caviae	South America	Wild guinea pigs	Cecum	Presumed ingestion of metacercaria	None	Not reported	141
Taxorchis ringueleti	South America	Wild guinea pigs	Cecum	Presumed ingestion of metacercaria	None	Not reported	140
Cestodes							
Anoplocephala sp.	South America	Guinea pigs	Intestine	Unknown	None	Not reported	143
Monoecocestus parcitesticulatus	South America	Guinea pigs	Intestine	Unknown	None	Not reported	105
Nematodes							
Heterakoidea							
Paraspidodera uncinata	Worldwide	Guinea pigs, other wild rodents	Cecum	Ingestion of embryonated egg	Weight loss, debilitation, diarrhea, bronchial eosinophilia	Not reported	91, 108

Trichostrongyloidea						
Graphidioides mazzai	South America	Wild guinea pigs, other wild rodents	Small intestine	Presumed ingestion of infective larvae	None	Not reported	91
Viannella travassosi	Brazil	Wild guinea pigs	Small intestine	Presumed ingestion of infective larvae	None	Not reported	91
Trichuroidea						
Capillaria hepatica	Peru	Wild guinea pigs	Liver	Presumed ingestion of embryonated egg	None	Reported	91
Trichuris gracilis	Brazil	Guinea pigs	Large intestine	Presumed ingestion of embryonated egg	None	Not reported	91

TABLE 14.2 Parasites of Guinea Pigs—Central Nervous System, Skin, Connective Tissue, Muscle, Urogenital System.

Parasite	Geographic distribution	Hosts	Location in host	Method of infection	Pathologic effects	Zoonosis	Reference
Flagellates							
Leishmania enriettii	South America	Guinea pigs	Skin	Presumed sandfly host	Cutaneous nodules and ulcers	Not reported	20
Trypanosoma cruzi	Americas	Guinea pigs, other mammals	Skin, cardiac muscle, other organs	Blood-sucking arthropod vector (Reduviids)	Unknown	Common	144
Coccidia							
Klossiella cobayae	Worldwide	Guinea pigs	Kidneys, lungs, spleen, other organs	Ingestion of sporocysts passed in urine	Variable nephritis	Not reported	64
Sarcocystis caviae	Unknown	Guinea pigs	Striated muscle	Ingestion of infective sporocyst from unknown definitive host	None	Not reported	69
Toxoplasma gondii	Worldwide	Guinea pigs, other mammals, birds	Many organ systems	Ingestion of sporulated oocyst in cat feces	Hepatitis, pneumonia, encephalitis, abortion	Common	1, 70
Microspora							
Encephalitozoon cuniculi	Worldwide	Guinea pigs, other mammals	Kidney, central nervous system	Ingestion of infective spores	Nephritis, encephalitis	Uncertain zoonotic potential of guinea pig strains	84, 85
Nematodes							
Rhabditoidea							
Pelodera strongyloides	Worldwide	Guinea pig, other mammals	Skin	Invasion through compromised skin, mucus membranes	Dermatitis	Reported	97
Ascaridoidea							
Baylisascaris procyonis	Worldwide	Guinea pigs, raccoons, other mammals	Central nervous system, other organs	Ingestion of embryonated egg in raccoon feces	Encephalitis	Reported	100
Filaroidea							
Ackertia borgosi	Argentina	Wild guinea pigs	Abdominal cavity	Presumed transmission by arthropod host	None	Not reported	143
Diptera (flies)							

Lucilia sericata, Calliphora vicina, Calliphora vomitoria	Europe	Guinea pigs, other mammals	Skin, deeper organs	Eggs deposited by adult fly	Myiasis	Reported	111, 112
Phthiraptera (lice)							
Gliricola porcelli	Worldwide	Guinea pigs, wild *Cavia* spp.	Pelage	Direct contact	Pruritus, unthriftiness, roughened coat, alopecia	Not reported	116
Gliricola spp.	South America	Wild Guinea pigs (*Cavia anolaine*)	Pelage	Direct contact	Unknown	Not reported	145
Gyropus ovalis	Worldwide	Guinea pigs, wild *Cavia* spp.	Pelage	Direct contact	Pruritus, unthriftiness, roughened coat, alopecia	Not reported	116
Pteropthirus spp.	South America	Wild guinea pigs	Pelage	Direct contact	Unknown	Not reported	118
Trimenopomhispidum	Worldwide	Wild guinea pigs	Pelage	Direct contact	Irritation	Not reported	116
Siphonaptera (fleas)							
Hectopsylla spp.	Unknown	Wild guinea pigs	Pelage	Direct contact	Unknown	Not reported	118
Leptopsylla seginis	Unknown	Wild guinea pigs	Pelage	Direct contact	Unknown	Not reported	91
Nosopsyllus fasciatus	Unknown	Wild guinea pigs	Pelage	Direct contact	Unknown	Not reported	118
Pulex irritans	Worldwide	Wild guinea pigs, other mammals	Pelage	Direct contact	Dermatitis	Common	118
Rhopalopsylla clavicola	Unknown	Wild guinea pigs	Pelage	Direct contact	Unknown	Not reported	118
Tiamastus cavicola	Unknown	Wild guinea pigs	Pelage	Direct contact	Unknown	Not reported	91
Arachnida							
Mites							
Astigmates							
Chirodiscoides caviae	Worldwide	Guinea pigs	Skin, pelage	Direct contact	Pruritus, alopecia	Not reported	120
Notoedres muris	Worldwide	Guinea pigs, other rodents	Skin	Direct contact	Dermatitis	Reported	146
Trixacarus caviae	Worldwide	Guinea pigs	Skin	Direct contact	Dermatitis	Transient zoonosis	125
Mesostigmates							
Ornithonyssus bacoti	Unknown	Wild guinea pigs	Skin	Direct contact	Dermatitis	Reported	118
Ornithonyssus braziliensis	Unknown	Wild guinea pigs	Skin	Direct contact	Unknown	Not reported	118
Ornithonyssus wernecki	Unknown	Guinea pigs	Skin	Direct contact	Unknown	Not reported	146
Prostigmates							
Demodex caviae	Unknown	Guinea pigs	Skin	Direct contact	Unknown	Not reported	147
Eutrombicula spp.	Unknown	Wild guinea pigs	Skin	Direct contact	Unknown	Probable	91, 146

REFERENCES

1. Vetterling, J.M. (1976) Protozoan parasites. In: Wagner, J.E. and Manning, P.J. (eds.) *The Biology of the Guinea Pig.* Academic Press, New York, 163–196.

2. Lee, J.L., Small, E.B., Lynn. D.H., and Bovee, E.C. (1985) Some techniques for collecting, cultivating and observing protozoa. In: Lee, J.J., Hutner, S.H., and Bovee, E.C. (eds.). *An Illustrated Guide to the Protozoa.* Society of Protozoologists, Lawrence, Kansas, 1–7.

3. Saxe, L.H. (1954) Transfaunation studies on the host specificity of the enteric protozoa of rodents. *J. Protozool.* **1,** 220–230.

4. Nie, D. (1950) Morphology and taxonomy of the intestinal protozoa of the guinea-pig, *Cavia porcella. J. Morphol.* **86,** 381–493.

5. Brugerolle, G. and Regnault, J-P. (2001) Ultrastructure of the enteromonad flagellate *Caviomonas mobilis. Parasitol. Res.* **87,** 662–665.

6. Saxe, L.H. (1954) The enteric protozoa of laboratory golden hamsters. *J. Parasitol.* **40**(Suppl.), 20.

7. Nie, D. (1948) The structure and division of *Chilomastix intestinalis* Kuczynski with notes of similar forms in man and other vertebrates. *J. Morphol.* **82,** 287–329.

8. Fantham, H.B. (1922) Some parasitic protozoa found in South Africa. V. *S. Afr. J. Sci.* **19,** 332–339.

9. Kofoid, C.A., McNeil, E., and Bonestell, A.E. (1935) A comparison of the distribution of the intestinal protozoa of the Norway rat, wood rat, and guinea pig with reference to the hydrogen ion concentrations as determined by the glass electrode. *U. Calif. Publ. No. 2001.* **41,** 1–8.

10. Hegner, R.W. (1923) Giardias from wild rats and mice and *Giardia caviae* sp. n. from the guinea pig. *Am. J. Hyg.* **3,** 345–349.

11. Fantham, H.B. (1923) Some parasitic protozoa found in South Africa. VI. *S. Afr. J. Sci.* **20,** 493–500.

12. Fujinami, F. and Iwasaki, H.O. (1984) (Giardiasis in guinea pigs: a case report.) *Exp. Anim.* **33,** 361–362.

13. Ballweber, L.R. (2001) *Veterinary Parasitology.* Butterworth Heinemann, Boston, Massachusetts.

14. Mohan, R. (1993) Evaluation of immunofluorescent and ELISA tests to detect *Giardia* and *Cryptosporidium* in birds. In: *Proceedings 1993 Annual Conference Association of Avian Veterinarians, August 31–September 4, 1993,* Nashville, Tennessee, 62–64.

15. Fremont, J.J. and Bowman, D.D. (2003) Parasites of guinea pigs. Document No. A0316.1003. In: Bowman, D.D. (ed.). *Companion and Exotic Animal Parasitology.* International Veterinary Information Service (www.ivis.org.), Ithaca, New York.

16. Zimmer, J.F., Miller, J.J., and Lindmark, D.G. (1988) Evaluation of the efficacy of selected commercial disinfectants in inactivating *Giardia muris* cysts. *J. Am. Anim. Hosp. Assoc.* **24,** 379–385.

17. Thompson, R.C.A., Hopkins, R.M., and Homan, W.L. (2000) Nomenclature and genetic groupings of *Giardia* infecting mammals. *Parasitol. Today* **16,** 210–213.

18. Lee, J.J. (1985). Order 5. Trichomonadida. In: Lee, J.J., Hutner, S.H., and Bovee, E.C. (eds.). *An Illustrated Guide to the Protozoa.* Society of Protozoologists, Lawrence, Kansas, 119–127.

19. Thomaz-Soccol, V., Pratlong, F., Langue, R., Castro, E., Luz, E, and Dedet, J.P. (1996) New isolation of *Leishmania enriettii* Muniz and Medina, 1948 in Paraná State, Brazil, 50 years after the first description, and isoenzymatic polymorphism of the *L. enriettii* taxon. *Ann. Trop. Med. Parastiol.* **90,** 491–495.

20. Lainson, R. (1997) On *Leishmania enriettii* and other enigmatic *Leishmania* species of the neotropics. *Mem. Inst. Oswaldo Cruz* **92,** 377–387.

21. Hertig, M. and McConnell, E. (1963) Experimental infection of Panamanian *Phlebotomus* sandflies with *Leishmania. Exp. Parasitol.* **14,** 92–106.

22. Luz, E., Biovannoni, M., and Borba, A.M. (1967) Infecção de *Lutzomyia monticola* por *Leishmania enrietti. An. Fac. Med. Univ. Fed. Paraná.* **9–10,** 121–128.

23. Monroy, A., Ridley, D.S., Heather, C.J., and Ridley, M.J. (1980) Histological studies of the elimination of *Leishmania enriettii* from skin lesions in the guinea pig. *Br. J. Exp. Pathol.* **61,** 601–610.

24. Behin, R., J. Mauel, and Rowe, D.S. (1977) Mechanisms of protective immunity in experimental cutaneous leishmaniasis of the guinea-pig. III. Inhibition of leishmanial lesion in the guinea-pig by delayed hypersensitivity reaction to unrelated antigens. *Clin. Exp. Immunol.* **29,** 320–325.

25. Wenrich, D.H. (1946) Culture experiments on intestinal flagellates. I. Trichomonad and other flagellates obtained from man and certain rodents. *J. Parasitol.* **32,** 40–53.

26. Hegner, R. and Schumaker, E. (1928) Some intestinal amoebae and flagellates from the chimpanzee, three-toed sloth, sheep and guinea-pig. *J. Parasitol.* **15,** 31–37.

27. Honigberg, B.M. (1963) Evolutionary and systematic relationships in the flagellate order Trichomonadida Kirby. *J. Protozol.* **10,** 20–63.

28. Faust, E.C. (1950) The intestinal protozoa of the guinea-pig. *Ann. Inst. Biol. Univ. Nac. Autonoma Mex.* **20,** 229–250.

29. Vincint, A.L., Porter, D.D., and Ash, L.R. (1975) Spontaneous lesions and parasites of the Mongolian gerbil, *Meriones unguiculatus. Lab. Anim. Sci.* **25,** 711–722.

30. Brugerolle, G. (2002) *Colpodella vorax:* ultrastructure, predation, life-cycle, mitosis, and phylo-genetic relationships. *Eur. J. Protistol.* **38,**113–125.

31. Simpson, A.G.B. and Patterson, D.J. (1996) Ultrastructure and identification of the predatory flagellate *Colpodella pugnax* Cienkowski (Apidomplexa) with a description of *Colpodella turpis* n. sp. and a review of the genus. *Syst. Parasitol.* **33,** 187–198.

32. Takamura, N., Shen, Y., and Xie, P. (2000) Species richness of protozoa in Japanese lakes. *Limnology* **1,** 91–106.

33. Watson, J.M. (1946) The bionomics of coprophilic protozoa. *Biol. Rev. Camb. Philos. Soc.* **21,** 121–139.

34. Prins, R.A. (1971) Isolation, culture, and fermentation characteristics of *Selenomonas ruminantium* var. *bryanti* var. n. from the rumen of sheep. *J. Bacteriol.* **105,** 820–825.

35. Robinson, I.M., Allison, M.J., and Bucklin, J.A. (1981) Characterization of the cecal bacteria of normal pigs. *Appl. Environ. Microbiol.* **41,** 950–955.

36. Lessel, E.F., Jr. and Breed, R.S. (1954) *Selenomonas boskamp,* 1922—a genus that includes species showing an unusual type of flagellation. Bacteriol. Rev. 18: 165–168.

37. Oxford, A.E. (1955) Some observations upon the status of the generic name *Selenomonas prowazek. Int. Bull. Bacteriol. Nomen. Taxon.* **5,** 131–132.

38. Orpin, C.G. (1976) Studies on the rumen flagellate *Sphaeromonas commmunis. J. Gen. Microbiol.* **94,** 270–280.

39. Hegner, R.W. (1926) *Endolimax caviae* n. sp. from the guinea-pig and *Endolimax janisae* n.sp. from the domestic fowl. *J. Parasitol.* **12,** 146–147.

40. Holmes, F.O. (1923) Observations on the cysts of *Entamoeba cobayae. Parasitology* **10,** 47–50.

41. Mudrow-Reichenow, L. (1956) Spontanes Vorkommen von Amöben und Ciliaten bei Laboratoriumstieren. *Z. Tropenmed. Parasitol.* **7,** 198–211.

42. Tilley, M., Upton, S.J., and Crisp, C.E. (1991) A comparative study on the biology of *Cryptosporidium* sp. from guinea pigs and *Cryptosporidium parvum* (Apicomplexa). *Can. J. Microbiol.* **37**, 949–952.

43. Xiao, L., Fayer, R., Ryan, U., and Upton, S.J. (2004) *Cryptosporidium* taxonomy: recent advances and implications for public health. *Clin. Microbiol. Rev.* **17**, 72–97.

44. Spano, F., Putignani, L., McLauchlin, J., Casemore, D.P., and Crisanti, A. (1997) PCR-RFLP analysis of the *Cryptosporidium* oocyst wall protein (COWP) gene discriminates between *C. wrairi* and *C. parvum,* and between *C. parvum* isolates of human and animal origin. *FEMS Microbiol. Let.* **150**, 209–217.

45. Sulaiman, I.M., Morgan, U.M., Thompson, R.C., Lal, A.A., and Xiao, L. (2000) Phylogenetic relationships of *Cryptosporidium* parasites based on the 70-kilodalton heat shock protein (HSP70) gene. *Appl. Environ. Microbiol.* **66**, 2385–2391.

46. Vetterling, J.M., Jervis, H.R., Merrill, T.G., and Sprinz, H. (1971) *Cryptoporidium wrairi* sp. n. from the guinea pig *Cavia procellus,* with an emendation of the genus. *J. Protozool.* **18**, 243–247.

47. Chrisp, C.E., Suckow, M.A., Fayer, R., Arrowood, M.J., Healey, M.C., and Sterling, C.R. (1992) Comparison of the host ranges and antigenicity of *Cryptosporidium parvum* and *Cryptosporidium wrairi* from guinea pigs. *J. Protozool.* **39**, 406–409.

48. Graczyk, T.K. and Cranfield, M.R. (1998) Experimental transmission of *Cryptosporidium* oocyst isolates from mammals, birds and reptiles to captive snakes. *Vet. Res.* **29**, 187–195.

49. Chrisp, C.E., Reid, W.C., Rusk, H.G., Suckow, M.A., Bush, A., and Thomann, M.J. (1990) Cryptosporidiosis in guinea pigs: an animal model. *Infect. Immun.* **58**, 674–679.

50. Jervis, H.R., Merrill, T.G., and Sprinz, H. (1966) Coccidiosis in the guinea pig small intestine due to a *Cryptosporidium.* *Am. J. Vet. Res.* **27**, 408–414.

51. Gibson, S.V. and Wagner, J.E. (1986) Cryptosporidiosis in guinea pigs: a retrospective study. *J. Am. Vet. Med. Assoc.* **120**, 1033–1034.

52. Cole, D.J., Snowden, K., Cohen, N.D., and Smith, R. (1999) Detection of *Cryptosporidium parvum* in horses: thresholds of acid-fast stain, immunofluorescence assay, and flow cytometry. *J. Clin. Microbiol.* **37**, 457–460.

53. Siefker, C., Rickard, L.G., Pharr, G.T., Simmons, J.S., and O'Hara, T.M. (2002) Molecular characterization of *Cryptosporidium* sp. isolated from northern Alaskan caribou (*Rangifer tarandus*). *J. Parasitol.* **88**, 213–216.

54. Fayer, R., C.A. Speer, and J.P. Dubey. (1997) The general biology of *Cryptosporidium.* In: Fayer, R. (ed). *Cryptosporidium and cryptosporidiosis.* CRC Press, Boca Raton, Florida, 1–4.

55. LaPage, G. (1940). The study of coccidiosis (*Eimeria caviae* [Sheather 1924]) in the guinea pig (continued). *Vet. J.* **96**, 190–202.

56. LaPage, G. (1940) The study of coccidiosis (*Eimeria caviae* [Sheather 1924]) in the guinea pig. Part I. *Vet. J.* **96**, 144–154.

57. Levine, N.D. and Ivens, V. (1965) *The Coccidian Parasites (Protozoa, Sporozoa) of Rodents.* Univ. Illinois Press, Urbana, IL.

58. Ryšavý, B. (1954) Příěvek k poznání kokcidií našich I dovezených obratlovcu. *Cesk. Parasitol.* **21**, 131–174.

59. Muto, T., Yusa, T., Sugisaki, M., Tanaka, K., Noguchi, Y., and Taguch, K. (1985) Studies on coccidiosis in guinea pigs. 2. Epizootiological survey. *Exp. Anim.* **34**, 31–39.

60. Ellis, P.A. and Wright, A.E. (1961) Coccidiosis in guinea pigs. *J. Clin. Pathol.* **14**, 394–396.

61. LaPage, G. (1940) The study of coccidiosis (*Eimeria caviae* [Sheather 1924]) in the guinea pig. Part II. *Vet. J.* **96**, 280–295.

62. Hankinson, G.J., Murphy, J.C., and Fox, J.G. (1982) Diagnostic exercise. *Lab Anim. Sci.* **32**, 35–36.

63. Calhoon, J.R. and Matthews, P.J. (1964) A method for initiating a colony of specific pathogen-free guinea pigs. *Lab. Anim. Care* **14**, 388–394.

64. Taylor, J.L., Wagner, J.E., Kusewitt, D.F., and Mann, P.C. (1979) *Klossiella* parasites of animals: a literature review. *Vet. Parasitol.* **5**, 137–144.

65. Pearce, L. (1916) *Klossiella* infection of the guinea pig. *J. Exp. Med.* **23**, 431–442.

66. Jackson, L. (1920) An intracellular protozoan parasite of the ducts of the salivary glands of the guinea-pig. *J. Infect. Dis.* **26**, 347–350.

67. Hofmann, H. and Hänichen, T. (1970) *Klossiella cobayae*—Nierenkokzidiose bei Meerschweinchen. *Berl. Münch. Tierärztl. Wochensch.* **83**, 151–153.

68. Stojanov, D.P. and Cvetanov, J.L. (1965) Über die Klossiellose bei Meerschweinchen. *Z. Parasitenkd.* **25**, 350–358.

69. Kean, B.H. and Grocott, R.G. (1945) Sarcosporidiosis or toxoplasmosis in man and guinea-pig. *Am. J. Pathol.* **21**, 467–483.

70. Green, L.E. and Morgan, K.L. (1991) *Toxoplasma* abortion in a guinea pig. *Vet. Rec.* **129**, 266–267.

71. Lainson, R. (1959) A note on the duration of *Toxoplasma* infection in the guinea-pig. *Ann. Trop. Med. Parasitol.* **53**, 120–121.

72. Markham, F.S. (1937) Spontaneous *Toxoplasma* encephalitis in the guinea pig. *Am. J. Hyg.* **26**, 193–196.

73. Hill, D. and Dubey, J.P. (2002) *Toxoplasma gondii:* transmission, diagnosis and prevention. *Clin. Microbiol. Infect.* **8**, 634–640.

74. Krishnan, R. (1968) Balantidiosis in a guinea pig. *Indian Vet J.* **45**, 917–920.

75. Clyti, E., Aznar, C., Couppie, P., el Guedj, M., Carme, B., and Pradinaud, R. (1998) Un cas de co-infection par *Balantidium coli* et VIH en Guyane Francaise. *Bull. Soc. Pathol. Exot.* **91**, 309–311.

76. Paulin, J.J. and Corliss, J.O. (1964) The somatic and oral infraciliature of the enigmatic ciliate *Cyathodinium piriforme. J. Protozool.* **11**, 438–444.

77. Kudo, R.R. (1966) *Protozoology.* 5th ed. Charles C. Thomas, Springfield, Illinois.

78. Fantham, H.B. (1925) Some parasitic protozoa found in South Africa. VIII. *S. Afr. J. Sci.* **22**, 346–354.

79. Lucas, M.S. (1932) A study of *Cyanthodinium piriforme.* An endozoic protozoan from the intestinal tract of the guinea pig. *Arch. Protistenkd.* **77**, 64–72.

80. Ito, A. and Imai, S. (2000) Ciliates from the cecum of capybara (*Hydrochoerus hydrochaeris*) in Bolivia I. The families Hydrochoerellidae n. fam., Protohallidae, and Pycnotrichidae. *Eur. J. Protistol.* **36**, 53–84.

81. Mathis, A. (2000) Microsporidia: emerging advances in understanding the basic biology of these unique organisms. *Int. J. Parasitol.* **30**, 795–804.

82. Illanes, O.G., Tiffani-Castiglioni, E., Edwards, J.F., and Shadduck, J.A. (1993) Spontaneous encephalitozoonosis in an experimental group of guinea pigs. *J. Vet. Diag. Invest.* **5**, 649–651.

83. Wasson, K. and Peper, R.L. (2000) Mammalian microsporidiosis. *Vet. Pathol.* **37**, 113–128.

84. Gannon, J. (1980) A survey of *Encephalitozoon cuniculi* in laboratory animal colonies in the United Kingdom. *Lab. Anim.* **14**, 91–94.

85. Wan, C-H, Franklin, C., Riley, L.K., Hook, R.R., Jr., and Besch-Williford, C. (1996) Diagnostic exercise: granulonatons encephalitis in guinea pigs. *Lab. Anim. Sci.* **46**, 228–230.

86. Harcourt-Brown, F.M. (2004) *Encephalitozoon cuniculi* infection in rabbits. *Sem. Avian Exotic Pet Med.* **13**, 86–93.

87. Xiao, L., Li, L., Visvesvara, G.S., Moura, H., Didier, E.S., and Lal, A.A. (2001) Genotyping *Encephalitozoon cuniculi* by multilocus analyses of genes with repetitive sequences. *J. Clin. Microbiol.* **39**, 2248–2253.

88. Piedrafita, D., Raadsma, H.W., Prowse, R., Spithill, T.W. (2004) Immunology of the host-parasite relationship in fasciolosis (*Fasciola hepatica* and *Fasciola gigantica*). *Can. J. Zool.* **82**, 233–250.

89. Strauss, J.M. and Heyneman, D. (1966) Fatal ectopic fascioliasis in a guinea pig breeding colony from Malacca. *J. Parasitol.* **52**, 413.

90. Gamarra, R.G. (1996) *Fasciola* infection in guinea-pigs in the Peruvian highlands. *Trop. Anim. Health Prod.* **28**, 143–144.

91. Dittmar, K. (2002) Arthropod and helminth parasites of the wild guinea pig, *Cavia aperea*, from the Andes and the Cordillera in Peru, South America. *J. Parasitol.* **88**, 409–411.

92. Mango, A.M., Mango, C.K.A., and Esamal, D.E. (1977) Further observations on the mortality, susceptibility, prepatency and recovery of *Fasciola gigantica* in rabbits and guinea pigs. *Bull. Anim. Hlth. Prod. Africa* **25**, 251–256.

93. Boray, J.C. (1969) Experimental fascioliasis in Australia. *Adv. Parasitol.* **7**, 95–210.

94. Srivastava, P.S. and Singh, K.S. (1972) Early migration of *Fasciola gigantica* Cobbold, 1855, in guinea-pig. *Indian J. Anim. Sci.* **42**, 63–71.

95. Srivastava, P.S. and Singh, K.S. (1972) Histopathological study of immature fascioliasis in guinea-pig. *Indian J. Anim. Sci.* **42**, 120–126.

96. Poiner, G.O. (1965) Life history of *Pelodera strongyloides* (Schneider) in the orbits of murid rodents in Great Britain. *Proc. Helminthol. Soc. Wash.* **32**, 158–161.

97. Todd, K.S., Jr., Seaman, W.J., and Gretschmann, K.W. (1982) *Pelodera strongyloides* dermatitis in a guinea pig. *Vet. Med. Small Anim. Clin.* **77**, 1400–1402.

98. Kazacos, K.R. (2001) *Baylisascaris procyonis* and related species. In: Samuel, W.M., Pybus, M.J., and Kocan, A.A. (eds.) *Parasitic Diseases of Wild Mammals.* 2nd ed. Iowa State University Press, Ames, Iowa, 301–341.

99. Sato, H., Kamiya, H., and Furuoka, H. (2003) Epidemiological aspects of the first outbreak of *Baylisascaris procyonis* larva migrans in rabbits in Japan. *J. Vet. Med. Sci.* **65**, 453–457.

100. van Andel, R.A., C.L. Franklin, C. Besch-Williford, L.K. Riley, R.R. Hook, Jr., and K.R. Kazacos. (1995) Cerebrospinal larva migrans due to *Baylisascaris procyonis* in a guinea pig colony. *Lab. Anim. Sci.* **45**, 27–30.

101. Craig, S.J., Conboy, G.A., and Hanna, P.E. (1995) *Baylisascaris* sp. infection in a guinea pig. *Lab. Anim. Sci.* **45**, 312–314.

102. Herlich, H. and Dixon, C.F. (1965) Growth and development of *Paraspidodera uncinata*, the cecal worm of the guinea pig. *J. Parasitol.* **51**, 300.

103. Herrera, N.I. (1967) Fauna helmintológica del Perú. *Paraspidodera uncinata* (Rudolphi, 1819), parásito intestinal de los cobayos. (Nematoda, Subuluroidea). *Bol. Chil. Parasitol.* **22**, 15–20.

104. Travassos, L. (1914) Contribuicão para o conhecimento da fauna helmintologica brazileira. *Mem. Inst. Oswaldo Cruz* **6**, 137–142.

105. Pinto, R.M., Gomes, D.C., Muniz-Pereira, L.C., and Noronha, D. (2002) Helminths of the guinea pig, *Cavia porcellus* (Linneaus), in Brazil. *Revta. Bras. Zool.* **19** (Suppl. 1), 261–269.

106. Sparrow, S. (1976) The microbiological and parasitological status of laboratory animals from accredited breeders in the United Kingdom. *Lab. Anim.* **10**, 365–373.

107. Lindquist, W.D. and Hitchcock, D.J. (1950) Studies on infections of a caecal worm, *Paraspidodera uncinata,* in guinea pigs. *J. Parasitol.* **36**, 37–38.

108. Conder, G.A., Richards, I.M., Jen, L-W., Marbury, K.S., and Oostneen, J.A. (1989) Bronchoalveolar eosinophilia in guinea pigs harboring unapparent infections of *Paraspidodera uncinata. J. Parasitol.* **75**, 144–146.

109. Eliazian, M., Shahlapour, A., and Tamiji, Y. (1975) Control of *Paraspidodera uncinata* in guinea-pigs with Levamisole. *Lab. Anim.* **9**, 381–382.

110. Betke, P., Nickel, S., and Wilhelm, A. (1982) Untersuchungen zu *Paraspidodera uncinata* (Nematoda, Heterakidae), einem Blinddarmparasitem von *Cavia porcellus. Angew. Parasitol.* **23**, 197–202.

111. Ribbeck, R., Schumann, H., and Bergmann, V. (1975) Calliphoirdenlarven als Erreger einer Myiasis bei Merrschweinchen. *Monat. Vet.* **30**, 584–587.

112. Hinaidy, H.K. and Niebauer, G.W. (1979) Fakultativmyiasis bei einem Kaninchen und einem Meerschiveinchen. *Wien. Tierärztl. Mschr.* **66**, 384–386.

113. Gorman, G.T., Zuniga, C.R., and Romero, M.S. (1986) Hallazgos de ectoparasitos en cobayos (*Cavia porcellus*). *Avan. Cien. Vet.* **1**, 63–64.

114. Ismail, S. and Ho, T.M. (1989) Ectoparasites of some laboratory animals. *Trop. Biomed.* **6**, 113–116.

115. Pequin, J. (1997) Phtiriose a *Trimenopon* chez un cobaye. *Point Vet.* **28**, 1309–1310.

116. White, S.D., Bourdeau, P.J., and Meredith, A. (2003) Dermatologic problems in guinea pigs. *Compend. Contin. Educ. Pract. Vet.* **25**, 690–697.

117. Ziomko, I. and Cencek, T. (1992) [Prevalence and control of mallophagen lice in guinea pigs in laboratory animal colonies]. (English summary) *Med. Weter.* **48**, 70–72.

118. Ronald, N.C. and Wagner, J.E. (1976) The arthropod parasites of the genus *Cavia.* In: Wagner, J.E., Manning, P.J. (eds.) *The Biology of the Guinea Pig.* Academic Press, New York, 201–109.

119. Hirst, S. (1922) Mites injurious to domestic animals. *Br. Mus. (Nat. Hist.) Econ. Ser.* **13**, 1–107.

120. Wagner, J.E., Al-Rabiai, S., and Rings, R.W. (1972) *Chirodiscorides caviae* infestation in guinea pigs. *Lab. Anim. Sci.* **22**, 750–752.

121. Collins, G.H., Pope, S., and Griffin, D.L. (1986) *Trixarcarus caviae* Fain et al. (Acari: Sarcoptidae): dimensions, population composition and development of infection in guinea pigs. *J. Aust. Entomol. Soc.* **25**, 17–22.

122. Fain, A., Hovell, G.J.R., and Hyatt, K.H. (1972) A new sarcoptid mite producing mange in albino guinea-pigs. *Acta Zool. Pathol. Antverpiensia* **56**, 73–82.

123. Kummel, B.A., Estes, S.A., and Arlian, L.G. (1980) *Trixacarus caviae* infestation of guinea pigs. *J. Am. Vet. Med. Assoc.* **177**, 903–908.

124. McDonald, S.E. and Lavoipierre, M.M.J. (1980) *Trixacarus caviae* infestation in two guinea pigs. *Lab Anim. Sci.* **30**, 67–70.

125. Donnelly, T.M. (2004) What's your diagnosis? Pruritus and alopecia in guinea-pigs. *Lab Animal* **33**, 21–23.

126. Rothwell, T.L.W., Pope, S.E., Rajczyk, Z.K., and Collins, G.H. (1991) Haematological and pathological responses to experimental *Trixacarus caviae* infection in guinea pigs. *J. Comp. Pathol.* **104**, 179–185.

127. Fuentealba, C. and Hanna, P. (1996) Mange induced by *Trixacarus caviae* in a guinea pig. *Can. Vet. J.* **37**, 749–750.

128. Beck, W. and Wrieg, H-H. (1998) *Trixacarus caviae*-Räude (Acari: Sarcoptidae) beim Meerschiveinchev—Erregerbiologie, Pathogenese, Klinik, Diagnose and Therapie. *Kleintierpraxis* **43**, 703–708.

129. Perraki, M., Saridomichelakis, M., Koutinas, C., Koutinas, A., and Papazahariadou, M. (2002) A case of *Trixacarus caviae* mange in a guinea pig (*Cavia porcellus*). *J. Hellenic Vet. Med. Soc.* **53,** 352–357.

130. Shipstone, M. (1997) *Trixacarus caviae* infestation in a guinea pig: failure to respond to ivermectin administration. *Aust. Vet. Pract.* **27,** 143–146.

131. Thoday, K.L. and Beresford-Jones, W.P. (1977) The diagnosis and treatment of mange in the guinea-pig caused by *Trixacarus* (*Caviacoptes*) *caviae* (Fain, Hovell, and Hyatt, 1972). *J. Small Anim. Pract.* **18,** 591–595.

132. Dorrestein, G.M. and van Bronswijk, J.E.M.H. (1979) *Trixarcarus caviae* Fain, Howell, and Hyatt 1972 (Acari: Sarcoptidae) as a cause of mange in guinea-pigs and papular urticaria in man. *Vet. Parasitol.* **5,** 389–398.

133. Harvey, R.G. (1987) Use of ivermectin for guinea pig mange. *Vet. Rec.* **120,** 351.

134. Hirsjärvi, P. and Phyälä, L. (1994) Ivermectin treatment of a colony of guinea pigs infested with fur mite (*Chirodiscoides caviae*). *Lab. Anim.* **29,** 200–203.

135. McKellar, Q.A., Midgley, D.M., Galbraith, E.A., Scott, E.W., and Bradley, A. (1992) Clinical and pharmacological properties of ivermectin in rabbits and guinea pigs. *Vet. Rec.* **130,** 71–73.

136. Ackerman, L. (1987) *Trixacarus caviae* infestation in a guinea pig. *Can. Vet. J.* **28,** 613.

137. Zenoble, R.D. and Greve, J.H. (1980) Sarcoptid mite infestation in a colony of guinea pigs. *J. Am. Vet. Med. Assoc.* **177,** 898–900.

138. Henderson, J.D. (1973) Treatment of cutaneous acariasis in the guinea pig. *J. Am. Vet. Med. Assoc.* **163,** 591–592.

139. Hafeli, W. (1989) Demodikose beim Meerschweinchen. *Kleintierpraxis* **34,** 337–338.

140. Sutton, C.A. (1975) Contribucion al conocimiento de la fauna parasitaria Argentina II. *Neotropica* **21,** 72–74.

141. Kawazoe, U., Cordeiro, N., and Artigas, P. (1981) *Taxorchis caviae* sp. n. (Trematoda: Parasmphistomidae), parasito intestinal de *Cavia aperea aperea* Erxleben, 1777 (Rodentia, Caviidae). *Mem. Inst. Oswaldo Cruz* **76,** 1–13.

142. Sutton, C.A. (1981) Contribucion al conocimiento de la fauna parasitaria Argentina IX. Nuevo digeneo en el roedir *Cavia aperea pamparum* Thomas. *Neotropica* **27,** 105–111.

143. Sutton, C.A. (1976) Contribucion al conocimiento de la fauna parasitaria Argentina III. Endoparasitos de *Cavia aperea pamparum* Thomas. *Neotropica* **22,** 33–40.

144. Herrer, A. (1964) Chagas' disease in Peru. I. The epidemiological importance of the guinea pig. *Trop. Georgr. Med.* **16,** 146–151.

145. Hopkins, G.H.E. (1949) The host association of the lice of mammals. *Zool. Soc. London* **119,** 387–604.

146. de la Cruz, K.D., Ribbeck, R., and Daugshies, A. (2003) Vorkommen and Verbreitung von ecktoparasiten bei meerschweinchen (*Cavia* spp.) in Peru, Sudamerika. *Berl. Munch. Tierarztl. Wschr.* **116,** 102–107.

147. Bacigalupo, J. and Roveda, R.J. (1954) *Demodex caviae* n. sp. *Rev. Med. Vet.* **36,** 149–153.

CHAPTER

15

Parasites of Rabbits

Trenton R. Schoeb, DVM, PhD; Samuel C. Cartner, DVM, MPH, PhD;
Robert A. Baker, DVM; and Lauretta W. Gerrity, DVM

INTRODUCTION

The domestic rabbit (*Oryctolagus cuniculus*) continues to serve as an important model of several human diseases and conditions. Most laboratory rabbits are purchased from commercial vendors and housed under modern conditions that prevent exposure to parasites common to feral lagomorphs. However, feral animals may be brought into the animal facility, researchers may occasionally purchase animals from smaller, "backyard" production units, or feral animals may contaminate feed and bedding stocks used within the modern animal facility. Each of these may result in parasite entry into the animal facility.

PROTOZOA

Phylum Sarcomastigophora

Class Mastigophora (Flagellates)

Enteromonas sp.

Trophozoites of *Enteromonas* sp. are round or pyriform and have four flagella, three of which extend from the anterior pole[1]. The fourth flagellum extends posteriorly along the surface of the trophozoite. *Enteromonas hominis* occurs in the cecum of several species, including cottontail rabbits (*Sylvilagus* sp.), as well as man, other primates, rats, and hamsters[1]. An *Enteromonas* sp. is described from domestic rabbits (*Oryctolagus cuniculus*)[2].

Giardia duodenalis

Several species of *Giardia* have been named after the host species in which they were found. Others recognize only five morphologically distinguishable species. These include *Giardia duodenalis* (Syn. *G. intestinalis, G. lamblia*), which infects humans and other mammals; *G. muris* of rodents; *G. psittaci* and *G. ardeae,* both of which infect birds; and *G. agilis,* which is found in amphibians[3]. Genetic analyses reveal considerable heterogeneity within *G. duodenalis,* such that some genotypes eventually may be designated as distinct species[3].

Morphology. *Giardia* spp. trophozoites are flattened, piriform, and bilaterally symmetrical, with an adhesive disk on one side, two anterior nuclei, four pairs of flagella, and two axostyles[1]. *G. duodenalis* trophozoites are 9 μ to 21 μ long, 5 μ to 15 μ wide, and 2 μ to 4 μ thick. Cysts are oval, have four nuclei, and are 8 μ to 12 μ long and 7 μ to 10 μ wide.

Hosts. *Giardia duodenalis* occasionally is found in rabbits. It also infects many other mammalian species, including dogs and cats, and is worldwide in distribution. It is one of the most common enteric parasites of humans and a frequent cause of diarrheal disease[4].

Life Cycle. *Giardia duodenalis* inhabits the proximal small intestine, where trophozoites adhere to the epithelial surface. Cysts are passed in the feces, and new hosts become infected by ingestion of cysts, commonly via contaminated water, but also via food and soil.

Pathologic Effects and Clinical Disease. It is uncertain whether *G. duodenalis* is pathogenic for rabbits, but it has been associated with diarrheal disease and mortality in domestic rabbits in a few cases[5].

Diagnosis, Treatment, and Prevention. Trophozoites and cysts are demonstrable in fecal smears or flotations. Levine[1] recommends zinc sulfate for flotation to avoid distortion of the cysts, fixation with Schaudinn's fluid, and staining with iron hematoxylin. The organisms also can be demonstrated by immunohistochemical and molecular methods[1,6]. Metronidazole in the drinking water has been used successfully to treat infected rabbits[5]. Prevention is by sanitary measures to prevent contamination of water, food, and the environment with cysts. Water treatment by filtration and chlorination is effective, but malfunctions can allow contamination of municipal water supplies.

Public Health Considerations. *Giardia duodenalis* is a common human pathogen, but the infectivity for humans of genotypes from rabbits is not clear[4]. There are no reports of human infection acquired from rabbits.

Monocercomonas cuniculi

Monocercomonas spp. have piriform cell bodies, an axostyle, and four flagella, three of which extend anteriorly and one of which is trailing[1]. *Monocercomonas cuniculi* occurs in the cecum of domestic rabbits, is 5 μ to 14 μ long, and is nonpathogenic.

Retortamonas cuniculi

Retortamonas spp. have pyriform to fusiform cell bodies with two flagella, one of which extends anteriorly, the other posteriorly[1]. *Retortamonas cuniculi* (Syn. *Embadomonas cuniculi*) inhabits the cecum and is nonpathogenic. Trophozoites are 5 μ to 10 μ by 7 μ to 13 μ and cysts are 3 μ to 4 μ by 5 μ to 7 μ.

Trypanosoma nabiasi

Trypanosoma nabiasi is a hemoflagellate found occasionally in wild European rabbits, but is very unlikely to occur in laboratory rabbits[5]. Trypomastigote forms measure 24 μm to 28 μm long. Cyclic development occurs in the flea, *Spilopsyllus cuniculi*.

Class Sarcodina (Amoebae)

Entamoeba cuniculi

Entamoeba cuniculi is a nonpathogenic commensal amoeba of the cecum and colon of rabbits throughout the world[1,5]. Morphologically it is similar to *Entamoeba muris*. The interested reader is directed to Chapter 11, Parasites of Rats and Mice for additional information. Trophozoites are 10 μ to 30 μ in diameter. Cysts have eight nuclei and are 7 μ to 21 μ in diameter.

Phylum Apicomplexa

Besnoitia oryctofelisi

The life cycle of *Besnoitia* spp. is associated with a predator-prey relationship. Definitive hosts of *Besnoitia* spp. are felids, and the intermediate hosts include a wide variety of prey species such as cattle, horses, goats, wildebeest, kudu, impala, opossums, rats, mice, and others[1]. The life cycle is similar to that of *Toxoplasma gondii,* and no disease occurs in definitive hosts. Cysts in tissues of intermediate hosts are large, have a thick wall, and have enlarged host cell nuclei at the periphery. *Besnoitia oryctofelisi* is reported from domestic rabbits in Argentina[7]. Infection with an unidentified *Besnoita* sp. was found in a domestic rabbit in Kenya that died suddenly and had suppurative bronchopneumonia[8]. Cysts measuring 127 μ to 185 μ in diameter were found in areas of the lungs not affected by bronchopneumonia and were associated with a mild mononuclear inflammatory reaction.

Cryptosporidium sp.

Morphology. Protozoa of the genus *Cryptosporidium* are intracellular extracytoplasmic parasites of the gastrointestinal tract. Replicative stages are located within the microvillus border of the host cell and protrude above its surface, rather than being located in the cytoplasm beneath the cell surface as is typical of coccidia in general[9]. Cryptosporidial oocysts contain four sporozoites, which are not contained within sporocysts[10]. Oocysts of *Cryptosporidium* spp. of mammals are similar in size and shape, ranging from 4.6 μ long by 4 μ wide (*C. felis*) to 8.4 μ long by 6.2 μ wide (*C. muris*)[11]. Dimensions of oocysts of rabbit cryptosporidia have not been reported.

Intracellular stages of rabbit *Cryptosporidium* have been described[12]. Light and electron microscopic features of *C. parvum* recently were reviewed[13], and excellent transmission electron micrographs have been published showing the intracellular stages of the life cycle and the characteristic "feeder" organelle[9].

Hosts. The species of *Cryptosporidium* that infects lagomorphs is not known, because the taxonomy of the cryptosporidia is unsettled and because most reports of cryptosporidia in rabbits appeared before the availability of molecular techniques. Based on genetic analysis, morphology, and host range, Xiao and co-workers[10] consider 13 species to be valid. Recently, a novel genotype was reported from European rabbits[14], suggesting the existence of a species or host-adapted strain specific for rabbits. The rabbit genotype was closely related to *C. hominis, C. meleagridis,* and other cryptosporidia known to affect humans. *Cryptosporidium* sp. infection has been reported in laboratory rabbits and a cottontail rabbit in the United States and in European rabbits[12-16].

Life Cycle. The life cycle of cryptosporidia of rabbits has not been described; however, it is presumed to be similar to that of *C. parvum*, which has been studied extensively[9]. Briefly, sporozoites released from ingested oocysts invade intestinal epithelial cells and undergo two generations of merogony. Second-generation merozoites develop into sexual stages which fuse to produce zygotes, which mature into unsporulated oocysts. Oocysts undergo two internal divisions to form four sporozoites each. The oocyst wall develops while still in the parasitophorous vacuole. About 20% of the oocysts are thin-walled and are capable of autoinfection, which is believed to allow the organism to persist in the host. The remaining thick-walled, environmentally resistant oocysts are shed in the feces and are infectious for new hosts.

Pathologic Effects. Intestinal lesions in most host species follow a pattern which includes loss of enterocytes and villus atrophy and fusion, accompanied by lamina propria edema and infiltration by inflammatory cells, which can be mixed or primarily mononuclear[9]. In rabbits, changes in the intestinal mucosa are minimal, and include a slightly decreased villus to crypt ratio, loss of microvilli from enterocytes where the organisms attached, and slight lamina propria edema (Figures 15.1 and 15.2)[12,15]. A broiler rabbit with diarrhea had villus atrophy[16].

Clinical Disease. Domestic rabbits in which *Cryptosporidium* sp. infection was identified were clinically normal[12,15]. Cryptosporidia have been identified in rabbits with diarrhea or other signs, but other possible etiologic agents also were present, making the role of *Cryptosporidium* infection impossible to determine with certainty[17]. Diarrheal disease in broiler rabbits in the Czech Republic was attributed to *C. parvum*[16]. The duration of illness was three to five days, and was accompanied by anorexia, lethargy, and dehydration.

Diagnosis. Methods for diagnosis of *Cryptosporidium* sp. infection have been published[18]. In laboratory animals, the diagnosis usually is based on histologic examination of the intestine. When numerous, oocysts are demonstrable in fecal wet mounts, but, in general, specimens should be concentrated by flotation. Staining of such preparations by methods such as Giemsa, safranin-methylene blue, Kinyoun, Ziehl-Neelsen, and DMSO-carbol fuchsin enhances visibility of oocysts. Immunofluorescent techniques also are used, but do not differentiate among oocysts of different cryptosporidia. Serologic methods such as ELISA also do not differentiate among cryptosporidia, but are useful to

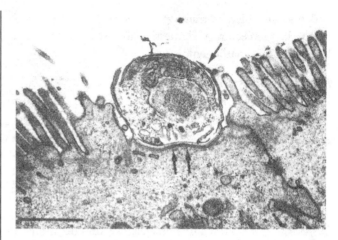

Fig. 15.2 *Cryptosporidium* sp. trophozoite within microvillus border, showing attachment zone (double arrows) and enveloping host cell membrane (single arrow). Bar = 1 μ. Reproduced from Rehg, J.E., Lawton, G.W., and Pakes, S.P. (1979) with permission.

assess exposure. Various polymerase chain reaction-based methods have been developed and have the advantage of both sensitive detection and specific identification[18–20].

Treatment. There is currently no treatment known to be effective against *Cryptosporidium* sp. infection in rabbits, but, because most reported cases have been subclinical, treatment is generally unwarranted. In the event of clinical disease, supportive therapy to maintain hydration and electrolyte balance probably would be sufficient.

Prevention. Prevention is by adherence to sanitary practices, which interrupt fecal-oral transmission of infectious oocysts. Oocysts may be widely distributed in the environment because of the broad host species distribution of cryptosporidia, the large numbers of oocysts shed during active infection, and the resistance of oocysts to environmental conditions and common disinfectants[9,18]. Waterborne transmission is a significant risk, because oocysts can find their way into water supplies, and only small numbers of oocysts are necessary to establish infection.

Public Health Considerations. Animals, especially calves, are frequent sources of human infection[9] but cryptosporidiosis acquired from rabbits has not been reported.

Eimeria stiedae

Morphology. Oocysts of *Eimeria* spp. have four sporocysts, each of which contains two sporozoites[1] (Figure 15.3). *Eimeria stiedae* oocysts are elongated ovoid or ellipsoidal, and measure 28 μ to 42 μ by 16 μ to 25 μ with a 6-μ to 10-μ micropyle[1,5] (Figure 15.4). The wall is smooth and colorless to red-orange. An oocyst residuum is present,

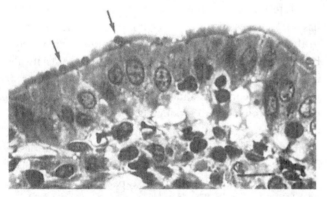

Fig. 15.1 *Cryptosporidium* sp. infection, small intestine. Organisms in microvillus border (arrows). Bar = 125 μ. Reproduced from Rehg, J.E., Lawton, G.W., and Pakes, S.P. (1979) with permission.

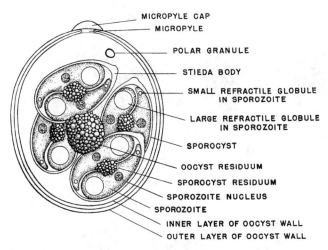

MICROPYLE CAP
MICROPYLE
POLAR GRANULE
STIEDA BODY
SMALL REFRACTILE GLOBULE
IN SPOROZOITE
LARGE REFRACTILE GLOBULE
IN SPOROZOITE
SPOROCYST
OOCYST RESIDUUM
SPOROCYST RESIDUUM
SPOROZOITE NUCLEUS
SPOROZOITE
INNER LAYER OF OOCYST WALL
OUTER LAYER OF OOCYST WALL

Fig. 15.3 Structure of sporulated *Eimeria* sp. oocyst. Reproduced from Levine, N.D. (1961) with permission.

but is small and difficult to see among the sporocysts. Sporocysts are 8 μ to 10 μ by 17 μ to 18 μ and contain a Stieda body.

Hosts. *Eimeria stiedae* (Syn. *M. stiedae, Coccidum oviforme, C. cuniculi, Psorospermium cuniculi*)[1] is common in domestic rabbits throughout the world, and also is reported from cottontail rabbits and hares[1,5]. Laboratory rabbits raised according to modern standards are generally free of the organism, but cases occasionally are reported[25].

Life Cycle. Ingested sporulated oocysts excyst in the duodenum. Sporozoites enter the intestinal mucosa and are carried to the liver by the portal veins, lymphatics, or both, possibly intracellularly in lymphatic monocytes. Upon reaching the liver, the sporozoites enter biliary epithelial cells, where they undergo an unknown number of generations of schizogony. Developing schizonts are evident three to six days after infection. Mature schizonts are 15 μ to 18 μ in diameter. Gametogeny can be evident by 11 days after infection. After the onset of gametogeny, developing and mature microgametes, macrogametes, and schizonts all are present concurrently. After fertilization, macrogametes develop an oocyst wall and exit the biliary epithelium and the liver. They then enter the intestine in the bile, pass out of the host, and undergo sporulation. The prepatent period is 14 to 18 days, and the patent period is 21 to 37 days[1,5].

Pathologic Effects. In severely affected rabbits, the liver is enlarged and all lobes contain discrete, yellow-gray bosselated or nodular lesions up to 2 cm in diameter (Figure 15.5). These are elevated above the capsular surface and tend to have a cord-like and sometimes tortuous

pattern. On the cut surface, these lesions are evident throughout the hepatic parenchyma and are hollow and filled with bile or inspissated exudate and debris. Depending on severity and duration, affected bile ducts can be fibrotic and difficult to cut. The gall bladder also can be affected. Ascites occurs occasionally. Lesions are correspondingly less severe in mildly affected rabbits.

Microscopic changes in the bile ducts and gall bladder are highly characteristic. The epithelium undergoes dramatic papilliferous hyperplasia, with numerous developing and mature schizonts, gametocytes, and oocysts within epithelial cells (Figure 15.6). Affected ducts often are distended, and the lumina contain oocysts, cell debris, and inflammatory cells. The inflammatory response is primarily lymphyocytic and plasmacytic, but in some cases there are significant numbers of neutrophils and macrophages. In severely affected ducts, mucosal destruction can result in leakage of the contents, which provokes severe granulomatous inflammation. In severe cases of sufficient duration, there can be a pronounced fibrotic response around affected ducts.

Mild peribiliary lymphoplasmacytic inflammation is common in domestic rabbits in which *E. stiedae* parasitism is not evident. Whether this represents resolved or treated infection is unclear.

Changes in serum components, including globulins, lipoproteins, enzymes, and bilirubin, are reported in hepatic coccidiosis. Metabolic acidosis[26] and vitamin E deficiency[27] have been reported in experimental disease.

Clinical Disease. Clinical signs are variable. Subclinical disease is common. Severe disease, which is more common in younger rabbits, is characterized by anorexia, lethargy, diarrhea, abdominal enlargement due to hepatomegaly, and icterus. The enlarged liver can comprise up to 20% of the body weight. Death can occur in young rabbits with very severe disease. Older rabbits are resistant.

Diagnosis. *Eimeria stiedae* infection can be detected by examining fecal specimens for oocysts in direct smears or flotations. However, oocysts may not be present in the feces in acute infection, and care must be taken in identifying oocysts, because those of some other *Eimeria* spp. of rabbits are similar. Demonstration of oocysts in bile at necropsy or of characteristic lesions with intraepithelial forms by histopathologic examination is definitive. Serologic tests have been developed but are not routinely used[5].

Treatment. Sulfonamides such as sulfamerazine and sulfaquinoxaline are widely used coccidiostats and are

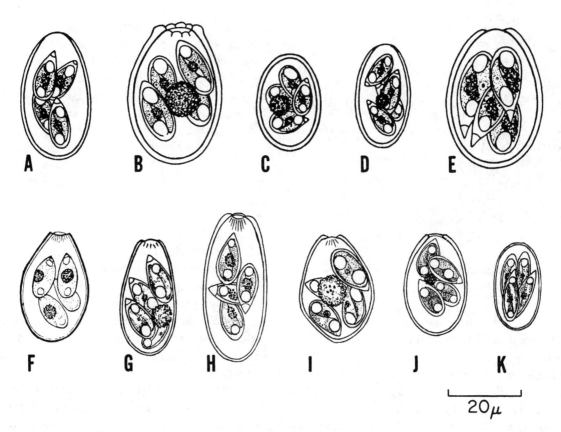

Fig. 15.4 *Eimeria* of the rabbit (sporulated oocysts). (A) *E. stiedae.* (B) *E. magna.* (C) *E. perforans.* (D) *E. media.* (E) *E. irresidua.* (F) *E. piriformis.* (G) *E. coecicola.* (H) *E. elongata.* (I) *E. intestinalis.* (J) *E. matsubayashii.* (K) *E. nagpurensis.* (A),(B),(C),(D),(E) reproduced from Carvalho, J.C.M. (1942); (F) reproduced from Kheisin, E.M. (1948); and (G),(H),(I),(J),(K) reproduced from Gill, B.S. and Ray, H.N. (1960) with permission.

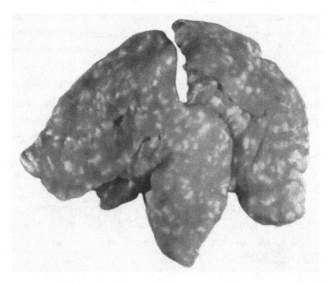

Fig. 15.5 Chronic proliferative cholangitis caused by *E. stiedae.* Courtesy of J.E. Harkness, Mississippi State University.

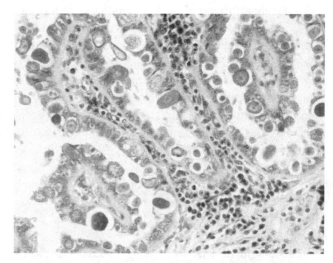

Fig. 15.6 Proliferated biliary epithelium with numerous intracellular *E. stiedae* forms and lymphoplasmacytic inflammatory cell response. Hematoxylin and eosin stain. Courtesy of J.E. Harkness, Mississippi State University.

effective inhibitors of *E. stiedai* at dosages of 0.02% to 0.10% in the drinking water or 0.03% to 1% in the feed[5]. Such treatments prevent disease and allow immunity to develop, which renders rabbits resistant to challenge. Other drugs reported to be effective include monensin, salinomycin, maduramycin, α-difluoromethylornithine, toltrazuril, methyl benzoquate and clopidol in combination, and narasin[23, 28–32].

Prevention. Control of hepatic coccidiosis is by preventing exposure to oocysts in feces or contaminated food or water[5]. Important measures include use of cages designed to facilitate efficient removal of droppings, frequent and thorough cleaning of cages and feeding and watering equipment with hot water and detergent, controlling vermin such as flies that could serve as mechanical vectors, educating personnel regarding the need for cleanliness and the risk of mechanical transmission by caretakers, and removing susceptible young rabbits from infected mothers as soon as possible.

Control is complicated by the resistance of oocysts to commonly used disinfectants, the difficulty of completely eliminating oocysts from the environment, shedding of oocysts from infected rabbits, and the direct life cycle of the organism. For these reasons prophylaxis with coccidiostats is a common practice. Rabbits free of *E. stiedae* are produced in colonies maintained according to strict barrier procedures. It is possible to substantially increase resistance by immunization[33]. However, no commercial vaccine is available.

Public Health Considerations. *Eimeria stiedae* does not infect humans.

Eimeria spp.

Morphology. More than a dozen *Eimeria* spp. are reported from the intestine of rabbits[1,5]. Distinguishing morphologic features of the oocysts of intestinal *Eimeria* spp. of rabbits are given in Table 15.1.

Hosts. Intestinal coccidia are common in wild and domestic *O. cuniculus* rabbits worldwide[5,34,35]. Intestinal coccidia also are common among cottontail rabbits and hares[36,37]. However, with the possible exception of *E. neoleporis*, it appears that intestinal coccidia of lagomorphs are host specific and that transmission to hosts of different genera does not occur[5].

Life Cycle. Oocysts passed in the feces undergo sporogony and become infective. Ingested infective oocysts release sporozoites in the intestine, where they invade the epithelium and undergo schizogony. Gametogony occurs after a number of generations of schizogony characteristic of each species. Fertilized macrogametes develop into oocysts, which are released from the host cells and passed from the host.

Pathologic Effects. Effects of coccidial infection vary[5]. In many cases the organisms provoke little or no reaction (Figure 15.7). In susceptible rabbits infected with virulent *Eimeria* spp., there can be extensive necrosis of epithelial cells, with edema, hemorrhage, and a mixed inflammatory cell response including neutrophils, macrophages, and lymphocytes. Affected areas can be grossly visible as multiple pale foci in the mucosa.

Clinical Disease. Severity of intestinal coccidiosis varies according to host susceptibility, infecting dose, and coccidial species. Infection with more than one *Eimeria* species is common. Many infections are subclinical[5]. In young rabbits, infection with more virulent *Eimeria* spp. can cause weight loss or failure to gain weight; diarrhea, which can be watery and bloody; dehydration; and death. In extreme cases, death can occur before oocysts are present in the feces.

Diagnosis. Diagnosis is by examination of fecal specimens, as described for *E. stiedae*, and by histologic examination of intestine.

Treatment. Treatments for *E. stiedae* generally are applicable to intestinal coccidia. Harkness and Wagner[38] recommend as coccidiostats sulfaquinoxaline (0.04% in water or 125 to 250 ppm in feed), sulfamethazine (0.077% in water or 0.5 to 1% in feed), sulfadimethoxine (75 to 100 mg/kg body weight), monensin (20 to 40 ppm in feed), decoquinate (62.5 ppm in feed), Rofenaid® (sulfadimethoxine + ormetoprim; 62.5 to 250 ppm in feed), lasalocid (120 ppm in feed), and diclazuril (1 ppm in feed). Polozowski[39] reported that salinomycin (25 to 50 ppm in feed), maduramycin (2 to 3 ppm), Lerbek® (clopidol + methylbenzoquate; 216.7 ppm), lasalocid (90 to 125 ppm), monensin (20 ppm), and robenidine (66 ppm) were highly effective in treating farmed rabbits in Europe that were infected with up to nine *Eimeria* species. Production was best in rabbits given salinomycin or maduramycin (2 ppm or 3 ppm). Narasin and maduramycin at 4.5 ppm was toxic, and robenidine was not effective against *E. stiedae*. Vanparijs and co-workers[40] recommend continuous treatment with 1 ppm diclazuril.

Prevention. Prevention is by the same measures as those for *E. stiedae*. McPherson and co-workers[41] reported eliminating intestinal *Eimeria* spp. from a breeding colony by rigorous sanitation, treatment with sulfaquinoxaline, and testing for infection and removing infected rabbits.

TABLE 15.1 Oocyst Morphology of Intestinal *Emeria* Species of Rabbits[1,5,34,184].

Species	Dimensions (μ)	Shape	Wall	Micropyle	Residual body
E. coccicola	23–40 × 15–21 (ave. 29 × 18)	Ellipsoid	Light yellow	Prominent	Variable
E. elongata	35–40 × 17–20	Elongate ellipsoid	Light gray	Prominent	None
E. exigua	12–21 × 10–18 (ave. 15 × 13)	Ovoid	Colorless	None	None
E. flavescens	25–37 × 14–24 (ave. 32 × 21)	Broad ellipsoid	Light yellow, bilayered	Prominent	None
E. intestinalis	21–36 × 15–21 (ave. 27 × 18)	Ellipsoid, piriform, or ovoid	Light yellow to light brown	Present	Large, granular
E. irresidua	35–42 × 19–28 (ave. 38 × 26)	Ovoid to ellipsoid	Light yellow, bilayered	Prominent	Small, variable
E. magna	27–41 × 17–29 (ave. 35 × 24)	Ovoid to ellipsoid	Dark yellow, orange, or brown; bilayered	Prominent, lipped	Large
E. matsubayashii	22–29 × 16–22 (ave. 25 × 18)	Ovoid	Light yellow	Present	Variable
E. media	19–37 × 13–22 (ave. 31 × 18)	Ovoid to ellipsoid	Light pink, thick	Present	Large
E. nagpurensis	20–27 × 10–15 (ave. 23 × 13)	Barrel-like	Colorless	None	None
E. neoleporis	33–44 × 16–23 (ave. 39 × 20)	Elongate ellipsoid	Light pink to yellow, bilayered	Present	Usually none
E. perforans	15–30 × 11–20 (ave. 21 × 15)	Ellipsoid	Colorless to light pink, bilayered	Indistinct	Small
E. piriformis	26–33 × 15–21	Piriform	Yellow-brown to dark brown, bilayered	Prominent	None
E. roobroucki	—	—	—	—	—
E. vejdovskyi	Ave. 29 × 18	—	—	—	—

458

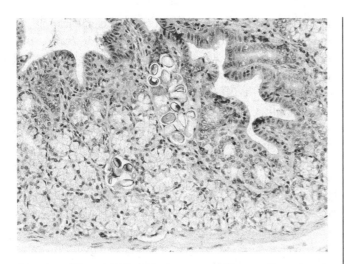

Fig. 15.7 *Eimeria* sp. in colonic mucosa. Hematoxylin and eosin stain. Courtesy of J.E. Harkness, Mississippi State University.

Public Health Considerations. *Eimeria* spp. of rabbits do not infect humans.

Hepatozoon cuniculi

Asexual stages of *Hepatozoon* (syn. *Leukocytogregarina*) spp. occur in the liver or other visceral organs of a vertebrate host, gametes develop in erythrocytes or leukocytes, and fertilization and sporogony occur in hematophagous arthropods[1]. There is one report from Italy of *Hepatozoon* sp. infection in domestic rabbits, in which gametocytes were found in leukocytes and schizonts in the spleen[5].

Sarcocystis cuniculi

Morphology. The morphologic features of *Sarcocystis* sp. oocysts are presented in Chapter 18, Parasites of Cats. In the rabbit, tissue cysts can be up to 5 mm long and can be grossly visible in affected muscle. Compartmentalization by thin internal septa is evident microscopically. Immature cysts contain round metrocytes 4 μ to 5 μ in diameter, whereas mature cysts contain curved, fusiform bradyzoites 11 μ to 16 μ long and 4 μ to 6 μ wide.

Hosts. *Sarcocystis cuniculi* infection occurs worldwide and is common in wild rabbits, but it is rare in domestic rabbits and has not been reported in laboratory rabbits[1,5].

Life Cycle. Felids are the definitive hosts of *S. cuniculi*. Rabbits become infected by ingestion of infective oocysts in cat feces. Sarcocysts develop in striated muscle and become infective for cats after about three months. Transmission to cats is via preying upon or scavenging infected rabbits.

Pathologic Effects. Sarcocysts occur in cardiac and skeletal muscle (Figures 15.8 and 15.9), in which they appear grossly as narrow pale streaks oriented parallel to the myofibers, although in mild infections they may not be readily visible. Intact cysts do not induce an inflammatory response. However, those that rupture or degenerate provoke severe myocarditis or myositis adjacent to the cysts, with accumulation of mixed inflammatory cells including lymphocytes, plasma cells, macrophages, and eosinophils, and with mineralization of degenerated myofibers. The lesions heal by scarring.

Clinical Disease. Infections in rabbits are usually subclinical, although severe infection can induce lameness[5].

Diagnosis, Treatment, and Prevention. In most cases the diagnosis is based on typical gross lesions with confirmation by histopathologic findings[5]. *Sarcocystis cuniculi* sarcocysts usually are septate and the wall contains densely packed fine projections visible at high magnification. Organisms can be demonstrated in smears of fresh muscle by phase microscopy or Giemsa staining. Treatment of *S. cuniculi* infection in rabbits has not been reported. Prevention is by sanitary husbandry practices to prevent exposure to cat feces.

Public Health Considerations. Human infection with *S. cuniculi* has not been reported.

Sarcocystis leporum

Sarcocystis leporum infection is common in cottontail rabbits[5]. Sexual stages occur in cats and raccoons[42]. The sarcocysts of *S. leporum* are similar to those of *S. cuniculis*[43]. The two organisms have been considered synonymous,

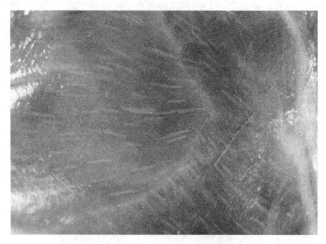

Fig. 15.8 Sarcocystosis, skeletal muscle. Pale streaks are grossly visible sarcocysts. Courtesy of J.E. Harkness, Mississippi State University.

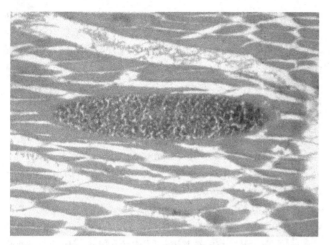

Fig. 15.9 *Sarcocystis* sp. cyst in skeletal muscle. Hematoxylin and eosin stain. Courtesy of J.E. Harkness, Mississippi State University.

but sporocysts from cats fed muscle from infected cottontail rabbits are not infective for domestic rabbits[42].

Toxoplasma gondii

Morphology. Morphologic characteristics of *Toxoplasma gondii* are presented in Chapter 18, Parasites of Cats.

Hosts. The interested reader is directed to Chapter 18, Parasites of Cats, for information on the host range of *T. gondii*. Briefly, definitive hosts are domestic and wild felids[1]. Intermediate hosts include numerous species of birds and mammals, including rabbits[1]. Toxoplasmosis in domestic rabbits was first reported in the early 1900s[5]. It has since been reported in rabbits from various locations around the world, and results of serologic surveys have suggested that subclinical infections were prevalent. There are only two reports of the disease in domestic rabbits in the United States[44,45], and no reports of toxoplasmosis in laboratory rabbits. Domestic rabbits may be relatively resistant, because they have been reported to develop only subclinical infection after experimental inoculation, whereas hares developed severe disseminated disease[46]. However, significant losses have occurred among domestic rabbits in Europe[47]. It is possible that experimental manipulation could activate latent infection[5].

Life Cycle. Rabbits become infected through ingestion of sporulated oocysts in cat feces. Parasitemia persists until circulating antibodies develop. Multiplication in sites of dissemination continues until the host dies or develops an effective immune response, in which case tachyzoites disappear, leaving bradyzoites in cysts. Cysts differ in persistence among different organs. They can persist in the brain and perhaps myocardium and skeletal muscle for long periods, possibly years, but disappear from other organs more rapidly. Cysts can contain many thousands of tightly packed bradyzoites and be up to 100 μ in diameter.

Pathologic Effects. Acute disseminated toxoplasmosis in rabbits is characterized by multifocal necrosis of affected organs[5,44,45]. Very acute lesions may lack an inflammatory cell response. The most prominent lesions occur in the spleen, lymph nodes, lungs, liver, and heart. Multiple pale foci of necrosis may be evident in the spleen, liver, and lungs. The spleen can be so severely affected as to be almost totally necrotic. Intra- and extracellular tachyzoites can be numerous in organs such as the lymph nodes and spleen. Acute severe disease is more frequent in young rabbits, whereas in older rabbits the course of the disease may be more prolonged. In such cases, inflammatory cell accumulation in lesions becomes increasingly prominent and can eventually become granulomatous, and contain progressively fewer organisms. Rabbits that recover have latent infection characterized by cysts primarily in the brain. There may be no reaction to the cysts, or there may be multifocal gliosis, granulomatous inflammation, and lymphocytic accumulations in the meninges and around blood vessels. Such lesions are similar to those of encephalitozoonosis.

Clinical Disease. Clinical toxoplasmosis is rare in rabbits. Reported clinical signs include fever, lethargy, oculonasal discharge, convulsions, tremors, ataxia, paraplegia, and quadraplegia[5]. Death can occur suddenly or within several days after the onset of signs. Some affected rabbits have recovered.

Diagnosis. In most cases, the diagnosis can be established from the type and distribution of lesions and the morphology and staining characteristics of the organisms. Transmission electron microscopic examination of affected tissues also can be helpful. In acute severe disease, the organisms may be demonstrable in smears of peritoneal inflammatory cells stained with Wright-Giemsa. *T. gondii* can be cultivated from affected tissues in cell culture or by intraperitoneal inoculation of cortisone-treated mice[48]. The organism also can be identified in tissues by immunohistochemistry[49] or polymerase chain reaction[50]. Serologic methods that have been used to test rabbit serum samples for antibodies to *T. gondii* include the Sabin-Feldman dye test, indirect immunofluorescence, and carbon immunoassay, but these rarely are used.

Treatment. Treatment of laboratory rabbits is generally not warranted. However, drugs such as tetracyclines, dihydrotriazones, pyrimethamine, sulfadiazine, and spiramycin have been used to treat human toxoplasmosis. Currently, combination therapy with sulfadiazine, pyrimethamine, and folinic acid is most commonly used and considered most effective[51].

Prevention. Toxoplasmosis is prevented by housing and husbandry practices that prevent contamination of facilities, equipment, food, and water with cat feces, including personnel education regarding hygiene practices to prevent introduction of oocysts from pet cats. Oocysts are resistant to many disinfectants, but are killed by heating and drying[5].

Public Health Considerations. *Toxoplasma gondii* infection is a significant health risk for pregnant women and AIDS patients[1,52]. However, the likelihood of acquiring the disease from laboratory rabbits is extremely low, because personnel would have to consume infected rabbit tissues.

Phylum Microspora

Encephalitozoon cuniculi

Morphology. Individual *Encephalitozoon cuniculi* (Syn. *Nosema cuniculi*) spores are 1.5 μ to 2 μ by 2.5 μ to 4 μ; oval, flattened on one side, or slightly curved; thick-walled; and have eccentric nuclei[5]. Characteristic of microsporidia, *E. cuniculi* spores have a polar filament coiled within the inner wall[53]. The polar filament can be seen by phase microscopic examination of wet mounts. Some spores may spontaneously extrude the filament, and the sporoplasm may be evident at the end of the filament. Treatments such as ether, hydrogen peroxide, or heat can induce extrusion of the filament.

Hosts. *Encephalitozoon cuniculi* occurs in wild and domestic mammals of many species throughout the world, including rabbits, mice, rats, hamsters, guinea pigs, dogs, foxes, cats, horses, pigs, squirrel monkeys, tamarins, and humans[54]. It is not present in most populations of specific pathogen-free rabbits, but is common in conventionally raised domestic rabbits. Rhesus monkeys have been experimentally infected with *E. cuniculi* from rabbits[55]. Serologic evidence suggests that infection also occurs in cattle[56] and goats[57], and the organism has been found in chicken embryos[58].

Isolates of *E. cuniculi* have been assigned to strains, based on the number of tetranucleotide repeats in the internal transcribed spacer region of the ribosomal RNA gene, and into karyotypes, based on variations in electrophoretically determined chromosome sizes[54]. Different strains have distinct host distributions. Strain I ("rabbit strain"), which includes karyotypes A, B, and C, infects rabbits, mice, and humans. Strain II ("mouse strain") occurs in mice and blue foxes, and includes karyotype F. Strain III ("dog strain") parasitizes domestic dogs and humans, and includes karyotypes D and E.

Life Cycle. Following infection, spores that come in contact with host cells extrude the polar filament through the host cell membrane, followed by expulsion of the sporoplast into the host cell[53]. The sporoplast proliferates and gives rise to meronts within a parasitophorous vacuole. Meronts differentiate into sporoblasts, which become sporonts and finally mature spores. Spores are discharged from the enlarging parasitophorous vacuole by rupture of the host cell, and may infect adjacent cells or be disseminated by the vascular system. New hosts become infected by ingestion, or possibly inhalation, of mature spores shed in excreta. In carnivores, transmission probably also occurs by consumption of infected prey.

The primary mode of transmission of *E. cuniculi* among rabbits is by ingestion of spores shed in the urine[5]. Rabbits can be infected by experimental inoculation via oral and other routes. It is unclear whether the organisms undergo initial multiplication in intestinal epithelial cells, but the organisms soon appear in many tissues. For the first 30 days after inoculation, they are most numerous in the kidneys, liver, and lungs; later, they are found mostly in the kidneys, brain, and heart[59]. Serum antibodies develop within three weeks after inoculation, but shedding can persist for 60 days.

Transplacental transmission of *E. cuniculi* has been documented in rabbits, mice, dogs, foxes, horses, and squirrel monkeys[54,60], and may also occur in guinea pigs[61]. The frequency of vertical transmission is unclear, but probably is less frequent in mildly affected hosts such as rabbits and more common in severely affected hosts such as dogs and foxes.

Pathologic Effects. The kidneys of infected rabbits commonly have multifocal, pale, slightly depressed foci that measure from pinpoint to a few mm in diameter in the capsular surfaces[5,59] (Figure 15.10). In acute disease, lesions may not be depressed and may be hemorrhagic. The microscopic features of the lesions include necrosis; pyogranulomatous, lymphocytic, and plasmacytic inflammation; and tubular loss with scarring, depending on their age (Figure 15.11). Surface incision reveals pale, linear, radiating streaks. In the brain, multifocal

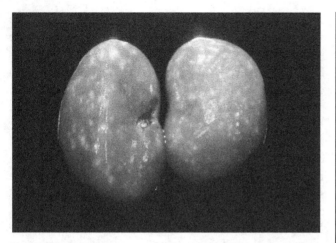

Fig. 15.10   Encephalitozoonosis lesions in capsular surface of kidneys.

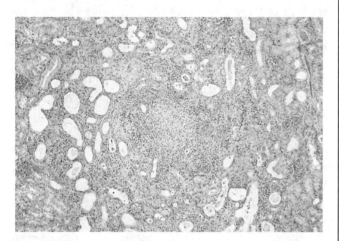

Fig. 15.11   Chronic tubulointerstitial nephritis in encephalitozoonosis. Hematoxylin and eosin stain.

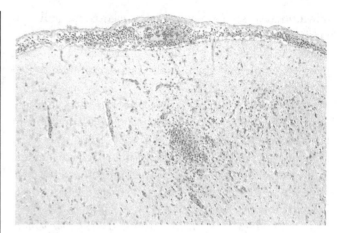

Fig. 15.12   Granulomatous encephalitis with lymphoplasmacytic leptomeningitis in encephalitozoonosis, cerebrum. Hematoxylin and eosin stain.

pyogranulomatous or granulomatous encephalitis, with perivascular and leptomeningeal accumulation of lymphocytes and plasma cells, is characteristic (Figure 15.12). Any part of the brain can be affected, but lesions are most prominent in the cerebral cortex and periventricular areas. Older lesions may be characterized only by glial nodules. Lesions in organs other than the brain and kidneys are uncommon. Organisms are most readily found in the brain and kidneys, but only in early stages of the disease.

Clinical Disease. Infection in rabbits usually is subclinical, but overt disease occasionally occurs[62]. Signs are neurological, and include ataxia, tremors, paresis, hyperesthesia, opisthotonos, torticollis, convulsions, and paralysis. One report describes an apparent epizootic of severe encephalitozoonosis that occurred after introduction of new rabbits into a rabbitry[63].

Diagnosis. Post-mortem diagnosis of encephalitozoonosis in rabbits is straightforward. Lesions are characteristic and sufficient for a presumptive diagnosis. Confirmation by use of special stains to demonstrate the organisms in tissue sections is adequate for routine diagnostic purposes. Organisms are difficult to locate in hematoxylin and eosin (HE) stained sections, but are easily identified using Brown and Brenn (Gram), Giemsa, and Goodpasture's carbol fuchsin stains (Figure 15.13). These stains also help differentiate encephalitozoonosis from toxoplasmosis, which is rare in domestic rabbits[44,45]. *Toxoplasma gondii* stains negative with Gram stain, and is not stained with Goodpasture's carbol fuchsin. In addition, *T. gondii* cysts have a distinct wall, whereas *E. cuniculi* pseudocysts do not. Differentiation of encephalitozoonosis from toxoplasmosis is described in detail by Shadduck and Pakes[64].

Serologic methods for detecting *E. cuniculi* antibodies have been reported, including indirect fluorescence antibody (IFA), carbon immunoassay, complement fixation, immunoperoxidase, indirect microagglutination, and enzyme-linked immunosorbent assay (ELISA) techniques[65]. Monitoring rabbit populations for *E. cuniculi* infection by serologic means was not widely practiced prior to availability of commercial testing, but inexpensive serologic testing using ELISA methods now is readily available commercially.

Other methods that have been used include a skin test; identification of spores by immunofluorescence, immunohistochemistry, or chitin-binding fluorescent dyes; and mouse inoculation[66]. *Encephalitozoon cuniculi*

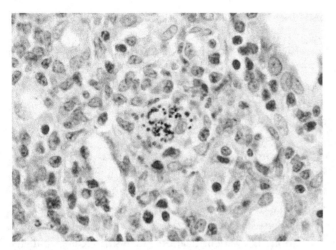

Fig. 15.13 *Encephalitozoon cuniculi* organisms in renal lesion. Brown and Brenn stain.

also can be isolated and grown in cell cultures[67]. Electron microscopy frequently is used to distinguish various microsporidia in human infections[59]. Highly sensitive and specific detection and identification of *E. cuniculi* can be accomplished using polymerase chain reaction (PCR) methods[60]. With appropriate sample preparation, PCR methods can be applied to samples of urine, feces, fresh or fixed embedded tissue, and cultured cells that contain the organism.

Treatment. Little information is available regarding treatment of encephalitozoonosis in rabbits, and treatment is unlikely to be indicated in a laboratory setting. In a trial in which serologically positive rabbits were given fenbendazole in the feed for four weeks, *E. cuniculi* was isolated from the brains of control rabbits but not from those of treated rabbits[68]. However, responses of pet rabbits to fenbendazole and albendazole have been variable[62].

Prevention. *Encephalitozoon*-free rabbits are commercially available, and are protected from re-infection by preventing exposure to viable spores in excreta of infected animals or contaminated environments. This is accomplished by adherence to building and husbandry standards that preclude contamination. Chlorination is effective against *E. cuniculi* in water[69]. Spores are susceptible to common disinfectants[70]. Thus, careful sanitation greatly reduces the likelihood of exposure to viable spores. Regular monitoring by serologic testing should be conducted to assure continued *E. cuniculi*-free status.

Elimination of *E. cuniculi* from breeding colonies may be achieved by combining sanitation measures with frequent serologic testing and eliminating seropositive rabbits. Breeding stock also can be obtained by Cesarean rederivation. Because of the possibility of transplacental transmission, rederived rabbits should be thoroughly tested by serologic methods or urine polymerase chain reaction assay.

Public Health Considerations. Microsporidia now are known to be significant opportunistic pathogenic fungi affecting immunosuppressed individuals. At least a dozen or more species have been identified. Of these, *E. cuniculi* appears to be among the most virulent. Zoonotic transmission from rabbits has not been reported, but without evidence to the contrary the possibility must be considered.

Enterocytozoon bieneusi

Enterocytozoon bieneusi has been demonstrated in farmed domestic rabbits in Spain[72]. Its spores have a single nucleus and are quite small, about 1 μ by 1.5 μ[54]. *Enterocytozoon bieneusi* is one of the most common microsporidian opportunists in humans with HIV disease, in which it parasitizes intestinal and biliary epithelium[71]. The risk of human infection from rabbits is unknown but is considered to be low.

TREMATODES

Fasciola hepatica

The biology of *Fasciola hepatica* is presented in Chapter 20, Parasites of Sheep and Goats. Briefly, *F. hepatica* infects many species of mammals, including humans, and is globally distributed. Infection in lagomorphs can be common in areas in which infected ruminants graze, and it is possible that lagomorphs could serve as a reservoir[73]. Rabbits become infected by ingesting metacercariae on vegetation or in water. Adult flukes inhabit the liver and bile ducts. Infection of rabbits is asymptomatic. Diagnosis is by finding eggs in feces. The need to treat *F. hepatica* infection in laboratory rabbits is extremely unlikely. Prevention is by preventing ingestion of infective metacercariae. *Fasciola hepatica* infects humans, but there are no reports of transmission from rabbits.

Hasstilesia tricolor

Morphology. *Hasstilesia tricolor* adults are very small, 350 μ to 640 μ long and 480 μ to 1,200 μ wide, and have ventral and oral suckers and a spinous cuticle[73]. The three color shades for which it is named are visible only in fresh, living specimens. The eggs are typical operculated trematode eggs and measure 20 μ to 22 μ long by 13 μ to 15 μ wide.

Hosts. *Hasstilesia tricolor* is common in wild rabbits in the United States[73], but has not been reported in domestic rabbits.

Life Cycle. Terrestrial snails serve as intermediate hosts[73]. Rabbits can become infected by ingesting either infected snails or free metacercariae. Adult trematodes develop in the small intestine with a prepatent period of 21 to 25 days.

Pathologic Effects and Clinical Disease. There is only one report of illness associated with *H. tricolor* infestation[74]. Thus, infestation appears to be subclinical in most cases.

Diagnosis, Treatment and Prevention. Diagnosis of *Hasstilesia* sp. infection is by demonstration of eggs in feces or of adults at necropsy. There are no reports of treatment. Prevention is by preventing ingestion of the intermediate host.

Public Health Considerations. There are no reports of *Hasstilesia* sp. infection in humans.

CESTODES

Domestic rabbits and other lagomorphs serve as hosts of cestodes of the order Cyclophyllidea. Cestodes of which lagomorphs are definitive hosts are of the families Anoplocephalidae or Davaineidae, whereas those of which lagomorphs are intermediate hosts are members of the family Taeniidae.

Adult Tapeworms of the Family Anoplocephalidae

Morphology. Members of the Anoplocephalidae lack a rostellum and hooks[73]. Among anoplocephalids of lagomorphs, the maximum size of *Cittotaenia variabilis* is up to 450 mm long by 10.5 mm wide; *Mosgovoyia* (Syn. *Cittotaenia*) *pectinata americana*, 240 mm by 11 mm; *Mosgovoyia perplexa*, 198 mm by 11 mm; *Mosgovoyia* (Syn. *Ctenotaenia*) *ctenoides*, 800 mm by 10.5 mm; and *Monoecocestus americana*, 47 mm long by 6.5 mm wide[75–77].

Hosts. Anoplocephalid cestodes are worldwide in distribution among lagomorphs. *Cittotaenia variabilis* has been found in domestic rabbits in the United States, and *C. variabilis*, *M. pectinata*, *M. perplexa*, *M. americana*, and *M. ctenoides* are reported from wild North American lagomorphs[78,79]. *Mosgovoyia perplexa*, *M. ctenoides*, *M. americana*, *Andrya cuniculi*, *M. pectinata*, *Cittotaenia denticulata*, and *Paranoplocephala wimerosa* are found in *O. cuniculus* rabbits in Europe[37,80–83]. *Mosgovoyia pectinata* has also been reported from scrub hares in South Africa[84],

and *Anoplocephaloides romerolagi* has been described from the volcano rabbit[85].

Life Cycle. The life cycles are incompletely known in most cases, but the usual intermediate hosts of anoplocephalid cestodes are orbatid mites. Cysticercoids develop in mites that ingest eggs passed from the definitive host, and new hosts become infected by ingesting infected mites. Adult cestodes of lagomorphs inhabit the small intestine.

Pathologic Effects and Clinical Disease. Most infections are subclinical, but large numbers of tapeworms have been associated with enteritis and intestinal obstruction and perforation[73].

Diagnosis, Treatment, and Prevention. Diagnosis in live rabbits is by identification of eggs in fecal specimens. Praziquantel is effective against adults, but incompletely effective against larvae[73]. The usual dose is 5 mg/kg, but higher doses can be used, because the oral toxic dose of praziquantel for rabbits is 1000 mg/kg[86]. Inasmuch as orbatid mites are non-parasitic mites that feed on plants, infection effectively is prevented by feeding properly stored commercial diets. Cestode infestation in research rabbits obtained from a poorly maintained conventional rabbitry is possible, but proper husbandry practices would prevent dissemination within the facility.

Public Health Considerations. Anoplocephalid cestodes of rabbits do not infect humans.

Adult Tapeworms of the Family Davaineidae

Several species of *Raillietina* occur in wild lagomorphs in North America, including *Raillietina salmoni* (Syn. *R. stilesiella*), *R. selfi*, *R. loeweni*, and *R. retractalis*[73]. Natural infection of domestic rabbits is not reported. Ants serve as intermediate hosts. Adult cestodes occupy the small intestine.

Larval Tapeworms of the Family Taeniidae

Taenia pisiformis

Morphology. Cysticerci of *Taenia pisiformis* occur in lagomorphs as thin-walled, fluid-filled cysts up to 18 mm in diameter attached to the surfaces of the abdominal viscera[73] (Figure 15.14).

Hosts and Life Cycle. Lagomorphs are intermediate hosts of *T. pisiformis* throughout the world[36,37,82,87]. Definitive hosts include dogs, foxes, and, less frequently, other carnivores. Domestic rabbits are susceptible to infection

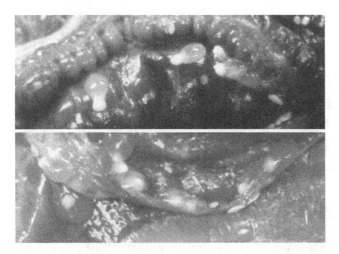

Fig. 15.14 *Taenia pisiformis* cysticerci in serosa of abdominal viscera (above) and peritoneum (below). Courtesy of J.E. Harkness, Mississippi State University.

via contamination of food or surroundings by feces of infected dogs or foxes.

Gravid proglottids passed from the definitive host contain infective eggs. Eggs ingested by the intermediate host hatch in the intestine. Larvae migrate via the portal veins to the liver and occasionally other viscera such as the mesenteric lymph nodes or lungs. Larval development occurs during migration in the liver. After about two to four weeks, larvae emerge from the liver, encyst on the liver capsule or other abdominal serosal surfaces, and develop into infective cysticerci. Definitive hosts become infected by consuming infected rabbits.

Pathologic Effects and Clinical Disease. Naturally occurring infections are seldom clinically evident. Metacestode migration in the liver can cause focal granulomatous inflammation and fibrosis. Severe infections, more typical of experimental inoculation, can result in severe hepatitis with chronic wasting or death[111].

Diagnosis, Treatment, and Prevention. Diagnosis of cysticercosis in laboratory rabbits usually occurs incidentally at necropsy. Microscopic examination of cyst fluid specimens collected by fine needle aspiration is diagnostic if parasite parts are present[88]. Cysts also can be detected by imaging techniques such as radiography and ultrasound[89,90]. Treatment rarely is indicated. Prevention is by proper husbandry to prevent contamination of the feed and environment with feces of domestic or wild canids. This includes thorough washing of fresh foods, if used, and insect control, because mechanical transmission by blowflies has been demonstrated[91].

Public Health Considerations. *Taenia pisiformis* is not known to affect humans.

Taenia serialis

Morphology. Coenuri of *Taenia serialis* are large, fluid-filled cysts up to 5 cm in diameter in the subcutis or connective tissue between skeletal muscles[73]. Numerous scolices may be present and may be arranged in rows (Figure 15.15).

Hosts and Life Cycle. Many species of lagomorphs can serve as intermediate hosts of *T. serialis*, adults of which occur in dogs and foxes[73]. Although *T. serialis* occurs in many locations throughout the world, it is less widely distributed and less common than *T. pisiformis*. Coenuri have been reported in laboratory and pet domestic rabbits[92]. The life cycle of *T. serialis* is similar to that of *T. pisiformis*[111].

Pathologic Effects and Clinical Disease. Coenuri in the subcutis typically have little effect on the host. Those located in the musculature can compromise mobility, especially if numerous.

Diagnosis, Treatment, and Prevention. Diagnosis, treatment, and prevention are as for *T. pisiformis*. The superficial location and size of the coenuri allow ready diagnosis in a living animal. Surgical removal of a cyst from a pet rabbit has been reported[90].

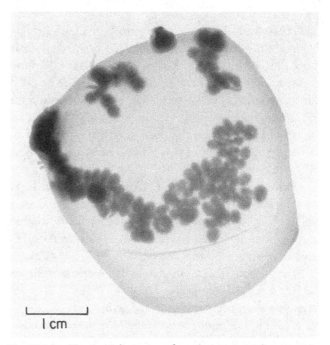

1 cm

Fig. 15.15 *Taenia serialis* coenurus from the intermuscular connective tissue of a rabbit. Note numerous buds. Courtesy of Marietta Voge, University of California.

Public Health Considerations. *Taenia serialis* causes rare cases of human coenurosis[93], but there is no risk of transmission from rabbits.

Other Taeniid Cestodes

Taenia polyacantha has been reported from rabbits and rodents in Europe and Alaska. Foxes are the definitive host[94]. In North America, hares (*Lepus americanus*) serve as intermediate hosts of *Taenia macrocystis,* whose definitive host is the lynx[95]. South American wild rabbits and hares have been reported as intermediate hosts of *Echinococcus* spp.[96,97].

NEMATODES

Superfamily Rhabditoidea

Strongyloides papillosus

Morphology. *Strongyloides* spp. are characterized by having both parasitic and free-living saprophytic forms. The esophagus of the free-living form is rhabditiform, with a distal bulb and valve, whereas that of the parasitic form has a long, cylindrical, filariform esophagus. Parasitic females of *Strongyloides papillosus* are 3.5 mm to 6 mm in length and 50 μ to 60 μ in diameter. Eggs are embryonated when passed from the host and measure 40 μ to 60 μ long by 20 μ to 25 μ in diameter.

Hosts and Life Cycle. *Strongyloides papillosus* primarily infects ruminants[111], but it also has been reported in European rabbits and hares[99]. Lagomorphs become infected upon ingestion of embryonated eggs or by larval skin penetration. Following hematogenous dissemination and pulmonary migration, adult parasitic females of *Strongyloides* sp. inhabit the small intestinal crypts and are parthenogenetic. Rabbits may also be infected experimentally with *S. papillosus*[100].

Pathologic Effects and Clinical Disease. Little information is available concerning pathologic effects in rabbits. Clinical disease in naturally infected wild rabbits and hares has not been reported[98,99]. Experimental infections can result in wasting and death[100,101].

Diagnosis, Treatment, and Prevention. Clinical diagnosis is by identification of eggs in fecal samples. Necropsy diagnosis usually is made by histopathologic examination, but adults also can be identified in mucosal scrapings. Treatment of rabbits is not reported. Control is by preventing contact with contaminated soil or feces of infected hosts.

Public Health Considerations. *Strongyloides papillosus* is not known to infect humans.

Superfamily Ascaridoidea

Baylisascaris procyonis

Morphology. The morphology of *Baylisascaris procyonis* is presented in Chapter 14, Parasites of Guinea Pigs. Further, Chitwood and Lichtenfels describe identification of ascarid larvae in sections[102]. Characteristic features include cervical or lateral alae, lateral chords, coelomyarian musculature, and paired lateral excretory gland cells.

Hosts and Life Cycle. *Baylisascaris procyonis,* of which the definitive host is the raccoon, has occasionally caused disease in domestic rabbits[103]. The life cycle of *B. procyonis* is presented in Chapter 14, Parasites of Guinea Pigs. Briefly, adult worms inhabit the small intestine of the raccoon definitive host. Environmentally resistant eggs become infective about 30 days after being passed in the feces. Rabbits become infected by ingesting infective eggs. The larvae leave the intestine and migrate extensively in the host's organs and tissues, including the central nervous system.

Pathologic Effects and Clinical Disease. Central nervous system lesions are characterized by necrosis, hemorrhage, and a mixed inflammatory response of lymphocytes and polymorphonuclear cells. Larvae can be evident in or near such lesions (Figure 15.16). Older lesions can be accompanied by gliosis and macrophages that contain hemosiderin. Multifocal granulomatous inflammation

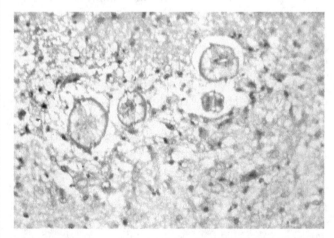

Fig. 15.16 *Baylisascaris* sp. larvae in the brain of a rabbit. Hematoxylin and eosin stain. Courtesy of J.E. Harkness, Mississippi State University.

occurs in affected visceral organs. Clinical signs are chiefly neurological, and include torticollis, ataxia, and circling[73]. The clinical course can be prolonged, with progressively increasing severity.

Diagnosis. Demonstration in tissue sections of nematodes with the characteristics of ascarid larvae[102] is sufficient for a presumptive diagnosis, although the larvae are not numerous in the brain and can be difficult to find. Distinctive characteristics are described for larvae of some ascarids in tissue sections[104], but for definitive determination of species, larvae should be examined by a qualified parasitologist. Specimens can be recovered from fresh tissues of affected animals using the Baermann method.

Treatment and Prevention. Treatment with 100 mg/kg mebendazole for three days is reported to be effective against migrating larvae[105]. Prevention is by husbandry that eliminates fecal contamination of feed, bedding, and cages by definitive hosts.

Public Health Considerations. Human larva migrans caused by *B. procyonis* appears to be very rare[106]. There is no risk to humans exposed to infected rabbits.

Superfamily Oxyuroidea

Passalurus ambiguus

Morphology. Adult male *Passalurus ambiguus* have a single spicule and are 3.8 mm to 5 mm long and 200 μ to 460 μ in diameter, whereas adult females are 5.3 mm to 11 mm long by 410 μ to 590 μ in diameter and have about 40 cuticular striations of the tail. Eggs are elongated, 93 μ to 105 μ long and 43 μ wide, and are flattened on one side (Figure 15.17).

Hosts. *Passalurus ambiguus* is the common pinworm of lagomorphs[73]. It infects domestic and wild rabbits and hares, and its distribution is worldwide. It was once common in laboratory rabbits, but modern husbandry practices and use of specific pathogen-free rabbits have greatly reduced its occurrence. Nonetheless, it still is encountered occasionally.

Life Cycle. *Passalurus ambiguus* has a direct life cycle. Adults inhabiting the cecum and colon produce embryonated eggs, which are infective when passed. Ingestion of infective eggs results in infection of new hosts. Young developing worms can be found in association with the mucosa of the small intestine and cecum.

Pathologic Effects and Clinical Disease. Fujiwara and co-workers[107] reported granulomatous appendicitis and lymphadenitis in which *P. ambiguus* larvae and

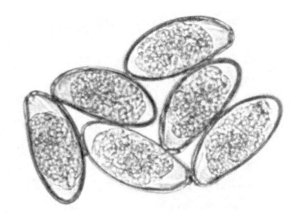

Fig. 15.17 *Passalurus ambiguus* ova. Courtesy of J.E. Harkness, Mississippi State University.

unidentified intracellular bacteria were found, but the role of the larvae in development of the lesions was unclear. No disease attributable to *P. ambiguus* has been reported, even though thousands of the nematodes can be present[73]. One report describes loss of condition and poor reproduction, which were improved by treatment, in rabbits infected with both *P. ambiguus* and *Obeliscoides cuniculi*[108].

Diagnosis, Treatment, and Prevention. Diagnosis is by demonstration of eggs in the feces or adults in the cecal and colonic contents. Juvenile worms can sometimes be found by histologic examination (Figure 15.18). Adult worms may be passed in the feces.

Recommended treatments include piperazine citrate at 1 g/L in the drinking water for one day; piperazine adipate for two days at 0.5 g/kg body weight/day for adults and 0.75 g/kg/day for young rabbits; phenothiazine at 1 g/50 g feed; fenbendazole at 50 ppm in the feed for five days; fenbendazole at 10 to 20 mg/kg orally, repeated in 14 days; and a single dose of thiabendazole at 400 mg/kg body weight[38,109]. Richardson[109] recommends ivermectin at 0.4 mg/kg, but Sovell and Holmes[110] report that ivermectin is poorly effective in treating *P. ambiguus* infection in snowshoe hares.

P. ambiguus is highly transmissible, inasmuch as the eggs are infective when passed from the host. Control is best accomplished by strict husbandry practices to prevent introduction of the parasite into the colony. Eliminating established infections requires treating the entire colony to eliminate egg-laying adult worms, combined with extremely thorough decontamination of the environment.

Public Health Considerations. *Passalurus ambiguus* does not infect humans.

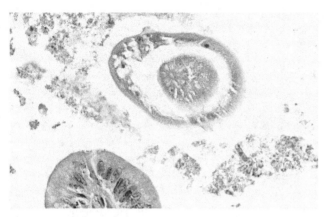

Fig. 15.18 *Passalurus ambiguus* larvae, cecum. Hematoxylin and eosin stain.

Other Oxyurids of Rabbits

Passalurus nonannulatus is morphologically similar to *P. ambiguus* and is found in wild North American lagomorphs[73]. *Dermatoxys veligera* also occurs in wild North American rabbits in the United States, and has been reported in domestic rabbits[73]. Adults inhabit the cecum. Females are 16 mm to 17 mm in length and 600 µ in diameter, and males are 8 mm to 11 mm long and 435 µ in diameter[111]. Spicules of the males measure 85 µ long, and the vulva of females is located 7 mm from the proximal end. Eggs are 50 µ by 110 µ, with one side somewhat flattened. Adults do not attach to the mucosa, but fourth stage larvae attach via hooks to the mucosa of the cecum, sometimes with formation of small ulcers. *Dermatoxys hispaniensis* has been reported in wild rabbits in Spain and the Spanish islands of Macaronesia[82]. *Dermatoxys vlakhaasi* occurs in scrub hares in South Africa[84].

Superfamily Trichostrongyloidea

Graphidium strigosum

Morphology. Adult male worms are 8 mm to 16 mm long and females 11 mm to 20 mm long[111]. Both are red and have fine longitudinal and transverse striations. Males have a prominent bursa and spicules that are 1.1 mm to 2.4 mm long. In females the vulva is located 1.1 mm to 3.3 mm from the end of the tail. Eggs measure 98 µ to 106 µ by 50 µ to 58 µ.

Hosts. *Graphidium strigosum* parasitizes domestic rabbits and wild lagomorphs in North America, Europe, Australia, and Macaronesia[73,80,82]. It is common in wild rabbits and hares, and is occasionally found in domestic

rabbits where husbandry practices are poor and permit exposure to feces of wild lagomorphs. It has not been reported in contemporary laboratory rabbits.

Life Cycle. Adults inhabit the stomach[73]. Eggs passed in the feces hatch and develop into infective third-stage larvae in four to six days. Transmission is by ingestion of infective larvae. The prepatent period is five weeks. The life span of adults is about six months.

Pathologic Effects and Clinical Disease. Infection is often subclinical. Severe infections can be associated with hemorrhagic or chronic catarrhal gastritis, anemia, weight loss, and, possibly, death[73,111].

Diagnosis, Treatment, and Prevention. Clinical diagnosis is by demonstration of eggs in fecal samples. Postmortem diagnosis is by identification of worms in scrapings of the gastric mucosa. Little information regarding treatment is available. Richardson[109] recommends oral treatment with fenbendazole at 10 to 20 mg/kg body weight or subcutaneous injection of ivermectin at 0.4 mg/kg body weight. Because larvae require several days to become infective, husbandry practices that include frequent and thorough sanitation and that prevent exposure to feces of wild lagomorphs are effective preventive measures.

Public Health Considerations. *Graphidium strigosum* is not known to infect humans.

Longistriata noviberiae

Longistriata noviberiae occurs in cottontail rabbits in the United States[36,73] and has been found in domestic rabbits in North Carolina[112]. It inhabits the small intestine. Adults are coiled and have transverse striations. The proximal end is slightly larger in diameter than the rest of the body. Males have a bursa and slender spicules 420 µ to 430 µ long. Males are 4 mm to 5 mm long and 55 mm to 65 mm in diameter; females are 5.5 mm to 6.5 mm long and 70 mm to 75 mm in diameter. Eggs measure 70 µ to 75 µ by 35 µ to 40 µ. The life cycle has not been described.

Nematodirus spp.

Nematodirus leporis, N. neomexicanus, N. arizonensis, and *N. triangularis* are reported from wild lagomorphs[73,113]. Among these, *N. leporis* is reported from *O. cuniculus*. Males measure 8 mm to 13 mm in length and have spicules 650 µ to 1,000 µ long. The bursa has rounded lobes and parallel posterolateral and mediolateral rays. Females are 16 mm to 20 mm in length. Eggs are oval and large, measuring 160 µ to 180 µ by 80 µ to 90 µ. *Nematodirus zembrae* occurs in rabbits in Spain[114].

Obeliscoides cuniculi

Morphology. Adult male *Obeliscoides cuniculi* measure 10 mm to 15 mm in length and 230 μ in diameter, and have paired spicules and a copulatory bursa (Figure 15.19). Females are 15 mm to 18 mm in length and average 546 μ in diameter, with the vulva located in the posterior segment of the body. Eggs are oval, thin-shelled, and measure 75 μ to 91 μ by 42 μ to 53 μ (Figure 15.20).

Hosts. Measures and Anderson[115] consider that *Obeliscoides cuniculi* comprises the subspecies *O. cuniculi cuniculi* that occurs in hares and *O. cuniculi multistriatus* that is found in cottontail rabbits. Domestic rabbits are susceptible to experimental infection with both subspecies[115]. *Obeliscoides cuniculi* is distributed worldwide[36,73,113]. There is one report of infection in a laboratory rabbit[116]. Guinea pigs can be infected experimentally. In laboratory settings, *O. cuniculi* is of little importance as a naturally occurring parasite.

Life Cycle. Adult worms inhabit the mucus adherent to the gastric mucosa[73,111] (Figure 15.21). Development of infective third-stage larvae after eggs are passed from the host requires about one week. Larvae ingested by susceptible hosts invade the gastric mucosa within about one day, develop to the fourth stage within three days, and undergo the final molt when they emerge from the mucosa. Adults can develop as early as 10 days after ingestion of larvae, and the prepatent period is 16 to 20 days. Some larvae can remain in arrested development in the mucosa and emerge later as previously emerged adults die.

Pathologic Effects. Gross lesions in the stomach consist of a thickened mucosa with a finely nodular or "cobblestone" surface, increased amounts of mucus, and, in some cases, petechiae. The mucosal thickening is the result of larval invasion of the mucosa, which induces epithelial hyperplasia of the gastric mucosal glands and a mixed inflammatory cell infiltrate in which lymphocytes and eosinophils predominate.

Clinical Disease. Most infections are subclinical[73,111]. Disease associated with natural infections is rare, but can result in diarrhea, anemia, and weight loss. Experimental infection with large numbers of larvae can induce similar signs, although they are transient and resolve within two weeks after inoculation.

Diagnosis. Clinical diagnosis is by demonstration of eggs in fecal samples. At necropsy, adult worms can be identified in scrapings of the mucus adherent to the gastric mucosa.

Treatment and Prevention. Information concerning efficacy of anthelminthic treatments is sparse[73]. Fenbendazole administered in the feed for five days at 50 ppm was reported to be effective[117]. Thiabendazole was only partially effective when given as a single dose of 250 mg/kg body weight[117], whereas dosing every four hours at 110 mg/kg body weight for the first dose and 70 mg/kg for eight additional doses was highly effective[118]. Prevention is by husbandry practices that prevent ingestion of infective larvae.

Public Health Considerations. *Obeliscoides cuniculi* does not infect humans.

Trichostrongylus affinis

Trichostrongylus affinis has been reported in cottontail rabbits and jackrabbits in the United States[36,73]. It inhabits the small intestine. Males measure 5 mm to 7.5 mm in length and 123 μ in average diameter, and have spicules measuring

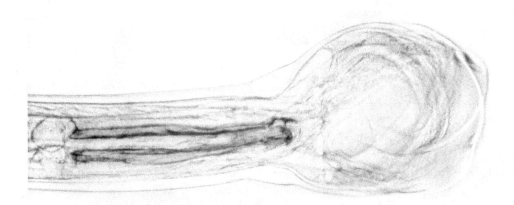

Fig. 15.19 Bursa of male *Obeliscoides cuniculi*. Courtesy of L. Measures, Maurice Lamontagne Institute, Quebec, Canada.

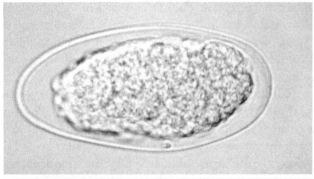

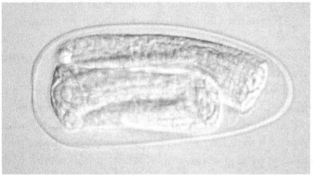

Fig. 15.20 *Obeliscoides cuniculi* eggs, fresh (above), larvated (below). Courtesy of L. Measures, Maurice Lamontagne Institute, Quebec, Canada.

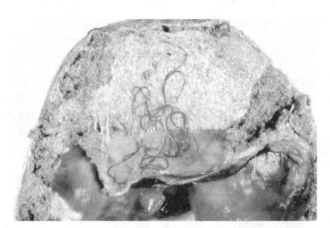

Fig. 15.21 *Obeliscoides cuniculi* adults in the stomach of a snowshoe hare (*Lepus americanus*). Courtesy of L. Measures, Maurice Lamontagne Institute, Quebec, Canada.

131μ to 156 μ in length and 29 μ in width. Females measure 8.7 mm to 9.2 mm in length and 106 μ to 177 μ in diameter. The vulva is located 1.6 mm to 1.7 mm from the end of the tail. Eggs are 57 μ to 66 μ by 33 μ to 40 μ. Eggs hatch and develop into infective larvae after exiting the host in feces. Transmission is by ingestion of infective larvae. The prepatent period is 10 to 11 days. Experimental infection with large numbers of larvae can result in weight loss.

Trichostrongylus calcaratus

Trichostrongylus calcaratus is common in wild cottontail rabbits and jackrabbits in the United States[36,73,87]. Adults inhabit the small intestine. Eggs passed in the feces develop into infective larvae in 16 to 18 days. Transmission is by ingestion of infective larvae. Natural infections often are subclinical, although large numbers of worms can be present. Severe experimental infections can be fatal.

Trichostrongylus ransomi

Trichostrongylus ransomi has been reported from cottontail rabbits in Louisiana, but appears to be uncommon[73]. Adults inhabit the small intestine. Males are 2.25 mm to 3 mm in length, and females are 3 mm to 3.5 mm. Eggs are 60 μ to 70 μ by 30 μ to 36 μ.

Trichostrongylus retortaeformis

Trichostrongylus retortaeformis is common in wild rabbits and hares in Europe and Australia[81,119–121], but has not been reported from North American lagomorphs. Adults inhabit the small intestine and rarely, the stomach. The cuticle has transverse and longitudinal grooves. Males measure 6.8 mm to 8.4 mm in length and 127 μ to 160 μ in diameter. The spicules are 145 μ and 172 μ long. Females are 9.6 mm to 10.4 mm in length and 104 μ to 112 μ in diameter. Eggs measure 86 μ to 87 μ by 41 μ to 46 μ.

The life cycle is direct, and typical of the superfamily[122]. Infective larvae exsheathed and were found in the small intestine within 12 hours after inoculation. The larvae underwent the third molt three to five days after inoculation and the final molt four to seven days after inoculation. The prepatent period was 12 to 13 days and the patent period 5.5 months. Some larvae invaded the small intestinal villi[123]. Infection has been associated with reduced populations of wild rabbits in Australia. Barker and Ford[124] described atrophic enteritis in infected rabbits.

Trichostrongylus spp.

Trichostrongylus colubriformis primarily parasitizes ruminants, but it has been reported in wild lagomorphs[73]. *Trichostrongylus axei* has been reported from mountain hares in Scotland[81]. The life cycle in experimental infection of domestic rabbits has been described[125]. *Trichostrongylus deflexu, T. falculatus,* and *T. thomasi* have been reported in South African scrub hares[84].

Superfamily Metastrongyloidea

Protostrongylus boughtoni

Morphology. Adult male *Protostrongylus boughtoni* measure 13 mm to 26 mm in length and 160 µ to 250 µ in diameter, have 260-µ to 320-µ spicules, and have a bursa[73]. Females measure 21 mm to 36 mm long and 200 µ to 300 µ in diameter, and the vulva is located about 200 µ from the distal end. The eggs are thin-shelled, elliptical, and 50 µ to 70 µ by 40 µ to 60 µ.

Hosts and Life Cycle. *Protostrongylus boughtoni* occurs in wild rabbits and hares in North America, especially the more northern areas of the continent[73]. Infection of domestic rabbits has not been reported. Adult worms inhabit the bronchi[73]. Eggs hatch into first-stage larvae while still in the airways. The larvae leave the host in the feces after being coughed up and swallowed. In the first stage, the larvae migrate into land snails, such as *Vallonia pulchella,* and develop into infective third-stage larvae. Although the larvae can leave the snail and establish infection after ingestion, most infections probably result from ingestion of the snail intermediate host.

Pathologic Effects and Clinical Disease. Gross lesions are small, discrete, firm nodules in the lungs. Microscopic changes are those of chronic bronchitis[126]. Lesions are reported to be more severe in cottontail rabbits than in hares[127]. Clinical signs of disease have not been sufficiently described.

Diagnosis, Treatment, and Prevention. Larvae can be isolated from feces using the Baermann procedure as described in Chapter 1, Collection, Preservation, and Diagnostic Methods. Ivermectin is reported to be only partially effective in clearing infection from snowshoe hares[110]. Prevention is by husbandry practices that prevent exposure to infected intermediate hosts.

Public Health Considerations. *Protostrongylus boughtoni* is not known to infect humans.

Protostrongylus spp.

Protostrongylus pulmonalis occurs in European hares[37,128]. Lesions are similar to those caused by *P. boughtoni,* with grossly evident pulmonary nodules characterized histologically by bronchiolitis, alveolitis, interstitial pneumonia, and intra-alveolar collections of larvae and eggs[128]. Such changes are also reported in European hares infected with *P. commutatus*[129].

Superfamily Spiruroidea

Gongylonema pulchrum

Morphology. Typical of the genus, *Gongylonema pulchrum* has distinctive round or oval cuticular thickenings, prominent cervical alae, small lips, and a short pharynx[111]. The tail of the male is asymmetrical. The right spicule is 84 µ to 180 µ long; the left, 4 µ to 23 µ long. Males measure up to 62 mm in length, and females can be up to 145 mm.

Hosts and Life Cycle. *Gongylonema pulchrum* occurs chiefly in sheep, goats, cattle, and pigs, but also has been reported from a variety of other species, including cottontail rabbits[79]. It has not been reported in domestic rabbits, but they are susceptible to experimental infection[130]. Adult worms reside in the esophageal mucosa[111]. Eggs passed in the feces are ingested by coprophagous beetles and develop into infective larvae in about 30 days. Definitive hosts are infected by ingestion of infected beetles. Cockroaches also can serve as intermediate hosts.

Pathologic Effects and Clinical Disease. Neither lesions nor clinical disease have been reported in rabbits infected with *G. pulchrum.*

Diagnosis, Treatment, and Prevention. Because *G. pulchrum* is considered nonpathogenic, diagnosis and treatment are usually not pursued. The worms are readily identified at necropsy by careful inspection of the esophageal mucosa, in which they are embedded in a characteristic serpentine pattern. Control is by preventing ingestion of beetle intermediate hosts.

Public Health Considerations. Human infection with *G. pulchrum,* in which the worm or larvae usually are found in the oral mucosa or subcutis, rarely occurs[131], but there is no evidence that such infections have been acquired from rabbits.

Superfamily Filarioidea

Brugia lepori

Brugia lepori has been reported from cottontail rabbits in Louisiana[132]. Adults occurred in the subcutis and abdominal lymphatic vessels. Males measured 11.7 mm to 18.6 mm long and 64 µ to 80 µ thick. Females measured 38.5 mm to 45.5 mm long by 125 µ to 134 µ wide. The microfilariae were sheathed and measured 275 µ to 330 µ long by 5 µ to 7 µ[132]. Circulating microfilariae of *Brugia* sp. were found in more than 60% of cottontail rabbits on Nantucket Island[133]. No manifestations of disease in rabbits were reported, and the life cycle has not been determined. Several cases of human *Brugia* sp. infection have been reported[134], but it is not known if any of these were of rabbit origin.

Dirofilaria scapiceps

Morphology. Adult *Dirofilaria scapiceps* (Syn. *Pelecitus scapiceps*) have a pre-esophageal cuticular ring and lateral alae, are spirally coiled, and have strongly tapered ends. Females average 28 mm long and 700 µ wide, with the vulva located about 1.5 mm from the anterior end of the worm. Males average 12.6 mm long and 431 µ wide, and have a right spicule that is 112 µ long and a left spicule that is 82 µ long.

Hosts. *Dirofilaria scapiceps* occurs in North America, in domestic and cottontail rabbits and hares[73]. Infection can be common among outdoor housed domestic rabbits.

Life Cycle. Adults inhabit the tendon sheaths of the hock joint, and less frequently, the fascia around the stifle joint[73]. Microfilariae circulate in the blood, but circadian periodicity is not evident. Intermediate hosts are mosquitoes of several species, in which ingested microfilariae develop to the third larval stage. New hosts become infected when fed upon by mosquitoes carrying infective larvae. Larvae first migrate to the subcutis, frequently that of the trunk, mature to the fifth stage, and then migrate to the area of hock joint and develop into adults. Prepatency is 137 to 234 days.

Pathologic Effects and Clinical Disease. Infection is usually subclinical, but can be associated with chronic tenosynovitis[135].

Diagnosis, Treatment, and Prevention. Infection can be detected by identifying microfilariae in the blood or adults in the tissues of the hock joint[73]. Treatment has not been reported. Prevention is by husbandry that excludes mosquitoes.

Public Health Considerations. *Dirofilaria scapiceps* is not known to infect humans.

Dirofilaria uniformis

Dirofilaria uniformis occurs in wild rabbits in the southern and southeastern United States[73]. It inhabits the subcutis of the trunk and is morphologically similar to *D. scapiceps*. Thus, it must be differentiated from immature *D. scapiceps* in that location. Adults are distinguished from *D. scapiceps* by the lack of a cuticular ring and lateral alae, and by having less tapered extremities. Females average 30 mm long by 496 µ in diameter, and males average 16 mm long by 347 µ in diameter. The spicules of males are 131 µ and 94 µ in length.

Superfamily Trichuroidea

Trichuris spp.

Morphology. *Trichuris leporis* and *Trichuris sylvilagi* are morphologically similar, and at times have been confused[73]. For both species, adult males measure 19 mm to 21 mm long while females measure 17.4 mm to 20.9 mm long. Ova measure 60 µ to 65 µ by 29 µ and have typical bipolar plugs. According to Tiner[136], *T. leporis* males have a spicule 1.6 mm to 3.2 mm long, whereas the spicule of *T. sylvilagi* is 6 mm to 8 mm in length. Kutzer, however, considers that Tiner's description of *T. sylvilagi* actually refers to *T. lepori*, and that Tiner's description of *T. lepori* refers to neither *T. lepori* nor *T. sylvilagi* but to another species[137].

Hosts. *Trichuris leporis* and *T. sylvilagi* have been reported in wild lagomorphs in Europe and the United States[82,87,113].

Life Cycle. Although not described in detail, the life cycle is direct[73]. Adults inhabit the cecum and large intestine, with the anterior end inserted into the mucosa. Eggs passed in the feces embryonate after roughly three weeks in the environment[111]. Transmission is by ingestion of infective embryonated eggs. The larvae penetrate the mucosa of the small intestine, and after two to 10 days migrate to the cecum and colon, where they mature.

Pathologic Effects and Clinical Disease. Lesions have not been described. Prevalence and intensity of *T. leporis* infection have been related to decreased body weight in snowshoe hares[113].

Diagnosis, Treatment, and Prevention. Diagnosis is by demonstration of trichurid eggs in fecal samples, or by finding adult worms at necropsy. Little information is available regarding treatment. Ivermectin is reportedly ineffective in snowshoe hares[110]. Control is by sanitary measures to prevent ingestion of infectious eggs from the feces of wild lagomorphs.

Public Health Considerations. Trichurids of lagomorphs are not known to infect humans.

ARTHROPODS

Class Insecta

Order Diptera

Family Cuterebridae

Botflies or warble flies, including *Cuterebra abdominalis* (Syn. *Cuterebra horripilum*), *C. buccata*, *C. cuniculi*, *C. jellisoni*, *C. lepivora*, *C. lepusculi*, and *C. ruficrus*, commonly parasitize wild lagomorphs in North America[36,73,138]. These are large flies with bee-like bodies about 20 mm long[111]. Females lay eggs near the entrance to the host's nest. Depending on the species, the larvae penetrate the skin directly, invade wounds, or enter natural body openings[73]. In some cases the larvae migrate via the trachea and body cavities to the subcutis, where they form painful cysts with a fistula through the skin. Cysts are 2 cm to 3 cm in diameter, and the overlying fur is moist with fluid oozing from the fistula.

Larvae are up to 25 mm long (Figure 15.22). Some species preferentially locate in specific areas of the body. Cysts in aberrant locations, such as the eye, occur occasionally. Larvae leave the host to pupate, leaving an open cyst that soon heals with scarring unless secondarily infected. One or a few cysts usually do not cause significant illness, but if they are numerous the host can become debilitated and possibly die.

Control is by preventing access of female flies to rabbit hosts. If necessary, larvae can be removed via minor surgery and topical treatment of the wound. *Cuterebra* spp. occasionally infest other host species, including humans, and may localize in aberrant locations such as the eye, trachea, and brain[139].

Order Phthiraptera

Haemodipsus spp.

Lice are uncommonly found infesting rabbits and hares. All of those known to parasitize lagomorphs are sucking lice (suborder Anoplura), which are distinguished by narrow heads and sturdy claws adapted for grasping hairs. *Haemodipsus ventricosus* (family Hoplopleuridae) is the most commonly reported rabbit louse. Other members of the genus affecting lagomorphs include *H. setoni* (wild rabbits, United States), *H. lyriocephalus* (wild hares, Europe), and *H. africanus* (wild hares, Africa) [78,87,140–142].

Haemodipsus ventricosus is widely distributed, occurring in the United States, Europe, Australia, New Zealand, and Africa[143]. It has a dorsoventrally flattened body with a pear- or teardrop-shaped outline, and is eyeless (Figure 15.23). Adults measure 1.2 mm to 2.5 mm long[111]. The first pair of legs has slender claws, but those of the second and third pairs are more robust.

Haemodipsus ventricosus parasitizes domestic rabbits and can be found anywhere on the body[143]. Light infestations can be manifested only by the presence of lice, nymphs, and eggs (or nits), which are attached to hairs near the base. Eggs are oval, 0.5 mm to 0.7 mm long, and have an operculum. Nymphs are morphologically similar to adults.

Heavy infestations can result in anemia, hair loss, and pruritic dermatitis on the dorsal and lateral parts of the body. Nymphal and adult lice suck blood. Transmission occurs only under conditions of prolonged close contact, such as from does to their litters.

Louse infestation among laboratory rabbits is extremely unlikely. Should treatment be required, lice are

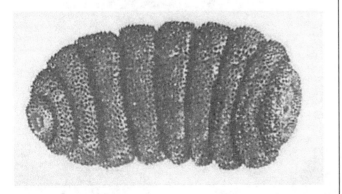

Fig. 15.22 *Cuterebra* sp. larva. Reproduced from Hofing, G.L. and Kraus, A.L. (1994) with permission.

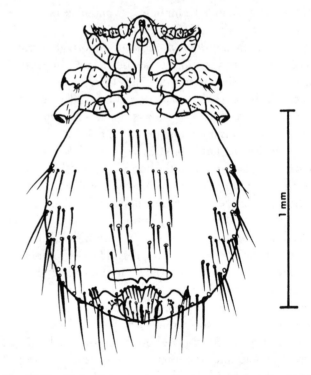

Fig. 15.23 *Haemodipsus ventricosus* female, ventral view. Courtesy of K.C. Kim, Pennsylvania State University.

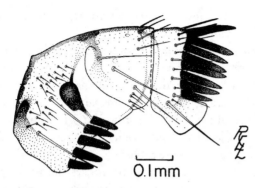

Fig. 15.24 Head of *Spilopsyllus cuniculi*. Courtesy of R.E. Lewis, Iowa State University.

susceptible to various topical treatments, including organophosphates and pyrethrins. Such treatments should be repeated at least once after 10 days to assure elimination of newly hatched nymphs. Ivermectin also should be effective at doses used for other ectoparasites. As a bloodsucker, *H. ventricosus* is a potential vector of infectious agents among rabbits. It is not known to bite humans.

Order Siphonaptera

Spilopsyllus cuniculi

Morphology. Adults of *Spilopsyllus cuniculi,* the European rabbit flea, are about 1 mm in length and have both genal and pronotal combs (Figure 15.24).

Hosts. *Spilopsyllus cuniculi* is an important vector of myxomatosis, and was introduced deliberately in Australia in an unsuccessful attempt to control populations of wild rabbits[73]. *Spilopsyllus cuniculi* occurs on wild rabbits and hares and on domestic rabbits in Europe and Australia[73,144,145]. It is not found in the United States.

Life Cycle. The reproductive cycle of *S. cuniculi* is synchronized with that of the host so that production of a new generation of fleas coincides with availability of new hosts. The ova of the flea mature only after the female feeds on a pregnant doe late in gestation[143]. Male and female fleas leave the doe to mate after parturition, and the females deposit their eggs in the nest. The environment of the nest protects the larvae from drying and allows them to obtain the blood-rich feces of adult fleas, which the larvae require. The warmth of the nest also allows the larvae to develop, pupate, and mature in as little as three weeks. Adult fleas preferentially feed on the top of the head and neck, and around the ears. Because of the stringent requirements of its life cycle, it is not likely to be found on laboratory rabbits.

Pathologic Effects and Clinical Disease. The bite of *S. cuniculi* is irritating, but usually does not result in lesions or clinical signs.

Diagnosis, Treatment, and Prevention. The diagnosis is made by identification of fleas collected from the host. Obtaining specimens can require some diligence, because there may be only a few fleas actually present on the host. Brushing or combing the rabbit over a light colored surface can help obtain specimens or identify feces. Rabbits that have died or been sacrificed recently enough to have maintained body temperature can be placed in bags to trap fleas that leave the body as it cools. Control in laboratory settings is accomplished by obtaining research rabbits from sources that preclude exposure to natural environments in which the flea can complete its life cycle. If wild rabbits are used in research, they should be quarantined, inspected, and, if necessary, treated. Treatments used for dog and cat fleas should be effective.

Public Health Considerations. Fleas serve as vectors to facilitate maintenance of reservoirs of infectious agents such as *Trypanosoma nabiasi,* and the etiologic agents of zoonotic diseases, including tularemia, plague, and Rocky Mountain spotted fever. However, rabbit fleas rarely bite humans, and the risk of transmission of zoonoses from rabbits to humans via flea bites is low[73].

Other fleas of rabbits

Numerous other species of fleas have been reported from lagomorphs, but only a few feed on domestic rabbits[143]. *Cediopsylla simplex,* the common eastern rabbit flea (Figure 15.25), and *Odontopsyllus multispinosus,* the giant eastern

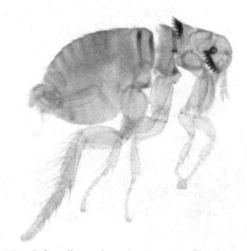

Fig. 15.25 *Cediopsylla simplex* male. Courtesy of J.E. Harkness, Mississippi State University.

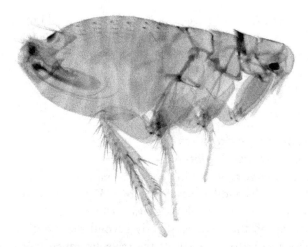

Fig. 15.26 *Odontopsyllus multispinosus* male. Courtesy of J.E. Harkness, Mississippi State University.

rabbit flea (Figure 15.26), are among the most common fleas affecting domestic rabbits in the United States, although both are primarily parasites of wild rabbits. *Cediopsylla simplex* is the more common of the two species, is morphologically similar to *Spilopsyllus cuniculi,* and occurs in a similar distribution on the host. Its life cycle also is similar to that of *S. cuniculi,* in that it is synchronized with the reproductive cycle of the host.

Other species of fleas that occur on wild rabbits of the United States include *C. inequalis, O. dentatus, Hoplopsyllus glacialis affinis,* and *Meringis* spp. Fleas of other hosts that occasionally are found on rabbits include *Echidnophaga gallinacea, Ctenocephalides canis,* and *Ctenocephalides felis. Echidnophaga myremecobii,* the Australian sticktight flea, is common among wild rabbits in Australia. *Hystrichopsylla talpae, Caenopsylla laptevi, Xenopsylla cunicularis, Echidnophaga iberica,* and *Pulex irritans* have been reported from European rabbits[145–147].

Class Arachnida

Ticks

Adult or immature stages of many species of both hard and soft ticks parasitize wild lagomorphs, including *O. cuniculi*[143]. Their chief importance is as vectors of zoonotic diseases, such as Rocky Mountain spotted fever, tularemia, and Lyme disease, though most ticks that feed on rabbits only rarely bite humans. Domestic rabbits are only occasionally affected by ticks, but laboratory rabbits are used in studies of immunity to ticks and tick-transmitted zoonoses[73].

Family Argasidae

Otobius lagophilus is the most common argasid tick that affects rabbits and hares; it occurs primarily in the Pacific Northwest[143]. Larvae and nymphs occur on the host, usually on the face, whereas the adults inhabit nesting areas and their surroundings. Other argasid ticks that affect rabbits include *O. megnini, Ornithodoros parkeri,* and *Ornithodoros turicata.*

Family Ixodidae
Haemaphysalis leporis-palustris **Morphology.** The body of the ixodid tick *Haemaphysalis leporis-palustris* is small and pear- or teardrop-shaped[143](Figure 15.27). It lacks eyes and is distinguished by its long hypostome, sharply angled lateral protrusions at the base of the mouthparts, and perianal grooves. Adult males are up to 2.2 mm long. Unengorged adult females can be up to 2.6 mm in length, whereas engorged females can measure as much as 1 cm.

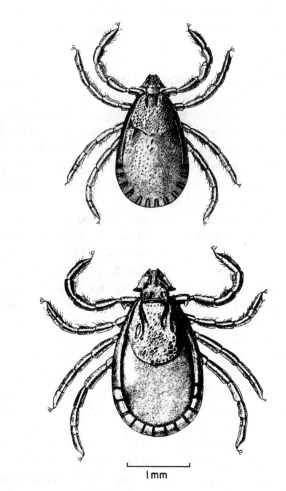

1 mm

Fig. 15.27 *Haemaphysalis leporis-palustris.* (Above) Male. (Below) Female. Courtesy of U.S. Department of Agriculture.

Hosts. *Haemaphysalis leporis-palustris* is commonly found on wild rabbits and hares throughout North America and elsewhere in the western hemisphere[73,148]. It occurs only occasionally on domestic rabbits, and is rarely encountered on laboratory rabbits. Immature stages also feed on other small mammals and birds.

Life Cycle. Rabbits and hares can host all stages of *H. leporis-palustris,* a three-host tick. Domestic rabbits are unlikely to be affected unless husbandry conditions are poor, inasmuch as each stage leaves the host after feeding and undergoes a period of development on the ground. Larvae and nymphs feed for four to 11 days and adult females feed for 19 to 25 days[111]. Unfed nymphs can survive up to one year, and unfed females up to 1.5 years[111].

Pathologic Effects and Clinical Disease. *Haemaphysalis leporis-palustris* usually attaches on the head, most commonly the inner or outer surface of the ear or back of the neck, but also under the chin and around the eyes and nose[73]. It also can be found occasionally on other parts of the body. Wild rabbits can be parasitized by such large numbers of ticks that anemia, emaciation, and even death can result.

Diagnosis, Treatment, and Prevention. The diagnosis is established by identification of the ticks. Treatment of laboratory rabbits is unlikely to be required, but individual ticks can be removed with care. If necessary, topical products such as sprays or dips should be effective. Control is by husbandry measures to prevent exposure to wild lagomorphs and birds and by controlling potentially infested vegetation near rabbit housing.

Public Health Considerations. Although humans are rarely bitten, *H. leporis-palustris* is a known vector of *Francisella tularensis, Rickettsia rickettsii* (Rocky Mountain spotted fever), *Borrelia burgdorferi* (Lyme disease), the Colorado tick fever virus, and other human pathogens[73,149–152]. Thus, personnel handling tick-infested rabbits should follow procedures to prevent transmission of such pathogens.

Other ixodid ticks of rabbits Ixodes dentatus and *Dermacentor parumapertus* are common among wild rabbits and hares[143]. *Ixodes dentatus* can harbor and transmit *B. burgdorferi* and other agents[152–154]. *Rickettsia rickettsii* has been recovered from *D. parumapertus* collected from black-tailed jackrabbits in Texas[155]. Other ixodid ticks infesting lagomorphs include *Amblyomma americana, A. cajennense, A. maculatum, Dermacentor andersoni, D. occidentalis, D. variabilis, I. angustus, I. muris, I. neotomae, I. ricinus californicus, I. sculptus,* *I. spinepalpis,* and *Rhipicephalus sanguineus.* Wild European rabbits are reported to be natural hosts of *Rhipicephalus pusillus,* an ixodid tick of the Mediterranean area that can carry rickettsiae[156]. Additional tick species are reported in wild lagomorphs of South Africa[157].

Mites

Suborder Astigmata

Leporacarus gibbus Leporacarus gibbus (Syn. *Listrophorus gibbus*) adult males average 440 μ long and 240 μ wide, and females, 560 μ by μ 310[73]. The bodies of both males and females are oval, with a rounded dorsal protrusion that extends slightly beyond the mouth parts (Figure 15.28). The legs of the male are much longer in relation to the body than those of the female, and extend well beyond the body margin. Males also have prominent adanal clasping organs.

Leporacarus gibbus has been reported from wild and domestic rabbits in Europe, North America, Australia, New Zealand, and elsewhere[142,144,158,159]. The mites cling to hair shafts and feed on epithelial cells and sebaceous secretions, and are most numerous on the back and abdomen. All stages are present, and the life cycle is completed on the host. It is considered nonpathogenic. Specimens can be obtained for diagnosis by plucking, brushing, or combing. Infestation can be treated topically with a carbamate acaricide or with ivermectin by subcutaneous injection at 400 μg/kg body weight weekly for three weeks[109,158]. *Leporacarus gibbus* only rarely parasitizes humans[160].

Notoedres cati Notoedres cati mainly parasitizes cats, but may also infest rabbits[111]. Disease is clinically and pathologically indistinguishable from that caused by *S. scabiei,* although it usually is less severe. Specific diagnosis must be made by identification of mites in skin scrapings. *Notoedres cati* is slightly smaller than *S. scabiei,* but the major differentiating feature is the position of the anus, which is dorsal in *N. cati* but terminal in *S. scabiei.* The dorsal spines are smaller than those of *S. scabiei.* Treatment and prevention are as for *S. scabiei. Notoedres cati* can transiently infest humans[161].

Psoroptes cuniculi **Morphology.** *Psoroptes cuniculi* (Syn. *Dermatodectes cuniculi, Psoroptes longirostris* var. *cuniculi, P. communis* var. *cuniculi, P. equi* var. *cuniculi*)[73] is a large, oval mite. Males measure 370 μ to 547 μ in length and 322 μ to 462 μ in width, and females measure 403 μ to 749 μ in length and 351 μ to 499 μ in width[73] (Figure 15.29)[162]. The chelicerae are long and pointed and the anus is

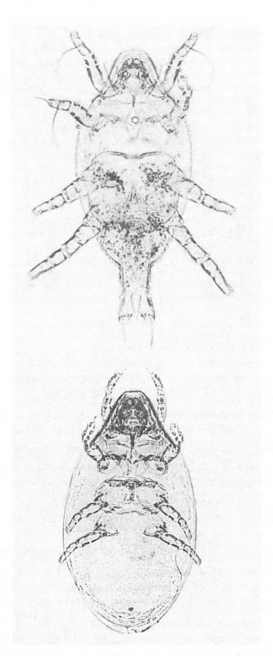

Fig. 15.28 *Leporacarus (Listrophorus) gibbus.* (Above) Male. (Below) Female. Reproduced from Hofing, G.L. and Kraus, A.L. (1994) with permission.

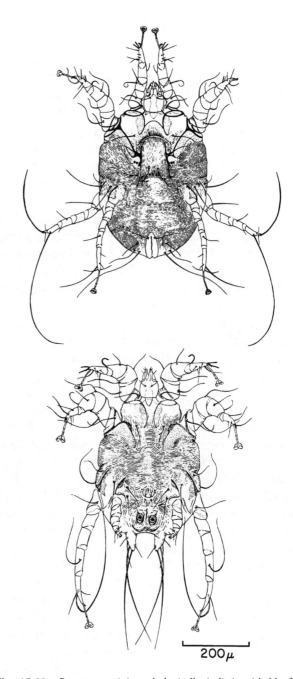

Fig. 15.29 *Psoroptes equi* (morphologically indistinguishable from *Psoroptes cuniculi*). (Above) Female. (Below) Male. Reproduced from Baker, E.W., Evans, T.M., Gould, D.J., Hull, W.B., and Keegan, H.L. (1956) with permission.

terminal. The legs are long, with five free segments and jointed pedicels. Both sexes have tarsal suckers on the first and second pairs of limbs. Males also have suckers on the third pair, whereas in females the third pair bears long setae and the fourth pair has suckers. The pedicels of the suckers are segmented. The posterior aspect of the idiosoma of males is bilobed, and each lobe bears two long and three short setae. That of females is striated and bears three pairs

of long setae, one lateral and two terminal. The female genital opening is U-shaped and located between the second pair of legs. The genitalia of males are heavily sclerotized and located between the fourth pair of legs, and a copulatory sucker is located on each side of the anus.

Hosts. *Psoroptes cuniculi* affects domestic rabbits worldwide but is rare on wild lagomorphs[73,111]. It was once common on laboratory rabbits, but improved husbandry practices and use of specific pathogen-free rabbits have greatly reduced its prevalence. The occurrence of mites of similar appearance on ruminants and horses[111,163] has contributed to uncertainty regarding both host range and taxomony. Based on taxonomic convention and results of molecular genetic analyses, *P. cuniculi, P. cervinus, P. natalensis,* and *P. ovis* are considered to be synonymous with *P. equi*[164]. However, single nucleotide polymorphisms in the second internal transcribed spacer of ribosomal DNA, as well as results of morphometric analysis of outer opisthosomal setae lengths, indicate that *P. cuniculi* parasitizing sheep and rabbits in the same area are distinct[165].

Life Cycle. *Psoroptes cuniculi* is nonburrowing, and primarily inhabits the inner surface of the pinnae and occasionally other areas of the body[73]. The life cycle requires about three weeks. All stages are found on the host and feed on tissue fluids obtained by piercing the epidermis or that exude from the inflamed surface. Epidermis and sebaceous secretions may also be ingested. Eggs hatch about four days after being laid, and the resulting larvae undergo two further immature stages of protonymph and tritonymph. Adult males attach to female tritonymphs, and copulation occurs after the female's final molt. Transmission is by direct contact. Mechanical transmission by houseflies has been demonstrated experimentally. Mites can survive off the host for up to three weeks at low temperature and high humidity, but survival is much shorter at low humidity and high temperature[166].

Pathologic Effects. *Psoroptes cuniculi* induces chronic proliferative dermatitis[73] (Figure 15.30). A variably thick accumulation of degenerated eosinophils, heterophils, desquamated epithelium, debris, and mites overlies the affected skin. The epidermis is hyperplastic and parakeratotic, and the dermis and epidermis are infiltrated with lymphocytes, eosinophils, and heterophils. Rabbits develop specific immune responses to mite antigens, and such responses are thought to be important in pathogenesis. *Psoroptes cuniculi* is reported to harbor *Staphylococcus aureus* and other bacteria[167]. The role of such bacteria in clinical disease is not known.

Clinical Disease. Otoacarisis (psoroptic mange, psoroptic scabies, ear mange, ear canker) is a highly pruritic condition caused by *P. cuniculi*[73]. Affected rabbits shake their heads and scratch their ears, in some cases to excoriation. In mild or early disease, the skin of the inner

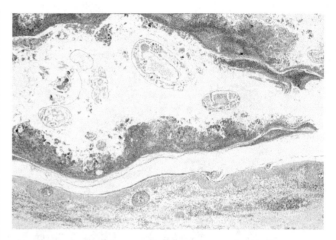

Fig. 15.30 Proliferative dermatitis caused by *Psoroptes cuniculi*. Sections of mites are present within layers of exudate and debris. Hematoxylin and eosin stain.

surface of the pinnae is reddened and covered by a thin layer of dry, light gray or tan crust. In advanced or severe disease, the ears are swollen and painful and have a foul odor. The crust becomes brown, flaky, and thicker, up to 2 cm thick in extreme cases (Figure 15.31), and the underlying skin is raw, red, and moist. The crust is composed of exuded tissue fluid, inflammatory cells, desquamated epithelial cells, and mite feces. Mites of all stages are present under and within the crust. Secondary bacterial infection can occur, and can lead to otitis externa or otitis media. Occasionally, lesions develop in other locations, such as the face, neck, legs, or trunk[168].

Diagnosis. Diagnosis is by identification of the mites, which are large and easily found. *Psoroptes* sp. may be distinguished from other mites of similar appearance, such as *Chorioptes* sp., by the jointed pedicels of the tarsal suckers.

Treatment. Topical treatment with mineral oil, either alone or containing an acaricide, was the standard treatment for *P. cuniculi* infection in the past. The treatment of choice is now ivermectin, administered by subcutaneous injection. Dosages of 100 to 440 μg/kg body weight have been reported to be effective, without observed adverse effects, although dosages as high as 500 μg/kg may be required[109]. The usual recommendation is to give a second dose after seven to 18 days. Topical selamectin at 6 to 18 mg/kg body weight[169] and orally administered injectable 1% moxidectin at 200 μg/kg given twice at an interval of 10 days[170] also are reported to eliminate *P. cuniculi*. Ivermectin administered in the drinking water was effective in treating clinically evident disease, but appeared not to

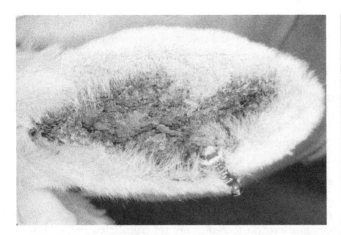

Fig. 15.31 Severe proliferative dermatitis caused by *Psoroptes cuniculi.*

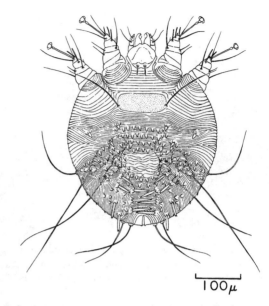

Fig. 15.32 *Sarcoptes scabiei* female, dorsal view. Reproduced from Baker, E.W., Evans, T.M., Gould, D.J., Hull, W.B., and Keegan, H.L. (1956) with permission.

eliminate the mites completely, because ear lesions reappeared after treatment was stopped[171].

Prevention. In modern research settings, it is feasible and highly effective to obtain rabbits free of *P. cuniculi* and maintain them free of mites. If rabbits are obtained from conventional sources, it is advisable to quarantine them and treat them prophylactically with ivermectin.

Public Health Considerations. *Psoroptes cuniculi* is not known to infest humans.

Sarcoptes scabiei **Morphology.** Adult female *Sarcoptes scabiei* mites measure only 300 μ to 600 μ long by 250 μ to 400 μ wide. Adult males are smaller, and measure 200 μ to 240 μ long by 150 μ to 200 μ wide[111] (Figure 15.32). The legs are short, and the third and fourth pairs do not extend to the body margin. The dorsal cuticle bears small triangular scales and has fine, primarily transverse grooves. The first and second pairs of legs of females and the first, second, and fourth pairs in males bear suckers on pedicels. The remaining limbs have terminal bristles. The anus is terminal.

Hosts. *Sarcoptes scabiei* parasitizes nearly all mammalian hosts, including humans. A few cases of infestation of domestic rabbits have been reported[172]. *Sarcoptes scabiei* from different host species are considered by many authors to be separate races, varieties, or species[173]. The validity of such classifications is unclear, and even approaches using molecular genetic analysis have been controversial[174].

Life Cycle. The life cycle of *S. scabiei* was described from human infestations, but the life cycle on other hosts is presumed to be similar[111]. Adult females burrow into the epidermis, where they lay eggs that hatch in three to five days. The six-legged larvae develop into eight-legged protonymphs, then deutonymphs. Some remain in the epidermis, whereas others exit the epidermis, move about, and either re-enter the epidermis or die. Mature males and females develop in about 17 days. Fertilized females may also move to new locations. All forms feed on epithelial cells and tissue fluid. Transmission is by contact with immature forms or fertilized females on the skin surface. The mites are not resistant to ordinary environmental conditions, and die within a few days if removed from the host.

Pathologic Effects. Lesions caused by *S. scabiei* are characterized microscopically by epidermal hyperplasia with orthokeratotic and parakeratotic hyperkeratosis and an overlying layer of keratinic and proteinaceous debris[172] (Figure 15.33). Mites and mite tunnels are in the debris and outer epidermal layers. The subjacent dermis contains an inflammatory cell infiltrate composed chiefly of lymphocytes and eosinophils. A suppurative response may be superimposed if there is secondary bacterial infection.

Clinical Disease. Signs of scabies infestation typically are first evident on the muzzle, later appearing around the eyes and on other areas of the face[73] (Figure 15.34). Other areas of the body can be affected, including the external genitalia. Early lesions are characterized by partial alopecia, hyperemia, and oozing of serous fluid. This progresses to a yellow-white or gray-white crust of epidermal cells and dried serum. The lesions are intensely pruritic, and the resultant scratching and rubbing increase their severity, as

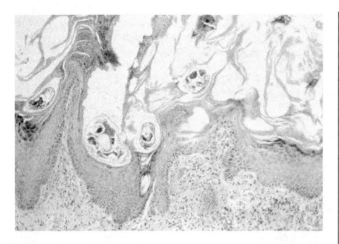

Fig. 15.33 *Sarcoptes scabiei* dermatitis, with dermal inflammatory cell accumulation, epidermal proliferation, and intradermal mites. Reproduced from Lin, S.L., Pinson, D.M., and Lindsey, J.R. (1984) with permission.

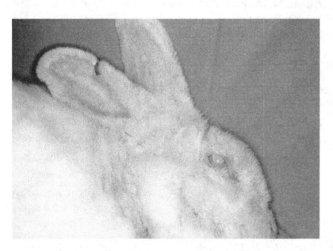

Fig. 15.34 *Sarcoptes scabiei* dermatitis. Reproduced from Lin, S.L., Pinson, D.M., and Lindsey, J.R. (1984) with permission.

do the secondary bacterial infections that occur in some cases. Severe disease can lead to debilitation and even death. An immunologic hypersensitivity reaction to the mites is thought to be the major pathogenetic mechanism of the dermatitis and pruritus.

Diagnosis. The diagnosis is made by examination of skin scrapings. Because these are burrowing mites, the specimen must be collected by adequately deep scraping. The position of the anus and the prominence of the dorsal scales distinguish *S. scabiei* from *Notoedres cati*. Clearing with potassium hydroxide solution may be required to adequately visualize these features.

Treatment and Prevention. There are no published studies evaluating treatment of sarcpotic mange in rabbits. Richardson recommends two doses of ivermectin, one week apart, at 400 µg/kg body weight by injection[109].

Public Health Considerations. Humans can be infested with *S. scabiei* mites from other hosts, especially dogs, and can develop significant dermatitis as a result[175], but there are no reported cases of human infestation acquired from rabbits.

Suborder Prostigmata

Cheyletiella parasitivorax **Morphology.** Adult *Cheyletiella parasitivorax* possess large, curved palpal claws which impart a distinctive appearance to this mite[111] (Figure 15.35). There is also a semicircular dorsal shield. The legs extend well beyond the body margins and bear feathered bristles and terminal tarsal combs. Adult males measure up to 320 µ long and 160 µ wide, whereas females measure 350 µ to 500 µ long and 200 µ wide.

Hosts. *Cheyletiella parasitivorax* parasitizes rabbits, dogs, and cats. It occurs throughout the world and is common in domestic rabbits[111,176,177]. Infestation among laboratory rabbits once was common, but probably is now rare. Several additional species of *Cheyletiella* have been described. Of these, *C. johnsoni*, *C. ochotonae*, and *C. takahasii* are reported to parasitize rabbits[178]. However, little or no information is available about infestation in rabbits with species other than *C. parasitivorax*.

Life Cycle. *Cheyletiella parasitivorax* is nonburrowing and inhabits the skin surface, where it feeds on tissue fluid. The mites primarily occur in the area over the scapulae, and eggs are attached to hair shafts 2 mm to 3 mm above the skin surface[111]. All stages can be found on the same host, and the life cycle is completed on the host. Transmission is by direct contact.

Pathologic Effects and Clinical Disease. In some cases there is partial alopecia and a fine gray-white scale on the skin surface, but the skin usually is not severely inflamed and may not be pruritic. Microscopic changes, when present, include mild epidermal hyperkeratosis and a mixed dermal inflammatory cell infiltrate of neutrophils, lymphocytes, plasma cells, and eosinophils. The area over the scapulae is most commonly affected (Figure 15.36), but other areas, including the face, also can be affected[179]. Infection is often subclinical.

Diagnosis. Mites can be collected by scraping, hair plucking, or use of a stiff brush. They are readily identified by their distinctive morphology, although if there are few

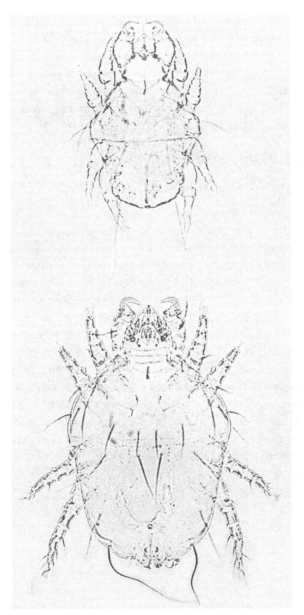

Fig. 15.35 *Cheyletiella parasitivorax.* (Above) Male. (Below) Female. Reproduced from Hofing, G.L. and Kraus, A.L. (1994) with permission.

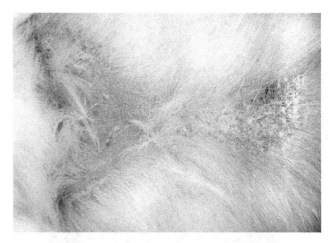

Fig. 15.36 *Cheyletiella parasitivorax* dermatitis over the scapulae.

mites in relation to the amount of epidermal debris, clearing with potassium hydroxide solution may be needed.

Treatment and Prevention. *Cheyletiella* mites are susceptible to a variety of acaricides, including benzyl benzoate, rotenone, pyrethrum, lindane, organophosphates, and avermectins[180]. Richardson[109] recommends ivermectin administered subcutaneously at a dosage of 300 μg/kg to 400 μg/kg body weight, repeated twice at two-week intervals.

Public Health Considerations. *Cheyletiella* mites can temporarily infest humans, resulting in severe dermatitis[181]. Typically, few mites are present, complicating diagnostic efforts.

Demodex cuniculi The follicle mite *Demodex cuniculi* occurs in rabbits[109]. It resembles *Demodex canis* morphologically. It is considered a normal resident of the skin, but there is one report of dermatitis attributed to it[182]. If necessary, infestation can be treated topically with a 0.01% solution of amitraz or by weekly subcutaneous injections of ivermectin at 500 μg/kg body weight until the condition resolves[109].

Trombiculids Mites of the family Trombiculidae (chiggers, red bugs, harvest mites) are found throughout the world. Only the larvae are parasitic. Adult mites are free-living in soil. Larvae hatch from eggs and climb onto plants, where they can survive up to 30 days awaiting a host. Upon reaching a host, the larvae attach to the skin, secrete saliva that digests a perforation in the epidermis called a stylostome, and feed on tissue fluid via the stylostome. Engorged larvae leave the host and undergo a period of development in the soil, emerge as nymphs, and feed on insects and insect eggs through the remainder of the life cycle. Larvae are deep red to pale yellow. When newly hatched, they are about 210 μ long and when engorged, about 400 μ long.

Trombiculid mites occur on wild lagomorphs and on domestic rabbits exposed to vegetation, but have not been reported on rabbits maintained in modern laboratory settings. The mites are not host specific, and several species have been found on lagomorphs. Among the more common are *Trombicula autumnalis, T. cavicola, T. irritans,* and *T. microti.* The saliva of the mites provokes a discrete focal

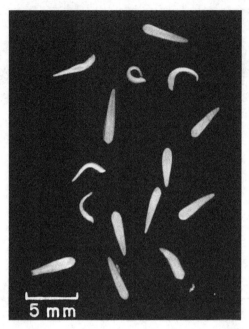

Fig. 15.37 *Linguatula serrata* nymphs. Courtesy of A. Fain, Institut de Médicine Tropicale Price Léopold.

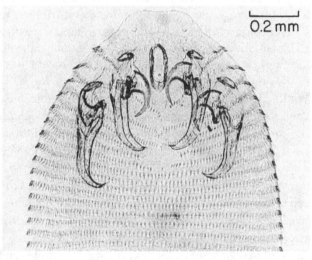

Fig. 15.38 *Linguatula serrata* nymph. Note spinous body rings and the two pairs of binate hooks. Courtesy of A. Fain, Institut de Médicine Tropicale Price Léopold.

irritant reaction with swelling and pruritus. Areas most commonly affected include the skin around the eyes and ears, the perineum, and the feet. Humans are commonly parasitized, acquiring the larvae from the environment in the same fashion as rabbits. Some species of trombiculid mites are reported to be capable of transmitting viral, rickettsial, and bacterial agents of zoonotic diseases[183].

Class Pentastomida

Linguatula serrata

Linguatula serrata occurs throughout the world. Many species of mammals, including wild lagomorphs, serve as intermediate hosts. Definitive hosts include canids, and in rare cases, humans. The interested reader is directed to Chapter 17, Parasites of Dogs, for information on the clinical aspects of adult infestations. Adults inhabit the respiratory tract. Eggs expelled in respiratory secretions into the environment are ingested by intermediate hosts. After hatching, larvae migrate from the intestine to mesenteric lymph nodes, undergo six to nine molts, and become infective nymphs, which are curved, 4 mm to 6 mm long, and located within small cysts (Figures 15.37 and 15.38). Transmission to definitive hosts occurs by ingestion of viscera containing nymphs. No clinical disease is evident in infected rabbits. Nymphs are found incidentally at necropsy.

TABLE 15.2 Parasites of Rabbits—Circulatory/Lymphatic System.

Parasite	Geographic distribution	Hosts	Location in host	Method of infection	Pathologic effects	Zoonosis	Reference
Flagellates							
Trypanosoma nabiasi	Europe, Turkey	Rabbits	Blood	Ingestion of flea vector or flea feces	None	Not reported	185
Trypanosoma sp.	US	Rabbits	Blood	Unknown	None	Not reported	186
Coccidia							
Hepatozoon cuniculi	Italy	Rabbits	Leucocytes, spleen	Unknown	Unknown	Not reported	187
Nematodes							
Filaroidea							
Dirofilaria immitis	Worldwide	Laboratory rabbits, dogs, other mammals	Pulmonary vasculature	Bite of mosquito intermediate host	Thrombus	Reported	194

TABLE 15-3 Parasites of Rabbits—Enterohepatic System.

Parasite	Geographic distribution	Hosts	Location in host	Method of infection	Pathologic effects	Zoonosis	Reference
Flagellates							
Chilomastix cuniculi	Worldwide	Lagomorphs	Cecum	Ingestion of organism in feces	None	Not reported	1
Enteromonas sp.	Worldwide	Lagomorphs	Cecum	Ingestion of organism in feces	None	Not reported	1
Giardia duodenalis	Worldwide	Lagomorphs, other mammals	Anterior small intestine	Ingestion of cysts in feces	Variable diarrhea	Not reported	1
Monocercomonas cuniculi	Worldwide	Rabbits	Cecum	Ingestion of organism in feces	None	Not reported	1
Retortamonas cuniculi	Worldwide	Rabbits	Cecum	Ingestion of organism in feces	None	Not reported	1
Amoebae							
Entamoeba cuniculi	Worldwide	Lagomorphs, rodents	Cecum, colon	Ingestion of cysts in feces	None	Not reported	1
Coccidia							
Cryptosporidium spp.	US, Europe	Lagomorphs	Small intestine	Ingestion of sporulated oocysts in feces	Enteritis	Uncertain	12
Eimeria coecicola	Europe, Asia	Rabbits	Jejunum, ileum, cecum	Ingestion of sporulated oocysts in feces	Severe enteritis	Not reported	1
Eimeria elongata	Europe	Rabbits	Intestine	Ingestion of sporulated oocysts in feces	Mild enteritis	Not reported	1
Eimeria exigua	Worldwide	Rabbits	Ileum	Ingestion of sporulated oocysts in feces	Mild enteritis	Not reported	1
Eimeria flavescens	Worldwide	Rabbits	Ileum, cecum, colon	Ingestion of sporulated oocysts in feces	Moderate to severe enteritis	Not reported	188
Eimeria intestinalis	Worldwide	Rabbits	Small intestine, colon	Ingestion of sporulated oocysts in feces	Severe catarrhal enteritis, sometimes death	Not reported	1
Eimeria irresidua	Worldwide	Rabbits	Small intestine	Ingestion of sporulated oocysts in feces	Moderate to severe hemorrhagic enteritis	Not reported	188
Eimeria magna	Worldwide	Rabbits	Jejunum, ileum	Ingestion of sporulated oocysts in feces	Moderate to severe enteritis, sometimes death	Not reported	1
Eimeria matsubayashii	Japan, India	Rabbits	Ileum, cecum	Ingestion of sporulated oocysts in feces	Mild to moderate fibrinonecrotic enteritis	Not reported	1
Eimeria media	Worldwide	Lagomorphs	Small intestine, colon	Ingestion of sporulated oocysts in feces	Mild to moderate enteritis	Not reported	184

484

Eimeria nagpurensis	India, Iran	Rabbits	Ingestion of sporulated oocysts in feces	Mild enteritis	Not reported	189
Eimeria neoleporis	Worldwide	Lagomorphs	Ingestion of sporulated oocysts in feces	Mild to severe enteritis in cottontail rabbits	Not reported	189
Eimeria perforans	Worldwide	Rabbits	Ingestion of sporulated oocysts in feces	Mild to moderate enteritis	Not reported	1
Eimeria piriformis	Worldwide	Rabbits	Ingestion of sporulated oocysts in feces	Moderate to severe enteritis	Not reported	1
Eimeria roobroucki	Europe	Rabbits	Ingestion of sporulated oocysts in feces	Unknown	Not reported	22
Eimeria stiedae	Worldwide	Lagomorphs	Ingestion of sporulated oocysts in feces	Hepatitis, biliary duct hyperplasia and fibrosis, icterus, enteritis, death	Not reported	1
Eimeria vejdovskyi	Europe	Rabbits	Ingestion of sporulated oocysts in feces	Unknown	Not reported	184
Microsporidia						
Enterocytozoon bieneusi	Europe	Rabbits, other mammals	Ingestion of spores	Unknown	Reported	72
Trematodes						
Dicrocoelium dendriticum	Americas, Asia, Europe	Lagomorphs, ruminants, humans	Ingestion of infected ants	Bile duct lesions, hepatic cirrhosis	Reported	37
Fasciola spp.	Worldwide	Lagomorphs, ruminants	Ingestion of metacercaria	Hepatitis	Reported	111
Hasstilesia spp.	US	Cottontail rabbits	Unknown	Catarrhal enteritis	Not reported	190
Cestodes						
Cyclophyllidea						
Andrya cuniculi	Europe	Rabbits	Ingestion of intermediate host (free-living mites)	None known	Not reported	80
Anoplocephaloides romerolagi	Europe	Rabbits	Ingestion of intermediate host (free-living mites)	None known	Not reported	85
Cittotaenia denticulata	Europe	Rabbits	Ingestion of intermediate host (free-living mites)	None known	Not reported	80
Cittotaenia variabilis	North America	Rabbits, cottontail rabbits	Ingestion of intermediate host (free-living mites)	None known	Not reported	75
Monoecocestus americana	Europe, North America	Lagomorphs	Ingestion of intermediate host (free-living mites)	Mild enteritis	Not reported	75
Mosgovoyia spp.	Europe, North America	Rabbits	Ingestion of intermediate host (free-living mites)	Mild enteritis, emaciation, sometimes death	Not reported	75, 84

(Continued)

TABLE 15-3 (Continued)

Parasite	Geographic Distribution	Hosts	Location in host	Method of infection	Pathologic effects	Zoonosis	Reference
Cyclophyllidea							
Paranoplocephala wimerosa	Europe	Rabbits	Small intestine	Ingestion of intermediate host (free-living mites)	None known	Not reported	80
Raillietina spp.	North America	Lagomorphs	Small intestine	Ingestion of intermediate host (ants)	None known	Not reported	73
Nematodes							
Rhabditoidea							
Strongyloides papillosus	Worldwide	Rabbits, hares, other mammals	Small intestine, lungs (larvae)	Ingestion of infective larva or penetration of skin or buccal mucosa by larva	None known	Not reported	99
Oxyuroidea							
Dermatoxys hispaniensis	Spain	Wild rabbits	Cecum, colon	Ingestion of embryonated egg	None	Not reported	82
Dermatoxys veligera	North America	Lagomorphs	Cecum, colon	Ingestion of embryonated egg	Mild typhlitis	Not reported	111
Dermatoxys vlakhaasi	Africa	Scrub hares	Cecum, colon	Ingestion of embryonated egg	None	Not reported	84
Passalurus ambiguus	Worldwide	Lagomorphs	Cecum, colon	Ingestion of embryonated egg	None	Not reported	82
Passalurus nonannulatus	North America	Cottontail rabbits, hares	Cecum, colon	Ingestion of embryonated egg	None	Not reported	111
Trichostrongyloidea							
Graphidium strigosum	Asia, Europe, North America	Lagomorphs	Stomach	Ingestion of infective larva	Gastritis, anemia, death	Not reported	111
Longistriata noviberiae	North America	Wild rabbits	Small intestine	Ingestion of infective larva	None	Not reported	112
Nematodirus spp.	Worldwide	Lagomorphs	Duodenum	Ingestion of infective larva	None	Not reported	113
Obeliscoides cuniculi	Worldwide	Lagomorphs	Stomach	Ingestion of infective larva	Hemorrhagic gastritis	Not reported	115, 116
Trichostrongylus calcaratus	North America	Lagomorphs, other mammals	Small intestine	Ingestion of infective larva	Anemia	Reported	87
Trichostrongylus ransomi	North America	Cottontail rabbits	Small intestine	Ingestion of infective larva	None	Not reported	73
Trichostrongylus retortaeformis	Asia, Europe, South America	Lagomorphs, goats	Duodenum, rarely stomach	Ingestion of infective larva	Enteritis	Not reported	124

Trichostrongylus spp.	Africa, Americas, Europe	Lagomorphs, other herbivores	Small intestine	Ingestion of infective larva	Variable, usually none	Not reported	36, 73, 81, 84, 125
Spiruroidea							
Gongylonema pulchrum	Worldwide	Cottontail rabbits, ruminants, swine	Esophageal mucosa	Ingestion of beetle or cockroach intermediate host	None	Rare	79, 111
Trichuroidea							
Trichuris spp.	Europe, North America	Lagomorphs, ground squirrels	Cecum, colon	Ingestion of embryonated egg	None	Not reported	136

TABLE 15-4 Parasites of Rabbits—Musculoskeletal System.

Parasite	Geographic Distribution	Hosts	Location in host	Method of infection	Pathologic effects	Zoonosis	Reference
Coccidia (Sporozoans)							
Besnoitia oryctofelisi	South America	Rabbits	Muscle	Ingestion of sporulated oocysts in feline feces	None	Not reported	7
Sarcocystis cuniculi	Worldwide	Cottontail rabbits	Striated and smooth muscle	Ingestion of sporulated oocysts in cat feces	Muscle cysts	Not reported	1
Sarcocystis leporum	Worldwide	Cottontail rabbits	Striated and smooth muscle	Ingestion of sporulated oocysts in cat or raccoon feces	Muscle cysts	Not reported	42

TABLE 15.5 Parasites of Rabbits—Nervous System.

Parasite	Geographic Distribution	Hosts	Location in host	Method of infection	Pathologic effects	Zoonosis	Reference
Coccidia							
Toxoplasma gondii	Worldwide	Lagomorphs, other mammals	Brain, myocardium, other organs	Ingestion of sporulated oocyst in cat feces	Organ-specific necrosis	Common	44–77
Microsporidia							
Encephalitozoon cuniculi	Worldwide	Rabbits, other mammals	Brain, kidneys, other tissues	Ingestion of spores, transplacental transmission	Encephalitis, nephritis	Reported	62–64
Nematodes							
Ascaridoidea							
Baylisascaris columnaris	North America	Rabbits, skunks	Central nervous system	Ingestion of embryonated eggs in skunk feces	Encephalitis	Rare	192
Baylisascaris procyonis	North America	Rabbits, other mammals	Central nervous system, other organs	Ingestion of embryonated eggs in raccoon feces	Encephalitis	Reported	103

489

TABLE 15.6 Parasites of Rabbits—Respiratory System.

Parasite	Geographic Distribution	Hosts	Location in host	Method of infection	Pathologic effects	Zoonosis	Reference
Nematodes							
Metastrongyloidea							
Protostrongylus boughtoni	North America	Cottontail rabbits, hares	Pulmonary bronchi	Ingestion of snail intermediate host	Pulmonary nodules	Not reported	127
Protostrongylus oryctolagi	Europe	Cottontail rabbits	Bronchi	Ingestion of mollusk intermediate host	Interstitial pneumonia, bronchiolitis	Not reported	111
Protostrongylus pulmonalis	Africa, Europe, North America	Lagomorphs, domestic animals	Lungs	Ingestion of snail intermediate host	Interstitial pneumonia	Not reported	198
Protostrongylus rufescens	Worldwide	Cottontail rabbits, ruminants	Pulmonary bronchioles	Ingestion of snail intermediate host	Interstitial pneumonia, bronchiolitis	Not reported	111
Protostrongylus sylvilagi	North America	Cottontail rabbits, hares	Lungs	Ingestion of mollusk intermediate host	Interstitial pneumonia	Not reported	111

490

TABLE 15-7 Parasites of Rabbits—Skin and Connective Tissue.

Parasite	Geographic Distribution	Hosts	Location in host	Method of infection	Pathologic effects	Zoonosis	Reference
Cestodes (Larval)							
Echinococcus granulosus	Worldwide	Lagomorphs, other mammals	Liver, lungs	Ingestion of hexacanth embryo in feces of canine definitive host	Larval cyst (hydatid cyst) formation	Common	191
Taenia macrocystis	North America	Hares	Back muscles, abdominal mesenteries, diaphragm, pericardium, liver	Ingestion of hexacanth embryo in feces of lynx definitive host	Larval cysts (strobilocerci) on muscles or in serous cavities	Not reported	191
Taenia polyacantha	Europe, North America	Lagomorphs, wild rodents	Peritoneal cavity, pleural cavity	Ingestion of hexacanth embryo in feces of fox definitive host	Larval cysts (cysticerci) in peritoneal cavity or pleural cavity	Not reported	191
Taenia pisiformis	Worldwide	Lagomorphs, wild rodents	Peritoneal cavity, liver	Ingestion of hexacanth embryo in feces of canine definitive host	Larval cysts (cysticerci) in peritoneal cavity, abdominal distention, liver damage	Not reported	191
Taenia serialis	Worldwide	Lagomorphs, wild rodents, dogs, primates	Subcutaneous tissues of thorax or limbs	Ingestion of hexacanth embryo in feces of canid definitive host	Subcutaneous larval cysts (coenuri)	Reported	191
Nematodes							
Filaroidea							
Brugia lepori	North America	Cottontail rabbits	Subcutis, abdominal lymphatic vessels	Transmitted by arthropod intermediate host	None	Unknown	132
Cercopithifilaria leporinua	North America	Snowshoe hares	Subcutis	Transmitted by arthropod intermediate host	None	Not reported	193
Dirofilaria scapiceps	North America	Cottontail rabbits, hares	Subcutis of trunk and later, the hock joint	Bite of mosquito intermediate host	Chronic tenosynovitis	Not reported	195
Dirofilaria uniformis	North America	Cottontail rabbits	Subcutis of trunk	Bite of mosquito intermediate host	None	Not reported	73
Micipsella numidica	Africa, Asia, Europe	Cottontail rabbits, hares	Subcutis	Transmitted by arthropod intermediate host	None	Not reported	196

(Continued)

491

TABLE 15-7 (Continued)

Arthropods

Diptera (flies)

Parasite	Geographic Distribution	Hosts	Location in host	Method of infection	Pathologic effects	Zoonosis	Reference
Ceratopogonidae (midges)	North America	Mammals	Skin	Direct contact	Dermatitis, pruritus	Common	199
Culicidae (mosquitoes)	Worldwide	Vertebrates	Skin	Direct contact	Pruritus, local inflammation, pathogen transmission	Common	111
Cuterebridae (bots)	North America	Lagomorphs, other mammals, birds	Subcutis	Egg deposited by female fly	Painful cysts	Reported	73, 138
Sarcophagidae (flesh flies)	Worldwide	Mammals, birds	Skin wounds	Larvae deposited by female fly	Dermal myiasis, fetid skin wounds	Reported	111
Simulidae (blackflies)	Worldwide	Mammals, birds	Skin	Direct contact	Irritation, pathogen transmission	Common	111

Phthiraptera (lice)

Parasite	Geographic Distribution	Hosts	Location in host	Method of infection	Pathologic effects	Zoonosis	Reference
Haemodipsus ventricosus	Worldwide	Rabbits	Pelage, especially dorsal and lateral trunk	Direct contact	Dermatitis, vector of *Francisella tularensis*	Not Reported	143
Haemodipsus spp.	Worldwide	Rabbits	Pelage	Direct contact	Dermatitis	Not Reported	140–142

Siphonaptera (fleas)

Parasite	Geographic Distribution	Hosts	Location in host	Method of infection	Pathologic effects	Zoonosis	Reference
Caenopsylla laptevi	Europe	Cottontail rabbits	Pelage	Direct contact	Dermatitis	Not reported	147
Cediopsylla simplex	North America	Cottontail rabbits	Pelage, bedding	Direct contact	Dermatitis	Not reported	143
Cediopsylla inequalis	North America	Cottontail rabbits	Pelage, bedding	Direct contact	Dermatitis	Not reported	143
Ctenocephalides spp.	Worldwide	Mammals	Pelage, bedding	Direct contact	Dermatitis	Common	145, 146
Echidnophaga gallinacea	Worldwide	Chickens, other birds, mammals	Pelage	Direct contact	Dermatitis	Common	145, 146
Echidnophaga iberica	Europe	Cottontail rabbits	Pelage	Direct contact	Dermatitis	Not reported	145, 146
Echidnophaga myrmecobii	Australia	Cottontail rabbits, other mammals	Pelage	Direct contact	Dermatitis	Not reported	145, 146
Hoplopsyllus glacialis affinis	North America	Cottontail rabbits	Pelage, bedding	Direct contact	Dermatitis	Not reported	143
Hystrichopsylla talpae	Europe	Wild rodents, cottontail rabbits	Pelage	Direct contact	Dermatitis	Not reported	145, 146
Meringis spp.	North America	Cottontail rabbits	Pelage, bedding	Direct contact	Dermatitis	Not reported	143
Odontopsyllus dentatus	North America	Cottontail rabbits	Pelage, bedding	Direct contact	Dermatitis	Not reported	143
Odontopsyllus multispinosus	North America	Cottontail rabbits	Pelage, bedding	Direct contact	Dermatitis	Not reported	143
Pulex irritans	Worldwide	Humans, other mammals	Pelage, bedding	Direct contact	Dermatitis	Common	145, 146

Species	Geographic distribution	Hosts	Location on host	Transmission	Effects	Human pathogen	Reference
Spilopsyllus cuniculi	Asia, Europe	Lagomorphs, hares, dog, cat	Pelage, bedding	Direct contact	Dermatitis, vector of myxomatosis virus and *Trypanosoma nabiasi*	Not reported	143
Xenopsylla cunicularis	Europe	Cottontail rabbits	Pelage	Direct contact	Dermatitis	Not reported	145, 146

Arachnida

Ticks (Soft)

Species	Geographic distribution	Hosts	Location on host	Transmission	Effects	Human pathogen	Reference
Ornithodoros parkeri	North America	Lagomorphs, wild rodents	Skin, bedding	Direct contact	Transmits relapsing fever, spotted fever	Reported; may transmit human pathogens	197
Ornithodoros turicata	Worldwide	Lagomorphs, other mammals	Skin, bedding	Direct contact	Transmits *F. tularensis* and other pathogens	Reported; may transmit human pathogens	197
Otobius lagophilus	North America	Cottontail rabbits, hares, cat	Skin (face), bedding	Direct contact	Transmits Colorado tick fever	Reported; may transmit Colorado tick fever	143, 197

Ticks (Hard)

Species	Geographic distribution	Hosts	Location on host	Transmission	Effects	Human pathogen	Reference
Amblyomma spp.	Worldwide	Lagomorphs, other mammals	Skin	Direct contact	Tick paralysis, local irritation, anemia, pathogen vector	Reported; transmits human pathogens	197
Dermacentor spp.	Worldwide	Lagomorphs, other mammals	Skin	Direct contact	Tick paralysis, local irritation, anemia, pathogen vector	Reported; transmits human pathogens	197
Haemaphysalis chordeilis	Americas	Cottontail rabbits, hares, small mammals	Skin	Direct contact	Anemia, emaciation, death, pathogen vector	Reported; transmits human pathogens	197
Haemaphysalis leporis-palustris	Americas	Cottontail rabbits, hares, small mammals, birds	Skin (head, neck)	Direct contact	Anemia, emaciation, death, pathogen vector	Reported; transmits human pathogens	197
Ixodes spp.	Worldwide	Lagomorphs, other mammals	Skin	Direct contact	Tick paralysis, local irritation, anemia, pathogen vector	Reported; transmits human pathogens	197
Rhipicephalus pusillus	Europe	Lagomorphs, other mammals	Skin	Direct contact	Anemia, emaciation, death, pathogen vector	Reported; transmits human pathogens	197

(Continued)

TABLE 15-7 (*Continued*)

Parasite	Geographic Distribution	Hosts	Location in host	Method of infection	Pathologic effects	Zoonosis	Reference
Ticks (Hard)							
Rhipicephalus sanguineus	Worldwide	Lagomorphs, dog, coyote, deer, cattle	Skin	Direct contact	Anemia, emaciation, death, pathogen vector	Reported; transmits human pathogens	197
Mites							
Astigmates							
Leporacarus gibbus	Worldwide	Lagomorphs	Pelage, back and abdomen	Direct contact	None	Reported	159
Psoroptes cuniculi	Worldwide	Domestic rabbits	External ear canal, pelage of face, neck, legs	Direct contact	Otitis externa and media, dermatitis, pruritus	Not reported	111
Notoedres cati	Worldwide	Cats, lagomorphs, other mammals	Skin	Direct contact	Dermatitis, pruritus	Reported	111
Sarcoptes scabiei	Worldwide	Mammals	Skin	Direct contact	Dermatitis, pruritus	Reported	111
Prostigmates							
Cheyletiella parasitivorax	Worldwide	Lagomorphs, dogs, cats	Pelage over scapulae	Direct contact	Alopecia, dermatitis, variable pruritus, hyperkeratosis	Reported	177
Cheyletiella spp.	Worldwide	Lagomorphs, other mammals	Pelage	Direct contact	Dermatitis	Not reported	178
Demodex cuniculi	Worldwide	Rabbits	Skin	Direct contact	Dermatitis	Not reported	182
Trombiculids (Chiggers)	Worldwide	Mammals	Skin	Direct contact	Dermatitis	Common	111
Arthropods							
Pentastomida (Tongue worms)							
Linguatula serrata	Worldwide	Lagomorphs, other mammals	Mesenteric lymph nodes	Ingestion of infective egg in canine feces	None	Reported	111

REFERENCES

1. Levine, N.D. (1985) *Veterinary Protozoology.* Iowa State University Press, Ames, IA.

2. Brugerolle, G. (1975) Ultrastructure of the genus *Enteromonas* da Fonseca (Zoomastigophorea) and revision of the order of Diplomonadida Wenyon (French). *J. Protozool.* **22,** 468–475.

3. Thompson, R.C., Hopkins, R.M., and Homan, W.L. (2000) Nomenclature and genetic groupings of *Giardia* infecting mammals. *Parasitol. Today* **16,** 210–213.

4. Ali, S.A. and Hill, D.R. (2003) *Giardia intestinalis. Curr. Opin. Infect. Dis.* **16,** 453–460.

5. Pakes, S.P. and Gerrity, L.W. (1994) Protozoal diseases. In: Manning, P.J., Ringler, D.H., and Newcomer, C.E. (eds.) *The Biology of the Laboratory Rabbit,* 2nd ed. Academic Press, San Diego, CA. 205–229.

6. Caccio, S.M. (2003) Molecular techniques to detect and identify protozoan parasites in the environment. *Acta Microbiol. Pol.* **52 (Suppl),** 23–34.

7. Venturini, L., Petruccelli, M., Piscopo, M., et al. (2002) Natural *Besnoitia* sp. infection in domestic rabbits from Argentina. *Vet. Parasitol.* **107,** 273–278.

8. Mbuthia, P.G., Gathumbi, P.K., Bwangamoi, O., and Wasike, P.N. (1993) Natural besnoitiosis in a rabbit. *Vet. Parasitol.* **45,** 191–198.

9. Tzipori, S. and Ward, H. (2002) Cryptosporidiosis: biology, pathogenesis and disease. *Microbes Infect.* **4,** 1047–1058.

10. Xiao, L., Fayer, R., Ryan, U., and Upton, S.J. (2004) *Cryptosporidium* taxonomy: Recent advances and implications for public health. *Clin. Microbiol. Rev.* **17,** 72–97.

11. Xiao, L., Morgan, U.M., Fayer, R., Thompson, R.C., and Lal, A.A. (2000) *Cryptosporidium* systematics and implications for public health. *Parasitol. Today* **16,** 287–292.

12. Rehg, J.E., Lawton, G.W., and Pakes, S.P. (1979) *Cryptosporidium cuniculus* in the rabbit (*Oryctolagus cuniculus*). *Lab. Anim. Sci.* **29,** 656–660.

13. Petry, F. (2004) Structural analysis of *Cryptosporidium parvum. Microsc. Microanal.* **10,** 586–601.

14. Ryan, U., Xiao, L., Read, C., Zhou, L., Lal, A.A., and Pavlasek, I. (2003) Identification of novel *Cryptosporidium* genotypes from the Czech Republic. *Appl. Environ. Microbiol.* **69,** 4302–4307.

15. Inman, L.R. and Takeuchi, A. (1979) Spontaneous cryptosporidiosis in an adult female rabbit. *Vet. Pathol.* **16,** 89–95.

16. Pavlasek, I., Lavicka, M., Tumova, E., and Skrivan, M. (1996) Spontaneous *Cryptosporidium* infection in weaned rabbits (Czech). *Vet. Med. (Praha)* **41,** 361–366.

17. Peeters, J.E., Geeroms, R., Carman, R.J., and Wilkins, T.D. (1986) Significance of *Clostridium spiroforme* in the enteritis-complex of commercial rabbits. *Vet. Microsc.* **12,** 25–31.

18. Fayer, R., Morgan, U., and Upton, S.J. (2000) Epidemiology of *Cryptosporidium:* Transmission, detection and identification. *Int. J. Parasitol.* **30,** 1305–1322.

19. Xiao, L., Lal, A.A., and Jiang, J. (2004) Detection and differentiation of *Cryptosporidium* oocysts in water by PCR-RFLP. *Methods Mol. Biol.* **268,** 163–176.

20. Limor, J.R., Lal, A.A., and Xiao, L. (2002) Detection and differentiation of *Cryptosporidium* parasites that are pathogenic for humans by real-time PCR. *J. Clin. Microbiol.* **40,** 2335–2338.

21. Levine, N.D. (1961) *Protozoan Parasites of Domestic Animals and Man.* Burgess, Minneapolis, 412 pages.

22. Carvalho, J.C.M. (1942) *Eimeria neoleporis* n. sp., occurring naturally in the cottontail and transmissible to the tame rabbit. *Iowa State Coll. J. Sci.* **16,** 409–410.

23. Kheisin, E.M. (1948) Development of two intestinal coccidia of the rabbit *Eimeria piriformis* Kotlan and Popesch and *Eimeria intestinalis* nom. nov. *Uch. Zap. Karelo-finsk. Univ.* **3,** 3.

24. Gill, B.S. and Ray, H.N. (1960) The coccidia of domestic rabbit and the common field hare of India. *Proc. Zool. Soc. Calcutta* **13,** 129–143.

25. Wilkinson, M.J., Bell, S., McGoldrick, J., and Williams, A.E. (2001) Unexpected deaths in young New Zealand white rabbits (*Oryctolagus cuniculus*). *Contemp. Top. Lab. Anim. Sci.* **40,** 49–51.

26. Fernandez, E., Roman, I.D., Cava, F., et al. (1996) Acid-base disturbances in the rabbit during experimental hepatic parasitosis. *Parasitol. Res.* **82,** 524–528.

27. Diehl, J.F. and Kistler, B.G. (1961) Vitamin E saturation test in coccidiosis infected rabbits. *J. Nutr.* **74,** 495–499.

28. San Martin-Nunez, B.V., Ordonez-Escudero, D., and Alunda, J.M. (1988) Preventive treatment of rabbit coccidiosis with alpha-difluoromethylornithine. *Vet. Parasitol.* **30,** 1–10.

29. Pakandl, M. (1986) Efficacy of salinomycin, monensin and lasalocid against spontaneous *Eimeria* infection in rabbits. *Folia Parasitol. (Praha)* **33,** 195–198.

30. Peeters, J.E. and Geeroms, R. (1986) Efficacy of toltrazuril against intestinal and hepatic coccidiosis in rabbits. *Vet. Parasitol.* **22,** 21–35.

31. Joyner, L.P., Catchpole, J., and Berrett, S. (1983) *Eimeria stiedai* in rabbits: The demonstration of responses to chemotherapy. *Res. Vet. Sci.* **34,** 64–67.

32. Peeters, J.E., Geeroms, R., Antoine, O., Mammerickx, M., Halen, P. (1981) Efficacy of narasin against hepatic and intestinal coccidiosis in rabbits. *Parasitology* **83,** 293–301.

33. Hanada, S., Umemoto, Y., Omata, Y., et al. (2003) *Eimeria stiedai* merozoite 49-kDa soluble antigen induces protection against infection. *J. Parasitol.* **89,** 613–617.

34. Gres, V., Voza, T., Chabaud, A., and Landau, I. (2003) Coccidiosis of the wild rabbit (*Oryctolagus cuniculus*) in France. *Parasite* **10,** 51–57.

35. Hobbs, R.P. and Twigg, L.E. (1998) Coccidia (*Eimeria* spp.) of wild rabbits in southwestern Australia. *Aust. Vet. J.* **76,** 209–210.

36. Lepitzki, D.A., Woolf, A., and Bunn, B.M. (1992) Parasites of cottontail rabbits of southern Illinois. *J. Parasitol.* **78,** 1080–1083.

37. Soveri, T. and Valtonen, M. (1983) Endoparasites of hares (*Lepus timidus* L. and *L. europaeus* Pallas) in Finland. *J. Wildl. Dis.* **19,** 337–341.

38. Harkness, J.E. and Wagner, J.E. (1995) *The Biology and Medicine of Rabbits and Rodents.* Williams and Wilkins, Baltimore, MD.

39. Polozowski, A. (1993) Coccidiosis of rabbits and its control (Polish). *Wiad. Parazytol.* **39,** 13–28.

40. Vanparijs, O., Desplenter, L., and Marsboom, R. (1989) Efficacy of diclazuril in the control of intestinal coccidiosis in rabbits. *Vet. Parasitol.* **34,** 185–190.

41. McPherson, C.W., Habermann, R.T., Every, R.R., and Pierson, R. (1962) Eradication of coccidiosis from large breeding colony of rabbits. *Proc. Anim. Care Panel* **12,** 133–140.

42. Fayer, R. and Kradel, D. (1977) *Sarcocystis leporum* in cottontail rabbits and its transmission to carnivores. *J. Wildl. Dis.* **13,** 170–173.

43. Munday, B.L., Smith, D.D., and Frenkel, J.K. (1980) Sarcocystis and related organisms in Australian Wildlife: IV. Studies on *Sarcocystis cuniculi* in European rabbits (*Oryctolagus cuniculus*). *J. Wildl. Dis.* **16,** 201–204.

44. Dubey, J.P., Brown, C.A., Carpenter, J.L., and Moore, J.J. III. (1992) Fatal toxoplasmosis in domestic rabbits in the USA. *Vet. Parasitol.* **44,** 305–309.

45. Leland, M.M., Hubbard, G.B., and Dubey, J.P. (1992) Clinical toxoplasmosis in domestic rabbits. *Lab. Anim. Sci.* **42,** 318–319.

46. Sedlak, K., Literak, I., Faldyna, M., Toman, M., and Benak, J. (2000) Fatal toxoplasmosis in brown hares (*Lepus europaeus*): Possible reasons of their high susceptibility to the infection. *Vet. Parasitol.* **93,** 13–28.

47. Bergmann, V., Heidrich, R., and Kiupel, H. (1980) Acute toxoplasmosis outbreak in rabbit flocks (German). *Angew. Parasitol.* **21,** 1–6.

48. Frenkel, J.K. (1971) Protozoal diseases of laboratory animals. In: Marcial-Rojas, R.A. (ed.) *Pathology of Protozoal and Helminthic Diseases.* Williams and Wilkins, Baltimore, MD, 318–369.

49. Bjerkas, I. and Landsverk, T. (1986) Identification of *Toxoplasma gondii* and *Encephalitozoon cuniculi* by immunoperoxidase techniques and electron microscopy in stored, formalin-fixed, paraffin-embedded tissues. *Acta Vet. Scand.* **27,** 11–22.

50. Jauregui, L.H., Higgins, J., Zarlenga, D., Dubey, J.P., and Lunney, J.K. (2001) Development of a real-time PCR assay for detection of *Toxoplasma gondii* in pig and mouse tissues. *J. Clin. Microbiol.* **39,** 2065–2071.

51. Remington, J.S., Thulliez, P., and Montoya, J.G. (2004) Recent developments for diagnosis of toxoplasmosis. *J. Clin. Microbiol.* **42,** 941–945.

52. Luft, B.J. and Remington, J.S. (1992) Toxoplasmic encephalitis in AIDS. *Clin. Infect. Dis.* **15,** 211–222.

53. Keeling, P.J. and Fast, N.M. (2002) Microsporidia: biology and evolution of highly reduced intracellular parasites. *Annu. Rev. Microbiol.* **56,** 93–116.

54. Didier, E.S., Didier, P.J., Snowden, K.F., and Shadduck, J.A. (2000) Microsporidiosis in mammals. *Microbes Infect.* **2,** 709–720.

55. Shadduck, J.A., Watson, W.T., Pakes, S.P., and Cali, A. (1979) Animal infectivity of *Encephalitozoon cuniculi.* *J. Parasitol.* **65,** 123–129.

56. Halanova, M., Letkova, V., Macak, V., Stefkovic, M., and Halan, M. (1999) The first finding of antibodies to *Encephalitozoon cuniculi* in cows in Slovakia. *Vet. Parasitol.* **82,** 167–171.

57. Cislakova, L., Literak, I., Balent, P., et al. (2001) Prevalence of antibodies to *Encephalitozoon cuniculi* (microsporidia) in Angora goats—a potential risk of infection for breeders. *Ann. Agric. Environ. Med.* **8,** 289–291.

58. Reetz, J. (1994) Natural transmission of microsporidia (*Encephalitozoon cuniculi*) by way of the chicken egg (German). *Tierarztl. Prax.* **22,** 147–150.

59. Wasson, K. and Peper, R.L. (2000) Mammalian microsporidiosis. *Vet. Pathol.* **37,** 113–128.

60. Baneux, P.J. and Pognan, F. (2003) *In utero* transmission of *Encephalitozoon cuniculi* strain type I in rabbits. *Lab. Anim.* **37,** 132–138.

61. Boot, R., van Knapen, F., Kruijt, B.C., and Walvoort, H.C. (1988) Serological evidence for *Encephalitozoon cuniculi* infection (nosemiasis) in gnotobiotic guinea pigs. *Lab. Anim.* **22,** 337–342.

62. Harcourt-Brown, F.M. and Holloway, H.K. (2003) *Encephalitozoon cuniculi* in pet rabbits. *Vet. Rec.* **152,** 427–431.

63. Kimman, T.G. and Akkermans, J.P. (1987) *Encephalitozoon cuniculi* in a rabbit-breeding colony (Dutch). *Tijdschr. Diergeneeskd.* **112,** 1405–1409.

64. Shadduck, J.A. and Pakes, S.P. (1971) Encephalitozoonosis (nosematosis) and toxoplasmosis. *Am. J. Pathol.* **64,** 657–671.

65. Aldras, A.M., Orenstein, J.M., Kotler, D.P., Shadduck, J.A., and Didier, E.S. (1994) Detection of microsporidia by indirect immunofluorescence antibody test using polyclonal and monoclonal antibodies. *J. Clin. Microbiol.* **32,** 608–612.

66. Conteas, C.N., Sowerby, T., Berlin, G.W., et al. (1996) Fluorescence techniques for diagnosing intestinal microsporidiosis in stool, enteric fluid, and biopsy specimens from acquired immunodeficiency syndrome patients with chronic diarrhea. *Arch. Pathol. Lab. Med.* **120,** 847–853.

67. Vavra, J., Bedrnik, P., and Cinatl, J. (1972) Isolation and in vitro cultivation of the mammalian microsporidian *Encephalitozoon cuniculi.* *Folia Parasitol. (Praha)* **19,** 349–354.

68. Suter, C., Muller-Doblies, U.U., Hatt, J.M., and Deplazes, P. (2001) Prevention and treatment of *Encephalitozoon cuniculi* infection in rabbits with fenbendazole. *Vet. Rec.* **148,** 478–480.

69. Johnson, C.H., Marshall, M.M., DeMaria, L.A., Moffet, J.M., and Korich, D.G. (2003) Chlorine inactivation of spores of *Encephalitozoon* spp. *Appl. Environ. Microbiol.* **69,** 1325–1326.

70. Waller, T. (1979) Sensitivity of *Encephalitozoon cuniculi* to various temperatures, disinfectants and drugs. *Lab. Anim.* **13,** 227–230.

71. Weiss, L.M. (2001) Microsporidia: Emerging pathogenic protists. *Acta Trop.* **78,** 89–102.

72. del Aguila, C., Izquierdo, F., Navajas, R., et al. (1999) *Enterocytozoon bieneusi* in animals: Rabbits and dogs as new hosts. *J. Eukaryot. Microbiol.* **46,** 8S–9S.

73. Hofing, G.L. and Kraus, A.L. (1994) Arthropod and helminth parasites. In: Manning, P.J., Ringler, D.H., and Newcomer, C.E. (eds.) *The Biology of the Laboratory Rabbit,* 2nd ed. Academic Press, San Diego, CA, 231–257.

74. Jacobson, H.A., Kirkpatrick, R.L., and Holliman, R.B. (1974) Emaciation and enteritis of cottontail rabbits infected with *Hasstilesia tricolor* and observations on a fluke to fluke attachment phenomenon. *J. Wildl. Dis.* **10,** 111–114.

75. Arnold, J.G. (1938) A study of the anoplocephaline cestodes of North American rabbits. *Zoologica (N.Y.)* **23,** 31–53.

76. Stunkard, H.W. (1941) Studies on the life history of the anoplocephaline cestodes of hares and rabbits. *J. Parasitol.* **27,** 299–325.

77. Honess, R.F. (1963) Unarmed cestodes of Wyoming rabbits. *Univ. Wyoming Publ.* **28,** 6–21.

78. Brittain, P.C. and Voth, D.R. (1975) Parasites of the black-tailed jackrabbit in north central Colorado. *J. Wildl. Dis.* **11,** 269–271.

79. Andrews, C.L. and Davidson, W.R. (1980) Endoparasites of selected populations of cottontail rabbits (*Sylvilagus floridanus*) in the southeastern United States. *J. Wildl. Dis.* **16,** 395–401.

80. Boag, B., Lello, J., Fenton, A., Tompkins, D.M., and Hudson, P.J. (2001) Patterns of parasite aggregation in the wild European rabbit (*Oryctolagus cuniculus*). *Int. J. Parasitol.* **31,** 1421–1428.

81. Boag, B. and Iason, G. (1986) The occurrence and abundance of helminth parasites of the mountain hare *Lepus timidus* (L.) and the wild rabbit *Oryctolagus cuniculus* (L.) in Aberdeenshire, Scotland. *J. Helminthol.* **60,** 92–98.

82. Foronda, P., Valladares, B., Lorenzo-Morales, J., Ribas, A., Feliu, C., and Casanova, J.C. (2003) Helminths of the wild rabbit (*Oryctolagus cuniculus*) in Macaronesia. *J. Parasitol.* **89,** 952–957.

83. Mead-Briggs, A.R. and Page, R.J. (1975) Records of anoplocephaline cestodes from wild rabbits and hares collected throughout Great Britain. *J. Helminthol.* **49,** 49–56.

84. Boomker, J., Horak, I.G., and Booyse, D.G. (1997) Parasites of South African wildlife. XV. Helminths of scrub hares, *Lepus saxatilis,* in the Kruger National Park. *Onderstepoort J. Vet. Res.* **64,** 285–290.

85. Kamiya, M., Suzuki, H., and Villa, R.-B. (1979) A new anoplocephaline cestode, *Anoplocephaloides romerolagi* sp. n. parasitic in the volcano rabbit, *Romerolagus diazi. Jpn. J. Vet. Res.* **27,** 67–71.

86. Arundel, J.H. (1986) Cestode infections of domestic animals. In: Campbell, W.C. and Rew, R.S. (eds.) *Chemotherapy of Parasitic Diseases.* Plenum, New York, NY, 479–494.

87. Clemons, C., Rickard, L.G., Keirans, J.E., and Botzler, R.G. (2000) Evaluation of host preferences by helminths and ectoparasites among black-tailed jackrabbits in northern California. *J. Wildl. Dis.* **36,** 555–558.

88. Arora, V.K., Gupta, K., Singh, N., and Bhatia, A. (1994) Cytomorphologic panorama of cysticercosis on fine needle aspiration. A review of 298 cases. *Acta Cytol.* **38,** 377–80.

89. Wolf, A., Rovira, A.R., Miller, K.L., and Widmer, W.R. (2002) What is your diagnosis? Two well-circumscribed, mineralized opacities in the left caudal quadrant of the abdomen. *J. Am. Vet. Med. Assoc.* **221,** 357–358.

90. O'Reilly, A., McCowan, C., Hardman, C., and Stanley, R. (2002) *Taenia serialis* causing exophthalmos in a pet rabbit. *Vet. Ophthalmol.* **5,** 227–230.

91. Lawson, J.R. and Gemmell, M.A. (1990) Transmission of taeniid tapeworm eggs via blowflies to intermediate hosts. *Parasitology* **100 (Pt 1),** 143–146.

92. Wills, J. (2001) Coenurosis in a pet rabbit. *Vet. Rec.* **148,** 188.

93. Ing, M.B., Schantz, P.M., and Turner, J.A. (1998) Human coenurosis in North America: Case reports and review. *Clin. Infect. Dis.* **27,** 519–523.

94. Tenora, F., Beranek, L., and Stanek, M. (1988) Larvocysts of the cestode *T. polyacantha* (Leucart, 1856) parasitizing *Oryctolagus cuniculus.* *Folia Parasitol. (Praha)* **35,** 21–22.

95. Bursey, C.C. and Burt, M.D. (1970) *Taenia macrocystis* (Diesing, 1850), its occurrence in Eastern Canada and Maine, U.S.A., and its life cycle in wild felines (*Lynx rufus* and *L. canadensis*) and hares (*Lepus americanus*). *Can. J. Zool.* **48,** 1287–1293.

96. Melendez, R.D., Yepez, M.S., and Coronado, A. (1984) *Echinococcus oligarthrus* cysts of rabbits in Venezuela. *J. Parasitol.* **70,** 1004–1005.

97. Schantz, P.M. and Lord, R.D. (1972) *Echinococcus* in the South American red fox (*Dusicyon culpaeus*) and the European hare (*Lepus europaeus*) in the Province of Neuquen, Argentina. *Ann. Trop. Med. Parasitol.* **66,** 479–485.

98. Epe, C., Coati, N., and Schnieder, T. (2004) Results of parasitological examinations of faecal samples from horses, ruminants, pigs, dogs, cats, hedgehogs and rabbits between 1998 and 2002 (German). *Dtsch. Tierarztl. Wochenschr.* **111,** 243–247.

99. Boag, B. (1972) Helminth parasites of the wild rabbit *Oryctolagus cuniculus* (L.) in north east England. *J. Helminthol.* **46,** 73–78.

100. Taira, N., Minami, T., and Smitanon, J. (1991) Dynamics of faecal egg counts in rabbits experimentally infected with *Strongyloides papillosus.* *Vet. Parasitol.* **39,** 333–336.

101. Nakamura, Y. and Motokawa, M. (2000) Hypolipemia associated with the wasting condition of rabbits infected with *Strongyloides papillosus.* *Vet. Parasitol.* **88,** 147–151.

102. Chitwood, M. and Lichtenfels, J.R. (1972) Identification of parasitic metazoa in tissue sections. *Exp. Parasitol.* **32,** 407–519.

103. Deeb, B.J. and DiGiacomo, R.F. (1994) Cerebral larva migrans caused by *Baylisascaris* sp. in pet rabbits. *J Am Vet Med Assoc* **205,** 1744–1747.

104. Bowman, D.D. (1987) Diagnostic morphology of four larval ascaridoid nematodes that may cause visceral larva migrans: *Toxascaris leonina, Baylisascaris procyonis, Lagochilascaris sprenti,* and *Hexametra leidyi.* *J. Parasitol.* **73,** 1198–1215.

105. Cuellar, C., Fenoy, S., Aguila, C., and Guillen, J.L. (1990) Evaluation of chemotherapy in experimental toxocarosis by determination of specific immune complexes. *J. Helminthol.* **64,** 279–289.

106. Rowley, H.A., Uht, R.M., Kazacos, K.R., et al. (2000) Radiologic-pathologic findings in raccoon roundworm (*Baylisascaris procyonis*) encephalitis. *AJNR Am. J. Neuroradiol.* **21,** 415–420.

107. Fujiwara, H., Uchida, K., and Takahashi, M. (1987) Occurrence of granulomatous appendicitis in rabbits (Japanese). *Jikken Dobutsu* **36,** 277–280.

108. Duwel, D. and Brech, K. (1981) Control of oxyuriasis in rabbits by fenbendazole. *Lab. Anim.* **15,** 101–105.

109. Richardson, V.C.G. (2000) *Rabbits. Health, Husbandry, and Diseases.* Blackwell Science, Oxford.

110. Sovell, J.R. and Holmes, J.C. (1996) Efficacy of ivermectin against nematodes infecting field populations of snowshoe hares (*Lepus americanus*) in Yukon, Canada. *J. Wildl. Dis.* **32,** 23–30.

111. Soulsby, E.J.L. (1982) *Helminths, Arthropods, and Protozoa of Domesticated Animals.* Williams and Wilkins, Baltimore, MD.

112. Stringer, R.P., Harkema, R., and Miller, G.C. (1969) Parasites in rabbits in North Carolina. *J. Parasitol.* **55,** 328.

113. Keith, I.M., Keith, L.B., and Cary, J.R. (1986) Parasitism in a declining population of snowshoe hares. *J. Wildl. Dis.* **22,** 349–363.

114. Audebert, F., Cassone, J., Kerboeuf, D., and Durette-Desset, M.C. (2002) The life cycle of *Nematodiroides zembrae* (Nematoda, Trichostrongylina) in the rabbit. *J. Parasitol.* **88,** 898–904.

115. Measures, L.M. and Anderson, R.C. (1983) New subspecies of the stomach worm, *Obeliscoides cuniculi* (Graybill), of lagomorphs. *Proc. Helminthol. Soc. Wash.* **50,** 1–14.

116. Jensen, L.J., Fox, J.G., Murphy, J.C., and Shalev, M. (1980) Natural infection of *Obeliscoides cuniculi* in a domestic rabbit. *Lab. Anim. Sci.* **30,** 231–233.

117. Worley, D.E. (1963) Experimental studies on *Obeliscoides cuniculi,* a trichostrongylid stomach worm of the rabbits. I. Host-parasite relationships and maintenance in laboratory rabbits. *J. Parasitol.* **49,** 46–50.

118. Watkins, A.R., Slocombe, J.O., and Fernando, M.A. (1984) The effects of single and multiple doses of thiabendazole on growing and arrested stages of the rabbit stomach worm *Obeliscoides cuniculi.* *Vet. Parasitol.* **16,** 295–302.

119. Soveri, T., Aarnio, M., Sankari, S., and Haukisalmi, V. (1992) Blood chemistry and endoparasites of the mountain hare (*Lepus timidus* L.) in high and low density populations. *J. Wildl. Dis.* **28,** 242–249.

120. Hobbs, R.P., Twigg, L.E., Elliot, A.D., and Wheeler, A.G. (1999) Evaluation of the association of parasitism with mortality of wild European rabbits *Oryctolagus cuniculus* (L.) in southwestern Australia. *J. Parasitol.* **85,** 803–808.

121. Foronda, P., Del Castillo, A., Abreu, N., Figueruelo, E., Pinero, J., and Casanova, J.C. (2003) Parasitic helminths of the wild rabbit, *Oryctolagus cuniculus,* in different bioclimatic zones in Tenerife, Canary Islands. *J. Helminthol.* **77,** 305–309.

122. Audebert, F., Hoste, H., and Durette-Desset, M.C. (2002) Life cycle of *Trichostrongylus retortaeformis* in its natural host, the rabbit (*Oryctolagus cuniculus*). *J. Helminthol.* **76,** 189–192.

123. Audebert, F., Vuong, P.N., and Durette-Desset, M.C. (2003) Intestinal migrations of *Trichostrongylus retortaeformis* (Trichostrongylina, Trichostrongylidae) in the rabbit. *Vet. Parasitol.* **112,** 131–146.

124. Barker, I.G. and Ford, G.E. (1975) Development and distribution of atrophic enteritis in the small intestines of rabbits infected with *Trichostrongylus retoartaeformis.* *J. Comp. Pathol.* **85,** 427–435.

125. Haupt, W. and Nickel, E.A. (1975) Course of the parasite phase of development of *Trichostrongylus axei* (Cobbold, 1879) Railliet et Henry, 1909, in the domestic rabbit (German). *Arch. Exp. Veterinarmed.* **29**, 129–134.

126. Goble, F.C. and Cheatum, E. (1944) Notes on the lungworms of North American Leporidae. *J. Parasitol.* **30**, 119–120.

127. Goble, F.C. and Dougherty, E.C. (1943) Notes on the lungworms (genus *Protostrongylus*) of varying hares (*Lepus americanus*) in eastern North America. *J. Parasitol.* **29**, 397–404.

128. Battisti, A., Di Paolo, M., and Di Guardo, G. (2000) Pulmonary protostrongyliasis in a mountain hare from Italy. *J. Wildl. Dis.* **36**, 367–369.

129. Pajersky, A., Svarc, R., and Medved'ova, M. (1992) Focal changes in the lungs of wild hares caused by the parasite *Protostrongylus commutatus* (Diesing, 1851). *Vet. Med. (Praha)* **37**, 249–255.

130. Kudo, N., Koneguchi, T., Ikadai, H., and Oyamada, T. (2003) Experimental infection of laboratory animals and sheep with *Gongylonema pulchrum* in Japan. *J. Vet. Med. Sci.* **65**, 921–925.

131. Jelinek, T. and Loscher, T. (1994) Human infection with *Gongylonema pulchrum*: A case report. *Trop. Med. Parasitol.* **45**, 329–330.

132. Eberhard, M.L. (1984) *Brugia lepori* sp. n. (Filarioidea: Onchocercidae) from rabbits (*Sylvilagus aquaticus, S. floridanus*) in Louisiana. *J. Parasitol.* **70**, 576–579.

133. Eberhard, M.L., Telford, S.R. III, and Spielman, A. (1991) A *Brugia* species infecting rabbits in the northeastern United States. *J. Parasitol.* **77**, 796–798.

134. Orihel, T.C. and Beaver, P.C. (1989) Zoonotic *Brugia* infections in North and South America. *Am. J. Trop. Med. Hyg.* **40**, 638–647.

135. Bartlett, C.M. (1984) Pathology and epizootiology of *Dirofilaria scapiceps* (Leidy, 1886) (Nematoda: Filarioidea) in *Sylvilagus floridanus* (J.A. Allen) and *Lepus americanus* Erxleben. *J. Wildl. Dis.* **20**, 197–206.

136. Tiner, J.D. (1950) Two new species of *Trichuris* from North America, with redescriptions of *Trichuris opaca* and *Trichuris leporis* (Nematoda: Aphasmidia). *J. Parasitol.* **36**, 350–355.

137. Kutzer, E. (1978) Notes to the hare-whipworm *Trichuris leporis* (Zeder, 1803) (German). *Z. Parasitenkd.* **56**, 69–72.

138. Baird, C.R. (1983) Biology of *Cuterebra lepusculi* Townsend (Diptera: Cuterebridae) in cottontail rabbits in Idaho. *J. Wildl. Dis.* **19**, 214–218.

139. Safdar, N., Young, D.K., and Andes, D. (2003) Autochthonous furuncular myiasis in the United States: Case report and literature review. *Clin. Infect. Dis.* **36**, e73–80.

140. Pfaffenberger, G.S. and Valencia, V.B. (1988) Ectoparasites of sympatric cottontails (*Sylvilagus audubonii* Nelson) and jack rabbits (*Lepus californicus* Mearns) from the high plains of eastern New Mexico. *J. Parasitol.* **74**, 842–846.

141. Broekhuizen, S. (1971) On the occurrence of hare lice, *Haemodipsus* spp. (Anoplura, Hoplopleuridae) on hares, *Lepus europaeus*, in the Netherlands. *Z. Parasitenkd.* **36**, 158–168.

142. Acevedo, P. (1990) Ectoparasites of wild rabbits (*Oryctolagus cuniculus*) from the Juan Fernandez archipelago. *Bol. Chil. Parasitol.* **45**, 29–31.

143. Kraus, A.L. (1974) Arthropod parasites. In: Weisbroth, S.H., Flatt, R.E., and Kraus, A.L. (eds.) *The Biology of the Laboratory Rabbit.* Academic Press, New York, NY, 287–310.

144. Pinter, L. (1999) *Leporacarus gibbus* and *Spilopsyllus cuniculi* infestation in a pet rabbit. *J. Small Anim. Pract.* **40**, 220–221.

145. Visser, M., Rehbein, S., and Wiedemann, C. (2001) Species of flea (Siphonaptera) infesting pets and hedgehogs in Germany. *J. Vet. Med. B Infect. Dis. Vet. Public Health* **48**, 197–202.

146. Osacar, J.J., Lucientes, J., Calvete, C., Peribanez, M.A., Garcia, M.J., and Castillo, J.A. (2001) Seasonal abundance of fleas (Siphonaptera: Pulicidae, Ceratophyllidae) on wild rabbits in a semiarid area of northeastern Spain. *J. Med. Entomol.* **38**, 405–410.

147. Cooke, B.D. (1999) Notes on the life-history of the rabbit flea *Caenopsylla laptevi ibera* Beaucournu and Marquez, 1987 (Siphonaptera: Ceratophyllidae) in eastern Spain. *Parasite* **6**, 347–354.

148. Keith, L.B. and Cary, J.R. (1990) Interaction of the tick (*Haemaphysalis leporispalustris*) with a cyclic snowshoe hare (*Lepus americanus*) population. *J. Wildl. Dis.* **26**, 427–434.

149. Fuentes, L., Calderon, A., and Hun, L. (1985) Isolation and identification of *Rickettsia rickettsii* from the rabbit tick (*Haemaphysalis leporispalustris*) in the Atlantic zone of Costa Rica. *Am. J. Trop. Med. Hyg.* **34**, 564–567.

150. Banerjee, S.N., Banerjee, M., Fernando, K., Dong, M.Y., Smith, J.A., and Cook, D. (1995) Isolation of *Borrelia burgdorferi*, the Lyme disease spirochete, from rabbit ticks, *Haemaphysalis leporispalustris*—Alberta. *Can. Commun. Dis. Rep.* **21**, 86–88.

151. Goethert, H.K. and Telford, S.R. III. (2003) Enzootic transmission of *Anaplasma bovis* in Nantucket cottontail rabbits. *J. Clin. Microbiol.* **41**, 3744–3747.

152. Goethert, H.K. and Telford, S.R. III. (2003) Enzootic transmission of *Babesia divergens* among cottontail rabbits on Nantucket Island, Massachusetts. *Am. J. Trop. Med. Hyg.* **69**, 455–460.

153. Telford, S.R. III, and Spielman, A. (1989) Competence of a rabbit-feeding *Ixodes* (Acari: Ixodidae) as a vector of the Lyme disease spirochete. *J. Med. Entomol.* **26**, 118–121.

154. Goethert, H.K. and Telford, S.R. III. (2003) Enzootic transmission of the agent of human granulocytic ehrlichiosis among cottontail rabbits. *Am. J. Trop. Med. Hyg.* **68**, 633–637.

155. Henke, S.E., Pence, D.B., Demarais, S., and Johnson, J.R. (1990) Serologic survey of selected zoonotic disease agents in black-tailed jack rabbits from western Texas. *J. Wildl. Dis.* **26**, 107–111.

156. Ciceroni, L., Pinto, A., Rossi, C., et al. (1988) Rickettsiae of the spotted fever group associated with the host-parasite system *Oryctolagus cuniculi/Rhipicephalus pusillus*. *Zentralbl. Bakteriol. Mikrobiol. Hyg. [A]* **269**, 211–217.

157. Horak, I.G., Spickett, A.M., Braack, L.E., and Penzhorn, B.L. (1993) Parasites of domestic and wild animals in South Africa. XXXII. Ixodid ticks on scrub hares in the Transvaal. *Onderstepoort J. Vet. Res.* **60**, 163–174.

158. Niekrasz, M.A., Curl, J.L., and Curl, J.S. (1998) Rabbit fur mite (*Listrophorus gibbus*) infestation of New Zealand White rabbits. *Contemp. Top. Lab. Anim. Sci.* **37**, 73–75.

159. Kirwan, A.P., Middleton, B., and McGarry, J.W. (1998) Diagnosis and prevalence of *Leporacarus gibbus* in the fur of domestic rabbits in the UK. *Vet. Rec.* **142**, 20–21.

160. Burns, D.A. (1987) Papular urticaria produced by the mite *Listrophorus gibbus*. *Clin. Exp. Dermatol.* **12**, 200–201.

161. Beck, W. (1996) Animal mite-induced epizoonoses and their significance in dermatology. *Hautarzt.* **47**, 744–748.

162. Baker, E.W., Evans, T.M., Gould, D.J., Hull, W.B., and Keegan, H.L. (1956) A Manual of Parasitic Mites of Medical or Economic Importance. *Tech. Publ. Natl. Pest Control Assoc., Inc.,* New York, NY, 170 pages.

163. Bates, P.G. (1999) Inter- and intra-specific variation within the genus *Psoroptes* (Acari: Psoroptidae). *Vet. Parasitol.* **83**, 201–217.

164. Zahler, M., Hendrikx, W.M., Essig, A., Rinder, H., and Gothe, R. (2000) Species of the genus *Psoroptes* (Acari: Psoroptidae): A taxonomic consideration. *Exp. Appl. Acarol.* **24**, 213–225.

165. Ochs, H., Mathis, A., and Deplazes, P. (1999) Single nucleotide variation in rDNA ITS-2 differentiates *Psoroptes* isolates from sheep and rabbits from the same geographical area. *Parasitology* **119** (Pt 4), 419–424.

166. Smith, K.E., Wall, R., Berriatua, E., and French, N.P. (1999) The effects of temperature and humidity on the off-host survival of *Psoroptes ovis* and *Psoroptes cuniculi*. *Vet. Parasitol.* **83**, 265–275.

167. Perrucci, S. and Rossi, G. (2002) Aerobic and microaerophilic bacteria isolated from *Psoroptes cuniculi*. *Parassitologia* **44**, 149–151.

168. Cutler, S.L. (1998) Ectopic *Psoroptes cuniculi* infestation in a pet rabbit. *J. Small. Anim. Pract.* **39**, 86–87.

169. McTier, T.L., Hair, J.A., Walstrom, D.J., and Thompson, L. (2003) Efficacy and safety of topical administration of selamectin for treatment of ear mite infestation in rabbits. *J. Am. Vet. Med. Assoc.* **223**, 322–324.

170. Wagner, R. and Wendlberger, U. (2000) Field efficacy of moxidectin in dogs and rabbits naturally infested with *Sarcoptes* spp., *Demodex* spp. and *Psoroptes* spp. mites. *Vet. Parasitol.* **93**, 149–158.

171. Koopman, J.P., Scholten, P.M., van Zutphen, T., and Hooghof, J.B. (1989) The effect of ivermectin on *Psoroptes* ear mange in rabbits (Dutch). *Tijdschr. Diergeneeskd.* **114**, 825–828.

172. Lin, S.L., Pinson, D.M., and Lindsey, J.R. (1984) Diagnostic exercise. Mange due to *Sarcoptes scabiei*. *Lab. Anim. Sci.* **34**, 353–355.

173. Lee, W.K. and Cho, B.K. (1995) Taxonomical approach to scabies mites of human and animals and their prevalence in Korea (Korean). *Korean J. Parasitol.* **33**, 85–94.

174. Skerratt, L.F., Campbell, N.J., Murrell, A., Walton, S., Kemp, D., and Barker, S.C. (2002) The mitochondrial 12S gene is a suitable marker of populations of *Sarcoptes scabiei* from wombats, dogs and humans in Australia. *Parasitol. Res.* **88**, 376–379.

175. Burroughs, R.F. and Elston, D.M. (2003) What's eating you? Canine scabies. *Cutis* **72**, 107–109.

176. Clark, J.D. and Ah, H.S. (1976) *Cheyletiella parasitivorax* (Megnin), a parasitic mite causing mange in the domestic rabbit. *J. Parasitol.* **62**, 125.

177. Akintunde, K.C., Pate, P., Lansdown, A.B., and Abraham, L. (1994) Cheyletid mite infection in laboratory rabbits. *Vet. Rec.* **134**, 560.

178. Bronswijk, J.E. and De Kreek, E.J. (1976) *Cheyletiella* (Acari: Cheyletiellidae) of dog, cat and domesticated rabbit, a review. *J. Med. Entomol.* **13**, 315–327.

179. Cloyd, G.G. and Moorhead, D.P. (1976) Facial alopecia in the rabbit associated with *Cheyletiella parasitivorax*. *Lab. Anim. Sci.* **26**, 801–803.

180. Curtis, C.F. (2004) Current trends in the treatment of *Sarcoptes*, *Cheyletiella* and *Otodectes* mite infestations in dogs and cats. *Vet. Dermatol.* **15**, 108–114.

181. Wagner, R. and Stallmeister, N. (2000) *Cheyletiella* dermatitis in humans, dogs and cats. *Br. J. Dermatol.* **143**, 1110–1112.

182. Harvey, R.G. (1990) *Demodex cuniculi* in dwarf rabbits *(Oryctolagus cuniculus)*: A case report. *J. Small Anim. Pract.* **31**, 204–207.

183. Saito, Y. (1962) Isolation of *Pasteurella tularensis* from ticks and chiggers parasitized on tularemic wild hares, with some tularemia transmission experiments. *Acta. Med. Biol. (Niigata)* **10**, 147–159.

184. Pakandl, M. (1988) Description of *Eimeria vejdovskyi* sp.n. and redescription of *Eimeria media* Kessel, 1929 from the rabbit. *Folia Parasitol. (Praha)* **35**, 1–9.

185. Grewal, M.S. (1956) Life cycle of the rabbit trypanosome, *Trypanosoma nabiasi* Railliet, 1895. *Trans. Roy. Soc. Trop. Med. Hyg.* **50**, 2–3.

186. Holliman, R.B. (1966) A *Trypanosoma lewisi*-like organism from the rabbit, *Sylvilagus floridanus*, in Virginia. *J. Parasitol.* **52**, 622.

187. Sangiorgi, G. (1914) *Leucocytogregarina cunuculi*, n. sp. *Giorn. Accad. Med. Torino.* **20**, 25–29.

188. Norton, C.C., Catchpole, J., and Joyner, L.P. (1979) Redescriptions of *Eimeria irresidua* Kessel and Jankiewicz, 1931 and *E. flavescens* Marotel and Guilhon, 1941 from the domestic rabbit. *Parasitology* **79**, 231–248.

189. Niak, A. (1967) *Eimeria* in laboratory rabbits in Teheran. *Vet. Record* **81**, 549.

190. Stringer, R.P., Harkema, R., and Miller, G.C. (1969) Parasites of rabbits on North Carolina. *J. Parasitol.* **55**, 328.

191. Jones, A. and Pybus, M.J. (2001) Taeniasis and Echinococcosis. In: Samuel, W.M., Pybus, M.J., and Kocan, A.A. (eds.). *Parasitic Diseases of Wild Mammals*, 2nd ed. Iowa State University Press. Ames, IA, 150–192.

192. Nettles, V.F. and Davidson, W.R. (1975) An epizootic of cerebrospinal nematodiasis in cottontail rabbits. *J. Am. Vet. Med. Assoc.* **167**, 600–602.

193. Bartlett, C.M. 1983. *Cercopithifilaria leporinus* n. sp. (Nematoda: Filarioidea) from the snowshoe hare (*Lepus americanus* Erxleben) (Lagomorpha) in Canada. Ann. Parasitol. Hum. Comp. **58**, 275–283.

194. Narama, I., Tsuchitani, M., Umemura, T. and Kamiya, H. (1982) Pulmonary nodule caused by *Dirofilaria immitis* in a laboratory rabbit (*Oryctolagus cuniculus domesticus*). *J. Parasitol.* **68**, 351–352.

195. Anderson, R.C. (2001) Filarioid Nematodes. In: Samuel, W.M., Pybus, M.J., and Kocan, A.A. (eds.). *Parasitic Diseases of Wild Mammals*, 2nd ed. Iowa State University Press. Ames, IA, 342–356.

196. Cancrini, G., Poglayen, G., and Vecchi, G. (1988) Report of *Micipsella numidica* (Seurat, 1917) in Italy (Italian). *Parassitologia* **30**, 219–224.

197. Allan, S.A. (2001) Ticks (Class Arachnida: Order Acarina). In: Samuel, W.M., Pybus, M.J., and Kocan, A.A. (eds.). *Parasitic Diseases of Wild Mammals*, 2nd ed. Iowa State University Press. Ames, IA, 72–106.

198. Battisti, A., Di Paolo, M., and Di Guardo, G. (2000) Pulmonary protostrongyliasis in a mountain hare from Italy. *J. Wildl. Dis.* **36**, 367–369.

199. Mullens, B.A. and Dada, C.E. (1992) Insects feeding on desert bighorn sheep, domestic rabbits, and Japanese quail in the Santa Rosa mountains of southern California. *J. Wildl. Dis.* **28**, 476–480.

CHAPTER

16

Parasites of Ferrets

Mary Patterson, MS, DVM, DACLAM;
and James G. Fox, DVM, MS, DACLAM

INTRODUCTION

Despite their increasing popularity as pets and their long-time use in biomedical research, including as experimental hosts for various parasitic infections[1], domestic ferrets (*Mustela putorius furo*) have been found to be naturally infected with relatively few species of parasites. This could result in part from the current husbandry practice of confined or indoor housing for most ferrets. Alternatively, some parasitisms may be underreported.

Regardless, the parasites that are commonly found in ferrets tend to be those that are also found in other carnivorous mammals, such as dogs and cats. Therefore, the interested reader will at times be referred to Chapter 17, Parasites of Dogs, and Chapter 18, Parasites of Cats, for additional information. Because of the dearth of naturally occurring parasites in ferrets, relatively little is known of their treatment. Veterinarians called upon to treat parasitic diseases in ferrets often must use drug guidelines developed in other host species, and should be aware that the administration of antiparasitic drugs to ferrets involves extralabel use.

PROTOZOA

Phylum Sarcomastigophora

Giardia sp.

Clinical cases of giardiasis have not been described in the literature. However, cysts and trophozoites have occasionally been identified in fecal specimens from ferrets. In addition, a recent publication reports the isolation and molecular characterization of a zoonotic genotype of *Giardia intestinalis* in a pet store ferret[38]. Although virtually nothing is known about *Giardia* sp. in ferrets, it is likely that the biology and clinical management would be similar to the same condition in dogs. Some have recommended that, if warranted, treatment be administered with oral metronidazole (50 mg/kg daily) for at least five days[2]. In dogs, oral fenbendazole (50 mg/kg daily) administered for three days, repeated in two weeks, has proven highly effective in treating giardiasis[3]. This regimen has not been evaluated in ferrets.

Phylum Apicomplexa

Cryptosporidium parvum

The reader is directed to Chapter 20, Parasites of Sheep and Goats, for information concerning the biology and management of *Cryptosporidium parvum*. Young ferrets can be infected with enteric *C. parvum* but the condition is usually subclinical and self-limiting, even in ferrets receiving immunosuppressive corticosteroids[4]. Diagnosis is made by identifying the very small (5 μm) oocysts in fresh fecal smears or concentrated fecal samples stained by acid-fast stains, auramine, or fluorescent antibodies[5]. Asexual and sexual stages can also be seen on the surface of microvilli by light microscopy (Figure 16.1).

No drug therapy for cryptosporidiosis is widely accepted as safe and efficacious at present, although paromomycin, an aminoglycoside antibiotic, has been shown to have potential use in humans and various animal species, including a cat that had cryptosporidian oocysts in its diarrheic feces[6]. However, caution must be advised in extrapolating the cat dosage used (165 mg/kg orally twice a day for five days) to ferrets, because a later report described acute renal failure in four cats treated with paromomycin at the same or a lower dosage level[7].

Recently, direct sequencing of polymerase chain reaction DNA products has been used to verify that the ferret

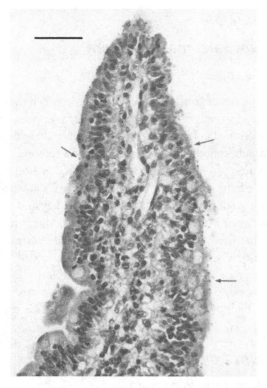

Fig. 16.1 Small intestinal villus of a ferret with numerous cryptosporidia (arrows) along the brush border. H & E stain, bar = 35 μ. Reproduced from Rehg, J.E., Gigliotti, F., and Stokes, D.C. (1988) with permission.

genotype of *C. parvum* is unique, and appears conserved among ferrets from different geographic areas[8]. It is unknown whether ferret isolates can infect humans, or if the ferret can be a reservoir for isolates of *C. parvum* recovered from other host species. The public health significance of ferret cryptosporidia will depend on evidence of interspecies transmission. In the meantime, ferret isolates of *C. parvum* should be considered zoonotic.

Eimeria spp. and *Isospora* sp.

Morphology, Hosts, and Life Cycle. Three species of coccidia, *Eimeria furonis, E. ictidea,* and *Isospora laidlawi,* were described in ferrets early in the last century[9,10]. In two case reports since then, ferrets have been found infected with coccidia morphologically consistent with *E. furonis*[11,12]. Oocysts of *E. furonis* measure 12.8 μm long by 12 μm wide. Those of *E. ictidea* measure 23.6 μm long by 17.5 μm wide, and those of *I. laidlawi* measure 34 μm long by 29 μm wide[9].

Sporulated oocysts of *E. furonis* and *E. ictidea* may also be differentiated from those of *I. laidlawi* by the number of sporocysts and sporozoites. Sporulated oocysts of *Eimeria* spp. contain four sporocysts, each of which contains two sporozoites, whereas oocysts of *Isospora* spp. contain two sporocysts, with four sporozoites each. Their life cycles are similar and direct[5]. Oocysts shed in the feces undergo sporulation to become infectious. Once these are ingested, sporozoites are released in the intestine to invade epithelial cells and become trophozoites. Asexual multiplication follows until merozoites form the sexual microgametes and macrogametes that fuse and mature to form oocysts. In addition to these, ferret kits raised on the same premises with puppies were found to shed oocysts of *I. ohioensis*. The ferrets exhibited no signs of disease[13].

Pathologic Effects and Clinical Disease. Healthy, young ferrets infected with coccidia typically have no ill effects, although diarrhea can occur when animals are stressed[2]. In one case, a four-month-old ferret presenting with diarrhea and lethargy was diagnosed post-mortem with enteric coccidiosis[14]. The inflamed and thickened intestinal villi contained coccidia in various stages of development (Figure 16.2). In another study, several ferrets with proliferative bowel disease were found to be coinfected with coccidia and *Lawsonia intracellularis,* but the contribution of the protozoa to the intestinal lesions in these cases could not be determined[11]. Hepatic coccidiosis was diagnosed in a weanling ferret which was emaciated, anorectic, and slightly icteric[12].

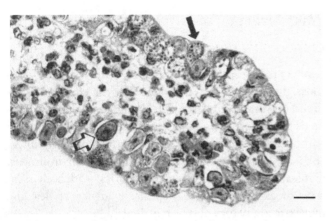

Fig. 16.2 Small intestinal villus of a ferret with enteric coccidiosis. A macrogamete (closed arrow) and oocyst (open arrow) are present within epithelial cells. Reproduced from Blankenship-Paris, T.L., Chang, J., and Bagnell, C.R. (1993) with permission.

Diagnosis. Fecal flotation techniques and direct smears are used to detect coccidian oocysts. The reader is referred to Chapter 1, Collection, Preservation, and Diagnostic Methods, for a description of methods.

Treatment and Prevention. Oral treatment regimens include any of the following: sulfadimethoxine at 30 mg/kg, cherry-flavored sulfadiazine-trimethoprim at 30 mg/kg, amprolium at 19 mg/kg, or decoquinate at 0.5 mg/kg[2]. The latter two coccidiostats are only commercially available in large volumes and thus are more practical for treating large groups of ferrets. Treatment should be administered for at least two weeks.

Ferrets should be placed in clean cages after the first treatment, at least once more during the first week of treatment, and again on the day before the period of treatment is concluded. One or more negative fecal examinations should be used to demonstrate treatment efficacy, regardless of the drug employed. Oocysts sporulate rapidly and thus can infect susceptible ferrets a few days after being shed. Therefore, prevention of oocyst transmission once an outbreak has occurred requires strict attention to sanitation, including thorough disinfection of cages and equipment.

Public Health Considerations. Coccidia of ferrets are not considered infectious to humans.

Toxoplasma gondii

The reader is referred to Chapter 18, Parasites of Cats, for a complete discussion of the biology and clinical aspects of toxoplasmosis. Like essentially all other mammals, ferrets may serve as intermediate hosts for *Toxoplasma gondii*. Ferrets become infected by ingesting raw meat that contains encysted stages or food contaminated by cat feces that contains sporulated oocysts. Infections are usually subclinical. In one report, ferrets used in a study on canine distemper were found to be infected with *Toxoplasma* by histological examination[15]. Elsewhere, congenital infection appeared to be responsible for *Toxoplasma*-like organisms in neonatal kits that died acutely with characteristic lesions of multifocal necrosis in the heart, liver, and lungs[16]. Antemortem diagnosis may be achieved serologically. Treatment of infected ferrets generally is not warranted; thus, guidelines are not available. Ferret food should be stored in sealed containers and protected from contamination with cat feces.

NEMATODES

Dirofilaria immitis

Ferrets are susceptible to infection with a variety of nematode parasites[17,18], but reports of these are rare. Related mustelids living in the wild are more commonly exposed to unusual nematode species; for example, gastric gnathosomiasis was recently documented in polecats (*Mustela putorius*) from Bulgaria[19]. The nematode of primary importance in laboratory ferrets is the heartworm, *Dirofilaria immitis*.

Morphology. The reader is referred to Chapter 17, Parasites of Dogs, for a morphologic description of *D. immitis*.

Hosts. Dogs and other canines are the most common definitive hosts of *D. immitis*. Cats, ferrets, harbor seals, and humans may also become infected.

Life Cycle. The life cycle of *D. immitis* in ferrets is similar to that described for dogs. Infection occurs when mosquitoes carrying infective third-stage larvae feed upon ferrets. The larvae migrate subcutaneously within the ferret host, reaching the heart as early as 70 days post-infection, where they become adult worms[20]. Adult worms copulate and the females release microfilaria into the bloodstream for ingestion by mosquitoes. Microfilaria develop to the infective third-stage larvae in the mosquito. Microfilaremia is not a consistent finding in ferrets.

Pathologic Effects and Clinical Disease. Adult worms are found in the right atrium and ventricle, pulmonary artery, and vena cavae of ferrets[21–24]. Cardiomegaly, pleural fluid, and ascites develop, and are accompanied by lethargy, anorexia, weakness, dyspnea, cyanosis, and persistent cough. Thoracic auscultation reveals normal to inaudible heart sounds and moist lung sounds.

Diagnosis. Dirofilariasis may be suspected with a history of exposure to mosquitoes, characteristic clinical signs, and radiographic or ultrasonographic evidence of thoracic changes. Because microfilaremia may not be present, definitive diagnosis requires heartworm antigen testing. At this time, heartworm test kits have not been thoroughly evaluated in ferrets[25].

Treatment. Because even one adult worm can be fatal, ferrets in heartworm-endemic areas should be maintained on a heartworm prevention program throughout the year. Monthly oral ivermectin formulated for dogs or cats is safe for ferrets. While the microfilaricidal dose of ivermectin is about 6 μg/kg, ferrets can tolerate much higher dosages[2]. A protocol for treatment of ferrets with dirofilariasis has been described[25]. The regimen combines melarsomine and ivermectin for treatment of adult worms and microfilaria, respectively. The adulticide melarsomine is given at 2.5 mg/kg intramuscularly once; one month later the same dosage of melarsomine is given twice, 24 hours apart.

Ancillary supportive care is also necessary, and includes diuretics for pleural effusion and oral prednisone at 0.5 mg/kg once or twice a day. Strict cage rest is recommended for four to six weeks after treatment. If animals have clinical signs and microfilaremia, 50 μg/kg ivermectin is administered subcutaneously every 30 days until signs and microfilaria are eliminated.

Prevention. Ferrets should be housed in such a way that they are not accessible to mosquitoes.

Public Health Considerations. Though uncommon, *D. immitis* will infect humans. However, most humans are at a greater risk of exposure as a result of mosquitoes feeding on infected dogs, versus those feeding on infected ferrets, especially because microfilaremia is uncommon in ferrets.

ARTHROPODS

Ferrets that live outdoors may become infested with a variety of arthropod parasites, including mites, ticks, and fly larvae[17,18]. In some cases, these may cause clinical disease. For example, abscesses, granulomatous masses, and fistulae have been reported due to myiasis[18]. The arthropod parasites most likely to be encountered in the laboratory setting are discussed below.

Class Insecta

Ctenocephalides sp.

Ferrets are susceptible to infestation with fleas similar to those that infest other mammals. In one survey of fleas found on various domestic pets brought to veterinary hospitals in Germany, the single ferret examined was infested with *Ctenocephalides felis*[26]. Flea transmission is by direct contact with a contaminated animal or environment. Clinical signs range from none to pruritus with scaly skin, areas of excoriation, and alopecia. Evidence of flea bite hypersensitivity may also be apparent[18].

The diagnosis is made when fleas or flea excreta are found on the animal. Adult fleas are most often located on ferrets in the area between the scapulae. Effective treatment requires eradicating fleas from the environment and from all potential hosts. Several products licensed for dogs and cats are safe and effective when used judiciously in ferrets[18,27]. For example, topical imidacloprid is efficacious and easily applied[28].

Class Arachnida

Demodex sp.

A potentially new species of *Demodex* was identified in skin scrapings and biopsies from two mildly pruritic adult ferrets. Presenting signs included discolored, yellowish skin and localized alopecia behind the ears, on the abdomen, in the inguinal region, and on the ventral aspect of the tail[29]. A potentially predisposing factor was that both ferrets had been repeatedly treated for ear mites with an ointment containing triamcinolone acetate, a glucocorticoid. Treatment with a series of amitraz dips (0.0125% to 0.0375%) was initiated, followed by multiple skin scrapings to confirm mite eradication. Ivermectin may represent an alternative acaricide.

Otodectes cynotis

The ear mite, *Otodectes cynotis,* that infests ferrets is the same species identified in dogs and cats[30,31]. The interested reader is referred to Chapters 17, Parasites of Dogs, and Chapter 18, Parasites of Cats, for additional information concerning this mite. The life cycle of *O. cynotis* is direct, and requires three weeks to complete. Transmission to a new host is via direct contact with contaminated animals or debris. Ferrets infested with ear mites usually show no clinical signs. However, secondary otitis interna may develop, and be accompanied by ataxia, circling, torticollis, and signs associated with Horner's syndrome[18,27,32,33].

Microscopic examination of ear canal debris reveals all life cycle stages of *O. cynotis*. Adult mites can often be observed moving in the auricular canal with the use of an otoscope. Uninfested ferrets routinely have dark waxy debris in their ear canals; therefore, microscopic or otoscopic evaluation is necessary for accurate diagnosis.

All affected or exposed animals should be simultaneously treated with an acaricide. In one clinical trial, topical ivermectin divided between the two ear canals was more efficacious than the same dosage given as a subcutaneous injection[33]. By topical or parenteral route, 1% ivermectin, diluted 1:10 in propylene glycol and administered at a dosage of 400 µg/kg, was given twice, two weeks apart. Ear canal debris was not removed prior to ivermectin administration; however, the cartilaginous canal was massaged after drug instillation.

Caution should be exercised when administering ivermectin to pregnant jills because congenital defects may develop in offspring of ferrets treated with 0.2 ml of 1% ivermectin during the first two to four weeks of gestation[18]. A combination of thiabendazole, dexamethasone, and neomycyin instilled topically in the ear canals once a day for two weeks with one intervening week without treatment is an alternative medication for pregnant animals. However, it has not been determined whether the cumulative dosage of dexamethasone could affect fetal development.

Sarcoptes scabiei

Sarcoptic mange is rare in all ferrets, but especially those housed indoors. *Sarcoptes scabiei* may be transmitted by direct contact with an infested host or via fomites. Two clinical syndromes have been described in ferrets with *S. scabiei* infestation[34]. In the pedal form, affected ferrets develop lesions on the toes and feet. These become swollen and encrusted. The claws can become necrotic if the condition goes untreated[35]. In the generalized form, ferrets become intensely pruritic, with focal or generalized alopecia. The face, pinnae, and ventrum may be affected[36]. Mite identification requires multiple skin scrapings from less excoriated areas, or examination of crusts that have been cleared with 10% potassium hydroxide. Acaricidal dips have been employed; however, ivermectin (200 to 400 µg/kg) given subcutaneously every two weeks until the mites are eradicated is effective and easily administered.

TABLE 16.1 Parasites of Ferrets.

Parasite	Geographic distribution	Hosts	Location in host	Method of infection	Pathologic effects	Zoonosis	Reference
Flagellates							
Giardia sp.	Worldwide	Ferrets	Small intestine	Ingestion of cyst in feces	Unknown	Unknown with ferret isolate but likely	2, 38
Coccidia							
Cryptosporidium parvum	Worldwide	Ferrets, other mammals	Small intestine	Ingestion of sporulated oocyst in feces	None	Unknown with ferret isolate but possible	4
Eimeria furonis	Worldwide	Mustelids	Intestine, liver	Ingestion of sporulated oocyst in feces	None	Not reported	9, 10, 12
Eimeria ictidea	Worldwide	Mustelids	Intestine	Ingestion of sporulated oocyst in feces	None	Not reported	9, 10
Isospora laidlawi	Worldwide	Mustelids	Intestine	Ingestion of sporulated oocyst in feces	None	Not reported	9, 10
Sarcocystis muris	Worldwide	Mustelids	Intestine	Ingestion of muscle cysts in infected rodents	None	Not reported	18
Toxoplasma gondii	Worldwide	Mammals	Heart, liver, lungs, other tissues	Ingestion of sporulated oocyst in cat feces or undercooked meat	Tissue specific	Common	16
Cestodes							
Ariotaenia procyonis	Americas, Asia, Europe	Mustelids, procyonids	Intestine	Ingestion of beetle intermediate host	None	Not reported	18
Dipylidium caninum	Worldwide	Canids, cats, mustelids, humans	Small intestine	Ingestion of flea intermediate host	None	Rare	18
Mesocestoides sp.	Worldwide	Carnivores	Small intestine, peritoneum	Ingestion of mite intermediate host	Peritonitis	Rare	18
Nematodes							
Ascaridoidea							
Toxascaris leonina	Worldwide	Canids, cats, mustelids	Small intestine	Ingestion of embryonated egg or paratenic host	Poor condition, alopecia, scaling	Not Reported	18
Toxocara cati	Worldwide	Canids, cats, mustelids	Small intestine	Ingestion of embryonated egg or paratenic host	Enteritis	Reported	18
Strongyloidea							
Ancylostoma sp.	Worldwide	Canids, cats, rodents, mustelids	Small intestine	Ingestion of embryonated egg or paratenic host	Enteritis	Reported	18
Metastrongyloidea							

Species	Geographic location	Host	Location in host	Transmission	Clinical signs	Frequency	Reference
Filaroides bronchialis	Russia	Mustelids	Lung	Unknown	None	Not reported	37
Spiruroidea							
Skrjabingylus (Spiroptera) nasicola	Europe	Mustelids	Frontal sinus	Ingestion of arthropod intermediate host	None	Not reported	37
Filaroidea							
Dirofilaria immitis	Worldwide	Canids, cats, ferrets, harbor seals, humans	Adult: right atrium and ventricle, pulmonary artery, vena, cava; Microfilaria: blood	Bite of mosquito	Cardiomegaly, pleural fluid, ascites	Rare	24
Trichuroidea							
Trichinella spiralis	Asia	Mammals	Adults: small intestine; larvae: muscles	Ingestion of undercooked meat	None	Potential	18
Arthropods							
Insecta							
Diptera							
Cuterebra sp.	Worldwide	Rodents, other mammals	Skin and underlying tissues	Deposition of eggs by adult fly	Cutaneous myiasis	Reported	18
Hypoderma bovis	Worldwide	Cattle, other mammals	Skin and underlying tissues	Deposition of eggs by adult fly	Cutaneous myiasis	Reported	18
Wohlfahrtia vigil	Worldwide	Mustelids	Skin and underlying tissues	Deposition of eggs by adult fly	Cutaneous myiasis, abscesses	Rare	18
Siphonaptera							
Ctenocephalides sp.	Worldwide	Mammals	Skin	Direct contact	Dermatitis	Common	28
Arachnida							
Mites							
Astigmatids							
Otodectes cynotis	Worldwide	Dogs, cats, ferrets, other mammals	Ear canal	Direct contact	Otitis interna	Not reported	32
Sarcoptes scabiei	Worldwide	Mammals	Skin	Direct contact, fomites	Dermatitis, crusting, alopecia	Common	35, 36
Prostigmatids							
Demodex sp.	Worldwide	Ferrets	Skin	Direct contact	Alopecia, scabby dermatitis	Not reported	29
Ticks							
Ixodes ricinus	Britain	Ferrets, other mammals	Skin	Direct contact	None	Reported	18

REFERENCES

1. Eberhard, M.L. (1998) Use of the ferret in parasitolgic research. In Fox, J.G (ed.). *Biology and Diseases of the Ferret,* 2nd ed. Williams and Wilkins, Baltimore, MD, 537–549.

2. Bell, J.A. (1994) Parasites of domesticated pet ferrets. *Compend. Cont. Educ. Pract. Vet.* **16,** 617–620.

3. Zajac, A.M., LaBranche, T.P., Donaghue, A.R., and Chu, T.C. (1998) Efficacy of fenbendazole in the treatment of experimental *Giardia* infection in dogs. *Am. J. Vet. Res.* **59,** 61–63.

4. Rehg, J.E., Gigliotti, F., and Stokes, D.C. (1988) Cryptosporidiosis in ferrets. *Lab. Anim. Sci.* **38,** 155–158.

5. Gardiner, C.H., Fayer, R., and Dubey, J.P. (1998) *An Atlas of Protozoan Parasites in Animal Tissues,* 2nd ed. Armed Forces Institute of Pathology, Washington, DC.

6. Barr, S.C., Jamrosz, G.F., Hornbuckle, W.E., Bowman, D.D., and Fayer, R. (1994) Use of paromomycin for treatment of cryptosporidiosis in a cat. *J. Am. Vet. Med. Assoc.* **205,** 1742–1743.

7. Gookin, J.L., Riviere, J.E., Gilger, B.C., and Papich, M.G. (1999) Acute renal failure in four cats treated with paromomycin. *J. Am. Vet. Assoc.* **215,** 1821–1823.

8. Abe, N. and Iseki, M. (2003) Identification of genotypes of *Cryptosporidium parvum* isolates from ferrets in Japan. *Parasitol. Res.* **89,** 422–424.

9. Hoare, C.A. (1927) On the coccidia of the ferret. *Ann. Trop. Med. Parasitol.* **21,** 313–321.

10. Hoare, C.A. (1935) The endogenous development of the coccidia of the ferret and the histopathological reaction of the infected intestinal villi. *Ann. Trop. Med. Parasitol.* **29,** 111–121.

11. Li, X., Pang, J., and Fox, J.G. (1996) Coinfection with intracellular *Desulfovibrio* species and coccidia in ferrets with proliferative bowel disease. *Lab. Anim. Sci.* **46,** 569–571.

12. Williams, B.H., Chimes, M.J., and Gardiner, C.H. (1996) Biliary coccidiosis in a ferret (*Mustela putorius furo*). *Vet. Pathol.* **33,** 437–439.

13. Scipioni-Ball, R.L. (2004) Personal communication.

14. Blankenship-Paris, T.L., Chang, J., and Bagnell, C.R. (1993) Enteric coccidiosis in a ferret. *Lab. Anim. Sci.* **43,** 361–363.

15. Coutelen, F. (1932) The existence of a natural generalized toxoplasma of the ferret. A new toxoplasma, *Toxoplasma laidlawi* n. sp., parasite of *Mustela (Putorius) putorius var. furo. C. R. Soc. Biol.* (Paris) **111,** 284–287.

16. Thornton, R.N. and Cook, T.G. (1986) A congenital toxoplasma-like disease in ferrets (*Mustela putorius furo*). *N.Z. Vet. J.* **34,** 31–33.

17. Cooper, J.E. (1990) Skin diseases of ferrets. *Vet. Ann.* **30,** 325–334.

18. Fox, J.G. (1998) Parasitic diseases. In: Fox, J.G. (ed.). *Biology and Diseases of the Ferret,* 2nd ed. Williams and Wilkins, Baltimore, MD, 375–391.

19. Tzvetkov, Y., Todev, I., Georgiev, B.B., and Biserkov, V.Y. (1999) Enzootic gnathostomiasis of the polecat, *Mustela putorius* L. in Bulgaria. *Bulg. J. Vet. Med.* **2,** 47–52.

20. Supakorndej, P., McCall, J.W., Lewis, R.E., Rowan, S.J., Mansour, A.E., and Holmes, R.A. (1992) Biology, diagnosis, and prevention of heartworm infection in ferrets. *Proc. Heartworm Symposium 1992.* 59–69.

21. Miller, W.R. and Merton, D.A. (1982) Dirofilariasis in a ferret. *J. Am. Vet. Med. Assoc.* **180,** 1103–1104.

22. Moreland, A.F., Battles, A.H., and Nease, J.H. (1986) Dirofilariasis in a ferret. *J. Am. Vet. Med. Assoc.* **188,** 864.

23. Parrott, T.Y., Greiner, E.C., and Parrott, J.D. (1984) *Dirofilaria immitis* infection in three ferrets. *J. Am. Vet. Med. Assoc.* **184,** 582–583.

24. Sasai, H., Kato, K., Sasaki, T., Kouama, S., Kotani, T., and Fukata, T. (2000) Echocardiographic diagnosis of dirofilariasis in a ferret. *J. Sm. Anim. Prac.* **41,** 172–174.

25. Petrie, J.P. and Morrisey, J.K. (2004) Cardiovascular and other diseases. In: Quesenberry, K.E. and Carpenter, J.W. (eds.). *Ferrets, Rabbits, and Rodents: Clinical Medicine and Surgery.* Saunders, St. Louis, MO, 58–71.

26. Visser, M., Rehbein, S., and Wiedemann, C. (2001) Species of flea (Siphonaptera) infesting pets and hedgehogs in Germany. *J. Vet. Med.* **48,** 197–202.

27. Orcutt, C. (2004) Dermatologic diseases. In: Quesenberry, K.E., Carpenter, J.W. (eds.). *Ferrets, Rabbits, and Rodents: Clinical Medicine and Surgery.* Saunders, St. Louis, MO, 107–114.

28. Hutchinson, M.J., Jacobs, D.E., and Mencke, N. (2001) Establishment of the cat flea (*Ctenocephalides felis felis*) on the ferret (*Mustela putorius furo*) and its control with imidacloprid. *Med. Vet. Entomol.* **15,** 212–214.

29. Noli, C., van der Horst, H.H.A., and Willemse, T. (1996) Demodicosis in ferrets (*Mustela putorius furo*). *Vet. Quart.* **18,** 28–31.

30. Lohse, J., Rinder, H., Gothe, R., and Zahler, M. (2002) Validity of species status of the parasitic mite *Otodectes cynotis. Med. Vet. Entomol.* **16,** 133–138.

31. Sweatman, G.K. (1958) Biology of *Otodectes cynotis,* the ear canker mite of carnivores. *Can. J. Zool.* **36,** 849–862.

32. Nie, I.A. and Pick, C.R. (1978) Infestation of a colony of ferrets with ear mite (*Otodectes cynotis*) and its control. *J. Inst. Anim. Tech.* **29,** 63–68.

33. Patterson, M.M. and Kirchain, S.M. (1999) Comparison of three treatments for control of ear mites in ferrets. *Lab. Anim. Sci.* **49,** 655–657.

34. Ryland, L.M. and Bernard. S.L. (1983) A clinical guide to the pet ferret. *Compend. Cont. Educ.* **5,** 25–32.

35. Phillips, P.H., O'Callaghan, M.G., Moore, E., and Baird, R.M. (1987) Pedal *Sarcoptes scabiei* infestation in ferrets (*Mustela putorius furo*). *Aust. Vet. J.* **64,** 289–290.

36. Scott, D.W., Miller, W.H., and Griffin, C.E. (2001) Dermatoses of pet rodents, rabbits, and ferrets. In: Scott, D.W., Miller, J.W., and Griffin, C. (eds.). *Muller and Kirk's Small Animal Dermatology,* 6th ed. WB Saunders Company, Philadelphia, PA, 1415–1458.

37. Petrow, A.M. (1928) Addition to the explanation of systematics of nematodes parasitic in the frontal sinus and lungs of Mustelidae. *Ann. Trop. Med. Parasitol.* **22,** 259–264.

38. Abe, N., Read, C., Thompson, R.C.A., and Iseki, M. (2005) Zoonotic genotype of *Giardia intestinalis* detected in a ferret. *J. Parasitol.* **91,** 179–182.

CHAPTER
17

Parasites of Dogs

Dwight D. Bowman, MS, PhD

PROTOZOA

Phylum Sarcomastigophora

Class Mastigophora (flagellates)

Hemoflagellates

Leishmania spp. **Morphology.** *Leishmania* organisms in the dog are ovoid and usually measure 2.5 μ to 5 μ long by 1.5 μ to 2 μ wide. The only stage present in the dog is the amastigote stage which is morphologically indistinguishable from that of *Trypanosoma cruzi*. Amastigotes contain a nucleus and a large kinetoplast, and are only found in macrophages, where they divide by binary fission (Figure 17.1). In culture and in the sand fly vector, amastigotes transform into a promastigote stage that is 14 μ to 20 μ long and 1.5 μ to 3.5 μ wide. The promastigotes have an anteriorly directed flagellum that exits the anterior end of the nucleus from the anteriorly placed kinetoplast. The promastigote stage does not have an undulating membrane.

Hosts. Dogs are susceptible to infection with *L. chagasi, L. infantum, L. mexicana, L. peruviana,* and *L. tropica*. Wild rodents serve as additional reservoir hosts. Humans are susceptible to infection with all of these species.

Life Cycle. *Leishmania* organisms are transmitted by the bite of a sand fly, *Phlebotomus* spp. in the Old World, and *Lutzomyia* spp. in the New World. When the fly bites

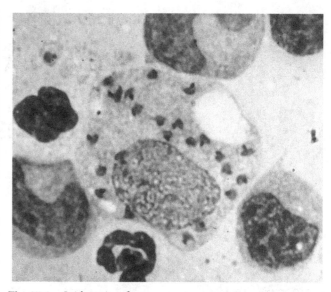

Fig. 17.1 *Leishmania infantum* amastigotes in a macrophage.

an infected host, it ingests macrophages in the skin that contain amastigotes. In the fly, the amastigotes transform into promastigotes that multiply by binary fission. Promastigotes migrate to the salivary glands and are inoculated during subsequent blood meals.

Pathologic Effects. *Leishmania* occurs in macrophages of the skin, liver, spleen, lymph nodes, mucosa, bone marrow, and elsewhere[1]. Strains differ in clinical signs, lesions, hosts, and epidemiologic features. *Leishmania infantum* and *L. chagasi* cause a visceral form of disease, while *L. tropica, L. peruviana,* and *L. mexicana* cause cutaneous lesions. Dogs may also develop cutaneous signs when infected with *L. infantum* or *L. chagasi*. It may be difficult to distinguish between cutaneous and visceral forms without tissue biopsy. In visceral leishmaniasis, the spleen is enlarged, congested, and purple or brown, and the liver and lymph nodes may be enlarged. Organ enlargement is due to local accumulation of infected macrophages. In cutaneous leishmaniasis, there may be scurfy desquamation of the skin and numerous cutaneous ulcers.

Clinical Disease. Visceral leishmaniasis results in anemia, alopecia, lymphadenopathy, cutaneous ulcers, hyperthermia, apathy, cachexia, and ulcerated mucosa[1]. Cutaneous leishmaniasis causes cutaneous ulcers that may be accompanied by alopecia and discoloration.

Diagnosis. Organisms can be found in stained smears of material from skin ulcers and in biopsy specimens collected from affected organs. *Leishmania* sp. promastigotes may be grown in culture of cutaneous lesions or deep biopsies using Novy, MacNeal, and Nicolle's medium, or other media supplemented with M199[2]. Molecular techniques are used to determine the species or strain of parasite present.

Treatment. Canine leishmaniasis may be treated with meglumine antimonate, allopurinol, and amphotericin B; or a combination of meglumine antimonate and allopurinol. Treatment may result in temporary clinical improvement and reduce anti-leishmanial antibody titers, but is usually ineffective in eradicating the organism[3]. For this reason there are concerns about the wide-scale treatment of dogs in endemic areas, because this approach could lead to drug resistance which may complicate treatment of human cases[4].

Prevention. Infection can be prevented by housing dogs in conditions that prevent or discourage sand fly bites, including housing dogs indoors, using screens, administering topical permethrin monthly[5], and using deltamethrin-impregnated collars[6].

Public Health Considerations. There have been reports of foxhounds in animal facilities and kennels developing visceral leishmaniasis[7]. In some cases, the source of infection and means of transmission could not be determined with certainty. In one U.S. outbreak, molecular typing of the species involved indicated that the organisms were the same as those in dogs in the Mediterranean[7]. Dogs in *Leishmania*-endemic areas are potential sources of human infection within the animal facility. Zoonotic transmission may occur if personnel do not protect broken skin from contamination.

Trypanosoma cruzi **Morphology.** Two forms of *Trypanosoma cruzi* infect mammals[8]. The trypomastigote form occurs in the blood (Figure 17.2). It is 16 µ to 20 µ long and has a pointed posterior end, a large stumpy body, a large terminal kinetoplast, a narrow undulating membrane, and a moderately long free flagellum. The large terminal kinetoplast is characteristic of this species of *Trypanosoma,* and the body is often found to be C-shaped rather than S-shaped in blood smears. The amastigote form occurs in groups in the cells of the skeletal muscle and the myocardium, and in fixed macrophages in the skin, liver, lungs, and spleen. The amastigote is 1.35 µ to 4 µ in diameter and characterized by a relatively large nucleus adjacent to the distinctive kinetoplast.

Hosts. *Trypanosoma cruzi* can be found in nearly all mammals within endemic areas, which include the southern United States, Mexico, and Central and South America. Reservoir hosts include rodents, opossums, raccoons, and similar wildlife species. Dogs, cats, and humans may also become infected.

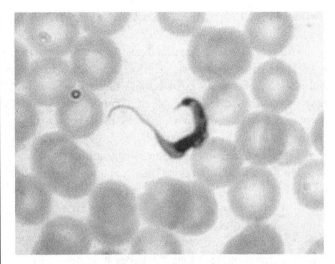

Fig. 17.2 *Trypanosoma cruzi* trypomastigote in a canine blood smear.

Life Cycle. Dogs become infected after consuming infected bugs, which serve as intermediate hosts, or after consuming other infected animals. Intrauterine infection also occurs[9]. Trypomastigotes cross the mucous membrane and enter the blood stream, then invade macrophages and striated muscle cells, especially those of the myocardium. There, trypomastigotes transform into amastigotes, which multiply by binary fission, destroying the infected cells as they form nests of organisms. Some amastigotes may revert to the trypomastigote form and re-enter the blood stream. Insect vectors become infected when they take a blood meal from an infected host. A period of development through promastigote and epimastigote forms in the insect ultimately produces the infective metacyclic trypomastigotes found in the insect's feces. The cycle in the bug takes 6 to 15 days.

Pathologic Effects. *Trypanosoma cruzi* causes either an acute or chronic disease in dogs. In acute disease, gross lesions include a diffusely pale myocardium with right ventricular enlargement, hepatomegaly, and a moderate amount of modified transudate in the abdominal cavity. Histology reveals severe diffuse granulomatous myocarditis with large numbers of pseudocysts. There may also be mild multifocal myositis[10] and pseudocysts in skeletal muscles and smooth muscles of the urinary bladder and small intestine. Some cases may develop multifocal encephalitis with pseudocysts in the cerebral cortex, cerebellum, and brain stem. The gross lesions develop into biventricular enlargement and thinning of the ventricular free walls as the disease becomes chronic. Histology reveals multifocal interstitial lymphohistiocytic cellular infiltrates, perivasculitis, and marked fibrosis in all areas of the myocardium.

Clinical Disease. Clinical signs may include ascites, respiratory distress, thoracic effusion, cyanosis, and weak pulse with ventricular arrhythmias. Electrocardiography may reveal first-degree heart block, chamber enlargement and ventricular-based arrhythmias. M-mode echocardiography can be used to confirm cardiac enlargement and possibly septal and left ventricular free wall thinning[11].

Diagnosis. Diagnosis is made by identifying the organisms in blood, by organ smears, or in tissue sections. Diagnosis can also be made through the culture of the blood in Novy, MacNeal, and Nicolle's medium. Another technique, known as xenodiagnosis, is to examine the intestinal tracts of clean bugs after they have been allowed to feed on suspected hosts.

Treatment. There is no effective treatment for *Trypanosoma cruzi* infections. Benznidazole effectivley clears dogs of infection in only up to two-thirds of cases[12].

Prevention. Preventing infection is difficult in dogs housed outdoors. Runs should be screened to prevent access of bugs or rodents. Bugs may be attracted to security lights adjacent to outdoor runs.

Public Health Considerations. Random-source dogs are often infected when acquired in *T. cruzi*-endemic areas. Animal workers may be infected through contact with the blood of an infected animal, needle sticks, or open wounds. Thus, blood and tissues of infected dogs must be handled with care. If fights occur between dogs, the blood from wounds is potentially infectious and should be handled with proper caution.

Enteric flagellates

Giardia canis **Morphology.** Trophozoites of *Giardia canis* measure 9 µ to 21 µ long, 5 µ to 15 µ wide, and 2 µ to 4 µ thick (Figure 17.3). Typical of the genus, the body is piriform with a broadly rounded anterior end, an extended posterior end, and a large sucking disc on the anterior ventral side. There are two anterior nuclei, two slender axostyles, eight flagella, and a median body. The cysts are ovoid and measure 8 µ to 12 µ long by 7 µ to 10 µ wide.

Hosts. *Giardia* is one of the most common parasites of the domestic dog. It is commonly found in laboratory-reared beagles, where many of the dogs from large commercial animal suppliers are routinely infected. *Giardia* is also commonly seen in animals visiting veterinary practices (7.2% overall in Canada, 7.5% in the United States, and

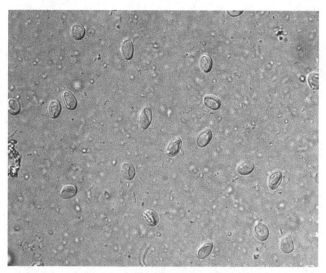

Fig. 17.3 *Giardia canis.* Cysts from the feces of an asymptomatic dog concentrated using zinc sulfate centrifugal flotation.

16.5% in Germany)[13–15]. Recent molecular biology studies suggest that the dog is host to its own species of *Giardia,* which is here designated as *Giardia canis*[16]. *Giardia canis* is morphologically similar to *G. intestinalis* of humans. Dogs can also occasionally be infected with *G. intestinalis.*

Life Cycle. Trophozoites colonize the proximal small intestine and reproduce by longitudinal binary fission. Trophozoites transform into cysts with passage through the intestinal tract. Transmission from host to host is through ingestion of cysts passed in the feces.

Pathologic Effects and Clinical Disease. There is very little anatomical pathology associated with *Giardia* infection[17]. Many infected dogs remain asymptomatic for months to years. Other dogs may have irregular bouts of diarrhea followed by asymptomatic periods. Some dogs develop chronic diarrhea, which persists until the parasites are removed by treatment.

Diagnosis. Diagnosis is by finding cysts in the feces, either with zinc sulfate flotation or a direct saline smear. The trophozoites and their flagella can be observed in motion in fresh feces. A fecal antigen detection test has been approved for the diagnosis of *Giardia* in dogs and cats.

Treatment. Treatments of choice for *Giardia* include metronidazole and fenbendazole[18]. Infected dogs may be treated with both products simultaneously for five days: metronidazole (25 mg/kg every 24 hours) and fenbendazole (50 mg/kg q.24 hours). Dogs that excrete cysts after treatment can be retreated for 10 days. Bathing dogs after treatment helps prevent re-infection[18].

Prevention. Preventing infection is difficult due to a high prevalence rate in the canine population. In situations where *Giardia*-free dogs are required, it may be necessary to use cesarean-derived pups. Even under these conditions, outbreaks may occur. If eradication of the parasite is attempted, all animals must be treated simultaneously. Also, dogs should be bathed and transferred to clean cages on each day of treatment.

Public Health Considerations. In most cases, humans become infected with human species of isolates of *Giardia*. Because dogs may also be infected with human strains, strict adherence to personal hygiene prevents infection of animal workers.

Pentatrichomonas hominis Morphology. Trophozoites measure 15 μ long and 5 μ wide (Figure 17.4)[19]. There is a single large nucleus at the anterior end, with four anterior flagella. A fifth flagellum exits the trophozoite anteriorly, then curves posteriorly. The latter flagellum is attached to the surface of the organism through an undulating membrane. The living trophozoite can be easily recognized by the movement of the anterior flagella and undulating membrane. No cyst stage is formed.

Hosts. Natural hosts of *P. hominis* include dogs and humans, where it lives as a commensal in the large intestine. It is not known whether canine and human isolates are cross-infective.

Life Cycle. Trophozoites are passed from host to host in the feces[20]. Trophozoites die rapidly in the environment, so successful transmission requires contact with fresh feces.

Pathologic Effects and Clinical Disease. Infection is not accompanied by pathologic changes or clinical signs.

Diagnosis, Treatment, and Prevention. Diagnosis is by finding trophozoites in the soft to liquid feces. Trophozoites are rarely found on fecal flotation. A diagnostic kit (In-Pouch Test) facilitates culturing of trichomonads in the feces of cats, but it has not been evaluated for use in dogs. Infections with *P. hominis* may be cleared with metronidazole. Preventing fecal oral contact between dogs, which can be difficult, prevents the infection from spreading. It is likely that puppies are infected from their mothers and that infections are routinely spread between littermates.

Public Health Considerations. Animal workers should practice good hygiene when working with potentially infected dogs.

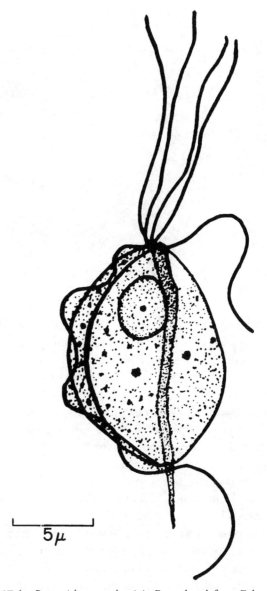

Fig. 17.4 *Pentatrichomonas hominis.* Reproduced from Fukushima, T., Mochizuki, K., Yamazaki, H., Watanabe, Y., Yamada, S., Aoyama, T,. et al. (1990) with permission.

Phylum Apicomplexa

Class Coccidia

Cryptosporidium canis

Morphology. The oocysts of *Cryptosporidium canis* are the smallest of the coccidial oocysts shed in dog feces. The oocysts are spheroid and 5 μ in diameter (Figure 17.5). The oocysts contain four sporozoites and are infectious when passed.

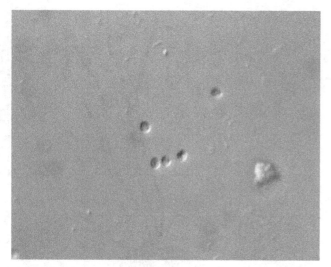

Fig. 17.5 *Cryptosporidium canis.* Oocysts from dog feces as they appear in a sugar flotation.

Hosts. What was once called *Cryptosporidium parvum* appears to actually be a group of morphologically indistinguishable species with distinct host restrictions. Thus, *C. canis* is considered to be restricted to dogs and other canids[21].

Life Cycle. Dogs become infected when they ingest sporulated oocysts passed in feces. Released sporozoites penetrate the epithelial cells of the small intestine and develop in an intracellular, extracytoplasmic location. There are two schizogonous cycles followed by gametogony and the formation of sporulated oocysts. Infection of the stomach has also been reported[22].

Pathologic Effects and Clinical Signs. Infection is associated with loss of ability to maintain water balance, but in most cases, epithelial damage is minimal. Clinical signs are typically restricted to mild diarrhea, unless the host is immune-suppressed or has another underlying condition such as viral infection or malignancy[23].

Diagnosis. Diagnosis is by identification of minute oocysts in feces, using a sugar flotation method. Human antigen detection tests for *Cryptosporidium* may be used for the detection of infections in animals. These tests have been routinely used and standardized in some diagnostic laboratories specifically for use with different animal hosts such as dogs and cattle.

Treatment. No drugs are approved for the treatment of *Cryptosporidium* sp. Dogs with chronic infections have been treated with paramomycin with various levels of success using a similar dosage regimen as that described for cats (165 mg/kg of body weight, per os, for five days)[24].

Prevention. *Cryptosporidium canis* is easily transmitted within the kennel environment, because oocysts are infectious when passed and are resistant to environmental extremes. Prevention is based on strict hygienic practices.

Public Health Considerations. *Cryptosporidium canis* does not infect immunologically competent people. Infection may occur in children, or in adults with immune deficiency[25]. Thus, animal workers should practice excellent hygiene when working with potentially infected dogs.

Hammondia heydorni

Morphology. *Hammondia heydorni* is one of the small coccidia of dogs. Oocysts are nearly spherical, measuring 10 µ to 13 µ in diameter. When sporulated, the oocysts contain two sporocysts, each with eight sporozoites.

Hosts. *Hammondia heydorni* has an obligatory two-host cycle. Dogs and other canines serve as definitive hosts, while rodents, deer, and other mammalian prey species serve as intermediate hosts.

Life Cycle. The intestinal stages of *H. heydorni* are found at the tips of the villi in the jejunum and ileum[26]. Oocysts are shed in the feces of dogs, and are infectious to rodents. Bradyzoite cysts form in rodent muscles, where they remain infective, awaiting consumption by a dog. The digestive process releases the bradyzoites, initiating infection.

Pathologic Effects and Clinical Disease. *Hammondia heydorni* is nonpathogenic in dogs. Intestinal infection in dogs causes little or no clinical signs.

Diagnosis, Treatment, and Prevention. Diagnosis is based on finding the small oocysts in dog fecal specimens. There is no approved treatment for the intestinal stages of *H. heydorni.* Prevention is by avoiding the feeding of raw meat to colony dogs. Cleaning kennels daily removes oocysts from the environment.

Public Health Considerations. *Hammondia heydorni* does not infect humans.

Hepatozoon americanum

Morphology. Life cycle stages of *Hepatozoon americanum* include gamonts and meronts. Gamonts are elongated, and measure 8 µ to 12 µ long and 5 µ in diameter. Meronts have a "wheel spoke" arrangement.

Hosts. Dogs and coyotes are the natural hosts of *H. americanum.* It is suspected that another wild animal may be a more typical host of this parasite in the United States. *Hepatozoon americanum* is restricted to the Americas, most prominently the southeastern and south-central United States[27].

Life Cycle. Dogs become infected through the ingestion of the infected hard ticks, such as nymphal or adult Gulf Coast ticks, *Amblyomma maculatum*[28]. Sporozoites are freed from the tick and initiate infection in the dog. Meronts develop in muscle cells, though initially, the host cell is a phagocytic cell located between muscle fibers[29]. A large, cystic structure called an "onion skin" cyst consists of concentric layers of a mucopolysaccharide that are laid down around this cell. Some meronts remain in the onion-skin cyst state, while others rupture and release merozoites that infect leukocytes. Ticks become infected when ingesting blood containing gamonts.

Pathologic Effects. Pathologic changes due to *H. americanum* infection may be severe in striated and cardiac muscle following rupture of mature meronts and formation of highly vascularized pyogranulomas. Infection is also often associated with a marked leukocytosis. Parasitemia may involve as few as 0.1% of circulating leukocytes.

Clinical Disease. *Hepatozoon americanum* causes a highly debilitating and often fatal disease. Clinical signs include fever, generalized pain, muscle atrophy, weakness, reluctance to rise, and bone proliferative lesions[30]. There may be gait abnormalities, stiffness, or recumbency. Without treatment, the chronic wasting will usually lead to death in about 12 months.

Diagnosis. Diagnosis is based on clinical signs, and on finding the rare gamont in blood smears. Muscle biopsy and serological testing are also used to assist in diagnosing this infection.

Treatment. Trimethoprim-sulfadiazine, clindamycin, and pyrimethamine, given daily for 14 days, is an approved and effective treatment for eliminating *H. americanum* in dogs. However, this only leads to a remission of clinical signs, typically with relapse in two to six months. Survival can be increased with long-term decoquinate treatment[31].

Prevention. Prevention consists of tick control, which is easier than with *H. canis,* because *A. maculatum* does not occur indoors.

Public Health Considerations. *Hepatozoon americanum* does not infect humans.

Hepatozoon canis

Morphology. Life cycle stages of *Hepatozoon canis* are morphologically similar to those of *H. americanum.*

Hosts. Dogs are the natural hosts of *H. canis,* which is found in Europe, Africa, and Asia, and is more benign than *H. americanum*[32].

Life Cycle. The life cycle is essentially similar to that of *H. americanum.* In Old World hepatozoonosis, the primary tick vector is *Rhipicephalus sanguineus*[33]. Meront formation occurs in the spleen, bone marrow, and liver. Gamonts circulate within neutrophils. Ticks become infected when ingesting blood that contains gamonts.

Pathologic Effects. Meronts can be found in the spleen, liver, bone marrow, and lymph nodes. Dogs with heavy infections develop neutrophilia, with nearly all neutrophils infected.

Clinical Disease. *Hepatozoon canis* usually causes no apparent signs, but fever, emaciation, anemia, splenomegaly, and death sometimes occur.

Diagnosis, Treatment, and Prevention. Diagnosis is by finding gamonts in peripheral blood smears. Occasionally, the meront stages are identified in biopsies, or in samples obtained at necropsy. Treatment consists of a course of imidocarb diprorionate and doxycycline for up to eight weeks. Infection may be prevented by incorporating a strict program of tick control[34]. Random-source dogs may introduce *H. canis* into the animal facility, but without the ticks, the infection is very unlikely to be spread between animals.

Public Health Considerations. *Hepatozoon canis* does not infect humans.

Isospora (= cystoisospora) canis

Morphology. *Isospora canis* is the large coccidian of dogs. The oocyst is broadly ellipsoidal to ovoid and measures 35 μ to 42 μ long by 27 μ to 33 μ wide (Figure 17.6). Sporulated oocysts contain two sporocysts, each of which encloses two sporozoites.

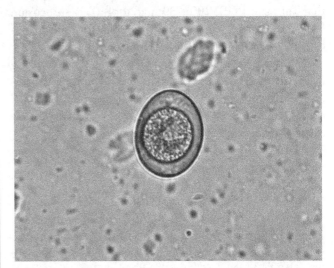

Fig. 17.6 *Isospora (= cystoisospora) canis.* Unsporulated oocyst from dog feces as it appears in a sugar flotation.

Hosts. Dogs are the only hosts of *I. canis* in which the life cycle is completed. Rodents and birds may become infected, and sporozoites remain encysted and viable in cells of the intestinal mucosa. These rodents and birds can serve as transport hosts if they are ingested by dogs, but the life cycle is not completed in these hosts.

Life Cycle. The life cycle is direct. Dogs become infected through the ingestion of sporulated oocysts, or infected rodents or birds[35]. After infection, asexual reproduction, followed by sexual reproduction, occurs in the intestinal mucosa, leading to the formation of oocysts. The prepatent period is six to nine days, and the patent period can be up to a month. Dogs can become infected through the ingestion of rodent or avian paratenic hosts that contain free sporozoites within various cells after the ingestion of oocysts.

Pathologic Effects and Clinical Disease. *Isospora canis* is moderately pathogenic[36]. Developmental stages are found in the intestinal lamina propria in the distal third of the small intestine[37]. Infection of pups with 50,000 to 80,000 oocysts resulted in clinical signs of coccidiosis by the eighth to ninth day after inoculation. Pups became dull and anorectic. As the infection increased in severity, the feces became watery, and occasionally, bloody. Pups became weak, anemic, emaciated, and febrile, and drank excessively. Clinical signs abated after a week.

Diagnosis. Diagnosis is by finding large oocysts in the feces.

Treatment. Dogs with clinical signs, or those at risk for severe infection, may be treated with sulfadimethoxine (55 mg/kg for the duration of the outbreak, but not longer than three weeks)[38]. More recently, others have reported that Toltrazuril (10, 20 or 30 mg/kg of a 5% suspension for three days) is also effective[39]. Supportive therapy is essential in heavily infected pups.

Prevention. Outbreaks can be prevented by removing feces daily. Dogs that are cesarean derived and maintained under barrier conditions remain coccidia-free. Coccidial oocysts are resistant to environmental extremes, and can be carried into a closed facility on shoes or clothing.

Public Health Considerations. Humans are not susceptible to infection with *I. canis*.

Isospora (= cystoisospora) spp.

Morphology. Dogs may be found infected with several species of small *Isospora* spp., including *I. neorivolta*, *I. ohioensis*, and *I. burrowsi*. Oocysts of these species measure 20 μ to 27 μ long by 15 μ to 24 μ wide, and are ellipsoid to ovoid in shape.

Hosts. *Isospora* spp. are common parasites of dogs throughout the world. A survey of random-source dogs in the United States showed an overall prevalence of around 5%[40]. Prevalence rates are lower in well-managed facilities.

Life Cycle. The life cycles of *Isospora* spp. are essentially similar to those of *I. canis*. Species differ in particular life cycle details. For example, *I. ohioensis* develops in epithelial cells of the jejunum, ileum, and colon[41], while the intracellular stages of *I. neorivolta* are found mainly in the lamina propria cells of the posterior small intestine[42], and *I. burrowsi* is found in the epithelial or lamina propria cells at the tips of the villi in the last half of the small intestine[43].

Pathologic Effects. Parasite stages that develop within the mucosa destroy the cells they parasitize. Thus, disease severity is largely determined by the size of the inoculum. Inoculation of six puppies with 10,000 oocysts of *I. ohioensis* resulted in the death of four of the puppies 12 days after infection[39].

Clinical Disease. Infections usually are not associated with clinical disease. Diarrhea, and occasionally, dysentery, develop in severe infections, such as occur in crowded conditions.

Diagnosis, Treatment, and Prevention. Diagnosis is by demonstration of oocysts in flotation preparations (Figure 17.7). Specific identification requires either molecular methods or histological examination of tissues. Treatment and prevention are as described for *I. canis*.

Public Health Considerations. *Isospora* spp. are not infective to humans.

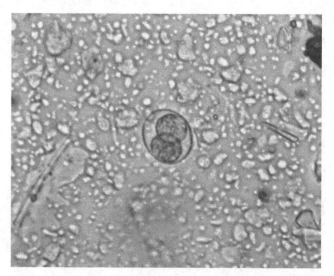

Fig. 17.7 *Isospora*(= *cystoisospora*) *ohioensis*. Sporulated oocyst from dog feces as it appears in a sugar flotation.

Neospora caninum

Morphology. Like *Hammondia heydorni*, *Neospora caninum* represents one of the small coccidia of dogs. Oocysts are nearly spherical, and measure 10 μ to 13 μ in diameter. When sporulated, the oocysts contain two sporocysts, each with eight sporozoites.

Hosts. Dogs serve as the definitive host. Several mammals, including goats, deer, horses, cattle, and others, serve as intermediate hosts[44].

Life Cycle. Oocysts are shed in the feces of dogs. Following ingestion by susceptible intermediate hosts, tissue cysts form and remain viable for long periods. Dogs become infected after consuming hosts bearing cysts. Transplacental transmission has also been reported[44].

Pathologic Effects. *Neospora caninum* may cause severe disseminated disease that is often associated with nonsuppurative meningoencephalomyelitis, myositis, myocarditis, hepatitis, dermatitis, and pneumonia[45].

Clinical Disease. The intestinal infection in dogs causes little or no signs in those that are shedding oocysts. Disseminated disease typically presents as progressive paralysis, which is more severe in the hind limbs. Signs include hind limb hyperextension, difficulty swallowing, jaw paralysis, muscle flaccidity, muscle atrophy, and heart failure[44]. Skin lesions present as patchy dermatitis with exudative skin pustules.

Diagnosis. Diagnosis is by finding the rare, small oocysts in dog fecal specimens. In cases of disseminated disease with paralysis, it is necessary to use immunologic or molecular methods to distinguish the organisms from *Toxoplasma gondii* and other potential causes of neurologic disease[46].

Treatment. The response to treatment depends upon the stage of the disease. A combination of trimethoprim, sulfadiazine, and pyrimethamine reversed *N. caninum*-associated paralysis in some dogs[44]. Cutaneous neosporosis has been successfully treated with clindamycin[44].

Prevention. Neosporosis may be prevented by avoiding the feeding of uncooked meat. Cleanliness is important to remove oocysts from the environment.

Public Health Considerations. *Neospora caninum* is not infectious to humans.

Class Piroplasmidia

Babesia canis

Morphology. The only stage of *Babesia canis* that is present in dogs is found within the red blood cells. These are typically pear-shaped and 4 μ to 5 μ in length, and often are found in pairs within erythrocytes (Figures 17.8 and 17.9)[18, 49].

Hosts. Dogs and other canids are the natural hosts of *B. canis*. *Babesia canis* is unlikely to be found in colony-bred dogs, but can be present in random-source dogs. Reports suggest that the seroprevalence in greyhounds from the southeastern United States is higher than that of the general pet population[49]. An examination of dogs in California shelters revealed a prevalence rate of 13%[50]. Three subspecies of *Babesia canis* are recognized: *Babesia canis canis*, which is found in Europe; *B. canis vogeli*, which is found in northern Africa and North America; and *B. canis rossi*, which is found in southern Africa[51,52].

Life Cycle. *Babesia canis canis* is transmitted by *Dermacentor reticulatus*, *B. canis vogeli* by *Rhipicephalus sanguineus*, and *B. canis rossi* by *Haemophysalis leachi*[52]. Sexual stages occur in the gut of the tick, and ultimately infective sporozoites are produced that can enter the mouthparts of the tick and be transferred by tick bite. Transovarial transmission can occur, and ticks may pass on the organism to offspring over several generations. In the greyhound, *B. canis* was found in

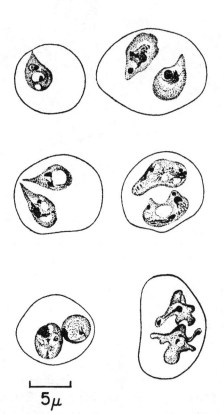

Fig. 17.8 *Babesia canis* in erythrocytes of the dog. Reproduced from Wenyon, C.M. (1926) with permission.

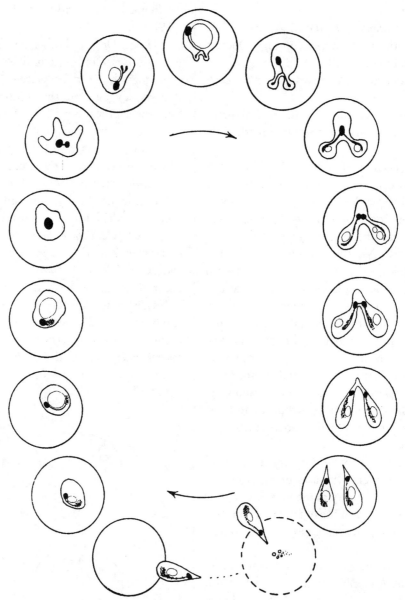

Fig. 17.9 *Babesia canis.* Reproductive cycle in circulating erythrocyte of the dog. Reproduced from Nuttall, G.H.F. and Graham-Smith, G.S. (1908) with permission.

11- to 18-day-old puppies, and it was suggested that they might have been infected transplacentally[53].

Pathologic Effects and Clinical Disease. All pathological manifestations are associated with hemolytic anemia caused by blood loss or autoimmune disease. Mild cases present with mild anemia, while severe cases present with an acute hemolytic crisis and life-threatening anemia[54]. Complications include acute renal failure, central nervous system signs, coagulopathies, icterus and hepatopathy, hemoglobinuria, immune-mediated hemolytic anemia, acute respiratory distress, hemoconcentration, and shock. Some dogs develop peracute signs, including collapsing, that are accompanied by severe intravascular hemolysis.

Diagnosis. Diagnosis is by detecting the organisms in blood smears within the erythrocytes along with the clinical signs of anemia. Some commercial laboratories also offer serologic testing and polymerase chain reaction assays.

Treatment. Diaminazine aceturate (3.5 mg/kg intramuscularly) is the drug of choice for uncomplicated babesiosis. Imidocarb (6 mg/kg intramuscularly or SQ) can be used for more complicated cases. Treatments may have severe side effects[54]. Trypan blue (10 mg/kg of a 1% solution IV) will suppress parasitemia, but will not clear infections. Clindamycin may be a useful drug when used in immunocompetent dogs[55].

Prevention. Prevention is based on tick control. A vaccine is available in Europe[56], but is likely to be useful only under specific conditions.

Public Health Considerations. *Babesia canis* does not infect humans.

Babesia gibsoni

Morphology. *Babesia gibsoni* is morphologically similar to *B. canis,* but the stages in the red blood cells are smaller.

Hosts. Dogs and other canids serve as natural hosts. *Babesia gibsoni* may actually represent several different strains, species, or subspecies[57]. A *Theileria*-like form infects dogs in California, and causes a relapsing form of infection. In the rest of the United States, the infection is mainly due to the classic *B. gibsoni* form common in pit bulls. In Europe, a *B. microti*-like species now appears to occasionally infect dogs. In one study, 3% of shelter dogs in California were infected with *B. gibsoni*[50].

Life Cycle. The life cycle is similar to that of *B. canis.* Tick vectors include *Rhipicephalus sanguineus* and *Haemaphysalis bispinosa*[54]. Interstadial and transovarial transmission occurs in ticks. Transplacental infection may explain infection in pups as young as three days of age[58].

Pathologic Effects and Clinical Disease. Pathologic manifestations are associated with chronic or acute hemolytic anemia[59]. Infected dogs develop mild to severe anemia. Surviving dogs become asymptomatic carriers. Dogs splenectomized before inoculation are likely to develop a fatal infection. Infected dogs undergoing splenectomy experience a worsening of the disease, but usually survive[59].

Diagnosis, Treatment, and Prevention. Diagnosis is by finding organisms in blood smears. Dogs intended for use as blood donors may be splenectomized to reveal latent infection. Treatment options are as described for *B. canis.* However, it is more difficult to eliminate infection with *B. gibsoni* because low levels of parasites seem to remain in the blood. Atovaquone plus azithromycin treatment seems somewhat more effective in clearing dogs of their infections than simple treatment with diaminazine aceturate[60]. Prevention is achieved through tick control.

Public Health Considerations. *Babesia gibsoni* does not infect humans.

TREMATODES

Family Opisthorchidae

Opisthorchis tenuicollis

Morphology. The morphology of the opisthorchid flukes is described in Chapter 3, Biology of Trematodes and Leeches. Adult *Opisthorchis tenuicollis* measure 7 mm to 18 mm long by 1.5 mm to 3 mm wide (Figure 17.10)[61]. The egg of *O. tenuicollis* measures 26 μ to 30 μ long by 11 μ to 15 μ wide.

Hosts. The range of definitive hosts includes dogs, cats, humans, and other fish-eating mammals. *Opisthorchis tenuicollis* occurs in North America, Europe, and Asia.

Life Cycle. Eggs passed in the feces hatch when ingested by a suitable snail. They develop in the snail to the cercarial stage, escape, and invade the flesh of a suitable freshwater fish. The endothermal host becomes infected by eating the fish. Metacercariae are released in the duodenum and migrate up the bile duct. Egg production occurs

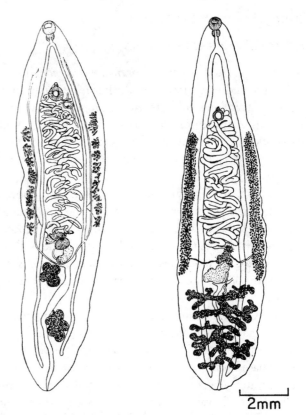

Fig. 17.10 (Left) *Opisthorchis tenuicollis.* (Right) *Clonorchis sinensis.* Reproduced from Lapage, G. (1962) with permission.

three to four weeks after infection; the complete life cycle requires about four months.

Pathologic Effects. *Opisthorchis tenuicollis* infection may result in catarrhal inflammation and epithelial desquamation of the bile duct, cirrhosis, and passive congestion of the liver, and rarely, pancreatitis.

Clinical Disease. Clinical signs are usually absent in mild infections, but the flukes can induce jaundice due to bile stasis.

Diagnosis. Diagnosis is based on identification of the eggs in the feces or the adult flukes in the bile duct at necropsy. The eggs are heavy and best recovered using sugar flotation or sedimentation procedures. Flukes can be visualized in dogs via computed tomography[62].

Treatment. Praziquantel (50 mg/kg) is the treatment of choice for infection with *Opisthorchis* spp. Multiple treatments may be required[63].

Prevention. There is little chance of transmission taking place in the laboratory. Dogs should not be fed raw fish.

Public Health Considerations. Dogs infected with this *O. tenuicollis* cannot transmit the infection to humans.

Family Schistosomatidae

Heterobilharzia americanum

Morphology. Adult *Heterobilharzia americanum* live in the hepatic and mesenteric veins. Adult male flukes measure up to 2 cm long. Adult females are much thinner than males, but may be longer, and may be found in the gynecophoral canal of the male. Eggs are round and spineless, measure 88 µ long by 74 µ wide, and are embryonated when passed[64].

Hosts. Natural definitive hosts include the bobcat, raccoon, nutria, swamp rabbit, opossum, and white-tailed deer in the southeastern United States. Infection of laboratory dogs is unlikely unless random-source dogs from endemic areas are used. *Heterobilharzia americanum* is the only schistosome of domestic animals naturally occurring in North America.

Life Cycle. The life cycle is indirect. Eggs passed in the feces hatch spontaneously when deposited in fresh water. Freshwater snails (*Lymnaea cubensis*) serve as the intermediate host. After several weeks, cercariae are shed into the water, where they penetrate the skin of the definitive host. The larval schistosome makes its ways to the lungs, before maturing in the mesenteric and hepatic veins in seven to nine weeks. Eggs passed by the female fluke

make their way to the intestinal lumen by eroding through host tissues. Adult worms can live four to 10 years.

Pathologic Effects. The migration of eggs through host tissues causes severe inflammation and granuloma formation. The bowel wall can become thickened and inflamed. Some eggs are also carried to the liver, where they cause the formation of granulomas and hepatic fibrosis. In heavy infections, the damage to the liver can be considerable, with marked collagen deposition[64].

Clinical Disease. Clinical signs of infection include diarrhea, dehydration, and anorexia. Chronic infection may also result in anemia, eosinophilia, hypoalbuminemia, edema[65], and hypercalcemia[66].

Diagnosis, Treatment, and Prevention. Diagnosis is based on history of geographical exposure, clinical signs, and the finding of the eggs in the feces. The eggs hatch spontaneously in fresh water, so if infections are suspected, initial mixing of the specimen prior to flotation should be in saline rather than tap water. Effective treatments include praziquantel (50 mg/kg)[64] and fenbendazole (50 mg/kg daily for 10 days)[67]. Infection in laboratory dogs is not likely to occur.

Public Health Considerations. Animal workers are not at risk of infection in the laboratory setting.

Family Troglotrematidae

Nanophyetus salmincola

Morphology. Adult *Nanophyetus salmincola* measure only 0.8 mm to 1.1 mm long and 0.3 to 0.5 mm wide (Figure 17.11). The egg is golden brown and has a small operculum at one end and a short blunt point at the other, and measures 64 µ to 80 µ long by 35 µ to 55 µ wide (Figure 17.12)[68].

Hosts. Definitive hosts of *N. salmincola* include many fish-eating endothermal animals such as dogs, raccoons, wild rodents, carnivores, and fish-eating birds. Prevalence rates may be high among feral animals on the west coast of North America and in eastern Siberia. Infection in laboratory dogs has not been reported.

Life Cycle. Eggs passed in the feces hatch after about three months. The first intermediate host is an aquatic snail and the second is a salmonid fish. The mammalian host is infected by eating the cercarial stages encysted in the fish. Mature worms develop in the small intestine of the definitive host in six to seven days.

Pathologic Effects and Clinical Disease. *Nanophyetus salmincola* is nonpathogenic in the dog. However, it is important because it harbors and transmits the

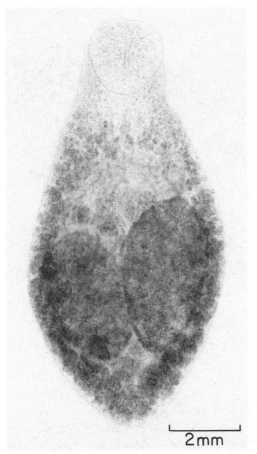

Fig. 17.11 *Nanophyetus salmincola* adult. Courtesy of Marietta Voge, University of California.

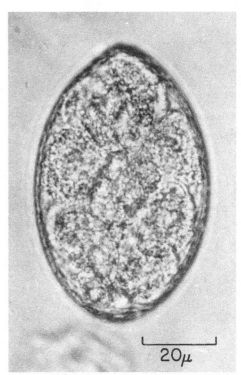

Fig. 17.12 *Nanophyetus salmincola* egg. Reproduced from Farrell, R.K. (1968) with permission.

rickettsial agent, *Neorickettsia helminthoeca,* the cause of salmon poisoning disease, and a second rickettsial-like agent that causes Elokomin fluke fever in dogs[69]. Dogs with salmon poisoning develop high fever, diarrhea, and vomiting, and platelet numbers are markedly reduced.

Diagnosis, Treatment, and Prevention. Diagnosis is based on identification of the eggs in the feces or the adult flukes in the intestine. Eggs can be found in flotations, sedimentations, or direct smears. Flukes can be eliminated with praziquantel (6 to 39 mg/kg intramuscularly or subcutaneously)[70]. Salmon poisoning disease requires treatment with doxycycline. Infection can be prevented by not feeding raw fish to dogs, particularly in the Pacific Northwest. Because of the complex life cycle, the infection cannot be transmitted in the laboratory, and no special control procedures are required.

Public Health Considerations. Natural infection in man has been reported. However, because of the complex life cycle, infected dogs are not a hazard to humans.

Paragonimus spp.

Morphology. Adult *Paragonimus* have brown, plump, ovoid bodies with spines protruding through the tegument. They measure 7.5 mm to 12 mm long and 4 mm to 6 mm wide, and are 3.5 mm to 5 mm thick (Figure 17.13). The oval eggs are golden brown, have a partly flattened operculum at one end, and measure 80 μ to 118 μ long by 48 μ to 60 μ wide (Figure 17.14)[71].

Hosts. *Paragonimus kellicotti* occurs in the lungs of dogs, cats, wild carnivores, domestic animals, and rarely humans in North America, particularly in the Great Lakes and Mississippi Valley regions. *Paragonimus westermanii* occurs in dogs, cats, monkeys, wild carnivores, domestic animals, and humans in Asia. In addition, minks, skunks, and wild cats may be infected in endemic areas.

Life Cycle. Eggs in the respiratory passages are coughed up, swallowed, and passed in the feces. Miracidia are infective to the first intermediate host, a snail, and then undergo asexual multiplication. Cercariae leave the snail and penetrate freshwater crabs or crayfish where they develop into metacercariae in the hemocoele of the crustacean. The mammalian host is infected by ingesting the infected crustacean. Young flukes are released in the

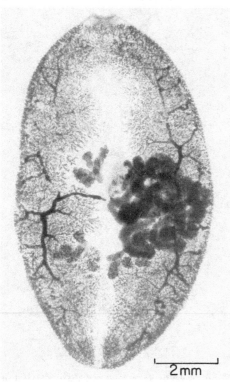

Fig. 17.13 *Paragonimus westermani* adult. Courtesy of Marietta Voge, University of California.

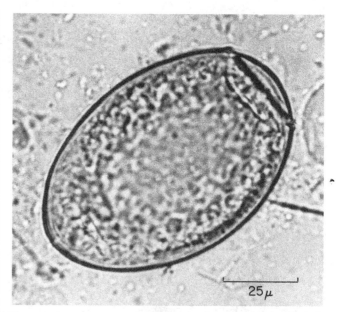

Fig. 17.14 *Paragonimus kellicotti* egg. Reproduced from Herman, L.H. and Helland, D.R. (1966) with permission.

duodenum, penetrate the intestinal wall, and migrate through the peritoneal cavity and diaphragm to the lungs, where they mature in five to six weeks (Figure 17.15).

Pathologic Effects. Gross lesions consist of focal areas of emphysema and soft, dark red to brown cysts, 2 cm to 3 cm in diameter, distributed throughout the parenchyma[72]. Incision of the cysts discloses the flukes, usually one to three in each cyst. Pleural adhesions sometimes occur. Histology of the lesion reveals hyperplasia of the bronchial epithelium and submucosal bronchial glands and focal areas of inflammation surrounding clusters of fluke eggs in the lung parenchyma.

Clinical Disease. Parasites in the lungs cause coughing, wheezing, moist rales, and progressive emaciation. Occasionally, young migrating flukes penetrate the pleura and cause pneumothorax[73]. This may also occur when a mature cyst ruptures. Rarely, flukes migrate to ectopic locations such as the brain or liver, and interfere with organ function.

Diagnosis, Treatment, and Prevention. Diagnosis is by demonstrating eggs in the feces or adult flukes in the lungs at necropsy. The eggs are heavy and are best recovered using sugar flotation or sedimentation techniques.

Treatments for paragonimiasis include fenbendazole (50 mg/kg/day for 14 days) or praziquantel (50 mg/kg/day for three days)[74]. Because of the complex nature of the life cycle, transmission within the animal facility is unlikely.

Public Health Considerations. *Paragonimus* spp. are known to infect humans. However, the lack of obligate intermediate hosts should preclude infection of animal facility personnel.

CESTODES

Pseudophyllidea

Diphyllobothrium latum

Morphology. The adult worm measures several meters in length. The scolex is elongated and flat, bears a groove on each side, and has no hooks. Proglottids are wider than they are long. Eggs are discharged continuously from the uterine pore, which is near the middle of the segment (Figure 17.16). Eggs are light brown and thin-shelled, and resemble those of trematodes in that they possess a small, inconspicuous operculum. They measure 59 μ to 71 μ long by 42 μ to 49 μ wide (Figure 17.17).

Hosts. *Diphyllobothrium latum* is commonly found in the small intestine of dogs, cats, wild carnivores, and humans in areas where certain freshwater fishes, such as pike, perch, and salmonids, occur. It is most prevalent in

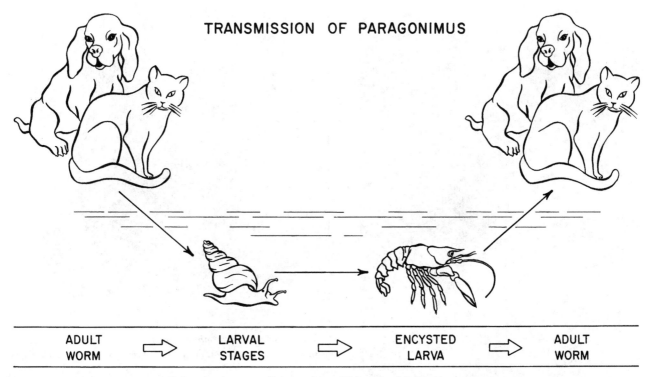

Fig. 17.15 *Paragonimus.* Diagram of life cycle. Courtesy of Marietta Voge, University of California.

the Great Lakes region of North America, the Baltic region of northern Europe, the lake regions of central Europe and southern Chile, and Japan. Infection may be common in random-source dogs in endemic areas. It does not occur in laboratory dogs reared on diets free of raw fish.

Life Cycle. The general life cycle of the pseudophyllidean tapeworms is described in Chapter 4, Biology of Cestodes. The definitive host is infected by ingesting raw or improperly cooked fish containing the infective larva (Figure 17.18). Eggs appear in the feces five to six weeks after infection.

Pathologic Effects and Clinical Disease. Natural infection in dogs is usually unapparent, and thus, usually asymptomatic.

Diagnosis, Treatment, and Prevention. Diagnosis is by finding the characteristic eggs in the feces examined following sugar flotation or sedimentation. Care must be taken to differentiate the eggs from those of the lung fluke (*Paragonimus*) and from the other species of Pseudophyllidean tapeworm, *Spirometra* spp., that infect dogs. Treatment with praziquantel (7.5 mg/kg) is curative[75]. Infection is unlikely in the animal facility, and can be prevented by avoiding the feeding of raw or improperly cooked fish.

Public Health Considerations. Infected dogs are not a direct hazard to humans.

Spirometra spp.

Morphology. *Spirometra* spp. are morphologically similar to *Diphyllobothrium*. The major difference is in the shape of the uterus, which is spiral in *Spirometra* and rosette-shaped in *Diphyllobothrium*. Eggs measure 41 µ by 67 µ and have an indistinct operculum and an abopercular bump (Figure 17.19).

Hosts. *Spirometra* spp. have been reported from dogs, cats, hyenas, and other carnivores around the world. Prevalence rates are high in wild felines and canines. *Spirometra mansoni* is common in the Far East and South America, and *S. mansonoides* is the species typically reported in North America.

Life Cycle. The life cycle is typical of the pseudophyllidean tapeworms. Adult worms live in the small intestine, and eggs are passed in the feces. Copepods of the genus *Cyclops* serve as intermediate hosts. Second intermediate hosts that feed on copepods include frogs, reptiles, birds, and mammals, but not fish[38]. The final host is infected when it eats the infected second intermediate host.

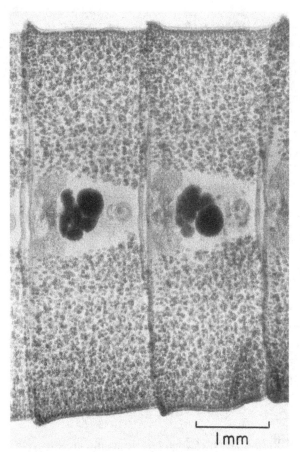

Fig. 17.16 *Diphyllobothrium latum,* mature proglottids. Note centrally located, coiled uterus. Courtesy of Marietta Voge, University of California.

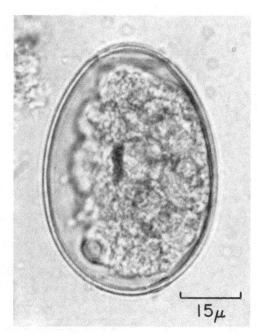

Fig. 17.17 *Diphyllobothrium latum,* embryonated egg. Note faint, inconspicuous operculum (top). Courtesy of Marietta Voge, University of California.

Pathologic Effects and Clinical Disease. Pathologic changes are not typically observed in dogs infected with *Spirometra* spp. There is usually no clinical disease, in spite of loss of large quantities of Vitamin B$_{12}$ to adult tapeworms[76].

Diagnosis, Treatment, and Prevention. Diagnosis is by finding characteristic eggs in sugar flotation or sedimentation preparations. The eggs are difficult to distinguish from those of *Diphyllobothrium,* which complicates diagnosis. Treatment has been successful with praziquantel (7.5 mg/kg)[76]. Infections are prevented by prohibiting access to paratenic hosts.

Public Health Considerations. Infected laboratory dogs are not a direct hazard to humans.

Cyclophyllidea

Dipylidium caninum

Morphology. Adult *Dipylidium caninum* are often 20 cm or more in length, but may be much shorter when large

numbers are present. Gravid proglottids are elongated, barrel-shaped, and filled with egg capsules (Figure 17.20). Each capsule contains three to 20 eggs (Figure 17.21). Individual eggs are spherical to oval and measure 31 μ to 50 μ long by 27 μ to 48 μ wide, with the size varying inversely with the number present in a capsule. When passed in the feces, gravid proglottids are white to pink and 8 mm to 12 mm long by 2 mm to 3 mm wide. They move about vigorously, expelling egg capsules and eggs.

Hosts. *Dipylidium caninum* occurs in the small intestine of dogs, cats, some wild carnivores, and rarely, humans (usually children) throughout the world. In fact, *D. caninum* may be the most common parasite of the dog, though increased use of highly effective flea products have markedly reduced its prevalence.

Life Cycle. The life cycle is indirect, and involves a flea intermediate host[77]. The dog louse (*Trichodectes canis*) and the human flea (*Pulex irritans*) may also serve as intermediate hosts (Figure 17.22). Dogs become infected by ingestion of the flea or louse. Development to the adult stage requires two to four weeks[38].

Pathologic Effects. Pathologic changes are limited to small intestinal mucosal lesions associated with insertion of the cestode rostellum. The worms move about throughout the day, so mucosal lesions may be numerous. Heavy infections may result in hemorrhagic enteritis.

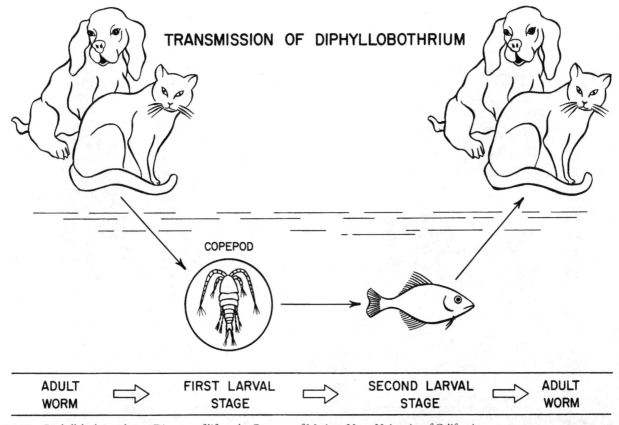

TRANSMISSION OF DIPHYLLOBOTHRIUM

COPEPOD

| ADULT WORM | ⇨ | FIRST LARVAL STAGE | ⇨ | SECOND LARVAL STAGE | ⇨ | ADULT WORM |

Fig. 17.18 *Diphyllobothrium latum.* Diagram of life cycle. Courtesy of Marietta Voge, University of California.

Clinical Disease. Infections are usually asymptomatic. Occasionally, heavy infections result in weakness, emaciation, vomiting, diarrhea, increased appetite, and convulsions. Heavily infected puppies may become impacted.

Diagnosis, Treatment, and Prevention. Diagnosis is by identifying gravid proglottids or egg capsules in the feces or perianal region. Infections may be cleared with praziquantel as per label instructions[78]. Elimination of fleas and lice from research animals prevents the completion of the life cycle and establishment of infection in laboratory colonies.

Public Health Considerations. *Dipylidium caninum* infection is uncommon in man and occurs only by accidental ingestion of an infected flea or louse.

Echinococcus granulosus

Morphology. Adult *Echinococcus granulosus* worms measure 2 mm to 9 mm long and have only three to four proglottids (Figure 17.23). The scolex bears a rostellum with hooks.

The eggs are ovoid, 32 μ to 36 μ long by 25 μ to 30 μ wide, and are indistinguishable from those of *Taenia*.

Hosts. *Echinococcus granulosus* occurs in the small intestine of dogs and wild canids. Larval stages are found in the liver, lungs, and peritoneal cavity of herbivores; and less commonly, in rabbits, rodents, dogs, cats, and primates, including humans[79]. The parasite is found throughout the world, particularly in areas where sheep are raised. It is most common in eastern and southern Europe, the Near East, southern South America, South Africa, southern Australia, New Zealand, and central Asia. There are small foci of the infection in the western United States.

Life Cycle. The life cycle is similar to that of *T. pisiformis.* Dogs become infected by ingestion of hydatid cysts in the viscera of the intermediate host. Each scolex develops into an adult worm. The prepatent period is about 56 days.

Pathologic Effects and Clinical Disease. Infection of dogs with *E. granulosus* is not associated with pathologic changes. Thus, there are no clinical signs of infection.

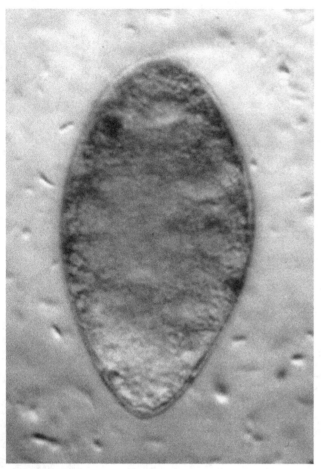

Fig. 17.19 *Spirometra mansonoides.* Egg passed in dog feces.

Diagnosis, Treatment, and Prevention. Diagnosis is by recognition of the small worms or gravid segments in the feces. The eggs cannot be differentiated from those of *Taenia*. Treatment is as described for *Taenia* sp. In areas where *E. granulosus* is endemic, newly acquired random-source dogs should be examined for *Taenia* eggs. If found, these dogs must be considered biohazardous, dewormed, and all fecal matter disposed of as biohazardous waste.

Public Health Considerations. The accidental ingestion of *E. granulosus* eggs from dog feces causes echinococcosis, or hydatid disease, in man[79]. This is a potentially life-threatening disease. Animal workers should be informed of the possible hazard and instructed in proper personal hygiene.

Taenia pisiformis

Morphology. Adult *Taenia pisiformis* measure up to 20 cm in length. The scolex bears a rostellum with two crowns of

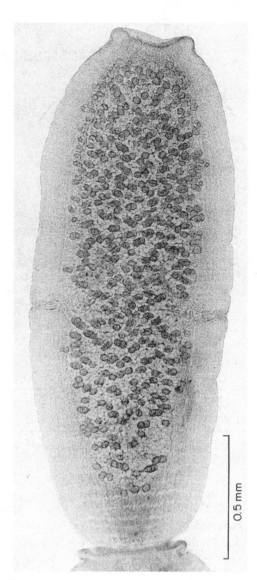

0.5 mm

Fig. 17.20 *Dipylidium caninum,* gravid proglottid. Courtesy of Marietta Voge, University of California.

hooks (Figure 17.24). Proximal segments are wider than they are long, mature segments almost square, and gravid segments are longer than they are wide. Gravid proglottids are white to cream colored, measure 8 mm to 11 mm long by 4 mm to 5 mm wide, and contain a uterus that has eight to 14 branches on each side of the medium stem (Figure 17.25). Eggs are typically taeniid, dark brown, spherical to subspherical, and 34 μ to 41 μ by 29 μ to 35 μ (Figure 17.26). The metacestode stage is described in Chapter 15, Parasites of Rabbits.

Hosts. *Taenia pisiformis* occurs in dogs throughout the world. Larval stages occur in lagomorphs and wild

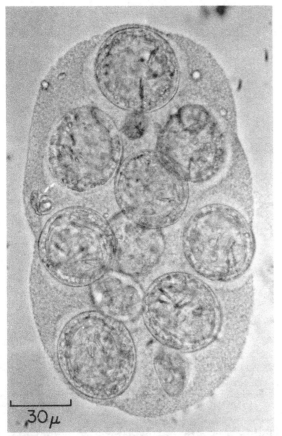

Fig. 17.21 *Dipylidium egg capsule* with eggs. Courtesy of Technical Sergeant R.R. Estes, U.S. Air Force School of Aerospace Medicine.

rodents. Infection is unlikely in laboratory animals, but may occur in random-source dogs.

Life Cycle. Dogs become infected after consuming lagomorph or rodent intermediate hosts. The wall of the cysticercus is digested away, freeing the larval cestode within. The worms grow to maturity in the small intestine in about two months, and gravid proglottids and eggs are passed in the feces.

Pathologic Effects and Clinical Disease. There are few pathologic effects associated with the presence of tapeworms in the canine small intestine[38]. Lesions form at the sites of small intestinal mucosal attachment. Light infections in the dogs are usually unapparent, whereas heavy infections may cause abdominal discomfort and enteritis.

Diagnosis, Treatment, and Prevention. Diagnosis is by finding eggs and proglottids in the feces. Dogs should be treated with praziquantel as per the labeled dose. Newly acquired dogs should be examined and treated if infected.

Public Health Considerations. This tapeworm is not known to infect humans.

Taenia serialis

Morphology. The adult worm is up to 70 cm long and 3 mm to 5 mm wide[38]. Scolices and proglottids are morphologically similar to *T. pisiformis*. Eggs measure 31 μ to 34 μ long by 27 μ to 30 μ wide.

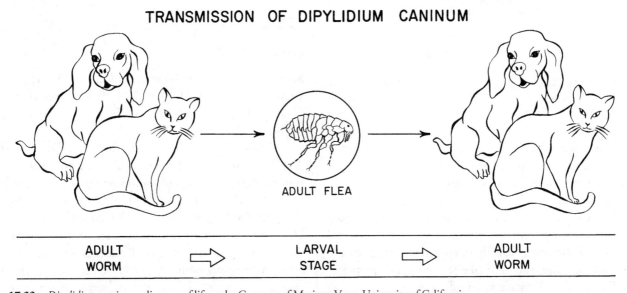

Fig. 17.22 *Dipylidium caninum,* diagram of life cycle. Courtesy of Marietta Voge, University of California.

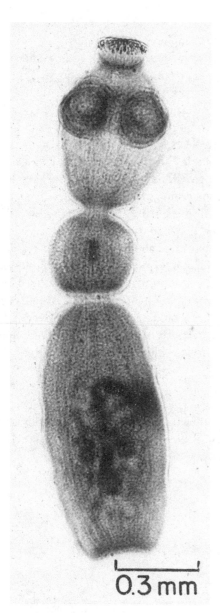

Fig. 17.23 *Echinococcus granulosus* adult. Courtesy of Marietta Voge, University of California.

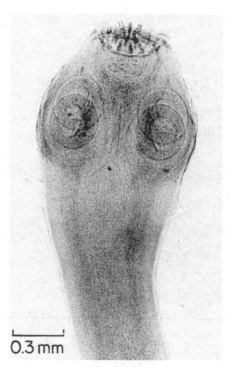

Fig. 17.24 *Taenia pisiformis* scolex. Courtesy of Marietta Voge, University of California.

Public Health Considerations. Humans may develop coenuri if infected with *T. serialis*. Thus, feces from infected dogs should be handled with caution, and laboratory personnel should be instructed in proper personal hygiene.

LEECHES

Limnatis nilotica

Morphology. This leech measures 8 cm to 15 cm long and 1 cm to 1.5 cm wide (Figure 17.27)[80]. It is green or brown on the ventral surface, with narrow orange stripes along the body ridges.

Hosts. Natural hosts include dogs, horses, other domestic animals, and humans in southern and central Europe, North Africa, and southwestern Asia. It is unlikely to occur in the laboratory except in random-source dogs.

Life Cycle. Leeches, like other members of the class Hirudinea, are hermaphroditic. The eggs are laid in cocoons and are characteristically attached to some object at the surface of a pond. Young leeches remain at the surface of the water following hatching. Infection of an endothermal host occurs while drinking. The young leech

Hosts and Life Cycle. Adult *T. serialis* occur in the small intestine of dogs and foxes[38]. Lagomorphs serve as natural intermediate hosts. The portion of the life cycle that occurs in the dog is similar to that of *T. pisiformis*.

Pathologic Effects and Clinical Disease. Pathologic changes are similar to those induced by *T. pisiformis*. Thus, infection of the dog is usually unapparent, though heavy infections may cause abdominal discomfort and enteritis.

Diagnosis, Treatment, and Prevention. These aspects are as described for *T. pisiformis*.

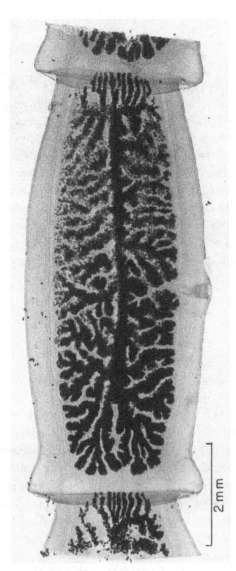

Fig. 17.25 *Taenia pisiformis,* gravid proglottid. Courtesy of Marietta Voge, University of California.

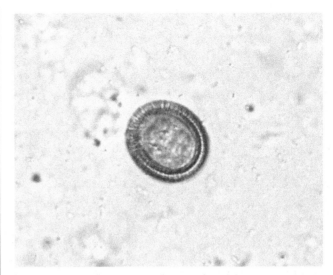

Fig. 17.26 *Taenia pisiformis* egg.

acquired dogs from endemic areas should be examined on arrival.

Public Health Considerations. Although this leech readily feeds upon humans[81], exposure under laboratory conditions is unlikely.

NEMATODES

Superfamily Rhabditoidea

Rhabditis strongyloides

Morphology. *Rhabditis strongyloides* larvae measure roughly 600 μ long. Characteristics of the order Rhabditida are described in Chapter 5, Biology of Nematodes and Acanthocephalans.

Hosts. *Rhabditis strongyloides* are free-living worms that live in manure or other decaying matter. However, third-stage larvae are capable of invading the follicles of the skin of dogs and other mammals maintained on unclean or moist bedding.

Life Cycle. The life cycle is direct. Dogs become infected by exposure to third-stage larvae in soiled bedding. Development to the adult stage does not occur on dogs.

Pathologic Effects and Clinical Disease. Infection results in localized dermatitis, which ranges in severity from mild erythema to severe pustular dermatitis. Clinical signs may include pruritus, alopecia, and crusting[82].

Diagnosis, Treatment, and Prevention. Diagnosis is by skin scraping, which often reveals large numbers of larvae. Larvae may also be cultured on agar plates. Affected

enters either the nose or the mouth, attaches to the mucosa of the upper respiratory tract, sucks blood for days or weeks, grows, detaches, and drops out through the nostrils. Adults are not parasitic.

Pathologic Effects and Clinical Disease. Attachment and feeding may result in edema of the glottis, dyspnea, and death from asphyxiation. Signs of infection include bleeding, or blood-tinged froth from the nose or mouth.

Diagnosis, Treatment, and Prevention. Diagnosis is by clinical signs and observation of the attached leech. Leeches rapidly detach when exposed to table salt. Newly

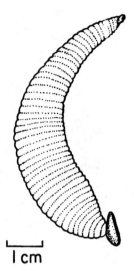

Fig. 17.27 *Limnatus nilotica.* Reproduced from Faust, E.C., Beaver, P.C., and Jung, R.C. (1968) with permission.

dogs should be shampoo and moved to clean and dry bedding. In some cases, dogs have been treated with ivermectin[83]. Dogs should be housed under clean, dry conditions.

Public Health Considerations. Humans are susceptible to *Rhabditis* dermatitis. However, such infections should not occur in the animal facility among personnel practicing personal hygiene.

Strongyloides stercoralis

Morphology. Adult female worms measure 2 mm to 5 mm long and 50 µ in diameter. The esophagus of the parthenogenetic female is about one-half of the total body length. The vulva of the female is near midbody, and the didelphic uterus has one branch that extends anteriorly and one branch that extends posteriorly. The ovaries fold back on the uterus but do not wrap around the uterus in a coiled fashion, as they do in other species such as *S. fuelleborni.* Parasitic males have not been found.

Hosts. Natural hosts of *S. stercoralis* include dogs and humans. Adult worms inhabit the small intestine.

Life Cycle. Dogs become infected through skin penetration by infective larvae (Figure 17.28)[84]. Larvae are carried to the lungs, coughed up, swallowed, and mature in the small intestine[85]. Eggs usually hatch in the intestine, so that first-stage larvae are released in the feces. The prepatent period is about two weeks. Larvae acquired from the skin can migrate into the mammary tissue and be passed to pups during nursing[86]. This route of infection is

more common when the bitch is infected just prior to, or during, lactation[87].

Pathologic Effects and Clinical Disease. Most infections with *S. stercoralis* are nonpathogenic. In heavy infections, the intestinal mucosa may contain thousands of worms threaded through the mucosa, resulting in extensive loss of intestinal surface. Migrating larvae may also damage lungs and other organs. Immune-compromised dogs may develop heavy infections in ectopic sites[88]. Most cases of canine infections with this worm are unapparent. Heavy infections of pups may cause mucoid diarrhea.

Diagnosis. Diagnosis is by finding larvae in the feces using the Baermann funnel technique or zinc-sulfate flotation. Larvae of *S. stercoralis* may be distinguished from those of hookworms by the size of the genital rudiment just posterior to midbody. In *S. stercoralis,* the structure is longer than the larva is wide[38].

Treatment. Ivermectin administration (200 µg/kg repeated in one week) has successfully cleared dogs of *S. stercoralis*[89]. All dogs in the facility should be treated simultaneously.

Prevention. Sanitation and management are the primary methods of control. Because first-stage larvae passed in the feces can develop into third-stage larvae within 48 hours, it is important that feces be removed daily and that food and water be kept free of contamination. Particular care must be taken to prevent the free-living stages from breeding in kennels, runs, or cages. Because moisture is essential to the survival of larvae, keeping surfaces dry greatly aids in controlling this parasite. Newly acquired dogs should be examined on arrival and treated if infected. Puppies should be examined to detect transmammary transmission.

Public Health Considerations. *Strongyloides stercoralis* is pathogenic for humans. An animal caretaker acquired the infection from dogs under his care in at least one case[90]. Animal care personnel should be made aware of this hazard and instructed in proper personal hygiene and safe methods of handling infected animals and excrement.

Superfamily Ascaridoidea

Toxascaris leonina

Morphology. Adult *Toxascaris leonina* are morphologically similar to *T. canis*[38]. They are differentiated from *T. canis* by their straight heads, conical tails lacking a protuberance, and heavy, wingless spicules in the male. Male worms measure 2 cm to 7 cm long, and females measure 2 mm to

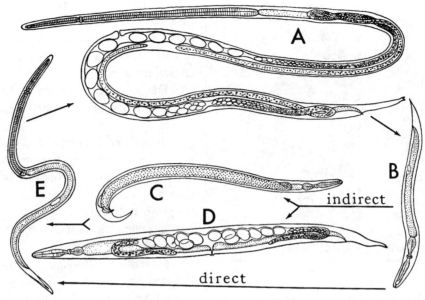

Fig. 17.28 *Strongyloides stercoralis* life cycle. The indirect cycle includes four rhabditiform stages (B), an adult male (C), or female (D), whose eggs hatch and pass through two rhabditiform stages and a filariform stage (E), to form the parthenogenetic female adult (A). The direct cycle does not pass through a free-living adult stage but passes through two rhabditiform stages (B), and a filariform stage (E), to form the parthenogenetic parasitic female adult (A). Reproduced from Chandler, A.C. and Read, C.P. (1961) with permission.

10 mm long. Eggs are smooth, with a nonpitted shell, and the zygote is lighter in color than that of *T. canis*. Eggs measure 75 μ to 85 μ long by 60 μ to 75 μ wide.

Hosts. Natural hosts of *T. leonina* include wild and domestic canines and felines. Random-source dogs are occasionally infected with *T. leonina,* but less commonly than with *T. canis*[40]. *Toxascaris leonina* is uncommon in animal facilities that practice good management and sanitation[91]. Neither transplacental or transmammary transmission occur. Thus, the infection is not easily maintained within colonies. Rodents and other mammals may serve as paratenic hosts[92].

Life Cycle. Eggs passed in the feces embryonate in three to six days[93]. Infection occurs either by ingestion of embryonated eggs or larvae in the musculature of paratenic hosts. Larvae develop in the wall of the intestine and return to the lumen to mature. The prepatent period is about 74 days. *Toxascaris leonina* does not migrate beyond the intestinal mucosa in the dog.

Pathologic Effects and Clinical Disease. *Toxascaris leonina* causes little pathology in dogs; thus, they typically do not develop clinical signs.

Diagnosis, Treatment, and Prevention. Diagnosis is by finding the eggs in the feces or identifying the worms passed in stools. The eggs are easily distinguished from those of *T. canis* because the external covering of the egg is smooth and the contained zygote is lighter in color than that of *T. canis* (Figure 17.29). Numerous products are approved for treatment of the *T. leonina* infection, including pyrantel pamoate, fenbendazole, and milbemycin oxime. Drug dosages may be found in the Appendix. Frequent removal of feces, good sanitation, treatment of infected dogs, and exclusion of paratenic hosts are the primary methods of prevention.

Public Health Considerations. Animal workers should exercise personal hygiene when working with dogs infected with *T. leonina*.

Toxocara canis

Morphology. Adult *Toxocara canis* are large, cream-colored worms that are curved ventrally at the anterior end and have narrow cervical alae (Figure 17.30). Males measure 4 cm to 10 cm long and have narrow, digitiform, terminal appendages, caudal alae, and winged spicules. The females measure 50 cm to 180 cm long with the vulva in the anterior quarter of the body. Eggs are subglobular to oval, measure 85 μ by 75 μ, and have a pitted surface[38] (Figure 17.29).

Hosts. *Toxocara canis* is one of the most common ascarid parasites of dogs throughout the world[96–97]. Infections are uncommon in laboratory colonies or kennels

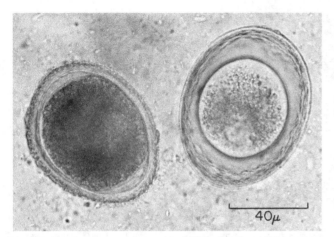

Fig. 17.29 Canine ascarids eggs. (Left) *Toxocara canis.* (Right) *Toxascaris leonina.* Reproduced from Ewing, S.A. (1967) with permission.

which practice good management and sanitation. Wild rodents, such as ground squirrels, serve as paratenic hosts. Larvae may be found in many vertebrate animals[98–99].

Life Cycle. Dogs often become infected in utero[100–101]. Pups less than three to five weeks old may also become infected by ingesting embryonated eggs. Adult dogs can also be infected by the ingestion of eggs, but these infections are light. Larvae undergo hepatotracheal migration and mature in the small intestine. Somatic larvae are activated during pregnancy, apparently by hormonal influence, and migrate to the fetus. Third-stage and fourth-stage larvae are found in the lungs, stomach, and intestine during the first postnatal week, and adults appear in the intestine by the end of the third week. Eggs appear in the feces as early as 23 days after parturition[102]. Rodents become infected by ingesting embryonated eggs. Larvae persist in the body without further development, and are infective to dogs if ingested.

Pathologic Effects. Dogs infected prenatally develop pulmonary lesions. Light infections result in mild petechial hemorrhaging, while heavy infections may cause pneumonia. Mature worms may be found in the stomach, bile duct, and peritoneal cavity. Heavily infected dogs can develop mucoid enteritis and intestinal impaction. Often the migrating larvae are arrested in the tissues, and granulomas form around them (Figure 17.31).

Clinical Disease. Clinical signs are only observed in young dogs[105]. Early signs include coughing and nasal discharge that usually subsides after about three weeks. Heavy infections frequently cause vomiting, anorexia, abdominal distension, mucoid diarrhea, debilitation, reduced growth

rate, allergic pruritus, and a characteristic foul oral odor. Less common signs include epileptiform seizures and death. Gut penetration by larvae can cause severe anemia as a prelude to death in pups. Adult dogs typically show no clinical signs.

Diagnosis. Diagnosis is by demonstrating eggs in the feces, worms in the intestine, or granulomatous lesions in tissues.

Treatment. Many products are approved for treating toxocariasis, including pyrantel pamoate, fenbendazole, and milbemycin oxime. Intrauterine infection can be minimized by the administering ivermectin or doramectin to the pregnant bitch[106]. In contrast, selamectin administered during pregnancy initially appeared effective, but it has not proven to be effective[107].

Prevention. Intrauterine transmission complicates efforts to prevent infection, making the condition difficult to control. Sanitation and frequent examination and treatment will usually prevent heavy infections and reduce the overall parasite burden. In many colonies, all dogs, including adults, are routinely dewormed, and females are treated with ivermectin before, during, and after pregnancy. Newly acquired dogs should be examined on arrival and treated if infected.

Public Health Considerations. *Toxocara canis* causes visceral larva migrans in humans[108]. Animal workers should handle infected animals and their excreta with caution. Infected dogs should be treated with anthelmintics to eliminate adult worms. Eggs require roughly two weeks to embryonate, and can remain infective for several years. Thus, routine cleaning of the facility and the use of runs with sealed floors reduce environmental contamination.

Superfamily Strongyloidea

Ancylostoma caninum

Morphology. Adult male *Ancylostoma caninum* measure 9 mm to 12 mm long, and females measure 15 mm to 18 mm long. Adults possess a subglobular buccal cavity with three well-developed teeth on each side[38]. The egg is ellipsoidal, thin-shelled, and measures 55 μ to 72 μ by 34 μ to 45 μ (Figure 17.32). The egg is usually in the two- to eight-cell stage when passed in the feces.

Hosts. Natural hosts include dogs and other canids throughout the world, especially in temperate and tropical zones. It is less common in cold climates. The prevalence of infection is high in random-source dogs living in endemic areas[40]. Infections are less common in well-managed laboratory animal facilities that practice good sanitation.

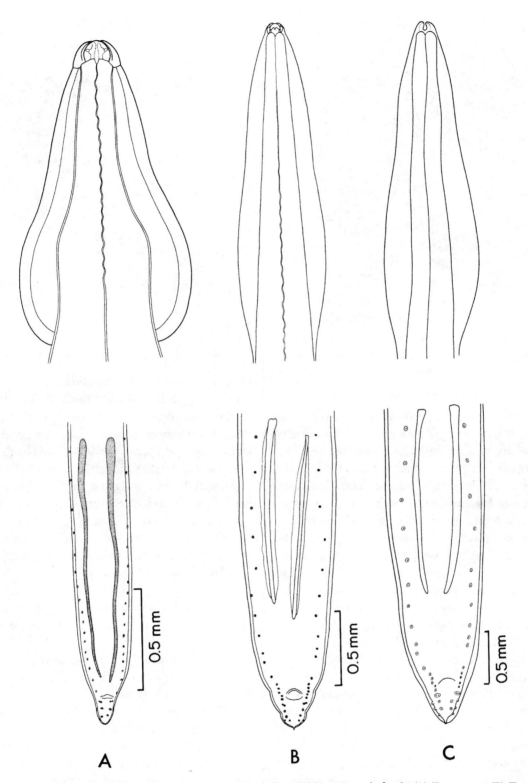

Fig. 17.30 Ascarids of the dog and cat. Ventral view. (Top) Anterior end. (Bottom) Posterior end of male. (A) *Toxocara cati*. (B) *Toxocara canis*. (C) *Toxascaris leonina*. Reproduced from Morgan, B.B. and Hawkins, P.A. (1949) with permission.

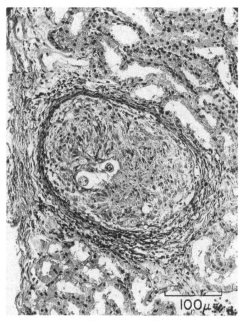

Fig. 17.31 Granuloma in the kidney of a dog with *Toxocara canis* larva in the center. Reproduced from Nobel, W.E.L., Robben, S.R.M., Dopfer, D., Hendrikx, W.M.L., Boersema, J.H., Fransen, F., et al. (2004) with permission.

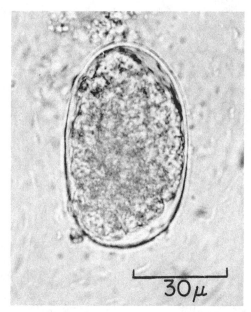

Fig. 17.32 *Ancylostoma caninum* egg. Reproduced from Ewing, S.A. (1967) with permission.

Life Cycle. The life cycle is direct. Eggs passed in the feces hatch in one to two days, and larvae reach the infective third stage in five to eight days. Desiccation and temperature extremes delay hatching and are lethal to larvae. Dogs become infected after ingesting third-stage larvae or through skin penetration. Ingested larvae develop in the gastrointestinal mucosa before maturing in the small intestine in about two weeks. Larvae penetrating the skin migrate to the lungs, are coughed up and swallowed, and mature in the intestine in three to five weeks. Larvae may persist within the tissues for prolonged periods. In lactating bitches, larvae undergo transmammary passage to nursing puppies[101,102]. Also, some larvae in the tissues make their way back to the intestine and resume development. This may occur in dogs previously cleared of adult worms. Dogs also may become infected through ingestion of paratenic hosts.

Pathologic Effects. Anemia and hypoproteinemia are common outcomes of hookworm infection. The primary lesion found is the small intestinal bleeding ulcer produced by the feeding activity of the adult worms (Figure 17.33). Focal pulmonary hemorrhages caused by migrating larvae also occur. Up to 0.2 ml of blood per worm per day may be lost.

Clinical Disease. Clinical signs caused by hookworm infection are associated with anemia. In young pups, especially those infected by the transmammary route, signs include mucosal pallor, diarrhea, weakness, progressive emaciation, cardiac failure, and death. Mature animals on an adequate diet often have no signs of infection other than mild hypochromic anemia, but heavily infected young animals, especially those infected by the transmammary route, develop more severe signs[109]. Less frequent signs include dermatitis and pruritus due to larval skin penetration in older, sensitized dogs and coughing and dyspnea due to larval migration in younger dogs.

Diagnosis. Diagnosis is by demonstrating eggs in the feces or mature worms in the intestine at necropsy.

Treatment. Numerous products are labeled to treat infections with the adult worms, including pyrantel pamoate, fenbendazole, and milbemycin oxime. Avermectins are most efficacious at preventing transmammary infections. Treatment of the bitch with ivermectin, doramectin, or moxidectin five to six days before whelping will either abrogate or markedly reduce infections of puppies receiving milk from their mother[110–112].

Prevention. Hookworm control is achieved by daily sanitation, elimination of harborage, provision of well-drained and sealed concrete runs, and regular treatment of infected animals. Bitches may transmit larvae to pups while nursing, though her feces remains negative by floatation. Newly acquired random-source dogs are likely to be infected and so should be checked and treated. Pups born from infected bitches should be tested for infection.

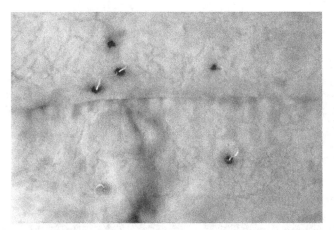

Fig. 17.33 *Ancylostoma caninum.* Adult worms attached to the small intestinal mucosa of a dog.

Public Health Considerations. Hookworm larvae are capable of penetrating the skin of people. Animal care personnel should exercise proper personal hygiene and safe methods of handling infected animals and excrement.

Uncinaria stenocephala

Morphology. Adult male *Uncinaria stenocephala* measure 5 mm to 8 mm long, and adult females measure 7 mm to 12 mm long. *Uncinaria stenocephala* differs from *Ancylostoma* in that *U. stenocephala* has a pair of cutting plates at the ventral border of the buccal cavity instead of teeth (Figure 17.34). Eggs measure 71 μ to 93 μ long by 37 μ to 55 μ wide (Figure 17.35).

Hosts. *Uncinaria stenocephala* occurs in the small intestine of dogs, cats, and foxes[113,114] in temperate zones throughout the world. It is most common in the northern United States, Canada, and Europe, and it is the only hookworm of importance in the British Isles. It is frequently seen in random-source dogs, and, to a lesser extent, in random-source cats in Europe. (The author has not seen this parasite in cats in the United States.) It is uncommon or absent in dogs and cats reared in the laboratory or in clean, well-managed kennels.

Life Cycle. The life cycle of *U. stenocephala* is similar to those of other hookworms[115,116]. Dogs are most commonly infected via the oral route. Adult worms are found in the small intestine. The prepatent period is 13 to 21 days. Following percutaneous infection, larvae migrate to the lungs and then return to the intestine via the tracheal route. Larvae can persist in the musculature of mice infected orally or through skin penetration. *Uncinaria*

stenocephala does not infect puppies via either transplacental or transmammary passage[117].

Pathologic Effects. *Uncinaria stenocephala* causes minimal damage to the intestine. Pathology is limited to petechial hemorrhages[115]. Skin penetration results in local dermatitis. Pulmonary larvae are likewise surrounded by focal areas of inflammation.

Clinical Disease. There is little to no clinical disease associated with this infection. Blood loss appears to be minimal in association with this infection, but experimentally infected greyhounds developed protein-losing enteropathy and suboptimum growth[118].

Diagnosis, Treatment, and Prevention. Diagnosis is by finding eggs in the feces or by the recovery of the worms at necropsy. Adult worms may be cleared with pyrantel pamoate or fenbendazole. Regular removal of feces and routine cage cleaning can prevent the transmission of this parasite. Dogs that are found to be infected should be treated.

Public Health Considerations. *Uncinaria stenocephala* is not considered to be a cause of cutaneous larva migrans in humans.

Superfamily Metastrongyloidea

Filaroides hirthi

Morphology. First-stage larval *Filaroides hirthi* passed in the feces measure 240 μ to 290 μ long (Figure 17.36). The

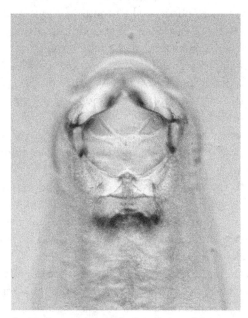

Fig. 17.34 *Uncinaria stenocephala.* Dorsal view of the anterior end.

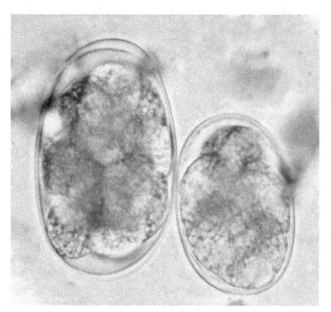

Fig. 17.35 Eggs of *Uncinaria* (left) and *Ancylostoma* (right).

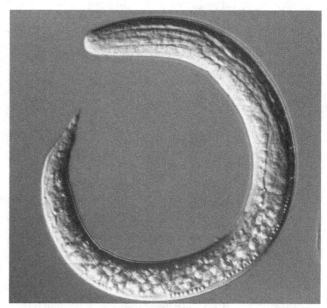

Fig. 17.36 *Filaroides hirthi*. First-stage larva.

esophagus measures 95 μ to 110 μ long. Larvae have a constriction and a kink just proximal to the end of the tail, and are virtually indistinguishable from those of *F. osleri*. They may be distinguished from other lung worm larvae because the first-stage larvae of *Filaroides* sp. lack the caudal spine present on the tail of larval *Angiostrongylus* sp. They also have rounded anterior ends that differentiate them from larval *Crenosoma vulpis*, which has a conical anterior end and a tail that ends in a sharp point without a constriction[119]. Adult *F. hirthi* are difficult to dissect out of fresh lung tissue[120]. However, in the adult male *F. hirthi*, the spicules are short and stout, and the cuticle appears inflated, but a bursa is not readily apparent. The vulva of the female is just anterior to the anus, and the uterus contains embryonated eggs.

Hosts. *Filaroides hirthi* inhabits the lung parenchyma of dogs and other canids (Figure 17.37). Dogs in research animal facilities have been found to be infected[121].

Life Cycle. The life cycle is direct, and is similar to that of *F. osleri*[122,123]. Ingested larvae arrive in the lungs within six hours via the hepatic portal circulation or mesenteric lymphatics. Larvae appear in the feces within five weeks of infection.

Pathologic Effects and Clinical Disease. Worms in lung parenchyma cause focal granulomatous reactions in the alveoli and bronchioles. Mild infections may be asymptomatic. Heavy infections cause dyspnea, coughing, and other

signs of respiratory distress, and may lead to radiographic changes[124]. Fatal cases of hyperinfection may develop in severely stressed and immunodeficient animals[125,126].

Diagnosis, Treatment, and Prevention. Diagnosis is by finding the larvae in the feces using a zinc-sulfate flotation. Larval *F. hirthi* are poorly motile, so the Baermann technique is less useful. Bronchoscopy can be used to distinguish infection with *F. hirthi* from that of *F. osleri*.

Eradication of infection is difficult. Ivermectin, albendazole, and others are among the drugs that have been used[127,128]. Cesarean derivation followed by barrier housing may be used to produce *Filaroides hirthi*-free dogs. Alternatively, treatment of dogs with albendazole (25 mg/kg/day for five days, repeated in four weeks) reduced the prevalence of infection in two kennels from 65% to 0.2% and 100% to 24%, respectively[127].

Public Health Considerations. *Filaroides hirthi* does not infect humans.

Filaroides osleri

Morphology. The male *Filaroides osleri* (Syn. *Oslerus osleri*) measures 5.6 mm to 7 mm long, and the female measures 10 mm to 13.5 mm long. Morphology is typical of the superfamily, and is described in Chapter 5, Biology of Nematodes and Acanthocephalans. In the male, the spicules are slightly unequal. In the female, the uterus extends anteriorly to the esophagus and is filled with embryonated eggs

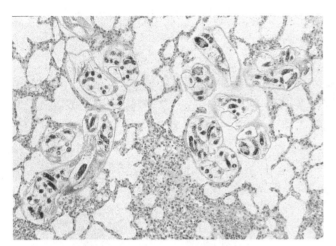

Fig. 17.37 *Filaroides hirthi.* Histologic section through adult females in lung of infected dog.

which measure 80 μ long by 50 μ wide. Larvae of *F. osleri* and *F. hirthi* are similar, and measure 300 μ long (Figure 17.38)[128, 129].

Hosts. Dogs and other canids throughout the world are the natural definitive hosts of *F. osleri*[130–133]. Thus, random-source dogs purchased for research may arrive infected[134].

Life Cycle. The life cycle is direct[135]. The first-stage larvae passed in the feces or in saliva are directly infective. Thus, infection follows the ingestion of relatively fresh feces, vomitus, or respiratory secretions. The prepatent period is six to seven months.

Pathologic Effects. Infection with *F. osleri* produces hemorrhagic or gray-white, granular, submucosal, wart-like nodules in the trachea and bronchi (Figure 17.39). These commonly occur at the bifurcation of the trachea, and may be observed two months after infection. Nodules may reach 18 mm in diameter. The coiled worms may be grossly visible within the nodules.

Clinical Disease. The principal clinical sign of infection is spasmodic dry cough brought on by exercise or exposure to cold air. Attacks are not induced by pressure upon the larynx. Young dogs are most severely affected and also develop respiratory distress, anorexia, and emaciation.

Diagnosis. The lesions observed by bronchoscope are pathognomonic. The infection can also be diagnosed by finding the larvae in fecal flotation using zinc-sulfate centrifugation[38].

Treatment. The infection can become endemic in breeding colonies and resist efforts to remove it from a colony. Anthelmintics used with mixed success include doramectin, ivermectin, albendazole, thiabendazole, and

others[136,137]. Parasite-free dogs may be derived by cesarean section, and raised in isolation from their dam and the rest of the colony. Some have recommended the removal of as many lesions as possible using an endoscope, followed by long-term anthelmintic treatment.

Prevention. Prevention requires cesarean derivation and barrier housing of *Filaroides osleri*-free pups. Random-source dogs from endemic areas should be examined and if found to be infected, treated or culled prior to incorporation into the breeding program[134,138].

Public Health Considerations. *Filaroides osleri* does not infect humans.

Superfamily Spiruroidea

Spirocerca lupi

Morphology. Adult *Spirocerca lupi* are bright red and usually coiled. Adult males measure 3 cm to 5.4 cm long, and females measure 5.4 cm to 8 cm long. The egg measures 30 μ to 37 μ long by 11 μ to 15 μ wide, has a thick shell,

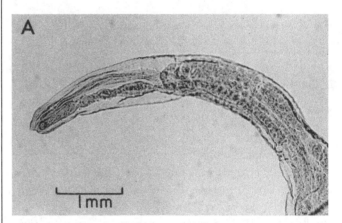

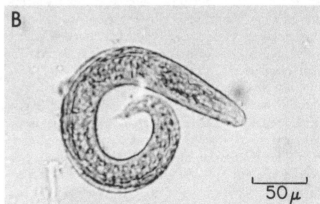

Fig. 17.38 *Filaroides osleri.* (A) Anterior end of adult female. Note embryonated eggs in the uterus. (B) First-stage larva. Reproduced from Mills, J.H.L. and Nielsen, S.W. (1966) with permission.

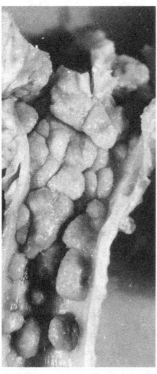

Fig. 17.39 *Filaroides osleri* lesions in the trachea of a dog. Reproduced from Mills, J.H.L. and Nielsen, S.W. (1966) with permission.

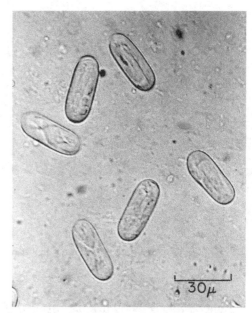

Fig. 17.40 *Spirocerca lupi* eggs. Reproduced from Bailey, W.S. (1963) with permission.

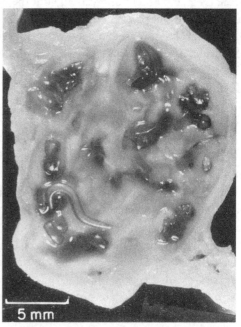

Fig. 17.41 *Spirocerca lupi* in the dog. Cross section of nodule in esophageal wall. Note adult worms. Reproduced from Bailey, W.S. (1963) with permission.

and usually contains a larva when passed in the feces (Figure 17.40)[139].

Hosts. Natural hosts include dogs and other canids, and large exotic cats, but not domestic cats. *Spirocerca lupi* occurs in tropical and subtropical regions of the world. It occurs in the southern United States, but is rare in the northern United States and does not occur in the British Isles. It may also be found in Africa, India, and in peninsular Malaysia[140–143]. Random-source dogs from endemic areas may be infected upon arrival at the animal facility. It does not occur in dogs raised in the laboratory, in kennels with good management and sanitation, or in cesarean-derived colonies.

Life Cycle. The life cycle is indirect. Adult *S. lupi* inhabit the wall of the esophagus or stomach (Figure 17.41). Eggs are excreted through a small opening in the infected tissue and are voided in the feces. Coprophagous beetles are the normal intermediate hosts, although cockroaches and many other insects have been infected experimentally. Following ingestion, eggs hatch and release larvae which encyst in the insect and are directly infective to the final host. If the insect is ingested by a paratenic host, larvae encyst in the mesentery or other tissue and

remain infective. Suitable paratenic hosts include many amphibians, reptiles, birds, and small mammals. Larvae ingested by the final host penetrate the stomach, migrate in the walls of the gastric artery to the aorta, and then pass through the connective tissue to the wall of the esophagus. The prepatent period is five to six months.

Pathologic Effects. Adult worms usually develop in the wall of the esophagus, but sometimes occur in the stomach, aorta, lungs, and other tissues[144,145]. *S. lupi* causes granulomatous inflammation and tumor-like nodules in these locations[145]. In addition to the worm, nodules may contain purulent, hemorrhagic fluid. Nodules in the aortic wall may result in aneurysm formation. These may rupture, causing fatal hemorrhage[146]. Malignant tumors often develop at the site of the nodules, either in the lumen of the esophagus or on the exterior wall[141,145,147]. Complications of tumor formation include pulmonary metastasis and hypertrophic pulmonary osteoarthropathy[148].

Clinical Disease. The scope and severity of clinical signs depend on nodule size. Small nodules are asymptomatic, whereas large pedunculated masses cause dyspnea and difficulty swallowing[149]. Vomiting may also occur.

Diagnosis. Diagnosis at necropsy is based on demonstrating worms within characteristic nodules. Lesions lacking worms are common in dogs in endemic areas, and are presumptive evidence of spirocercosis. Antemortem diagnosis is based on clinical signs, gastroscopic or radiological examination, or identification of eggs in the feces. Care must be taken to differentiate eggs of *S. lupi* from those of *Physaloptera* sp., which are similar. Sugar flotation is the best method for egg detection[150].

Treatment. Ivermectin or doramectin are effective treatments[151,152]. In addition, doramectin may prevent infection when administered at 30-day intervals[153].

Prevention. Because the life cycle is indirect, infection is unlikely in a research facility that practices good management and sanitation. Newly acquired animals with signs of infection or eggs in the feces should be treated.

Public Health Considerations. *Spirocerca lupi* does not infect humans.

Superfamily Filaroidea

Dipetalonema reconditum

Morphology. Adult *Dipetalonema reconditum* are small. Males measure 11.5 mm to 15 mm long and females measure 17.5 mm to 32 mm long. The microfilariae are superficially similar to those of *D. immitis*. The presence of a curved tail is diagnostic for *D. reconditum,* but this occurs in only one-third of the microfilariae, and does not rule out the possibility of a mixed infection. Microfilariae of *D. reconditum* measure 258 μ to 292 μ long and 4.7 μ to 5.8 μ

wide (Figure 17.42)[154], and have a rectangular anterior end, versus the tapered anterior end of *D. immitis*[155].

Hosts. The dog is the definitive host of *D. reconditum*. Infections occur globally, but are common in North America and Europe, and are important because the microfilariae of *D. reconditum* are frequently confused with those of *D. immitis*.

Life Cycle. The life cycle is indirect. Fleas serve as the intermediate host of *D. reconditum*[156]. The microfilariae are in the blood of the dog and are transmitted by the bite of the flea. It has also been shown that the louse, *Heterodoxus spiniger,* can serve as an intermediate host of *Dipetalonema reconditum*[38].

Pathologic Effects and Clinical Disease. Infection with *D. reconditum* is not associated with pathology or clinical signs.

Diagnosis, Treatment, and Prevention. Microfilariae are found in the circulating blood, and can be differentiated from those of *D. immitis* (Figure 17.43)[157]. Likewise, antigen detection assays can distinguish between heartworm and *D. reconditum*-infected dogs. No treatment is warranted. Flea control reduces the incidence of infection.

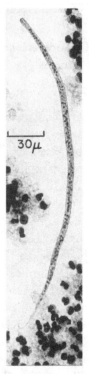

Fig. 17.42 *Dipetalonema reconditum* microfilaria. Reproduced from Lindsey, J.R. (1965) with permission.

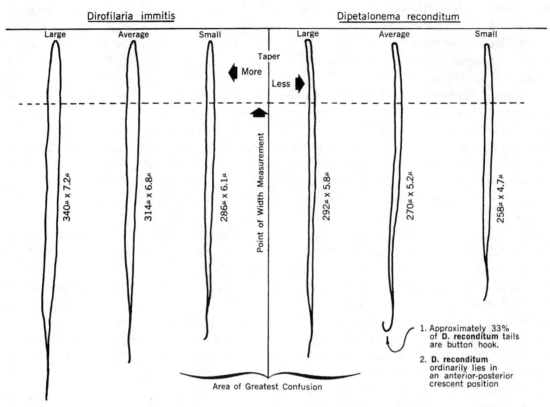

Fig. 17.43 Differential morphologic characteristics of *Dirofilaria immitis* and *Dipetalonema reconditum*. Reproduced from Morgan, H.C. (1966) with permission.

Public Health Considerations. *Dipetalonema reconditum* does not infect humans.

Dirofilaria immitis

Morphology. Adult *Dirofilaria immitis* are long, white, and slender[158]. Adult males measure 12 cm to 20 cm long and have a spirally coiled, blunt tail, small caudal alae, five pre-anal and six postanal pairs of papillae, unequal spicules, and no bursa or gubernacula. Adult females measure 25 cm to 31 cm long, and have the vulva near the posterior end of the esophagus (Figure 17.44). Microfilariae measure 286 µ to 340 µ long and 6.1 µ to 7.2 µ wide[159], and have a straight tail with no terminal hook (Figure 17.45).

Hosts. The dog heartworm occurs in the pulmonary arteries, right ventricle, and vena cava (Figure 17.46)[160] of dogs, other canids, ferrets, sea lions, cats, and humans. It is found throughout the world, especially in the tropics and subtropics, but cases have occurred in all 50 of the United States.

Life Cycle. The life cycle is indirect. Adult worms in the dog release microfilariae, which circulate in the blood and are ingested by blood-feeding mosquitoes. Developmental stages are found in the Malpighian tubules of the mosquito for about 15 to 16 days (eight to 10 days in the tropics). Larvae then enter the body cavity of the mosquito and migrate to the thorax and head, concentrating in the cavity of the labia or cephalic spaces of the head. Infective larvae are deposited by the mosquito while feeding and penetrate the skin through the feeding site. Further development occurs in the deep fascia, and possibly in the subcutaneous tissue, viscera, or lymphatics. Young adult worms arrive in the lungs in three to four months. The prepatent period is six to eight months[161].

Pathologic Effects. Infection with heartworm results in mechanical interference with blood flow, leading to hypertrophy and enlargement of the right ventricle, dilatation of the pulmonary arteries, and passive congestion of the lungs, liver, and spleen, accompanied by ascites[162]. Worms in the pulmonary arteries cause villous proliferation of the vascular intima. Worms also cause lysis of red blood cells moving past them within the artery. Hemoglobin released from ruptured erythrocytes is taken up by

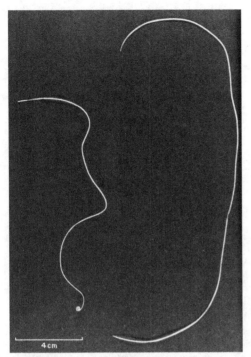

Fig. 17.44 *Dirofilaria immitis* adults. (Left) Male. (Right) Female. Courtesy of S.H. Abadie, Louisiana State University.

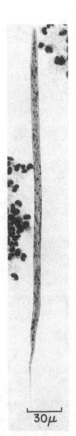

Fig. 17.45 *Dirofilaria immitis* microfilaria. Reproduced from Lindsey, J.R. (1965) with permission.

pulmonary macrophages, imparting a brown color to the lungs of heartworm-infected dogs. These changes decrease blood flow and tissue perfusion, leading to organ ischemia[163].

In contrast to adult worms, circulating microfilariae produce little damage. However, when microfilariae die, small granulomas form around them. The presence of circulating antigen antibody complexes and their deposition in the kidney can lead to renal disease in chronically infected dogs[164].

Clinical Disease. Signs vary with the worm load and duration of infection. The usual signs are lack of endurance, cough, ascites, and heart failure. Other signs include dry hair coat, anorexia, weight loss, increased respiration, rales, and hematuria.

Diagnosis. Microfilariae circulate in the bloodstream of most dogs infected with canine heartworm, but up to 20% of dogs may have occult infections because of single sex infections, past anthelmintic treatment, or immune clearance of microfilariae. Therefore, tests should be performed for both circulating microfilariae and circulating antigen.

Treatment. Adult heartworms may be cleared by the administration of melarsomine dihydrochloride (Immiti-cide). For up-to-date treatment recommendations, one should examine the treatment guidelines of the American Heartworm Society.

Prevention. Random-source dogs entering animal facilities are often infected in areas of high prevalence. Infection not only compromises the health of the laboratory dog, but may also render animals unfit for studies involving cardiac and pulmonary physiology[165]. Elimination of mosquitoes prevents infection. Dogs housed outdoors should be placed on monthly heartworm preventive medication.

Public Health Considerations. Dirofilariasis has been reported in people, but is uncommon[166]. Laboratory personnel who work with infected dogs in areas where the mosquito vector is present should be aware of this potential hazard.

Superfamily Trichuroidea

Eucoleus aerophilus

Morphology. Adult *Eucoleus aerophilus* (Syn. *Capillaria aerophila*) are long and thin[167]. Adult males measure 1.5

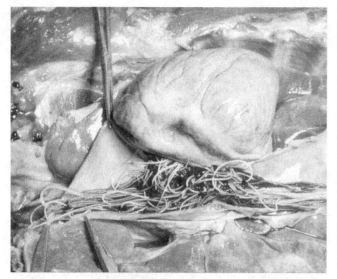

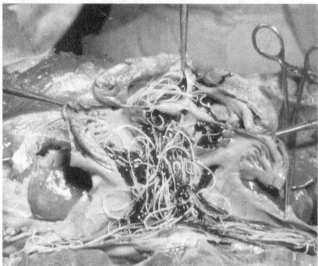

Fig. 17.46 *Dirofilaria immitis* in the dog. (Top) Worms in the right auricle and anterior and posterior vena cavae. (Bottom) Heart opened, also showing worms in the right ventricle. Reproduced from Jackson, R.F., von Lichtenberg, F., and Otto, G.F. (1962) with permission.

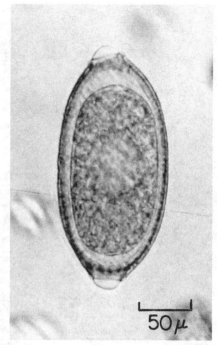

Fig. 17.47 *Eucoleus aerophilus* egg. Reproduced from Burrows, R.B. (1965) with permission.

cm to 2.5 cm long and females measure 2 cm to 4 cm long. The male has two caudal lobes and a single spicule with a spiny sheath. The vulva of the female is near the posterior end of the esophagus. The egg is brown, oval, measures 58 μ to 70 μ long by 29 μ to 40 μ wide, and has a granular shell and bipolar plugs (Figure 17.47)[168].

Hosts. *Eucoleus aerophilus* is primarily a parasite of the respiratory tract of the fox, but has also been reported from the dog, cat, and other carnivores in North America, South America, and Europe[132,169,170]. Infections are uncommon in laboratory-reared dogs, but may be seen in random-source animals.

Life Cycle. The life cycle is direct[171]. Eggs are passed in the sputum or feces and embryonate in 30 to 50 days. Infection occurs when embryonated eggs are ingested. The larvae hatch in the small intestine, penetrate the mucosa, and travel hematogenously to the lungs. Larvae penetrate the alveoli, migrate up the air passages as they develop, and reach maturity about 40 days after infection. The adult worms inhabit the epithelium of the bronchioles, bronchi, and trachea, where their thin bodies are threaded through the epithelial surface.

Pathologic Effects. Heavy infections result in tracheobronchitis, pulmonary edema, hemorrhage, and sometimes pneumonia. Larvae, adult worms, and eggs may be present in histologic sections of affected tissues.

Clinical Disease. Young animals are the most susceptible to pulmonary disease caused by *E. aerophilus*. Light infections are usually unapparent. Heavily infected dogs develop a cough, nasal discharge, dyspnea, and anorexia, and become debilitated[172].

Diagnosis, Treatment, and Prevention. Diagnosis is by identifying eggs in the sputum or feces. The eggs in the feces must be differentiated from those of *T. vulpis* (larger), *E. boehmi* (partially embryonated when passed), and *Pearsonema plica* (in feces contaminated with urine). Parasites may be eliminated with ivermectin or benzimidazoles.

Sanitation and the treatment of infected animals are the primary methods of control. Newly acquired dogs and cats should be examined on arrival and treated if infected. Because the eggs do not embryonate for 30 to 50 days, frequent and complete cleaning of cages, pens, and runs prevents the dissemination of the parasite.

Public Health Considerations. Humans have occasionally been found to be infected. Therefore, animal workers should exercise personal hygiene when working with infected dogs or cats.

Eucoleus boehmi

Morphology. Adult *Eucoleus boehmi* resemble adults of *E. aerophilus*[173]. The surface of the egg of *E. boehmi* is pitted, while that of *E. aerophilus* is covered with anastomosing ridges. The egg of *E. boehmi* is passed partially embryonated, and the developing morula in the egg often appears square or rectangular.

Hosts. *Eucoleus boehmi* inhabits the nasal cavity and paranasal sinuses of dogs and related canids around the world. It was originally described from the frontal sinus of a fox. The worms are found threaded through the mucosa of the sinuses.

Life Cycle. The life cycle is thought to be similar to that of *E. aerophilus*.

Pathologic Effects and Clinical Disease. Infection results in sinusitis. Most cases are asymptomatic; however, heavy infections result in rhinitis[174]. Infected dogs may develop chronic serous nasal discharge and occasional sneezing. The discharge can become purulent if secondary infection occurs.

Diagnosis, Treatment, and Prevention. Diagnosis is by finding the characteristic egg in the nasal sinuses or feces, or detecting worms in the sinuses at necropsy[175]. Ivermectin and fenbendazole have both been used effectively for treatment[174,176]. Strategies for prevention are as described for *E. aerophilus*.

Public Health Considerations. *Eucoleus boehmi* does not infect people.

Pearsonema plica

Morphology. Adult *Pearsonema plica* (Syn. *Capillaria plica*) are long, thin, and finely striated. Adult males measure 1.3 cm to 3 cm long and females measure 3 cm to 6 cm long. The spicular sheath of the male lacks spines. The egg is colorless to yellow, measures 60 µ long by 30 µ wide, and has bipolar plugs (Figure 17.48)[177].

Hosts. *Pearsonema plica* is the urinary capillarid of dogs, foxes, and other animals[178–181]. Infection is cosmopolitan in distribution and common in hunting dogs in Europe, but it is seldom reported in dogs elsewhere.

Life Cycle. The life cycle is indirect. Eggs passed in the urine are ingested by an earthworm[182]. The eggs hatch in the intestine of the earthworm, and the larvae burrow through the intestinal wall into the connective tissue. They are infective to the dog in about 24 hours, and are released when a dog eats the earthworm. After two molts in the dog's intestinal mucosa, third-stage larvae enter the portal circulation; pass through the liver, heart, lungs, and the general circulation to the kidneys; and migrate through the renal glomeruli, tubules, pelvis, and ureter to the bladder, where they develop to adults. The prepatent period is 58 to 63 days.

Pathologic Effects and Clinical Disease. Infection with *P. plica* is usually unapparent and causes little pathology[183]. Dogs may have leukocytes in the urine, and sometimes develop haematuria[184,185].

Diagnosis, Treatment, and Prevention. Diagnosis is by recognition of the adults in the urinary tract or the characteristic eggs in the urine. The eggs must be differentiated from those of fecal capillarids, which may contaminate

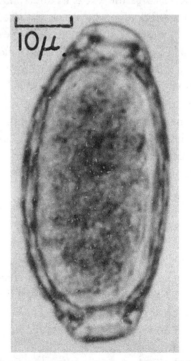

Fig. 17.48 *Pearsonema plica* egg. Reproduced from Habermann, R.T. and Williams, F.P. Jr. (1958) with permission.

urine samples. The infection may be eliminated with fenbendazole or ivermectin[185,186]. Prevention is by sanitation and exclusion of earthworms.

Public Health Considerations. *Pearsonema plica* does not affect humans.

Trichuris vulpis

Morphology. Adult *Trichuris vulpis* are characterized by a long, slender esophageal portion that occupies three-fourths of the body length, and a thick, blunted posterior section up to 1.3 mm wide, which contains the reproductive organs[167]. Both sexes measure 4.5 mm to 7.5 mm long, but females are wider posteriorly. The male posterior end is coiled dorsally with a single spicule enclosed in a terminal sheath, which evaginates where the spicule protrudes. The vulva is near the junction of the thin and thick portions of the body. The eggs are brown and oval, measure 70 μ to 80 μ long by 32 μ to 40 μ wide, and have a thick wall with bipolar plugs (Figure 17.49).

Hosts. *Trichuris vulpis* occurs in the cecum and colon of dogs, foxes, and other canids throughout the world. Infection is common in random-source dogs. Infections are uncommon in kennel-raised dogs routinely given anthelmintics, and in cesarean-derived, barrier-maintained colonies.

Life Cycle. The life cycle is direct. Dogs become infected by ingesting eggs which have embryonated in the environment. Eggs may embryonate in as few as nine days under optimal environmental conditions. Following ingestion, the larva emerges from the egg and enters the anterior small intestinal mucosa, aided by a retractable lancet. The larva returns to the lumen in two to 10 days, passes to the cecum, and matures in 70 to 90 days. Adults inhabit the cecum and less commonly, the colon (Figure 17.50)[187]. The prepatent period is about three months. Adult worms live for 16 months[188].

Pathologic Effects. Larval migration is restricted to the intestinal mucosa, causing little effect on the host. The adults in the cecum and colon embed deeply in the mucosa (Figure 17.51)[189]. These sometimes cause thickening and inflammation but usually produce little or no reaction. Large numbers of parasites are often seen in older dogs.

Clinical Disease. Clinical signs are only observed in heavily infected dogs, and include weight loss, abdominal pain, and mild to severe diarrhea that sometimes contains blood[190].

Diagnosis, Treatment, and Prevention. Diagnosis is based on identification of the eggs in the feces or adults in

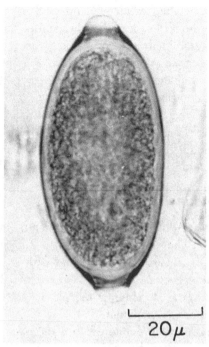

Fig. 17.49 *Trichuris vulpis* egg. Reproduced from Burrows, R.B. (1965) with permission.

the large intestine. Effective anthelmintics include fenbendazole, Febantel, or milbemycin oxime[191]. Complete elimination of *T. vulpis* from a research colony can be achieved by raising cesarean-derived progeny in isolation. Control in a conventional kennel is achieved by sanitation and routine treatment of infected animals. Eggs tolerate temperature extremes but not desiccation. Sunlight and concentrated saline solutions are lethal to unhatched larvae. Newly acquired dogs should be examined on arrival and treated if infected.

Public Health Considerations. *Trichuris vulpis* does not infect humans.

Superfamily Dioctophymatoidea

Dioctophyma renale

Morphology. Adult *Dioctophyma renale* are bright red. The females measure up to 1 m in length and about 12 mm in diameter. The smaller males measure 0.14 mm to 0.4 mm long and 4 mm to 6 mm in diameter, and have a fleshy, bell-shaped terminal copulatory bursa with a single, bristle-like spicule. The egg is ellipsoid, about 74 μ long by 47 μ wide. It is yellow-brown and has a thick shell that is covered with funnel-shaped pits except at the ends (Figure 17.52)[192].

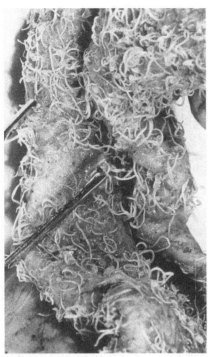

Fig. 17.50   *Trichuris vulpis* in the colon of a dog. Reproduced from Gaafar, S.M. (1964) with permission.

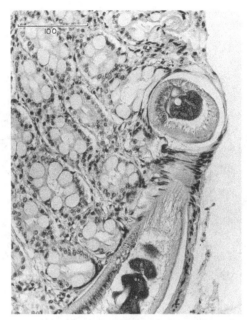

Fig 17.51   *Trichuris vulpis* embedded in the mucosa of the colon of a dog. Reproduced from Smith, H.A. and Jones, T.C. (1966) with permission.

Hosts. *Dioctophyma renale* infects dogs, wild carnivores, domestic animals, and humans[193–197], and is the largest nematode of terrestrial animals. It has been reported globally, and is frequently found in mink in North America[193].

Life Cycle. The life cycle is indirect. Eggs passed in the urine embryonate in water and require seven to nine months to develop, depending on environmental temperature[198]. Oligochaetes serve as first intermediate hosts, while fish and frogs become second intermediate hosts when they consume infected oligochaetes[199]. Salamanders serve as paratenic hosts[200]. Infective larvae freed by digestion penetrate the intestinal wall of the definitive host, enter the abdominal cavity, and mature in the renal pelvis, often in the right kidney. Aberrant development may occur in the abdominal cavity. The prepatent period is four months.

Pathologic Effects. Pathologic changes include hydronephrosis and progressive destruction of the parenchyma of infected kidneys, culminating in a fibrotic capsule that contains the worm and hemorrhagic fluid. Noninfected kidneys can hypertrophy to twice their normal size. Worms that develop in the abdominal cavity may cause peritonitis and adhesions.

Clinical Disease. Infection with *D. renale* may cause hematuria or other evidence of kidney disease, but is often unapparent until necropsy[201].

Diagnosis, Treatment, and Prevention. Diagnosis is by demonstrating the parasite in the kidney or the abdominal cavity. Finding eggs in the urine is also diagnostic. However, single sex infections, or worms in the abdominal cavity, will not be detected by urinalysis. Contrast radiography and ultrasonography may facilitate diagnosis. Treatment is usually by surgical removal of the worm. A nephrectomy may also be necessary. Because the life cycle is indirect, infection in the laboratory is self-limiting, and no control procedures are necessary.

Public Health Considerations. *Dioctophyma renale* occurs sporadically in humans[202]. However, animal workers cannot be directly infected from dogs.

ACANTHOCEPHALA

Oncicola canis

Morphology. Adult *Oncicola canis* have a conical body, tapered posteriorly, and are flat, gray, and wrinkled. The male measures 6 mm to 13 mm long (Figure 17.53)[203], and the female measures 7 mm to 14 mm long. The proboscis has hooks arranged in rows. The egg is brown, oval, and 60 μ to 70 μ long by 40 μ to 50 μ wide (Figure 17.54)[204]. It contains an embryo that has several spines at the anterior end.

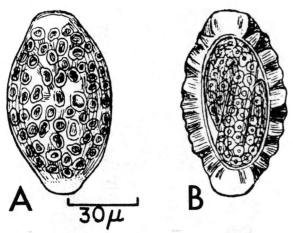

Fig. 17.52 *Dioctophyma renale* egg. (A) Superficial view. (B) Optical section of embryonated egg. Reproduced from Yorke, W. and Maplestone, P.A. (1926) with permission.

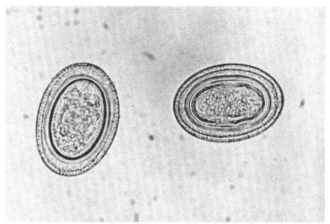

Fig. 17.54 *Oncicola canis* egg. Reproduced from Benbrook, E.A. and Sloss, M.W. (1961) with permission.

Pathologic Effects and Clinical Disease. Adult worms attach to the wall of the canine small intestine. The proboscis is usually deeply embedded and sometimes penetrates the peritoneal surface. Clinical signs may be absent or include mild enteritis.

Diagnosis, Treatment, and Prevention. Diagnosis is by identifying eggs in the feces or adult worms in the intestine at necropsy. Experience gained from treating primates infected with acanthocephalans suggests that ivermectin, fenbendazole, and albendazole may be effective when used in various regimens for extended periods; however, clearing a large number of infected animals may be very difficult and require several treatments and fecal examinations. All have seemed to be successful. Prevention is by keeping facilities free of insects which may serve as intermediate hosts.

Public Health Considerations. *Oncicola canis* does not infect humans.

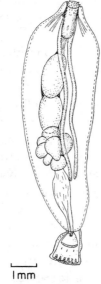

Fig. 17.53 *Oncicola canis* male. Reproduced from Wehr, E.E. (1965) with permission.

Hosts. *Oncicola canis* occurs in the dog, and is found in the United States, particularly Texas, and northeastern Mexico. It is locally common and likely to occur only in random-source dogs in endemic areas.

Life Cycle. The life cycle is indirect, and is generally described in Chapter 5, Biology of Nematodes and Acanthocephalans. A cockroach serves as the first intermediate host. Armadillos and turkeys may serve as paratenic hosts containing cystacanths[205].

ARTHROPODS

Class Insecta

Order Diptera

Family Calliphoridae

The Calliphoridae includes the blow flies (*Chrysomyia, Lucilia, Phormia*), bottle flies (*Calliphora* and *Phaenicia*), tumbu fly (*Cordylobia anthropophaga*), and others. Most of these develop in carrion and only accidentally or facultatively cause myiasis in dogs and other animals. Adults are attracted to decaying organic matter, such as fetid, purulent sores or soiled pelage. Their maggots feed primarily on dead or gangrenous tissue and only secondarily invade adjacent healthy tissue.

Other calliphorids of veterinary importance include the screwworm flies (*Cochliomyia, Chrysomyia bezziana,* and others), which cause primary myiasis. *Cochliomyia hominivorax,* the New World screwworm fly, occurs in the Americas south of Panama, while *Chrysomyia bezziana,* the Old World screwworm, occurs in Africa and southern Asia. Both are obligate myiasis producers and will seek any fresh open wound regardless of host species[206]. Debilitated animals are especially susceptible to attack. Screwworm fly larvae could be encountered in random-source dogs in endemic areas and can attack dogs in kennels if they are not maintained in screened facilities. The interested reader is directed to Chapter 6, Biology of Arthropods, for a description of the life cycle.

Prognosis in untreated cases is grave, because secondary myiasis-producing flies follow the primary screwworm invasions with fatal results. Lesions in dogs with long hair coats may initially go undetected. Infested dogs may present as debilitated or depressed. Shaving of the hair coat often reveals the lesion, which may be swarming with maggots of various sizes. Some may have penetrated deeply into the tissue. It may also be difficult to observe lesions when they occur in the ears[207]. Lesions must be cleaned and topical insecticides applied. Dogs may also be treated with systemic avermectins. Recently, nitempyram was used in a series of dogs with maggots of *C. hominivorax,* and within 24 hours, almost all the maggots within the lesions were dead[208]. Although humans are susceptible to infection[206], infected laboratory animals are not a direct hazard to human health.

Family Culicidae

Important mosquito genera include *Anopheles, Aedes,* and *Culex.* Mosquitoes occur throughout the world and attack all endothermal animals, including dogs. Their importance relates to their annoying and sometimes painful feeding habits, and their ability to act as vectors of many pathogens. In dogs, these include the canine heartworm, *Dirofilaria immitis.* Additional information is presented in Chapter 6, Biology of Arthropods. Salivary secretions introduced while taking a blood meal cause local inflammation and pruritus. The degree of insult varies with the species of mosquito and the susceptibility of the individual animal. However, most dogs react only mildly to the bites of mosquitoes, unless they receive large numbers of bites. Mosquito feeding can be prevented by screening (18-mesh-per-inch) outdoor dog

housing areas. Mosquitoes also transmit human pathogens and so may place animal workers in facilities where blood-borne pathogens are studied at risk.

Family Muscidae

The interested reader is referred to Chapter 10, Parasites of Birds, for information on muscid flies of veterinary importance. Among the most bothersome is *Stomoxys calcitrans,* a globally distributed blood-sucking fly that will attack any endothermal animal, including dogs. Adults resemble the housefly but are distinguished by their darker color, more robust appearance, and modified skin-piercing mouthparts[206]. Eggs are deposited deep in decaying vegetation or in urine-soaked feed or bedding. Adult flies usually attack the ears and legs, causing severe, painful bites, and sometimes local inflammation. These flies can serve as mechanical vectors of some protozoa, bacterial, rickettsial, and viral diseases as they move from host to host until they are full. Dogs occasionally present with bleeding edges to their ears or muzzle. Dogs should be treated with topical repellants, and fly bites attended to, where fly activity is heavy. Large numbers of flies indicate the presence of a nearby collection of decaying vegetation or urine-soaked bedding. Its removal may markedly reduce the number of flies.

Family Psychodidae

The phlebotomine sand flies, *Phlebotomus* sp. and *Lutzomyia* sp., occur in temperate and tropical regions throughout the world. *Phlebotomus* is found in the Old Word and *Lutzomyia* is found in the New World[206]. Sand flies resemble mosquitoes, but are smaller, hairier, have short mouthparts, and the wings tend to lack scales and have straight venation extending from the base to the tip[206]. Many species of sand fly prefer to feed on rodents, but some readily feed on dogs. Sand flies breed in crevices, cracks in kennel walls, and rodent burrows, under conditions of moderate temperature, high relative humidity, and darkness[206].

Larval stages feed on detritus and pupate in the soil. Adults feed at dusk and dawn, tearing small holes in the flesh and lapping up blood and tissue fluid from the wound[209]. Sand flies serve as efficient vectors of *Leishmania* sp., because macrophages attracted to skin lesions readily become infected and are themselves ingested by other sand flies. The bites of sand flies do not normally cause clinical disease. Netting used to protect dogs from sand flies must have openings smaller than that used to exclude mosquitoes. Several pesticides are marketed to prevent sand fly attack[5,6,210,211]. Phlebotomine sand flies are significant vectors of human leishmaniasis, but there is little risk to personnel working within animal facilities unless *Leishmania* sp. is under study in the facility.

Family Sarcophagidae

Flesh flies of importance include the *Sarcophaga* sp. and *Wohlfahrtia* sp. The larvae of sarcophagid flies produce dermal myiasis in a range of hosts, including the dog. Infestation with maggots of these species is uncommon and only likely to occur in random-source dogs. Adults are medium-to-large gray and black flies. Larvae are recognized by their characteristic posterior spiracular slits that slant away from the midventral line. Gravid females deposit larvae instead of eggs on open wounds, fetid sores, and serous discharges[206]. Larvae develop in four to seven days, and pupation occurs on the soil in four days. The full cycle takes about two weeks to complete in temperate areas.

The maggots of these species are usually scavengers but become facultative parasites when they occur in wounds of endothermal animals. The larvae are voracious and often actively invade healthy tissue, producing deep lesions. Affected dogs may appear moribund and listless. They are likely to have matted and soiled hair coats that attract flies. Under the matted hair may be large areas of tissue destruction resulting from the flies excavating through the skin and deeper tissues. Lesions should be clipped and groomed, and a pesticide applied. Fly strike can be prevented by screening outdoor animal rooms. Skin wounds should be kept clean. These flies attack humans and often produce severe mutilation[206], but infected laboratory animals are not a direct hazard to personnel.

Order Phthiraptera

Linognathus setosus

Morphology. *Linognathus setosus* is a large louse (Figure 17.55). Adults appear slightly blue when fully engorged. The head is blunt, rounded anteriorly, and about as wide as it is long. The mouthparts are anteriorly directed. The abdomen is oval and covered with numerous long hairs. Six spiracles are located on each side, but no plates are evident. The thoracic spiracles are large. The total length of the female is about 2 mm and the male is about 1.75 mm[212].

Hosts. *Linognathus setosus* is a sucking louse occasionally found on dogs and wild canids[213–215]. Infestation is more common on long-haired breeds throughout the world, and is often localized to the shoulders and neck, especially underneath the collar. Rabbits and chickens are also susceptible.

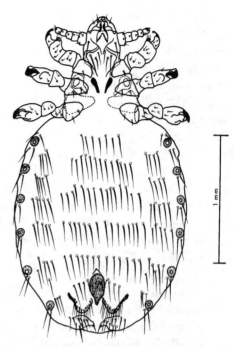

Fig. 17.55 *Linognathus setosus* female, ventral view. Courtesy of K.C. Kim, Pennsylvania State University.

Life Cycle. Eggs are deposited on hairs and hatch in five to 12 days. Lice develop through three nymphal stages to the adult stage. Transmission is by direct contact, and by fomites, including brushes and combs. Immature stages do not survive off of the host.

Pathologic Effects and Clinical Disease. Heavy infestations cause dermatitis, alopecia, restlessness, and pruritus.

Diagnosis, Treatment, and Prevention. Diagnosis is based on clinical signs and on finding lice or eggs. Lice may be eliminated by treating dogs with insecticides[216,217]. Treated dogs should be placed in clean disinfected cages, and treatment should be repeated to eliminate recently hatched nymphs. Newly acquired dogs should be examined and treated as necessary.

Public Health Considerations. *Linognathus setosus* does not infest humans.

Trichodectes canis

Morphology. *Trichodectes canis* is a short, broad louse, approximately 2 mm long (Figure 17.56), and is yellow with dark markings[38]. The head is quadrangular and broader than it is long. The antennae are short, stout, three-segmented, and fully exposed. The antennae of the male have a much enlarged basal segment. Each leg has

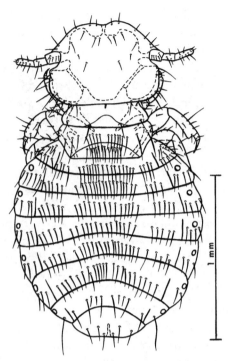

Fig. 17.56 *Trichodectes canis* female, dorsal view. Courtesy of R.D. Price, University of Minnesota.

only one tarsal claw. The abdomen is oval and has one dorsal transverse row of medium-length hairs across each segment and six pairs or spiracles. The mouthparts are located ventrally on the head of the louse.

Hosts. *Trichodectes canis* is a chewing louse found on the dog and wild canids throughout the world. Once common on random-source and kennel-reared puppies, it is now less prevalent, especially in the United States.

Life Cycle. After fertilization, the female lays several eggs daily for the rest of her life, which is about 30 days[38]. Eggs are cemented near the base of the hair, hatch in one to two weeks, molt three times, and develop into mature lice in about two additional weeks. The louse feeds on tissue debris and survive only three to seven days if separated from the host. Transmission is by direct contact and fomites, including grooming equipment. Immature stages do not survive off of the host.

Pathologic Effects. Effects on the hair or skin are usually minimal, though heavy infestations may cause dermatitis. The eggs and nits can be seen on the hair and may give it a scruffy appearance. More importantly, *T. canis* may serve as a vector of the dog tapeworm, *Dipylidium caninum*.

Clinical Disease. *Trichodectes canis* is usually found on the head, neck, and tail, attached by its claws or mandibles to the base of a hair. Lice may congregate near body openings or skin abrasions, in an effort to remain in a moist environment. Common signs include irritation, rubbing, scratching, biting of infested areas, sleeplessness, nervousness, alopecia, and a rough matted coat. Infestations are more prevalent on dogs that are very young, old, debilitated, or maintained in unsanitary conditions.

Diagnosis, Treatment, and Prevention. Diagnosis is based on clinical signs and demonstration of lice or louse eggs. *Trichodectes canis* is highly susceptible to treatment with imidacloprid, selamectin, fipronil, and topical permethrins[217–220]. Treated dogs should be placed in clean, disinfected cages, and treatment repeated to eliminate recently hatched nymphs. Newly acquired dogs should be examined and isolated and treated if infested. In the tropics, dogs can be infested with another mallophagan louse, *Heterodoxus spiniger*.

Public Health Considerations. *Trichodectes canis* does not feed on humans. However, *Dipylidium caninum* may be transmitted to people by ingestion of an infected louse.

Class Arachnida

Ticks

Family Argasidae
Otobius megnini *Otobius megnini,* the spinose ear tick, is a soft tick commonly found in the ears of large, domestic animals, including dogs. The interested reader is directed to Chapter 20, Parasites of Sheep and Goats, for additional information. The original range of the spinose ear tick was the semiarid regions of the southwestern United States and Mexico. More recently, it has also been reported throughout the continental United States, Hawaii, western Canada, South America, Africa, Madagascar, India, and Australia. It was probably introduced into these areas on transported livestock.

Immature stages of this tick attach deep in the external auditory canal of the host, causing extreme irritation, edema, hemorrhage, and pain. The ear canal is sometimes completely filled with ticks and debris. Secondary effects include trauma of the external ear, secondary infection of the auditory canal, deafness, and sometimes death. Otitis externa, with severe head shaking and scratching, are common clinical signs. Some dogs have been observed to engage in frantic head shaking and vocalization[221]. Newly acquired dogs should be examined and treated if ticks are discovered. Because of the location of the parasite deep in the ear canal, the ticks can be very difficult to remove. Immature stages of the spinose ear tick also invade the external ear of humans and cause severe pain, but such infestations are very rare.

Family Ixodidae

Amblyomma americanum *Amblyomma americanum,* the lone star tick, is abundant in wooded and brushy areas throughout the Americas[206]. Susceptible hosts include wild rodents, dogs, wild carnivores, domestic animals, some ground-inhabiting birds, and humans. The interested reader is directed to Chapter 20, Parasites of Sheep and Goats, for additional information. The bite of *Amblyomma americanum* is particularly annoying because the mouthparts are elongated. The wound caused by the bite of *A. americanum* may be invaded by screwworm maggots. Heavy infestations can lead to severe anemia and debilitation.

Ticks may be eliminated with acaricidal treatments such as permethrins[222]. Newly acquired dogs should be checked and treated for tick infestations. Underbrush, tall grass, and weeds should be removed from around dog kennels, and reservoir hosts should be prevented access to buildings that house dogs.

Special care must be taken when manually removing ticks. By inserting a needle or scalpel under the mouthparts and applying slow, gentle traction, the tick can usually be detached intact.

This tick is a vector of *Rickettsia rickettsii, Francisella tularensis, Ehrlichia* sp., and *Hepatozoon americanus,* and is a reservoir, if not a vector, of *Coxiella burnetii*[28,223]. People handling infested dogs should be particularly careful. Care should also be taken to prevent contamination of open wounds or mucous membranes with fluids from engorged or crushed ticks.

Dermacentor variabilis **Morphology.** *Dermacentor variabilis,* the American dog tick, is a large, ornate tick. The adult male measures 4 mm to 5 mm long and has a gray, enameled appearance. The adult female is slightly larger and has a scutum which is mostly gray. This tick is differentiated from *D. andersoni* by the scutal ornamentation and the smaller, more numerous goblets in its spiracular plates.

Hosts. Immature stages feed on many species of wild rodents and lagomorphs, especially deer mice, voles, cotton rats, rice rats, and cottontail rabbits. Adults are common on the dog and wild carnivores, and they sometimes bite humans[224]. Although this tick seldom invades research animal facilities, adults may be found on random-source dogs. It is not likely to be encountered on laboratory dogs obtained from kennels that practice good sanitation and parasite control.

Life Cycle. The life cycle of *Dermacentor* sp. is presented in Chapter 20, Parasites of Sheep and Goats.

Pathologic Effects. The bite of *D. variabilis* causes local inflammation, edema, and hemorrhage. Large numbers of feeding ticks can cause severe anemia, irritability, debilitation, and tick paralysis.

Diagnosis, Treatment, and Prevention. Diagnosis is based on clinical signs and on identification of the tick on the host. Acaricides effective against other members of the Ixodidae will eliminate *D. variabilis.* Newly acquired dogs should be checked and treated for tick infestations. Underbrush, tall grass, and weeds should be removed from around laboratory dog kennels, and reservoir hosts should be excluded from areas housing research dogs.

Public Health Considerations. The American dog tick is a known vector of human and canine pathogens, including *Rickettsi rickettsii* and *Francisella tularensis,* and its bite may cause tick paralysis in humans. Infested research dogs should be handled with caution, and care should be taken to prevent the contamination of open wounds or mucous membranes with fluids from crushed ticks.

Ixodes spp. Several of the *Ixodes* parasitize endothermal animals, including dogs. The most common species in North America are *Ixodes scapularis* (the black-legged tick) in the eastern United States and Mexico, and *I. pacificus* (the California black-legged tick) along the west coast of North America from California to British Columbia. *Ixodes ricinus* (the castor-bean tick) is the most common species in Europe; *I. persulcatus* is most common in Eastern Europe and northern Asia; *I. canisuga* (the British dog tick) is common in the British Isles; *I. holocyclus* is common in Australia; and *I. pilosus, I. rubicundus, I. rasus,* and *I. schillingsi* are common in Africa.

The bite of *Ixodes* causes irritation, trauma, and sometimes paralysis. In addition, this tick is a major vector of *Borrelia, Ehrlichia,* and *Babesia* from rodents to dogs and humans[206]. *Ixodes* are characterized by anal groves that join anterior to the anus. The mouthparts are long, and the scutum lacks eyes, festoons, and ornamentation. *Ixodes* species are three-host ticks. The life cycle is presented in Chapter 6, Biology of Arthropods. Because of the long hypostome, the mouthparts may detach and remain in the host after the tick is removed, resulting in persistent, severe irritation, often with secondary bacterial invasion.

The mouthparts can be removed as described for *Amblyomma*. Ticks may be eliminated with fipronil or permethrin[225–227]. Newly acquired dogs should be checked and treated for tick infestations. Brush, tall grass, and weeds should be removed from around dog kennels, and reservoir hosts excluded from areas where dogs are housed. Animal workers should exercise care in handling ticks which may be carriers of human pathogens.

Rhipicephalus sanguineus **Morphology.** Male *Rhipicephalus sanguineus* (brown dog tick, kennel tick) measure 2.2 mm to 3.2 mm long, and females measure 2.4 mm to 2.7 mm long when unengorged, but up to 1.5 mm long after feeding[206]. Both sexes have eyes and inornate, dark brown scuta. The posterior of the body bears festoons. The basis capitulum is hexagonal (Figure 17.57).

Hosts. *Rhipicephalus sanguineus* is found on dogs, and less commonly, other mammals, in the southwestern United States, Mexico, Central and South America, southern Europe, and Africa. In warm climates, it occurs outdoors and indoors. In cool climates it is generally confined to heated buildings.

Life Cycle. *Rhipicephalus sanguineus* is a three-host tick. The life cycle is described in Chapter 6, Biology of Arthropods. Adult females feed for about a week, while males remain attached for weeks to months. Immature ticks are common in the pelage of the neck, whereas adults attach almost anywhere, frequently between the digits of the feet.

Pathologic Effects and Clinical Disease. The bite of *R. sanguineus* causes irritation, inflammation, hyperemia, edema, hemorrhage, and thickening of the skin. This tick also transmits many pathogens of dogs, including *Babesia canis* and *B. vogeli, Hepatozoon canis, Ehrlichia canis,* and the filarial nematode *Dipetalonema reconditum*[206].

Diagnosis, Treatment, and Prevention. Diagnosis is based on identification of the tick on the host. Infested dogs should be treated with fipronil, selamectin, or permethrins[228–230]. Laboratory animal facilities should be designed so that cracks and crevices are minimized. Cages and pens should be constructed of metal, concrete, or other material that can be readily cleaned and disinfected. High pressure cleaning of facilities with hot water or steam when empty can eliminate ticks. Newly acquired animals should be examined on arrival and treated if infested.

Public Health Considerations. The brown dog tick is a vector of several important pathogens of humans[206], including *Rickettsia rickettsii* (the cause of Rocky Mountain spotted fever), *R. siberica* (the cause of Siberian tick typhus), *R. conori* (the cause of boutonneuse fever), and *Francisella tularensis* (the cause of tularemia). Laboratory

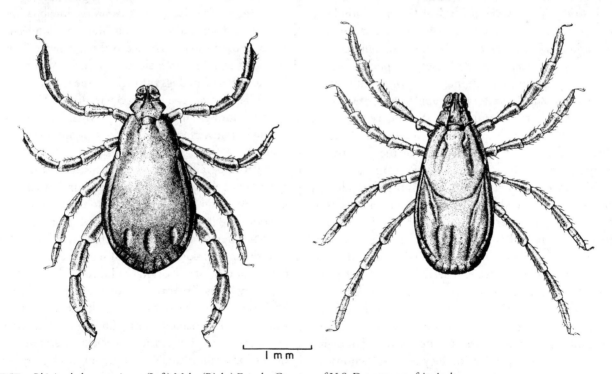

1 mm

Fig. 17.57 *Rhipicephalus sanguineus.* (Left) Male. (Right) Female. Courtesy of U.S. Department of Agriculture.

animals infested with this tick should be handled with caution, and care should be taken when removing ticks manually to prevent the contamination of open wounds or mucous membranes with fluids from crushed ticks.

Mites

Suborder Astigmata

Sarcoptes scabiei **Morphology.** *Sarcoptes scabiei* is a burrowing mite. The morphology of *S. scabiei* is presented in Chapter 15, Parasites of Rabbits. Briefly, adult females measure 380 µ long by 270 µ wide[206,231]. The male is similar to the female but smaller, measuring 220 µ long by 170 µ wide, and is further distinguished from the female and immature forms by the presence of an ambulacral sucker on the fourth pair of legs and a sclerotized, bell-shaped genital opening between this pair of legs.

Hosts. Dogs, foxes, and other canids around the world are host to the subspecies *S. scabiei canis*[232]. Although cross-infestation occurs between hosts and their subspecies, such infestations are usually transient and mild. *Sarcoptes scabiei* is sometime present on random-source dogs.

Life Cycle. The life cycle is direct, requires 10 to 14 days, and is presented in Chapter 15, Parasites of Rabbits. Transmission is by direct contact, but the mites are capable of living off the host for a number of hours and will respond to host cues to find a new host[233].

Pathologic Effects and Clinical Disease. Pathologic effects of infestation include hyperkeratosis and parakeratosis, and within the epidermis, burrows containing mites and mite eggs. *Sarcoptes scabiei* causes sarcoptic mange, or scabies. Clinical signs include intense pruritus, self-mutilation, generalized alopecia, and papular dermatitis with subsequent rupture and crusting[234]. Secondary pyoderma is not uncommon, and heavily infested dogs may become cachetic and die. Early lesions occur in the inguinal or axillary regions, or along the margins of the pinnae.

Diagnosis. A tentative diagnosis is based on clinical signs, and is confirmed by demonstrating mites or eggs in deep skin scrapings. Lesions should be scraped vigorously with a sharp curved knife until the skin is roseate. Scrapings are transferred to a microscope slide with a drop of glycerin, mineral oil, or water; covered with a cover glass; and examined under low power light microscopy. Scrapings from the tips of the ears often yield mites even though the ear may be free of lesions. If burrows are evident in intact skin, adult female mites can often be teased out with a needle. Diagnosis by histopathology requires demonstration of mites in section[235].

Treatment. Approved treatments for scabies include amitraz and selamectin[236,237]. Other effective acaricides include moxidectin, milbemycin oxime, and fipronil[238–240]. The mites are also susceptible to avermectins, which are commonly used.

Prevention. While mites do not travel far from the canine host[241], dogs should be held in isolation and all past and current housing areas disinfected.

Public Health Considerations. *Sarcoptes scabiei canis* causes mild, transient infestations in humans[233]. These are, however, intensely pruritic, and involve papular eruptions. For these reasons, infected dogs should be handled with caution.

Suborder Mesostigmata

Pneumonyssoides caninum **Morphology.** Adult *Pneumonyssoides caninum* (Syn. *Pneumonyssus caninum*) measure 1 mm to 1.5 mm long[242]. Both sexes have palps of five segments, a small, irregular dorsal shield, an irregular sternal plate that is wider than it is long, and a small, ovoid anal plate. The sternal plate of the female has two pairs of setae and that of the male has three pairs. The female genital opening is a transverse slit between the fourth pair of legs, and there is no epigynial plate. The first leg of both sexes has a large pair of naked, sessile, tarsal claws, dissimilar from those of the other legs[243] (Figure 17.58).

Hosts. *Pneumonyssoides caninum* inhabits the nasal cavities and sinuses of canids in the United States, South Africa, Europe, and Australia. Although generally uncommon and of unknown incidence in the laboratory, it might be encountered in dogs throughout the world.

Life Cycle. The life cycle is direct. Dogs become infected through direct contact[244]. Mites have been experimentally transferred to other dogs by intranasal inoculation[245].

Pathologic Effects and Clinical Disease. Infestations are generally nonpathogenic and asymptomatic. Usually, clinical signs are limited to excessive mucus production and hyperemia of the nasal mucosa. However, heavily infested dogs may develop a bronchial cough, rhinitis, lacrimation, listlessness, inappetence, sudden loss of consciousness, and orbital cellulites[242, 245, 246, 247].

Diagnosis, Treatment, and Prevention. Diagnosis is by direct observation of mites near the external nares, often while the dog is sleeping, or by finding the mite or its eggs in nasal washings[244]. *Pneumonyssoides caninum* has been successfully eliminated by treatment with ivermectin or milbemycin oxime[248]. Prevention is by isolation and

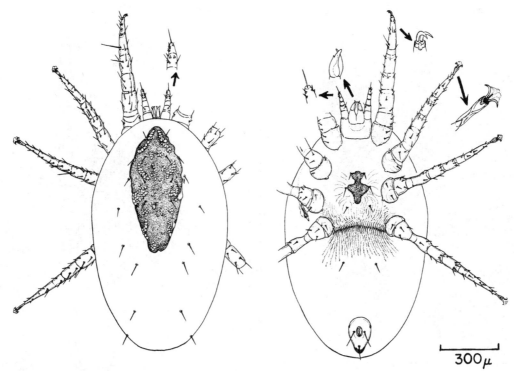

Fig. 17.58 *Pneumonyssoides caninum* female. (Left) Dorsal view. (Right) Ventral view. Reproduced from Baker, K.P., Evans, T.M., Gould, D.J., Hull, W.B., and Keegan, H.L. (1956) with permission.

treatment of dogs known to be infected, prior to release into the research animal colony.

Public Health Considerations. *Pneumonyssoides caninum* does not infest humans.

Suborder Prostigmata
Cheyletiella yasguri **Morphology.** Female *Cheyletiella yasguri* are oval and measure 350 µ to 500 µ in length, and are larger than the males (Figure 17.59). Both sexes have a single semicircular dorsal shield and a large gnathosoma. The palpal tibia has a curved claw that is dentate on its inferior margin and is diagnostic for comparing this to other mites found on dogs. Tarsal claws are absent from the legs.

Hosts. *Cheyletiella yasguri* infests dogs, and probably other carnivores.

Life Cycle. The life cycle is direct. All stages, including the egg, larva, first nymph, second nymph, and adult male and female, may be found on the host or in the bedding[249]. The eggs are glued to the hairs.

Pathologic Effects. *Cheyletiella yasguri* causes a mild form of mange, with exfoliative dermatitis, mild alopecia, hyperemia, pruritus, serous exudation, and thickening of the skin. A subacute, nonsuppurative dermatitis with cellular infiltration and mild hyperkeratosis is seen in tissue section.

Clinical Disease. Typical clinical signs include exfoliative dermatitis with flaky, branlike squames, principally on the backs of puppies. The disease is called "walking dandruff" because when the skin is examined with a hand lens, the flakes on the skin appear to move due to the mites walking amidst the dander.

Diagnosis, Treatment, and Prevention. Diagnosis is by identifying mites in skin scrapings or on tufts of hair. Effective acaricides include selamectin, fipronil, permethrin, ivermectin, and milbemycin oxime[250–254]. Because these mites might inhabit litter and bedding, it is advisable that cages, equipment, and rooms be treated with steam or pressure washed with soapy water at the same time animals are treated.

Public Health Considerations. *Cheyletiella yasguri* is known to transiently infest humans, typically after holding infested dogs[255]. Thus, infested dogs should be handled with caution.

Demodex canis **Morphology.** Adult *Demodex canis* measure 200 µ to 400 µ long and are vermiform in shape (Figure

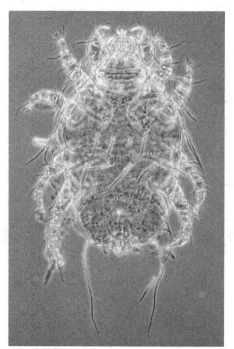

Fig. 17.59 *Cheyletiella yasguri.*

17.60). They have four pairs of short, stumpy legs, small mouthparts, and no setae. A small, blunt rostrum contains minute stylet-like chelicerae and compressed palpal segments. The penis of the male is dorsal and anterior; the female genital opening lies between the fourth pair of legs.

Hosts. *Demodex canis* is the common follicle-inhabiting mite of the dog and is the cause of demodectic mange. It occurs throughout the world, in all dog breeds. In one survey, 53% of skin sections from 208 apparently normal dogs were found infested[256]. Prevalence is not affected by age, sex, or length of hair, but clinical signs are more common in dogs under one year of age, and are more likely to be recognized in short-haired breeds. Only barrier-reared dogs derived from cesarean-section-derived stock are free of this mite.

Life Cycle. The life cycle is direct. Mites are commonly found in the sebaceous glands and hair follicles. Eggs hatch in six days, and the entire life cycle, which can be completed in a skin pustule, takes about 24 days[257]. The mode of transmission is unknown, but involves some form of direct contact. Neonatal transmission from the nursing bitch to her offspring has been suggested[258], and this may represent the usual route.

Pathologic Effects. Two forms of cutaneous lesions have been reported in dogs infested with *D. canis*. Both

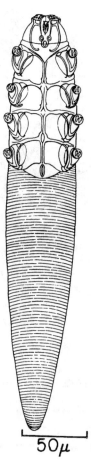

50μ

Fig. 17.60 *Demodex canis* female, ventral view. Reproduced from Baker, K.P., Evans, T.M., Gould, D.J., Hull, W.B., and Keegan, H.L. (1956) with permission.

types may be present concurrently. Squamous lesions are characterized by dry, scaly dermatitis, alopecia, and mild induration. Early lesions commonly appear on the head. Pustular lesions occur independently of, or may follow, the squamous type, and are generally associated with secondary bacterial infection. Pustular lesions are characterized by chronic, moist dermatitis, and purulent exudates. The term "red mange" is applied to a generalized hyperemia with little or no pustule formation.

Histologic lesions include capillary dilatation, epidermal acanthosis, and hyperplasia and distension of the sebaceous glands[259]. Distended hair follicles rupture and hairs released into the dermis induce foreign-body reactions and secondary bacterial infection with pustule formation.

Clinical Disease. Approximately 90% of demodicosis cases are localized, with coin-sized lesions on the head, flank, or legs. Ten percent of cases will progress to generalized demodicosis with alopecia and pyoderma.

Diagnosis. Diagnosis is based on clinical signs and microscopic identification of mites in skin scrapings. However, demonstration of mites in association with lesions is not conclusive, because *D. canis* is common in apparently normal dogs. Thus, other causes of skin lesions should be considered.

Treatment. The only approved and effective therapy for demodicosis is amitraz, which may be associated with side effects[236]. When secondary pyoderma is present, antibiotics such as enrofloxacin may also be necessary[260]. Other common treatments include the avermectins, such as doramectin, ivermectin, moxidectin, and milbemycin oxime[261].

Prevention. Most dogs are asymptomatic carriers of *D. canis*. If *Demodex*-free dogs are required, they must be generated through cesarean section followed by barrier mainenance[258].

Public Health Considerations. *Demodex canis* does not naturally infest humans. However, transient dermatitis may result from prolonged contact with infested dogs.

Class Pentastomida

Linguatula serrata

Morphology. Adult *Linguatula serrata* have a transparent, tongue-shaped body with approximately 90 annuli[262] (Figure 17.61). The anterior end has two pairs of simple retractile hooks. The female measures 8 cm to 13 cm long and 1 cm wide. Reddish-orange eggs are visible along the median line of the body. The male measures 2 cm long and 0.3 cm to 0.4 cm wide. The egg is oval, 70 µ to 90 µ in diameter, and is individually enclosed in a thin, bladder-like envelope containing clear fluid. It has a thick chitinous shell containing an embryo with rudimentary mouthparts and four short legs, each bearing two claw-like hooks. The so-called dorsal organ or facette is on the back of the embryo.

Hosts. The adult stage is found in the nasal passages of dogs, foxes, and wolves, and less commonly in horses, goats, sheep, and humans. Nymphs occur in rats, guinea pigs, rabbits, primates, and livestock. *Linguatula serrata* is found throughout the world. It is most common in eastern Europe[263], and has been reported from the Americas[264], South Africa, Middle East[265], and Australasia[266]. *Linguatula serrata* is unlikely to be encountered except in an occasional random-source dog.

Life Cycle. The life cycle is indirect. Eggs are expelled from the definitive host in the nasal mucus or are swallowed and passed in the feces[267]. That portion of the life

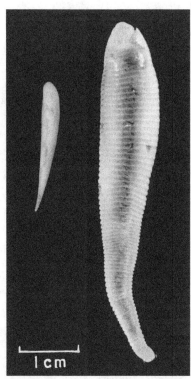

Fig. 17.61. *Linguatula serrata.* (Left) Male. (Right) Female. Courtesy of A. Fain, Institut de Médecine Tropicale Prince Léopold.

cycle occurring in intermediate hosts is presented in Chapter 15, Parasites of Rabbits. Dogs are infected by ingesting viscera containing the infective stage[268]. The means by which nymphs reach the nasal cavity is unknown, but may occur while contaminated food is being masticated, or later during emesis. Adults survive about two years in the dog, feeding on nasal mucus, nasal secretions, and occasionally blood.

Pathologic Effects. Pathologic effects depend on the number of worms present[269]. Changes observed range from catarrhal and hemorrhagic sinusitis to sinus ulcers and osteoporosis of the turbinates. Parakeratosis of the mucosa, hypertrophy of the submucosal glands of the glandular acini, and hemosiderin particles in the gland cells are also observed. Chronic ulcers on the mucosa are characterized by infiltration of lymphocytes and histiocytes, and by small hemorrhages. Associated cytolysis produces a dense hyaline crust.

Clinical Disease. Most dogs show no signs of infection, but a severe catarrhal or suppurative rhinitis and epistaxis may occur. Restlessness, sneezing, and difficulty breathing are occasionally seen. The sense of smell is often reduced or abolished.

Diagnosis. Diagnosis is based on clinical signs and the presence of *L. serrata* eggs in the feces or nasal mucus.

Treatment Prevention, and Public Health Considerations. In one report, treatment with ivermectin resulted in the expulsion of the adult worm[263]. More commonly, treatment involves the physical removal of the worms from the nasal passages. Infection will not occur in the animal facility. Random-source dogs found to be infected upon entry should be treated or culled. The risk of human infection is low, but the nymph is capable of developing in people following ingestion of eggs passed in feces[270].

TABLE 17.1 Parasites of Dogs—Circulatory/Lymphatic System.

Parasite	Geographic distribution	Hosts	Location in host	Method of infection	Pathologic effects	Zoonosis	Reference
Flagellates							
Trypanosoma brucei, T. congolense	Africa	Dogs, other mammals	Blood, cerebro-spinal fluid	Bite of infected tsetse fly (Glossina)	Fever, anemia, edema, emaciation, muscular atrophy, incoordination, paralysis, death	Not reported	8
Trypanosoma evansi	Africa, Americas, Asia	Dogs, other mammals	Blood, cerebro-spinal fluid	Bite of infected fly (Tabanus, Stomoxys, Haematopota, Lyperosia)	Fever, anemia, edema, emaciation, muscular atrophy, incoordination, paralysis, death	Not reported	8
Trypanosoma rangeli	Central and South America	Dogs, cats, primates	Blood	Bite of Reduviid bug or contamination with bug feces	None	Reported	8
Coccidia							
Hepatozoon canis	Africa, Asia, Europe	Dogs, cats, wild carnivores	Spleen, lymph nodes, liver, bone marrow, neutrophils	Ingestion of infected ticks (Rhipicephalus sanguineus)	Splenomegaly, anemia	Not reported	32
Pyroplasmids							
Babesia canis	Africa, Asia, Europe, North America	Canids	Erythrocytes	Transmitted during feeding of hard tick; possible transplacental transmission	Anemia, splenomegaly, hepatomegaly, fever, icterus	Not reported	57
Babesia gibsoni	Africa, Asia, North America	Canids	Erythrocytes	Transmitted during feeding of hard tick; possible transplacental transmission	Anemia	Not reported	57
Babesia vogeli	Africa, Asia	Dogs	Erythrocytes	Transmitted during feeding of hard tick	Anemia, fever, icterus	Not reported	8
Trematodes							
Heterobilharzia americanum	Southeastern US	Dogs, bobcats, raccoons, other mammals	Hepatic and mesenteric veins	Skin penetration by cercariae released from snail intermediate host	Granuloma formation in multiple tissues, enteritis, hepatic fibrosis, anemia	Reported	65

(Continued)

557

TABLE 17.1 (*Continued*)

Parasite	Geographic distribution	Hosts	Location in host	Method of infection	Pathologic effects	Zoonosis	Reference
Trematodes							
Schistosoma japonicum	Asia	Dogs, cats, humans, other mammals	Mesenteric vein, portal veins	Skin penetration by cercaria	Hemorrhagic diarrhea, thickened intestinal wall, microscopic granulomas in various organs	Common	271
Schistosoma spindale	Africa, Asia	Dogs, ruminants, other mammals	Mesenteric vein, portal veins	Skin penetration by cercaria	Intestinal nodules, hepatic cirrhosis	Reported	285
Nematodes							
Metastrongyloidea							
Angiostrongylus vasorum	Worldwide	Dogs, foxes, other carnivores	Heart, pulmonary artery	Ingestion of mollusk intermediate host	Pulmonary consolidation, thrombus formation, cardiac dilatation, hepatic congestion	Not reported	277
Filaroidea							
Brugia ceylonensis	Ceylon	Dogs	Lymphatic system	Bite of mosquito intermediate host	None	Reported	286
Brugia pahangi	Africa, Malay Peninsula	Dogs, cats, wild carnivores, primates	Lymphatic system	Bite of mosquito intermediate host	None	Not reported	287
Dirofilaria immitis	Worldwide	Canids, cats, wild carnivores, humans	Right ventricle, pulmonary artery, vena cava	Bite of mosquito intermediate host	Cardiac enlargement, pulmonary congestion, ascites	Reported	161

TABLE 17.2 Parasites of Dogs—Enterohepatic System.

Parasite	Geographic distribution	Hosts	Location in host	Method of infection	Pathologic effects	Zoonosis	Reference
Flagellates							
Giardia canis	Worldwide	Dogs	Anterior small intestine	Ingestion of cysts in feces	Steatorrhea	Possible	13
Pentatrichomonas hominis	Worldwide	Dogs, humans	Large intestine	Ingestion of trophozoites in feces	None	Common	20
Trichomonas canistomae	Europe, North America	Dogs	Oral cavity	Direct contact	None	Not reported	8
Amoebae							
Entamoeba hartmanni	Worldwide	Dogs, also found in rhesus monkeys, humans	Cecum, colon	Ingestion of cysts passed in feces	None	Reported	8
Coccidia							
Cryptosporidium canis	Worldwide	Dogs	Small intestine, stomach	Ingestion of sporulated oocysts	Mild enteritis, diarrhea	Reported	21, 22
Hammondia heydorni	Worldwide	Dogs and other canids	Small intestine	Ingestion of intermediate host (rodents, deer, other prey species)	None	Not reported	26
Isospora canis	Worldwide	Dogs	Small intestine	Ingestion of sporulated oocysts in feces or infected paratenic hosts (rodents and birds)	Moderate enteritis, diarrhea	Not reported	37
Isospora spp.	Worldwide	Dogs (also found in cats, other carnivores)	Small intestine, sometimes cecum, colon	Ingestion of sporulated oocysts in feces	Enteritis, diarrhea	Not reported	41, 42, 43
Neospora caninum	Worldwide	Dogs	Intestine	Ingestion of intermediate host, transplacental transmission	Meningoencephalitis, myositis, myocarditis, hepatitis, dermatitis, pneumonia	Not reported	46
Sarcocystis sp.	Worldwide	Dogs	Small intestine	Ingestion of bradyzoites in muscle cysts of intermediate host (livestock)	None	Not reported	8
Trematodes							
Alaria sp.	Europe, North America	Canids	Small intestine	Ingestion of intermediate host (frog) or paratenic host (snake)	Catarrhal enteritis	Reported	288
Amphimerus pseudofelineus	Americas	Dogs, cats	Bile duct	Ingestion of metacercaria in fishes	Hepatic cirrhosis, pancreatitis	Reported	289

(Continued)

559

TABLE 17.2 *(Continued)*

Trematodes

Parasite	Geographic distribution	Hosts	Location in host	Method of infection	Pathologic effects	Zoonosis	Reference
Apophallus sp.	Europe, North America	Canids, cats, birds	Small intestine	Ingestion of metacercaria encysted in fishes	None known	Not reported	290
Clonorchis sinensis	Asia	Dogs, also cats, humans, other mammals	Bile duct, pancreatic duct, duodenum	Ingestion of metacercaria encysted in fishes	Inflammation of bile duct, hepatic cirrhosis, rarely pancreatitis	Common	282
Cryptocotyle sp.	Europe, North America	Dog, other carnivores, fish-eating birds	Small intestine	Ingestion of metacercaria encysted in fishes	Enteritis	Not reported	291
Echinochasmus perfoliatus	Asia, Europe	Dogs, cats, foxes, swine, other mammals	Small intestine	Ingestion of infected fishes	Enteritis	Reported	292
Echinostoma sp.	Asia	Dogs, rats, swine, primates, other mammals	Small intestine	Ingestion of intermediate host (infected mollusk)	None known	Reported	293
Heterophyes heterophyes	Asia, Greece, Northern Africa	Dogs, other carnivores, fish-eating birds	Small intestine	Ingestion of metacercaria encysted in fishes	Mild enteritis	Reported	294
Metagonimus yokogawai	Asia, Eastern Europe	Dogs, other mammals, fish-eating birds	Small intestine	Ingestion of metacercaria encysted in fishes	Mild enteritis	Reported	295
Metorchis conjunctus	North America	Canids, other carnivores	Bile duct, gallbladder	Ingestion of metacercaria encysted in fishes	Inflammation of bile duct, hepatic cirrhosis, pancreatitis	Reported	296
Nanophyetus salmincola	West coast of North America, eastern Siberia	Dogs, other fish-eating mammals and birds	Small intestine	Ingestion of metacercaria in salmonid fishes	Vector of *Neorickettsia helminthoeca*	Reported	69
Opisthorchis tenuicollis	Asia, Europe, North America	Dogs (also cats, other fish-eating mammals, humans)	Bile duct, pancreatic duct, duodenum	Ingestion of metacercaria in fishes	Inflammation of bile duct; sometimes hepatic cirrhosis; rarely pancreatitis	Reported	283
Phagicola sp.	Americas, Europe, Israel	Canids, cats, other carnivores	Small intestine	Ingestion of metacercaria encysted in fishes	None known	Reported	297
Pseudamphistomum truncatum	Asia, Europe	Canids, other carnivores	Bile duct	Ingestion of metacercaria encysted in fishes	None known	Reported	298
Pygidiopsis genata	Asia, Israel, northern Africa	Dogs, cats, rodents	Small intestine	Ingestion of metacercaria in fishes	None known	Not reported	299
Stictodora sawakinensis	Africa, Asia	Dogs	Small intestine	Ingestion of metacercaria in fishes	None known	Not reported	300

Cestodes

560

Pseudophyllidea

Species	Geographic distribution	Definitive host	Location in host	Mode of infection	Pathology	Zoonosis	Reference
Diphyllobothrium latum	Asia, Americas, Europe	Dogs, cats, wild carnivores	Small intestine	Ingestion of intermediate host (freshwater fishes)	None	Reported	30
Diphyllobothrium cordatum	Greenland, Iceland, Japan, North America	Pinnipeds, dogs	Small intestine	Probably ingestion of unknown intermediate host	None known	Reported	301
Spirometra mansoni	Asia, South America	Dogs, cats, other carnivores	Small intestine	Ingestion of intermediate host (small vertebrates, except fishes)	None	Reported	76
Spirometra mansonoides	North America	Dogs, cats, other carnivores	Small intestine	Ingestion of intermediate host (small vertebrates, except fishes)	None	Reported	76

Cyclophyllidea

Species	Geographic distribution	Definitive host	Location in host	Mode of infection	Pathology	Zoonosis	Reference
Diplopylidium nolleri	Southern Europe, southwestern Asia	Dogs, foxes, cats	Intestine	Ingestion of transport or intermediate host (reptiles)	None known	Not reported	302
Dipylidium caninum	Worldwide	Dogs, cats, other carnivores	Small intestine	Ingestion of intermediate host (fleas, lice)	Enteritis, anal pruritus	Reported	77
Echinococcus granulosis	Worldwide	Dogs, wild canids	Adult: small intestine Metacestode: visceral organs	Ingestion of intermediate host or eggs in feces	Adult: none Metacestode: abdominal distention, organ cysts	Intermediate host	79
Echinococcus multilocularis	Europe, North America, Siberia	Foxes, other canids, cats	Adult: small intestine Metacestode: Liver	Ingestion of intermediate host or eggs in feces	Adult: None Metacestode: liver cysts	Intermediate host	274
Joyeuxiella pasqualei	Africa, southern Europe	Dogs, cats, other carnivores	Intestine	Ingestion of transport or intermediate host (reptiles)	None known	Not reported	302
Taenia hydatigena	Worldwide	Dogs, other carnivores	Small intestine	Ingestion of viscera of intermediate host (ruminants, swine)	Mild enteritis	Reported	303
Taenia multiceps	Worldwide	Canids	Small intestine	Ingestion of neural tissue of intermediate host (sheep, goats)	None	Reported	304
Taenia ovis krabbei	Northern Europe, South America	Dogs	Small intestine	Ingestion of muscle of intermediate host (reindeer)	None	Not reported	305
Taenia ovis ovis	Worldwide	Canids	Small intestine	Ingestion of viscera of intermediate host (sheep, goats)	None	None known	306
Taenia pisiformis	Worldwide	Dogs	Small intestine	Ingestion of intermediate host (lagomorphs, wild rodents)	None	Not reported	38

(Continued)

TABLE 17.2 (Continued)

Parasite	Geographic distribution	Hosts	Location in host	Method of infection	Pathologic effects	Zoonosis	Reference
Taenia serialis	Worldwide	Dogs, foxes	Small intestine	Ingestion of intermediate host (lagomorphs)	None	Reported	38
Nematodes							
Rhabditoidea							
Strongyloides stercoralis	Worldwide	Dogs (also cats, primates)	Adult: Duodenum, jejunum Larva: lungs, pericardium	Ingestion of infective larva or penetration of skin or oral mucosa by larva	Enteritis, broncho pneumonia	Common	82
Ascaridoidea							
Toxascaris leonina	Worldwide	Dogs, cats	Small intestine	Ingestion of embryonated egg or rodent paratenic host	Mild enteritis	Reported	91, 93
Toxocara canis	Worldwide	Dogs	Small intestine	Transplacental, transmammary, ingestion of embryonated egg or rodent or avian paratenic host	Enteritis, pulmonary hemorrhages, pneumonia	Common	103
Strongyloidea							
Ancylostoma braziliense	Africa, Americas, Asia	Dogs, cats, other carnivores	Small intestine	Ingestion of infective larva or paratenic hosts; skin penetration	Mild diarrhea	Common	275
Ancylostoma caninum	Worldwide	Dogs, other canids	Small intestine	Ingestion of infective larva or paratenic host, skin penetration or transmammary infection	Anemia, enteritis, pulmonary hemorrhages	Common	101, 102
Ancylostoma ceylanicum	Africa, Asia, South America	Dogs, cats, other carnivores	Small intestine	Ingestion of infective larva or paratenic hosts; skin penetration	Enteritis, anemia	Reported	276
Uncinaria stenocephala	Worldwide	Dogs, foxes, cats	Small intestine	Skin penetration or ingestion of infective larva	Enteritis, dermatitis	Reported	118
Spirurida							
Gnathostoma spinigerum	Africa, Asia, Europe	Dogs, other carnivores	Stomach wall	Ingestion of second intermediate host (small vertebrates)	Tumor-like nodules in stomach wall	Reported	307

Organism	Distribution	Definitive host	Location	Transmission	Clinical signs	Zoonotic	Page
Physaloptera sp.	Worldwide	Dogs, cats, other carnivores	Stomach, duodenum	Ingestion of intermediate host (insects)	Gastritis	Reported	308
Spirocerca lupi	Worldwide in tropical and subtropical regions	Canids, large exotic felids	Esophagus, stomach, aorta, lungs, other organs	Ingestion of intermediate host (cockroaches, dung beetles); or paratenic host (small vertebrates)	Esophageal nodules, aortic aneurysm, tumor formation	Not reported	149
Trichuroidea							
Trichuris vulpis	Worldwide	Canids	Cecum, colon	Ingestion of embryonated egg	Enteritis	Not reported	188
Acanthocephala							
Oncicola canis	Americas	Dogs, coyotes, felids	Small intestine	Ingestion of intermediate host (cockroaches) or paratenic host (armadillos, turkeys)	Enteritis, intestinal perforation	Not reported	205
Macracanthorhynchus ingens	North America	Raccoons, dogs, other carnivores	Small intestine	Ingestion of intermediate host (millipede, *Narceus*)	Mild enteritis	Rare	281

563

TABLE 17.3 Parasites of Dogs—Respiratory System.

Parasite	Geographic distribution	Hosts	Location in host	Method of infection	Pathologic effects	Zoonosis	Reference
Trematodes							
Paragonimus kellicotti	North America	Dogs, cats, wild carnivores, domestic animals	Lungs (also found in brain, liver, other organs)	Ingestion of crustacean intermediate host (crab, crayfish)	Focal emphysema, lung cysts	Reported	72
Paragonimus westermanii	Asia	Dogs, wild carnivores, domestic animals, primates	Lungs (also found in brain, liver, other organs)	Ingestion of crustacean intermediate host (crab, crayfish)	Focal emphysema, lung cysts	Reported	284
Leeches							
Limnatis nilotica	Asia, Africa, Europe	Dogs, horses, other domestic animals	Mucosa of upper respiratory tract	Direct contact while drinking; enters through nose or mouth	Edema of the glottis, dyspnea, epistaxis	Reported	81
Diestecostoma mexicanum	Central America	Dogs	Upper respiratory tract	Invasion of mouth or nares while drinking	Dyspnea, anemia	Not reported	309
Nematodes							
Metastrongyloidea							
Crenosoma vulpis	Asia, Europe, North America	Foxes, dogs, cats	Bronchi, trachea	Ingestion of intermediate host (slugs, snails)	Mild bronchitis, persistent cough	Not reported	280
Filaroides hirthi	Europe	Dogs, other canids	Lungs	Ingestion of infective larvae	None	Not reported	123
Filaroides milksi	Europe, North America	Dogs, other carnivores	Lungs, bronchioles	Ingestion of infective larvae	Small white foci in lungs	Not reported	129
Filaroides osleri	Worldwide	Canids	Trachea, bronchi	Ingestion of infective larvae	Hemorrhagic granular nodules	Not reported	129
Trichuroidea							
Eucoleus aerophila	Americas, Europe	Foxes, dogs, cats, other carnivores	Bronchioles, bronchi, trachea	Ingestion of embryonated egg	Bronchitis, tracheitis, pneumonia	Reported	173
Eucoleus boehmi	Worldwide	Canids	Nasal cavity, paranasal sinuses	Ingestion of embryonated egg	Sinusitis	Not reported	173
Arachnida							
Mites							
Mesostigmates							

Species	Distribution	Hosts	Location	Transmission	Clinical signs	Zoonotic	Reference
Pneumonysoides caninum	Worldwide	Dogs	Nasal cavities, sinuses	Direct contact	Hyperemia of nasal mucosa, excessive mucus production	Not reported	244
Pentastomids							
Linguatula serrata	Worldwide	Canids, other domestic animals	Nasal cavity	Ingestion of nymphs in viscera of intermediate host (rodents, lagomophs)	Rhinitis, epistaxis, dyspnea	Reported	263

TABLE 17.4 Parasites of Dogs—Central Nervous System, Musculoskeletal System, Skin and Connective Tissue, and Urogenital System.

Parasite	Geographic distribution	Hosts	Location in host	Method of infection	Pathologic effects	Zoonosis	Reference
Flagellates							
Leishmania spp.	Worldwide	Dogs, wild rodents, humans	Macrophages of skin and visceral and lymphoid organs	Bite of sand fly host	Skin ulceration, organ enlargement	Common	7
Trypanosoma cruzi	Americas	Dogs, other mammals, humans	Myocardium, skeletal muscle, smooth muscle	Ingestion of infected bugs (Hemiptera)	Myocarditis, myositis	Common	9
Coccidia							
Hepatozoon americanum	Americas	Dogs, coyotes	Striated and cardiac muscle	Ingestion of infected ticks (*Amblyomma maculatum*)	Myositis, myocarditis	Not reported	32
Cestodes							
Larval							
Mesocestoides corti	North America, Central America	Dogs, other carnivores, rodents	Adult: small intestine Larva: peritoneal cavity	Ingestion of intermediate hosts	Cysts in liver, other abdominal organs	Rare	310
Mesocestoides lineatus	Africa, Asia, Europe	Dogs, other mammals	Adult: small intestine Larva: Peritoneal cavity, pleural cavity	Ingestion of intermediate hosts	Cysts in abdominal organs	Rare	273
Spirometra erinacei	Asia, Europe, South America	Dogs, other carnivores, rodents, chickens	Adult: small intestine Larva: subcutis, muscle	Ingestion of intermediate hosts	Cysts in subcutis, muscle	Reported	311
Nematodes							
Metastrongyloidea							
Parastrongylus (Angiostrongylus) cantonensis	Australasia, Southern US	Dogs (Natural hosts: rats)	Central nervous system	Ingestion of snail intermediate host	Meningoencephalitis	Reported	278, 279
Spiruroidea							
Thelazia californiensis	Mexico, US	Dogs, other carnivores, wild ruminants	Lacrimal ducts, conjunctival sacs, nictitating membrane	Larva deposited by fly (*Fannia, Musca*) feeding on conjunctival fluids	Scleral congestion, lacrimation, keratoconjunctivitis, photophobia	Reported	312
Thelazia callipaeda	Asia, Europe	Dogs, lagomorphs	Lacrimal ducts, conjunctival sacs, nictitating membrane	Larva deposited by fly feeding on conjunctival fluids	Scleral congestion, lacrimation, keratoconjunctivitis, photophobia	Reported	313
Filaroidea							

Organism	Distribution	Host	Location in host	Transmission	Clinical signs	Zoonotic	Reference
Dipetalonema dracunculoides	Africa, Asia, Europe	Canids	Peritoneal cavity	Transmitted by infected arthropod during feeding	None known	Not reported	314
Dipetalonema grassii	Africa, Europe	Dogs, cats	Subcutis, peritoneal cavity	Transmitted by infected tick during feeding	None known	Not reported	315
Dipetalonema reconditum	Worldwide	Dogs	Subcutis	Transmitted by infected flea or tick during feeding	None	Not reported	156
Dirofilaria repens	Africa, Asia, Europe	Dogs, other carnivores	Subcutis	Transmitted by infected mosquito during feeding	Dermatitis, pruritus, alopecia	Reported	316
Nematodes							
Trichuroidea							
Pearsonema plica	Worldwide, especially Europe	Dogs, cats, foxes, other mammals	Urinary bladder	Ingestion of intermediate host (earthworm)	Cystitis	Not reported	184
Dioctophymatoidea							
Dioctophyma renale	Worldwide	Dogs, other carnivores	Kidneys, abdominal cavity	Ingestion of uncooked viscera of fish	Hydronephrosis, renal hypertrophy, peritonitis	Reported	198
Dracunculoidea							
Dracunculus insignis	North America	Dogs, wild carnivores	Skin, subcutis, viscera	Ingestion of intermediate host (copepods) or paratenic host (frogs)	Skin papules, erythema, pruritus	Not reported	317
Dracunculus medinensis	Asia, eastern Europe, New Guinea	Dogs, other mammals	Skin, subcutis, viscera	Ingestion of intermediate host (copepods)	Skin papules, erythema, pruritus	Reported	318
Diptera (flies)							
Calliphoridae (blow flies, bottle flies, screwworm flies)	Worldwide	Dogs, other mammals, birds	Skin wounds	Eggs deposited by female fly	Dermal myiasis, fetid skin wounds	Reported	207
Ceratopogonidae (midges)	Worldwide	Dogs, other mammals, birds	Skin	Direct contact	Irritation, pathogen transmission	Common	206
Culicidae (mosquitoes)	Worldwide	Dogs, other mammals, birds	Skin	Direct contact	Pruritus, local inflammation, pathogen transmission	Common	206
Muscidae (filth flies)	Worldwide	Dogs, other mammals, birds	Skin	Direct contact	Irritation, pathogen transmission, accidental myiasis	Common	206
Psychodidae (sand flies)	Worldwide	Dogs, other mammals, birds	Skin	Direct contact	Pathogen transmission	Common	206, 209

(Continued)

TABLE 17.4 (Continued)

Parasite	Geographic distribution	Hosts	Location in host	Method of infection	Pathologic effects	Zoonosis	Reference
Diptera (flies)							
Sarcophagidae (flesh flies)	Worldwide	Dogs, other mammals, birds	Skin wounds	Larvae deposited by female fly	Dermal myiasis, fetid skin wounds	Reported	206
Simulidae (blackflies)	Worldwide	Dogs, other mammals, birds	Skin	Direct contact	Irritation, pathogen transmission	Common	206
Phthiraptera (lice)							
Heterodoxus spiniger	Worldwide in tropical climates	Canids	Pelage	Direct contact	Irritation, alopecia, debilitation	Not reported	319
Linognathus setosus	Worldwide	Canids, also rabbits, chickens	Pelage, plumage, especially of neck and shoulders	Direct contact	Dermatitis, alopecia, pruritus	Not reported	215
Trichodectes canis	Worldwide	Canids	Pelage, especially near body openings	Direct contact	Dermatitis, alopecia; vector of Dipylidium caninum	Not reported	218
Siphonaptera (fleas)							
Ctenocephalides sp.	Worldwide	Dogs, other mammals	Pelage, bedding	Direct contact	Allergic dermatitis, pruritus, ruffled coat, self-induced trauma, weight loss; intermediate host for Dipylidium caninum	Reported	206
Arachnida							
Ticks (Soft)							
Otobius megnini	Worldwide	Large, domestic animals	Ears	Direct contact	Otitis externa, irritation, edema	Reported	221
Ticks (Hard)							
Amblyomma spp.	Worldwide	Dogs, other mammals, birds	Skin	Direct contact	Local inflammation, anemia, tick paralysis; vectors of canine pathogens	Common	206
Dermacentor spp.	Worldwide	Dogs, other mammals, birds	Skin	Direct contact	Local inflammation, anemia, tick paralysis; vectors of canine pathogens	Common	224
Ixodes spp.	Worldwide	Dogs, other mammals, birds	Skin	Direct contact	Local inflammation, anemia, tick paralysis; vectors of canine pathogens	Common	206

Species	Distribution	Hosts	Location	Effects	Prevalence	
Rhipicephalus sanguineus	Africa, Americas, Europe	Dogs, other mammals	Skin	Local inflammation, anemia, tick paralysis; vectors of canine pathogens	Common	206
Mites						
Astigmates						
Otodectes cynotis	Worldwide	Dogs, other carnivores	External ear canal, sometimes skin of feet, tail	Otitis, dermatitis, pruritus, self-ulceration of auditory canal, auricular hematoma	Not reported	320
Sarcoptes scabiei	Worldwide	Canids, other mammals	Skin	Papular dermatitis, pruritus, self-inflicted trauma, alopecia, thickening of skin, emaciation, death	Common	234
Prostigmates						
Demodex canis	Worldwide	Dogs	Hair follicles	Dermatitis, alopecia	Not reported	261
Cheyletiella yasguri	Europe, North America	Dogs, other carnivores	Skin, pelage	Alopecia, scaly dermatitis, pruritus, thickening of skin	Common	249

569

REFERENCES

1. Mattos Junior, D.G., Pinheiro, J.M., Menezes, R.C., and Costa, D.A. (2004) Clinical and laboratorial aspects of seropositive dogs to leishmaniosis. *Arq. Bras. Med. Vet. Zootec.* **56,** 119–122.

2. Debrabant, A., Joshi, M.B., Pimenta, P.F.P., and Dwyer, D.M. (2004) Generation of *Leishmania donovani* axenic amastigotes: their growth and biological characteristics. *Int. J. Parasitol.* **34,** 205–217.

3. Baneth, G. and Shaw, S.E. (2002) Chemotherapy of canine leishmaniosis. *Vet. Parasitol.* **106,** 315–324.

4. Lamothe, J. (2004) Use of meglumine antimonate in canine leishmaniasis. *Vet. Rec.* **154,** 378.

5. Mencke, N., Volf, P., Volfova, V., and Stanneck, D. (2003) Repellent efficacy of a combination containing imidacloprid and permethrin against sand flies (*Phlebotomus papatasi*) on dogs. *Parasitol. Res.* **90,** S108–111.

6. Reithinger, R., Teodoro, U., and Davies, C.R. (2001) Topical insecticide treatments to protect dogs from sand fly vectors of leishmaniasis. *Emerg. Infect. Dis.* **7,** 872–876.

7. Lindsay, D.S., Zajac, A.M. and Barr, S.C. (2002) Leishmaniasis in American foxhounds: an emerging zoonosis? *Compend. Contin. Educ. Pract. Vet.* **24,** 304–313.

8. Levine, N.D. (1985) *Veterinary Protozoology.* Iowa State University Press, Ames, IA. 414 pages.

9. Barr, S.C., Beek, O.V., Carlisle Nowak, M.S., Lopez, J.W., Kirchhoff, L.V., Allison, N. et al. (1995) *Trypanosoma cruzi* infection in Walker Hounds from Virginia. *Am. J. Vet. Res.* **56,** 1037–1044

10. Barr, S.C., Schmidt, S.P., Brown, C.C., and Klei, T.R. (1991) Pathologic features of dogs inoculated with North American *Trypanosoma cruzi* isolates. *Am. J. Vet. Res.* **52,** 2033–2039.

11. Barr, S.C. (1991) American trypanosomiasis in dogs. *Compend. Contin. Educ. Pract. Vet.* **13,** 745–754.

12. Guedes, P.M., Veloso, V.M., Tafuri, W.L., Galvao, L.M., Carneiro, C.M., and Lana, M.D. et al. (2002) The dog as model for chemotherapy of the Chagas' disease. *Acta Tropica* **84,** 9–17.

13. Jacobs, S.R., Forrester, C.P.R., Yang, J., Olson, B.E., Olson, M.E., and Wallis, P.M. (2002) A survey of prevalence of *Giardia* in dogs presented to Canadian veterinary practices. In *Giardia: The Cosmopolitan Parasite.* CABI Publishing, Oxford, England, 81–85.

14. Zislin, A., Goldstein, M., Hustead, D., Olson, B.E., Olson, M.E., and Wallis, P.M. (2002) Prevalence of *Giardia* in companion animal populations in the USA. In *Giardia: The Cosmopolitan Parasite,.* CABI Publishing, Oxford, England, 87–90.

15. Barutzki, D., Olson, B.E., Olson, M.E., and Wallis, P.M. (2002) Prevalence of *Giardia* spp. in dogs in Germany. In *Giardia: The Cosmopolitan Parasite.* CABI Publishing, Oxford, England, 91–95.

16. Abe, N., Kimata, I., and Iseki, M. (2003) Identification of genotypes of *Giardia intestinalis* isolates from dogs in Japan by direct sequencing of the PCR amplified glutamate dehydrogenase gene. *J. Vet. Med. Sci.* **65,** 29–33.

17. Buret, A.G., Scott, K.G.E., Chin, A.C., Olson, B.E., Olson, M.E., and Wallis, P.M. (2002) Giardiasis: pathophysiology and pathogenesis. In *Giardia: The Cosmopolitan Parasite.* CABI Publishing, Oxford, England, 109–125.

18. Decock, C., Cadiergues, M.C., Roques, M., and Franc, M. (2003) Evaluation of four treatments of canine giardiasis. *Rev. Med. Vet.* **154,** 763–766.

19. Wenrich, D.H. (1930) Intestinal flagellates of rats. In: Hegner, R. and Andrews, J. (eds.) *Problems and Methods of Research in Protozoology.* Macmillan, New York, 124–142.

20. Fukushima, T., Mochizuki, K., Yamazaki, H., Watanabe, Y., Yamada, S., Aoyama, T,. et al. (1990) *Pentatrichomonas hominis* from beagle dogs—detection method, characteristics and route of infection. *Exper. Anim.* **39,** 187–192.

21. Fayer, R., Trout, J.M., Xiao, L., Morgan, U.M., Lal, A.A., and Dubey, J.P. (2001) *Cryptosporidium canis* n. sp. from domestic dogs. *J. Parasitol.* **87,** 1415–1422.

22. Miller, D.L., Liggett, A., Radi, Z.A., and Branch, L.O. (2003) Gastrointestinal cryptosporidiosis in a puppy. *Vet. Parasitol.* **115,** 199–204.

23. Turnwald, G.H., Barta, O., Taylor, H.W., Kreeger, J., Coleman, S.U., and Pourciau, S.S. (1988) Cryptosporidiosis associated with immunosuppression attributable to distemper in a pup. *J. Am. Vet. Med. Assoc.* **192,** 79–81.

24. Barr, S.C., Jamrosz, G.F., Hornbuckle, W.E., Bowman, D.D., and Fayer, R. (1994) Use of paromomycin for treatment of cryptosporidiosis in a cat. *J. Am. Vet. Med. Assoc.* **205,** 1742–1743.

25. Gatei, W., Suputtamongkol, Y., Waywa, D., Ashford, R.W., Bailey, J.W., Greensill, J. et al. (2002) Zoonotic species of *Cryptosporidium* are as prevalent as the anthroponotic in HIV-infected patients in Thailand. *Ann. Trop. Med. Parasitol.* **96,** 797–802.

26. Matsui, T. (1987) Studies on *Isospora heydorni. Bull. Nippon Vet. Zootech. Coll.* **36,** 144–145.

27. Vincent Johnson, N.A., Macintire, D.K., Lindsay, D.S., Lenz, S.D., Baneth, G., Shkap, V. et al. (1997) A new *Hepatozoon* species from dogs: description of the causative agent of canine hepatozoonosis in North America. *J. Parasitol.* **83,** 1165–1172.

28. Ewing, S.A., DuBois, J.G., Mathew, J.S., and Panciera, R.J. (2002) Larval Gulf Coast ticks (*Amblyomma maculatum*) (Acari: Ixodidae) as host for *Hepatozoon americanum* (Apicomplexa: Adeleorina). *Vet. Parasitol.* **103,** 43–51.

29. Panciera, R.J., Mathew, J.S., Cummings, C.A., Duffy, J.C., Ewing, S.A., and Kocan, A.A. (2001) Comparison of tissue stages of *Hepatozoon americanum* in the dog using immunohistochemical and routine histologic methods. *Vet. Pathol.* **38,** 422–426.

30. Macintire, D.K., Vincent Johnson, N., Dillon, A.R., Blagburn, B., Lindsay, D., Whitley, E.M., et al. (1997) Hepatozoonosis in dogs: 22 cases (1989–1994). *J. Am. Vet. Med. Assoc.* **210,** 916–922.

31. Macintire, D.K., Vincent Johnson, N.A., Kane, C.W., Lindsay, D.S., Blagburn, B.L., and Dillon, A.R. (2001) Treatment of dogs infected with *Hepatozoon americanum*: 53 cases (1989–1998). *J. Am. Vet. Med. Assoc.* **218,** 77–82.

32. Baneth, G., Mathew, J.S., Shkap, V., Macintire, D.K., Barta, J.R., and Ewing, S.A. (2003) Canine hepatozoonosis: two disease syndromes caused by separate *Hepatozoon* spp. *Trends Parasitol.* **19,** 27–31.

33. Baneth, G., Samish, M., Alekseev, E., Aroch, I., and Shkap, V. (2001) Transmission of *Hepatozoon canis* to dogs by naturally-fed or percutaneously-injected *Rhipicephalus sanguineus* ticks. *J. Parasitol.* **87,** 606–611.

34. Calmon, J.P. (1995) Canine hepatozoonosis: study of an infested kennel. *Point Veterinaire* **27,** 85–90.

35. Markus, M.B. (1983) The hypnozoite of *Isospora canis. S. Afr. J. Sci.* **79,** 117.

36. Becker, C., Heine, J., and Boch, J. (1981) Experimental *Cystoisospora canis* and *C. ohioensis* infections in dogs. *Tierarztl. Umsch.* **36,** 336–341.

37. Nemeseri, L. (1960) Beitrage sur Atiologie der Coccidiose der Hunde. I. *Isospora canis* sp. n. *Acta Vet. Bud.* **10,** 95–99.

38. Georgi, J.R. and Georgi, M.E. (1991) *Canine Clinical Parasitology,* Lea and Febiger, Philadelphia, PA, 227 pages.

39. Daugschies, A., Mundt, H.C., and Letkova, V. (2000) Toltrazuril treatment of cystoisosporosis in dogs under experimental and field conditions. *Parasitol. Res.* **86,** 797–799.

40. Blagburn, B.L., Lindsay, D.S., Vaughan, J.L., Rippey, N.S., Wright, J.C., Lynn, R.C., et al. (1996) Prevalence of canine parasites based on fecal flotation. *Compend. Cont. Educ. Pract. Vet.* **18,** 483–509.

41. Dubey, J.P. (1978) Life-cycle of *Isospora ohioensis* in dogs. *Parasitology* **77,** 1–11.

42. Dubey, J.P. and Mahrt, J.L. (1978) *Isospora neorivolta* sp.n. from the domestic dog. *J. Parasitol.* **64,** 1067–1073.

43. Trayser, C.V. and Todd, K.S., Jr. (1978) Life cycle of *Isospora burrowsi* n.sp. (Protozoa: Eimeriidae) from the dog *Canis familiaris. Am. J. Vet. Res.* **39,** 95–98.

44. Linsday, D.S. and Dubey, J.P. (2000) Canine neosporosis. *J. Vet. Parasitol.* **14,** 1–11.

45. Dubey, J.P., Carpenter, J.L., Speer, C.A., Topper, M.J., and Uggla, A. (1988) Newly recognized fatal protozoan disease of dogs. *J. Am. Vet. Med. Assoc.* **192,**1269–1285.

46. Dubey, J.P., Barr, B.C., Barta, J.R., Bjerkas, I., Bjorkman, C., Blagburn, B.L., et al. (2002) Redescription of *Neospora caninum* and its differentiation from related coccidia. *Int. J. Parasitol.* **32,** 929–946.

47. Wenyon, C.M. (1926) Protozoology: A manual for medical men, veterinarians and zoologists. Ballière, Tindall, and Cox, London.

48. Nuttall, G.H.F. and Graham-Smith, G.S. (1908) The mode of multiplication of *Piroplasma bovis, P. pitheci* in the circulating blood compared with that of *P. canis,* with notes on other species of *Piroplasma. Parasitology* **1,** 134–142.

49. Taboada, J., Harvey, J.W., Levy, M.G., and Breitschwerdt, E.B. (1992) Seroprevalence of babesiosis in Greyhounds in Florida. *J. Am. Vet. Med. Assoc.* **200,** 47–50.

50. Yamane, I., Gardner, I.A., Ryan, C.P., Levy, M., Urrico, J., and Conrad, P.A. (1994) Serosurvey of *Babesia canis, Babesia gibsoni* and *Ehrlichia canis* in pound dogs in California, USA. *Prevent. Vet. Med.* **18,** 293–304.

51. Carret, C., Walas, F., Carcy, B., Grande, N., Precigout, E., Moubri, K., et al. (1999) *Babesia canis canis, Babesia canis vogeli, Babesia canis rossi:* differentiation of the three subspecies by a restriction fragment length polymorphism analysis on amplified small subunit ribosomal RNA genes. *J. Eukaryot. Microbiol.* **46,** 298–303.

52. Uilenberg, G., Franssen, F.F.J., Perie, N.M., and Spanjer, A.A.M. (1989) Three groups of *Babesia canis* distinguished, and a proposal for nomenclature. *Vet. Quart.* **11,** 33–40.

53. Breitschwerdt, E.B., Malone, J.B., MacWilliams, P., Levy, M.G., Qualls, C.W., Jr., and Prudich, M.J. (1983) Babesiosis in the Greyhound. *J. Am. Vet. Med. Assoc.* **182,** 978–982.

54. Lobetti, R.G. (1998) Canine babesiosis. *Compend. Cont. Educ. Pract. Vet.* **20,** 418–431.

55. Wulansari, R., Wijaya, A., Ano, H., Horii, Y., Nasu, T., Yamane, S., et al. (2003) Clindamycin in the Treatment of *Babesia gibsoni* Infections in Dogs. *J. Am. Anim. Hosp. Assoc.* **39,** 558–562.

56. Moreau, Y., Vidor, E., Bissuel, G., and Dubreuil, N. (1989) Vaccination against canine babesiosis: an overview of field observations. *Malaria and Babesiosis: 3rd International Congress on Malaria and Babesiosis* (France on September 7–11, 1987), **83,** 95–96.

57. Boozer, A.L. and Macintire, D.K. (2003) Canine babesiosis. *Vet. Clin. N. Am., Sm. Anim. Pract.* **33,** 885–904.

58. Farwell, G.E., LeGrand, E.K., and Cobb, C.C. (1982) Clinical observations on *Babesia gibsoni* and *Babesia canis* infections in dogs. *J. Am. Vet. Med. Assoc.* **180,** 507–511.

59. Groves, M.G. and Dennis, G.L. (1972) *Babesia gibsoni;* field and laboratory studies on canine infections. *Exp. Parasitol.* **31,** 153–159.

60. Birkenheuer, A.J., Levy, M.G., and Breitschwerdt, E.B. (2004) Efficacy of combined atovaquone and azithromycin for therapy of chronic *Babesia gibsoni* (Asian genotype) infections in dogs. *J. Vet. Int. Med.* **18,** 494–498.

61. Lapage, G. (1962) Mönnig's veterinary helmintology and entomology. 5th ed. Williams and Wilkins, Baltimore, MD. 600 pages.

62. Lee, K., Hong, S., Han, J., Yoon, C., Lee, S., Kim, S. et al. (2003) Experimental clonorchiasis in dogs: CT findings before and after treatment. *Radiology* **228,** 131–138.

63. Hong, S., Lee, S., Lee, S., Kho, W., Lee, M., Li, S. et al. (2003) Sustained-release praziquantel tablet: pharmacokinetics and the treatment of clonorchiasis in beagle dogs. *Parasitol. Res.* **91,** 316–320.

64. Slaughter, J.B., II, Billups, L.H., and Acor, G.K. (1988) Canine heterobilharziasis. *Compend. Cont. Educ. Pract. Vet.* **10,** 606–612.

65. Flowers, J.R., Hammerberg, B., Wood, S.L., Malarkey, D.E., Dam, G.J.V., Levy, M.G., et al. (2002) *Heterobilharzia americana* infection in a dog. *J. Am. Vet. Med. Assoc.* **220,** 193–196.

66. Fradkin, J.M., Braniecki, A.M., Craig, T.M., Ramiro Ibanez, F., Rogers, K.S., and Zoran, D.L. (2001) Elevated parathyroid hormone-related protein and hypercalcemia in two dogs with schistosomiasis. *J. Am. Anim. Hosp. Assoc.* **37,** 349–355.

67. Ronald, N.C. and Craig, T.M. (1983) Fenbendazole for the treatment of *Heterobilharzia americana* infection in dogs. *J. Am. Vet. Med. Assoc.* **182,** 172.

68. Farrell, R.K. (1968) Rickettsial diseases, In: Catcott, E.J. (ed.) *Canine Medicine.* American Veterinary Publications, Santa Barbara, CA., 164–169.

69. LeJeune, J.T. and Hancock, D.D. (2001) Public health concerns associated with feeding raw meat diets to dogs. *J. Am. Vet. Med. Assoc.* **219,** 1222–1225.

70. Foreyt, W.J. and Gorham, J.R. (1988) Evaluation of praziquantel against induced *Nanophyetus salmincola* infections in coyotes and dogs. *Am. J. Vet. Res.* **49,** 563–565.

71. Herman, L.H. and Helland, D.R. (1966) Paragonimiasis in a cat. *J. Am. Vet. Med. Assoc.* **149,** 753–757.

72. Dubey, J.P., Toussant, M.J., Hoover, E.A., Miller, T.B., Sharma, S.P., and Pechman, R.D. (1979) Experimental *Paragonimus kellicotti* infection in dogs. *Vet. Parasitol.* **5,** 325–337.

73. van Rensburg, I.B.J., Vester, A., and Hiza, M.H. (1987) Parasitic pneumonia in a dog caused by a lung fluke of the genus *Paragonimus. J. S. Afr. Vet. Assoc.* **58,** 203–206.

74. Bowman, D.D., Frongillo, M.K., Johnson, R.C., Beck, K.A., Hornbuckle, W.E., and Blue, J.T. (1991) Evaluation of praziquantel for treatment of experimentally induced paragonimiasis in dogs and cats. *Am. J. Vet. Res.* **52,** 68–71.

75. Kirkpatrick, C.E., Knochenhauer, A.W., and Jacobson, S.I. (1987) Use of praziquantel for treatment of *Diphyllobothrium* sp. infection in a dog. *J. Am. Vet. Med. Assoc.* **190,** 557–558.

76. Little, S. and Ambrose, D. (2000) *Spirometra* infection in cats and dogs. *Compend. Contin. Educ. Pract. Vet.* **22,** 299–303.

77. Boreham, R.E. and Boreham, P.F.L. (1990) *Dipylidium caninum:* life cycle, epizootiology, and control. *Comp. Cont. Educ. Pract. Vet.* **12,** 667–675.

78. Hopkins, T.J., Gyr, P., and Hedemann, P.M. (1988) Nematocidal and cesticidal efficacy of a tablet formulation containing febantel, pyrantel embonate and praziquantel in dogs. *Vet. Med. Rev.* **59,** 71–75.

79. Eckert, J. and Deplazes, P. (2004) Biological, epidemiological, and clinical aspects of echinococcosis, a zoonosis of increasing concern. *Clin. Microbiol. Rev.* **17**, 107–135.

80. Faust, E.C., Beaver, P.C., and Jung, R.C. (1968) Animal agents and vectors of human disease. 3rd ed. Lea and Febiger, Philadelphia, PA. 461 pages.

81. Cheikh Rouhou, F., Besbes, M., Makni, F., Chaabouni, M., and Ayadi, A. (2000) *Limnatis nilotica* causing severe anaemia in an infant. *Med. Trop.* **60**, 100–101.

82. Horton, M.L. (1980) Rhabditic dermatitis in dogs. *Mod. Vet. Pract.* **61**, 158–159.

83. Cagnasso, A. and Peirone, B. (1988) Dermatitis due to *Pelodera strongyloides* in a dog. *Summa* **5**, 74.

84. Chandler, A.C. and Read, C.P. (1961) Introduction to parasitology, with special reference to the parasites of man. 10th ed. John Wiley, New York, NY. 822 pages.

85. Schad, G.A., Aikens, L.M., and Smith, G. (1989) *Strongyloides stercoralis:* is there a canonical migratory route through the host? *J. Parasitol.* **75**, 740–749.

86. Shoop, W.L., Michael, B.F., Eary, C.H., and Haines, H.W. (2002) Transmammary transmission of *Strongyloides stercoralis* in dogs. *J. Parasitol.* **88**, 536–539.

87. Mansfield, L.S. and Schad, G.A. (1995) Lack of transmammary transmission of *Strongyloides stercoralis* from a previously hyperinfected bitch to her pups. *J. Helm. Soc. Wash.* **62**, 80–83.

88. Genta, R.M., Schad, G.A., and Hellman, M.E. (1986) *Strongyloides stercoralis:* parasitological, immunological and pathological observations in immunosuppressed dogs. *Tran. Roy. Soc. Trop. Med. Hyg.* **80**, 34–41.

89. Mansfield, L.S. and Schad, G.A. (1992) Ivermectin treatment of naturally acquired and experimentally induced *Strongyloides stercoralis* infections in dogs. *J. Am. Vet. Med. Assoc.* **201**, 726–730.

90. Georgi, J.R. and Sprinkle, C.L. (1974) A case of human strongyloidosis apparently contracted from asymptomatic colony dogs. *Am. J. Trop. Med. Hyg.* **23**, 899–901.

91. Fisher, M.A., Murphy, M.G., and Siedek, E.M. (2002) Epidemiology of *Toxascaris leonina* infection post-weaning within a colony of dogs. *J. Helminthol.* **76**, 27–29.

92. Smith, H.V., Quinn, R., Bruce, R.G., and Girdwood, R.W.A. (1982) Development of the serological response in rabbits infected with *Toxocara canis* and *Toxascaris leonina. Trans. Roy. Soc. Trop. Med. Hyg.* **76**, 89–94.

93. Sprent, J.F.A. (1959) The life history and development of *Toxascaris leonina* (von Linstow 1902) in the dog and cat. *Parasitology* **49**, 330–371.

94. Ewing, S.A. (1967) Examination for parasites. In: Coles, E.H. (ed.) *Veterinary Clinical Pathology.* W.B. Saunders, Philadelphia, PA. 331–391.

95. Morgan, B.B. and Hawkins, P.A. (1949) *Veterinary Helminthology.* Burgess, Minneapolis, MN. 400 pages.

96. Turkowicz, M. and Cielecka, D. (2002) Prevalence of intestinal nematodes in dogs from Warsaw Region. *Wiad. Parazytol.* **48**, 407–411.

97. Coggins, J.R. (1998) Effect of season, sex, and age on prevalence of parasitism in dogs from southeastern Wisconsin. *J. Helm. Soc. Wash.* **65**, 219–224.

98. Pahari, T.K. and Sasmal, N.K. (1990) Infection of Japanese quail with *Toxocara canis* larvae and establishment of patent infection in pups. *Vet. Parasitol.* **35**, 357–364.

99. Acharya, S., Sasmal, N.K., Jana, D.N., and Roy, S. (2002) Migratory behaviour of *Toxocara canis* larvae in piglets and establishment of patent infection in pups. *J. Vet. Parasitol.* **16**, 157–161.

100. Burke, T.M. and Roberson, E.L. (1985) Prenatal and lactational transmission of *Toxocara canis* and *Ancylostoma caninum:* experimental infection of the bitch at midpregnancy and at parturition. *Int. J. Parasitol.* **15**, 485–490.

101. Burke, T.M. and Roberson, E.L. (1985) Prenatal and lactational transmission of *Toxocara canis* and *Ancylostoma caninum:* experimental infection of the bitch before pregnancy. *Int. J. Parasitol.* **15**, 71–75.

102. Douglas, J.R. and Baker, N.F. (1959) The chronology of experimental intrauterine infections with *Toxocara canis* (Werner, 1782) in the dog. *J. Parasitol.* **45**, 43.

103. Nobel, W.E.L., Robben, S.R.M., Dopfer, D., Hendrikx, W.M.L., Boersema, J.H., Fransen, F., et al. (2004) Infections with endoparasites in dogs in Dutch animal shelters. *Tijdschr. Diergeneeskd.***129**, 40–44.

104. Bloom, F. (1965) Spontaneous renal lesions. In: Ribelin W.E. and McCoy J.R (eds.) *The Pathology of Laboratory Animals.* Charles C. Thomas, Springfield, IL, 93–123.

105. Vossmann, T. and Stoye, M. (1986) Clinical, haematological and serological findings in puppies after prenatal infection with *Toxocara canis. J. Vet. Med. B. Infect. Dis. Vet. Public Health* **33**, 574–585.

106. Epe, C., Pankow, W.R., Hackbarth, H., Schnieder, T., and Stoye, M. (1995) A study on the prevention of prenatal and galactogenic *Toxocara canis* infections in pups by treatment of infected bitches with ivermectin or doramectin. *Appl. Parasitol.* **36**, 115–123.

107. Payne Johnson, M., Maitland, T.P., Sherington, J., Shanks, D.J., Clements, P.J.M., Murphy, M.G., et al. (2000) Efficacy of selamectin administered topically to pregnant and lactating female dogs in the treatment and prevention of adult roundworm (*Toxocara canis*) infections and flea (*Ctenocephalides felis felis*) infestations in the dams and their pups. *Vet. Parasitol.* **91**, 347–358.

108. Despommier, D. (2003) Toxocariasis: clinical aspects, epidemiology, medical ecology, and molecular aspects. *Clin. Microbiol. Rev.* **16**, 265–272.

109. Gottstein, B. (1987) Clinical, haematological and serological findings in puppies after different intensity of milk-borne challenge with *Ancylostoma caninum*. Thesis, Tierarztliche Hochschule Hannover, 86 pages.

110. Meyer, O.K.H. (1988) Trials of ivermectin treatment of bitches for the prevention of galactogenic infection of puppies with *Ancylostoma caninum*. Thesis, Tierarztliche Hochschule Hannover, 112 pages.

111. Rosler, K. (1998) Efficacy of moxidectin on reactivated somatic larvae of *Ancylostoma caninum* Ercolani 1859 (Ancylostomatidae) in pregnant bitches. Thesis, Tierarztliche Hochschule Hannover, 90 pages.

112. Schnieder, T., Lechler, M., Epe, C., Kuschfeldt, S., and Stoye, M. (1996) The efficacy of doramectin on arrested larvae of *Ancylostoma caninum* in early pregnancy of bitches. *J. Vet. Med. Ser. B* **43**, 351–356.

113. Smith, G.C., Gangadharan, B., Taylor, Z., Laurenson, M.K., Bradshaw, H., Hide, G., et al. (2003) Prevalence of zoonotic important parasites in the red fox (*Vulpes vulpes*) in Great Britain. *Vet. Parasitol.* **118**, 133–142.

114. Vanparijs, O., Hermans, L., and Flaes, L.V.D. (1991) Helminth and protozoan parasites in dogs and cats in Belgium. *Vet. Parasitol.* **38**, 67–73.

115. Gibbs, H.C. (1958) On the gross and microscopic lesions produced by the adults and larvae of *Dochmoides stenocephala* (Railliet, 1884) in the dog. *Can. J. Comp. Med. Vet. Sci.* **22**, 382–385.

116. Gibbs, H.C. (1961) Studies on the life cycle and developmental morphology of *Dochmoides stenocephala* (Railliet, 1884) (Ancylostomidae: Nematoda). *Can. J. Zool.* **39**, 325–348.

117. Feilke, M. (1985) Studies on the possibility of prenatal and lactogenic infections of *Uncinaria stenocephala* in beagles. Thesis, Tierarztliche Hochschule Hannover, 66 pages.

118. Walker, M.J. and Jacobs, D.E. (1985) Pathophysiology of *Uncinaria stenocephala* infections of dogs. *Vet. Ann.* **25**, 263–271.

119. Greve, J.H. (1985) Identifying nematode larvae in feces of dogs and cats. *Iowa State Univ. Vet.* **47**, 98–101.

120. Georgi, J.R. and Anderson, R.C. (1975) *Filaroides hirthi* sp.n. (Nematoda: Metastrongyloidea) from the lung of the dog. *J. Parasitol.* **61**, 337–339.

121. Vajner, L., Vortel, V., and Brejcha, A. (2000) Lung filaroidosis in the beagle dog breeding colony. *Vet. Med.* **45**, 25–30.

122. Georgi, J.R., Georgi, M.E., Fahnestock, G.R., and Theodorides, V.J. (1979) Transmission and control of *Filaroides hirthi* lungworm infection in dogs. *Am. J. Vet. Res.* **40**, 829–831.

123. Georgi, J.R., Fahnestock, G.R., Bohm, M.F.K., and Adsit, J.C. (1979) The migration and development of *Filaroides hirthi* larvae in dogs. *Parasitology* **79**, 39–47.

124. Rendano, V.T., Georgi, J.R., Fahnestock, G.R., and King, J.M. (1979) *Filaroides hirthi* lungworm infection in dogs: its radiographic appearance. *J. Am. Vet. Rad. Soc.* **20**, 2–9.

125. Genta, R.M. and Schad, G.A. (1984) *Filaroides hirthi:* hyperinfective lungworm infection in immunosuppressed dogs. *Vet. Pathol.* **21**, 349–354.

126. Carrasco, L., Hervas, J., Gomez Villamandos, J.C., Chacon, M.D.L.F., and Sierra, M.A. (1997) Massive *Filaroides hirthi* infestation associated with canine distemper in a puppy. *Vet. Rec.* **140**, 72–73.

127. Erb, H.N. and Georgi, J.R. (1982) Control of *Filaroides hirthi* in commercially reared Beagle dogs. *Lab. Anim. Sc.* **32**, 394–396.

128. Bauer, C. and Bahnemann, R. (1996) Control of *Filaroides hirthi* infections in beagle dogs by ivermectin. *Vet. Parasitol.* **65**, 269–273.

129. Mills, J.H.L. and Nielsen, S.W. (1966) Canine *Filaroides osleri* and *Filaroides milksi* infection. *J. Am. Vet. Med. Assoc.* **149**, 56–63.

130. Bredal, W., Gjerde, B., Heiene, R., and Press, C. (1999) First verified case of *Oslerus osleri* infection in a dog from Norway. *Eur. J. Comp. Anim. Pract.* **9**, 77–82.

131. Dunsmore, J.D. and Burt, R.J. (1972) *Filaroides osleri* in dingoes in south-eastern Australia. *Aust. Vet. J.* **48**, 548–551.

132. Henke, S.E., Pence, D.B., and Bryant, F.C. (2002) Effect of short-term coyote removal on populations of coyote helminths. *J. Wildl. Dis.* **38**, 54–67.

133. Kotani, T., Horie, M., Yamaguchi, S., Tsukamoto, Y., Onishi, T., Ohashi, F., et al. (1995) Lungworm, *Filaroides osleri,* infection in a dog in Japan. *J. Vet. Med. Sci.* **57**, 573–576.

134. Weston, R. (1975) Endoparasites in dogs supplied for laboratory use. 1. The incidence of infestation. 2. Effectiveness of quarantine. *Anim. Technol.* **26**, 69–77.

135. Dorrington, J.E. (1968) Studies on *Filaroides osleri* infestation in dogs. *Onderstepoort J. Vet. Res.* **35**, 225–286.

136. Levitan, D.M., Matz, M.E., Findlen, C.S., and Fister, R.D. (1996) Treatment of *Oslerus osleri* infestation in a dog: case report and literature review. *J. Am. Anim. Hosp. Assoc.* **32**, 435–438.

137. Gahlod, B.M., Kolte, S.W., and Kurkure, N.V. (2002) Treatment of canine *Oslerus osleri* infection with doramectin—a case report. *Indian Vet. J.* **79**, 168–169.

138. Auro de Ocampo, A. and Dominguez, O.J. (1978) The findings of *Filaroides osleri* in dogs used for research. A description of 6 cases. *Vet. Mexico* **9**, 105–110.

139. Bailey, W.S. (1963) Parasites and cancer: Sarcoma in dogs associated with *Spirocerca lupi. Ann. N.Y. Acad. Sci.* **108**, 890–923.

140. Minnaar, W.N., Krecek, R.C., and Fourie, L.J. (2002) Helminths in dogs from a peri-urban resource-limited community in Free State Province, South Africa. *Vet. Parasitol.* **107**, 343–349.

141. Harmelin, A., Perl, S., Yakobson, B., Markovics, A., and Orgad, U. (1991) *Spirocerca lupi*—review and occurrence in Israel. *Israel J. Vet. Med.* **46**, 69–73.

142. Oliveira Sequeira, T.C.G., Amarante, A.F.T., Ferrari, T.B., and Nunes, L.C. (2002) Prevalence of intestinal parasites in dogs from Sao Paulo State, Brazil. *Vet. Parasitol.* **103**, 19–27.

143. Choo, L.N. (1987) Gastrointestinal helminths of dogs and cats in Singapore. *Singapore Vet. J.* **10–11**, 12–24.

144. Gupta, V.P. and Pande, B.P. (1962) A note on pulmonary spirocercosis in a dog. *J. Parasitol.* **48**, 505–506.

145. Johnson, R.C. (1992) Canine spirocercosis and associated esophageal sarcoma. *Comp. Contin. Educ. Pract. Vet.* **14**, 577–580.

146. Ivoghli, B. (1977) Fatal aortic aneurysm and rupture caused by *Spirocerca lupi* in a dog. *J. Am. Vet. Med. Assoc.* **170**, 834.

147. Ranen, E., Lavy, E., Aizenberg, I., Perl, S., and Harrus, S. (2004) Spirocercosis-associated esophageal sarcomas in dogs: a retrospective study of 17 cases (1997–2003). *Vet. Parasitol.* **119**, 209–221.

148. Brodey, R.S. (1971) Hypertrophic osteoarthropathy in the dog: a clinicopathologic survey of 60 cases. *J. Am. Vet. Med. Assoc.* **159**, 1242–1256.

149. Michal Mazaki, T., Baneth, G., Itamar, A., Harrus, S., Kass, P.H., Tomer, B.A., et al. (2002) Canine spirocercosis: clinical, diagnostic, pathologic, and epidemiologic characteristics. *Vet. Parasitol.* **107**, 235–250.

150. Markovics, A. and Medinski, B. (1996) Improved diagnosis of low intensity *Spirocerca lupi* infection by the sugar flotation method. *J. Vet. Diag. Invest.* **8**, 400–401.

151. Mylonakis, M.E., Rallis, T.S., Koutinas, A.F., Ververidis, H.N., and Fytianou, A. (2004) A comparison between ethanol-induced chemical ablation and ivermectin plus prednizolone in the treatment of symptomatic esophageal spirocercosis in the dog: a prospective study on 14 natural cases. *Vet. Parasitol.* **120**, 131–138.

152. Lavy, E., Aroch, I., Bark, H., Markovics, A., Aizenberg, I., Mazaki Tovi, M., et al. (2002) Evaluation of doramectin for the treatment of experimental canine spirocercosis. *Vet. Parasitol.* **109**, 65–73.

153. Lavy, E., Harrus, S., Mazaki Tovi, M., Bark, H., Markovics, A., Hagag, A. et al. (2003) *Spirocerca lupi* in dogs: prophylactic effect of doramectin. *Res. Vet. Sci.* **75**, 217–222.

154. Lindsey, J.R. (1965) Identification of canine microfilariae. *J. Am. Vet. Med. Assoc.* **146**, 1106–1114.

155. Morgan, H.C. (1966) Canine blood parasites: Filariasis. *Vet. Med.* **61**, 829–841.

156. Lindemann, B.A. and McCall, J.W. (1984) Experimental *Dipetalonema reconditum* infections in dogs. *J. Parasitol.* **70**, 167–168.

157. Morgan, H.C. (1966) Canine blood parasites: Filariasis. *Vet. Med.* **61**, 829–841.

158. Lok, J.B., Boreham, P.F.L., and Atwell, R.B. (1988) *Dirofilaria* sp.: taxonomy and distribution. In: *Dirofilariasis,* CRC Press, Boca Raton, FL, 1–28.

159. Lindsey, J.R. (1965) Identification of canine microfilariae. *J. Am. Vet. Med. Assoc.* **146**, 1106–1114.

160. Jackson, R.F., von Lichtenberg, F., and Otto, G.F. (1962) Occurrence of adult heartworms in the venae cavae of dogs. *J. Am. Vet. Med. Assoc.* **141,** 117–121.

161. Kotani, T. and Powers, K.G. (1982) Developmental stages of *Dirofilaria immitis* in the dog. *Am. J. Vet. Res.* **43,** 2199–2206.

162. Otto, G.F. and Jackson, R.F. (1969) Pathology of heartworm disease. *J. Am. Vet. Med. Assoc.* **154,** 370–373.

163. Rawlings, C.A. (2002) Effect of monthly heartworm preventatives on dogs with young heartworm infections. *J. Am. Anim. Hosp. Assoc.* **38,** 311–314.

164. Grauer, G.F., Culham, C.A., Dubielzig, R.R., Longhofer, S.L., and Grieve, R.B. (1989) Experimental *Dirofilaria immitis*-associated glomerulonephritis induced in part by in situ formation of immune complexes in the glomerular capillary wall. *J. Parasitol.* **75,** 585–593.

165. Godfrey, W.D., Neely, W.A., Elliott, R.L., and Grogan, J.B. (1966) Canine heartworms in experimental cardiac and pulmonary surgery. *J. Surg. Res.* **6,** 331–336.

166. Ciferri, F. (1982) Human pulmonary dirofilariasis in the United States: a critical review. *Am. J. Trop. Med. Hyg.* **31,** 302–308.

167. Levine, N.D. (1980) *Nematode Parasites of Domestic Animals and Man,* Burgess Publishing Co., Minneapolis, MN, 477 pages.

168. Burrows, R.B. (1965) *Microscopic Diagnosis of the Parasites of Man.* Yale University Press, New Haven, CT. 328 pages.

169. Segovia, J.M., Torres, J., and Miquel, J. (2004) Helminth parasites of the red fox (*Vulpes vulpes* L., 1758) in the Iberian Peninsula: an ecological study. *Acta Parasitol.* **49,** 67–79.

170. Sauerland, D., Monrad, J., and Spohr, A. (2001) Incidence of *Trichuris vulpis* and *Capillaria aerophila* in Danish kennel dogs. *Dan. Veterinaertidsskrift* **84,** 6–9.

171. Christenson, R.O. (1938) Life history and epidemiological studies on the fox lungworm, *Capillaria aerophila* (Creplin, 1839). *Livro jub. Lauro Travassos Instituto Oswaldo Cruz,* 119–136.

172. Packova, I. (1998) Case reports: diagnosis, therapy. A chronic cough outbreak in a breeding kennel—pulmonary *Capillaria* infection. *Veterinarstvi* **48,** 516.

173. Romashov, B.V. (2000) Three capillariid species (Nematoda, Capillariidae) of carnivores (Carnivora) and discussion of system and evolution of the nematode family Capillariidae. 1. Redescription of *Eucoleus aerophilus* and *E. boehmi. Zool. Zhurnal* **79,** 1379–1391.

174. Schoning, P., Dryden, M.W., and Gabbert, N.H. (1993) Identification of a nasal nematode (*Eucoleus boehmi*) in greyhounds. *Vet. Res. Commun.* **17,** 277–281.

175. Campbell, B.G. and Little, M.D. (1991) Identification of the eggs of a nematode (*Eucoleus boehmi*) from the nasal mucosa of North American dogs. *J. Am. Vet. Med. Assoc.* **198,** 1520–1523.

176. Evinger, J.V., Kazacos, K.R., and Cantwell, H.D. (1985) Ivermectin for treatment of nasal capillariasis in a dog. *J. Am. Vet. Med. Assoc.* **186,** 174–175.

177. Habermann, R.T. and Williams, F.P. Jr. (1958) The identification and control of helminths in laboratory animals. *J. Natl. Cancer Inst.* **20,** 979–1009.

178. Sreter, T., Szell, Z., Marucci, G., Pozio, E., and Varga, I. (2003) Extraintestinal nematode infections of red foxes (*Vulpes vulpes*) in Hungary. *Vet. Parasitol.* **115,** 329–334.

179. Torres, J., Miquel, J., and Motje, M. (2001) Helminth parasites of the eurasian badger (*Meles meles* L.) in Spain: a biogeographic approach. *Parasitol. Res.* **87,** 259–263.

180. Thiess, A., Schuster, R., Nockler, K., and Mix, H. (2001) Helminth findings in indigenous raccoon dogs *Nyctereutes procyonoides* (Gray, 1834). *Berl. Munch. Tierarztl. Wochenschr.* **114,** 273–276

181. Segovia, J.M., Torres, J., Miquel, J., Llaneza, L., and Feliu, C. (2001) Helminths in the wolf, *Canis lupus,* from north-western Spain. *J. Helminthol.* **75,** 183–192.

182. Enigk, K. (1950) Die biologie von *Capillaria plica* (Trichurioidea, Nematodes). *Zeitschrift Tropenmed. Parasitol.* **1,** 560–571.

183. Veen, L.V. (2002) *Capillaria plica* infection of the bladder of a shetland sheepdog. *Tijdschr. Diergeneeskd.* **127,** 393–394.

184. Senior, D.F., Solomon, G.B., Goldschmidt, M.H., Joyce, T., and Bovee, K.C. (1980) *Capillaria plica* infection in dogs. *J. Am. Vet. Med. Assoc.* **176,** 901–905.

185. Gillespie, D. (1983) Successful treatment of canine *Capillaria plica* cystitis. *Vet. Med. Sm. Anim. Clin.* **78,** 681–682.

186. Kirkpatrick, C.E. and Nelson, G.R. (1987) Ivermectin treatment of urinary capillariasis in a dog. *J. Am. Vet. Med. Assoc.* **191,** 701–702.

187. Gaafar, S.M. (1964) Internal parasitism of small animals. *Vet. Med.* **59,** 907–913.

188. Kirkova, Z. (2003) Studies on the life cycle of *Trichuris vulpis. Bulg. J. Vet. Med.* **6,** 35–42.

189. Smith, H.A. and Jones, T.C. (1966) *Veterinary Pathology.* 3rd ed. Lea and Febiger, Philadelphia, PA. 1192 pages.

190. Ruckstuhl, N., Deplazes, P., and Reusch, C. (2002) Clinical signs and course of disease in dogs with *Trichuris vulpis*-infection. *Kleintierpraxis* **47,** 19–26.

191. Bowman, D.D., Legg, W., and Stansfield, D.G. (2002) Efficacy of moxidectin 6-month injectable and milbemycin oxime/lufenuron tablets against naturally acquired *Trichuris vulpis* infections in dogs. *Vet. Ther.* **3,** 286–289.

192. Yorke, W. and Maplestone, P.A. (1926) The nematode parasites of vertebrates. Blakiston, Philadelphia, PA. 536 pages.

193. Mech, L.D. and Tracy, S.P. (2001) Prevalence of giant kidney worm (*Dioctophyma renale*) in wild mink (*Mustela vison*) in Minnesota. *Am. Midl. Nat.* **145,** 206–209.

194. Carvalho, C.T.D. and Vasconcellos, L.E.M. (1996) Disease, food and reproduction of the maned wolf—*Chrysocyon brachyurus* (Illiger) (Carnivora, Canidae) in southeast Brazil. (1995) *Rev. Bras. Zool.* **12,** 627–640.

195. Seville, R.S. and Addison, E.M. (1995) Nongastrointestinal helminths in marten (*Martes americana*) from Ontario, Canada. *J. Wildl. Dis.* **31,** 529–533.

196. Cersosimo, F., Soccol, V.T., Ohi, M., and Busetti, E.T. (1984) *Dioctophyma renale* in cats in Curitiba, Parana. In *First veterinary research meeting, State University of Londrina, Brazil, 26–30 Nov. 1984. 1984,* 38; Supp. to Semina 5, (16). Dep. de Med. Vet. Univ. Est. de Londrina.

197. Unruh, D.H.A., King, J.E., Eaton, R.D.P., and Allen, J.R. (1973) Parasites of dogs from Indian settlements in northwestern Canada: a survey with public health implications. *Can. J. Comp. Med.* **37,** 25–32.

198. Woodhead, A.E. (1950) Life history of the giant kidney worm, *Dioctophyma renale* (Nematoda), of man and many other mammals. *Trans. Am. Microscop. Soc.* **69,** 21–46.

199. Measures, L.N. and Anderson, R.C. (1985) Centrarchid fish as paratenic hosts of the giant kidney worm, *Dioctophyma renale* (Goeze, 1782), in Ontario, Canada. *J. Wildl. Dis.* **21,** 11–19.

200. Hasegawa, H., Doi, T., Tochimoto, T., and Myata, A. (2002) Parasitic helminths collected from the Japanese giant salamander, *Andrias japonicus* (Temminck, 1837) (Amphibia: Cryptobranchidae), in Japan. *Comp. Parasitol.* **69,** 33–42.

201. Gargili, A., Firat, I., Toparlak, M., and Cetinkaya, H. (2002) First case report of *Dioctophyme renale* (Goeze, 1782) in a dog in Istanbul, Turkey. *Turk Veterinerlik ve Hayvancilik Dergisi* **26,** 1189–1191.

202. Gutierrez, Y., Cohen, M., and Machicao, C.N. (1989) *Dioctophyme* larva in the subcutaneous tissues of a woman in Ohio. *Am. J. Surg. Pathol.* **13**, 800–802.

203. Wehr, E.E. (1965) Nematodes and acanthocephalids of poultry. In: Biester, H.E. and Schwarte, L.H. (eds.) *Diseases of Poultry.* 5th ed. Iowa State University Press, Ames IA. 965–1005.

204. Benbrook, E.A. and Sloss, M.W. (1961) *Veterinary Clinical Parasitology.* 3rd ed. Iowa State University Press, Ames, IA. 240 pages.

205. Martinez, F.A. (1986) Acanthellae of *Oncicola canis* in armadilloes in Argentina. *Vet. Argentina* **3**, 272–275.

206. Goddard, J. (2003) *Physician's Guide to Arthropods of Medical Importance,* CRC Press, Boca Raton, FL. 444 pages.

207. Chermette, R. (1989) A case of canine otitis due to screwworm, *Cochliomyia hominivorax,* in France. *Vet. Rec.***124**, 641.

208. Machado, M.L. da S. and Rodrigues, E.M.P. (2002) Use of nitenpyram as a larvicide in canine myiasis caused by larvae of *Cochliomyia hominivorax. Acta Scientiae Veterinariae* **30**, 59–62.

209. Agrela, I., Sanchez, E., Gomez, B. and Feliciangeli, M.D. (2002) Feeding behavior of *Lutzomyia pseudolongipalpis* (Diptera: Psychodidae), a putative vector of visceral leishmaniasis in Venezuela. *J. Med. Entomol.* **39**, 440–445.

210. David, J.R., Stamm, L.M., Bezerra, H.S., Souza, R.N., Killick Kendrick, R., and Lima, J.W.O. (2001) Deltamethrin-impregnated dog collars have a potent anti-feeding and insecticidal effect on *Lutzomyia longipalpis* and *Lutzomyia migonei. Mem. Inst. Oswaldo Cruz* **96**, 839–847.

211. Mercier, P., Jasmin, P., and Sanquer, A. (2003) Prevention of sand fly attack by topical application of a permethrin/pyriproxyfen combination on dogs. *Vet. Ther.* **4**, 309–316.

212. Kim, K.C., Pratt, H.D., and Stojanovich, C.J. (1986) *The Sucking Lice of North America. An Illustrated Manual for Identification,* Pennsylvania State University Press, University Park, PA. 241 pages.

213. Christensson, D., Zakrisson, G., Holm, B., and Gunnarsson, L. (1998) Lice on dogs in Sweden. *Sven. Vet.* **50**, 189–191.

214. Saito, T., Hashiguchi, M., Utsnomiya, K., Yamaashi, K., Yoshida, K., Ikeda, F., et al. (2003) Prevalence of ectoparasitoses in domestic dogs and cats in Fukuyama City, Hiroshima Prefecture in 2002 (January-December). *J. Vet. Med. Japan* **56**, 801–804.

215. Gonzalez, A., del Castro , C., and Gonzalez, S. (2004) Ectoparasitic species from *Canis familiaris* (Linne) in Buenos Aires province, Argentina. *Vet. Parasitol.* **120**, 123–129.

216. Beck, C.W. (2000) The efficacy of fipronil (Frontline R) against ectoparasites: control of lice, mites and mallophages in diverse small animals. *Tierarztl. Umsch.* **55**, 244–250.

217. Hanssen, I., Mencke, N., Asskildt, H., Ewald Hamm, D., and Dorn, H. (1999) Field study on the insecticidal efficacy of Advantage against natural infestations of dogs with lice. *Parasitol. Res.* **85**, 347–348.

218. Shanks, D.J., Gautier, P., McTier, T.L., Evans, N.A., Pengo, G., and Rowan, T.G. (2003) Efficacy of selamectin against biting lice on dogs and cats. *Vet. Rec.***152**, 234–237.

219. Pollmeier, M., Pengo, G., Jeannin, P., and Soll, M. (2002) Evaluation of the efficacy of fipronil formulations in the treatment and control of biting lice, *Trichodectes canis* (De Geer, 1778) on dogs. *Vet. Parasitol.* **107**, 127–136.

220. Endris, R.G., Reuter, V.E., Nelson, J., and Nelson, J.A. (2001) Efficacy of a topical spot-on containing 65% permethrin against the dog louse, *Trichodectes canis* (Mallophaga: Trichodectidae). *Vet. Ther.* **2**, 135– 139.

221. White, S.D., Scott, K.V., and Cheney, J.M. (1995) *Otobius megnini* infestation in three dogs. *Vet. Dermatol.* **6**, 33–35.

222. Endris, R.G., Hair, J.A., Anderson, G., Rose, W.B., Disch, D., and Meyer, J.A. (2003) Efficacy of two 65% permethrin spot-on formulations against induced infestations of *Ctenocephalides felis* (Insecta: Siphonaptera) and *Amblyomma americanum* (Acari: Ixodidae) on beagles. *Vet. Ther.* **4**, 47–55.

223. Steiert, J.G. and Gilfoy, F. (2002) Infection rates of *Amblyomma americanum* and *Dermacentor variabilis* by Ehrlichia chaffeensis and Ehrlichia ewingii in Southwest Missouri. *Vector Borne Zoonotic Dis.* **2**, 53–60.

224. Goldberg, M., Rechav, Y., and Durden, L.A. (2002) Ticks parasitizing dogs in Northwestern Georgia. *J. Med. Entomol.* **39**, 112–114.

225. Jacobson, R., McCall, J., Hunter, J., III, Alva, R., Irwin, J., Eschner, A., et al. (2004) The ability of fipronil to prevent transmission of *Borrelia burgdorferi,* the causative agent of lyme disease to dogs. *J. Appl. Res. Vet. Med.* **2**, 39–45.

226. Hellmann, K., Knoppe, T., Krieger, K., and Stanneck, D. (2003) European multicenter field trial on the efficacy and safety of a topical formulation of imidacloprid and permethrin (AdvantixTM) in dogs naturally infested with ticks and/or fleas. *Parasitol. Res.* **90**, S125–126.

227. Endris, R.G., Matthewson, M.D., Cooke, D., and Amodie, D. (2002) Repellency and efficacy of 65% permethrin and 9.7% fipronil against *Ixodes ricinus. Tierarztl. Umsch.* **57**, 556–566.

228. McCall, J.W., Alva, R., Irwin, J.P., Carithers, D., and Boeckh, A. (2004) Comparative efficacy of a combination of fipronil/(S)-methoprene, a combination of imidacloprid/permethrin, and imidacloprid against fleas and ticks when administered topically to dogs. *J. Appl. Res. Vet. Med.* **2**, 74–77.

229. Young, D.R., Arther, R.G., and Davis, W.L. (2003) Evaluation of K9 AdvantixTM vs. Frontline Plus(R) topical treatments to repel brown dog ticks (*Rhipicephalus sanguineus*) on dogs. *Parasitol. Res.* **90**, S116– 118.

230. Jernigan, A.D., McTier, T.L., Chieffo, C., Thomas, C.A., Krautmann, M.J., Hair, J.A., et al. (2000) Efficacy of selamectin against experimentally induced tick (*Rhipicephalus sanguineus* and *Dermacentor variabilis*) infestations on dogs. *Vet. Parasitol.* **91**, 359–375.

231. Fain, A. (1968) Etude de la variabilite de *Sarcoptes scabiei* avec une revision des Sarcoptidae. *Acta Zool. Pathol. Antverp.* **47**, 3–196.

232. Walton, S.F., Choy, J.L., Bonson, A., Valle, A., McBroom, J., Taplin, D., et al. (1999) Genetically distinct dog-derived and human-derived *Sarcoptes scabiei* in scabies-endemic communities in northern Australia. *Am. J. Trop. Med. Hyg.* **61**, 542–547.

233. Arlian, L.G., Runyan, R.A., Achar, S., and Estes, S.A. (1984) Survival and infestivity of *Sarcoptes scabiei* var. *canis* and var. *hominis. J. Am. Acad. Dermatol.* **11**, 210–215.

234. Arlian, L.G., Morgan, M.S., Rapp, C.M., and Vyszenski Moher, D.L. (1995) Some effects of sarcoptic mange on dogs. *J. Parasitol.* **81**, 698–702.

235. Morris, D.O. and Dunstan, R.W. (1996) A histomorphological study of sarcoptic acariasis in the dog: 19 cases. *J. Am. Anim. Hosp. Assoc.* **32**, 119–124.

236. Hugnet, C., Bruchon Hugnet, C., Royer, H., and Bourdoiseau, G. (2001) Efficacy of 1.25% amitraz solution in the treatment of generalized demodicosis (eight cases) and sarcoptic mange (five cases) in dogs. *Vet. Dermatol.* **12**, 89–92.

237. Hoh, W., Jeong, A., Jeong, H., Eom, K., Oh, T., Hoh, W.P., et al. (2002) Efficacy of twice a week selamectin application as a treatment for mixed canine scabies and ear mite infestation in a dog. *J. Vet. Clin.* **19**, 401–404.

238. Koutinas, A.F., Saridomichelakis, M.N., Soubasis, N., Bornstein, S., and Koutinas, C.K. (2001) Treatment of canine sarcoptic mange with fipronil spray: a field trial. *Aust. Vet. Pract.* **31**, 115–119.

239. Fourie, L.J., Rand, C.D., Heine, J., and du Rand, C. (2003) Evaluation of the efficacy of an imidacloprid 10%/moxidectin 2.5% spot-on against *Sarcoptes scabiei* var canis on dogs. *Parasitol. Res.* **90,** S135–136.

240. Bensignor, E. (2000) Treatment of canine scabies with bi-weekly administrations of milbemycin oxime. *Ann. Med. Vet.* **144,** 409–414.

241. Arlian, L.G., ChannaBasavanna, G.P., and Viraktamath, C.A. (1989) Host-parasite interaction of *Sarcoptes scabiei* (Acari). *Progress in Acarology.* **123,** 131.

242. Marks, S.L., Moore, M.P., and Rishniw, M. (1994) *Pneumonyssoides caninum:* the canine nasal mite. *Comp. Contin. Educ. Pract. Vet.***16,** 577–583.

243. Baker, K.P., Evans, T.M., Gould, D.J., Hull, W.B., and Keegan, H.L. (1956) A manual of parasitic mites of medical or economic importance. In *Technical Publication of the national Pest Control Association., Inc. New York,* 170 pages.

244. Saeki, H., Song, K., Pak, T., Uchida, A., Hayasaki, M., Song, K.H., et al. (2004) Larvae of canine nasal mites (*Pneumonyssoides caninum*) detected in a domestic dog. *J. Jap. Vet. Med. Assoc.* **57,** 245–248.

245. Gunnarsson, L., Zakrisson, G., Lilliehook, I., Christensson, D., Rehbinder, C., and Uggla, A. (1998) Experimental infection of dogs with the nasal mite *Pneumonyssoides caninum.* *Vet. Parasitol.* **77,** 179–186.

246. Papazoglou, L.G., Plevraki, K., and Diakou, A. (2000) Rhinitis due to *Pneumonyssoides caninum* in a dog. *Aust. Vet. Pract.* **30,** 79–82.

247. Gunnarsson, L.K., Zakrisson, G., Egenvall, A., Christensson, D.A., and Uggla, A. (2001) Prevalence of *Pneumonyssoides caninum* infection in dogs in Sweden. *J. Am. Anim. Hosp. Assoc.* **37,** 331–337.

248. Rehbinder, C. and Karlsson, T. (2003) Treatment of canine nasal mite infection. *Sven. Vet.* **55,** 19–22.

249. Foxx, T.S. and Ewing, S.A. (1969) Morphologic features, behavior, and life history of *Cheyletiella yasgur*i. *Am. J. Vet. Res.* **30,** 269–285.

250. White, S.D., Rosychuk, R.A.W., and Fieseler, K.V. (2001) Clinicopathologic findings, sensitivity to house dust mites and efficacy of milbemycin oxime treatment of dogs with *Cheyletiella* sp. infestation. *Vet. Dermatol.* **12,** 13–18.

251. Mueller, R.S. and Bettenay, S.V. (2002) Efficacy of selamectin in the treatment of canine cheyletiellosis. *Vet. Rec.* **151,** 773.

252. Endris, R.G., Reuter, V.E., Nelson, J.D., and Nelson, J.A. (2000) Efficacy of 65% permethrin applied as a topical spot-on against walking dandruff caused by the mite, *Cheyletiella yasguri,* in dogs. *Vet. Ther.* **1,** 273–279.

253. Chadwick, A.J. (1997) Use of a 0.25% fipronil pump spray formulation to treat canine cheyletiellosis. *J. Sm. Anim. Pract.* **38,** 261–262.

254. Paradis, M. and Villeneuve, A. (1988) Efficacy of ivermectin against *Cheyletiella yasguri* infestation in dogs. *Can. Vet. J.* **29,** 633–635.

255. Wagner, R. and Stallmeister, N. (2000) *Cheyletiella* dermatitis in humans, dogs and cats. *Br. J. Dermatol.* **143,** 1110–1112.

256. Koutz, F.R., Groves, H.F., and Gee, C.M. (1960) A survey of *Demodex canis* in the skin of clinically normal dogs. *Vet. Med.* **55,** 52–53.

257. Unsworth, K. (1946) Studies on the clinical and parasitological aspects of canine demodectic mange. *J. Comp. Pathol. Ther.* **56,** 114–127.

258. Greve, J.H. and Gaafar, S.M. (1966) Natural transmission of *Demodex canis* in dogs. *J. Am. Vet. Med. Assoc.***148,** 1043–1045.

259. Baker, K.P. (1969) The histopathology and pathogenesis of demodecosis of the dog. *J. Comp. Pathol.* **79,** 321–327.

260. Solcan, G., Carp Carare, M., Guguianu, E., Timofte, D., Carp Carare, C., and Solcan, C. (2001) Updates in therapy of canine secondary deep pyoderma. *Lucrai Stiinifice Medicina Veterinara, Universitatea de Stiinte Agricole si Medicina Veterinara "Ion Ionescu de la Brad" Iasi* **44,** 329–334.

261. Mueller, R.S. (2004) Treatment protocols for demodicosis: an evidence-based review. *Vet. Dermatol.***15,** 75–89.

262. Sambon, L.W. (1922) A synopsis of the family Linguatulidae. *J. Trop. Med.Hyg.* **25,** 188–206, 391– 428.

263. Paoletti, B., Peli, A., Traversa, D., and Ragaini, L. (2003) Linguatulosis in dogs. Review of the literature and report of a case in Abruzzo. *Obiettivi e Documenti Veterinari* **24,** 37–43.

264. Lombardero, O.J. and Santa Cruz, A.M. (1986) Parasites of stray dogs in the city of Corrientes (Argentina). Changes over a 25 year-period. *Vet. Argentina* **3,** 888–892.

265. Meshgi, B. and Asgarian, O. (2003) Prevalence of *Linguatula serrata* infestation in stray dogs of Shahrekord, Iran. *J. Vet. Med. Ser.B* **50,** 466–467.

266. Egelund, T. and Dietz, H.H. (2002) Nasal worms in dogs. Detection of the nasal worm *Linguatula serrata* (Frohlich 1789) in 2 dogs imported from Nepal. *Dan. Vet.* **85,** 22–23.

267. Hobmaier, A. and Hobmaier, M. (1940) On the life-cycle of *Linguatula rhinaria. Am. J. Trop. Med.* **20,** 199–210.

268. Tavasouli, M., Javadi, S., and Hadian, M. (2001) Experimental infection and study of life cycle of *Linguatula serrata* in dogs. *J. Fac. Vet. Med. Univ. Tehran* **56,** 1–3.

269. Negrea, O., Miclaus, V., Rotaru, O., and Cozma, V. (1998) Histopathological aspects of nasal *Linguatula* infection in dogs. *Rev. Rom. Med. Vet.* **8,** 51–58.

270. Maleky, F. (2001) A case report of *Linguatula serrata* in human throat from Tehran, central Iran. *Indian J. Med. Sci.* **55,** 439–441.

271. Xiao, S., Yang, Y., Zhang, C. and You, J. (1996) Microscopic observations on livers of rabbits and dogs infected with *Schistosoma japonicum* cercariae and early treatment with artemether or praziquantel. *Acta Pharmacol. Sinica* **17,** 167–170.

272. Rim, H.J. (2005) Clonorchiasis: an update. *J. Helminthol.* **79,** 269–281.

273. Padgett, K.A. and Boyce, W.M. (2004) Life-history studies on two molecular strains of *Mesocestoides* (Cestoda: Mesocestoididae): identification of sylvatic hosts and infectivity of immature life stages. *J. Parasitol.* **90,** 108–113.

274. Deplazes, P., Hegglin, D., Gloor, S., and Romig, T. (2004) Wilderness in the city: the urbanization of *Echinococcus multilocularis. Trends Parasitol.* **20,** 77–84.

275. Bowman, D.D. (1992) Hookworm parasites of dogs and cats. *Comp. Contin. Educ. Pract. Vet.* **14,** 585–595.

276. Vetter, J.C.M. and Linden, M.E.L. (1977) Skin penetration of infective hookworm larvae. III. Comparative studies on the path of migration of the hookworms *Ancylostoma braziliense, Ancylostoma ceylanicum,* and *Ancylostoma caninum. Zeitschr. Parasitenkd* **53,** 155–158.

277. Costa, J.O., Costa, H.M. de A., and Guimaraes, M.P. (2003) Redescription of *Angiostrongylus vasorum* (Baillet, 1866) and systematic revision of species assigned to the genera *Angiostrongylus* Kamensky, 1905 and *Angiocaulus* Schulz, 1951. *Rev. Med. Vet.* **154,** 9–16.

278. Kelly, W.R., Waddell, A.H., and Mason, K.V. (1977) Naturally acquired *Angiostrongylus cantonensis* infection: a cause of ascending paralysis in pups in the Brisbane area. II. Clinical pathology and post mortem findings. In *Proceedings of the 54th Annual Conference, Perth, 9–13 May 1977,* 73–74.

279. Kim, D.Y., Stewart, T.B., Bauer, R.W., and Mitchell, M. (2002) *Parastrongylus (=Angiostrongylus) cantonensis* now endemic in Louisiana wildlife. *J. Parasitol.* **88,** 1024–1026.

280. McGarry, J.W., Martin, M., Cheeseman, M.T., and Payne Johnson, C.E. (1995) *Crenosoma vulpis,* the fox lungworm, in dogs. *Vet. Rec.* **137,** 271–272.

281. Pearce, J.R., Hendrix, C.M., Allison, N., and Butler, J.M. (2001) *Macracanthorhynchus ingens* infection in a dog. *J. Am. Vet. Med. Assoc.* **219,** 194–196.

282. Rim, H.J. (2005) Clonorchiasis: an update. *J. Helminthol.* **79,** 269–281.

283. Upatham, E.S. and Viyanant, V. (2003) *Opisthorchis viverrini* and opisthorchiasis: a historical review and future perspective. *Acta Trop.* **88,** 171–176.

284. Willie, S.M. and Snyder, R.N. (1977) The identification of *Paragonimus westermanii* in bronchial washings. Case report. *Acta Cytol.* **21,** 101–102.

285. Sumanth, S., D'Souza, P.E., and Jahannath, M.S. (2004) A study of nasal and visceral schistosomosis in cattle slaughtered at an abattoir in Bangalore, South India. *Rev. Sci. Tech.* **23,** 937–942.

286. Jayewardene, L.G. (1962) On two filarial parasites from dogs from Ceylon, *Brugia ceylonensis* n. sp. and *Dipetalonema* sp. *J. Helminthol.* **36,** 269–280.

287. Snowden, K.F. and Hammerberg, B. (1989) The lymphatic pathology of chronic *Brugia pahangi* infection in the dog. *Trans. R. Soc. Trop. Med. Hyg.* **83,** 670–678.

288. Craig, H.L. and Craig, P.S. (2005) Helminth parasites of wolves (*Canis lupus*): a species list and an analysis of published prevalence studies in Nearctic and Palearctic populations. *J. Helminthol.* **79,** 95–103.

289. Todd, K.S. Jr., Bergeland, M.E., and Hickman, G.R. (1975) *Amphimerus pseudofelineus* infection in a cat. *J. Am. Vet. Med. Assoc.* **166,** 458–459.

290. Robinson, R.D., Thompson, D.L., and Lindo, J.F. (1989) A survey of intestinal helminths of well-cared-for dogs in Jamaica, and their potential public health significance. *J. Helminthol.* **63,** 32–38.

291. Wootton, D.M. (1957) The life history of *Cryptocotyle concavum* (Creplin, 1825) Fischoeder, 1903 (Trematoda: Heterophyidae). *J. Parasitol.* **43,** 271–279.

292. Sahai, B.N. and Srivastava, H.D. (1970) Studies on *Echinochasmus perfoliatus* (Ratz, 1908) Dietz, 1909: incidence in dogs and development of the miracidium. *J. Helminthol.* **44,** 315–330.

293. Macpherson, C.N. (2005) Human behaviour and the epidemiology of parasitic zoonoses. *Int. J. Parasitol.* **35,** 1319–1331.

294. Himonas, C.A. (1964) *Heterophyes heterophyes* from dogs in Greece. *J. Parasitol.* **50,** 799.

295. Cho, S.Y., Kim, S.I., Earm, Y.E., and Ho, W.K. (1985) A preliminary observation on watery content of small intestine in *Metagonimus yokogawai* infected dog. *Kisaengch'unghak Chapchi.* **23,** 175–177.

296. Jordan, H.E. and Ashby, W.T. (1957) Liver fluke (*Metorchis conjunctus*) in a dog from South Carolina. *J. Am. Vet. Med. Assoc.* **131,** 239–240.

297. Manfredi, M.T. and Oneto, M. (1997) *Phagicola longa* (Heterophyidae) in dogs from Chile: morphological findings and taxonomical problems. *Parasitologia* **39,** 9–11.

298. Simpson, V.R., Gibbons, L.M., Khalil, L.F., and Williams, J.L. (2005) Cholecystitis in otters (*Lutra lutra*) and mink (*Mustela vison*) caused by the fluke *Pseudamphistomum truncatum. Vet. Rec.* **157,** 49–52.

299. Mansour, N.S., Youssef, M. Awadalla, H.N., Hammouda, N.H., and Boulos, L.M. (1981) Susceptibility of small laboratory animals to *Pygidiopsis genata* (Trematoda: Heterophydae). *J. Egypt. Soc. Parasitol.* **11,** 225–234.

300. Mahmoud, N.M., Abdel-Salam, F.A., Abdel-Gawad, A.F., and el-Assaly, T.M. (1988) Heterophyid metacercarial cysts in Mugil at Cairo with reference to *Stictodora sawakinensis* (Looss, 1899*). J. Egypt. Soc. Parasitol.* **18,** 591–597.

301. Stroud, R.K. (1978) Parasites and associated pathology observed in pinnipeds stranded along the Oregon coast. *J. Wildl. Dis.* **14,** 292–298.

302. Haralabidis, S.T., Papazachariadou, M.G., Koutinas, A.F., and Rallis, T.S. (1988) A survey on the prevalence of gastrointestinal parasites of dogs in the area of Thessaloniki, Greece. *J. Helminthol.* **62,** 45–49.

303. Featherston, D.W. (1969) *Taenia hydatigena.* 1. Growth and development of adult stage in the dog. *Exp. Parasitol.* **25,** 329–338.

304. Edwards, G.T. and Herbert, I.V. (1981) Some quantitative characters used in the identification of *Taenia hydatigena, T. ovis, T. pisiformis* and *T. multiceps* adult worms, and *T. multiceps* metacestodes. *J. Helminthol.* **55,** 1–7.

305. Flueck, W.T. and Jones, A. (2005) Potential existence of a sylvatic cycle of *Taenia ovis krabbei* in Patagonia, Argentina. *Vet. Parasitol.* **135,** 381–383.

306. Coman, B.J. and Rickard, M.D. (1975) The location of *Taenia pisiformis, Taenia ovis* and *Taenia hydatigena* in the gut of the dog and its effect on net environmental contamination with ova. *Z. Parasitenkd.* **47,** 237–248.

307. Daengsvang, S. (1981) Gnathostomiasis in Southeast Asia. *Southeast Asian J. Trop. Med. Public Health.* **12,** 319–332.

308. Theisen, S.K., LeGrange, S.N., Johnson, S.E., Sherding, R.G. and Willard, M.D. (1998) *Physaloptera* infection in 18 dogs with intermittent vomiting. *J. Am. Anim. Hosp. Assoc.* **34,** 74–78.

309. Hatherhill, C.W. (1967) *Diestecostoma mexicanum* infestation of dogs. *Vet. Rec.* **81,** 262.

310. Schmidt, J.M. and Todd, K.S. (1978) Life cycle of *Mesocestoides corti* in the dog (*Canis familiaris*). *Am. J. Vet. Res.* **39,** 1490–1493.

311. Huang, Y.Y., Ikeuchi, H., and Yuda, K. (1970) Case of *Sparganum mansoni* infection and distribution of *Diphyllobothrium erinacei* in cats and dogs in Miyagi Prefecture. *Igaku To Seibutsugaku* **80,** 121–124.

312. Doezie, A.M., Lucius, R.W., Aldeen, W., Hale, D.V., Smith, D.R., and Mamalis, N. (1996) *Thelazia californiensis* conjunctival infestation. *Opthalmic Surg. Lasers* **27,** 716–719.

313. Otranto, D., Lia, R.P., Buono, V., Traversa, D., and Giangaspero, A. (2004) Biology of *Thelazia callipaeda* (Spirurida, Thelaziidae) eyeworms in naturally infected definitive hosts. *Parasitology* **129,** 627–633.

314. Bolio, M.E., Montes, A.M., Alonso, F.D., Gutierrez, C., Bernal, L.J., Rodriguez-Vivas, R.I., et al. (2004) Prevalence of *Dipetalonema dracunculoides* in dogs in Murcia, Spain. *Vet. Rec.* **154,** 726–727.

315. Tarello, W. (2004) Identification and treatment of *Dipetalonema grassii* microfilariae in a cat from central Italy. *Vet. Rec.* **155,** 565–566.

316. Tarello, W. (2003) Dermatitis associated with *Dirofilaria repens* microfilariae in a dog from Rome. *Vet. J.* **165,** 175–177.

317. Beyer, T.A., Pinckney, R.D., and Cooley, A.J. (1999) Massive *Dracunculus insignis* infection in a dog. *J. Am. Vet. Med. Assoc.* **214,** 366–368.

318. Tirgari, M. and Radhakrishnan, C.V. (1975) A case of *Dracunculus medinensis* in a dog. *Vet. Rec.* **96,** 43–44.

319. Zlotorzycka, J., Modrzejewska, M., and Saxena, A.K. (1995) *Heterodoxus spiniger* (Boopiidae, Mallophaga) from *Canis familiaris* from India in the light of scanning electron microscopes. *Wiad Parazytol.* **41,** 455–462.

320. Kraft, W., Kraiss-Gothe, A., and Gothe, R. (1988) *Otodectes cynotis* infestation of dogs and cats: biology of the agent, epidemiology, pathogenesis and diagnosis and case description of generalized mange in dogs. *Tierarztl. Prax.* **16,** 409–415.

CHAPTER
18

Parasites of Cats

Dwight D. Bowman, MS, PhD

PROTOZOA

Phylum Sarcomastigophora

Class Mastigophora (flagellates)

Hemoflagellates

Leishmania spp. **Morphology.** *Leishmania* organisms in the cat are ovoid and measure 2.5 μ to 5 μ long by 1.5 μ to 2 μ wide. The amastigote stage is present in the cat and is morphologically indistinguishable from that of *T. cruzi*. The amastigotes contain a nucleus and a large kinetoplast, are found only in macrophages, and divide by binary fission.

Hosts. Cats are susceptible to *Leishmania* spp. associated with both visceral and cutaneous forms of the disease[1]. Dogs, opossums, sloths, primates, small rodents, and other animals are the primary reservoirs of *Leishmania* spp. Infection by strains causing visceral disease have been reported in cats from Europe, northern Africa, and the Middle East[1,2,3]. Infection by strains causing cutaneous disease have been reported in cats from Texas and South America[4,5].

Life Cycle. *Leishmania* organisms are transmitted between hosts by the bite of a sand fly, *Phlebotomus* spp. in the Old World and *Lutzomyia* spp. in the New World. When the flies bite an infected host, they ingest macrophages in the skin that contain amastigotes (Figure 18.1). In the fly, amastigotes transform into promastigotes that multiply by binary fission. Promastigotes migrate to the salivary glands

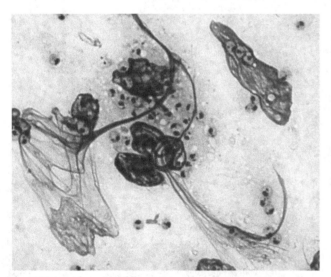

Fig. 18.1 *Leishmania infantum.* Amastigotes in impression smear.

———

Tables are placed at the ends of chapters.

of the fly and are inoculated when the fly bites the next host. In the cat, these transform back into amastigotes.

Pathologic Effects and Clinical Disease. Naturally occurring visceral leishmaniasis has not been studied in cats. Organisms have been seen in the spleen and bone marrow of experimentally infected cats[2,6]. In cutaneous disease, parasites develop at the site of deposition by the fly, such as on the nose and ears. Lesions present as non-healing, chronically expanding dermal ulcers that do not respond to therapies that target bacterial or fungal infections.

Diagnosis. Organisms can be found in stained smears of material from ulcers or in biopsy specimens collected from the affected organs. For a specific diagnosis, molecular techniques are used to determine the species or strain of parasite present.

Treatment and Prevention. Treatment of visceral leishmaniasis is difficult in all cases, and there have been few attempts to treat infected cats. One cat was treated successfully with 20 injections of antimony compound (Glucantime) over a period of 55 days[7]. In one case, cutaneous lesions were excised by surgical removal of the affected pinna. However, cutaneous lesions returned two years later at the stump of the ear, and eventually, on the nose and muzzle[8]. Housing cats in conditions that preclude the bites of sand flies can prevent infection.

Public Health Considerations. Transmission of infection from cats to animal workers requires the transfer of infective material through broken skin. Proper personal protection should greatly reduce the risk of transmission.

Trypanosoma cruzi. **Morphology, Host, and Life Cycle.** The morphology, host distribution, and life cycle of *Trypanosoma cruzi* are presented in Chapter 17, Parasites of Dogs. Cats are commonly found infected in Latin America. Prevalence rates of 2% to 50% have been reported[9,10].

Pathologic Effects and Clinical Disease. *Trypanosoma cruzi* has only been reported on one occasion to cause disease in a cat that presented with convulsions and posterior paralysis[11]. However, it is possible that this is due to little attention being paid to the feline as a host of these parasites in the areas where it is common.

Diagnosis. Diagnosis is by identifying the organisms in blood or organ smears or in tissue sections. Diagnosis can also be made through the culture of the blood in liver infusion tryptose (LIT) medium, or the use of xenodiagnosis, in which the intestinal tracts of clean bugs are examined after feeding on suspected hosts. Additional diagnostic methods include serology and polymerase chain reaction (PCR) assay.

Treatment and Prevention. There is no effective treatment for *Trypanosoma cruzi* infection in cats. Preventing infection is difficult to impossible in cats that are allowed to dwell outside or hunt. Bugs should not gain access to most animal facilities under laboratory conditions. If cats have access to the outside, the facility should be screened to exclude bugs and wild rodents.

Public Health Considerations. Random-source cats acquired from areas enzootic for *T. cruzi* may arrive infected. Animal workers could become infected through contact with the blood of an infected animal, either through a needle stick or by blood entering a wound. If fights occur between cats, the blood from wounds must be considered potentially infectious and handled with due caution to protect personnel.

Enteric flagellates

Giardia felis. **Morphology.** The morphologic features of the trophozoites and cysts of *Giardia felis* are similar to those of *G. canis,* and are described in Chapter 17, Parasites of Dogs.

Hosts. Formerly, it was thought that a single species of *Giardia* infected most mammals, but recent molecular evidence suggests that cats are host to a species different from that found in humans or dogs[12]. *Giardia felis* lives in the proximal small intestine of the host, and is one of the most common parasites of the domestic cat. Prevalence rates range from 1% to 50%, with infections seemingly higher in cattery-housed, versus free-ranging, animals[13].

Life Cycle. The life cycle is similar to that described for *G. canis.* Cysts are infectious when passed in the feces.

Pathologic Effects and Clinical Disease. There is little pathology associated with *Giardia.* Thus, the mechanisms underlying the clinical signs have yet to be determined. Most cats remain asymptomatic, though infections may persist for months to years. Others develop intermittent to chronic diarrhea that is amenable to treatment.

Diagnosis. Fecal cysts are easily demonstrated in zinc sulfate flotation. The motile trophozoites can be observed in direct saline smears made from fresh, diarrheic feces. An antigen detection test has been approved for the diagnosis of the infection in the feces of cats[13].

Treatment. Treatments effective against *Giardia* include metronidazole and fenbendazole[14,15]. Cats should be treated with both products simultaneously for five days. If the cat remains positive after treatment, it is suggested that the treatment be repeated for 10 days.

Prevention. Preventing infection is difficult because so many cats are infected, and re-infection appears common. In those situations where *Giardia*-free cats are required, it may be necessary to use cesarean rederivation and barrier housing. Treatment to eradicate *G. felis* from a colony should include simultaneous treatment of all animals, along with daily bathing and transfer to clean cages.

Public Health Considerations. *Giardia felis* from cats has been found in humans. However, most human *Giardia* carriers are infected with the human species, *G. lamblia.* Cats can also be infected with *G. lamblia,* but less commonly than dogs[16]. Animal workers should practice personal hygiene when cleaning or during handling and disposal of cat feces.

Tetratrichomonas felistomae. **Morphology.** Trophozoites of *Tetratrichomonas felistomae* measure 6 μ to 11 μ long and 3 μ to 5 μ wide. An axostyle runs the length of the trophozoite, causing the posterior end to appear pointed. Trophozoites bear four anteriorly directed free-flagella, and a posteriorly directed flagellum attached by an undulating membrane. The posterior flagellum may terminate at the end of the undulating membrane or extend further as a short, unattached portion.

Hosts and Life Cycle. *Tetratrichomonas felistomae* inhabits the gingival border of cats. It remains uncertain whether organisms of similar appearance in dogs are the same or different species[17]. The life cycle is direct. Trophozoites represent the only stage present, and divide by binary fission. Transmission is by passage through saliva.

Pathologic Effects and Clinical Disease. *Tetratrichomonas felistomae* has been found in cats with gingivitis and in normal cats. Thus, the pathogenic potential of *T. felistomae* is uncertain. It is possible that *T. felistomae* is a commensal, and has simply been found in the mouths of cats undergoing oral examination, or that the organisms increase in number along areas of gingival inflammation. It should be noted that cats with gingivitis often have underlying viral infections such as FIV, FeLV, and FIP[18].

Diagnosis. The organisms can be found by placing a small quantity of material from along the gum-line of a suspect cat on a slide with saline and examining it with a microscope. The trichomonads move with a jerky, rapid, movement of the flagella. The undulating can occasionally be observed.

Treatment and Prevention. Improved dental hygiene will probably remove *T. felistomae.* Prevention of transmission is very difficult in group-housed cats.

Public Health Considerations. *Tetratrichomonas felistomae* does not infect humans.

Tritrichomonas foetus. **Morphology.** Trophozoites of *Tritrichomonas foetus* resemble those of *Pentatrichomonas hominis,* and measure 15 μ long and 5 μ wide. There are three anteriorly directed flagella and a posterior flagellum that trails free. The undulating membrane runs nearly the full length of the trophozoite. The costa at the anterior end is prominent, and the axostyle is thick throughout its length. There is no cyst stage.

Hosts and Life Cycle. Recent evidence suggests that natural hosts of *T. foetus* also include cats and swine, in addition to cattle, the traditional host[19]. The life cycle is direct. Transmission is fecal-oral, with trophozoites passing between hosts. Trophozoites survive for short periods in fresh feces.

Pathologic Effects and Clinical Disease. Cats infected with *T. foetus* develop large bowel diarrhea and typically produce loose, pasty ("cow-pie") feces that soils the hair coat[19]. Diarrhea may be sporadic or persistent, and does not always respond to therapy[20].

Diagnosis. Trophozoites can be observed in fecal smears prepared in saline rather than water. The trophozoites are seen to swim with a directional motion which is easily distinguished from the falling-leaf motion of *G. felis* trophozoites. Infections in cats have also been diagnosed using the In-Pouch TF kit (BioMed Diagnostics Inc.), typically used for diagnosing trichomoniasis in cattle[21]. The kit facilitates culture of the agent and does not require the preparation of special media or the use of special incubators. *T. foetus* may be detected using single-tube polymerase chain reaction assay[22].

Treatment and Prevention. In those cases where treatment is deemed necessary, some, but not all, infections may be cleared by treatment with metronidazole. Routine cleaning and fecal disposal clears areas where cats may become infected with trophozoites passed in the feces.

Public Health Considerations. It is unlikely that humans are susceptible to infection with *T. foetus.* An unusual and fatal case of meningoencephalitis in a human has been reported. The patient had recently undergone bone marrow transplantation and was immune suppressed. *Tritrichomonas foetus* was recovered at autopsy. However, the source of the infection was not identified[23].

Phylum Apicomplexa

Class Coccidia

Cryptosporidium felis

Morphology. The oocysts of *Cryptosporidium felis* are the smallest of the coccidial-like oocysts shed in cat feces.

Oocysts are spheroid and 5 μ in diameter. They contain four sporozoites, and are infectious when passed.

Hosts. Cats serve as the natural host of *C. felis*[24]. Infections are common throughout the world[25–27].

Life Cycle. The life cycle of *C. felis* is direct. Cats become infected upon ingestion of sporulated oocysts in cat feces. Oocysts release sporozoites in the small intestine, and the free sporozoites then penetrate the epithelial cells of the small intestine. Development occurs just under the membrane of the infected cell. There are two schizogonous cycles, followed by gametogony and oocyst production.

Pathologic Effects and Clinical Disease. Infection causes loss of water balance in intestinal epithelial cells, resulting in diarrhea[28]. Most cats actually show few signs of infection unless they have been immunosuppressed or have other underlying conditions such as a malignancy.

Diagnosis, Treatment, and Prevention. The small fecal oocysts are best demonstrated using sugar flotation. Antigen detection kits developed for use in human medicine have also proven useful for diagnosing infections in other animals. No drugs are effective against *C. felis.* Cats have been treated with paromomycin, but this is not always successful, and there are sometimes complications[29]. *Cryptosporidium felis* is ideally suited for survival and transmission within animal facilities. The oocysts are infectious when passed and are moderately resistant to environmental extremes. Most infections are asymptomatic; thus, the entire colony may eventually become infected.

Public Health Considerations. Humans are not natural hosts of *C. felis.* Rarely, however, infections have been reported in immunocompromised humans[30]. Thus, animal workers should exercise personal hygiene when working with potentially infected cats.

Isospora (= Cystoisospora) felis

Morphology. Ocysts of *Isospora felis* are broadly ellipsoidal to ovoid and measure 38 μ to 51 μ long by 27 μ to 39 μ wide. The oocyst is not sporulated when passed in the feces. After the oocyst sporulates, it contains two sporocysts, each containing four sporozoites (Figure 18.2). The sporocysts tend to be spheroid and measure 20 μ to 26 μ long by 17 μ to 22 μ wide. The sporulated sporocyst contains a prominent residuum and four sporozoites. The sporocysts are 10 μ to 15 μ long.

Hosts. Cats are the only hosts of the sexual stages of *I. felis. Isospora felis* has been found in the feces of cats around the world[27,31,32]. Rodents, cows, and dogs have been shown to be capable of serving as paratenic hosts[33–35],

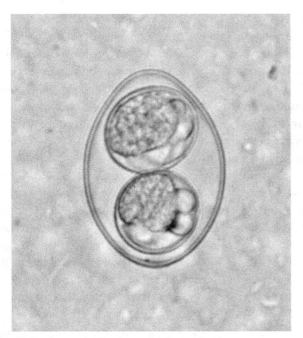

Fig. 18.2 *Isospora* (= *Cystoisospora*) *felis* sporulated oocyst.

therefore, some investigators place *I. felis* in the genus *Cystoisospora*.

Life Cycle. Typically, the life cycle is direct[35]. Cats become infected through ingestion of sporulated oocysts. Cats can also be infected through the ingestion of rodents or birds that harbor sporozoites. After ingesting an oocyst or an infected paratenic host, schizogony and gametogony occur in the duodenal or jejunal epithelium[36]. Oocysts appear in the feces seven to 11 days after infection, and the patent period is 10 to 11 days.

Pathologic Effects and Clinical Disease. *Isospora felis* is moderately pathogenic in kittens older than six weeks of age[35,37,38]. After infection, there is erosion of the superficial epithelial cells, and then later destruction of the mucosa. Clinical signs include soft, mucoid feces. In younger kittens, the infection can induce enteritis, emaciation, blood-tinged feces, and death.

Diagnosis. The oocyst in the feces of cats is easily identified after floatation by its large size and distinctly ovoid shape.

Treatment. Toltrazuril (10 to 30 mg/kg daily for three days) or ponazuril (20 mg/kg daily for one to three days) should clear animals of their infections[39]. However, the shedding of any oocysts that are already formed will not be affected by the administration of anticoccidials, because these cannot penetrate the oocyst wall.

Prevention. The oocysts require time in the external environment to sporulate and become infectious. Sporulation time ranges from eight hours at 38°C to 40 hours at 20°C, and several days at lower temperatures. The oocysts are resistant to environmental extremes. Thus, animal workers should take care not to bring oocysts into the animal facility on their shoes or clothing.

Public Health Considerations. *Isospora felis* is not infectious to humans.

Isospora (= Cystoisospora) rivolta

Morphology. Oocysts of *Isospora rivolta* measure 23 μ to 29 μ long by 20 μ to 26 μ wide and are nearly spherical in shape. There is no micropyle present, and inclusions, the so-called "hazy bodies," may be observed between the sporont and the wall of the oocyst in freshly passed feces. The hazy bodies degenerate as the sporont sporulates, and the mature sporulated oocysts do not contain a residuum. Each sporulated oocyst contains two sporocysts, and each sporocyst contains four sporozoites.

Hosts. Cats are the only hosts for the sexual stages of *I. rivolta*. *Isospora rivolta* has been found in the feces of cats around the world[27,31,32]. Mice and other rodents, as well as cows and opossums, have been found to serve as paratenic hosts[35,40]. Thus, like *I. felis*, *I. rivolta* has been placed in the genus *Cystoisospora*.

Life Cycle. The life cycle is similar to that of *I. felis*[35,40]. The prepatent period is four to seven days, and the patent period is usually greater than two weeks.

Pathologic Effects. Infections with *Isospora rivolta* are capable of causing disease in newborn, but not weaned, kittens[40]. The lesions consist of congestion, erosion of the intestinal epithelium, and villous atrophy.

Clinical Disease. Diarrhea can occur three to four days after oocyst inoculation in newborn animals. Heavily infected kittens may die. Animals inoculated at 10 to 13 weeks of age or older typically show no signs of infection.

Diagnosis, Treatment, and Prevention. The oocysts can be found using flotation procedures, and are identified by size. Treatment is as described for *I. felis*. The oocysts require time in the external environment (24 hours at 24°C, 12 hours at 30°C, and 8 hours at 37°C) to sporulate and become infectious. Thus, the removal of the feces on a very regular basis prevents the oocysts from becoming infectious. The oocysts are resistant to environmental extremes; thus, it is important that animal workers take care not to transport oocysts into the facility on shoes or clothing.

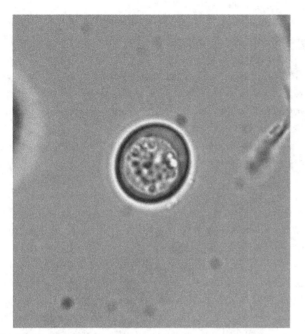

Fig. 18.3 *Toxoplasma gondii* unsporulated oocyst.

Public Health Considerations. Humans are not susceptible to infection with *I. rivolta*.

Toxoplasma gondii

Morphology. Oocysts of *Toxoplasma gondii* are spherical to subspherical, and measure 11 μ to 13 μ in diameter (Figure 18.3). Sporulated oocysts contain a residuum and two sporocysts, both of which contain four sporozoites. Oocysts of *T. gondii* are morphologically indistinguishable from the other small oocysts passed in cat feces, i.e., *Hammondia hammondi* and *Besnoitia darlingi*. The asexual stages, the tachyzoites and bradyzoites, are crescent- or banana-shaped and measure 4 μ to 8 μ long by 2 μ to 4 μ wide.

Hosts. Cats and other felids are the only hosts in which sexual reproduction of the parasite occurs. Many, if not most, warm-blooded animals may serve as paratenic hosts. Serological surveys reveal that a history of exposure to *T. gondii* depends on the population of cats sampled, that exposure is common, and that the percentage of cats with a history of exposure increases as cats age[41–44]. Cats from specific pathogen free (SPF) colonies are typically free of infection with *T. gondii*. Other than very young kittens, cats from random-source facilities should be assumed to be infected until serological tests indicate otherwise.

Life Cycle. The life cycle of *T. gondii* may be direct or indirect. Cats become infected by ingesting sporulated oocysts (direct) or infected paratenic hosts (indirect)[45,46]. Following ingestion of oocysts, the prepatent period is 18 days[47], but is only three to 10 days for cats consuming paratenic hosts. The patent period ranges from seven to 20 days. Only about 20% of cats that ingest oocysts will produce oocysts, while about 97% of cats fed tissues that contain bradyzoites will produce oocysts. Cats may also be congenitally infected, but the frequency of this mode of infection is unknown[48].

Pathologic Effects. Cats with disseminated disease develop pathologic changes specific to the organ systems involved[49]. Lesions are most commonly seen in the lungs, and include diffuse edema and congestion, failure to collapse, and discoloration. The liver may also be affected, and diffuse necrotizing hepatitis may be visible grossly. Ocular lesions, including uveitis and retinochoroiditis, may occur commonly. The development of central nervous system disease is rare, and results in glial nodules and necrotizing abscesses. In contrast, cats undergoing the intestinal enteroepithelial cycle typically do not develop intestinal pathology[50] unless there is concurrent visceral disease.

Clinical Disease. Cats with disseminated disease can develop fever (40°C to 42°C), dyspnea, polypnea, icterus, anorexia, lethargy, hypothermia, and sudden death[51,52]. Rare central nervous system involvement results in neurologic signs. As noted above, intestinal infection is generally asymptomatic.

Diagnosis. Diagnosis is by demonstration of the oocysts in the feces using routine flotation methods. Specific determination of *T. gondii*, if required, can be done by mouse inoculation or polymerase chain reaction (PCR) techniques. A diagnosis of disseminated disease must meet three criteria, including: (1) clinical signs consistent with the toxoplasmosis, (2) serologic evidence of recent or active infection, and (3) positive response to anti-*Toxoplasma* treatment or have organisms demonstrated in biopsy specimens or body fluids. Typically, a high IgM titer and low IgG titer indicate active infection. Organisms can be detected in tissues by mouse inoculation, immunohistochemistry, PCR assay, or microscopic examination of stained bronchiolar lavage or peritoneal aspirate material.

Treatment. The current drug of choice for disseminated toxoplasmosis in cats is clindamycin hydrochloride, administered orally at 10 to 12 mg/kg twice daily for four weeks. Ponazuril and toltrazuril may also be effective[53,54].

Prevention. The best means of prevention in the animal care facility is the routine cleaning of litter pans, especially in the case of cats that have been acquired recently[55]. Oocysts sporulate within 24 hours at 25°C. Oocysts survive well at 4°C, but cannot tolerate freezing, and are killed within 24 hours at 37°C and within minutes at 50°C.

Public Health Considerations. *Toxoplasma gondii* is a significant zoonosis. Pregnant and immune-suppressed people are at increased risk for serious disease. Under most circumstances cats that have once shed oocysts of *T. gondii* do not shed again[56]. However, immune suppression with high daily doses of corticosteroids (10 to 80 mg/kg prednisolone) can cause chronically infected cats to resume oocyst shedding, but typical clinical doses of 5 to 20 mg/kg corticosteroid given weekly for four weeks do not cause oocyst excretion.

Infection with *I. felis* may facilitate a resumption of excretion of *T. gondii* oocysts, while cats that become infected with feline immunodeficiency virus do not resume oocyst shedding. Animal workers should exercise proper personal hygiene when working with potentially infected cats. Regular cage cleaning and hand washing are important and help prevent infections. Most laboratory infections have resulted from accidental self-inoculation via needle sticks. Thus, researchers should exercise extreme caution when handling infectious material.

Class Piroplasmidia

Cytauxzoon felis

Morphology. Two life cycle stages of *Cytauxzoon felis* occur in the cat[57]. Schizonts occur within histiocytes, and macrophages present in the bone marrow, veins, and venules of various organs, including the lungs, liver, spleen, lymph nodes, brain, and kidneys (Figure 18.4). Merozoites are produced later in the infection, and are found in circulating red blood cells. Thus, merozoites may not be found in the blood of cats with acute disease.

Hosts. The bobcat is the natural definitive host of *C. felis*. Other large exotic cats, as well as small domestic cats, may also become infected. The prevalence of infection is high in the southeastern United States. Infections have also been reported from cats in Mongolia, Spain, Zimbabwe, and South Africa[58–60]. *C. felis* is transmitted by ticks, and therefore is rare in research colony cats.

Life Cycle. Cats become infected through the bite of the tick vector *Dermacentor variabilis*[61]. Schizonts develop within macrophages, which become markedly enlarged. If the cat survives for more than six days, erythrocytes become

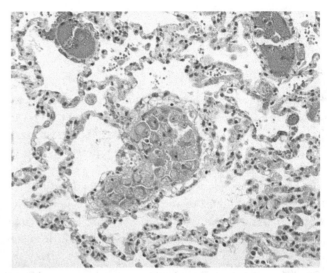

Fig. 18.4 *Cytauxzoon felis* schizonts in macrophages occluding the lumen of a blood vessel in the lung of a naturally infected cat.

infected and the merozoite stage develops. It is thought that blood-feeding ticks become infected as nymphs and transmit the parasite to the next host as adults.

Pathologic Effects and Clinical Disease. Cats with acute disease typically develop anemia, depression, fever, dehydration, and icterus. The majority of cats die within nine to 15 days of inoculation[62,63]. The cause of death is occlusion of veins and venules with schizont-laden macrophages. Hematologic changes may be severe, and result from displacement of hematopoietic tissue within the bone marrow. If the cat survives acute infection, the small merozoites can be found in the red blood cells. Typically, no more than 1% to 4% of the red blood cells are infected. Other pathologic findings include splenomegaly and hepatomegaly. Some cats survive the infection without treatment[64].

Diagnosis, Treatment, and Prevention. During the acute phase of the disease, organisms can be identified in smears of bone marrow or in biopsy specimens. Chronic disease is diagnosed by finding the merozoites in red blood cells. There are no treatments that are consistently efficacious during the acute stage of the disease. Antiprotozoals can be administered but the prognosis is poor. Supportive care should be provided, and includes antibiotics to prevent secondary bacterial infections. Exclusion of ticks from the animal facility prevents the spread of infection from random-source cats harboring *C. felis* at the time of entry into the facility.

Public Health Considerations. *Cytauxzoon felis* does not appear to be infectious to humans.

TREMATODES

Family Dicrocoeliidae

Platynosomum fastosum

Morphology. Adult *Platynosomum fastosum* flukes are lanceolate and measure 4 mm to 8 mm long by 1.2 mm to 2.5 mm wide (Figure 18.5)[65, 66]. The egg is brown, oval, thick-shelled, and operculated. The egg measures 34 μ to 50 μ long by 20 μ to 35 μ wide.

Hosts. *Platynosomum fastosum* occurs in the gallbladder and bile duct of the cat in most regions of the world[67–71]. It is common in the Caribbean, and in one survey, the prevalence in the Bahamas was 50%. It is less common in the United States. *Platynosomum fastosum* has also been reported from the American opossum, *Didelphis virginiana.*

Life Cycle. Eggs passed in the feces release miracidia, which develop into cercariae in a snail intermediate host. Cercariae leaving the snail are ingested by second intermediate hosts, terrestrial isopods ("pill bugs"), which are in turn eaten by a paratenic host. These include lizards and occasionally, frogs or toads, where the immature trematodes encyst in the common bile duct or gallbladder. Cats become infected by the ingestion of the paratenic host. If fact, it is for this reason that infection with *P. fastosum* is sometimes called "lizard poisoning." The prepatent period is eight weeks[66].

Pathologic Effects and Clinical Disease. With infection, the gallbladder and bile duct are distended, the wall of the bile duct is thickened, and the liver is enlarged[72–74]. Histologic lesions include hyperplasia of the biliary epithelium, cellular infiltration of the lamina propria, and fibrosis of the duct wall (Figure 18.6)[75]. In heavy infections, clinical signs include vomiting, diarrhea, emaciation, jaundice, and death[72–74].

Diagnosis and Treatment. Diagnosis is by demonstrating the eggs in the feces or flukes in the gallbladder or bile duct during surgery or necropsy, or in histologic sections. Praziquantel (20 mg/kg) markedly reduces the number of eggs shed by infected cats. For complete resolution, worms may be surgically removed from the gallbladder.

Prevention. Because of the need for multiple intermediate hosts for completion of the life cycle, there is little chance of the infection cycling within a facility. However, in areas where the disease is common, random-source cats are likely to be infected. It is important in those areas to prevent the access of lizards to any outside pens where animals may be held.

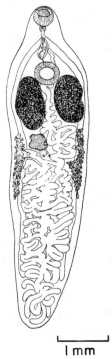

|— 1 mm —|

Fig. 18.5 *Platynosomum fastosum* adult. Reproduced from Lapage, G. (1962) with permission.

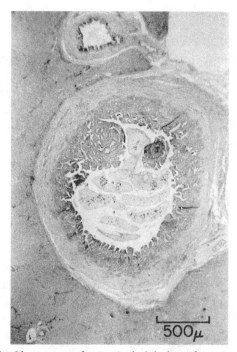

500μ

Fig. 18.6 *Platynosomum fastosum* in the bile duct of a cat. Reproduced from Greve, J.H. and Leonard, P.O. (1966) with permission.

Public Health Considerations. *Platynosomum fastosum* does not infect humans.

Family Opisthorchidae

Clonorchis sinensis

Morphology. Adult *Clonorchis sinensis* are lanceolate, have a smooth tegument, and measure 10 mm to 35 mm long by 3 mm to 5 mm wide[76]. The ventral sucker is small, the vitellaria are lateral, and the egg-filled uterus fills the middle of the anterior half of the body between the intestinal ceca. The paired testes are in the posterior of the body and are highly branched. The eggs have a thick shell with a distinct, convex operculum, contain an asymmetrical miracidium when passed in the feces, and measure 27 μ to 35 μ long by 12 μ to 20 μ wide (Figure 18.7).

Hosts. *Clonorchis sinensis* is capable of developing in many fish-eating mammals, birds, and reptiles in Japan and Southeast Asia[77]. Cats, dogs, and humans are commonly infected in endemic areas. The adults of these flukes occur in the gall bladder, bile duct, and sometimes the pancreatic ducts and small intestine.

Life Cycle. Eggs passed in the feces hatch following ingestion by a suitable snail. They develop in the snail to the cercarial stage, escape, and invade the flesh of a suitable freshwater fish. The endothermal host becomes infected by eating the fish. Metacercariae are released in the duodenum and migrate up the bile duct. Egg production occurs three to four weeks after infection; the complete life cycle requires about four months.

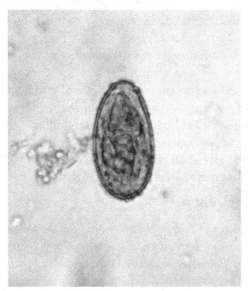

Fig. 18.7 *Clonorchis sinensis* egg.

Pathologic Effects and Clinical Disease. In heavy infections, *C. sinensis* causes catarrhal inflammation and epithelial desquamation of the bile duct, variable cirrhosis, passive congestion of the liver, and rarely, pancreatitis. Clinical signs are usually absent in mild infections, but the flukes can induce jaundice associated with bile stasis.

Diagnosis, Treatment, and Prevention. Diagnosis is based on identification of the eggs in the feces or adult worms in the bile duct at necropsy. Adult worms may also be visualized with computed tomography. Infection with *C. sinensis* can be eliminated with praziquantel (50 mg/kg). Treatment is likely to require more than one dose[78]. There is little chance of transmission taking place in the laboratory. Animals should not be fed raw fish.

Public Health Considerations. While humans are susceptible to infection by *C. sinensis,* there is no concern of transmission from cats to humans.

Opisthorchis tenuicollis

Opisthorchis tenuicollis closely resembles *C. sinensis* morphologically and biologically. Thus, the reader is directed to the preceding section on *C. sinensis* for information equally applicable to *O. tenuicollis*. Adult flukes measure 7 mm to 18 mm long by 1.5 mm to 3 mm wide. The paired testes are in the posterior of the body and are globular. The eggs measure 26 μ to 30 μ long by 11 μ to 15 μ wide. *Opisthorchis tenuicollis* occurs in North America, Europe, and Asia[77,79]. Pathologic changes, clinical findings, diagnosis, treatment, prevention, and public health considerations are similar to those of *C. sinensis*.

Family Troglotrematidae

Paragonimus sp.

Cats are susceptible to infection with *Paragonimus kellicotti* and *P. westermanii*. The interested reader is directed to Chapter 17, Parasites of Dogs, for general information concerning these flukes. In the cat, gross lesions consist of focal areas of emphysema and soft, dark red-to-brown cysts, 2 cm to 3 cm in diameter, that are distributed throughout the lung parenchyma (Figure 18.8)[80]. Incision of the cysts discloses the flukes, usually one to three in each cyst (Figure 18.9). Pleural adhesions sometimes occur. Histology of the lesions reveals hyperplasia of the bronchial epithelium and submucosal bronchial glands and focal areas of inflammation in the lung parenchyma with clusters of fluke eggs (Figure 18.10). Parasites in the lungs cause coughing, wheezing, moist rales, and progressive emaciation. Occasionally, the young

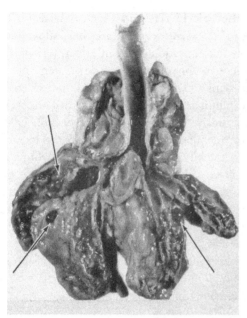

Fig. 18.8 *Paragonimus kellicotti* cysts (arrows) in the lungs of a cat. Reproduced from Herman, L.H. and Helland, D.R. (1966) with permission.

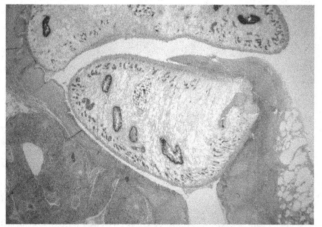

Fig. 18.9 *Paragonimus kellicotti* histological section through two worms in a nodule in the lung of a naturally infected cat.

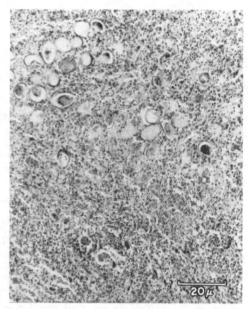

Fig. 18.10 *Paragonimus kellicotti* in the lung of a cat. Note inflammatory cells and fluke eggs. Reproduced from Herman, L.H. and Helland, D.R. (1966) with permission.

CESTODES

Pseudophyllidea

Diphyllobothrium latum

The biology of *Diphyllobothrium latum* is presented in Chapter 17, Parasites of Dogs. Infections are common in the small intestine of cats, other wild carnivores, and humans in areas where pike, perch, and salmonid fishes are found. It is most prevalent in the Great Lakes region of North America, the Baltic region of northern Europe, the lake regions of central Europe and southern Chile, and in Japan[83–85]. Infection in random-source cats is common in endemic areas and absent in others. It does not occur in laboratory cats reared on diets free of raw fish. Natural infections of cats are usually unapparent. Human infections are associated with eosinophilia and anemia due to worm competition for vitamin B_{12}. Similar effects have not been reported in cats. Praziquantel is effective, although it may require dosages as high as 7.5 mg/kg.

Spirometra spp.

The biology of *Spirometra mansoni* and *S. mansonoides* is presented in Chapter 17, Parasites of Dogs. These tapeworms are parasites of cats and other carnivores around the world[67,77,84]. Pathologic effects in cats are variable, and when present, are usually minimal[86]. Likewise, clinical

migrating flukes penetrate the pleura and cause pneumothorax. This will also occasionally happen when a mature cyst ruptures. On rare occasions, the flukes migrate to ectopic locations such as the brain or liver, and these infections are associated with the disruption of function of the organ involved. Infections can be treated through the administration of fenbendazole (50 mg/kg/day for 14 days) or praziquantel (50 mg/kg/day for three days)[81,82].

disease is usually absent. Some of the early workers believed that infections of cats with *S. mansonoides* caused severe anemia and weight loss in spite of cats developing a voracious appetite. However, these observations have not been confirmed. Treatment has been successful with praziquantel (7.5 mg/kg). Because cats acquire infections through the ingestion of infected intermediate hosts, transmission should not occur in the animal facility.

Cyclophyllidea

Dipylidium caninum

The biology of *Dipylidium caninum* is presented in Chapter 17, Parasites of Dogs. Cats are commonly infected in many parts of the world[87,88]. However, improved flea control has markedly decreased the prevalence of infection. Still, random-source cats may be infected upon entry into the animal facility. There are few pathologic effects associated with the presence of tapeworms in the small intestine. The worms attach with their rostellum to the intestinal mucosa and cause slight wounds at the attachment site. They move about throughout the day, so the small wounds are greater in number than the actual number of adult worms that are present. Infections in cats are usually asymptomatic, though heavy infections may cause weakness, emaciation, vomiting, diarrhea, a voracious appetite, convulsions, and chronic enteritis which may be hemorrhagic. Praziquantel is effective at removing the flukes. Flea control must be instituted to break the life cycle.

Taenia taeniaeformis

Morphology. The adult worm measures 15 cm to 60 cm long and 5 mm to 6 mm wide[76]. The scolex bears a rostellum with two crowns of claw-hammer-shaped hooks. The gravid segments contain an egg-filled uterus composed of a central, longitudinal stem with 16 to 18 lateral branches on each side. The posterior segments are characteristically bell-shaped (Figure 18.11). Eggs are typical taeniid; they are spherical, measure 24 μ to 31 μ long by 22 μ to 27 μ wide, and have a striated capsule (Figure 18.12).

Hosts. Adult *Taenia taeniaeformis* (Syn. *Taenia infantis*) occurs in the small intestine of wild and domestic cats throughout the world[32,76,77]. Random-source cats are often infected. The larva is common in the liver of mice, rats, black rats, cotton rats, voles, and other wild rodents.

Life Cycle. The larval stage, a strobilocercus, is found in the liver of the intermediate host. Following ingestion by a cat, the larval tapeworm matures in the cat intestine

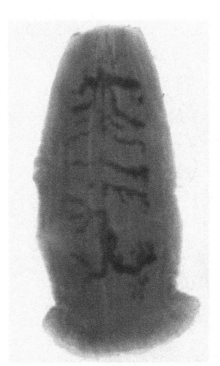

Fig. 18.11 *Taenia taeniaeformis* segment. Note the bell shape. Courtesy of J.R. Georgi, Cornell University.

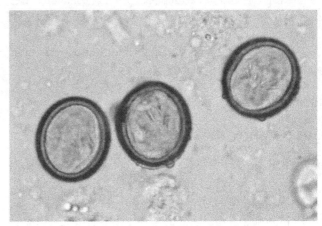

Fig. 18.12 *Taenia taeniaeformis* eggs. Courtesy of J.R. Georgi, Cornell University.

within a few weeks. Gravid proglottids and eggs are then passed in the feces (Figure 18.13).

Pathologic Effects and Clinical Disease. Pathologic changes are limited to focal areas of necrosis associated with embedding of the scolex into the wall of the intestinal mucosa. There are no clinical signs associated with the infection.

Diagnosis, Treatment, and Prevention. Diagnosis is based on finding the adult worm in the intestine or the eggs or

TRANSMISSION OF TAENIA TAENIAEFORMIS

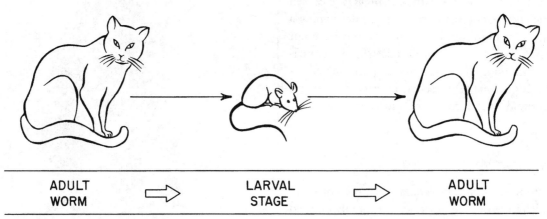

ADULT
WORM ⇨ LARVAL
STAGE ⇨ ADULT
WORM

Fig. 18.13 Life cycle of *Taenia taeniaeformis*. Note that the entire life cycle can be completed in the laboratory. Courtesy of Marietta Voge, University of California.

gravid proglottids in the feces. If a taeniid segment is found in the feces of a cat, the chances are very good that the species is *T. taeniaeformis*. However, in areas where *Echinococcus multilocularis* is prevalent, it might be difficult to ascertain whether the host is infected with *Taenia* or *Echinococcus* if only a taeniid egg is found in a fecal preparation. Praziquantel effectively eliminates the infection[89]. Newly acquired cats should be examined and treated if infected.

Public Health Considerations. Humans have occasionally become infected with *T. taeniaeformis,* this is quite rare[90].

NEMATODES

Superfamily Ascaridoidea

Toxascaris leonina

The biology of *Toxascaris leonina* is presented in Chapter 17, Parasites of Dogs. *Toxascara leonina* is common in the small intestine of cats and other carnivores throughout the world[83,84]. Random-source cats are occasionally found to be infected with *T. leonina,* but less commonly than with *Toxocara cati*. *Toxascaris leonina* is uncommon in laboratory cat colonies with good management and sanitation practices. Neither transplacental nor transmammary transmission occur. Thus, the life cycle is not easily maintained within colonies. Pathologic changes are absent in cats infected with *T. leonina*. Likewise, clinical signs are absent.

Toxocara cati

Morphology. Adults of *Toxocara cati* (Syn. *Toxocara mystax*) are large, cream-colored worms that are curved ventrally at

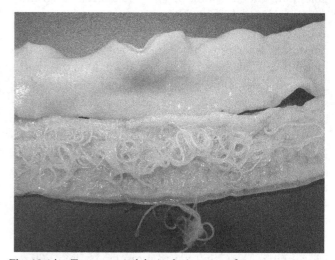

Fig. 18.14 *Toxocara cati* adults in the intestine of a cat at necropsy.

the anterior end and have cervical alae[76]. The adults are similar to those of *T. canis,* from which they can be differentiated by their short, broad, cervical alae that end abruptly, and by the long spicules of the male (Figure 18.14). The male measures 3 cm to 7 cm long and has a narrow, digitiform, terminal appendage; caudal alae; and winged spicules. The female is 4 cm to 10 cm long and has its vulva in the anterior quarter of the body. The egg, which is smaller and more finely pitted than that of *T. canis,* measures 70 μ long by 65 μ wide (Figure 18.15).

Hosts. *Toxocara cati* is found in the small intestine of cats and other felids throughout the world[32,77,83,91]. It is the most common ascarid of cats and is frequently a serious pathogen in young animals. Random-source laboratory

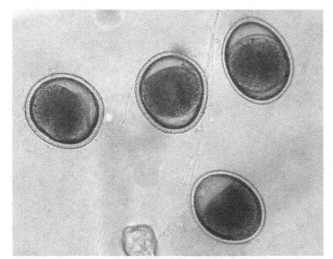

Fig. 18.15 *Toxocara cati* eggs. Courtesy of J.R. Georgi, Cornell University.

cats are frequently infected, but infections are uncommon in laboratory colonies.

Life Cycle. The life cycle differs from that of *T. canis* in that infection is commonly by ingestion of larvae encysted in earthworms, cockroaches, birds, rodents, and a variety of other paratenic hosts[76]. Larvae thus ingested develop in the cat intestine without undergoing parenteral migration. Larvae enter the stomach wall and begin their final development, eventually returning to the small intestinal lumen for the patent adult phase. Infection can also occur through the ingestion of embryonated eggs. Larvae obtained by this route likewise do not typically undergo somatic migration, but develop within the wall of the stomach and intestine. Some worms ingested as embryonated eggs undergo migration to deeper tissues. Kittens routinely become infected with *T. cati* through transmammary transmission of larvae. When kittens are infected via this route, the worms do not migrate outside of the gastrointestinal tract[92]. Transplacental transmission does not occur.

Pathologic Effects and Clinical Disease. Occasionally, infected kittens develop thickened bowel loops. Typically, infected kittens develop neither pathologic changes nor clinical signs of infection, though frequently infected kittens can develop pronounced medial hypertrophy of the pulmonary vessels.

Diagnosis, Treatment, and Prevention. Diagnosis is based on demonstration of eggs in the feces or worms in the intestine. Many products are approved for treating infections with *T. cati*[93,94]. Little research has been done to develop methods of preventing transmammary transmission.

Sanitation and frequent examination and treatment greatly reduce environmental contamination and usually prevent heavy infections. Newly acquired cats should be examined on arrival and treated as necessary.

Public Health Considerations. The larvae of *Toxocara cati* are capable of causing visceral larva migrans in people[95]. It has long been believed that most infections in people have been due to the larvae of *T. canis,* but recent serological evidence suggests that *T. cati* is another common cause of human infections.

Superfamily Strongyloidea

Ancylostoma braziliense

Morphology. Adult male *Ancylostoma braziliense* measure 7.8 mm to 8.5 mm long and females measure 9 mm to 10.5 mm long. There are two teeth on each side of the buccal cavity; the outer pair is large and the inner pair is very small (Figure 18.16). The eggs are indistinguishable from those of *A. caninum* and *A. tubaeforme,* but are smaller than those of *Uncinaria stenocephala.*

Hosts. *Ancylostoma braziliense* occurs in the small intestine of wild and domestic felids and canids throughout the Caribbean coastal areas of the Americas and along eastern coastal areas of South America[96,97]. *Ancylostoma braziliense* is frequently identified in random-source cats in endemic areas, but is uncommon in laboratory facilities.

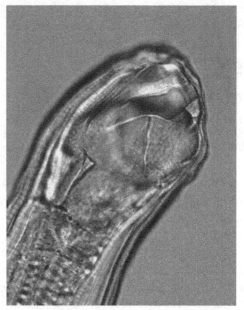

Fig. 18.16 *Ancylostoma braziliense* buccal capsule, lateral view.

Larvae may persist in rodent paratenic hosts for up to 18 months[98].

Life Cycle. The life cycle of *Ancylostoma braziliense* is similar to that of *A. tubaeforme.* Ingested larvae enter the intestinal mucosa and mature to the fourth larval stage before final maturation to the adult stage within the lumen of the small intestine. Skin-penetrating larvae migrate to the lungs and are later coughed up and swallowed, and complete their maturation in the intestinal lumen. The prepatent period is 14 to 16 days after oral inoculation, and 14 to 27 days after skin penetration. It appears that neither transplacental nor transmammary transmission occur in kittens.

Pathologic Effects and Clinical Disease. Compared to infection with other hookworms, infection with *A. braziliense* causes relatively mild hemorrhage at feeding sites within the intestine. Blood loss from worm feeding is only 1 to 2 μl/worm/day. Infection of kittens does not usually affect hemoglobin levels or weight gain. However, heavily infected kittens could eventually become anemic from chronic blood loss.

Diagnosis, Treatment, and Prevention. Diagnosis is based on finding eggs in the feces or mature worms in the intestine at necropsy. Eggs can be specifically identified by modern molecular methods[99]. There are products approved for use against adult *A. braziliense,* and most of the formulations effective against *A. tubaeforme* are also likely to be efficacious. Protective measures for a facility are as described for *A. tubaeforme.*

Public Health Considerations. *Ancylostoma braziliense* is the major cause of cutaneous larva migrans in humans[100]. Larvae can develop to the infective stage in a few days in moist environments with temperatures around 30°C. Therefore, animal caretakers should practice excellent personal hygiene and remove cat feces daily.

Ancylostoma tubaeforme

Morphology. For many years, *Ancylostoma tubaeforme,* the common hookworm of the cat, was considered to be synonymous with *A. caninum,* the common hookworm of the dog. However, the two are now considered to be distinct species. Adult *A. tubaeforme* measure 7 mm to 12 mm long. Both males and females possess a subglobular buccal cavity with three well-developed teeth on each side. *Ancylostoma tubaeforme* can be distinguished from *Uncinaria stenocephala* by the presence of sharp teeth rather than cutting plates in the buccal capsule. The adults of *A. braziliense* only have two well-developed teeth on each

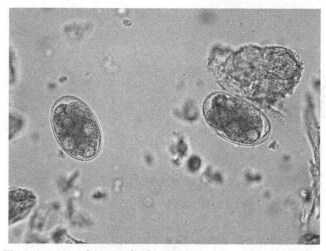

Fig. 18.17 *Ancylostoma tubaeforme* eggs.

side of the buccal capsule. The egg is ellipsoidal, thin-shelled, and measures 55 μ to 72 μ long by 34 μ to 45 μ wide. The egg is usually in the two to eight-celled stage when passed in the feces (Figure 18.17). The eggs are smaller than those of *U. stenocephala,* but are indistinguishable from those of *A. caninum.*

Hosts. The hosts are cats and other felids. The parasite can be common in random-source cats, but is uncommon in colony-bred animals. Rodents can serve as paratenic hosts but little is known of potential transmission from rodents to cats.

Life Cycle. The life cycle is direct[76]. Infection occurs either by ingestion of infective larvae or by larval penetration of the skin. After oral inoculation, the larvae enter the wall of the stomach and small intestine where they remain for 10 to 12 days as they mature into adult worms. After larvae penetrate the skin, they migrate through the lungs, are coughed up and swallowed, and then spend less time in the wall of the gastrointestinal tract. The prepatent period is 18 to 28 days following oral infection, and 19 to 25 days following skin penetration. The adult worms can survive for 18 months to two years. Neither transplacental nor transmammary transmission occur, which partially explains the low prevalence of infection in animal colonies.

Pathologic Effects and Clinical Disease. *Ancylostoma tubaeforme* feeds on host blood, leading to weight loss and development of regenerative anemia. Heavy infections may cause death.

Diagnosis, Treatment, and Prevention. Diagnosis is based on the clinical signs of anemia and the demonstration of eggs in the feces or mature worms in the intestine at necropsy. Several anthelmintics are approved for treating hookworm disease. All are efficacious against adult worms, and many are also effective against larval stages within the wall of the intestinal tract[93,101,102]. Complete elimination of *A. tubaeforme* is possible with anthelmintic treatment and good sanitation. Random-source cats are likely to be infected upon entry, and so should be evaluated and treated.

Public Health Considerations. The infective-stage larvae of *A. tubaeforme* can penetrate human skin and cause cutaneous larva migrans. Thus, animal caretakers should practice excellent personal hygiene and keep cat cages and litter pans clean.

Superfamily Trichostrongyloidea

Ollulanus tricuspis

Morphology. The male worm measures 0.7 mm to 0.8 mm long and 35 μ wide and has stout spicules. The female worm measures 0.8 mm to 1 mm long and 40 μ wide[76] (Figure 18.18)[103]. The vulva is located in the posterior part of the body. The eggs in the female are few in number and relatively large compared to the size of the female worm.

Hosts. This minute nematode occurs in the stomach of cats, other carnivores, and pigs. It has been found in cats in Europe, the Americas, Egypt, and Australia[104,105].

Life Cycle. *Ollulanus tricuspis* is ovoviviparous. Thus, the eggs embryonate and hatch within the female. First-stage larvae measure 350 μ long. Second- and third-stage larvae also develop within the female. Thus, female worms give birth to infective third-stage larvae. The infective larvae are passed by emesis; infection is by ingestion of the vomitus. Larvae mature within the lumen of the stomach.

Pathologic Effects and Clinical Disease. Infections with *O. tricuspis* are usually unapparent and are recognized only at necropsy. The worms in the stomach cause increased mucous secretion, and in heavy infections, can cause hemorrhagic gastritis. In severe cases, lesions include hyperplasia of the stomach epithelium, inflammation, cellular infiltration, and sclerosis of the epithelium. Infected cats may present with a history of chronic vomiting with or without wasting. Cats may become anorexic and dehydrated.

Diagnosis, Treatment, and Prevention. Antemortem diagnosis is difficult, and requires the careful examination of vomitus and stomach irrigation fluids. Post-mortem diagnosis is made by examining washings or scrapings of the stomach wall. Treatment with tetramisole has been efficacious and without side effects. In areas where the infection is

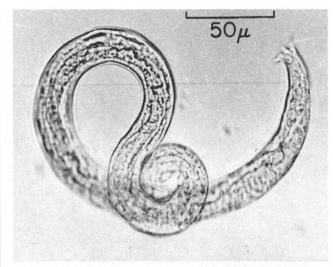

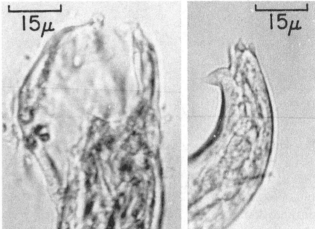

Fig. 18.18 *Ollulanus tricuspis.* (Top) Young female. (Bottom) Posterior ends of adult male (left) and adult female (right). Reproduced from Burrows, R.B. (1965) with permission.

common, dissemination of the infection can be prevented by housing cats individually. Most outbreaks occur in large catteries where animals are housed in groups.

Public Health Considerations. *Ollulanus tricuspis* does not infect humans.

Superfamily Metastrongyloidea

Aelurostrongylus abstrusus

Morphology. The female worm measures 9 mm long and the male measures 4 mm to 7 mm long. The female vulva lies anterior to the anus, and the tail ends bluntly. The male spicules are sub-equal. The eggs measure 70 μ long by 80 μ wide. The first-stage larvae passed in the feces measures 360 μ to 400 μ long and 20 μ wide and has an undulating tail with a dorsal spine (Figure 18.19).

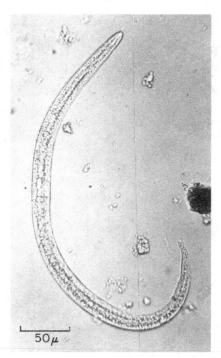

Fig. 18.19 *Aelurostrongylus abstrusus* larva. Reproduced from Burrows, R.B. (1965) with permission.

Hosts. *Aelurostrongylus abstrusus* is common in cats around the world[106,107]. Wild rodents, frogs, toads, snakes, lizards, and small birds serve as paratenic hosts. *Aelurostrongylus abstrusus* is likely to occur in laboratory cats obtained from random-source cat suppliers but not from cats raised in the laboratory animal facility or in catteries that practice good management and sanitation.

Life Cycle. Eggs passed by adult worms hatch in the lungs, and the larvae pass up the trachea, are swallowed, and pass out in the feces. Snails and slugs serve as intermediate hosts, but the cat is probably more frequently infected by eating paratenic hosts. The ingested larvae are liberated in the intestine, penetrate the mucosa, and migrate to the lungs. Adult worms are found in the alveolar ducts and terminal bronchioles eight to nine days after infection. Egg laying begins about four weeks after infection, and first-stage larvae are found in the feces about six weeks after infection. Adult worms live nine months or longer.

Production of larvae by *A. abstrusus* following infection and re-infection has been studied[107]. The pre-patent period was 35 to 48 days (mean 38 days). Peak larval production occurred 60 to 120 days from the time of infection. Two infected cats continued to produce larvae for more than one year. When all 17 cats were re-infected 390 days after primary infection, 56% of the cats produced larvae

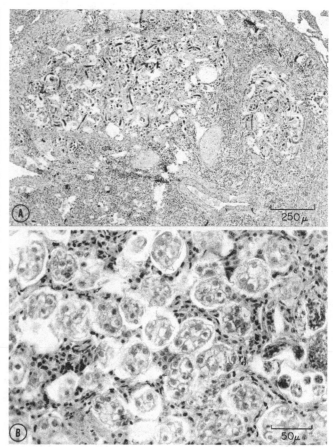

Fig. 18.20 *Aelurostrongylus abstrusus* in the lung of a cat. (A) Larvae in a small bronchus. (B) Clusters of embryonating eggs in the alveoli and larvae in an alveolar duct. Reproduced from Smith, H.A. and Jones, T.C. (1966) with permission.

within 90 days, and larval output for two animals persisted until the 660th day of the study with the larvae in the feces probably being derived from the secondary infection.

Pathologic Effects and Clinical Disease. Gross lesions consist of gray nodules, 1 mm to 10 mm in diameter, either scattered over the surface of the lungs or arranged in clusters[76]. The nodules, when incised, exude a milky fluid that contains many eggs and larvae. Mature worms are found at the terminal parts of the bronchioles. In microscopic sections, the embryonating eggs and larvae are seen in the alveoli, alveolar ducts, and bronchioles (Figure 18.20)[108]. Lesions in wild rodents consist of larval cysts, usually in the omentum. Clinical signs are usually absent. Heavy infections may lead to chronic cough, progressive dyspnea, anorexia, and emaciation.

Diagnosis, Treatment, and Prevention. Presumptive diagnosis is based on clinical signs, and is confirmed by demonstration of the first-stage larvae in the feces. At necropsy, larvae may be demonstrated in wet mounts made from pulmonary lesions. The infection may be eliminated by long-term treatment with fenbendazole. Because mollusks are obligatory intermediate hosts, the life cycle cannot be completed in well-managed research animal facilities. Infected, incoming cats should be treated.

Public Health Considerations. *Aelurostrongylus abstrusus* does not infect humans.

Superfamily Spiruroidea

Physaloptera spp.

Morphology. Cats are susceptible to infection with several species of *Physaloptera*, including *Physaloptera rara, P. pacitae, P. pseudopraeputialis,* and *P. praeputialis.* These worms are thick and muscular and resemble ascarids[76]. Males measure 13 mm to 45 mm long, and females measure 15 mm to 60 mm long. The eggs are embryonated when passed, have a clear, thick shell, and measure 43 µ to 60 µ long by 29 µ to 42 µ wide (Figure 18.21).

Hosts. *Physaloptera* spp. occur in the stomach and duodenum of cats, dogs, and related carnivores[97,105,109]. *Physaloptera rara* occurs in the United States. It is common in the Midwest, but uncommon in other areas. *Physaloptera pacitae* has been found in the Philippines. *Physaloptera pseudopraeputialis* has also been found in the Philippine

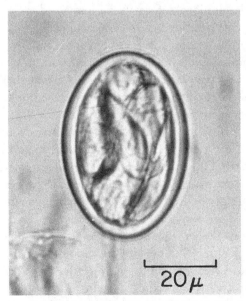

Fig. 18.21 *Physaloptera rara* egg. Reproduced from Burrows, R.B. (1965) with permission.

Islands, and in the United States. *Physaloptera praeputialis* has been found in most regions of the world, and is common in Hawaii, South Africa, Venezuela, and peninsular Malaysia. These nematodes are likely to be found in laboratory cats and dogs obtained from random-source animal suppliers in endemic areas. They are unlikely to occur in animals raised in the laboratory or in catteries with good management and sanitation.

Life Cycle. The life cycles of the *Physaloptera* spp. are incompletely understood, but an arthropod intermediate host, such as a cockroach, cricket, or beetle, is always required[76]. Paratenic hosts include amphibians, reptiles, or small mammals.

Pathologic Effects and Clinical Disease. *Physaloptera* spp. attach firmly to the stomach or duodenal wall, and cause focal necrotic lesions at these sites. Early clinical signs include vomiting and anorexia. Later signs include debilitation and dark, tarry feces.

Diagnosis, Treatment, and Prevention. Diagnosis is by finding the embryonated eggs in the feces or the adult worms in the stomach or duodenum at necropsy. Treatment has been attempted with ivermectin and pyrantel pamoate, but the outcome of these clinical treatments has varied. Because of the need for intermediate hosts, infections within the laboratory setting are self-limiting.

Public Health Considerations. *Physaloptera* spp. do not infect humans.

Superfamily Trichuroidea

Eucoleus aerophilus

The biology of *Eucoleus aerophilus* is presented in Chapter 17, Parasites of Dogs. Infections are uncommon in laboratory-reared cats, but may be found in random-source cats upon entry into the animal facility[110]. Infected cats may develop tracheobronchitis, pulmonary edema, hemorrhage, and pneumonia. Larvae, adult worms, and eggs are present in sections of affected tissues (Figure 18.22)[111]. Young animals are the most susceptible to disease caused by *E. aerophilus.* Light infections are usually unapparent. Heavy infections are associated with coughing, nasal discharge, dyspnea, anorexia, and debilitation. Infected cats may be treated with ivermectin or a benzimidazole. Newly acquired cats should be examined on arrival and treated if infected. Because the eggs do not embryonate for 30 to 50 days, frequent and complete cleaning of cages, pens, and runs prevents the dissemination of the parasite[112].

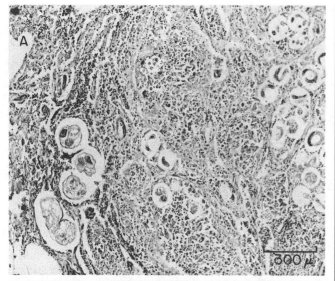

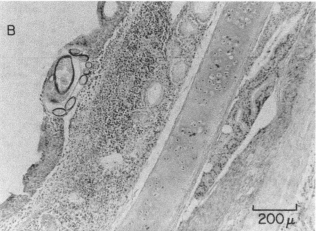

Fig. 18.22 *Eucoleus aerophilus* infection. (A) Larvae and adults in the lung of a cat. (B) Adult and eggs in the tracheal mucosa of a cat. (A) reproduced from Habermann, R.T. and Williams, F.P. (1958) with permission. (B) reproduced from Herman, L.H. (1967) with permission.

Pearsonema feliscati

Morphology. Adult *Pearsonema feliscati* are long, thin, and finely striated. Males measure 1.3 cm to 3 cm long and females measure 3 cm to 6 cm long. The spicular sheath of the male lacks spines. The egg is colorless to yellow, and measures approximately 60 µ long by 30 µ wide, and has bipolar plugs.

Hosts. *Pearsonema feliscati* is the urinary capillarid of the cat[113,114]. It is considered by some to be synonymous with *P. plica. Pearsonema feliscati* has been recovered from the urinary bladder and renal pelvises of cats around the world, and is more common in older, versus younger, cats. Reports of infection in laboratory cats are rare.

Life Cycle. The life cycle of *P. feliscati* is likely similar to that of *P. plica*, with earthworms serving as intermediate hosts. It has not been determined whether the life cycle can also be direct or whether paratenic hosts play a role in natural infections[76]. The prepatent period is 58 to 63 days.

Pathologic Effects and Clinical Disease. The worms inhabit the bladder epithelium. Inflammation of the mucous membranes is evident histologically, and includes vasodilation, extravasated blood, separating transitional epithelium, and inflammatory cells. Urinary protein content increases with increasing worm burdens. Clinical signs are usually absent, but heavily infected cats may develop signs of post-renal obstruction.

Diagnosis, Treatment, and Prevention. Diagnosis is based on recognition of the adults in the urinary tract or the characteristic eggs in the urine. Elimination of the worms has been achieved with fenbendazole and with ivermectin. Prevention is primarily by sanitation.

Public Health Considerations. *Pearsonema feliscati* does not infect humans.

ARTHROPODS

Class Insecta

Order Diptera

Family Cuterebridae

The family Cuterebridae occurs only in the Americas[76,115]. All species are obligatory parasites that produce primary myiasis. Additional information is presented in Chapter 6, Biology of Arthropods. Typical hosts include rodents and lagomorphs, but cats are also susceptible to infestation as they hunt around rodent burrows. Infestations tend to be seasonal in temperate regions because the adult flies lay eggs for only a short time. However, in more tropical areas, infestations may occur throughout the year.

Cats are dead-end hosts. Maggots develop from the larva to the third instar just under the skin of the cat (Figure 18.23). However, even if the instar matures to its full size, it will usually not develop to an adult. Clinical signs depend on where the larvae migrate within the cat. In uncomplicated cases, the large "bots" are located in lesions under the dermis, frequently in the head region. Treatment is by surgical removal of the maggot. Cats suspected of harboring migrating larvae may be treated with ivermectin[116,117]. In other cases, larvae migrate through the central nervous system and cause severe neurologic disease (Figure 18.24). Larval migration

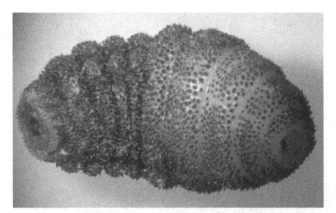

Fig. 18.23 *Cuterebra* third-stage larva from a warble in the cheek of a cat.

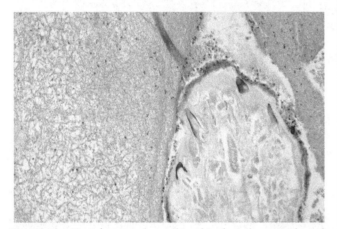

Fig. 18.24 *Cuterebra* second-stage larva histological section through larvae in the tissue of the central nervous tissue. Note the large dark spines and the tracheal tissue in the maggot.

may be the cause of feline ischemic encephalopathy, a condition that is diagnosed seasonally in cats in New England[118]. Infestations should not occur in animal facilities, but random-source cats may be infested upon entry into the facility.

Family Psychodidae

Cats are susceptible to attack by phlebotomine sand flies[119]. Information on the biology of the sand flies is presented in Chapter 17, Parasites of Dogs. Sand flies are important as vectors of leishmaniasis in both the Old and New Worlds. There are usually no clinical signs directly associated with the feeding activities of sand flies unless many flies are involved. In these cases, cats may develop lesions on the muzzle or ear pinnae. Treatment consists of cleansing the wounds and applying topical antibiotics, followed by fly control.

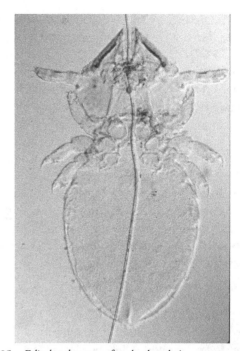

Fig. 18.25 *Felicola subrostratus* female, dorsal view.

Order Phthiraptera

Felicola subrostratus

Morphology. *Felicola subrostratus* has a triangular head, which is pointed anteriorly, and a median longitudinal ventral groove[76] (Figure 18.25). The antennae are three-segmented, fully exposed, and similar in both sexes. The adults measure 1 mm to 1.5 mm long and are yellow to tan. There is one tarsal claw on each leg. The abdomen is short and broad and has three pairs of spiracles and a sparse, fine, transverse row of minute dorsal hairs across each segment.

Hosts. *Felicola subrostratus* can be found in large numbers on aged or diseased cats and some wild felids. It occurs in North and South America, Europe, and Africa, and is probably cosmopolitan in location[120]. Although this louse is the most common cause of louse infestation of cats, infestation often goes unnoticed. Consequently, the true prevalence is unknown. It can occur on random-source cats. Another chewing louse of cats occurring in the tropics is *Heterodoxus spiniger*.

Life Cycle. The eggs are laid on the fur of the cat where they are glued to individual hair shafts[76]. The eggs hatch in 10 to 20 days and reach the adult stage in two to three weeks. The complete life cycle requires three to six weeks. The louse feeds on skin debris. Adults live two to three weeks but cannot survive off the host for more than a few days. Transmission is primarily by direct contact.

Pathologic Effects and Clinical Disease. Effects on the hair or skin are usually minimal or absent. The eggs and nits can be seen on the hair and may give it a scruffy appearance. Heavy infestations cause restlessness, pruritus, scratching, a ruffled coat, and sometimes alopecia.

Diagnosis, Treatment, and Prevention. Diagnosis is based on clinical signs and on demonstration of the parasite or parasite eggs. *Felicola subrostratus* is easily eradicated with a variety of products[121,122]. Newly acquired cats should be examined and isolated and treated if infested. The treated cat should be placed in a clean, disinfected cage. Treatment should be repeated to ensure that any nymphs that hatch from eggs are also killed.

Public Health Considerations. *Felicola subrostratus* does not infest humans.

Order Siphonaptera

Ctenocephalides spp.

Morphology. Cats are susceptible to infestation with *Ctenocephalides felis* and *C. canis* (Figure 18.26). Both species are somewhat variable in size. Females may exceed 2.5 mm in length while males can be less than 1 mm long, with size overlap between the two sexes. Both species are dark brown and possess distinctly characteristic genal and pronotal combs. *Ctenocephalides felis* usually has an elongated head, especially in the female, a single subapical bristle on the dorsal margin of the hind tibia, and three setae in the lateral metanotal area. *Ctenocephalides canis* has a short, blunt head (Figure 18.27), two small subapical bristles on the dorsal margin of the hind tibia, and usually only two setae on the lateral metanotal area. The larvae are small, white, and maggot-like, with a sclerotized head

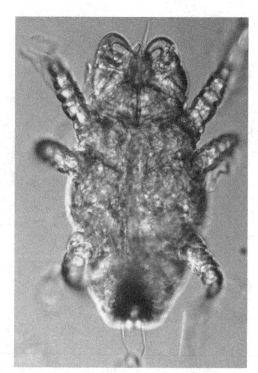

Fig. 18.27 *Cheyletiella blakei.* Note the large palpal claws.

capsule and chewing mouthparts. The larvae are legless but have a pair of caudal processes called anal struts. The eggs are small, white, and ovoid.

Hosts. Recently, *C. felis* appears to have displaced *C. canis* to the point where the latter has become difficult to find. *Ctenocephalides felis* infests cats and dogs, and occasionally other endothermal animals such as opossums, raccoons, and people. *Ctenocephalides canis* tends to be restricted to dogs and wild canids. *Ctenocephalides felis* has been assigned to four distinct subspecies: *C. felis felis,* which occurs throughout the world; *C. felis strongylus,* which is found over most of Africa, except in the Sahara region and in southwestern Africa, where *C. felis damarensis* occurs; and *C. felis orientis* in India, Ceylon, southwestern Asia, and New Guinea[123]. Fleas are common on random-source dogs and cats, but are not usually found on those raised for research.

Life Cycle. Only adult fleas are found on the host, where mating and oviposition occur[124]. The eggs fall quickly from the pelage and collect in the bedding. The incubation period is two to four days under optimum conditions of 25°C and 80% relative humidity. There are three larval instars, but active feeding takes place only during the first and second instars. The larvae ingest organic material of both plant and animal origin, including pellets

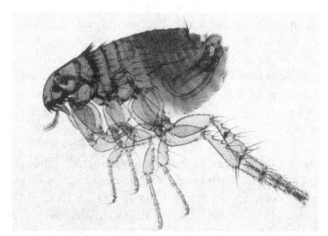

Fig. 18.26 *Ctenocephalides felis* male.

of dried blood that have been excreted by the adults. Shortly after molting, the third instar larva becomes quiescent and spins a cocoon, which is oval and inconspicuous. The pupa is formed within a few days, and is followed by maturation to the adult stage in two weeks. The life cycle from egg to adult is completed in 18 to 21 days under optimum conditions of temperature and humidity, but it probably requires a longer period in nature. The lifespan also depends on the temperature, humidity, and the presence of a suitable host. Desiccation is as important as starvation in causing death. Fleas can best survive harsh environmental conditions in the pupal stage. Cats become infested by direct contact with other infested animals, or by entering an area where hungry adult fleas are awaiting a new host or where fleas in pupal cases are awaiting a host to stimulate their eclosion.

Pathologic Effects. Histologic changes vary with the degree of self-induced trauma and immune reactivity. Initially, the affected skin undergoes a predominantly eosinophilic and neutrophilic inflammatory infiltration. Later, there is increased proliferation of fibroblasts and connective tissue. Acanthosis, parakeratosis, and degeneration of the pilosebaceous system often follow. In addition, fleas serve as intermediate hosts of *Dipylidium caninum* and can serve as vectors of *Bartonella henselae*, the agent of cat scratch fever; feline leukemia virus; and some rickettsial agents[125,126].

Clinical Disease. Flea infestation sometimes causes only minor clinical response in affected cats. More frequently, restlessness, irritability, weight loss, ruffled coat, biting, scratching, and self-induced trauma are seen. Flea saliva causes allergic dermatitis. Wheals and erythema occur at the site of the bite, but these are often not recognized in long-haired breeds. Sometimes, small raised papules occur. Other lesions depend on the degree of self-inflicted trauma and often consist of excoriations, ulcerations, and alopecia. These lesions are usually located at the base of the tail and over the lower back. In chronic cases, the skin becomes thickened and indurated. *C. felis* on cats appear to prefer the area of the head and neck more than other parts of the body. The fewest fleas are typically found on the legs and tail[127].

Diagnosis, Treatment, and Prevention. Infestation is diagnosed by finding fleas or flea excrement on the host. The excrement is seen as small, dark, gritty particles in the pelage. It is important to distinguish dermatosis caused by fleas from that of other sources. Remission of signs and lesions after the parasites have been eliminated supports

a diagnosis of flea-induced dermatitis. Several highly efficacious products have been approved for treatment of flea infestation[123]. All random-source cats entering a facility should be treated and quarantined for several days.

Public Health Considerations. *Ctenocephalides felis* and *C. canis* readily feed on humans. Recent reports indicate that *Bartonella henselae*, the agent of cat-scratch fever, may be transmissible to humans through contaminated flea feces[124,126].

Class Arachnida

Mites

Suborder Prostigmata
Cheyletiella blakei. Morphology. *Cheyletiella blakei* resembles *C. yasguri* of the dog[128]. Both sexes have a single semi-circular dorsal shield and a large gnathosoma. The palpal tibia has a heavy curved claw that is dentate on its inferior margin, which is diagnostic (Figure 18.27).

Hosts and Life Cycle. *Cheyletiella blakei* is a parasite of cats. These mites are nonburrowing, obligatory parasites[128]. The life cycle is similar to that of *C. yasguri* of dogs. All stages occur on the host. The eggs are glued to the hairs.

Pathologic Effects and Clinical Disease. *Cheyletiella blakei* causes a mild form of mange, with exfoliative dermatitis, mild hair loss, hyperemia, pruritus, serous exudation, and thickening of the skin. A subacute, nonsuppurative dermatitis with cellular infiltration and mild hyperkeratosis is seen in tissue section. Clinical signs include flaky, bran-like material in the pelage. The condition is referred to as "walking dandruff" because when the pelage is examined with a hand lens, the flakes on the skin appear to move due to the mites walking about amidst the dander.

Diagnosis, Treatment, and Prevention. Diagnosis is by identifying the mites in skin scrapings or tufts of hair. The mites can be eliminated with selamectin, fipronil, permethrin, ivermectin, or milbemycin oxime[129,130]. Because *C. blakei* survives off of the host, cages, equipment, and rooms should be treated with steam or pressure and washed with soapy water at the same time animals are treated.

Public Health Considerations. Humans may develop transient dermatitis after handling infested cats[131].

Demodex cati. Morphology. The morphology of *Demodex cati* is similar to *D. canis*, and typical of the genus. Mites are cigar shaped with very short legs[132]. The male measures roughly 180 μ long and the female measures about 200 μ long. The eggs are elongated and measure 70 μ long (Figure 18.28). The short legs are on the anterior portion of the

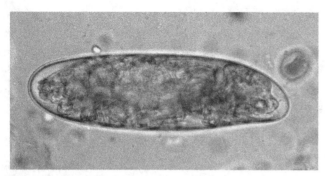

Fig. 18.28 *Demodex cati* egg.

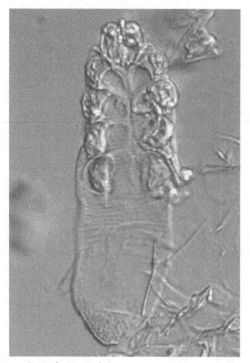

Fig. 18.29 *Demodex gatoi* adult.

body, and the posterior (opisthoma) region comprises about two-thirds of the total body length. The shorter and less common species found on cats, *D. gatoi,* bears an opisthoma which is much shorter by comparison (Figure 18.29).

Hosts and Life Cycle. *Demodex cati* has been found on cats from most parts of the world. The mites live in the hair follicles. There is another shorter version of *Demodex* that occurs on cats[133], *D. gatoi,* that has been described, but it is relatively rare in comparison with *D. cati.* The life cycle is similar to that described for *D. canis* in Chapter 17, Parasites of Dogs[132].

Pathologic Effects and Clinical Disease. Cats may develop both localized and generalized demodicosis[132]. The localized form is typically associated with acne or erythematous patches of alopecia on the eyelids, face, chin, or neck. The generalized form is diagnosed when cats have more than five localized lesions. In either form, the hair follicles become inflamed and may be associated with follicular and perifollicular dermatitis. Severe cases may be facilitated by some other underlying condition[134,135].

Diagnosis, Treatment, and Prevention. Diagnosis is by scraping the lesions to reveal large numbers of mites. Most cases of demodicosis in cats can be treated with ivermectin, although generalized disease may require multiple treatments. Doramectin has also been used with some success[136]. Because asymptomatic infestation with *D. cati* is common, purposeful prevention is not generally practiced.

Public Health Considerations. *Demodex cati* does not usually infest humans. However, transient dermatitis may develop after extended close contact with severely affected cats.

Suborder Astigmata
Lynxacarus radovskyi. **Morphology.** *Lynxacarus radovskyi* mites are laterally compressed[137]. They are small, measuring only about 0.5 mm long. They are typically found clinging to the hairs of the host (Figure 18.30). The eggs measure 200 µ long.

Hosts and Life Cycle. *Lynxacarus radovskyi* has been reported only from cats. The species on the bobcat has been described as a separate species, *L. morlani*[138]. The eggs are glued to the hair shaft by the female mite[139]. There is a larva, a nymph, and adult males and females. Transmission is by direct contact.

Pathologic Effects and Clinical Disease. Infestation with *L. radovskyi* is accompanied by minimal pathologic

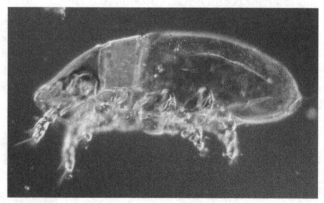

Fig. 18.30 *Lynxacarus radovskyi.*

changes[140]. When present, clinical signs include dry, dull, and rust-colored hair-coat that can feel granular due to the mites and eggs on the hairs[139].

Diagnosis, Treatment, and Prevention. Mites can be visualized on the skin with a magnifying glass. Microscopic examination of the hairs likewise reveals mites and eggs. Treatment with pyrethrin-based shampoos has been found to be efficacious, as has parenteral treatments with ivermectin[139]. Infested cats should be housed separately and treated upon entry into the facility.

Public Health Considerations. Humans who handle infested cats are susceptible to transient infestation with *L. radovskyi*.

Notoedres cati. **Morphology.** Adult female *Notoedres cati* measure 275 μ by 230 μ and resemble *N. muris* except that it has scale-like, middorsal integumental striations, a single pair of paragenital setae, and large perianal setae (Figure 18.31). The male and immature stages resemble those of *Sarcoptes scabiei*. Adults can be differentiated from those of *S. scabiei* because on *N. cati*, the anus is dorsally located, versus ventrally located on *S. scabiei*.

Hosts. *Notoedres cati* infests cats, rabbits, and the coatimundi. Infestations are common in North America, Europe, Africa, and possibly elsewhere. It is likely to be encountered in laboratory cats obtained as random-source animals, but unlikely to be found otherwise.

Life Cycle. Transmission is by direct contact and spread of larvae and nymphs. The life cycle is similar to that described for *S. scabiei* in Chapter 17, Parasites of Dogs. Adults appear within five days of egg hatching.

Pathologic Effects and Clinical Disease. Infested cats develop epidermal penetration of the skin by mites and acanthotic and hyperkeratotic lesions[141]. Common sites of infestation include the ears, neck, and face (Figure 18.32); and less commonly, the legs, ventral abdomen, and genital region, especially in younger animals[142]. Clinical signs include persistent pruritus, alopecia, and self-inflicted trauma. A grayish yellow crust develops on the ears, face, and neck, and the skin becomes thickened and wrinkled. Involvement of the entire body sometimes occurs, with subsequent dehydration, debilitation, and death.

Diagnosis. Other diseases that must be distinguished from notoedric mange include dermatomycosis, superficial pyoderma, and chronic eczematous dermatitis. The presence of the parasite or eggs in deep skin scrapings is diagnostic for mange. In the cat, notoedric mange must be distinguished from mange caused by *Otodectes cynotis*, the ear mite. The two mites can be differentiated morphologically.

Treatment and Prevention. Infestation with *N. cati* can be eliminated with ivermectin or other avermectin products[143]. Cats with evidence of infestation at the time of entry into the animal facility should be examined and treated if infested.

Public Health Considerations. *Notoedres cati* sometimes causes transient dermatitis in people[144]; therefore, animals should be handled with caution.

Otodectes cynotis. **Morphology.** The adult female has a small fourth pair of legs, whereas the male possesses large, stalked ambulacral suckers on the fourth pair of legs

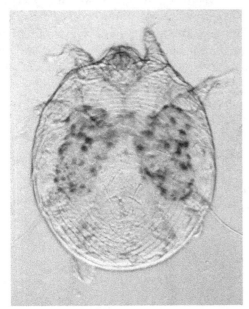

Fig. 18.31 *Notoedres cati* adult female, dorsal view.

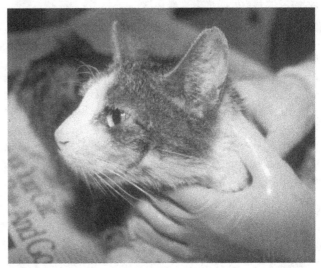

Fig. 18.32 *Notoedres cati* mange on a cat.

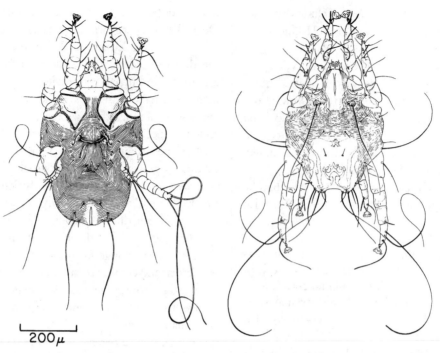

Fig. 18.33 *Otodectes cynotis.* (Left) Female, ventral view. (Right) Male, dorsal view. Reproduced from Baker, E.W., Evans, T.M., Gould, D.J., Hull, W.B., and Keegan, H.L. (1956) with permission.

(Figure 18.33)[145]. In addition, the ambulacral suckers of both sexes arise from short, unsegmented stalks.

Hosts and Life Cycle. *Otodectes cynotis* is common on wild and random-source cats and rabbits and coatimundi[146,147], but is uncommon in laboratory-reared cats. Transmission from is by direct contact[128]. The female mite glues eggs to the ear canal. The eggs develop and hatch in four days. The life cycle includes a larva and two nymphal stages. Each stage requires three to five days to mature before molting. The life cycle is completed in 18 to 28 days.

Pathologic Effects. Infested cats develop crusty waxy material that overlays the epithelial surface, the epithelium becomes hyperkeratotic and hyperplastic, the ceruminous and sebaceous glands appear to undergo dramatic reactive hyperplasia, mast cells and macrophages become greatly increased in number, and there is a dilation of underlying blood vessels[128]. In heavy infestations, ears contain a dry, waxy, parchment-like material that occurs as sheets throughout the ear canal.

Clinical Disease. The mites are usually found deep in the external auditory meatus, where they cause intense irritation because of accumulation of inflammatory exudates and cerumen. Infested cats engage in head shaking and ear scratching. Ulceration of the auditory canal is common. Auricular hematoma, otitis media with torticollis and circling, and convulsions sometimes occur.

Diagnosis, Treatment, and Prevention. Diagnosis is based on clinical signs and lesions, and is confirmed by identification of the mites. *Otodectes cynotis* is often visible with the aid of an otoscope, but microscopic examination of scrapings may be more rewarding. Many effective products are approved for the treatment of *O. cynotis* infestation[129,148,149]. Because infestation is common, random-source cats should be treated upon entry into the animal facility.

Public Health Considerations. *Otodectes cynotis* does not persist on human hosts.

TABLE 18.1   Parasites of cats—circulatory/lymphatic system.

Parasite	Geographic Distribution	Hosts	Location in Host	Method of Infection	Pathologic Effects	Zoonosis	Reference
Piroplasmids							
Babesia cati	India	Cats	Erythrocytes	Bite of tick host	Unknown	Not reported	76
Babesia felis	Africa	Cats	Erythrocytes	Bite of tick host (*Haemaphysalis leachi*)	Anemia, listlessness	Not reported	161
Babesia herpailuri	South Africa, South America	Cats	Erythrocytes	Bite of tick host	Unknown	Not reported	76
Cytauxzoon felis	Worldwide	Cats	Erythrocytes; venules of visceral organs, brain, lymph nodes	Bite of tick host (*Dermacentor variabilis*)	Vascular occlusion	Not reported	62
Nematodes							
Metastrongyloidea							
Gurltia paralysans	South America	Cats	Veins of lumbar leptomeninges	Unknown	Thrombosis of veins, posterior paralysis	Not reported	76
Filaroidea							
Brugia beaveri	Southeast Asia	Cats, raccoons	Adult: lymphatics, lymph nodes Microfilaria: blood	Bite of mosquito	Unknown	Not reported	163
Brugia malayi	Southeast Asia	Cats, primates	Adult: lymphatics, lymph nodes Microfilaria: blood	Bite of mosquito	Unknown	Reported	76
Brugia pahangi	Indonesia, Malaysia, Thailand	Cats, dogs	Adult: lymphatics, lymph nodes Microfilaria: blood	Bite of mosquito	Lymphangitis	Reported	162
Brugia patei	Kenya	Cats, dogs	Adult: lymphatics, lymph nodes Microfilaria: blood	Bite of mosquito	Unknown	Not reported	76

TABLE 18.2 Parasites of cats—enterohepatic system.

Parasite	Geographic Distribution	Hosts	Location in Host	Method of Infection	Pathologic Effects	Zoonosis	Reference
Flagellates							
Giardia felis	Worldwide	Cats	Anterior small intestine	Ingestion of cyst in feces	Mild enteritis, diarrhea	Reported	13
Tetratrichomonas felistomae	US	Cats	Mouth	Oral contact	Uncertain. Possible gingivitis	Not reported	18
Tritrichomonas foetus	Worldwide	Cats, cattle, swine	Large intestine	Ingestion of trophozoites in feces	Enteritis, diarrhea	Not reported	20
Coccidia							
Besnoitia caprae	Africa	Cats	Intestine	Ingestion of tissue cysts in intermediate host (goats)	None	Not reported	154
Besnoitia besnoiti	Africa, Asia, South America, Southern Europe	Cats	Intestine	Ingestion of tissue cysts in intermediate host (cattle)	None	Not reported	153
Besnoitia darlingi	Americas	Cats	Intestine	Ingestion of tissue cysts in intermediate host (opossums)	None	Not reported	150
Besnoitia jellisoni	Americas	Cats	Intestine	Ingestion of tissue cysts in intermediate host (rodents, opossums)	None	Not reported	155
Besnoitia tarandi	Alaska, Canada, Finland	Cats	Intestine	Ingestion of tissue cysts in intermediate host (reindeer)	None	Not reported	156
Besnoitia wallacei	Africa, Australia	Cats	Intestine	Ingestion of tissue cysts in intermediate host (rats, mice)	None	Not reported	151
Cryptosporidium felis	Worldwide	Cats	Small intestine	Ingestion of sporulated oocysts	Enteritis, diarrhea	Reported in immune-compromised humans	28
Hammondia hammondi	Worldwide	Cats	Intestine	Ingestion of tissue cysts in intermediate host (rodents, goats)	None	Not reported	152
Isospora felis	Worldwide	Cats (dogs, rodents, cattle, and birds as paratenic hosts)	Intestine	Ingestion of sporulated oocyst or paratenic host	Enteritis, diarrhea	Not reported	37, 38
Isospora rivolta	Worldwide	Cats (rodents, cattle, and opossums as paratenic hosts)	Intestine	Ingestion of sporulated oocyst or paratenic host	Enteritis, diarrhea	Not reported	40

604

Organism	Geographic distribution	Host	Site	Transmission	Lesions		Reference
Sarcocystis spp.	Worldwide	Cats (mammals as intermediate hosts)	Intestine	Ingestion of tissue cysts in intermediate hosts	None	Not reported	76
Toxoplasma gondii	Worldwide	Cats (mammals and birds as paratenic hosts)	Intestine, visceral organs, brain, lymph nodes	Ingestion of tissue cysts in paratenic hosts or sporulated oocysts in feces; transplacental transmission	Often unapparent; lesions specific to affected organs	Common	50
Trematodes							
Alaria marcianae	Greenland, Iceland, North America	Cats, coyotes	Small intestine	Ingestion of infected snake (*Thamnophis maricanus*)	None	None known	76
Clinostomum spp.	Africa	Cats	Oral cavity	Ingestion of intermediate host (unknown)	None	Not reported	76
Clonorchis sinensis	Asia	Cats, dogs; fish-eating mammals, birds, and reptiles	Gall bladder, bile duct, pancreatic duct, small intestine	Ingestion of intermediate host (fishes)	Bile duct inflammation, hepatic congestion, pancreatitis	Reported	76
Echinochasmus perfoliatus	Africa, Asia	Cats	Small intestine	Ingestion of intermediate host (fishes)	None	Not reported	76
Eurytrema procyonis	North America	Cats, raccoons, foxes	Pancreatic duct, gall bladder	Ingestion of intermediate host (unknown)	Pancreatic atrophy and fibrosis	Not reported	157
Mesostephanus milvi	Africa, Japan, India	Cats	Small intestine	Ingestion of intermediate host (unknown)	None	Not reported	76
Opisthorchis tenuicollis	Asia, Europe, North America	Cats	Gall bladder, bile duct, pancreatic duct, small intestine	Ingestion of intermediate host (fishes)	Bile duct inflammation, hepatic congestion, pancreatitis	Reported	76
Platynosomum fastosum	Americas, Asia, Western Africa	Cats	Gallbladder, bile duct	Ingestion of infected intermediate host (lizards, frogs, toads)	Biliary obstruction, diarrhea, hepatic enlargement	Not reported	158
Prohemistomum vivax	Egypt	Cats	Small intestine	Ingestion of second intermediate host (fishes)	None	Not reported	76
Pygidiopsoides spindalis	North America	Cats	Small intestine	Ingestion of second intermediate host (fishes)	None	Not reported	76
Cestodes							
Pseudophyllidea							
Diphylobothrium latum	Asia, Americas, Europe	Cats, dogs, wild carnivores	Small intestine	Ingestion of intermediate host (fresh-water fishes)	None	Reported	76
Spirometra erinaceieuropaei	Africa, Australia, Europe	Cats, dogs	Small intestine	Ingestion of infected intermediate host (small marine vertebrates)	None	Reported	160

(Continued)

TABLE 18.2 (Continued)

Parasite	Geographic Distribution	Hosts	Location in Host	Method of Infection	Pathologic Effects	Zoonosis	Reference
Spirometra mansoni	Asia, South America	Cats, dogs, other carnivores	Small intestine	Ingestion of intermediate host (small vertebrates, except fishes)	None	Reported	76
Spirometra mansonoides	Americas	Cats, dogs, other carnivores	Small intestine	Ingestion of intermediate host (small vertebrates, except fishes)	None	Reported	76
Cyclophyllidea							
Diplopylidium spp.	Africa, southern Europe	Cats	Small intestine	Ingestion or transport or intermediate host (reptiles)	None	Not reported	76
Dipylidium caninum	Worldwide	Cats, dogs	Small intestine	Ingestion of intermediate host (fleas)	Enteritis, anal pruritus	Reported	159
Echinococcus multilocularis	Europe, Japan, North America	Cats, canids	Small intestine	Ingestion of intermediate host (rodents)	None	Reported	76
Mesocestoides lineatus	Worldwide	Cats, canids	Small intestine; larva in abdominal cavity	Ingestion of intermediate host (amphibians, reptiles, birds, small mammals)	None	Reported	76
Taenia taeniaeformis	Worldwide	Cats	Small intestine	Ingestion of strobilocercus in intermediate host (rodents)	Focal intestinal mucosal necrosis at attachment sites	Reported	76
Nematodes							
Rhabditoidea							
Strongyloides felis	Australia	Cats	Small intestine	Penetration of skin or buccal mucosa by larva	Adenomatous-metaplasia of glandular epithelium of intestinal crypts	Not reported	165
Strongyloides tumefaciens	US	Cats	Large intestine	Unknown	Nodular lesions in colon	Not reported	164
Ascaridoidea							
Toxascaris leonina	Worldwide	Cats, dogs	Small intestine	Ingestion of embryonated egg or paratenic host	Mild enteritis	Reported	76
Toxocara cati	Worldwide	Cats	Small intestine	Ingestion of embryonated egg or infected paratenic host; transmammary	Enteritis, pulmonary vascular hypertrophy	Reported	92
Strongyloidea							
Ancylostoma braziliense	Africa, Americas	Cats, canids	Small intestine	Ingestion of infective larva or paratenic hosts; skin penetration	Focal hemorrhaging at feeding sites, anemia	Common	98
Ancylostoma ceylanicum	Asia, southern Africa	Cats, canids	Small intestine	Ingestion of infective larva or paratenic hosts; skin penetration	Focal hemorrhaging at feeding sites, anemia	Reported	98

Species	Geographic distribution	Host	Location	Transmission	Pathology	Zoonosis	Reference
Uncinaria stenocephala	Worldwide, mostly north of the equator	Cats, dogs	Small intestine	Ingestion of infective larva or paratenic hosts; skin penetration	Mild focal hemorrhaging at feeding sites	Reported	98
Trichostrongyloidea							
Ollulanus tricuspis	Americas, Australia, Europe, Northern Africa	Cats, other carnivores, swine	Stomach	Ingestion of larva passed by emesis	Gastritis	Not reported	76
Spirurida							
Abbreviata gemina	Egypt	Cats, wild carnivores, chickens	Stomach	Ingestion of intermediate host (insects)	Unknown	Not reported	76
Cyathospirura seurati	Worldwide	Cats, foxes, rats	Stomach	Ingestion of intermediate host (arthropods)	Unknown	Not reported	76
Cylicospirura felineus	Australia, India, New Zealand, North America	Cats	Stomach	Ingestion of intermediate host (arthropods)	Purulent gastric cysts	Not reported	76
Cylicospirura subaequalis	Africa, India, South America	Cats, wild carnivores	Stomach	Ingestion of intermediate host (arthropods)	Purulent gastric cysts	Not reported	76
Physaloptera brevispiculum	Ceylon	Exotic felids	Stomach	Ingestion of intermediate host (insects)	Unknown	Not reported	76
Physaloptera praeputialis	Worldwide	Cats	Stomach	Ingestion of intermediate host (insects)	Gastritis	Reported	76, 109
Physaloptera pseudopraeputialis	Philippine Islands, US	Cats	Stomach	Ingestion of intermediate host (insects)	Gastritis	Not reported	76, 109
Physaloptera pacitae	Central America, Philippine Islands	Cats	Stomach	Ingestion of intermediate host (insects)	Unknown	Not reported	76
Physaloptera rara	US	Cats, dogs, other carnivores	Stomach, duodenum	Ingestion of intermediate host (insects)	Gastritis	Unknown	76, 109
Trichuroidea							
Trichuris spp.	Americas, Australia, Europe	Cats	Cecum, colon	Ingestion of embryonated egg	None	Not reported	76
Dioctophymatoidea							
Soboliphyme baturini	North America, Asia	Martens (*Martes americana*), cats	Stomach wall	Unknown	None	Not reported	166
Acanthocephala							
Oncicola canis	Americas	Canids, cats	Small intestine	Ingestion of intermediate host (cockroaches) or paratenic host (armadillos, turkeys)	Enteritis, intestinal perforation	Not reported	168
Oncicola companulatus	South America	Cats	Small intestine	Ingestion of intermediate or transport host	Enteritis, intestinal perforation	Not reported	168

TABLE 18.3 Parasites of cats—respiratory system.

Parasite	Geographic Distribution	Hosts	Location in Host	Method of Infection	Pathologic Effects	Zoonosis	Reference
Trematodes							
Paragonimus kellicotti	North America	Cats, dogs, wild carnivores, domestic animals	Lungs, occasionally other organs	Ingestion of crustacean intermediate host (crab, crayfish)	Focal emphysema, lung cysts, pneumothorax	Reported	80
Paragonimus westermanii	Asia	Cats, dogs, wild carnivores, domestic animals	Lungs, occasionally other organs	Ingestion of crustacean intermediate host (crab, crayfish)	Focal emphysema, lung cysts, pneumothorax	Reported	80
Nematodes							
Strongylida							
Mammomonogamus spp.	Asia, Caribbean, South America	Cats	Nares, nasopharynx, trachea	Indirect; otherwise unknown	Inflammation of the nasopharynx	Reported	169
Metastrongyloidea							
Aelurostrongylus abstrusus	Worldwide	Cats	Lungs (omentum in rodents)	Ingestion of paratenic host (small vertebrates)	Focal areas of pulmonary consolidation	Not reported	106
Anafilaroides rostratus	Asia, Israel, North America	Cats, wild rodents	Lungs	Ingestion of intermediate or transport host (rodents)	Unknown	Not reported	170, 171
Troglostrongylus spp.	Africa, North America	Cats	Lungs	Ingestion of intermediate host or transport host (rodents)	Unknown	Not reported	173
Vogeloides spp.	Asia, Eastern Europe, North America	Cats	Lungs	Unknown	Unknown	Not reported	76, 167
Trichuroidea							
Eucoleus aerophilus	Europe, North and South America	Cats, foxes, dogs	Lungs	Ingestion of embryonated eggs	Tracheobronchitis, pulmonary edema, hemorrhage, pneumonia	Reported	110

TABLE 18.4 Parasites of cats—skin and connective tissue; musculoskeletal, urogenital, and central nervous systems.

Parasite	Geographic Distribution	Hosts	Location in Host	Method of Infection	Pathologic Effects	Zoonosis	Reference
Flagellates							
Leishmania spp.	Americas (cutaneous form), Europe, Middle East, northern Africa (visceral form)	Cats, dogs, sloths, rodents, primates, other mammals	Macrophages, spleen, bone marrow, skin	Bite of infected sand fly vector	Visceral or cutaneous lesions	Reported	1
Trypanosoma cruzi	Americas	Cats, other mammals	Muscle, skin, visceral organs, blood	Ingestion of infected bug vector	Myocarditis	Common	11
Nematodes							
Strongyloidea							
Mammomonogamus auris	China	Cats	Middle ear	Indirect, otherwise unknown	Hemorrhagic middle ear mucosa	Not reported	76
Trichuroidea							
Pearsonema feliscati	Worldwide	Cats	Urinary bladder	Ingestion of intermediate host (earthworms) or paratenic host	Cystitis	Not reported	114
Diptera (flies)							
Cuterebridae (bot flies)	Americas	Cats, rodents, lagomorphs	Subcutaneous, nasal passages	Direct contact	"warbles," feline ischemic encephalopathy	Reported	115, 118
Psychodidae (sand flies)	Worldwide	Cats, dogs, other mammals, birds	Skin	Direct contact	None	Common	119
Phthiraptera (lice)							
Felicola subrostratus	Probably worldwide	Cats	Pelage	Direct contact	Mild dermatitis, alopecia	Not reported	122
Siphonaptera (fleas)							
Ctenocephalides spp.	Worldwide	Cats, dogs, other mammals	Pelage, skin	Direct contact	Dermatitis, pathogen transmission	Common	123

(Continued)

TABLE 18.4 *(Continued)*

Parasite	Geographic Distribution	Hosts	Location in Host	Method of Infection	Pathologic Effects	Zoonosis	Reference
Arachnida							
Mites							
Astigmates							
Lynxacarus radovskyi	Australia, US	Cats	Pelage	Direct contact	Dry, dull, rust-colored coat	Reported	140
Notoedres cati	Africa, Europe, North America	Cats, rabbits, coatimundi	Skin (ears, head, neck)	Direct contact	Scaly dermatitis, alopecia, excoriation	Reported	142
Otodectes cynotis	Worldwide	Cats, rabbits, coatimundi	Auditory canal	Direct contact	Inflammation, torticollis	Reported	147
Prostigmates							
Cheyletiella blakei	Worldwide	Cats	Skin	Direct contact	Dermatitis, crusting	Common	128
Demodex cati	Worldwide	Cats	Skin	Direct contact	Dermatitis, alopecia	Not reported	132
Demodex gatoi	Unknown	Cats	Epidermal surface	Direct contact	Dermatitis, alopecia in immune-compromised cat	Not reported	132

610

REFERENCES

1. Simoes-Mattos, L., Bevilaqua, C.M.L., Mattos, M.R.F., and Pompeu, M.M.d.-L. (2004) Feline leishmaniasis: uncommon or unknown? *Rev. Port. Cienc. Vet.* **99**, 79–87.

2. Pennisi, M.G., Venza, M., Reale, S., Vitale, F., and Giudice, S.l. (2004) Case report of leishmaniasis in four cats. *Vet. Res. Commun.* **28**, 363–366.

3. Savani, E.S.M.M., Camargo, M.C.G.d.-O., Carvalho, M.R.d., et al. (2004) The first record in the Americas of an autochthonous case of *Leishmania* (*Leishmania*) *infantum chagasi* in a domestic cat (*Felix catus*) from Cotia County, Sao Paulo State, Brazil. *Vet. Parasitol.* **120**, 229–233.

4. Morsy, T.A. and El-Seoud, S.M.F.A. (1994) Natural infection in two pet cats in a house of a zoonotic cutaneous leishmaniasis patient in Imbaba Area, Giza Governorate, Egypt. *J. Egypt. Soc. Parasitol.* **24**, 199–204.

5. Schubach, T.M.P., Figueiredo, F.B., Pereira, S.A., et al. (2004) American cutaneous leishmaniasis in two cats from Rio de Janeiro, Brazil: first report of natural infection with *Leishmania* (*Viannia*) *braziliensis*. *Trans. Royal Soc. Trop. Med. Hyg.* **98**, 165–167.

6. Hervas, J., Lara, F.C.M.d., Sanchez-Isarria, M.A., et al. (1999) Two cases of feline visceral and cutaneous leishmaniosis in Spain. *J. Feline Med. Surg.* **1**, 101–105.

7. Durao, J.F.C., Rebelo, E., Peleteiro, M.C., Correia, J.J., and Simoes, G. (1994) First case of leishmaniosis in a domestic cat reported in Portugal. *Rev. Port. Cienc. Vet.* **89**, 140–144.

8. Barnes, J.C., Stanley, O., and Craig, T.M. (1993) Diffuse cutaneous leishmaniasis in a cat. *J. Am. Vet. Med. Assoc.* **202**, 416–418.

9. Balderrama, F., Romero, A., Garcia, J.A., et al. (1981) Epidemiological study of Chagas' disease in the Trigal Department of Santa Cruz, Bolivia. *Bol. Inform. CENETROP* **7**, 16–22.

10. Wisnivesky-Colli, C., Gurtler, R.E., Solarz, N.D., Lauricella, M.A., and Segura, E.L. (1985) Epidemiological role of humans, dogs and cats in the transmission of *Trypanosoma cruzi* in a central area of Argentina. *Rev. Instit. Med. Trop. Sao Paulo* **27**, 346–352.

11. Talice, R.V. (1938) Primeras observationes en el Uruguay de gatos espontaneamente infectados por el *Trypanosoma cruzi*. *Arch. Urug. Med. Chir. Espesiald.* **13**, 61–65.

12. Read, C.M., Monis, P.T., and Thompson, R.C.A. (2004) Discrimination of all genotypes of *Giardia duodenalis* at the glutamate dehydrogenase locus using PCR-RFLP. *Infect. Genet. Evol.* **4**, 125–130.

13. Bianciardi, R., Papini, R., Giuliani, G., and Cardini, G. (2004) Prevalence of *Giardia* antigen in stool samples from dogs and cats. *Rev. Med. Vet.* **155**, 417–421.

14. Keith, C.L., Radecki, S.V., and Lappin, M.R. (2003) Evaluation of fenbendazole for treatment of *Giardia* infection in cats concurrently infected with *Cryptosporidium parvum*. *Am. J. Vet. Res.* **64**, 1027–1029.

15. Scorza, A.V. and Lappin, M.R. (2004) Metronidazole for the treatment of feline giardiasis. *J. Feline Med. Surg.* **6**, 157–160.

16. Berrilli, F., Di Cave, D., De Liberato, C., Franco, A., Scaramozzino, P., and Orecchia, P. (2004) Genotype characterisation of *Giardia duodenalis* isolates from domestic and farm animals by SSU-rRNA gene sequencing. *Vet. Parasitol.* **122**, 193–199.

17. Cielecka, D., Borsuk, P., Grytner-Ziecina, B., and Turkowicz, M. (2000) First detection of *Trichomonas tenax* in dog and cat by PCR-RFLP. *Acta Parasitologica* **45**, 350–352.

18. Gothe, R., Beelitz, P., Schol, H., and Beer, B. (1992) Trichomonad infections of the oral cavity of cats in southern Germany. *Tierarztl. Prax.* **20**, 195–198.

19. Levy, M.G., Gookin, J.L., Poore, M., Birkenheuer, A.J., Dykstra, M.J., and Litaker, R.W. (2003) *Tritrichomonas foetus* and not *Pentatrichomonas hominis* is the etiologic agent of feline trichomonal diarrhea. *J. Parasitol.* **89**, 99–104.

20. Foster, D.M., Gookin, J.L., Poore, M.F., Stebbins, M.E., and Levy, M.G. (2004) Outcome of cats with diarrhea and *Tritrichomonas foetus* infection. *J. Am. Vet. Med. Assoc.* **225**, 888–892.

21. Gookin, J.L., Foster, D.M., Poore, M.F., Stebbins, M.E., and Levy, M.G. (2003) Use of a commercially available culture system for diagnosis of *Tritrichomonas foetus* infection in cats. *J. Am. Vet. Med. Assoc.* **222**, 1376–1379.

22. Gookin, J.L., Birkenheuer, A.J., Breitschwerdt, E.B., and Levy, M.G. (2002) Single-tube nested PCR for detection of *Tritrichomonas foetus* in feline faeces. *J. Clin. Microbiol.* **40**, 4126–4130.

23. Okamoto, S., Wakui, M., Kobayashi, H., et al. (1998) *Trichomonas foetus* meningoencephalitis after allogeneic peripheral blood stem cell transplantation. *Bone Marrow Trans.* **21**, 89–91.

24. Sargent, K.D., Morgan, U.M., Elliot, A., and Thompson, R.C.A. (1998) Morphological and genetic characterisation of *Cryptosporidium* oocysts from domestic cats. *Vet. Parasitol.* **77**, 221–227.

25. McGlade, T.R., Robertson, I.D., Elliot, A.D., Read, C., and Thompson, R.C.A. (2003) Gastrointestinal parasites of domestic cats in Perth, Western Australia. *Vet. Parasitol.* **117**, 251–262.

26. McReynolds, C.A., Lappin, M.R., Ungar, B., et al. (1999) Regional seroprevalence of *Cryptosporidium parvum*-specific IgG of cats in the United States. *Vet. Parasitol.* **80**, 187–195.

27. Ragozo, A.M.A., Muradian, V., Ramos-e-Silva, J.C., et al. (2002) Occurrence of gastrointestinal parasites in feces of cats from the cities of Sao Paulo and Guarulhos. *Braz. J. Vet. Res. Anim. Sci.* **39**, 244–246.

28. Lappin, M.R., Dowers, K., Taton-Allen, G., and Cheney, J. (1997) Cryptosporidiosis and inflammatory bowel disease in a cat. *Feline Pract.* **25**, 10–13.

29. Barr, S.C., Jamrosz, G.F., Hornbuckle, W.E., Bowman, D.D., and Fayer, R. (1994) Use of paromomycin for treatment of cryptosporidiosis in a cat. *J. Am. Vet. Med. Assoc.* **205**, 1742–1743.

30. Pieniazek, N.J., Bornay-Llinares, F.J., Slemenda, S.B., et al. (1999) New *Cryptosporidium* genotypes in HIV-infected persons. *Emerg. Infect. Dis.* **5**, 444–449.

31. Razmi, G.R. (2000) Prevalence of feline coccidia in Khorasan province of Iran. *J. Appl. Anim. Res.* **17**, 301–303.

32. Robben, S.R.M., Nobel, W.E.L., Dopfer, D., et al. (2004) Infections with helminths and/or protozoa in cats in animal shelters in the Netherlands. *Tijdschr. Diergeneeskd.* **129**, 2–6.

33. Freire, R.B. and Lopes, C.W.G. (1996) Distribution of hypnozoites of *Cystoisospora felis* (Wenyon, 1923) Frenkel, 1977 (Apicomplexa: Sarcocystidae) in experimentally infected albino mice. *Rev. Bras. Parasitol. Vet.* **5**, 23–27.

34. Melo, P.S., Carvalho-Filho, P.R.d., Oliveira, F.C.R.d., Flausino, W., and Lopes, C.W.G. (2003) Hypnozoites of *Cystoisospora felis* (Apicomplexa: Cystoisosporinae) in swine visceras: a new intermediate host. *Rev. Bras. Parasitol. Vet.* **12**, 103–107.

35. Dubey, J.P. and Streitel, R.H. (1976) *Isospora felis* and *I. rivolta* infections in cats induced by mouse tissue or oocysts. *Br. Vet. J.* **132**, 649–651.

36. Gobel, E. and Schonweitz, W. (1982) Development of *Cystoisospora felis* in the cat. *Fortschr. Veterinarmed. Beihefte Zentralb. Veterinarmed.* **35**, 278–281.

37. Loss, Z.G. and Lopes, C.W.G. (1992) Some clinical aspects of *Cystoisospora felis* (Wenyon, 1926) Frenkel, 1976 (Apicomplexa:

Cystoisosporinae) experimentally infected in cats. *Arq. Univ. Fed. Rural Rio de Janeiro* **15**, 79–84.

38. Loss, Z.G. and Lopes, C.W.G. (1992) Pathology of a *Cystoisospora felis* (Wenyon, 1926) Frenkel, 1976 (Apicomplexa: Cystoisosporinae) experimental infection in cats. *Arq. Univ. Fed. Rural do Rio de Janeiro* **15**, 113–119.

39. Lloyd, S. and Smith, J. (2001) Activity of toltrazuril and diclazuril against *Isospora* species in kittens and puppies. *Vet. Rec.* **148**, 509–511.

40. Dubey, J.P. (1979) Life cycle of *Isospora rivolta* (Grassi, 1879) in cats and mice. *J. Protozool.* **26**, 433–443.

41. Dubey, J.P., Navarro, I.T., Sreekumar, C., et al. (2004) *Toxoplasma gondii* infections in cats from Parana, Brazil: seroprevalence, tissue distribution, and biologic and genetic characterization of isolates. *J. Parasitol.* **90**, 721–726.

42. Dubey, J.P., Saville, W.J.A., Stanek, J.F., and Reed, S.M. (2002) Prevalence of *Toxoplasma gondii* antibodies in domestic cats from rural Ohio. *J. Parasitol.* **88**, 802–803.

43. Gauss, C.B.L., Almeria, S., Ortuno, A., Garcia, F., and Dubey, J.P. (2003) Seroprevalence of *Toxoplasma gondii* antibodies in domestic cats from Barcelona, Spain. *J. Parasitol.* **89**, 1067–1068.

44. Salant, H. and Spira, D.T. (2004) A cross-sectional survey of anti-*Toxoplasma gondii* antibodies in Jerusalem cats. *Vet. Parasitol.* **124**, 164–177.

45. Dubey, J.P. (1979) Direct development of enteroepithelial stages of *Toxoplasma* in the intestines of cats fed cysts. *Am. J. Vet. Res.* **40**, 1634–1637.

46. Dubey, J.P. (2001) Oocyst shedding by cats fed isolated bradyzoites and comparison of infectivity of bradyzoites of the VEG strain *Toxoplasma gondii* to cats and mice. *J. Parasitol.* **87**, 215–219.

47. Dubey, J.P. (1997) Tissue cyst tropism in *Toxoplasma gondii*: a comparison of tissue cyst formation in organs of cats, and rodents fed oocysts. *Parasitology* **115**, 15–20.

48. Dubey, J.P., Mattix, M.E., and Lipscomb, T.P. (1996) Lesions of neonatally induced toxoplasmosis in cats. *Vet. Pathol.* **33**, 290–295.

49. Parker, G.A., Langloss, J.M., Dubey, J.P., and Hoover, E.A. (1981) Pathogenesis of acute toxoplasmosis in specific-pathogen-free cats. *Vet. Pathol.* **18**, 786–803.

50. Dubey, J.P. and Carpenter, J.L. (1993) Histologically confirmed clinical toxoplasmosis in cats: 100 cases (1952–1990). *J. Am. Vet. Med. Assoc.* **203**, 1556–1566.

51. Last, R.D., Suzuki, Y., Manning, T., Lindsay, D., Galipeau, L., and Whitbread, T.J. (2004) A case of fatal systemic toxoplasmosis in a cat being treated with cyclosporin A for feline atopy. *Vet. Dermatol.* **15**, 194–198.

52. Powell, C.C. and Lappin, M.R. (2001) Clinical ocular toxoplasmosis in neonatal kittens. *Vet. Ophthalmol.* **4**, 87–92.

53. Haberkorn, A. (1996) Chemotherapy of human and animal coccidioses: state and perspectives. *Parasitol. Res.* **82**, 193–199.

54. Rommel, M., Schnieder, T., Krause, H.D., and Westerhoff, J. (1987) Trials to suppress the formation of oocysts and cysts of *Toxoplasma gondii* in cats by medication of the feed with toltrazuril. *Vet. Med. Rev.* **2**, 141–153.

55. Lindsay, D.S., Blagburn, B.L., and Dubey, J.P. (1997) Feline toxoplasmosis and the importance of the *Toxoplasma gondii* oocyst. *Compend. Contin. Educ. Pract. Vet.* **19**, 448–461, 506.

56. Dubey, J.P. (1976) Reshedding of *Toxoplasma* oocysts by chronically infected cats. *Nature* **262**, 213–214.

57. Meier, H.T. and Moore, L.E. (2000) Feline cytauxzoonosis: a case report and literature review. *J. Am. Anim. Hosp. Assoc.* **36**, 493–496.

58. Criado-Fornelio, A., Gonzalez-del-Rio, M.A., Buling-Sarana, A., and Barba-Carretero, J.C. (2004) The "expanding universe" of piroplasms. *Vet. Parasitol.* **119**, 337–345.

59. Ketz-Rilev, C.J., Reichard, M.V., Bussche, R.A.v.-d., Hoover, J.P., Meinkoth, J., and Kocan, A.A. (2003) An intraerythrocytic small piroplasm in wild-caught Pallas's cats (*Otocolobus manul*) from Mongolia. *J. Wildl. Dis.* **39**, 424–430.

60. Glenn, B.L. and Stair, E.L. (1984) Cytauxzoonosis in domestic cats: report of two cases in Oklahoma, with a review and discussion of the disease. *J. Am. Vet. Med. Assoc.* **187**, 822–825.

61. Blouin, E.F., Kocan, A.A., and Kocan, K.M. (1992) Development and transmission of *Cytauxzoon felis* by *Dermacentor variabilis*. In *First International Conference on Tick Borne Pathogens at the Host Vector Interface: An Agenda for Research:* Proceedings and Abstracts, September 15–18, 1992, University of Minnesota College of Agriculture, Department of Entomology, and Minnesota Extension Service, Saint Paul, Minnesota, USA. pages 75–81.

62. Hoover, J.P., Walker, D.B., and Hedges, J.D. (1994) Cytauxzoonosis in cats: eight cases (1985–1992). *J. Am. Vet. Med. Assoc.* **205**, 455–460.

63. Meinkoth, J., Kocan, A.A., Whitworth, L., Murphy, G., Fox, J.C., and Woods, J.P. (2000) Cats surviving natural infection with *Cytauxzoon felis*: 18 cases (1997–1998). *J. Vet. Intern. Med.* **14**, 521–525.

64. Walker, D.B. and Cowell, R.L. (1995) Survival of a domestic cat with naturally acquired cytauxzoonosis. *J. Am. Vet. Med. Assoc.* **206**, 1363–1365.

65. Lapage, G. (1962) *Mönnig's Veterinary Helminthology and Entomology.* 5th ed. Williams and Wilkins, Baltimore, MD. 600 pages.

66. Foley, R.H. (1994) *Platynosomum concinnum* infection in cats. *Compend. Contin. Educ. Pract. Vet.* **16**, 1271–1285.

67. Amin, B. (1978) Parasites of the domestic cat in Selangor, Malaysia. *Kajian Veterinar.* **10**, 107–114.

68. Chung, N.Y., Miyahara, A.Y., and Chung, G. (1977) The prevalence of feline liver flukes in the city and county of Honolulu. *J. Am. Anim. Hosp. Assoc.* **13**, 258–262.

69. Ferreira, A.M.R., Almeida, E.C.P.D., and Labarthe, N.V. (1999) Liver fluke infection (*Platynosomum concinnum*) in Brazilian cats: prevalence and pathology. *Feline Pract.* **27**, 19–22.

70. Hitt, M.E. (1981) Liver fluke infection in south Florida cats. *Feline Pract.* **11**, 26–29.

71. Ikede, B.O., Losos, G.J., and Isoun, T.T. (1971) *Platynosomum concinnum* infection in cats in Nigeria. *Vet. Rec.* **89**, 635–638.

72. Bielsa, L.M. and Greiner, E.C. (1985) Liver flukes (*Platynosomum concinnum*) in cats. *J. Am. Anim. Hosp. Assoc.* **21**, 269–274.

73. Jenkins, C.C., Lewis, D.D., Brock, K.A., Hager, D.A., and Meyer, D.J. (1988) Extrahepatic biliary obstruction associated with *Platynosomum concinnum* in a cat. *Compend. Contin. Educ. Pract. Vet.* **10**, 628–632.

74. Newell, S.M., Graham, J.P., Roberts, G.D., et al. (2001) Quantitative hepatobiliary scintigraphy in normal cats and in cats with experimental cholangiohepatitis. *Vet. Radiol. Ultrasound* **42**, 70–76.

75. Greve, J.H. and Leonard, P.O. (1966) Hepatic flukes (*Platynosomum concinnum*) in a cat from Illinois. *J. Am. Vet. Med. Assoc.* **149**, 418–420.

76. Bowman, D.D., Hendrix, C.M., Lindsay, D.S., and Barr, S.C. (2002) *Feline Clinical Parasitology*, Iowa State University Press, Ames, Iowa.

77. Scholz, T., Uhlirova, M., and Ditrich, O. (2003) Helminth parasites of cats from the Vientiane Province, Laos, as indicators of the occurrence of causative agents of human parasitoses. *Parasite* **10**, 343–350.

78. Hong, S., Lee, S., Lee, S., et al. (2003) Sustained-release praziquantel tablet: pharmacokinetics and the treatment of clonorchiasis in beagle dogs. *Parasitol. Res.* **91**, 316–320.

79. Hering-Hagenbeck, S. and Schuster, R. (1996) A focus of opisthorchiidosis in Germany. *Appl. Parasitol.* **37**, 260–265.

80. Herman, L.H. and Helland, D.R. (1966) Paragonimiasis in a cat. *J. Am. Vet. Med. Assoc.* **149**, 753–757.

81. Bowman, D.D., Frongillo, M.K., Johnson, R.C., Beck, K.A., Hornbuckle, W.E., and Blue, J.T. (1991) Evaluation of praziquantel for treatment of experimentally induced paragonimiasis in dogs and cats. *Am. J. Vet. Res.* **52**, 68–71.

82. Nicanor-Ibanez, H. and Cesar-Jara, C. (1992) Experimental paragonimiasis: therapeutical tests with praziquantel—first report. *Mem. Inst. Oswaldo Cruz* **87**, 107.

83. Barutzki, D. and Schaper, R. (2003) Endoparasites in dogs and cats in Germany 1999–2002. *Parasitol. Res.* **90**, 148–150.

84. Mar, P., Su, Y., Fei, A.C.Y., and Bowman, D.D. (1999) A survey of endoparasitic zoonoses of stray dogs and cats in Taipei city. *Asia Season. Rep. Env. Microbiol.* **8**, 77–86.

85. Tanaka, H., Watanabe, M., and Ogawa, Y. (1985) Parasites of stray dogs and cats in the Kanto region, Honshu, Japan. *J. Vet. Med., Japan* **771**, 657–661.

86. Uga, S., Goto, M., Matsumura, T., and Kagei, N. (1986) Natural infection of *Sparganum mansoni* in cats captured in Hyogo Prefecture, Japan. *Jap. J. Parasitol.* **35**, 153–159.

87. Dalimi, A., Sadraeii, J., and Tabaeii, S.J. (1996) A study on three cestode species of subfamily Dipylidinae from stray cats of Tehran. *J. Fac. Vet. Med. Univ. Tehran* **50**, 89–96.

88. Hinaidy, H.K. and Jahn, J. (1998) Morphometric observations on *Dipylidium caninum* from dogs and cats in Austria. *Wien. Tierarztl. Monatsschr.* **85**, 424–428.

89. Bauditz, R. and Sachs, H. (1979) Droncit injectable: new possibilities of tapeworm control. *Vet. Med. Rev.* **2**, 129–133.

90. Ekanayake, S., Warnasuriya, N.D., Samarakoon, P.S., Abewickrama, H., Kuruppuarachchi, N.D., and Dissanaike, A.S. (1999) An unusual 'infection' of a child in Sri Lanka, with *Taenia taeniaformis* of the cat. *Ann. Trop. Med. Parasitol.* **93**, 869–873.

91. Martinez-Barbabosa, I., Vazquez-Tsuji, O., Romero-Cabello, R., Gutierrez-Cardenas, E.M., and Amancio-Chasin, O. (2003) The prevalence of *Toxocara cati* in domestic cats in Mexico City. *Vet. Parasitol.* **114**, 43–49.

92. Coati, N., Schnieder, T., and Epe, C. (2004) Vertical transmission of *Toxocara cati* Schrank 1788 (Anisakidae) in the cat. *Parasitol. Res.* **92**, 142–146.

93. Genchi, C., Basano, F.S., Mortarino, M., et al. (2003) Selamectin (StrongholdReg., Pfizer): one year-use in the dog and in the cat in Italy. *Vet. Cremona* **17**, 51–59.

94. Reinemeyer, C.R. and Charles, S. (2003) Evaluation of the efficacy of a combination of imidacloprid and moxidectin against immature *Toxocara cati* in cats. *Parasitol. Res.* **90**, S140–141.

95. Fisher, M. (2003) *Toxocara cati*: an underestimated zoonotic agent. *Trends Parasitol.* **19**, 167–170.

96. Anderson, T.C., Foster, G.W., and Forrester, D.J. (2003) Hookworms of feral cats in Florida. *Vet. Parasitol.* **115**, 19–24.

97. Labarthe, N., Serrao, M.L., Ferreira, A.M.R., Almeida, N.K.O. and Guerrero, J. (2004) A survey of gastrointestinal helminths in cats of the metropolitan region of Rio de Janeiro, Brazil. *Vet. Parasitol.* **123**, 133–139.

98. Bowman, D.D. (1992) Hookworm parasites of dogs and cats. *Compend. Contin. Educ. Pract. Vet.* **14**, 585–595.

99. Traub, R.J., Robertson, I.D., Irwin, P., Mencke, N., and Thompson, R.C.A. (2004) Application of a species-specific PCR-RFLP to identify *Ancylostoma* eggs directly from canine faeces. *Vet. Parasitol.* **123**, 245–255.

100. Heukelbach, J., Wilcke, T., and Feldmeier, H. (2004) Cutaneous larva migrans (creeping eruption) in an urban slum in Brazil. *Int. J. Dermatol.* **43**, 511–515.

101. Humbert-Droz, E., Buscher, G., Cavalleri, D., and Junquera, P. (2004) Efficacy of milbemycin oxime against fourth-stage larvae and adults of *Ancylostoma tubaeforme* in experimentally infected cats. *Vet. Rec.* **154**, 140–143.

102. McTier, T.L., Shanks, D.J., Wren, J.A., et al. (2000) Efficacy of selamectin against experimentally induced and naturally acquired infections of *Toxocara cati* and *Ancylostoma tubaeforme* in cats. *Vet. Parasitol.* **91**, 311–319.

103. Burrows, R.B. (1965) *Microscopic Diagnosis of the Parasites of Man.* Yale University Press, New Haven, 328 pages.

104. Ayaz, E., Deger, S., Gul, A., and Yuksek, N. (2001) The distribution of helminths in Van cats and their importance in public health. *Turkiye Parazitoloji Dergisi* **25**, 166–169.

105. Pomroy, W.E. (1999) A survey of helminth parasites of cats from Saskatoon. *Can. Vet. J.* **40**, 339–340.

106. Burgu, A. and Sarmehmetoglu, O. (2004) *Aelurostrongylus abstrusus* infection in two cats. *Vet. Rec.* **154**, 602–604.

107. Ribeiro, V.M. and Lima, W.S. (2001) Larval production of cats infected and re-infected with *Aelurostrongylus abstrusus* (Nematoda: Protostrongylidae). *Rev. Med. Vet.* **152**, 815–820.

108. Smith, H.A. and Jones, T.C. (1966) *Veterinary Pathology*, 3rd ed., Lea and Febiger, Philadelphia, PA, 1192 pages.

109. Campbell, K.L. and Graham, J.C. (1999) *Physaloptera* infection in dogs and cats. *Compend. Contin. Educ. Pract. Vet.* **21**, 299–314.

110. Foster, S.F., Martin, P., Allan, G.S., Barrs, V.R., and Malik, R. (2004) Lower respiratory tract infections in cats: 21 cases (1995–2000). *J. Feline Med. Surg.* **6**, 167–180.

111. Habermann, R.T. and Williams, F.P. (1958) The identification and control of helminths in laboratory animals. *J. Natl. Cancer Inst.* **20**, 979–1009.

112. Herman, L.H. (1967) *Capillaria aerophila* infection in a cat. *Vet. Med.* **62**, 466–468.

113. Harris, L.T. (1981) Feline bladderworm. *Vet. Med. Small Anim. Clin.* **76**, 844.

114. Wilson-Hanson, S. and Prescott, C.W. (1982) *Capillaria* in the bladder of the domestic cat. *Aust. Vet. J.* **59**, 190–191.

115. Sabrosky, C.W. (1986) *North American Species of Cuterebra: The Rabbit and Rodent Bot Flies (Diptera: Cuterebridae)*, Entomology Society of America, 240 pages.

116. Dvorak, L.D., Bay, J.D., Crouch, D.T., and Corwin, R.M. (2000) Successful treatment of intratracheal cuterebrosis in two cats. *J. Am. Anim. Hosp. Assoc.* **36**, 304–308.

117. Harris, B.P., Miller, P.E., Bloss, J.R., and Pellitteri, P.J. (2000) Ophthalmomyiasis interna anterior associated with *Cuterebra* spp in a cat. *J. Am. Vet. Med. Assoc.* **216**, 352–355.

118. Glass, E.N., Cornetta, A.M., deLahunta, A., Center, S.A., and Kent, M. (1998) Clinical and clinicopathologic features in 11 cats with *Cuterebra* larvae myiasis of the central nervous system. *J. Vet. Int. Med.* **12**, 365–368.

119. Dias, F.d.-O.P., Lorosa, E.S., and Rebelo, J.M.M. (2003) Blood feeding sources and peridomiciliation of *Lutzomyia longipalpis* (Lutz and Neiva, 1912) (Psychodidae, Phlebotominae). *Cad. Saude Publica* **19**, 1373–1380.

120. Akucewich, L.H., Philman, K., Clark, A., et al. (2002) Prevalence of ectoparasites in a population of feral cats from north central Florida during the summer. *Vet. Parasitol.* **109**, 129–139.

121. Shanks, D.J., Gautier, P., McTier, T.L., Evans, N.A., Pengo, G., and Rowan, T.G. (2003) Efficacy of selamectin against biting lice on dogs and cats. *Vet. Rec.* **152**, 234–237.

122. Pollmeier, M., Pengo, G., Longo, M., and Jeannin, P. (2004) Effective treatment and control of biting lice, *Felicola subrostratus* (Nitzsch in Burmeister, 1838), on cats using fipronil formulations. *Vet. Parasitol.* **121**, 157–165.

123. Georgi, J.R. and Georgi, M.E. (1991) *Canine Clinical Parasitology,* Lea and Febiger, Malvern, PA, 227 pages.

124. Rust, M.K. and Dryden, M.W. (1997) The biology, ecology, and management of the cat flea. *Ann. Rev. Entomol.* **42**, 451–473.

125. Vobis, M., D'-Haese, J., Mehlhorn, H., and Mencke, N. (2003) Evidence of horizontal transmission of feline leukemia virus by the cat flea (*Ctenocephalides felis*). *Parasitol. Res.* **91**, 467–470.

126. Kelly, P.J., Meads, N., Theobald, A., Fournier, P.E., and Raoult, D. (2004) *Rickettsia felis, Bartonella henselae,* and *B. clarridgeiae* in New Zealand. *Emerg. Infect. Dis.* **10**, 967–968.

127. Hsu, M., Hsu, T., and Wu, W. (2002) Distribution of cat fleas (Siphonaptera: Pulicidae) on the cat. *J. Med. Entomol.* **39**, 685–688.

128. Foley, R.H. (1991) Parasitic mites of dogs and cats. *Compend. Contin. Educ. Pract. Vet.* **13**, 783–800.

129. Beck, C.W. (2000) The efficacy of fipronil (FrontlineReg.) against ectoparasites: control of lice, mites and mallophages in diverse small animals. *Tierarztl. Umsch.* **55**, 244–250.

130. Chailleux, N. and Paradis, M. (2002) Efficacy of selamectin in the treatment of naturally acquired cheyletiellosis in cats. *Can. Vet. J.* **43**, 767–770.

131. Wagner, R. and Stallmeister, N. (2000) *Cheyletiella* dermatitis in humans, dogs and cats. *Br. J. Dermatol.* **143**, 1110–1112.

132. Foley, R.H. (1995) Feline demodicosis. *Compend. Contin. Educ. Pract. Vet.* **17**, 481–487.

133. Desch, C.E., Jr. and Stewart, T.B. (1999) *Demodex gatoi:* new species of hair follicle mite (Acari: Demodecidae) from the domestic cat (Carnivora: Felidae). *J. Med. Entomol.* **36**, 167–170.

134. Guaguere, E., Olivry, T., Delverdier-Poujade, A., Denerolle, P., Pages, J.P., and Magnol, J.P. (1999) *Demodex cati* infestation in association with feline cutaneous squamous cell carcinoma *in situ:* a report of five cases. *Vet. Dermatol.* **10**, 61–67.

135. Poucke, S.V. (2001) Ceruminous otitis externa due to *Demodex cati* in a cat. *Vet. Rec.* **149**, 651–652.

136. Johnstone, I.P. (2002) Doramectin as a treatment for canine and feline demodicosis. *Aust. Vet. Pract.* **32**, 98–103.

137. Tenorio, J.M. (1974) A new species of *Lynxacarus* (Acarina: Astigmata: Listrophoridae) from *Felis catus* in the Hawaiian Islands. *J. Med. Entomol.* **11**, 599–604.

138. Greve, J.H. and Gerrish, R.R. (1981) Fur mites (*Lynxacarus*) from cats in Florida. *Feline Pract.* **11**, 28–30.

139. Foley, R.H. (1991) An epizootic of a rare fur mite in an island's cat population. *Feline Pract.* **19**, 17–19.

140. Craig, T.M., Teel, P.D., Dubuisson, L.M., and Dubuisson, R.K. (1993) *Lynxacarus radovskyi* infestation in a cat. *J. Am. Vet. Med. Assoc.* **202**, 613–614.

141. Foley, R.H. (1991) A notoedric mange epizootic in an island's cat population. *Feline Pract.* **19**, 8–10.

142. Leone, F., Albanese, F., and Fileccia, I. (2003) Feline notoedric mange: a report of 22 cases. *Prat. Med. Chir. Anim. Compagnie.* **38**, 421–427.

143. Itoh, N., Muraoka, N., Aoki, M., and Itagaki, T. (2004) Treatment of *Notoedres cati* infestation in cats with selamectin. *Vet. Rec.* **154**, 409.

144. Hatsushika, R., Miyoshi, K., and Shimizu, M. (1979) Five human cases of feline scabies, *Notoedres cati,* infestation. *Jap. J. San. Zool.* **30**, 289–291.

145. Baker, E.W., Evans, T.M., Gould, D.J., Hull, W.B., and Keegan, H.L. (1956) *A Manual of Parasitic Mites of Medical or Economic Importance.* Technical Publications of the National Pest Control Association, Inc., New York. 170 pages.

146. Itoh, N. and Itoh, S. (2002) Prevalence of *Otodectes cynotis* infestation in household cats. *J. Jap. Vet. Med. Assoc.* **55**, 155–158.

147. Lohse, J., Rinder, H., Gothe, R., and Zahler, M. (2002) Validity of species status of the parasitic mite *Otodectes cynotis. Med. Vet. Entomol.* **16**, 133–138.

148. Blot, C., Kodjo, A., Reynaud, M.C., and Bourdoiseau, G. (2003) Efficacy of selamectin administered topically in the treatment of feline otoacariosis. *Vet. Parasitol.* **112**, 241–247.

149. Fourie, L.J., Kok, D.J., and Heine, J. (2003) Evaluation of the efficacy of an imidacloprid 10%/moxidectin 1% spot-on against *Otodectes cynotis* in cats. *Parasitol. Res.* **90**, S112–113.

150. Smith, D.D. and Frenkel, J.K. (1984) *Besnoitia darlingi* (Apicomplexa, Sarcocystidae, Toxoplasmatinae): transmission between opossums and cats. *J. Protozool.* **31**, 584–587.

151. Frenkel, J.K. (1977) *Besnoitia wallacei* of cats and rodents: with a reclassification of other cyst-forming isosporoid coccidia. *J. Parasitol.* **63**, 611–628.

152. Dubey, J.P. and Sreekumar, C. (2003) Redescription of *Hammondia hammondi* and its differentiation from *Toxoplasma gondii. Int. J. Parasitol.* **33**, 1437–1453.

153. Diesing, L., Heydorn, A.O., Matuschka, F.R., et al. (1988) *Besnoitia besnoiti:* Studies on the definitive host and experimental infections in cattle. *Parasitol. Res.* **75**, 114–117.

154. Njenga, J.M., Bwangamoi, O., Kangethe, E.K., Mugera, G.M., and Mutiga, E.R. (1995) Comparative ultrastructural studies on *Besnoitia besnoiti* and *Besnoitia caprae. Vet. Res. Commun.* **19**, 295–308.

155. Ernst, J.V, Chobotar, B., Oaks, E.C., Hammond, D.M. (1968) *Besnoitia jellisoni* (Sporozoa: Toxoplasmea) in rodents from Utah and California. *J. Parasitol.* **54**, 545–549.

156. Dubey, J.P., Sreekumar, C., Rosenthal, B.M., et al. (2004) Redescription of *Besnoitia tarandi* (Protozoa: Apicomplexa) from the reindeer (*Rangifer tarandus*). *Int. J. Parasitol.* **34**, 1273–1287.

157. Anderson, W.I., Georgi, M.E., and Car, B.D. (1987) Pancreatic atrophy and fibrosis associated with *Eurytrema procyonis* in a domestic cat. *Vet. Rec.* **120**, 235–236.

158. Rodriguez-Vivas, R.I., Williams, J.J., Quijano-Novelo, A.G., Bolio, G.M., and Torres-Acosta, J.F. (2004) Prevalence, abundance, and risk factors of live fluke (*Platynosomum concinnum*) infection in cats in Mexico. *Vet. Rec.* **154**, 693–694.

159. Gadre, D.V., Kumar, A., and Mathur, M. (1993) Infection by *Dipylidium caninum* through pet cats. *Indian J. Pediatr.* **60**, 151–152.

160. Ooi, H.K., Chang, S.L., Huang, C.C., Kawakami, Y., and Uchida, A. (2000) Survey of *Spirometra erinaceieuropaei* in frogs in Taiwan and its experimental infection in cats. *J. Helminthol.* **74**, 173–176.

161. Penzhorn, B.L., Schoeman, T., and Jacobson, L.S. (2004) Feline babesiosis in South Africa: a review. *Ann. N.Y. Acad. Sci.* **1026**, 183–186.

162. Denham, D.A. and Fletcher, C. (1987) The cat infected with *Brugia pahangi* as a model of human filariasis. *CIBA Found. Symp.* **127**, 225–235.

163. Harbut, C.L. and Orihel, T.C. (1995) *Brugia beaveri:* microscopic morphology in host tissues and observations on its life history. *J. Parasitol.* **81**, 239–243.

164. Hendrix, C.M., Blagburn, B.L., and Lindsay, D.S. (1987) Whipworms and intestinal threadworms. *Vet. Clin. North Am. Small Anim. Pract.* **17**, 1355–1375.

165. Speare, R. and Tinsley, D.J. (1987) Survey of cats for *Strongyloides felis. Aust. Vet. J.* **64**, 191–192.

166. Zarnke, R.L., Whitman, J.S., Flynn, R.W., and Ver Hoef, J.M. (2004) Prevalence of *Soboliphyme baturini* in marten (*Martes americana*) populations from three regions of Alaska, 1990–1998. *J. Wildl. Dis.* **40**, 452–455.

167. Pence, D.B., Tewes, M.E., and Laack, L.L. (2003) Helminths of the ocelot from southern Texas. *J. Wildl. Dis.* **39**, 683–689.

168. Soulsby, E.J.L. (1982) *Helminths, Arthropods and Protozoa of Domesticated Animals,* 7th ed., Lea and Febiger, Philadelphia, PA, 809 pages.

169. Cuadrado, R., Maldonado-Moll, J.F., and Segarra, J. (1980) Gapeworm infection of domestic cats in Puerto Rico. *J. Am. Vet. Med. Assoc.* **176**, 996–997.

170. Seneviratna, P. (1959) Studies on *Anafilaroides rostratus* Gerichter, 1949 in cats. I. The adult and its first stage larva. *J. Helminthol.* **33**, 99–108.

171. Seneviratna, P. (1959) Studies on *Anafilaroides rostratus* Gerichter, 1949 in cats. II. The life cycle. *J. Helminthol.* **33**, 109–122.

172. Watson, T.G., Nettles, V.F., and Davidson, W.R. (1981) Endoparasites and selected infectous agents in bobcats (*Felis rufus*) from West Virginia and Georgia. *J. Wildl. Dis.* **17**, 547–554.

CHAPTER

19

Parasites of Swine

T. Bonner Stewart, PhD

INTRODUCTION

Parasites must be considered as variables in biomedical research. Parasitic infections can spread quickly through a herd and are often easily recognized by the presence of moribund or dead pigs. However, loss of appetite, reduction in rate of gain, poor feed utilization, potentiation of other pathogens, and interference with research are the more common results of parasitism in the research animal facility. Parasite prevalence rates vary greatly, depending on geographic region, type of housing, management, nutrition, pig breed and strain, and species of parasite. The parasites

_____

Tables are placed at the ends of chapters.

discussed in this chapter are those more likely to be encountered in the research environment, while the tables at the end of the chapter also include less common parasites.

PROTOZOA

Phylum Sarcomastigophora

Class Mastigophora (flagellates)

Isospora suis
Morphology. Oocysts are large, oval to subspherical, and measure 24.6 μ to 31.9 μ long by 23.2 μ to 29 μ wide[1].

Hosts and Life Cycle. *Isospora suis* has been identified in pigs throughout the world. The life cycle is direct.

Oocysts released in the feces sporulate in the environment in four days. Sporozoites are released following ingestion. These undergo schizogony, followed by gametogony, in the small intestine. The prepatent period is six to eight days.

Pathologic Effects and Clinical Disease. Typically, only young pigs are affected, while adults are asymptomatic carriers. The predominant clinical sign is profuse diarrhea. Other signs include emaciation, terminal constipation, and death.

Diagnosis, Treatment, and Prevention. Presumptive diagnosis is by finding large numbers of characteristic oocysts in diarrheic feces. The diagnosis is confirmed histologically. The condition can be treated with Amprolium. Supplemental fluids and electrolytes may facilitate recovery. Prevention is based on improved hygiene and eliminating overcrowding.

Public Health Considerations. *Isospora suis* does not infect humans.

Phylum Ciliophora

Balantidium coli

The ciliated protozoan *Balantidium coli* is a common, commensal organism found globally in the cecum and anterior colon of swine, including those used in research. It also infects guinea pigs, dogs, rats, and primates, including humans. The motile trophozoite is pleomorphic and measures 30 μ to 150 μ long by 25 μ to 120 μ in diameter. Trophozoites are covered with longitudinal rows of cilia. A subterminal cytostome is present. Cysts measure 40 μ to 60 μ in diameter. A kidney-shaped macronucleus and a smaller micronucleus are present in both trophozoites and cysts.

Reproduction is by binary fission. Environmentally resistant cysts are released into the environment. In the intestinal tract, *B. coli* feeds on starch, bacteria, ingesta, and nematode eggs. It is a secondary invader into mucosal lesions, following other invaders, and produces hyaluronidase, which enlarges lesions.

Humans, other primates, and dogs have been found clinically affected in zoos and in areas near hog farms. *B. coli* may cause an explosive bloody diarrhea in these species. Treatment is generally not warranted, though *B. coli* can be eliminated with oxytetracycline[1]. It is probably impractical to attempt to keep swine free of *B. coli*. However, strict adherence to sanitation protocols minimizes infections. Animal care personnel should practice excellent personal hygiene when working with pigs.

CESTODES

Cyclophyllidea

Taenia solium

Swine serve as the natural intermediate host for *Taenia solium* (Syn. *Cysticercus cellulosae*), while humans serve as the natural definitive host. Larval forms (cysticerci) develop in the skeletal and cardiac muscles of the pig following ingestion of proglottids in human feces. Cysticerci measure up to 18 mm in diameter, and are infective by two to three months and remain so for two years.

Following ingestion of infected muscle tissue by humans, tapeworms mature to the adult stage in the small intestine. Cysticercosis in swine is usually of no clinical significance, though very heavy infections may cause myocarditis. Humans may also serve as intermediate hosts of *T. solium,* and may develop life-threatening infections of the central nervous system. Infections in swine are generally diagnosed incidentally at necropsy. Thus, treatment is typically not attempted. Infections in swine can be prevented by prohibiting access to human feces. While cysticercosis is a life-threatening condition for humans, it is not likely that animal workers will contract the disease from research swine, unless carcasses are made available for human consumption.

NEMATODES

Superfamily Rhabditoidea

Strongyloides ransomi

Morphology. Only parthenogenetic females are present in the parasitic generation. Adults are practically microscopic, measuring just 3.3 mm to 4.5 mm in length. The filariform esophagus occupies about a third of the total body length. The vulva is located near the middle of the body. The thin-shelled eggs passed in the feces contain larvae and measure 45 μ to 55 μ long by 26 μ to 35 μ wide (Figure 19.1).

Hosts. *Strongyloides ransomi,* the small-intestinal threadworm, parasitizes swine, primarily in the warmer climatic regions, where it is an important parasite of suckling pigs.

Life Cycle. Larvated eggs passed in the feces hatch in a few hours into first-stage rhabditiform larvae. These may develop either directly into infective larvae (homogonic cycle) or into males and females (heterogonic cycle), which in turn produce infective larvae. In the homogonic cycle, infective larvae can appear in a little more than a day. In the heterogonic cycle, infective larvae can appear in 2.5 days.

Swine become infected through several routes. Percutaneous penetration by larvae produce patent infections in six to 10 days. Larvae enter the bloodstream, proceed to the lungs, undergo tracheal migration, and are swallowed. Oral infections occur when ingested larvae penetrate the mucous membranes and migrate to the lungs. Third-stage larvae arriving in the stomach are killed by gastric secretions. Transcolostral infection may also occur by four days after birth. This is considered the primary means of infection of neonates in the southeastern United States. Larvae in the sow colostrum differ physiologically from infective larvae in the environment, and pass through the stomach and develop into adults in the small intestine without migration. Larvae responsible for infection of

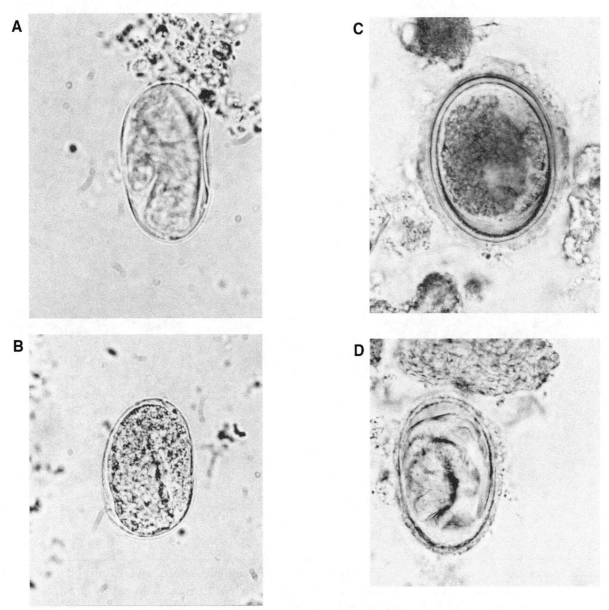

Fig. 19.1 Eggs of common swine parasites. (A) *Strongyloides* egg is thin-shelled, lacking one of three layers, and larvated; (B) *Ascarops* egg is larvated and similar to that of *Physocephalus* and *Gongylonema;* (C) *Ascaris* egg has an outer proteinaceous layer which is often missing; (D) *Metastrongylus* egg; (E) *Oesophagostomum* egg; (F) *Hyostrongylus* egg; (G) *Globocephalus* egg; (H) *Stephanurus dentatus* egg passed in the urine; (I) *Trichuris* egg; (J) *Macracanthorhynchus* egg. All eggs photographed at the same magnification. Reproduced from Corwin, R.M. and Stewart, T.B. (1999) with permission.

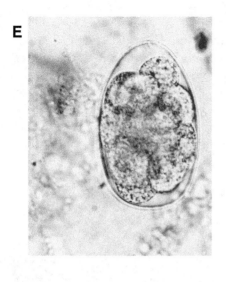

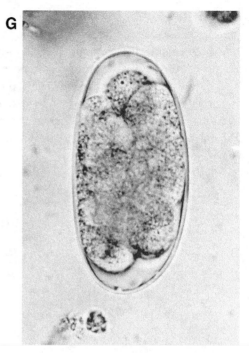

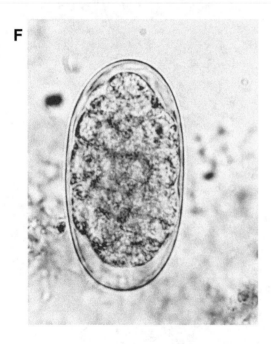

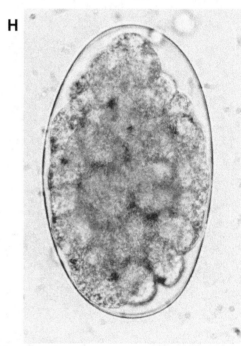

Fig. 19.1   *(Continued)*

neonates are sequestered in the mammary fat of the sow and apparently are mobilized and included in the colostrum[3,4]. Prenatal infection results in patent infections in suckling pigs as early as two to three days after birth. Larvae from the sow accumulate in various tissues of the fetus during the latter part of pregnancy, and complete migration to the small intestine of the newborn rapidly after birth.

Pathologic Effects and Clinical Disease. Infected pigs develop diarrhea, followed by progressive dehydration. In heavy infections, death generally occurs before pigs are 10 to 14 days old, but stunting and unthriftiness are the more usual sequelae of *S. ransomi* infection[5]. Larvae can be distributed throughout most tissues of the body, and lesions depend on the number of larvae and host

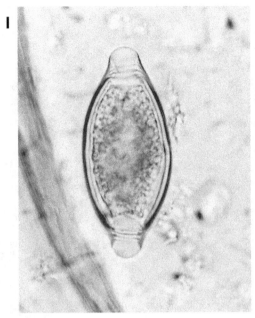

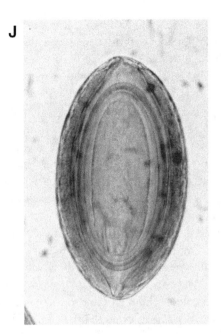

Fig. 19.1   *(Continued)*

response[6]. In this regard, Duroc pigs are less susceptible to the effects of infection than Hampshire pigs, and the F$_1$ cross of the two breeds is intermediate in response[7].

Diagnosis, Treatment, and Prevention. Diagnosis is by identification of eggs in feces or finding the adults in the small intestine at necropsy, when there is a history of diarrhea and unthriftiness. However, care must be taken because clinical disease can be confused with colibacillosis and coccidiosis. Infections with somatic and adult worms may be treated with ivermectin (injectable or feed additive), doramectin, thiabendazole, and levamisole[2]. Infective larvae are susceptible to environmental extremes, particularly dessication. Thus, infections can be prevented by providing clean, dry housing for research swine.

Public Health Considerations. *Strongyloides ransomi* does not infect humans.

Superfamily Ascaridoidea

Ascaris suum

Morphology. Ascarids are large, stout-bodied, pinkish-yellow nematodes with three prominent lips surrounding the mouth (Figure 19.2). Females measure 20 cm to 40 cm long, and the males measure 15 cm to 25 cm long. The male tail is conical and bent ventrally. Males have two stout spicules. The female vulva is anterior to the middle of the body. Eggs are thick-shelled and brownish-yellow with a mammillated proteinaceous coating on the exterior and

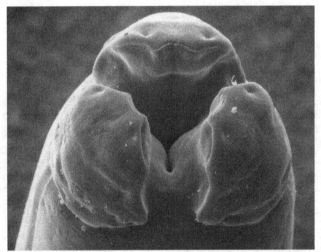

Fig. 19.2   The three lips of *Ascaris suum*. Reproduced from Corwin, R.M. and Stewart, T.B. (1999) with permission.

measure 50 μ to 80 μ long by 40 μ to 60 μ wide. The eggs are unsegmented when passed (Figure 19.1).

Hosts. *Ascaris suum* infects swine and is found worldwide. It is the most common gastrointestinal worm parasite in pigs, with typical prevalence rates of 50% to 75%. It is more common in growing pigs than in mature pigs. Although now recognized as a separate species, the large roundworm of humans, *A. lumbricoides,* was once thought to represent human infections with *A. suum.*

Life Cycle. The life cycle of *A. suum* is direct, and involves a hepatotracheal migration route. Eggs are laid in the intestine of the pigs and pass out in the feces. At room temperature, infective, third-stage larvae develop in about a month[8]. Eggs remain infective for seven years or longer if protected from environmental extremes. Following ingestion, eggs hatch in the digestive tract. The liberated third-stage larvae penetrate the intestinal wall and generally pass via the hepatic portal system to the liver. A few, however, may pass via the lacteals to the mesenteric lymph nodes. Still others may be found in the peritoneal cavity. Most larvae arrive at the liver by the first or second day after ingestion, and are in the lungs by days four to seven. Beginning on day eight, larvae penetrate the bronchioles, are coughed up into the trachea, and are swallowed. By 10 to 15 days after infection, larvae have returned to the small intestine and molted to the fourth larval stage. At this time, some larvae move from the small intestine into the cecum and colon. The final molt to the young adult stage occurs 21 to 30 days after ingestion of eggs. The prepatent period is 40 to 53 days.

Female ascarids are phenomenal egg producers, capable of laying hundreds of thousands to nearly 2 million eggs per day. The eggs are sticky and are easily transported by cockroaches and other arthropods, birds, boots, etc. Most disinfectants have no effect on the eggs, but heat (steam) and direct sunlight render them nonviable.

Most adult *A. suum* live in pigs only about six months, at which time acquired immunity causes them to begin to be expelled. Thereafter, pigs may continue to carry a light infection for a year or longer. In foreign hosts such as humans or other animals, larvae may migrate, but are generally unable to develop to adults in the intestine and are expelled in the feces if they reach the digestive system. Thus, the life cycle is not completed in these aberrant hosts.

Pathologic Effects. Following ingestion, larvae migrate through the liver and cause focal lesions that consist of eosinophilic infiltration, lymphoid nodules in portal areas, and hemorrhaging. On repeated exposure there is an increase in connective tissue, infiltrating eosinophils, and dilation of lymphatics, which grossly appear as whitish spots, commonly referred to as "milk spots." Such lesions disappear within 25 days.

In the lungs, migrating larvae cause verminous pneumonia, which may result in death if large numbers of larvae are involved. Clinical signs are those of pneumonia. Pigs have an asthmatic cough ("thumps") and may breathe with difficulty. Hemorrhagic foci are present in the lungs. In addition, there may be an exudate, edema, and emphysema with secondary bacterial pneumonia. Migration of

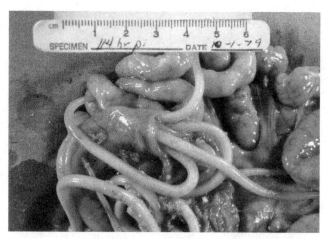

Fig. 19.3 *Ascaris* emerging from a tear in the gut wall. Photo by Mark Martinez. Reproduced from Corwin, R.M. and Stewart, T.B. (1999) with permission.

A. suum larvae markedly enhances the pathogenicity of swine influenza virus and other respiratory pathogens.

Adult worms also compete with the host for nutrients and interfere with absorption of nutrients by the host. They may occlude and rupture the small intestine (Figure 19.3). Adult worms may also migrate into the common bile duct and occlude it, causing icterus.

Diagnosis. Diagnosis is by finding the characteristic eggs in fecal flotation or milk spot liver lesions at necropsy. In heavy infections the adult worms can be seen and felt in the intact intestine. In areas where the kidney worm is endemic, liver lesions must be differentiated because early lesions caused by *Stephanurus dentatus* can be confused with those caused by *A. suum*.

Treatment. Feeding pyrantel tartrate for several weeks can be helpful under lot or pasture conditions to control infections and reduce lesions from ascarids. Prophylactic use of pyrantel or repetitive treatments with fenbendazole reduce worm populations and also appear to stimulate immunity against *A. suum*[9,10]. Anthelmintics effective against adult worms include ivermectin (injectable or feed additive), doramectin, moxidectin, levamisole, dichlorvos, and piperazine[2].

Prevention. Eggs are remarkably resistant to common disinfectants that are used in the animal facility. Thus, it is extremely important to prevent the buildup of ascarid eggs in the animal facility environment. Eggs can be killed with steam.

Public Health Considerations. *Ascaris suum* causes visceral larva migrans in humans. Animal workers should practice excellent personal hygiene when working with potentially infected pigs.

Superfamily Strongyloidea

Globocephalus urosubulatus

The hookworm of swine, *Globocephalus urosubulatus*, may be found in feral and pastured swine throughout the world, but is uncommon in laboratory swine. Adult worms measure 4.5 mm to 5.5 mm long and the females measure 5 mm to 6 mm long. The mouth opens subdorsally, and the buccal capsule is globular or funnel-shaped (Figure 19.4)[11]. The eggs are typically strongyloid and measure 52 μ to 56 μ long by 26 μ to 35 μ wide (Figure 19.1). Pigs become infected by ingestion or skin penetration of infective larvae. Adults mature in the small intestine. Little is known of the pathology caused by *G. urosubulatus*, but it is likely similar to hookworm diseases of other animals.

Anthelmintics useful for treating canine hookworm disease may also be effective for treating swine infected with *G. urosubulatus*. Ivermectin is not effective[12]. Because *G. urosubulatus* survives best in moist environments, such as pastures, housing research pigs indoors or on concrete greatly decreases opportunities for infection. *Globocephalus urosubulatus* has not been reported to infect humans.

Oesophagostomum spp.

Morphology. Adult female *Oesophagostomum* have stout, slightly curved bodies, and measure 1 cm to 2 cm long. Males are slightly shorter. Species differentiation is by shape of the esophagus and buccal capsule and the length of the tail and spicules (Figure 19.5). The eggs measure 70 μ long by 40 μ wide; they are morulated when passed, thin-shelled, and typically strongyloid (Figure 19.1).

Hosts. Swine are the natural hosts to at least three species of *Oesophagostomum*. Of these, *O. dentatum* and *O. quadrispinulatum* are the most common and occur throughout the world. Another species, *O. brevicaudum*, occurs in the southeastern United States and Asia. Two additional named species, *O. granatensis* in Europe and *O. georgianum* in the southeastern United States, are probably morphovariants of *O. dentatum*[13,14].

Life Cycle. Eggs are deposited in the environment. First-stage larvae emerge and molt to the infective third larval stage by one week, and can survive on pastures for up to 12 months. Swine are infected by ingesting third-stage larvae in pens or on pasture, by mechanical transmission by flies, or by ingesting rats harboring encysted larvae[15]. After ingestion, larvae enter the mucosa of the cecum and colon and molt to the fourth larval stage, and then return to the intestinal lumen for the final molt to adult. The prepatent period is three weeks.

Pathologic Effects and Clinical Disease. Mucosal larvae induce the formation of nodules in the cecum and rectum[16,17]. These may be associated with focal petechiation[18]. Locally, there is also focal thickening of the mucosa due to inflammation consisting of lymphocytes,

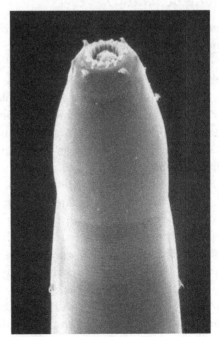

Fig. 19.5 Scanning electron micrograph of anterior of *Oesophagostomum brevicaudum*. Reproduced from Corwin, R.M. and Stewart, T.B. (1999) with permission.

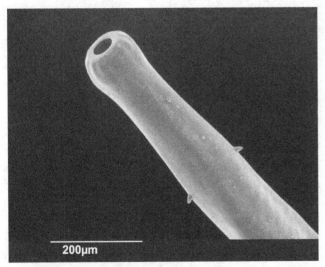

200μm

Fig. 19.4 Scanning electron micrograph of anterior end of adult female *Globocephalus* sp.

macrophages, and eosinophils. By one week after infection, nodules may measure up to 8 mm in diameter and be filled with yellow to black necrotic debris. The wall of the cecum and colon become edematous from extensive thrombosis of lymphatics, with the possible formation of localized fibrinonecrotic membranes. Resolution begins the second week, with ultimate scarring at the former sites of nodule formation.

Secondary infections may occur and exacerbate the clinical signs, which include depression, anorexia, and scouring. Pigs older than three months of age are more susceptible to disease[19]. A periparturient rise in fecal egg count is maintained through lactation, with subsequent expulsion of worms[19,20].

Diagnosis, Treatment, and Prevention. Diagnosis is by finding characteristic eggs in feces. Feeding pyrantel tartrate for several weeks can be helpful under lot or pasture conditions to control infections and reduce lesions caused by nodular worms. Other effective anthelmintics include ivermectin (injectable or feed additive), doramectin, moxidectin, fenbendazole, and piperazine[2].

Public Health Considerations. Humans may become infected with *Oesophagostomum* spp. of pigs[21]. Animal workers should practice excellent personal hygiene when working with infected swine.

Stephanurus dentatus

Morphology. Adult *Stephanurus dentatus,* swine kidney worms, are thick-bodied with black and white mottling from contents of the reproductive and intestinal tracts showing through the cuticle. Adult worms measure 1 cm to 3 cm long by 2 mm in diameter. The eggs are typical of the superfamily. They are ellipsoidal, thin-walled, and morulated, and measure 120 µ long by 70 µ wide (Figure 19.1).

Hosts. Domestic and feral pigs raised on soil in warm climates are most often infected. In North America, *S. dentatus* is found from the Carolinas to southern Missouri in the United States; interstate transport accounts for the worm's appearance as far north as Canada[22].

Life Cycle. Adult worms may be found in the kidneys and in cysts within the perirenal fat, with fistulous openings into the ureters. Worms may also be found in ectopic sites, including the pancreas, lumbar muscles, spinal cord, and lungs. Eggs are voided in the urine, with the greatest numbers found at first urination from overnight accumulation in the bladder. Eggs hatch in one to two days, molt to the infective third larval stage in three to five days, and survive for several months in warm, moist, shaded conditions.

Infection occurs through ingestion or skin penetration of infective larvae or by ingestion of infected earthworm paratenic hosts[23,24]. Prenatal infection sometimes occurs[25]. Following infection, larvae migrate from the small intestine to the mesenteric lymph nodes and molt to the fourth larval stage, which move through portal veins to the liver[26]. Other larvae migrate to the bronchioles, pancreas, or spleen[27]. In the liver, fourth-stage larvae undergo a final molt to the young adult stage, leave the liver, and migrate through the body cavity to perirenal and mesenteric fat[26]. The prepatent period is typically nine to 12 months, and eggs may be shed for up to three years[25].

Pathologic Effects and Clinical Disease. Larval migration is associated with pathological changes. Thus, mesenteric lymph nodes may be edematous and swollen. Hepatic changes include inflammation, eosinophilia, abscess formation, and extensive fibrosis, making this infection easily differentiated from ascarid migration. Similar lesions can be seen in other organs. Nodules are formed in perirenal fat, and fistulous tracts are present along the ureters. Posterior paralysis has been associated with migration around the spinal cord.

Diagnosis, Treatment, and Prevention. Diagnosis is by finding eggs in the urine or adult worms at necropsy. Infections can be treated with ivermectin, doramectin, fenbendazole, and levamisole[2]. Where research swine are bred on site, a management system in which only gilts are used as breeders and boars are kept separate from gilts will effectively eliminate kidney worms. This is due to the long prepatent period, and because only animals two years old or older pass kidney worm eggs in significant numbers. Swine breeders that provide animals to local research facilities should use this management system[2].

Public Health Considerations. *Stephanurus dentatus* has not been reported to infect humans.

Superfamily Trichostrongyloidea

Hyostrongylus rubidus

Morphology. Adult *Hyostrongylus rubidus* are slender, red worms with cuticular striations (Figure 19.6). Males measure 4 mm to 7 mm long and females measure 5 mm to 9 mm long. Males have a pair of short spicules and a bursa. The female vulva is located on the mid posterior half of the body. Cervical papillae are present. The eggs are typical strongyle type and are in the 16- to 32-cell stage when passed in the feces. They are thin-shelled and measure 60 µ to 76 µ long by 30 µ to 38 µ wide (Figure 19.1).

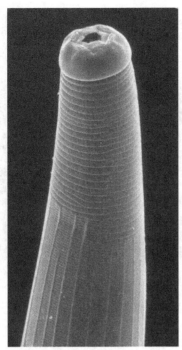

Fig. 19.6 Scanning electron micrograph of anterior of *Hyostrongylus rubidus* showing cuticular striations. Reproduced from Corwin, R.M. and Stewart, T.B. (1999) with permission.

Hosts. *Hyostrongylus rubidus* is the red stomach worm of pigs. Worms are commonly found in the lesser curvature of the stomach.

Life Cycle. Eggs develop on the ground into infective third-stage larvae in about seven days. After ingestion, the infection becomes patent in about 21 days. Larvae enter the gastric glands, where they remain for about two weeks where they molt twice, returning to the lumen as young adults. Larvae can remain in the mucosa for several months in a histotrophic stage similar to that of *Ostertagia* sp. of cattle and sheep, and cause formation of small nodules.

Pathologic Effects and Clinical Disease. Infections are typically nonpathogenic. Heavily infected pigs may develop hyperemia, catarrhal gastritis, submucosal edema, hyperplasia of the gastric gland area, erosion of the mucosa, and gastric ulcers[28–30]. *Hyostrongylus rubidus* is a blood sucker, and in herds with clinical hyostrongylosis, emaciation and pallor of the skin and mucous membranes may be apparent in adult animals[31,32]. Clinically unapparent infections can lead to reduced weight gains and feed conversion as well as nitrogen imbalance[33,34].

Diagnosis, Treatment, and Prevention. The eggs are nearly indistinguishable from those of *Oesophagostomum* spp. in both size and morphology, although *H. rubidus*

eggs are more advanced in development. The two can be differentiated by larval culture[35]. Several anthelmintics are effective against *H. rubidus,* including ivermectin (injectable or feed additive), doramectin, fenbendazole, thiabendazole, dichlorvos, and pyrantel tartrate[2]. Because *H. rubidus* survives best in moist environments, such as on pasture, housing research pigs indoors or on concrete greatly decreases opportunities for infection.

Public Health Considerations. *Hyostrongylus rubidus* does not infect humans.

Superfamily Metastrongyloidea

Metastrongylus spp.

Morphology. Adult *Metastrongylus* spp. are slender and white, with females measuring 50 mm in length and males 25 mm in length. Males have paired spicules. Mucoid deposits around adults make it difficult to separate individuals. Eggs are embryonated and thick-shelled and measure 40 μ to 50 μ in diameter (Figure 19.1).

Hosts. Species found in swine include *M. apri* (Syn. *Metastrongylus elongatus*), *M. confusus*, *M. pudendotectus*, *M. madagascariensis,* and *M. salmi.* These occur exclusively in the bronchi and bronchioles, especially the diaphragmatic lobes, of swine. *Metastrongylus* spp. occur worldwide and natural infections often consist of two species. *M. apri* is the most common of the known species.

Life Cycle. Embryonated eggs are released by female worms, coughed up and swallowed, and pass out with the feces. Earthworms ingest these eggs, which then hatch, and first-stage larvae migrate to the heart of the earthworm host. Infective larvae develop within 10 days. Infected earthworms are consumed by rooting swine. In the pig, third-stage larvae penetrate the wall of the intestine and are transported to the mesenteric lymph nodes, where they molt to the fourth larval stage. These are then transported via the circulation, to the lungs (Figure 19.7), where they undergo their final molt. The prepatent period is four weeks.

Pathologic Effects and Clinical Disease. Dissection of the bronchioles reveals mucoid plugs in the diaphragmatic lobes of the lungs, representing accumulations of adult worms and eggs. Parasites, mucus, and cellular exudate cause airway occlusion and induce atelectasis, observed as coughing or "thumps."

Diagnosis. The eggs of *Metastrongylus* spp. may be difficult to find in fecal flotations. Recognition may be facilitated by examining mucous aggregates for entrapped eggs. At necropsy, lungworms can be extruded by clipping

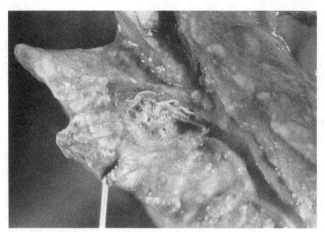

Fig. 19.7 Cluster of *Metastrongylus* worms in a terminal bronchiole of the diaphragmatic lobe of the lung. Photo by Blaise Brazos. Reproduced from Corwin, R.M. and Stewart, T.B. (1999) with permission.

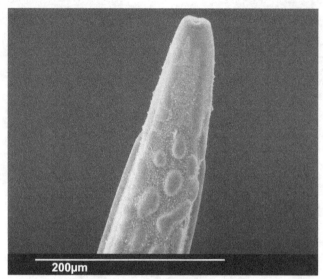

Fig. 19.8 Scanning electron micrograph of anterior end of adult female *Gongylonema* sp.

the posteroventral margins or the tip of the diaphragmatic lobes of the lungs.

Treatment and Prevention. Lungworm infections may be treated with ivermectin (injectable or feed additive), doramectin, moxidectin, fenbendazole, and levamisole. Infection can be prevented by eliminating sources of earthworm intermediate hosts. This requires housing research pigs indoors or on concrete.

Public Health Considerations. *Metastrongylus* spp. do not infect humans.

Superfamily Spiruroidea

Ascarops strongylina

Ascarops strongylina is found in the stomach of pigs worldwide. Wild rodents have also been found to be infected[36]. Adult male worms measure 10 mm to 15 mm long and the females measure 16 mm to 22 mm long. Adult worms are red and the buccal capsule bears a pair of teeth anteriorly[11]. The eggs are thick-shelled and measure 34 μ to 40 μ long by 18 μ to 22 μ wide (Figure 19.1). The life cycle of *A. strongylina* is indirect. Pigs become infected by consuming coprophagus beetles. *Ascarops strongylina* may cause gastritis when present in large numbers. Infections are best treated with dichlorvos or fenbendazole[2]. Infection can be prevented by eliminating sources of beetle intermediate hosts. *Ascarops strongylina* does not infect humans.

Gongylonema pulchrum

Gongylonema pulchrum inhabits the epithelial layer of the esophagus and tongue of swine and ruminants and less

commonly, rabbits, deer, bears, squirrels, horses, camels, and primates, including humans, throughout the world. Adult male worms measure up to 62 mm long and females measure up to 145 mm long[11]. Anteriorly, the cuticle bears numerous round or oval thickenings, and cervical alae are prominent (Figure 19.8). The spicules are unequal in length. The eggs are thick-shelled and measure 57 μ to 59 μ long by 30 μ to 34 μ wide.

The life cycle is indirect. Eggs released in the feces are ingested by coprophagus beetles, in which the eggs hatch and larvae develop to the infective stage in 30 days. Pigs become infected after consuming infected beetles. Larvae migrate anteriorly from the stomach to the esophagus and oral cavity of the definitive host. Adult worms are not highly pathogenic, though mild inflammatory reactions do occur. When chronic, these may lead to hypertrophy of the epithelium.

Diagnosis is by finding the characteristic eggs in fecal samples. There are no effective anthelmintic treatments reported for pigs infected with. *G. pulchrum*. Infection can be prevented by eliminating sources of arthropod intermediate hosts. Rarely, humans have become infected with *G. pulchrum*. Animal workers should practice excellent personal hygiene when working with infected pigs.

Physocephalus sexalatus

Physocephalus sexalatus is found in the stomach of pigs throughout the world. It has also been found in lagomorphs and other mammals. Adult male worms measure 6 mm to 13 mm long and females measure 13 mm to 22.5 mm long. The cuticle of the anterior end is slightly inflated in the region of the pharynx, and the inflation is followed by three cervical alae on either side[11]. The mouth is small and lacks teeth. The eggs are thick-shelled and measure 31 μ to 39 μ long by 12 μ to 17 μ wide. The life cycle is similar to that of *Ascarops strongylina*. Heavily infected animals develop gastritis, including inappetence, excessive thirst, growth retardation, and death.

Diagnosis is by finding the characteristic eggs in the feces. Infections may be eliminated with dichlorvos or fenbendazole[2]. Infection can be prevented by eliminating sources of arthropod intermediate hosts. *Physocephalus sexalatus* does not infect humans.

Superfamily Trichuroidea

Trichinella spiralis

Morphology. First-stage larval *Trichinella spiralis* cysts in muscle tissue measure 400 μ to 600 μ long and 250 μ in diameter. Adult female worms are found in small intestinal lamina propria. They have a stichosome-type esophagus, produce larvated eggs *in utero,* and measure 3 mm to 4 mm long and 60 μ in diameter. Adult males are rarely seen, but are about one-half the size of females.

Hosts. All mammalian species are probably susceptible to infection with *T. spiralis,* though climate appears to influence natural cycles. For example, in temperate zones, the natural cycle typically includes swine and bears as natural hosts[37], while in the arctic zone polar bears, grizzly bears, and walruses are natural hosts[38,39]. Other species, including humans, become infected incidentally. Trichinellosis is found less frequently in tropical zones. Regulation of garbage feeding to swine, public health programs, and recently improved trichinoscopic and serodiagnostic techniques have reduced the prevalence of this infection.

Life Cycle. Muscle cysts are ingested and digested in the stomach and small intestine, and first-stage larvae are liberated into the small intestine. Molting from first stage through the young adult stage occurs in two to six days. Males die soon after mating and females burrow into lymph spaces, where they deposit larvae. Larvae circulate in the blood from eight to 25 days postinfection, then penetrate the sarcolemma of skeletal muscle fibers throughout the body and become encysted by three months (Figure 19.9). Although calcification of cysts begins at six to nine months, first-stage larvae remain viable for up to 11 years, demonstrating the symbiotic

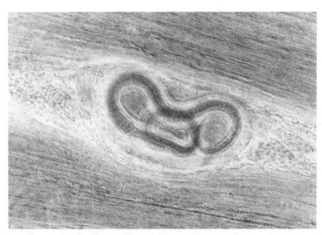

Fig. 19.9 *Trichinella* larvated cyst. Photo by Blaise Brazos. Reproduced from Corwin, R.M. and Stewart, T.B. (1999) with permission.

relationship between the larvae and the host muscle fiber, or "nurse cell"[40].

Modes of transmission in swine herds include cannibalism, tail biting, scavenging on carcasses of dead animals (cats, foxes, raccoons), and direct or indirect feeding of raw garbage. Some hog lots are built on covered garbage dumps[41–44].

Pathologic Effects and Clinical Disease. *Trichinella* is much less pathogenic for swine than for rats and humans. Experimental infections in pigs cause decreased weight gains and intense muscle pain, but most pigs recover with rapid weight gain[45]. Experimentally infected miniature pigs develop eosinophilia and hypergammaglobulinemia[46]. Clinical illness has not been described in naturally infected pigs.

Diagnosis. Diagnosis is by digestion of muscle at necropsy, or by enzyme-linked immunosorbent assay (ELISA) for detection of *Trichinella*-specific antibodies[47]. A pooled-sample digestion method using 5-gram to 6-gram diaphragm samples from lots of 20 pig carcasses has been adopted by several European countries but not by the U.S. Department of Agriculture[48]. Pooled samples are digested and homogenized using 1% pepsin/1% HCL and a mixing action which simulates peristaltic motion of the stomach. Analysis of pooled samples can be accomplished in 1.5 hours[49]. An ELISA test using an excretory antigen for diagnosis of trichinosis was evaluated in the field with sera from herds with ongoing transmission of *T. spiralis*[50]. Results showed a sensitivity of 93% to 96% with sera from infected pigs. Of those that were false-negative, most had fewer than five larvae per gram of tissue.

Treatment and Prevention. Ivermectin has no anthelmintic activity against *T. spiralis,* whereas excellent efficacy was reported for albendazole[2]. Calf thymus extract, cyclosporin A, and the experimental compound luxabendazole have also been proven to be efficacious[51].

Public Health Considerations. While trichinosis remains an important zoonotic disease, animal workers cannot become infected as a result of working with infected research swine.

Trichuris suis

Morphology. Adult female *Trichuris suis* measure 6 cm to 8 cm long while males measure about half that length. The anterior or esophageal portion of the worm measures 0.5 mm in diameter and extends two thirds the length of the body. The esophagus is a stichosome-type, consisting of a column of spiraling stichocytes, one cell layer in thickness. A microscopic lancet protrudes from the stoma in all stages. Glandular and muscular components are interspersed along the esophagus. The posterior third of the body is thicker, measuring 0.65 mm in diameter, and contains the midgut of the worm and the reproductive tract.

Bipolar, thick-shelled eggs may be seen in the uterus of the female, and a single copulatory spicule is present in the male. Eggs measure 60 μ long by 25 μ wide, are yellow to brown, and are released in the one-cell stage (Figure 19.1).

Hosts. Wild and domestic swine are the natural hosts of *Trichuris suis,* the swine whipworm. However, primates, including humans, may also be infected[52]. Whipworms are globally distributed and are common in endemic areas.

Life Cycle. Eggs passed in the feces require three to four weeks to embryonate to the infective, first larval stage. They can remain infective for as long as six years. After ingestion, infective eggs hatch in the small intestine and cecum, where the released larvae penetrate cells lining the crypts. A histotrophic phase persists for two weeks with gradual larval migration from the deeper lamina propria to the submucosa. Luminal development through four molts begins the third week postinfection with the posterior body coming into view and the anterior end remaining buried in the mucosa (Figure 19.10)[53]. The prepatent period is six to seven weeks and the life span is four to five months[54].

Pathologic Effects and Clinical Disease. *Trichuris* infections cause enterocyte destruction, ulceration of the intestinal mucosal lining, capillary erosion and blood loss, mucosal edema, formation of fibrinonecrotic membranes, anemia, hypoalbuminemia, and possibly secondary bacterial infection. Thus, trichuriosis must be considered in the differential diagnosis of swine dysentery complex that does not respond to antibiotic therapy.

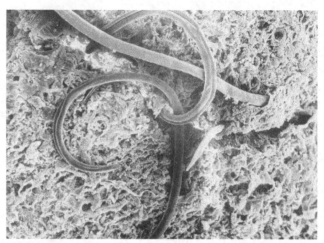

Fig. 19.10 *Trichuris* worm. Note intracellular penetration. Reproduced from Batte, E.G., McLamb, R.D., Muse, K.E., Tally, S.D., and Vestal, T.J. (1977) with permission.

Clinical signs include anorexia, mucoid to bloody diarrhea, dehydration, and death. Swine less than six weeks of age are more susceptible, though adult swine may show clinical infection when stressed. Light infections persist, allowing intermittent shedding of eggs. Infection of pigs with *T. suis* was shown to induce suppression of mucosal immunity to resident bacteria and is linked to the pathogenesis of necrotic proliferative colitis[55].

Diagnosis, Treatment, and Prevention. A presumptive diagnosis can be made based on clinical signs, including bloody scouring. Confirmation is by finding eggs in the feces and adult worms at necropsy. Trichurids are sporadic egg shedders. Thus, little significance can be given to the number of eggs per gram of feces. Infections may be eliminated with dichlorvos or fenbendazole. Other commonly used anthelmintics give variable results against whipworms[2]. Infections can be prevented by frequently cleaning pens to minimize parasite load in the environment. Research swine should not be housed on soil.

Public Health Considerations. Controlled studies suggest that humans are susceptible to infection with *T. suis*[52]. Animal workers should practice excellent personal hygiene when working with infected research swine.

ACANTHOCEPHALA

Macracanthorhynchus hirudinaceus is the thorny-headed worm of swine. Infections are common in most swine-raising regions of the world. Incidental hosts include muskrats (*Ondatra zibethicus*), squirrels, and humans. Adult male worms measure up to 10 cm in length and

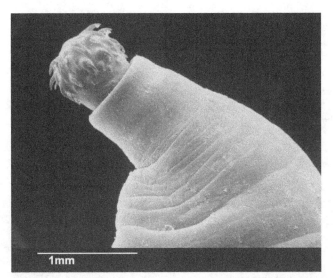

Fig. 19.11 Scanning electron micrograph of anterior end of adult *Macracanthorhynchus hirudinaceus.*

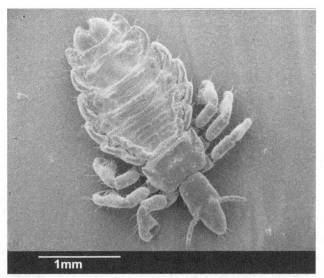

Fig. 19.12 Scanning electron micrograph of dorsal view of adult *Haematopinus suis.*

females measure up to 35 cm in length. Eggs measure 110 μ long by 65 μ wide, are brown, and have a three-layered shell (Figure 19.1). Adult worms are pale red in color and the cuticle is transversely wrinkled. The proboscis is small and bears six rows of hooks (Figure 19.11)[11].

The life cycle is indirect, with dung beetles serving as intermediate hosts. Larval beetles become infected by feeding on embryonated worm eggs. Pigs become infected through ingestion of infected larval or adult beetles[56]. In the pig, worms develop to the adult stage in two to three months. Adult worms attach to the ileal portion of the small intestine and cause nodular lesions, which are sometimes invaded by secondary organisms. Occasionally the gut wall is perforated by the proboscis, and peritonitis results.

Diagnosis is by finding the characteristic eggs in fecal flotation samples. Eliminating the parasite with anthelmintics is difficult. For example, in one study, doramectin eliminated only 62.1% of *M. hirudinaceus*[57]. In a limited study, others have found the antidiarrheal drug loperamid effective when administered orally at 1 to 1.5 mg/kg twice per day for three consecutive days[58].

Infection can be prevented by housing research pigs indoors or on concrete, and eliminating beetles. As noted above, humans are susceptible to infection with *M. hirudinaceus,* though patent infections do not develop. Animal workers should practice excellent personal hygiene when working with infected research pigs.

ARTHROPODS

Class Insecta

Order Phthiraptera

Haematopinus suis

Haematopinus suis is the sucking louse of pigs. Infestations are common globally. Adult *H. suis* lack eyes, the paratergal plates are prominent, and there is one row of spines on each abdominal segment (Figure 19.12)[11]. The tarsal claws are of equal size. Lice are highly host-specific. Thus, infestations are limited to swine. Mild infestations are generally of no consequence, but heavy infestations can lead to severe anemia.

Lice can be eliminated with ivermectin or doramectin[2]. Infestations can be prevented by purchasing research swine from reputable dealers, and if necessary, treating swine at the time of entry into the animal colony. *Haematopinus suis* does not infect humans.

TABLE 19.1 Parasites of swine—circulatory and lymphatic systems.

Parasite	Geographic Distribution	Hosts	Location in Host	Method of Infection	Pathologic Effects	Zoonosis	Reference
Flagellates							
Trypanosoma simiae	East and Central Africa	Warthogs, other swine, other mammals	Blood, lymphoid tissue in many organs	Transmitted by tsetse fly (*Glossina*)	Encephalitis, myocarditis, pneumonia, death	Not reported	59
Trypanosoma suis	Central Africa	Warthogs, other swine	Blood	Transmitted by tsetse fly (*Glossina*)	Systemic illness, death	Not reported	60
Piroplasmids							
Babesia perroncitoi	Africa, Asia, Europe	Wild and domestic swine	Blood	Transmitted by tick	Anemia, dependent edema, icterus	Not reported	61
Babesia trautmanni	Central Africa, Europe	Wild and domestic swine	Blood	Transmitted by tick	Anemia, icterus, dependent edema	Not reported	62
Trematodes							
Schistosoma incognitum	Asia	Swine, dogs, rats, primates	Mesenteric veins	Skin penetration by cercariae	Phlebitis, granulomatous reactions	Not reported	63
Schistosoma japonicum	Asia	Swine, other mammals	Hepatic portal vessels	Skin penetration by cercariae, transplacental transmission	Phlebitis, granulomatous reactions	Common	64

TABLE 19.2 Parasites of swine—enterohepatic system.

Parasite	Geographic Distribution	Hosts	Location in Host	Method of Infection	Pathologic Effects	Zoonosis	Reference
Flagellates							
Chilomastix mesnili	Worldwide	Primates, swine	Cecum, colon	Ingestion of cyst	None	Common	1
Enteromonas suis	India	Swine	Cecum	Ingestion of cyst	None	Not reported	1
Giardia duodenalis	Worldwide	Mammals	Small intestine	Ingestion of cyst	Mild enteritis	Common	65
Tetratrichomonas buttreyi	Europe, US	Swine, cattle	Cecum, colon	Ingestion of trophozoite	None	Not reported	66
Trichomitus rotunda	North America	Swine	Cecum, colon	Ingestion of trophozoite	None	Not reported	1
Tritrichomonas suis	Worldwide	Swine, cattle	Stomach, cecum, small intestine	Ingestion of trophozoite	None	Not reported	67
Amoebae							
Entamoeba suis	Worldwide	Swine	Cecum, colon	Ingestion of cyst	None	Not reported	68
Iodamoeba butschlii	Worldwide	Swine, primates	Cecum, colon	Ingestion of cyst	None	Common	1
Coccidia							
Eimeria spp.	Worldwide	Swine	Large intestine	Ingestion of sporulated oocyst	None	Not reported	1, 11
Isospora almaataensis	Eastern Europe	Swine	Unknown	Unknown	None	Not reported	11
Isospora suis	Worldwide	Swine	Small intestine	Ingestion of sporulated oocyst in feces	Enteritis	Not reported	69
Ciliates							
Balantidium coli	Worldwide	Swine, primates, dogs, rats	Large intestine	Ingestion of cyst	Secondary invader: enteritis	Reported	70
Trematodes							
Brachylaemus suis	Africa	Swine	Intestine	Ingestion of second intermediate host (rabbits, rodents, pigeons)	None	Not reported	72
Clonorchis sinensis	Asia	Swine, cats, dogs, primates, other mammals	Liver, gallbladder, bile duct, pancreatic duct, small intestine	Ingestion of second intermediate host (fishes)	Cholangitis, hepatic cirrhosis	Reported	11
Dicrocoelium dendriticum	Worldwide	Livestock, swine, dogs, lagomorphs, humans	Liver	Ingestion of second intermediate host (ants)	Hepatic cirrhosis, bile duct distension	Reported	11
Echinochasmus perfoliatus	Asia, Europe	Swine, dogs, cats, foxes	Intestine	Ingestion of second intermediate host (fishes)	Enteritis	Reported	11
Eurytrema pancreaticum	Asia, Eastern Europe, South America	Swine, ruminants, humans	Pancreas, bile duct, duodenum	Ingestion of second intermediate host (grasshoppers, crickets)	Pancreatitis	Reported	73

(Continued)

631

TABLE 19.2 (Continued)

Parasite	Geographic Distribution	Hosts	Location in Host	Method of Infection	Pathologic Effects	Zoonosis	Reference
Fasciola hepatica	Worldwide	Ruminants, swine, other mammals	Hepatic bile ducts	Ingestion of metacercaria on herbage	Hepatitis	Reported	74
Fasciolopsis buski	Asia, US	Swine, humans	Small intestine	Ingestion of metacercaria on tubers	Enteritis	Common	75
Gastrodiscus aegyptiacus	Africa, India	Equids, swine	Intestines	Ingestion of metacercaria on herbage	Unknown	Not reported	76
Gastrodiscoides hominis	Africa, Asia, Australia	Swine, humans	Cecum, colon	Ingestion of metacercaria on herbage	Enteritis caused by juvenile flukes	Common	77
Metagonimus yokogawai	Asia, Balkans	Swine, dogs, cats, humans, pelicans	Small intestine	Ingestion of second intermediate host (fishes)	Mild enteritis	Reported	78
Opisthorchis tenuicollis	Asia, Europe	Swine, cats, dogs, foxes, cetaceans	Hepatic bile ducts, intestine, pancreas	Ingestion of second intermediate host fishes	Cholangitis, hepatic cirrhosis	Reported	11
Postharmostomum suis	Tunisia	Swine	Small intestine	Ingestion of intermediate host (snails)	Mild anemia	Not reported	11
Cestodes							
Larval							
Echinococcus granulosus	Worldwide	Sheep, swine, primates, other mammals	Liver	Ingestion of egg in feces of definitive host (dogs)	Hydatid cyst	Common	79
Adult							
Diphyllobothrium latum	Eastern Europe, North and South America	Swine, dogs, cats, polar bears, other fish-eating mammals	Small intestine	Ingestion of second intermediate host (fishes)	None	Reported	11
Nematodes							
Rhabditoidea							
Strongyloides ransomi	Worldwide	Swine	Small intestine	Ingestion, skin penetration, transmammary, transplacental transmission	Enteritis	Not reported	4
Ascaridoidea							
Ascaris suum	Worldwide	Swine	Small intestine	Ingestion of embryonated egg	Enteritis, focal hepatitis, pneumonia	Reported	80
Strongyloidea							

632

Organism	Geographic distribution	Host(s)	Location	Mode of infection	Pathology	Zoonosis	Ref.
Ancylostoma duodenale	Africa, Asia, Europe	Humans, wild carnivores, swine	Small intestine	Ingestion, skin penetration of infective larvae	Enteritis, anemia, cutaneous larva migrans	Common	11
Bourgelatia diducta	Asia	Swine	Cecum, colon	Ingestion of embryonated eggs	Unknown	Not reported	11
Globocephalus spp.	Worldwide	Swine	Small intestine	Ingestion, skin penetration	Enteritis, anemia	Not reported	81
Necator americanus	Africa, Americas, Asia	Humans, swine, dogs	Small intestine	Ingestion, skin penetration of infective larvae	Enteritis, anemia	Common	11
Oesophagostomum brevicaudum	Americas, Asia	Swine	Cecum, colon	Ingestion of infective larvae or paratenic hosts (rodents)	Enteritis, intestinal nodules	Reported	11
Oesophagostomum dentatum	Asia, Americas, Europe	Swine	Cecum, colon	Ingestion of infective larvae or paratenic hosts (rodents)	Enteritis, intestinal nodules	Reported	17
Oesophagostomum quadrispinulatum	Americas, Asia, Europe	Swine	Cecum, colon	Ingestion of infective larvae or paratenic hosts (rodents)	Enteritis	Reported	11
Oesophagostomum spp.	Worldwide	Swine	Cecum, colon	Ingestion of infective larvae or paratenic hosts (rodents)	Enteritis, intestinal nodules	Reported	11
Trichostrongyloidea							
Hyostrongylus rubidus	Worldwide	Swine	Stomach	Ingestion of infective larvae	Gastritis, anemia	Not reported	28, 30
Mecistocirrus digitatus	Central America	Ruminants, swine	Stomach	Ingestion of infective larvae	Unknown	Reported	82, 83
Ollulanus tricuspis	Americas, Australia, Europe, northern Africa	Cats, other carnivores, swine	Stomach	Ingestion of larva passed by emesis	Catarrhal gastritis	Not reported	11
Trichostrongylus axei	Worldwide	Ruminants, swine, equids	Stomach	Ingestion of infective larvae	None	Reported	11
Trichostrongylus colubriformis	Worldwide	Ruminants, rabbits, dogs, swine	Small intestine	Ingestion of infective larvae	None	Reported	84
Spiruroidea							
Ascarops strongylina	Worldwide	Swine, rodents, camels	Stomach	Ingestion of intermediate host (coprophagus beetles)	Gastritis	Not reported	85
Gnathostoma doloresi	Asia	Swine	Stomach	Ingestion of intermediate host (copepod)	Hepatitis, gastritis	Not reported	86
Gnathostoma hispidum	Asia, Europe	Swine, other mammals, snakes	Stomach	Ingestion of intermediate host (copepod)	Hepatitis, gastritis	Reported	87
Gongylonema pulchrum	Worldwide	Swine, other mammals	Tongue, esophagus	Ingestion of intermediate host (coprophagus beetles)	Mild glossitis, esophagitis	Reported	88

(Continued)

TABLE 19.2 (*Continued*)

Parasite	Geographic Distribution	Hosts	Location in Host	Method of Infection	Pathologic Effects	Zoonosis	Reference
Physocephalus sexalatus	Worldwide	Swine, lagomorphs, other mammals	Stomach	Ingestion of intermediate host (coprophagus beetles)	Gastritis	Not reported	11
Simondsia paradoxa	Asia, Australia, Europe	Swine	Stomach	Unknown	Gastric nodules, gastritis	Not reported	89
Trichuroidea							
Trichuris suis	Worldwide	Swine	Cecum, colon	Ingestion of embryonated egg	Anemia, enteritis	Not reported	11
Acanthocephala							
Macracanthorhynchus hirudinaceus	Worldwide	Swine, muskrats, squirrels	Small intestine	Ingestion of intermediate host (coprophagus beetles)	Intestinal nodules	Reported	56
Arthropods							
Diptera (flies)							
Larval							
Gastrophilus spp.	Worldwide	Swine, other mammals	Tongue, mouth, stomach, rectum	Ingestion, skin penetration of larvae	Gastritis, localized inflammation	Reported	11

634

TABLE 19·3 Parasites of swine—skin and connective tissue and musculoskeletal system.

Parasite	Geographic Distribution	Hosts	Location in Host	Method of Infection	Pathologic Effects	Zoonosis	Reference
Coccidia							
Sarcocystis miescheriana	Worldwide	Swine	Hepatic venules, myocardium	Ingestion of sporulated sporocysts in feces of definitive host (canid)	Abortion, myositis, dyspnea, purpura of the skin	Not reported	1, 90
Sarcocystis porcifelis	Worldwide	Swine	Muscle	Ingestion of sporulated sporocysts in feces of definitive host (cat)	Myositis, lameness, diarrhea	Not reported	1, 90
Sarcocystis porcihominis	Worldwide	Swine	Muscle	Ingestion of sporulated sporocysts in feces of definitive host (human)	Usually none	Common	1, 90
Cestodes							
Larval							
Taenia hydatigena	Worldwide	Ruminants, swine	Abdominal cavity, liver	Ingestion of eggs in feces of definitive host (canids)	Cysticercus	Not reported	11
Taenia solium	Worldwide	Swine, dogs, primates	Heart, muscle, subcutis, brain	Ingestion of embryonated eggs passed by definitive host (man)	Myocarditis	Common	11
Nematodes							
Filaroidea							
Setaria congolensis	Africa	Swine	Peritoneal cavity	Bite of intermediate host (arthropod)	None	Not reported	11
Suifilaria suis	Africa	Swine	Subcutaneous and muscle tissue	Unknown	Skin nodules	Not reported	11
Trichuroidea							
Trichinella spiralis	Worldwide	Swine, bears, rats, other mammals	Muscle, small intestine	Ingestion of encysted larvae in muscle tissue	Myositis, enteritis	Common	91
Arthropods							
Phthiraptera (lice)							
Haematomyzus hopkinsi	Africa	Warthogs	Skin	Direct contact	Unknown	Not reported	93
Haematopinus suis	Worldwide	Swine	Skin	Direct contact	Anemia	Not reported	92

(Continued)

TABLE 19-3 *(Continued)*

Siphonaptera (fleas)

Parasite	Geographic Distribution	Hosts	Location in Host	Method of Infection	Pathologic Effects	Zoonosis	Reference
Pulex irritans	Worldwide	Humans, swine, goats, badgers, dogs, cats, rats	Skin	Direct contact	Dermatitis	Common	11
Tunga spp.	Worldwide	Swine, primates	Skin	Direct contact	Agalactia	Common	94, 95, 96
Ticks (soft)							
Ornithodorus moubata	Africa	Swine, porcupines, humans	Skin	Direct contact	Vector of viral and rickettsial pathogens	Reported, vector of pathogenic spirochetes	97
Mites							
Astigmates							
Sarcoptes scabiei var suis	Worldwide	Swine, other mammals	Skin	Direct contact	Papular dermatitis, self-inflicted trauma, skin thickening, emaciation, death	Common	98
Prostigmates							
Demodex phylloides	Worldwide	Swine	Hair follicles	Direct contact	Dermatitis	Not reported	11

636

TABLE 19.4   Parasites of swine—central nervous, respiratory, and urogenital systems.

Parasite	Geographic Distribution	Hosts	Location in Host	Method of Infection	Pathologic Effects	Zoonosis	Reference
Trematodes							
Paragonimus kellicotti	North America	Dogs, cats, swine, wild carnivores, domestic animals	Lung	Ingestion of crustacean intermediate host (crab, crayfish)	Focal emphysema, lung cysts	Reported	99
Paragonimus westermanii	Asia	Dogs, swine, wild carnivores, domestic animals, primates	Lung, other organs	Ingestion of crustacean intermediate host (crab, crayfish)	Focal emphysema, lung cysts	Reported	11
Nematodes							
Strongyloidea							
Stephanurus dentatus	Worldwide	Swine, cattle, donkeys	Kidney, ureter, other organs	Ingestion of infective larvae or paratenic host (earthworm), skin penetration, transplacental transmission	Dermal nodules, lymphadenopathy, hepatitis, hepatic cirrhosis, renal cysts, thickened and occluded ureters	Not reported	27, 28
Metastrongyloidea							
Metastrongylus spp.	Worldwide	Swine	Lung	Ingestion of intermediate host (earthworm)	Bronchitis, pneumonia	Not reported	11, 100
Spiruroidea							
Thelazia ershowi	Eastern Europe	Swine	Conjunctival sac	Transmitted by intermediate host (fly)	Unknown	Not reported	11
Dioctophymatoidea							
Dioctophyma renale	Worldwide	Dogs, swine, other mammals	Kidney	Ingestion of intermediate host (annelid) or paratenic host (fish, frog)	Destruction of kidney parenchyma	Reported	11

REFERENCES

1. Levine, N.D. (1985) *Veterinary Protozoology.* Iowa State University Press, Ames, IA. 414 pages.

2. Corwin, R.M. and Stewart, T.B. (1999) Internal Parasites. In: *Diseases of Swine,* 8th ed. Straw, B.S., D'Allaire, S., Mengeling, W.L., and Taylor, D.J. (eds.). Iowa State University Press, Ames, IA. 713–730.

3. Moncol, D.J. (1975) Supplement to the life history of *Strongyloides ransomi* Schwartz and Alicata,1930 (Nematoda: Strongyloididae) of pigs. *Proc. Helminthol. Soc. Wash.* **42,** 86–92.

4. Stewart, T.B., Stone, W.M., and Marti, O.G. (1976) *Strongyloides ransomi:* Prenatal and transmammary infection of pigs of sequential litters from dams experimentally exposed as weanlings. *Am. J. Vet. Res.* **37,** 541–544.

5. Stewart, T.B., Schroeder, W.F., Shalkop, W.T., and Stone, W.M. (1968) Strongyloidiosis: Natural infection of suckling pigs with *Strongyloides ransomi. Vet. Med. Small Anim. Clin.* **63,** 1145–1150.

6. Stone, W.M. and Simpson, C.F. (1967) Larval distribution and histopathology of experimental *Strongyloides ransomi* infection in young swine. *Can. J. Comp. Med. Vet. Sci.* **31,** 197–202.

7. Johnson, J.C. Jr., Stewart, T.B., and Hale, O.M. (1975) Differential response of Duroc, Hampshire, and crossbred pigs to a superimposed infection with the intestinal threadworm, *Strongyloides ransomi. J. Parasitol.* **61,** 517–524.

8. Geenen P.L., Bresciani, J., Boes, J. et al. (1999) The morphogenesis of *Ascaris suum* to the infective third stage larvae within the egg. *J. Parasitol.* **85,** 616–622.

9. Southern, L.L., Stewart, T.B., Bodak-Koszalka, E., Leon, D.L., Hoyt, P.G., and Bessette, M.E. (1989) Effect of fenbendazole and pyrantel tartrate on the induction of protective immunity in pigs naturally or experimentally infected with *Ascaris suum. J. Anim. Sci.* **67,** 628–634.

10. Stankiewicz, M. and Jeska, E.L. (1990) Evaluation of pyrantel-tartrate abbreviated *Ascaris suum* infections for development of resistance in young pigs against migrating larvae. *Int. J. Parasitol.* **20,** 77–81.

11. Soulsby, E.J.L. (1982) *Helminths, Arthropods and Protozoa of Domesticated Animals,* 7th ed., Lea and Febiger, Philadelphia, PA. 809 pages.

12. Fernandez-de-Mera, I.G., Vicente, J., Gortazar, C., Hofle, U., and Fierro, Y. (2004) Efficacy of an in-feed preparation of ivermectin against helminths in the European wild boar. *Parasitol. Res.* **92,** 133–136.

13. Raynaud, J.P., Graber, M., and Euzeby, J. (1974) Experiments in the biology of 3 species of *Oesophagostomum quadrispinulatum, granatensis* or *dentatum:* Attempts to validate those 3 species. *Proc. Int. Congr. Pig Vet. Soc.,* Sec. P, **3,** 5.

14. Stewart, T.B. and Gasbarre, L.C. (1989) The veterinary importance of nodular worms (*Oesophagostomum* spp.). *Parasitol. Today* **5,** 209–213.

15. Jacobs, D.E. and Dunn, A.M. (1968) The epidemiology of porcine oesophagostomiasis. *Nord. Vet. Med.* **20,** 258–266.

16. Tafts, L.F. (1966) Helminths in the pig. *Vet. Rec.* **79,** 671.

17. McCracken, R.M. and Ross, J.G. (1970) The histopathology of *Oesophagostomum dentatum* infection in pigs. *J. Comp. Pathol.* **80,** 619–623.

18. Jacobs, D.E. (1969) Experimental infections of guinea pigs with *Oesophagostomum* spp. of porcine origin: Pathogenesis and parasitology of a single infection. In *Pathology of Parasitic Diseases. Purdue University Studies,* 231.

19. Hass, D.K., Brown, L.J., and Young, R. Jr. (1972) Infectivity of *Oesophagostomum dentatum* larvae in swine. *Am. J. Vet. Res.* **33,** 2527–2534.

20. Connan, R.M. (1967) Observations on the epidemiology of parasitic gastroenteritis due to *Oesophagostomum* spp. and *Hyostrongylus rubidus* in the pig. *Vet. Rec.* **80,** 424–429.

21. Polderman, A.M. and Blotkamp, J. (1995) *Oesophagostomum* infections in humans. *Parasitol. Today* **11,** 451–456.

22. Smith, H.J. and Hawkes, A.B. (1978) Kidney worm infection of feral pigs in Canada with transmission to domestic swine. *Can. Vet. J.* **19,** 30–43.

23. Tromba, F.G. (1955) The role of the earthworm, *Eisenia foetida,* in the transmission of *Stephanurus dentatus. J. Parasitol.* **41,** 157–161.

24. Batte, E.G., Harkema, R., and Osborne, J.C. (1960) Observations on the life cycle and pathogenicity of the swine kidney worm (*Stephanurus dentatus*). *J. Am. Vet. Med. Assoc.* **136,** 622–625.

25. Batte, E.G., Moncol, D.J., and Barber, C.W. (1966) Prenatal infection with the swine kidney worm (*Stephanurus dentatus*) and associated lesions. *J. Am. Vet. Med. Assoc.* **149,** 758–765.

26. Lichtenfels, J.R. and Tromba, F.G. (1972) The morphogenesis of *Stephanurus dentatus* (Nematoda: Strongylina) in swine with observations on larval migration. *J. Parasitol.* **58,** 757–766.

27. Waddell, A.H. (1969) The parasitic life cycle of the swine kidney worm *Stephanurus dentatus. Diesing. Aust. Vet. J. Zool.* **17,** 607–618.

28. Porter, D.A. (1940) Experimental infections of swine with the red stomach worm, *Hyostrongylus rubidus. Proc. Helminthol. Soc. Wash.* **7,** 20–27.

29. Kendall, S.B., Thurley, D.C., and Pierce, M.A. (1969) The biology of *Hyostrongylus rubidus.* I. Primary infection in young pigs. *J. Comp. Pathol.* **79,** 87–95.

30. Stockdale, P.H.G. (1974) Pathogenesis of *Hyostrongylus rubidus* in growing pigs. *Br. Vet. J.* **130,** 366–373.

31. Davidson, J.B., Murray, M., and Sutherlan, I.H. (1968) *Hyostrongylus rubidus:* A field study of its pathogenesis, diagnosis and treatment. *Vet. Rec.* **23,** 582–588.

32. Appert, A. and Taranchon, P. (1969) Existence et frequence en France de *Hyostrongylus rubidus* (Hassal et Stiles 1892) chez le porc. *Bull. Acad. Vet.* **42,** 249–253.

33. Dey-Hazra, A., Kolm, H.P., Enigk, K., and Giese, W. (1972) Gastrointestinal loss of plasma proteins in *Hyostrongylus* infected pigs. *Z. Parasitenkd.* **38,** 14–20.

34. Stewart, T.B., Hale, O.M., and Marti, O.G. (1985) Experimental infections with *Hyostrongylus rubidus* and the effects on performance of growing pigs. *Vet. Parasitol.* **17,** 219–227.

35. Honer, M.R. (1967) The routine differentiation of the ova and larvae of two parasites of swine: *Hyostrongylus rubidus* (Hassall and Stiles 1892) and *Oesophagostomum dentatum* (Rud 1803). *Z. Parasitenkd.* **29,** 40.

36. Ganzorig, S., Batsaikhan, N., Samiya, R., Morishima, Y., Oku, Y., and Kamiya, M. (1999) A second record of adult *Ascarops strongylina* (Rudolphi, 1819) (Nematoda: Spirocercidae) in a rodent host. *J. Parasitol.* **85,** 283–285.

37. Schad, G.A., Leiby, D.A., and Murrell, K.D. (1984) Distribution, prevalence and intensity of *Trichinella spiralis* infection in furbearing mammals of Pennsylvania. *J. Parasitol.* **70,** 372–377.

38. Kim, W.C. (1983) Geographic distribution and prevalence. In: *Trichinella and Trichinosis,* Campbell, W.C. (ed.). Plenum Press, New York, NY. 445–500.

39. McLean, J.P., Vialett, J., Law, C., and Staudt, M. (1989) Trichinosis in the Canadian Arctic: Report of five outbreaks and a new clinical syndrome. *J. Inf. Dis.* **160,** 513–520.

40. Despommier, D.D. (1990) *Trichinella spiralis:* The worm that would be a virus. *Parasitol. Today* **6,** 193–196.

41. Kazacos, K.R. (1986) Trichinosis. *J. Am. Vet. Med. Assoc.* **188,** 1272–1275.

42. Campbell, W.C. (1988) Trichinosis revisited—Another look at modes of transmission. *Parasitol. Today* **4,** 83–86.

43. Hanbury, R.D., Doby, B.P., Miller, H.O., and Murrell, K.D. (1986) Trichinosis in a herd of swine: Cannibalism as a major mode of transmission. *J. Am. Vet. Med. Assoc.* **188,** 1155–1159.

44. Zimmerman, W.J., Hubbard, E.D., Schwarte, L.H., and Biester, H.E. (1962) Trichinosis in Iowa swine with further studies on modes of transmission. *Cornell Vet.* **52,** 156–163.

45. Scholtens, R.G., Kagan, I.G., Quist, K.D., and Norman, L.G. (1966) An evaluation of tests of the diagnosis of trichinosis in swine and observations. *Am. J. Epidemiol.* **83,** 489–500.

46. Beck, J.W. and Anfinson, T.A. Jr. (1965) Some host responses of miniature pigs to infection with *Trichinella spiralis. J. Parasitol.* **51,** 60–62.

47. Gamble, H.R., Anderson, W.R., Graham, C.E., and Murrell, K.D. (1983) Diagnosis of swine trichinosis by enzyme-linked immunosorbent assay (ELISA) using an excretory-secretory antigen. *Vet. Parasitol.* **13,** 349–361.

48. Zimmerman, W.J. (1967) A pooled sample method for post slaughter detection of trichiniasis in swine. *Proc. U.S. Livest. Sanit. Assoc.* **72,** 358–366.

49. Oliver, D.G., Hanbury, R.D., and Van Houwellin, C.D. (1985) *Proc 89th Ann. Meet. U.S. Anim. Health Assoc.,* Milwaukee, WI.

50. Murrell, K.D., Anderson, W.R., Schad, G.A., et al. (1986) Field evaluation of the enzyme-linked immunosorbent assay for swine trichinosis: Efficacy of the excretory-secretory antigen. *Am. J. Vet. Res.* **47,** 1046–1049.

51. James, E.R. (1989) ICT7: The 1988 *Trichinella* Olympics. *Parasitol. Today* **5,** 66–67.

52. Beer, R.J. (1976) The relationship between *Trichuris trichiura* (Linnaeus 1758) of man and *Trichuris suis* (Schrank 1788) of the pig. *Res. Vet. Sci.* **20,** 47–54.

53. Batte, E.G., McLamb, R.D., Muse, K.E., Tally, S.D., and Vestal, T.J. (1977) Pathophysiology of swine trichuriasis. *Am. J. Vet. Res.* **38,** 1075–1079.

54. Beer, R.J.S. (1973) Studies on the biology of the life cycle of *Trichuris suis* Schrank 1788. *Parasitology* **67,** 253–262.

55. Mansfield, L.S. and Urban, J.F. The pathogenesis of necrotic proliferative colitis in swine is linked to whipworm induced suppression of mucosal immunity to resident bacteria. *Vet. Immunol. Immunopathol.* **50,** 1–17.

56. Daynes, P. (1966) Note on the biological cycle of *Macracanthorhynchus hirudinaceus* (Pallas 1781) in Madagascar. *Rev. Elev. Med. Vet. Pays Trop.* **19,** 277–282.

57. Yazwinski, T.A., Tucker, C., Featherston, H., Johnson, Z., and Wood-Huels, N. (1997) Endectocidal efficacies of doramectin in naturally parasitized pigs. *Vet. Parasitol.* **70,** 123–128.

58. Mehlhorn, H., Taraschewski, H., Zhao, B., Raether, W., and Dunagan, T.T. (1990) Loperamid, an efficacious drug against the acanthocephalan *Macracanthorhynchus hirudinaceus* in pigs. *Parasitol. Res.* **76,** 624–626.

59. Moloo, S.K., Zweygarth, E., and Sabwa, C.L. (1992) Virulence of *Trypanosoma simiae* in pigs infected by *Glossina brevipalpis, G. pallidipes* or *G. morsitans centralis. Ann. Trop. Med. Parasitol.* **85,** 681–683.

60. Peel, E. and Chardome, M. (1953) Preliminary note on *Trypanosoma suis,* developing in the salivary glands of *Glossina brevipalpis. Ann. Soc. Belg. Med. Trop.* **33,** 457–458.

61. Vercruysse, J. and Parent, R. (1981) Porcine babesiosis epizootic due to *Babesia perroncitoi,* Cerruti 1939 in Senegal. *Ann. Soc. Belg. Med. Trop.* **61,** 125–131.

62. Dipeolu, O.O., Otesile, E.B., Adetunji, A., and Fagbemi, B.O. (1983) Studies on blood parasites of pigs in Nigeria: pathogenicity of *Babesia trautmanni* in experimentally infected pigs. *Zentralbl. Veterinarmed. B.* **30,** 97–102.

63. Sinha, P.K. and Srivastava, H.D. (1965) Studies on *Schistosoma incognitum* Chandler, 1926 on the host specificity of the blood fluke. *Indian Vet. J.* **42,** 335–341.

64. Willingham, A.L. 3rd, Hurst, M., Bogh, H.O., et al. (1998) *Schistosoma japonicum* in the pig: the host-parasite relationship as influenced by the

65. Fortess, E. and Meyer, E.A. (1976) Isolation and axenic cultivation of *Giardia* trophozoites from the guinea pig. *J. Parasitol.* **62,** 689.

66. Castella, J., Munoz, E., Ferrer, D., and Gutierrez, J.F. (1997) Isolation of the trichomonad *Tetratrichomonas buttreyi* (Hibler et al., 1960) Honigberg, 1963 in bovine diarrhoeic faeces. *Vet. Parasitol.* **70,** 41–45.

67. Lun, Z.R., Chen, X.G., Zhu, X.Q., Li, X.R., and Xie, M.Q. (2005) Are *Tritrichomonas foetus* and *Tritrichomonas suis* synonyms? *Trends Parasitol.* **21,** 122–125.

68. Das, N. and Ray, H.N. (1968) A hyperparasite of *Entamoeba suis* from the Indian domestic pig *Sus scrofa. J. Protozool.* **15,** 383–385.

69. Mundt, H.C., Joachim, A., Becka, M., and Daugschies, A. (2006) *Isospora suis:* an experimental model for mammalian intestinal coccidiosis. *Parasitol Res.* **98,** 167–175.

70. Hindsbo, O., Nielsen, C.V., Andreassen, J., et al. (2000) Age-dependent occurrence of the intestinal ciliate *Balantidium coli* in pigs at a Danish research farm. *Acta Vet. Scand.* **41,** 79–83.

71. Permin, A., Yelifari, L., Bloch, P., Steenhard, N., Hansen, N.P., and Nansen, P. (1999) Parasites in cross-bred pigs in the Upper East region of Ghana. *Vet. Parasitol.* **87,** 63–71.

72. Yamaguti, S. (1958) The digenetic trematodes of vertebrates, vol. 1 part 1. In: *Systema Helminthum.* Interscience Publishers, Inc., New York, NY. 909.

73. Jang, D.H. (1969) Study on the *Eurytrema pancreaticum:* II. Life Cycle. *Kisaengchunghak Chapchi.* **7,** 178–200.

74. Horchner, F. and Dalchow, W. (1972) Experimental *Fasciola hepatica* infection in swine. *Berl. Munch. Tierarztl. Wochenschr.* **85,** 184–188.

75. Kuntz, R.E. and Lo, C.T. (1967) Preliminary studies on *Fasciolopsis buski* (Lankester, 1857) (giant Asian intestinal fluke) in the United States. *Trans. Am. Microsc. Soc.* **86,** 163–166.

76. Malek, E.A. (1971) The life cycle of *Gastrodiscus aegyptiacus* (Cobbold, 1876) Looss, 1896 (Trematoda: Paramphistomatidae: Gastrodiscinae). *J. Parasitol.* **57,** 975–979.

77. Dutt, S.C. and Srivastava, H.D. (1972) The life history of *Gastrodiscoides hominis* (Lewis and McConnel, 1876) Leiper, 1913—the amphistome parasite of man and pig. *J. Helminthol.* **46,** 35–46.

78. Rim, H.J., Kim, K.H., and Joo, K.H. (1996) Classification and host specificity of *Metagonimus* spp. from Korean freshwater fish. *Korean J. Parasitol.* **34,** 7–14.

79. Eckert, J. and Thompson, R.C. (1988) *Echinococcus* strains in Europe: a review. *Trop. Med. Parasitol.* **39,** 1–8.

80. Boes, J., Slotved, H.C., Murrell, K.D., et al. (2002) Alternative migration routes of *Ascaris suum* in the pig. *J. Parasitol.* **88,** 180–183.

81. Hartwich, G. (1986) Type identity of the swine parasites *Globocephalus longemucronatus* and *G. urosubulatus* (Nematoda, Strongyloidea). *Angew. Parasitol.* **27,** 207–214.

82. Fernando, S.T. (1965) Morphology, systematics, and geographic distribution of *Mecistocirrus digitatus,* a trichostrongylid parasite of ruminants. *J. Parasitol.* **51,** 149–155.

83. Fernando, S.T. (1965) The life cycle of *Mecistocirrus digitatus,* a trichostrongylid parasite of ruminants. *J. Parasitol.* **51,** 156–163.

84. Mullee, M.T. and Cox, D.D. (1967) A naturally acquired infection of *Trichostrongylus colubriformis* in a hog in the United States. *J. Parasitol.* **53,** 325.

85. de la Muela, N., Hernandez de Lujan, S., and Ferre, I. (2001) Helminths of wild boar in Spain. *J. Wildl. Dis.* **37,** 840–843.

86. Ishiwata, K., Diaz Camacho, S.P., Amrozi, Horii, Y., Nawa, N., and Nawa, Y. (1998) Gnathostomiasis in wild boars from Japan. *J. Wildl. Dis.* **34,** 155–157.

intensity and duration of experimental infection. *Am. J. Trop. Med. Hyg.* **58,** 248–256.

87. Daengsvang, S. (1972) An experimental study on the life cycle of *Gnathostoma hispidum* Fedchenko 1872 in Thailand with special reference to the incidence and some significant morphological characters of the adult and larval stages. *Southeast Asian J. Trop. Med. Public Health.* **3,** 376–389.

88. Naem, S., Seifi, H., and Simon, G.T.(2000) Scanning electron microscopy of adult *Gongylonema pulchrum* (Nematoda: Spirurida). *J. Vet. Med. B Infect. Dis. Vet. Public Health.* **47,** 249–255.

89. Spratt, D.M. and Pavlov, P.M. (1996) *Simondsia paradoxa:* newly recorded nematode parasite from feral pigs in Australia. *Aust. Vet. J.* **74,** 394–395.

90. Dubey, J.P. (1976) A review of *Sarcocystis* of domestic animals and of other coccidia of cats and dogs. *J. Am. Vet. Med. Assoc.* **169,**1061–1078.

91. Murrell, K.D., Lichtenfels, R.J., Zarlenga, D.S., and Pozio, E. (2000) The systematics of the genus *Trichinella* with a key to species. *Vet. Parasitol.* **93,** 293–307.

92. Davis, D.P. and Williams, R.E. (1986) Influence of hog lice, *Haematopinus suis,* on blood components, behavior, weight gain and feed efficiency of pigs. *Vet. Parasitol.* **22,** 307–314.

93. Rodhain, F. (1976) Presence of *Haematomyzus hopkinsi* Clay, 1963, in Ethiopia. *Ann. Parasitol. Hum. Comp.* **51,** 473–475.

94. Pampiglione, S., Trentini, M., Fioravanti, M.L., Onore, G., and Rivasi, F. (2000) Additional description of a new species of *Tunga* (Siphonaptera) from Ecuador. *Parasite* **10,** 9–15.

95. Cooper, J.E. (1976) Letter: *Tunga penetrans* infestation in pigs. *Vet. Rec.* **98,** 472.

96. Verhulst, A. (1976) *Tunga penetrans* (*Sarcopsylla penetrans*) as a cause of agalactia in sows in the Republic of Zaire. *Vet. Rec.* **98,** 384.

97. Walton, G.A.(1953) *Ornithodorus moubata* in wart-hog and porcupine burrows in Tanganyika territory. *Trans. R. Soc. Trop. Med. Hyg.* **47,** 410–411.

98. Jensen, J.C., Nielsen, L.H., Arnason, T., and Cracknell, V. (2002) Elimination of mange mites *Sarcoptes scabiei* var. *suis* from two naturally infested Danish sow herds using a single injection regime with doramectin. *Acta Vet. Scand.* **43,**75–84.

99. Ishii, Y. (1966) Differential morphology of *Paragonimus kellicotti* in North America. *J. Parasitol.* **52,** 920–925.

100. Ewing, S.A. and Todd, A.C. (1961) Association among members of the genus *Metastrongylus* Molin, 1861 (Nematoda: Metastrongvlidae). *Am. J. Vet. Res.* **22,** 1077–1080.

CHAPTER
20

Parasites of Sheep and Goats

Thomas M. Craig, DVM, PhD

INTRODUCTION

Sheep and goats are often used as laboratory animals. They have a number of parasites that they may bring with them to the laboratory. The way in which the animals are kept in the laboratory environment will to a large extent determine which parasites they encounter. Loosely housed animals are more likely to become infected with parasites, compared to those confined in individual stanchions. Housing in a dry-lot does not preclude parasite acquisition. Vegetation at the edges of the pens may harbor infective nematode larvae. Excessive moisture from water troughs and lack of adequate drainage provide optimal conditions for protozoan development. Overcrowding, common to animal maintenance in a dry-lot, exacerbates ectoparasite infestation.

PROTOZOA

Phylum Sarcomastigophora

Class Mastigophora (flagellates)

Hemoflagellates
Salivarian trypanosomes. **Morphology.** Salivarian trypanosomes include *Trypanosoma brucei, T. congolense, T. evansi,* and *T. vivax. Trypanosoma brucei* has two morphologically distinguishable forms, the long, slender form (20 µ to 40 µ long) and the stumpy form (15 µ to 25 µ long). The free flagellum is long and the kinetoplast is

---

Tables are placed at the ends of chapters.

subterminal in the slender form, while the free flagellum is short and the kinetoplast terminal in the stumpy form. *Trypanosoma evansi* appears as a long slender form (15 to 33 µ long) with a free flagellum identical to that of *T. brucei. Trypanosoma congolense* is small (12 µ to 18 µ long) with an inconspicuous undulating membrane and a marginal kinetoplast. *Trypanosoma vivax* is 20 µ to 30 µ long with a rounded posterior and a large kinetoplast. The undulating membrane is inconspicuous and the parasite is extremely active.

Hosts. Except for *T. evansi,* salivarian trypanosomes are transmitted to sheep, goats and other mammals by the tsetse fly (*Glossina* spp.) in Central Africa. The prevalence of infection by salivarian trypanosomes in small ruminants is low but may be significant at times. The range of *T. vivax* has extended to South America as well as outside of the tsetse belt in Africa. *Trypanosoma evansi* is found in northern Africa, southern Asia, and South America, where it infects horses and ruminants.

Life Cycle. Trypomastigotes circulating in the blood are ingested by tsetse flies. They multiply in the gut of the fly, then move to the salivary glands where they become epimastigotes. Approximately three weeks post exposure some of the organisms become metacyclic trypomastigotes, the infective stage to the vertebrate host. The metacyclic trypomastigotes are injected into the host. The parasite reproduces by binary fission at the injection site, then moves into the blood stream, where there are reproducing slender trypomastigotes and the stumpy forms that are infective to tsetse flies.

T. vivax is also transmitted mechanically, as well as by the tsetse fly. The trypomastigotes of *Trypanosoma evansi* are mechanically transmitted from an infected host by horse flies, stable flies and other biting arthropods, as well as vampire bats[1].

Pathologic Effects. An area of swelling, the "chancre," occurs where the parasites are introduced into the body. The chancre contains the metacyclic trypomastigotes. Lymph node enlargement, splenomegaly, and hypergammaglobulinemia, along with increased susceptibility to other diseases, are signs of the subversion of the immune system by the proliferation of trypomastigotes. Anemia and inflammation of the tissues, including myocarditis, lead to wasting and weakness[2].

Clinical Disease. Sheep and goats are susceptible to Nagana, the disease caused by these parasites. Depending on the subspecies of *T. brucei*, small ruminants may be infected without showing clinical signs or suffer from chronic disease characterized by fever, anemia photophobia, and enlarged lymph nodes[3]. Fever, anemia and wasting are the common signs associated with *T. congolense*. *Trypanosoma vivax* infections may have central nervous signs as well as anemia and wasting. The disease may be acute or chronic, depending upon the strain of parasite encountered[4]. Although sheep and goats that are infected with *T. evansi* are not considered at risk for disease, they may serve as reservoirs[5,6]. Dwarf African breeds of sheep and goats possess varying degrees of trypanotolerance[7,8] and are able to survive in the tsetse belt when other breeds succumb to disease.

Diagnosis. Rarely, trypomastigotes may be found on thin blood films. However, examination of thick blood films or the buffy coat recovered from a microhematocrit tube enhances the probability of finding organisms because the parasites are concentrated with these techniques[9]. *Trypanosoma vivax* may be recovered from lymph nodes, and, along with the other salivarian trypanosomes, may be found in spinal fluid.

Treatment and Prevention. Treatment guidelines for infected ruminants are available from the World Health Organization. Animals arriving from endemic areas should be tested and treated or culled prior to entering the colony herd.

Public Health Considerations. Two subspecies of *T. brucei* cause sleeping sickness in humans but require tsetse transmission or blood inoculation for transmission.

Stercorarian trypanosomes. **Morphology.** Stercorarian trypanosomes include *Trypanosoma melophagium* and *T. theodori*. The trypomastigote of *T. melophagium* is curved, approximately 50 μ long, and has a sharply pointed posterior and a short flagellum. The large, rod-shaped kinetoplast lies near the nucleus. *Trypanosoma theodori* is morphologically similar.

Hosts. *Trypanosoma melophagium* occurs in the blood of sheep in temperate areas of the world. Sheep and the sheep ked *Melophagus ovinus* are the only apparent hosts. *Trypanosoma theodori* occurs in the goat. The vector of *T. theodori* is the hippoboscid *Lipotena caprina*.

Life Cycle. The epimastigote stage reproduces by binary fission in the hindgut of the ked. Some of the organisms become trypomastigotes. Sheep become infected by ingesting the infected ked, with penetration of the oral mucous membranes by metacyclic trypomastigotes. The parasite apparently reproduces by binary fission in the sheep, but the parasitemia is so low it is usually not detected. The life cycle of *T. theodori* is apparently the same.

Pathologic Effects and Clinical Disease. No deleterious effects are reported in infections of sheep by *T. melophagium*. Likewise, *T. theodori* does not cause disease in goats[10].

Diagnosis. Diagnosis is by culture of blood at 22°C to 28°C to induce the development of epimastigotes similar to those in the ked[11]. The culture used is a biphasic blood agar medium. If *T. melophagium* is similar to the nonpathogenic cattle *T. theileri*, it can also grow in a cell culture medium at 37°C.

Treatment and Prevention. Treatment is not considered to be necessary. Controlling keds prevents infection.

Public Health Considerations. These parasites are not infective to humans.

Enteric flagellates

Chilomastix caprae. *Chilomastix caprae* has been reported from the rumen of a goat. It is thought to be the same organism as *C. bettencourti*, an organism found in the cecum of rodents. The organism appears to be a harmless commensal but the speciation and possible importance are unresolved[12].

Giardia duodenalis. **Morphology.** *Giardia duodenalis* (Syn, *Giardia intestinalis*, *G. lamblia*) trophozoites bear eight flagella and a large, adhesive disk; are binucleated; and measure 13 μ by 7 μ long. The cyst is ellipsoidal, measures 10 μ by 8 μ long, and contains four nuclei following binary fission. The flagella, median body, and axostyle may be seen when the cyst is stained.

Hosts. The host specificity of *G. duodenalis* is unresolved. It is likely that most mammalian species, including humans, are susceptible, even if there are specific strains or species of the organism. *Giardia* is a common parasite of small ruminants in some geographic localities.

Life Cycle. Trophozoites attach to enterocytes that line the host's duodenum. Some trophozoites encyst and binary fission occurs, forming two daughter trophozoites within. The cyst is the environmentally resistant stage and is ingested by the next host in contaminated food or water.

Pathologic Effects and Clinical Disease. The presence of the parasite adhered to the microvillus border of enterocytes prevents the upper intestine from absorbing nutrients, primarily fats and fat-soluble vitamins. This leads to fermentation in the bowel, resulting in steatorrhea and diarrhea. *Giardia duodenalis* may cause diarrhea in goat kids and decrease production in lambs[13,14].

Diagnosis, Treatment, and Prevention. Diagnosis is by observing trophozoites in fresh feces or recovering cysts, preferably by flotation in zinc sulfate solution (specific gravity 1.18). Immune assay for coproantigens or polymerase chain reaction (PCR) techniques can detect low numbers of organisms in feces.

Because clinical signs are lacking in most small ruminants it is doubtful that treatment is warranted. However, metronidazole or one of the benzimidazoles (albendazole or fenbendazole) may be effective in treating these hosts. The cysts of *Giardia* are resistant to many disinfectants.

High levels of hypochlorite solutions or quaternary ammonia compounds may kill cysts, but steaming or flaming quarters that were previously occupied by infected animals may be the best approach. Filtering contaminated water supplies removes cysts.

Public Health Considerations. Humans may share the organism with sheep and goats and therefore animal workers may be at risk from exposure to cysts.

Tetratrichomonas ovis. Tetratrichomonas ovis is a common inhabitant of the rumen of sheep. There are four anterior flagella with an undulating membrane, axostyle, and trailing flagellum. *Tetratrichomonas ovis* is considered non-pathogenic[15].

Class Sarcodina (amoebae)

Balamuthia mandrillaris

A naturally infected sheep was identified with an amoeba in its brain that cross-reacted serologically with the amoeba, *B. mandrillaris,* found in the brain of a mandrill. The lesions were those of an inflammatory infiltration near the olfactory tract. The sheep had dermal lesions of the poll and was pregnant at the time of infection, which may have increased its susceptibility to disease[16]. The organism

is associated with human deaths previously thought to have been due to *Acanthamoeba* spp.[17].

Phylum Apicomplexa

Class Coccidia

Besnoitia caprae

Morphology, Hosts, and Life Cycle. *Besnoitia caprae* produces large cysts measuring 0.5 mm in diameter. Wild and domestic cats are the definitive hosts of *Besnoitia* spp. *Besnoitia caprae* infects goats but not sheep[18]. The taxonomy of the *Besnoitia* in goats is uncertain, as are details of the life cycle. It is likely that ruminants are infected when they ingest sporulated oocysts from cat feces. Blood-feeding flies may also serve as mechanical vectors. Cats are infected when they ingest tissues of intermediate hosts that contain bradyzoite cysts.

Pathologic Effects and Clinical Disease. Cysts are found in the skin and other tissues of the intermediate host[18]. Hyperkeratosis was seen in the skin of naturally infected goats[19]. Others have reported finding cysts in the conjunctiva, or thickening of the skin of the scrotum and legs in infected goats[18,19].

Diagnosis, Treatment, and Prevention. Histological examination of lesions reveals large cysts in the skin and other tissues. There is no satisfactory treatment of the infection. Absolute recommendations cannot be made until the complete life cycle is elucidated. Preventing animal waste from contaminating feed and controlling biting flies may aid prevention efforts. A live vaccine against *B. besnoiti* reduces clinical disease but does not prevent infection[20].

Public Health Considerations. *Besnoitia* is not infectious to humans.

Cryptosporidium parvum

Morphology, Hosts, and Life Cycle. The morphology and life cycle of *Cryptosporidium* is discussed in Chapter 15, Parasites of Rabbits. *Cryptosporidium parvum* inhabits the microvillous border of enterocytes and other epithelial cells in a variety of mammalian hosts, including sheep and goats.

Pathologic Effects and Clinical Disease. Host enterocytes are not disrupted as with other coccidia, but they appear to be functionally impaired. The villi are stunted and fused and may not produce membrane-bound enzymes. Infected young kids and lambs may develop signs of diarrhea[21,22]. The age of the neonate at the time of exposure largely determines the course of disease; younger animals are more adversely affected.

Cryptosporidium can cause major problems in a laboratory colony. Most disinfectants are ineffective, and the ability of the sporulated oocyst to infect immediately upon being passed from the host, combined with autoinfection, lead to easy spread within the laboratory environment. Signs will dissipate in a few days to two weeks in hosts with fully functional immune systems[23], but may continue indefinitely in immune-compromised hosts.

Diagnosis. Diagnosis is by observation of the oocysts by acid fast or immunofluorescence staining of fecal smears, or by concentration of oocysts by centrifugal sugar flotation techniques. Antigen detection indicates infection in a high percentage of diarrheic stools[24]. Previously infected individuals have specific antibody levels to the organisms. Finding organisms is not proof of disease, and in some situations nearly the entire population will be infected from time to time and yet not show signs of disease. Large numbers of organisms and clinical signs are indicative of disease.

Treatment. There is no specific treatment available for food-producing animals. Palliative treatment, including maintaining hydration and preventing hypothermia, is sufficient in most cases, providing that a functional immune system is present.

Prevention. Sanitation by steam or flame treatment is usually necessary to kill oocysts. Vacating the premises for a week to several months, depending on the environment, allows oocysts to desiccate. Ammonia or formol saline are active against the oocysts.

Public Health Considerations. The parasite causes diarrhea in humans and other mammals. The organism shows a great diversity in the genetic makeup of various populations, often leading to confusion as to whether or not it is a single species that infects a wide range of hosts, or if a number of related but distinct species cause similar disease in their hosts[25]. Regardless, animal workers should practice excellent personal hygiene and wear personal protective equipment when working with infected sheep or goats.

Eimeria spp.

Morphology. Sheep and goats are susceptible to several *Eimeria* spp. (Figures 20.1 and 20.2), including *E. alijevi, E. ahsata, E. arlongi, E. caprina, E. capriovina, E. crandallis, E. christenseni, E. faurai, E. hirici, E. intracata, E. ninakohlyakimovae, E. ovina, E. ovinoidalis,* and *E. parva.* The morphology of *Eimeria* is discussed in Chapter 15, Parasites of Rabbits.

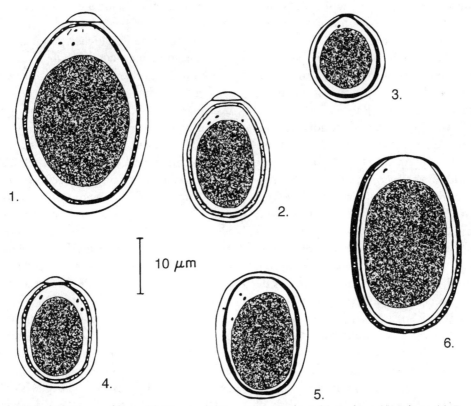

Fig. 20.1 Unsporulated *Eimeria* oocysts of goats. (1) *Eimeria christenseni,* (2) *E. arlongi,* (3) *E. alijevi,* (4) *E. hirici,* (5) *E. ninakohlyakimovae,* and (6) *E. caprina.* Courtesy of Catherine G. Wade.

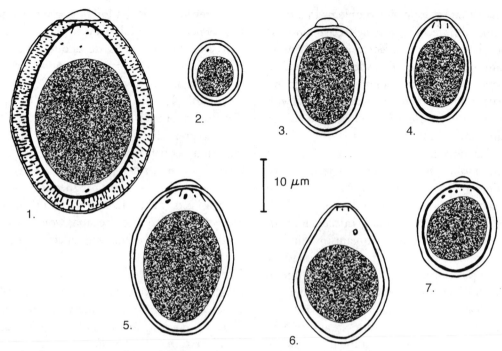

10 μm

Fig. 20.2   Unsporulated *Eimeria* oocysts of sheep. (1) *Eimeria intricata*, (2) *E. parva*, (3) *E. ovina*, (4) *E. ovinoidalis*, (5) *E. ahsata*, (6) *E. faurai*, (7) *E. crandalis*. Courtesy of Catherine G. Wade.

Hosts and Life Cycle. *Eimeria* are host-specific and they inhabit distinct regional niches within the gastrointestinal tract of the host. The species of *Eimeria* found in small ruminants are specific to the host. That is, goat coccidia do not occur in sheep and vice versa, with the exception of *E. caprovina*[26–28]. The life cycle of *Eimeria* spp. is discussed in Chapter 15, Parasites of Rabbits.

Pathologic Effects. Most species of coccidia are nonpathogenic; therefore, large numbers of oocysts may be passed in the feces of asymptomatic hosts. Coccidiosis is seldom associated with a single *Eimeria* species. Animals concurrently infected with both small- and large-intestinal *Eimeria* spp. are more adversely affected than those with two species in the same organ[29]. Highly pathogenic species include *E. crandallis* and *E. ovoidalis* in sheep[30,31], and *E. ninakohlyakimovae* and *E. arlongi* in goats[32]. However, most of the reports of coccidiosis in small ruminants do not indicate which species are involved and it seems reasonable that almost any species of *Eimeria* can cause disease under crowded, unsanitary conditions.

Clinical Disease. Coccidiosis caused by *Eimeria* spp. is a common disease of sheep and goats in confinement systems. Infection with *Eimeria* is nearly universal in sheep and goats, whereas clinical coccidiosis is a disease of stressed or naïve animals. The signs of coccidiosis are those of diarrhea, with production of mucus and/or blood in the feces, rough hair coat, weakness, chronic "poor-doers," and death. There is a higher prevalence and intensity of infection in young than in adults[33,34]. While diarrhea is a common sign, other causes of diarrhea should be considered. Fortunately, small ruminants develop immunity to disease caused by *Eimeria* but the immunity is not sterile and immune hosts pass oocysts. Very young lambs are resistant to infection and then have increased susceptibility after the first month[35,36]. Lambs exposed to oocysts during the early resistant phase are resistant to re-infection[37].

Diagnosis. The diagnosis of coccidiosis is by observation of clinical signs such as diarrhea with or without blood, excessive mucus in the stool, and large numbers of oocysts in the stool identified by fecal flotation techniques. Finding oocysts in the feces by flotation methods is the usual method of determining if infection is present. Most coccidial oocysts float in a medium with a specific gravity of 1.17 or greater. A few species require a higher specific gravity (sp. gr. 1.26), and centrifugal sugar flotation may be the most efficient means of detecting oocysts. However, unless there is are more than several thousand oocysts per gram of feces, the presence of oocysts is unlikely to be diagnostic for coccidiosis. Lambs or kids may suffer from disease during the prepatent period and have signs of disease with low oocyst counts. However, this situation will not last for long because most clinical cases have large numbers of oocysts passed[38].

Identifying species of coccidia may be aided by examining sporulated oocysts. Sporulation requires one to two days. Oocysts should be separated from fecal material by flotation after straining through a sieve to remove large particulate matter. The oocysts are then placed in a petri dish—for adequate oxygenation—in a solution of tap water with 2% potassium dichloride or 2% sulfuric acid added to limit bacterial or fungal proliferation. The identification of sporulated oocysts is aided by consulting texts[27,39,40].

Treatment. Coccidiostats inhibit the development of coccidia within the host's gut. When these drugs are used prophylactically, they prevent disease. However, most of the coccidia have developed beyond the point where the coccidiostat is likely to exert its influence when an animal is already showing clinical signs of disease, and therefore a clinical response does not occur. If there is a clinical response, it is largely because immunity has developed. It appears desirable for a few parasites to develop in the host while on coccidiostats[38]. This allows protective immunity to develop while the host is protected against disease. However, this approach also selects for parasites that are resistant to the drug[41]. Therefore, specific coccidiostats may lose their effectiveness and it may become necessary to periodically evaluate drugs at the flock level.

One practice that leads to drug resistance and/or susceptible hosts is the use of coccidiostats year 'round. When the number of oocysts to which the animals are exposed becomes very low, it may fall below the threshold exposure necessary to stimulate a protective response. Then the host population is at risk when the coccidia become resistant to the coccidiostat. A better approach is to use coccidiostats at times of risk (i.e. parturition, inclement weather, shipping, weaning), and then allow resistance to protect the animal from disease.

Even with the best treatment, once an animal has developed signs of coccidiosis, there are likely to be some permanent effects on its continued growth, resulting in runty, "poor-doing" kids or lambs. Reducing exposure by spreading out animals lowers the magnitude of infection[42]. Keeping the environment clean, dry, and uncrowded reduces stress and the level of exposure; however, chemicals are the basis of coccidia control.

Prevention. Coccidiosis is a disease brought on by poor management and other sources of stress. Contaminated feed, water, or bedding provides heavy exposure, and there are direct relationships between the level of exposure acquired immunity, and the onset of disease.

Public Health Considerations. *Eimeria* do not infect humans.

Neospora caninum

Morphology, Hosts, and Life Cycle. The morphology and life cycle of *Neospora caninum* are discussed in Chapter 17, Parasites of Dogs. Canids serve as definitive hosts, and may also serve as intermediate hosts of *N. caninum*. Cattle are commonly infected with the organism. Sheep and goats have been naturally and experimentally infected. Following ingestion of sporulated oocysts, bradyzoite cysts form in the central nervous system. Transmission to canids is by the ingestion of tissues or placenta. Vertical transmission between intermediate hosts is an important means of sustaining the infection. This transmission can go from generation to generation without any apparent clinical signs.

Pathologic Effects and Clinical Disease. The most important outcomes of neosporosis are abortion and neonatal death. Aborted lambs or kids have myositis and cysts in the brain[43,44]. Animals that survive the infection become asymptomatic carriers.

Diagnosis, Treatment, and Prevention. Histological findings of the thick-walled cyst, which are distinct from the cysts of *T. gondii,* or the immunohistological identification of tachyzoites in the tissues of the aborted fetus are diagnostic[45]. The presence of antibody indicates infection, but does not prove that abortion was due to *N. caninum.* While clindamycin has been used in dogs infected with the tissue phase of the organism, it is doubtful that any drug will benefit ruminants. Avoiding the contamination of feed with fecal material from canids prevents horizontal transmission. A vaccine has been evaluated in sheep[46] and has shown partial protection against abortion, but infection of lambs still occurred.

Public Health Considerations. Humans are not susceptible to infection with *N. caninum.*

Sarcocystis spp.

Morphology. Sheep and goats are susceptible to infection with several species of *Sarcocystis*, including *S. arieticanis, S. capracanis, S. gigantea, S. hircicanis, S. medusiformis, S. moulei,* and *S. tenella.* Cysts in the musculature of sheep (*S. tenella, S. arieticanis, S. gigantea,* and *S. medusi- formis*) or goats (*S. capracanis, S. hircicanis,* and *S. moulei*) vary in size and shape. The size and shape of the cyst, including the cyst wall, is diagnostic for the various species. Canids and felids are the definitive hosts for specific *Sarcocystis* species, and sporulated sporocysts, each containing four sporozoites, are found in their feces. The oocyst wall is a thin membrane and may still be intact, or the sporocysts may be separate.

Hosts and Life Cycle. All *Sarcocystis* infections involve predator-prey relationships. Canids are the definitive hosts of *S. tenella, S. arieticanis, S. capricanis,* and *S. hircicanis,* and felids are the definitive hosts of *S. gigantea, S. medusiformis,* and *S. moulei*[47]. The general life cycle of *Sarcocystis* that infect sheep and goats is similar to that described for rodents in Chapter 11, Parasites of Rats and Mice.

Pathologic Effects and Clinical Disease. *Sarcocystis* pathogenicity depends on parasite species, dose, and the age of the infected intermediate host. Anorexia, weight loss, anemia, depressed wool production, hind limb ataxia or paresis, myositis, and abortion have all been observed with *S. tenella* in sheep. Abortion is accompanied by focal placental necrosis and fetal brain lesions[48]. Non-suppurative encephalomyelitis has been seen in natural disease outbreaks[49]. On many farms, most animals become infected by one year of age and show no clinical signs.

Diagnosis, Treatment, and Prevention. Diagnosis is based on necropsy findings. Cysts and meronts can be identified in tissue by immunochemistry. Positive serology only indicates exposure; it does not demonstrate etiology. No treatment is likely to be of value in infected sheep or goats. Preventing carnivores from consuming carcasses of sheep or goats lowers the numbers of sporocysts in the environment. Amprolium has been used experimentally to reduce the severity of disease in lambs[50].

Public Health Considerations. The *Sarcocystis* species in sheep and goats are not infective to humans.

Toxoplasma gondii

Morphology and Life Cycle. The morphology and life cycle of *Toxoplasma gondii* are discussed in Chapter 18, Parasites of Cats.

Hosts. Felids are the only definitive hosts for *T. gondii*. The tissue forms of the organism can infect avian and mammalian species, including sheep and goats.

Pathologic Effects and Clinical Disease. Abortion and neonatal death are the most important effects of *T. gondii* on sheep and goats. The lamb or kid may die in the uterus, be stillborn, or succumb within a few days of birth. Young animals that survive it have apparently normal

lives as chronic carriers of tissue cysts. There is necrosis of the placental cotyledons with white nodules visible on gross examination. Nodules may be seen in the liver and brain of the fetus. Goats are highly sensitive to clinical toxoplasmosis with as few as 1,000 oocysts causing death[51]. In adult goats, organisms are found in muscle and the liver, kidney, brain, and placenta. If ewes are infected early in gestation the fetus is likely to be absorbed. During the later stages the fetus dies in the uterus or soon after birth. A significant number of asymptomatic lambs are born with the infection[52]. Adult sheep rarely show clinical signs of disease.

Diagnosis. A diagnosis of toxoplasmosis may be suggested by a history of animals having a primary exposure to *Toxoplasma* during pregnancy, or the finding of white foci on the cotyledons or tissues of aborted fetuses. Serology indicates exposure to the parasite and elevated IgM or rising IgG titers suggest *Toxoplasma* abortion. Serologic activity by the fetus indicates the organism crossed the placenta, because maternal antibody does not cross the ruminant placenta. Observation of the organisms in tissues confirms infection. Mouse inoculation using greater quantities of tissue than visualized by histology is a more sensitive test.

Treatment. There is little reason to treat sheep or goats with normal functioning immune systems because they will become chronically infected but not have clinical disease, and are resistant to new infection. However, in animals recently exposed for the first time, treatment for three days with a combination of sulfamezathine and pyrimethamine was successful in increasing the number of viable lambs produced compared to untreated ewes[53].

Prevention. A live incomplete tachyzoite vaccine protects against challenge for 18 months[54]. Abortion is rare in ewes that have previously aborted due to toxoplasmosis, so infection of ewes before breeding may actually prevent disease. Adding replacement ewes to the flock before breeding on properties where toxoplasmosis has been diagnosed may expose the replacements to oocysts before they become pregnant. Sanitary procedures that prevent the contamination of feed by cat feces or bodies of infected rodents reduces the risk of infection.

Public Health Considerations. Toxoplasmosis is a serious disease in immune-compromised humans or in cases of congenital transmission. Handling placentas of infected does or ewes without gloves, or ingesting undercooked tissues or milk are the primary sources of infection to humans. Therefore, animal workers should practice excellent hygiene when handling placentas known or suspected to contain *T. gondii*.

Class Piroplasmida

Babesia spp.

Morphology. Sheep and goats are susceptible to infection with *Babesia capreoli*, *B. motasi*, and *B. ovis*. Babesias are obligate red blood cell parasites, and are classified as large or small, depending on the size of the intraerythrocytic piroplasms. In sheep and goats, *B. motasi* (2.5 μ to 4 μ long by 2 μ wide) is the large species. When paired, the large pear-shaped organisms lie at an acute angle. The small *B. ovis* piroplasms, which measure 1 μ to 2.5 μ long, are at an obtuse angle[55].

Hosts. *Babesia* of sheep and goats are cross-infective. *Babesia capreoli* normally infects deer, but can infect sheep. Ticks serve as definitive hosts. *Rhipicephalus bursa* is a vector of both *B. motasi* and *B. ovis*, and *Haemaphysalis punctata* transmits *B. ovis* in northern Europe[56]. *Ixodes ricinus* is the vector of *B. capreoli* in sheep and deer in Great Britain[57].

Life Cycle. Piroplasms reproduce by binary fission within erythrocytes. Gametogony and fertilization occur in the tick gut. Several generations of asexual reproduction then occur in the tick haemocoel. Transovarian and transstadial transmission occur. The organisms invade the salivary glands of ticks, where they undergo sporulation. Sporozoites are infective to the vertebrate host, where they become merozoites or piroplasms in the erythrocytes.

Pathologic Effects. In general, small *Babesia* are more virulent than large strains. For example, *B. ovis* is highly virulent to sheep, while *B. motasi* is only moderately so. Erythrocyte destruction caused by rapidly dividing parasites causes anemia, fever, hemoglobinemia, and hemoglobinuria. There may be a sequestration of infected cells in capillary beds and hypotensive shock may occur. The liver and spleen become enlarged and the tissues and mucous membranes become jaundiced.

Clinical Disease. Clinical signs in sheep include anemia, fever, anorexia, diarrhea, depression, and icterus. The signs seen in a flock vary with the age of the animals involved. Young animals become infected but are often asymptomatic carriers because of premunity. Older animals exposed for the first time, or following reexposure after a long period of being *Babesia*-free, may exhibit clinical disease.

Diagnosis. Geographic locality and history of the flock are useful for a presumptive diagnosis. Finding the piroplasms in thick or thin blood films is proof of infection. The level of parasitemia is too low to detect in chronic carriers, so observation is strong evidence of disease. Serologic tests and PCR are useful for evaluating flock exposure and carrier status.

Treatment and Prevention. Imidocarb dipropionate is effective in treating ovine babesiosis[58]. A flock consisting of chronic carriers will not show clinical signs. *Babesia*-free animals in endemic areas can be purposefully inoculated when young, to induce a carrier state. However, the administration of blood from carriers does carry risk because high parasitemia may cause disease or other pathogens may be transmitted. Older animals administered blood from carriers can be treated with imidocarb when they begin to show signs of disease. This provides protection from future natural exposures so long as adequate antibody titers remain. Disease can also be prevented by the prophylactic use of imidocarb so that as serum levels decline and the sheep are exposed, the infection will be moderated sufficiently to allow survival while premunity develops.

Area-wide tick control programs are unlikely to prevent infections where three-host ticks are present.

Public Health Considerations. Infection of humans with small ruminant *Babesia* has not been reported.

Theileria spp.

Morphology. Piroplasms of *Theileria hirci* and *T. ovis* are found in erythrocytes, and measure 1 μ to 2 μ. They are round to rod-shaped but are never paired like *Babesia*.

Hosts. *Theileria hirci* is the agent of malignant theileriosis of sheep and goats in Eastern Europe, the Middle East, and North Africa, and it is transmitted by *Hyalomma* spp.[59]. *Theileria ovis* is a benign parasite of sheep in Europe, Asia, and Africa.

Life Cycle. Sporozoites are inoculated into the host during tick feeding. The sporozoites enter into lymphocytes in lymph nodes and undergo schizogony, ultimately producing micromerozoites, which enter erythrocytes and form piroplasms. The piroplasms are infective to larval or nymphal ticks. Sexual reproduction occurs in the tick, producing sporozoites that are transmitted to the host after several days of feeding.

Pathologic Effects and Clinical Disease. Infection with *T. hirci* results in lymphadenopathy followed by lymphocytolysis, hemorrhages on mucous membranes and serosal surfaces, anemia, icterus, and pulmonary edema. Animals become febrile, weak, and lethargic. Mortality rates are high.

Diagnosis, Treatment, and Prevention. History and clinical signs are indicative of theileriosis. Finding meronts (schizonts) in the lymphocytes obtained by lymph node biopsy, or the presence of piroplasms in erythrocytes, confirms infection. Once clinical signs have been seen it is probably too late to successfully treat an infected host. Tick control may be successful because the organism is transmitted several days after attachment. This treatment approach has been used against bovine theileriosis in eastern Africa, where animals were dipped twice weekly during the season of greatest tick activity.

Public Health Considerations. *Theileria* infections have not been reported in humans.

TREMATODES

Family Dicrocoeliidae

Dicrocoelium spp.

Morphology. Sheep and goats are susceptible to infection with *Dicrocoelium dendriticum* and *D. hospes*. These are small (<1 cm long), lancet-shaped flukes with simple caeca. The uterus is large and branched. The eggs are brown, measure 45 µ by 30 µ long, and contain a miracidium when passed.

Hosts. Natural definitive hosts include sheep, goats, cattle, deer, and rabbits. Several species of terrestrial snails serve as the first intermediate host and *Formica* ants serve as the second intermediate host of *D. dendriticum*. Likewise, *Campanotus* ants serve as the second intermediate host of *D. hospes*. *Dicrocoelium dendriticum* is found in many parts of the temperate world and *D. hospes* is found in sub-Saharan Africa.

Life Cycle. Adult flukes inhabit the bile ducts, from which they expel eggs that are immediately infective to snails. Two generations of asexual development occur within the snail. Cercarial development takes three months and cercariae are expelled from the snail in pulmonary exudates (the slime ball). Ants ingest slime balls and the cercariae form metacercariae in the body cavity or brain. Metacercariae in the brain cause the ant to grasp forage and hang on until ingested by a grazing herbivore. The immature flukes travel directly from the small intestine up the bile ducts with no migration in the liver parenchyma. The prepatent period is 10 to 12 weeks.

Pathologic Effects and Clinical Disease. Light infections are asymptomatic. In contrast, extremely heavy infections (thousands of flukes) may result in fibrosis of the small bile ducts and subsequent cirrhosis, edema, and emaciation.

Diagnosis, Treatment, and Prevention. Diagnosis is by finding the small brownish eggs on fecal examination, or the adult worms in the bile ducts. Benzimidazoles given

at higher rates than for other helminths, or praziquantel at double the dose for tapeworms, are effective. Netobimin at 20 mg/kg may be effective[59]. Prevention is complicated by the long-term survival of eggs and the presence of infected snails in the environment. In these cases, sheep should be treated regularly to prevent egg shedding. In endemic areas, research sheep should be housed on dry lots.

Public Health Considerations. The infection has been reported in humans following ingestion of infected ants.

Family Fasciolidae

Fasciola gigantica

Morphology. Adult *Fasciola gigantica* measure 7.5 cm long and are leaf shaped, with a short conical anterior end. In other ways it resembles *F. hepatica*. The operculated eggs are golden colored and measure 190 µ long by 100 µ wide.

Hosts and Life Cycle. The host distribution and life cycle are similar to *F. hepatica*. The parasite is found in tropical and semitropical regions. The prepatent period is 13 to 16 weeks. Metacercariae may not encyst on vegetation but may be found on the water surface, so drinking, in addition to grazing, facilitates transmission[59].

Pathologic Effects and Clinical Disease. The disease is similar to that caused by *F. hepatica* but fewer flukes are required to cause clinical disease. Goats are more likely to suffer adverse reactions than sheep[60].

Diagnosis, Treatment, and Prevention. Diagnosis, treatment and prevention recommendations are as for *F. hepatica*.

Public Health Considerations. Ingesting metacercariae from contaminated vegetation or water infects humans. Thus, animal workers cannot be directly infected from animals.

Fasciola hepatica

Morphology. Adult flukes are measure 3.5 cm by 1 cm long and are thin, leaf-shaped, gray brown, with a conical anterior end. There are shoulders behind the anterior cone. One sucker surrounds the mouth, and another, ventral sucker, used as a holdfast, can be seen with the naked eye. The internal organs are branched and the cuticle is covered with small spines. The operculated eggs are light yellow to gold and measure 150 µ long by 90 µ wide.

Hosts. Domestic ruminants are the natural definitive hosts, though other mammals may become infected. Adult flukes are found in the hepatic bile ducts. The intermediate hosts are amphibious snails of the genus *Lymnaea*. *Fasciola* *hepatica* occurs in temperate and sub-tropical areas of the world.

Life Cycle. Eggs passed in the feces hatch in one to two weeks. Eggs only hatch in water during daylight and when free from fecal material. The miracidium has only a few hours to find a suitable snail, which it penetrates. Each miracidium reproduces asexually in the snail, resulting in up to 600 cercariae, which leave the snail in water and encyst on submerged grass. Encysted metacerariae are ingested during grazing. They exit the cyst in the small intestine and penetrate the intestinal wall into the peritoneal cavity. They penetrate the capsule of the liver and begin migration through the parenchyma for six to eight weeks. The immature flukes enter the bile ducts and mature, producing eggs in eight to 12 weeks. Adult flukes are long-lived.

Pathologic Effects. The acute disease is manifested in sheep and goats by severe hepatic enlargement and hemorrhagic tracts during migration two to six weeks post infection. Fibrinous tags are seen on the liver capsule. Affected sheep have pale mucous membranes, are weak, and may have ascites. Subacute disease is seen when the exposure is low and over a longer time span. Some of the flukes reach the bile ducts and cause cholangitis and tracts in the liver. Anemia and hypoalbuminemia are seen with jaundiced or pale mucous membranes, ascites, and bottle jaw (intermandibular edema). Chronic fascioliosis typically results in fibrous proliferation surrounding the hyperplastic bile ducts and a blockage of blood vessels in the liver, causing local fibrosis. The liver is pale and firm with the ventral lobe reduced in size[61].

Clinical Disease. Acute disease results in sudden death or weak animals with pale mucous membranes similar to that seen with acute hemonchosis. Clinical signs develop more slowly with chronic disease. Animals are pale, lose condition, and show signs of hypoproteinemia, weight loss, wool break, and nonresponsive anemia.

Diagnosis. No eggs are found in the feces during the acute or subacute disease. Thus, diagnosis is by postmortem examination. Serologic tests have been developed and are reliable as early as two weeks post infection[62]. Serum levels of glutamate dehydrogenase rise early in fluke migration and gamma glutamyl transpeptidase levels rise when the flukes reach the bile ducts[59]. Chronic cases are diagnosed by finding eggs in feces. Daily fecal egg counts may vary greatly.

Treatment and Prevention. Triclabendazole is the most effective drug for *Fasciola* infections because it has the capacity to kill flukes as early as one week into migration. Other drugs that are effective in removing later migratory stages are rafoxinide, closantel, nitroxynil, and clorsulon[59]. Albendazole is effective in removing adult flukes. However, local populations of worms may be resistant to specific anthelmintics. Research sheep and goats should be kept off of pastures harboring lymnaed snails.

Public Health Considerations. Humans acquire infection of *F. hepatica* by ingesting metacercariae from vegetation. Thus, animal workers cannot be directly infected from animals.

Family Paramphistomatidae

Morphology. Sheep and goats are susceptible to infection with several paramphistomes, including *Calicophoron calicophorum*, *C. microbothrium*, *Cotylophoron cotylphorum*, *C. panamensis*, *Paramphistomum cervi*, *P. ichikawai*, *Ornithocoelium* spp., and others. These are robust, 1-cm-long, conical flukes with a large ventral sucker, smaller oral sucker, and in some species, a genital sucker. The eggs are large (150 μ long by 90 μ wide), operculated, and unlike those of *F. hepatica*, are clear.

Hosts. Adult paramphistomes inhabit the reticulum of ruminants. Larval stages use aquatic snails of the genera *Planorbis* or *Bulinus* as intermediate hosts[59] or amphibious snails of the genus *Lymnaea*[63]. Fluke and host species vary depending on the geographic locality.

Life Cycle. The life cycles are generally similar to that of *F. hepatica*. Ingested metacercariae excyst in the small intestine and the immature flukes feed on plugs of mucosa in the duodenum for approximately six weeks. They then migrate to the reticulum and attach as adults. The prepatent period is seven to 10 weeks.

Pathologic Effects and Clinical Disease. The most acute damage occurs during the histophagic phase in the duodenum. The host becomes emaciated with a thickened, corrugated, gelatinous anterior small intestine. Immature flukes burrow into the intestinal wall as far as the muscularis mucosa, drawing tissue into the oral sucker. The mucosa lifts from the muscularis in heavy infections and there is diffuse cellular proliferation around the flukes[64,65]. Most infections are asymptomatic. In heavy infections, diarrhea and emaciation coincide with the activity of immature flukes in the intestine.

Diagnosis, Treatment, and Prevention. Flukes may be observed at necropsy. Speciation is difficult but only one or two species of rumen flukes are likely to occur in a given geographic region. Sedimentation or differential sieving may recover the eggs. Resorantel and oxyclozanide are the drugs of choice against adult and immature rumen flukes[59]. Research sheep and goats should not be housed on pastures known to flood regularly.

Public Health Considerations. There are none.

CESTODES

Order Cyclophyllidea

Echinococcus granulosus

Morphology. The morphology of the adult tapeworm is presented in Chapter 17, Parasites of Dogs. The metacestode (larval) stage of *Echinococcus granulosus* is the hydatid cyst, a thick-walled, fluid-filled structure that varies in size with anatomic location and age of the cyst. Each cyst contains thousands of protoscoleces.

Hosts and Life Cycle. Several species of mammals have been identified with hydatid cysts, including sheep, other ruminants, swine, and humans. Gravid proglottids are passed in the feces of canids. The eggs are distributed in the environment, where they may survive for as long as two years, then are consumed by an intermediate host. The embryo penetrates the gut, where it is carried to the liver, lungs, or occasionally other organs. The hydatid cyst grows slowly and matures in six to 12 months in sheep. The mature cyst is consumed by canids, resulting in the establishment of hundreds to thousands of adult worms in the small intestine.

Pathologic Effects and Clinical Disease. In sheep, approximately 70% of the cysts are found in the lungs and 25% are found in the liver[66]. The diameter and shape of the cyst varies with location, but 20-cm diameter cysts are not unusual. The presence of the space-occupying cyst is usually well tolerated by sheep, because there is little host reaction to the cyst. Thus, most infections are asymptomatic.

Diagnosis, Treatment, and Prevention. Diagnosis is by finding cysts at necropsy. The eggs passed in the stool of canids are indistinguishable from those of *Taenia* spp. No treatment is warranted in ruminant hosts. Praziquantel and other anthelmintics are effective in dogs. Sheep and goats used in research must be prevented from grazing pastures contaminated by feral dogs. Treatment of dogs is effective but the proper disposal of carcasses is essential because wild canids are not amenable to treatment.

Public Health Considerations. Hydatid disease is a locally important condition in humans. However, humans become infected through ingestion of eggs from canids, not through contact with infected ruminants.

Moniezia expansa

Morphology. Adult *Moniezia expansa* measure up to 2 m long and 1.5 cm wide. The rostellum is unarmed. The eggs are variable in shape but usually triangular, approximately 60 μ long, and contain a pyriform apparatus with a hexacanth embryo.

Hosts. *Moniezia expansa*, the "broad" tapeworm, is a member of the family Anoplocephalidae and is found primarily in sheep, goats, and a wide variety of deer and antelope. A closely related species, *M. benedeni*, is found primarily in cattle but has been reported in small ruminants.

Life Cycle. Gravid proglottids and eggs are expelled in the feces. Forage mites in the family Oribatidae ingest the eggs. The hexacanth embryos migrate into the body cavity of the mites and form cysticercoids. The cysticercoid is infective in one to four months and the sheep or goat ingests the mite while grazing. The scolex attaches in the small intestine. The prepatent period is six weeks. Adult worms only live about three months.

Pathologic Effects and Clinical Disease. *Moniezia expansa* rarely causes disease, even in kids and lambs, though some have reported diarrhea, ill thrift, and intestinal obstruction due to *M. expansa*[59].

Diagnosis, Treatment, and Prevention. Diagnosis is by finding proglottids in the feces, adult worms on postmortem examination, or eggs in fecal floatation preparations. Benzimidazoles may be effective if administered at doses higher than recommended for nematodes. Praziquantel, niclosamide, or bunamidine may be used for treatment or prevention by treating lambs or kids in the late spring when mite populations are greatest.

Public Health Considerations. Humans are not susceptible to infection with *Moniezia* sp.

Taenia spp.

Morphology. Only metacestode stages of *Taenia* are found in the tissues of sheep or goats. Larval *T. ovis* was at one time named *Cysticercus ovis*. The metacestode stage of *T. hydatigena* was called *C. tenuicollis*. The cyst of *T. multiceps* was named *Coenurus cerebrallis*, with each cyst containing numerous protoscoleces.

Hosts and Life Cycle. Canids serve as definitive hosts for all of these tapeworms. Sheep are the most common intermediate host for all three species. Cattle and swine are often also infected with *T. hydatigena*.

Proglottids are passed in the feces of canids. The eggs are distributed in the environment. After ingestion by the intermediate host the hexacanth embryo tears through the intestine and is picked up in the blood and transported to the muscle, liver, or central nervous system. Development occurs in the muscle with *T. ovis*. After migration through the liver, the cyst of *T. hydatigena* is formed on the liver surface or in the peritoneal cavity. The coenurus of *T. multiceps* matures in the brain or spinal cord of the infected intermediate host. After a dog or wild canid eats the intermediate host, adult tapeworms mature in the small intestine.

Pathologic Effects and Clinical Disease. Cysticerci of *T. ovis* are nonpathogenic in muscle and therefore asymptomatic. Larval *T. hydatigena* cause a condition known as "hepatitis cysticercosa," in which migration tracts in the liver resemble those caused by *Fasciola hepatica*. Affected sheep may become anemic and hypoproteinemic. Coenuri of *T. multiceps* in the brain or spinal cord may cause pathology, depending on their location. Large space-occupying cysts lead to clinical signs, including softening of the skull over the lesion, circling, blindness, paraplegia, and hyperaesthesia. In addition, the sheep develops a high-stepping gait, a condition known as "gid."

Diagnosis, Treatment, and Prevention. Postmortem diagnosis is by finding cysts at necropsy. Infections with *T. multiceps* may be diagnosed antemortem based on radiographic evidence and central nervous signs in sheep living in endemic areas. Cysts of *T. multiceps* may be removed surgically[66]. Sheep and goats used in research must be prevented from grazing on pastures contaminated by feral dogs. Treatment of dogs is effective but the proper disposal of carcasses is essential because wild canids are not amenable to treatment.

Public Health Considerations. Humans are not susceptible to infection with *T. ovis* or *T. hydatigena,* although rare infections with *T. multiceps* have been reported as a result of accidental consumption of eggs in canid feces.

Thysanosoma actinioides

Morphology. *Thysanosoma actinioides,* the "fringed" tapeworm, is a member of the family Thysanosomidae. The fringed tapeworm bears a series of papillae on the posterior of each proglottid. Adults measure 15 cm to 30 cm long by 8 mm wide, and produce triangular to square eggs without a pyriform apparatus.

Hosts. The primary definitive host is the sheep but other ruminants in the western United States and South America may be infected. The parasite is normally an inhabitant of the small intestine[83] but is frequently found in the common bile duct.

Life Cycle. Gravid proglottids and eggs are expelled in the feces. Psocids (book lice) ingest the eggs. The hexacanth embryos migrate into the body cavity of the psocids, where cysticercoids are formed. Sheep or others ingest psocids while grazing. The worms do not remain attached in any one location within the small intestine or bile ducts, but move about quite readily.

Pathologic Effects and Clinical Disease. The presence of the worms in the bile ducts has caused some to associate *T. actinioides* with several hepatic diseases; however, evidence for this is lacking. The primary importance of infection is liver condemnation due to the presence of the parasite[67].

Diagnosis, Treatment, and Prevention. Diagnosis is by finding eggs in the feces or adult worms at necropsy. Infections may be treated with Niclosamide[59] or albendazole[68]. Housing research sheep indoors or on dry lot may prevent infections.

Public Health Considerations. *Thysanosoma actinioides* does not infect humans.

LEECHES

Morphology. *Limnatis nilotica,* the "horse leech," is a member of the class Hirudinea. *Limnatis nilotica* is a flattened, segmented worm with a triangular anterior sucker. The posterior segments are dark brown or greenish, with longitudinal rows of dark spots, and form a large sucker. The ventral surface of the leech is darker than its dorsal surface.

Hosts and Life Cycle. Sheep and other mammals are susceptible to leech attack. The leech is widespread in Europe and northern Africa. Adult hermaphroditic leeches produce egg packets that develop in pools of water that contain vegetation. Young leeches inhabit the water surface, whereas adults live in the muddy bottom. Vibrations associated with approaching animals attract the leeches to the host, which then ingests them. Leeches attach to the pharynx and nasal cavities where they suck blood for days to weeks, eventually leaving while the host is drinking.

Pathologic Effects and Clinical Disease. Pathologic changes associated with leech infection include blood loss anemia, severe edema in the head region, and resulting dyspnea. Affected animals extend the head, breathe through an open mouth, and exhale bloody froth. Death may result from asphyxiation[69].

Diagnosis, Treatment, and Prevention. Diagnosis is based on clinical signs and by direct observation of attached leeches in the nasal cavity or throat. Treatment is by extracting the leeches with gentle traction. Chloroform water or cocaine preparations may be used to paralyze the leech and facilitate removal[70]. Prevention is by watering livestock from clean water troughs or troughs that have been treated with copper sulfate. The chances of exposure are much greater when watering ponds are low, rather than when the pools are full.

Public Health Considerations. Humans represent suitable hosts for leeches. However, animal workers cannot become infected from sheep or goats, unless the leech attaches to the surgeon after it is removed.

NEMATODES

Most nematodes that affect sheep and goats are acquired via grazing and are not transmitted within the laboratory animal facility. However, sheep and goats intended for research may arrive at the facility already infected. Treatment with suitable anthelmintics on arrival may not be completely effective because of anthelmintic resistance, lack of efficacy against hypobiotic larvae, or improper administration of the compound. The latter may include use of an improper anthelmintic for the parasite species or improper dose rate of the correct anthelmintic for the specific host.

Superfamily Rhabditoidea

Strongyloides papillosus

Morphology. Adult parasitic female *Strongyloides papillosus* measure 3.5 mm to 6 mm long. Parasitic males have not been reported. The genus is readily identified by the rhabditiform esophagus, which extends roughly one-third the length of the body. The uterus and digestive tract are braided and the female produces thin-shelled, larvated eggs measuring 40 μ to 60 μ long by 20 μ to 36 μ wide[71]. The tail is blunt.

Hosts. *Strongyloides papillosus* inhabits the duodenum of sheep and goats, as well as other ruminants, including cattle and deer. Rabbits may also become infected.

Life Cycle. Eggs produced by the parasitic female worms hatch in the environment and develop into infective larvae (homogonic life cycle) or free-living adults of both sexes (heterogonic life cycle). Most eggs develop into infective larvae at 20°C; at 30°C eggs develop into free-living larvae[72]. Sheep and goats are infected through skin penetration by third-stage larvae found in moist organic material. Transmammary infection also occurs, so that *S. papillosus* is often the first nematode found in lambs or kids. In the absence of new exposure, arrested larvae in the tissues provide a source of infection to replace adults lost from the intestine[73]. The prepatent period is six to 14 days.

Pathologic Effects and Clinical Disease. Skin penetration by larval worms results in dermatitis. Dermatitis may progress to foot rot in sheep[74]. Diarrhea may occur, but there is only weak correlation between clinical signs and worm burden, which is represented by fecal egg count[59]. Sudden deaths due to cardiac arrhythmias (ventricular fibrillation preceded by sinus tachycardia) may occur in lambs and calves housed in heavily contaminated environments[75,76].

Diagnosis, Treatment, and Prevention. Diagnosis is by finding worms in the duodenum and possibly the jejunum. Larvated eggs passed in the feces are readily recovered by flotation techniques and can be easily differentiated from the eggs of other gastrointestinal nematodes.

Benzimidazoles and macrolides are effective against most populations of adult worms. These drugs may be effective against larvae in the tissues when the larvae are metabolically active but they do not appear to have activity against hypobiotic larvae.

Research animals should be housed in clean, dry environments unsuitable for survival of free-living larvae. Treatment of dams at parturition reduces transmammary transmission.

Public Health Considerations. *Strongyloides papillosus* does not infect humans.

Superfamily Oxyuroidea

Skrjabinema ovis

Morphology. Adult male *Skrjabinema ovis* measure 2.5 mm to 3.5 mm long and bear a single spicule measuring 120 μ long. Adult females measure 5 mm to 10 mm long and the eggs measure 50 μ to 30 μ long, with a slightly flattened side. They are embryonated when passed[71].

Hosts and Life Cycle. *Skrjabinema ovis* is found in the colon of sheep and goats. A separate species, *S. caprae*, was described for the goat but is likely synonymous[77]. The life cycle is direct. Embryonated eggs are deposited in the perianal region before falling to the ground, where grazing sheep and goats ingest them. Larvae migrate from the small intestine to the colon, where they mature. The prepatent period is 24 days.

Pathologic Effects and Clinical Disease. *Skrjabinema ovis* is not known to cause clinical disease.

Diagnosis, Treatment, and Prevention. Diagnosis is by finding adult worms in the colon. The eggs may be found on the hair, wool, or skin, or adhered to inanimate objects in the environment such as feed racks. Occasionally, eggs may be recovered from the surface of a fecal pellet.

Treatment is usually not indicated, though modern anthelmintics are effective against adult worms in the colon. Infections may be minimized by treating animals for adult worms and immediately moving them to a clean environment after thoroughly washing the infected animal. Three treatments at biweekly intervals prevent development of newly acquired larvae. It is unlikely that eggs survive in the environment longer than a month.

Public Health Considerations. *Skrjabinema ovis* does not infect humans.

Superfamily Strongyloidea

Bunostomum trigonocephalum

Morphology. *Bunostomum trigonocephalum* belongs to the family Ancylostomatidae. Unlike many other hookworms, *B. trigonocephalum* possesses two cutting plates at the margin of the buccal cavity, and a tooth near the esophagus. Adult worms measure 12 mm to 26 mm long. The spicules measure 600 µ to 640 µ long. The female has a blunt tail and the vulva is mid-body. The eggs are thick shelled and the internal cells are darker than most strongyle eggs, and often have debris clinging to the eggshell.

Hosts and Life Cycle. Sheep and goats are natural hosts of *B. trigonocephalum*. Other natural hosts include antelope. Eggs are passed in the feces and hatch in the environment. Sheep and goats become infected through skin penetration or ingestion of infective, third-stage larvae. Larvae follow a skin-tracheal migration pattern, molting in the lungs and again in the small intestine. The prepatent period varies but is greater than 40 days. Adult worms survive in the intestine for more than a year[71]. Larval development may be delayed, with larvae instead entering hypobiosis under the influence of host immunity. Thus, clinical disease may occur more commonly at the end of the dry season when the host immunity is at its lowest[59].

Pathologic Effects and Clinical Disease. Infections in young animals result in anemia, hypoproteinemia, diarrhea, and weight loss. Foot stamping or other activities indicating local irritation may be seen when larvae are penetrating the skin.

Diagnosis, Treatment, and Prevention. Diagnosis is by finding adult worms in the small intestine. Coproculture and larval identification are necessary to distinguish infection with *B. trigonocephalum* from infection with other strongyles.

Any of the modern anthelmintics used in sheep and goats are effective against *Bunostomum*. Strategic use of anthelmintics that are effective against hypobiotic larvae during the dry season may prevent the accumulation of larvae in the environment. Frequent removal of manure from the pens in which young animals are confined reduces contact. Because larvae do not leave the fecal pellet before skin penetration, areas heavily soiled with feces increase the risk of infection. Therefore, *B. trigonocephalum* is common in poorly kept confinement facilities.

Public Health Considerations. *Bunostomum trigonocephalum* does not infect humans.

Chabertia ovina

Morphology. *Chabertia ovina*, the large-mouthed bowel worm, is a robust worm that measures 13 mm to 20 mm long. The buccal cavity is large, and is slightly hooked at the anterior end. The eggs are typical of the superfamily, and measure 90 µ long by 51 µ wide.

Hosts. Natural hosts include sheep and goats, as well as other ruminants such as cattle, antelope, deer, and camels.

Life Cycle. *Chabertia* has a direct life cycle. Eggs passed in the feces embryonate and hatch in hours to days, depending on the temperature. Both the eggs and larvae can survive freezing weather conditions. The larvae are ingested during grazing. The parasite is found in cool temperate climates and may be transmitted during the winter. Development occurs in the wall and lumen of the colon. The prepatent period is approximately 50 days.

Pathologic Effects and Clinical Disease. The larvae and immature adult worms are voracious bloodsuckers, whereas adults are plug feeders. The bowel becomes edematous, fibrotic, and hemorrhagic. The most severe lesions correspond to the period of larval development. Bloody diarrhea may be observed roughly three weeks after infection, and persist for up to two months. Decreased wool production is a sequella to the infection[71].

Diagnosis, Treatment, and Prevention. Diagnosis is by finding worms in the colon at necropsy. Eggs passed in the feces are not distinguishable from the eggs of other strongyles. However, the infective third-stage larva obtained by coproculture can be differentiated from those of other gastrointestinal nematodes. Most commonly used anthelmintics are effective against *C. ovina*. As a result, the parasite is now rare. Infections may be prevented by treatment of adults and maintenance of young animals indoors, on dry lot, or on clean pastures.

Public Health Considerations. *Chabertia ovina* does not infect humans.

Oesophagostomum columbianum

Morphology. *Oesophagostomum columbianum,* the "nodular" worm, is a white, robust worm measuring 12 mm to 18 mm in length. The cephalic vesicle is not inflated. There are 20 to 24 elements in the external leaf crown and 40 to 48 elements in the internal leaf crown. The cervical papillae are well developed. The spicules measure 750 μ to 850 μ long. The female has a long, tapering tail. The eggs are typical for the superfamily, and measure 70 μ to 80 μ long by 50 μ wide[71].

Hosts and Life Cycle. Natural hosts include sheep, goats, and camelids. Adult worms live in the lumen of the colon and the eggs are passed in the feces. Hatched larvae feed on bacteria and develop in the fecal pellet to the infective third-stage in approximately one week. The larvae are ingested during grazing and encyst in the wall of the small intestine approximately three days following infection. These larvae molt to the fourth stage, emerge from the cysts, and are carried to the colon for maturation to the adult stage[78]. The prepatent period is approximately 45 days. In immune hosts, small intestinal larvae may be trapped in the cyst for up to a year, and eventually die[59].

Pathologic Effects. Pathologic effects are due to the reaction surrounding the larvae within the nodule in the intestine, or during the time of emergence of the fourth-stage larvae from the wall of the intestine. Lesions consist of eosinophilic, caseous nodules, which ulcerate as larvae emerge from the mucosa. Ulceration may result in anemia[79]. Fourth-stage larvae are plug feeders and the adult worms imbibe blood.

Clinical Disease. Clinical signs include anemia, diarrhea, weight loss, and anorexia in the presence of only a few adult worms. The nodules occasionally perforate the intestine, resulting in peritonitis. Worm burdens decline with advancing age and repeated exposure, though inflammation and nodule formation resulting from encystment of third-stage larvae may remain marked[79].

Diagnosis, Treatment, and Prevention. Diagnosis is by finding nodules in the small intestine or adults in the large intestine. Eggs are readily found on fecal flotation but cannot be differentiated from other strongyle eggs. However, infective third-stage larvae can be differentiated from other genera of nematodes.

Modern anthelmintics are effective against the adult and luminal larval worms. Treatment of animals in which the parasite has been identified should rid the flock of the infection. The parasite has become rare in recent years in areas where anthelmintic treatment is commonly practiced.

Public Health Considerations. Humans are not susceptible to infection with *O. columbianum.*

Oesophagostomum venulosum

Oesophagostomum venulosum is a robust, bursate worm measuring 12 mm to 24 mm in length and 300 μ to 600 μ wide, with an inflated cephalic vesicle. The external leaf crown has 18 elements and the internal leaf crown has 36. The spicules measure 1.1 mm to 1.5 mm long, and the eggs are typical of the superfamily[59]. The biology of *O. venulosum* is similar to that of *O. columbianum.* Likewise, lesions consist of intestinal nodules, petechial hemorrhages, and ulcers. Clinical signs include decreased weight gain, diarrhea, and excessive mucous production. Other aspects of infection with *O. venulosum* are similar to *O. columbianum.*

Superfamily Trichostrongyloidea

Cooperia curticei

Morphology. The head of adult *Cooperia curticei* (Syn. *Cooperia surnabada*) is bulbous, with transverse striations running the length of the body. There are 14 to 16 longitudinal striations. Adult worms measure 5 mm to 6 mm long. The spicules measure 140 μ long, and are stout and curvaceous.

Hosts and Life Cycle. *Cooperia curticei* is a parasite of the small intestine of sheep, goats, and occasionally, wild ruminants. The life cycle is similar to that of other trichostrongylid nematodes. Larvae are inactive during the winter on pasture but rapidly develop in the summer. The prepatent period can be as short as 12 to 14 days[77].

Pathologic Effects and Clinical Disease. The parasite is a mild pathogen. Softening of the stool at the time of patency was the only sign seen in lambs[80].

Diagnosis, Treatment, and Prevention. Diagnosis, treatment, and prevention strategies are similar to those of *Teladorsagia circumcincta.*

Public Health Considerations. *Cooperia curticei* does not infect humans.

Dictyocaulus filaria

Morphology. Adult male *Dictyocaulus filaria* measure 25 mm to 80 mm long, with short, stubby, bursal rays. The spicules are stout and curved, and measure 400 µ to 500 µ long. The females measure 50 mm to 100 mm long with embryonated eggs in the uterus.

Hosts and Life Cycle. *Dictyocaulus filaria* inhabits the trachea and bronchi of sheep and goats. Eggs released by the females hatch in the lungs of the host. First-stage larvae are coughed up, swallowed, and passed in the feces. The larvae do not feed in the fecal pellets but develop to the infective stage in a minimum of five days. Infective larvae are passively dispersed by rain, or by crawling onto *Philobus* sporangophores, which burst, thereby propelling spores and larvae onto the pasture. Larvae are ingested and penetrate the intestinal wall, and are carried to the mesenteric lymph nodes. Here, they molt to the fourth larval stage, are carried by lymph and blood to the lungs, and break out of the capillaries and enter the alveoli. Larvae then ascend to the bronchioles where they molt to the adult stage and mature. The prepatent period is five weeks.

Pathologic Effects and Clinical Disease. Pathologic effects include damage to the alveoli, bronchioles, and bronchi due to cellular infiltration and a plugging of the smaller air passages. Bronchitis occurs due to production of excessive mucus, entrapment of eggs and larvae, and development of a foreign body reaction, with the influx of massive numbers of eosinophils, macrophages, and giant cells. Interstitial emphysema and edema occur, and opportunistic bacteria may invade areas of inflammation around dead and dying worms[59]. Clinical signs include coughing and ill thrift in young animals. Goats are more adversely affected than sheep. Dyspnea and nasal discharge are seen in heavily infected individuals.

Diagnosis. Diagnosis is by finding characteristic first-stage larvae in the feces. The first-stage larva bears a knob at the anterior end of the sheath and has a straight tail. The protoplasmic knob is a useful characteristic to differentiate the larvae from those of other lungworms found in small ruminants.

Treatment. The modern anthelmintics (levamisole, macrolides, or benzimidazoles) effectively eliminate *D. filaria*. Supportive treatment may be necessary to supplement oxygen, kill bacterial invaders, and reduce inflammation. Parenterally administered macrolides are effective against incoming larvae for a month or longer so that infected animals may remain on contaminated pasture while possibly gaining immunity to the parasite.

Prevention. Infection with *D. filaria* can be prevented by not allowing susceptible animals to graze where disease outbreaks have occurred in the present or previous year's grazing season. Use of residual anthelmintics or feeding of anthelmintics may protect susceptible animals from infection, though experience with tissue-migrating larvae is necessary for the development of immunity. Thus, chronically medicated animals remain susceptible to disease and to infection with parasite strains that have developed anthelmintic resistance.

Public Health Considerations. Humans are not susceptible to infection with *D. filaria*.

Haemonchus contortus

Morphology. Adult male worms measure 10 mm to 20 mm long, and females measure 18 mm to 30 mm long. A lancet in the buccal cavity is used to cut small blood vessels so the worms can imbibe large quantities of blood. The blood-filled intestine causes freshly collected worms to appear red. The ovaries and uterus, which are white, wrap around the intestine, giving a "barber's pole" or candy cane appearance to the females. The spicules are less than 440 µ long and have a hook at the distal end. The female usually has a flap or swelling near the vulva. The size of this structure is influenced by the host immune system, with large linguiform flaps in susceptible hosts, and small knobs in resistant hosts. Differences among *Haemonchus* species are based on spicule length and cuticular ridge morphology[81] or differences in ribosomal DNA[82].

Hosts. Sheep and goats are the primary hosts, but antelope, deer, camelids, and cattle may be infected. Gerbils can be infected experimentally, and have been a useful laboratory animal host[83].

Life Cycle. The life cycle is direct, and typical of the superfamily. Sheep and goats are infected through ingesting third-stage larvae while grazing. Worm development occurs in the abomasums, where larvae enter gastric pits and molt to the fourth larval stage, which feeds on blood. Final development to patent infection requires approximately three weeks. Adult worms live for months in susceptible hosts. Adult female worms produce 5,000 to 6,000 eggs per day, ensuring the survival of offspring even under unfavorable environmental conditions. The resumption of more favorable weather conditions may result in the ingestion of massive numbers of infective larvae previously dormant in fecal pats. Arrested development (hypobiosis) within the host is common in *Haemonchus* infections and occurs within the abomasum during the early fourth larval stage. Resumption of development of arrested larvae also occurs during more favorable external conditions, or when host immunity wanes, such as occurs during the periparturient period.

Pathologic Effects. Pathologic changes accompanying infection with *H. contortus* are related to the loss of blood and protein. Edema may be generalized, and the body cavities become filled with fluid. Bone marrow changes suggest the duration of the disease. Abomasal lesions may be absent, though hosts undergoing an immune response to the worms may develop increased mucosal cellularity, with mast cells, eosinophils, or globular leukocytes.

Clinical Disease. *Haemonchus* is the most pathogenic nematode parasite of sheep and goats in the tropics or temperate areas. Diarrhea is seldom seen with haemonchosis, although the stool may be soft. The clinical presentation varies depending on the physiologic status of the host and parasite burden. Peracute disease is characterized by sudden death with few warning signs, except that the stool may be soft and the packed cell volume falls below 10. Only a few individuals in the flock are affected. The anemia is responsive, and immature erythrocytes are seen in the survivors. Acute disease is seen in more individuals in the flock, and the most common signs are anemia, pale mucous membranes, hypoproteinemia, and intermandibular edema (bottle jaw). The host may be constipated or have a normal stool. A common sequela to acute haemonchosis is wool break, in which wool sheds off a few weeks following the acute signs of disease. Chronic disease is characterized by unresponsive anemia. Affected animals show signs of ill thrift, poor-quality wool, weight loss, or failure to gain.

Diagnosis. A diagnosis of haemonchosis may be suspected as erythrocyte and hemoglobin levels become depressed. Macrocytic, normochromic anemia is typical of acute haemonchosis. Chronic haemonchosis occurs when iron, cobalt, and copper levels are depleted (microcytic, hypochromic anemia). Serum protein levels are low. Because protein loss occurs through the gastrointestinal tract, both albumin and globulin levels are lowered.

Fecal flotation using a saline or sugar flotation medium with a specific gravity of 1.18 or greater will float the eggs of *Haemonchus* and other nematodes. Fecal examination reveals thin-shelled, segmented eggs. Eggs are not diagnostic for *Haemonchus* because other genera of strongylids produce identical eggs. A quantitative test such as the modified McMaster method helps the clinician determine whether there is evidence of sufficient numbers of worms to cause disease. There is a somewhat linear relationship between fecal egg count and worm burden. Egg counts greater than 4,000 eggs per gram of feces are associated with haemonchosis.

Treatment. Most modern anthelmintics are effective against *Haemonchus*. However, *H. contortus* is prone to anthelmintic resistance[84–86]. Goats metabolize anthelmintics differently than sheep[87] and resistance is seen in goats before it is seen in sheep. Therefore, anthelmintic dosages suitable for sheep may be insufficient for treating goats. Some have found that sheep dosages should be doubled for goats.

Animals intended for research may be managed differently than those intended as breeders. Research subjects should be free of gastrointestinal nematodes.

Breeding animals remaining on pasture can be managed in a variety of ways. For example, animals can be treated after they have been exposed to large numbers of worms. Treatment two weeks after a rain should remove many of the recently acquired worms before they can begin passing eggs. Housing indoors or on dry lot after a disease outbreak may enable the host to recover both immunity as well as erythrocyte volume and serum protein levels. In addition, individual animals that have a greater number of worm eggs in their feces than the remainder of the population can be identified by determining egg counts or by measuring the color of the ocular mucous membranes (for instance, FAMACHA carding). Treating high shedders rather than the entire host population can reduce pasture contamination nearly as much as treating the entire flock, and will ensure the survival of susceptible worms, because those in the untreated animals will not be selected. A corollary to individual treatment is the culling of those animals that are treated most often. Not only are they not resistant to worms, their offspring will likely have similar traits.

Prevention. Lessening exposure of susceptible hosts is a critical component of control programs. Reducing pasture contamination should be attempted in the early spring or at the onset of the rainy season. This can be accomplished in a several ways, such as rotating pastures so that pastures are vacated for at least 30 days in warm wet periods. Using pastures that have been used for crops, especially in the last half of the grazing season, is an effective measure for reducing exposure. Alternate or co-grazing with other species of livestock may harvest *Haemonchus* larvae from the pasture. In general, the *Haemonchus* in sheep and goats are poorly adapted to cattle and vice versa, though recent observations question this assumption because some populations of *H. contortus* may thrive in calves.

Pastures with plants that are high in condensed tannins are beneficial for hosts because the incoming larvae may be adversely affected and proteins are able to bypass the rumen[88]. The physical structure of some plants may challenge larvae to ascend vegetation or may provide protection from adverse pasture conditions[89]. If animals are allowed to browse their chances of acquiring larvae diminishes as the distance from the ground increases. Most infective larvae are found within two inches (50 mm) of the soil surface.

Predaceous fungi which kill larvae in pastures, have been evaluated as agents. One species, *Duddingtonia flagrans,* is able to traverse the digestive tract and is present in the fecal pat when the larvae hatch. Feeding spores or incorporating them in ruminal boluses can lower pasture contamination in specific circumstances[90].

Strategic deworming to remove arrested or recently emerged larvae before they contaminate the pasture has a great impact on pasture contamination. For example, treating the ewe or doe in the periparturient relaxation of resistance greatly reduces pasture contamination. Protein is vital during the periparturient and early growth periods. Increased protein levels may lessen worm egg production and provide a level of tolerance for worms.

Selecting individual animals with some resistance to *Haemonchus,* those that have the capacity to rebound from the effects of parasitism, may be beneficial, because the offspring of resistant hosts are also likely to be resistant[91,92].

Public Health Considerations. Humans are rarely infected by *Haemonchus*[71], probably because grazing is the means of infection. Therefore, normal associations with infected animals do not represent a risk.

Nematodirus battus

Morphology. *Nematodirus battus* is a slender, twisted worm with an anterior inflation and transverse striations. Adult males measure 10 mm to 13 mm. The spicules measure 850 μ to 950 μ long and are united at the posterior end. Female worms measure 17 mm to 22 mm long and have a pointed tail. The large eggs measure 195 μ long by 95 μ wide, and are brownish in color with parallel sides.

Hosts and Life Cycle. Sheep are the natural hosts of *N. battus.* The parasite is found in the ileum of sheep in cool, moist, temperate areas. The life cycle is direct. Eggs passed in the feces embryonate in the environment and must undergo a period of prolonged cooling followed by warm temperatures to hatch. Infective third-stage larvae hatch from the eggs in the summer following the one in which they were deposited. Lambs ingest larvae while grazing. There is no migration into the intestine; development occurs on the surface of the intestine. The prepatent period is 15 days.

Pathologic Effects and Clinical Disease. Pathologic effects include villous atrophy with disruption of the mucosa of the ileum. The intestine is unable to absorb fluids or nutrients and the lamb develops diarrhea and rapidly becomes dehydrated and anorexic, and loses weight.

Diagnosis, Treatment, and Prevention. Diagnosis is by finding larval and/or adult worms at necropsy. Because the clinical signs and death occur during the larval stages, eggs may be scarce or absent. A history of young animals grazing the first season, time of year, and pasture history may facilitate diagnosis. The infection may be eliminated by administering levamisole, benzimidazoles, or macrolides[59]. Research animals can be housed indoors or on dry lot to prevent infection. Lambs housed on pasture should not be grazed on those that held lambs in the previous year. If this is not possible, prophylactic treatment prior to the onset of clinical signs can be effective.

Public Health Considerations. *Nematodirus battus* does not infect humans.

Nematodirus spp.

Morphology. Sheep and goats are susceptible to infection with *Nematodirus abnormalis, N. filicollis,* and *N. spathiger. Nematodirus* are thin, twisted worms up to 2 cm in length. *Nematodirus filicollis* males are 10 mm to 15 mm in length with a large bursa and large bosses on the underside of the bursa. The spicules are 700 μ to 900 μ long with a pointed terminal membrane where the spicules fuse. The females measure 15 mm to 20 mm long and have a blunt tail end with a single spine. The eggs measure 150 μ long by 90 μ wide and have six to eight cells when passed from the host. *Nematodirus abnormalis* males measure 11 mm to 17 mm long with spicules that are 900 μ to 1250 μ long and have an asymmetrical posterior. The females are similar to those of *N. filicollis,* with eggs measuring 210 μ long by 100 μ wide. *Nematodirus spathiger* males measure 10 mm to 19 mm long with a relatively small bursa and small bosses on the underside. The spicules are 700 μ to 1100 μ long with spoon-shaped terminal ends. The females measure 15 mm to 29 mm long with a blunt tail and clear, colored eggs measuring 200 μ long by 100 μ wide.

Hosts and Life Cycle. Sheep, goats, camels, camelids, and wild ruminants are the primary hosts. The life cycle is direct. Larvae develop within the egg and can survive conditions unsuitable to other trichostrongylids. They are often found in hot, dry, or sub-arctic environments[66]. Transmission occurs when conditions are favorable for the infective larvae to hatch from the eggs. Many of the incoming larvae become hypobiotic within the small intestine of the host. All development occurs within the lumen of the intestine. The prepatent period for most *Nematodirus* spp is approximately three weeks, but it is only two weeks for *N. spathiger*[77].

Pathologic Effects and Clinical Disease. Pathologic changes include worms encircling the villi and distorting the mucosa in the anterior small intestine. Fourth-stage *N. spathiger* larvae penetrate into the mucosa and may be associated with clinical disease, including poor weight gain, and may contribute to parasitic gastroenteritis when found with other nematode species.

Diagnosis, Treatment, and Prevention. Diagnosis is by finding the eggs in the feces or worms in the intestine. Levamisole, fenbendazole, oxfendazole, albendazole, and macrolides should be effective against *Nematodirus* spp. Prevention is difficult because *Nematodirus* eggs may hatch at any time when conditions are right in the environment, for up to two years after being passed[66]. Lambs develop a strong resistance to re-infection but may carry arrested larvae for a considerable time. Strategic treatment early in the season that is favorable for transmission may lessen pasture contamination by removing the newly arriving worms before they can reproduce[59].

Public Health Considerations. Humans are not susceptible to infection with *Nematodirus* spp.

Teladorsagia circumcincta

Morphology. *Teladorsagia* (*Ostertagia*) *circumcincta* (Syn. *Teladorsagia davtiani*, *T. trifurcata*) adult males measure approximately 8 mm long. The spicules measure 300 μ and bear three points on the distal end. Adult females measure 10 mm to 12 mm long with a vulvar flap near the curled tail. The eggs are thin shelled, segmented, and measure 90 μ long by 50 μ wide[93,94]. Sheep and goat strains are biochemically and morphologically distinct, which may explain observed differences between the two host species[95].

Hosts. Natural hosts include sheep, goats, camelids, deer, and antelope. Marmots and rabbits may also become infected. Infections of sheep and goats are common in temperate, moist climates throughout the world.

Life Cycle. The life cycle is typical of the superfamily. Larvae in pastures are susceptible to hot, dry conditions, so disease is most often seen in cooler, moist seasons[96]. Ingested larvae may develop directly to the adult stage in the abomasum or may arrest at the early fourth larval stage and remain in a state of hypobiosis for several months.

Pathologic Effects. The primary damage to the host occurs when the early adult emerges from the gastric glands. Gastric pH rises from the normal 2 up to 7, which allows secondary bacterial invasion. Umbilicated nodules develop in the abomasal mucosa, giving the tissue the appearance of Moroccan leather. Abomasal folds become edematous, and the mucosa may slough. Regional lymph nodes enlarge and there is movement of fluids and macromolecules through open cell junctions resulting in protein loss, including hypoalbuminemia and hyperpepsinogenemia[59].

Clinical Disease. Clinical signs include anorexia, diarrhea, dehydration, intermandibular edema, and weight loss. Small intestinal trichostrongyles may exacerbate clinical signs. Infection with *T. circumcincta* is more severe in goats than sheep, possibly because of the goat's failure to mount an adequate immune response.

Diagnosis, Treatment, and Prevention. Diagnosis is by identification of adult worms in the abomasum. Elevated serum pepsinogen and low serum albumin are suggestive of disease, especially when associated with the age of animal, time of year, and clinical signs. Adult and immature worms are generally susceptible to benzimidazole or macrolide anthelmintics; however, resistance has developed to these compounds. Anthelmintics must be evaluated at the local level to determine their relative value against specific parasite populations.

Because the free-living stages of the parasite are susceptible to heat and desiccation, grazing lambs in pastures not occupied by weanlings the previous autumn will reduce parasite burdens. Treatment of does or ewes near the time of parturition negates the effects of the periparturient relaxation of resistance, and lowers the pasture contamination when the lambs or kids begin to graze.

Public Health Considerations: *Teladorsagia circumcincta* does not infect humans.

Trichostrongylus axei

Morphology. *Trichostrongylus axei* is a small, slender worm with an anterior excretory notch that is diagnostic for the genus. Adult male worms measure 2.5 mm to 6 mm in length with dissimilar spicules, one greater than 100 μ long and the other less than 100 μ long. The females measure 3 mm to 8 mm in length with approximately 12 eggs in the uterus. The eggs are typical of the superfamily.

Hosts. Natural hosts of *T. axei* include sheep, goats, cattle, antelope, deer, swine, rabbits, rodents, and horses. Cattle are the primary host, and other livestock become infected when grazing with or following cattle in a rotational grazing system.

Life Cycle. The life cycle is direct, with eggs passed in the feces. Hatched first-stage larvae feed on fecal bacteria and molt twice to the infective third stage. Infection occurs by ingestion of third-stage larvae during grazing. Development occurs in the abomasum (stomach) with the larvae penetrating the mucosal crypts and emerging as adult worms approximately 15 days post-infection. The prepatent period is approximately three weeks.

Pathologic Effects and Clinical Disease. Changes in the gastric mucosa include hyperplasia, increased abomasal pH, and increased permeability of the mucosa, leading to an edematous abomasum and subsequent diarrhea. Hemoconcentration and anemia were seen in artificially infected lambs[97]. In the natural setting *T. axei* is just one of the parasites in the abomasum and is seldom a primary pathogen. However, heavy infections may result in weight loss, diarrhea, dehydration, and death[98].

Diagnosis Treatment, and Prevention. Diagnosis is by recovery of adult worms from the abomasum. Fecal egg counts are low and thus are of little diagnostic value. The eggs of *T. axei* are not easily distinguished from those of other trichostrongyles. Coproculture and larval identification are useful. Increased serum gastrin levels suggest abomasal nematode infection, but are not diagnostic in themselves[99].

Any of the modern anthelmintics are effective against *T. axei*. Because cattle are the primary hosts, treating cattle or preventing co-grazing or rotational grazing with cattle should lower exposure. However, controlling more important parasites may be facilitated by mixed grazing practices.

Public Health Considerations. *Trichostrongylus axei* has been reported in humans but is not associated with disease[100].

Trichostrongylus colubriformis

Morphology. Adult male *Trichostrongylus colubriformis* measure 4.5 mm to 7 mm long, with a large bursa and subequal spicules that are 125 μ to 165 μ in length, with a spade-like posterior. The gubernaculum is boat-shaped. Adult females measure 5 mm to 8 mm long and possess a well-developed ovijector. The eggs are typical of the superfamily.

Hosts. Sheep and goats are the most common hosts. However, *T. colubriformis* has been found in the abomasum and/or small intestine of deer, antelope, camelids, cattle, rodents, and primates, including humans. The anterior small intestine is the primary habitat of the parasite. There may be sheep- and goat-adapted strains of *T. colubriformis*[77].

Life Cycle. The life cycle is direct, and is similar to that of *T. axei*. Uningested larvae survive for prolonged periods in the environment, with moderate temperatures and moisture[101]. The periparturient relaxation of resistance to nematodes in ewes' results in resumed development of hypobiotic larvae so that their offspring will be in the pasture when the lambs begin to graze[102].

Pathologic Effects. Infection results in villus atrophy and increased mucosal permeability in the anterior portion of the small intestine. The emergence of the immature worms from the mucosa into the lumen is associated with the most significant tissue damage[59]. The endothelial cells lining the blood vessels are separated and there is infiltration of mast cells and neutrophils[103]. There is protein loss and failure to absorb specific nutrients, which may lead to skeletal changes in lambs[104,105].

Clinical Disease. Lambs infected with *T. colubriformis* may develop anorexia, weight loss, diarrhea, dehydration, lethargy, and abdominal pain[71]. The diarrhea is often dark in color, hence one of the common names, "black scours worm," is descriptive. Infections are most evident in the spring and autumn when there is sufficient moisture to support larval development[106]. Lambs or kids are at higher risk than adults.

Diagnosis, Treatment, and Prevention. Diagnosis is by recovery of adult worms from the lumen of the small intestine. The eggs of *T. colubriformis* are not sufficiently distinct to allow for accurate species identification. Coproculture and identification of third-stage larvae may be used to identify the worms. Modern anthelmintics are effective; however, anthelmintic resistance may develop. Therefore, anthelmintic efficacy should be monitored. Strategic deworming practices minimize worm burdens.

Public Health Considerations. Humans may become infected with *T. colubriformis*.

Trichostrongylus longispicularis

Trichostrongylus longispicularis resembles *T. colubriformis* except the spicules are long and slender and do not have the step-like feature near the posterior end. Although it is probably a valid species[107] it is similar to *T. colubriformis* in biology, range, and host effects.

Trichostrongylus vitrinus

Trichostrongylus vitrinus resembles *T. colubriformis* except that the spicules have sharply pointed posterior ends. The natural hosts, biology, and life cycle are similar to *T. colubriformis* except that *T. vitrinus* is more tolerant of cold temperatures and has adapted to cool moist climates[106]. *Trichostrongylus vitrinus* causes more severe erosions of the intestine and a greater decline in serum albumin levels than does *T. colubriformis*[108]. Infected lambs are anorexic, diarrheic, and exhibit reduced weight gains. The disease is more severe than that caused by *T. colubriformis* in lambs. Diagnosis, treatment, and prevention are as described for *T. colubriformis*. Human infections have been reported.

Superfamily Metastrongyloidea

Muellerius capillaris

Morphology. Male worms measure 11 mm to 13 mm long with a spiral, coiled tail and a rudimentary bursa. The females measure 20 mm long and are brownish in color.

Hosts and Life Cycle. *Muellerius capillaris* is a common parasite found in the pulmonary alveoli of sheep and goats. Female worms produce strongyle-type eggs that hatch, releasing larvae which are coughed up, swallowed, and passed in the feces. Snails and slugs serve as intermediate hosts. The first-stage larva penetrates the snail's foot and develops to the infective larval stage in 20 to 50 days. Snails are consumed by the definitive host while browsing. Larvae migrate through the mesenteric lymph nodes and are carried by lymph and blood to the lungs. The larvae then enter the alveoli and ascend to the bronchioles, where they mature. The prepatent period is five to six weeks. First-stage larvae survive for months in the environment. Snails remain infected for life and adult worms may live for two years in the definitive host[59].

Pathologic Effects and Clinical Disease. Worms occupy the alveoli and incite a tissue reaction consisting of round cells, giant cells, and connective tissue, resulting in nodule formation in the pulmonary parenchyma. Nodules eventually calcify[71]. Clinical signs are usually absent.

Diagnosis, Treatment, and Prevention. Nodules, which are readily palpable, are pathognomonic for the infection. The larvae may be recovered by Baermann technique. Larvae lack an anterior knob and have a dorsal spine on the kinked tail. Modern anthelmintics, including benzimidazoles, levamisole, or macrolides, eliminate the infection. Infection may be prevented by eliminating the snail intermediate host or by housing research animals indoors or on dry lot.

Public Health Considerations. *Muellerius capillaris* does not infect humans.

Parelaphostrongylus tenuis

Morphology. Adult *Parelaphostrongylus tenuis* are slender, yellowish-brown to black, and measure 6 cm to 9 cm long.

Hosts. The normal host of *P. tenuis* is the white-tailed deer, in which worms are found in the meningeal venous sinus. Other ruminants, including mule deer, wapiti, llamas, sheep, and goats, may be infected. The parasite is widespread in many areas in the eastern half of North America.

Life Cycle. Adult female worms release unembryonated eggs into the venous blood where they are carried to the lungs of the white-tailed deer. The eggs become trapped in the alveolar capillaries. Larvae develop within the egg and hatch into the alveoli, then ascend the bronchiolar escalator and are swallowed and pass into the environment on the surface of the fecal pellet. The larvae exit the fecal pellet and penetrate or are eaten by terrestrial snails or slugs. Development to the infective stage takes four weeks or longer within the gastropod.

Ingestion of the gastropod during browsing is the means of infection by deer or other abnormal hosts. Within the definitive host the larvae penetrate the wall of the abomasum and migrate into the peritoneal cavity, then to the central nervous system following the spinal nerves. Larvae migrate into the lumbar spinal canal in approximately 10 days, enter the spinal cord in the dorsal gray matter, and begin an anterior migration. During the migration they molt twice and leave the spinal cord approximately 40 days post-infection. Larvae continue migration in the subdural space and enter the venous sinuses. The prepatent period is 12 to 20 weeks[69].

Pathologic Effects. White-tailed deer seldom show more than transient signs of infection. In contrast, infections are pathogenic in abnormal hosts such as sheep, goats, and others. Lesions are found in the spinal cord due to larval migration, and include necrosis, perivascular infiltration, and loss of myelin.

Clinical Disease. Goats appear to be more susceptible to disease than sheep, but this may simply reflect differences in dietary preference. Clinical signs vary from mild ataxia or head tilt to paraplegia or tetraplegia. The signs are greater than can be accounted for by just mechanical damage to the spinal cord during migration.

Diagnosis. The history of grazing in an area frequented by white-tailed deer should alert the veterinarian that meningeal worm could be implicated in nervous manifestations of research sheep or goats housed out-of-doors. Post-mortem finding of nematodes in the central nervous system is the confirmatory diagnosis.

Treatment. Anthelmintics probably have little influence on the progress of disease once clinical signs occur. Some affected animals recover completely or partially regardless of treatment. Anti-inflammatory drugs and supportive care may facilitate recovery. Macrocyclic lactones and some benzimidazoles are extremely effective in killing *P. tenuis* but these drugs do not traverse the undamaged blood-brain barrier. Perhaps some apparent response to treatment is due to local leakage of the drug in levels high enough to kill the larvae but below the toxicity tolerance of the host.

Prevention. White-tailed deer should not be housed in areas where the disease has not been reported. Fencing out deer from enclosures for at least a year to allow the death of larvae in the soil or for two or three years for the death of infected snails or slugs may render a property free of infection. Treatment with effective anthelmintics during the migration from intestine into the spinal cord gives a level of protection. Macrolides have residual effects and prophylactic treatment at monthly intervals may prevent disease but will probably ensure the selection of resistant gastrointestinal worms such as *Haemonchus*. Treatment of white-tailed deer with drugs such as ivermectin lowers the number of larvae passed in the feces but does nothing to affect adult worms.

Public Health Considerations. Humans are not susceptible to infection with *Parelaphostrongylus tenuis*.

Protostrongylus spp.

Morphology. Sheep and goats are susceptible to infection with lungworms in the genus *Protostrongylus,* including *Protostrongylus davtiani, P. rufescens, P. skrjabini,* and *P. stilesi.* The adults are reddish and measure 20 mm to 60 mm long. The male reproductive organs are important taxonomic features.

Hosts and Life Cycle. *Protostrongylus* are found in wild and domestic sheep and goats. The life cycle is similar to that of *Muellerius capillaris.*

Pathologic Effects and Clinical Disease. Pathologic changes include occlusion of small bronchioles with debris consisting largely of worms and eggs. The changes are usually seen as an incidental finding at necropsy. Clinical signs are seldom seen with *Protostrongylus* spp. When present, they include respiratory distress, weight loss, and diarrhea[109].

Protostrongylus stilesi is transmitted to bighorn lambs in utero[110], and may result in secondary bacterial infection and fatal pneumonia by six weeks of age[77].

Diagnosis, Treatment, and Prevention. Diagnosis is by finding adult worms in the small bronchi. Larvae recovered by the Baermann technique have a kinked tail and lack a terminal spine and anterior knob. Modern anthelmintics such as benzimidazoles, levamisole, or macrolides should successfully eliminate infection with *Protostrongylus*. Reducing the snail population on pasture lowers the prevalence of lungworm infection in the flock.

Public Health Considerations. *Protostrongylus* does not infect humans.

Superfamily Spiruoidea

Gongylonema spp.

Morphology. Sheep and goats may become infected with *Gongylonema pulchrum, G. monnigi,* and *G. verrucosum,* the "stitch worm." *Gongylonema* spp. are long, slender worms measuring 3 cm to 9 cm in length. The anterior end of the worm bears cuticular plaques (bosses) arranged in longitudinal rows. The spicules are uneven in length with a curved end. The uterus contains embryonated eggs.

Hosts and Life Cycle. The parasites are found in the mucosa of the rumen, esophagus, or tongue of sheep, goats, deer, camels, cattle, swine, equids, bears, and primates. Embryonated eggs are passed in the feces and are consumed by coprophagus beetle larvae or cockroaches. The infective larva becomes encapsulated in beetle muscles and develops to the infective third larval stage in about a month. Ingestion of the beetle frees the third-stage larva, which ascends the esophageal mucosa and matures to the adult stage. The prepatent period is two months.

Pathologic Effects and Clinical Disease. The sinuous migratory pattern of the "stitch worm" is a pathognomonic lesion. Esophagitis may result from mechanical damage caused by migration of the adult female during egg release[111]. Infections are typically asymptomatic.

Diagnosis, Treatment, and Prevention. The sinuous esophageal worm migration tracts are diagnostic. The embryonated eggs are not easily found by standard parasitological techniques. Effective treatment strategies have not been reported. Because adult beetles may fly considerable distances, prevention of infection is difficult.

Public Health Considerations. Human infections by *G. pulchrum* are rare because transmission requires ingestion of infected beetles.

Superfamily Trichuroidea

Capillaria spp.

Adult *Capillaria* spp. are long, thin worms with a sticho-some esophagus. Unlike *Trichuris,* the posterior portion of the worm is not broader than the anterior portion. Adult *Capillaria bovis* measure 11 mm to 25 mm long while *C. brevipes* measures 8 mm to 12 mm long. *Capillaria bovis* has been identified in cattle, sheep, goats, and other ruminants and *C. brevipes* has been identified in cattle and sheep[71]. The life cycle is unknown but is apparently similar to that of *Trichuris.* There are no reports of disease caused by *Capillaria.* Treatment and prevention strategies are similar to *Trichuris. Capillaria* spp. do not infect humans.

Trichuris spp.

Morphology. Sheep and goats are susceptible to infection with *Trichuris discolor, T. ovis,* and *T. skrjabini.* The esophagus is of the stichosome type, and runs three-fourths the length of the worm. The neck resembles a whip, while the posterior region is broad. Adult male worms have a curled tail while that of the female is blunt. Species are differentiated by reproductive morphology. *Trichuris ovis* has a spicule greater than 5 mm in length. In contrast, the spicule of *T. discolor* measures less than 3.1 mm long and the spicule of *T. skrjabini* measures less than 1.6 mm long. The vulva of *T. discolor* is not everted nor are there spines on the vulva, while the vulva of *T. ovis* is everted, measures 50 µ to 100 µ wide, and bears papilla-like spines. Lastly, the everted vulva of *T. skrjabini* is narrower and the spines are acutely pointed[112]. The eggs are barrel-shaped and yellow to brown with a plug in each end.

Hosts. *Trichuris* are found in the cecum and colon of wild and domestic ruminants, including sheep and goats. However, worms are rarely speciated. Thus, information concerning host specificity and distribution of worm species is lacking.

Life Cycle. The life cycle is direct. Eggs are passed in the feces and embryonate in the environment in one to two months. The eggs of *Trichuris* are resistant to the environment and are viable several years after being passed. Eggs hatch, releasing larvae that enter the glands of the cecal mucosa where they remain during development. The adults lie on the mucosal surface with the esophagus embedded in the mucosa. The prepatent period is approximately 12 weeks.

Pathologic Effects and Clinical Disease. Intestinal mucosal damage results from the frequent movement of large numbers of worms. While sheep and goats seldom develop clinical signs, sloughed mucosa containing blood and mucus may occasionally be observed in the feces. Diarrhea, weight loss, and anorexia may also occur following massive exposure in sheep[113].

Diagnosis, Treatment, and Prevention. Diagnosis is by finding the characteristic eggs in the feces. Speciation requires recovery of adult worms. All of the currently used anthelmintics have some effect against the worm. However, the efficacy may not be as good against immature worms so repeated treatment may be necessary. Whipworm eggs persist in the environment. Disinfectants are of little if any value so steam or flame may be necessary to kill eggs. Treatment and quarantine of newly arrived animals may aid in the control of the infection. Research animals should be housed indoors or on dry lot, with frequent removal of feces.

Public Health Considerations. *Trichuris* spp. from ruminants are not infectious to humans.

ARTHROPODS

The biology and general morphology of the arthropods is presented in Chapter 6, Biology of Arthropods. The interested reader is directed to that material for more in-depth coverage.

Class Insecta

Order Diptera (flies)

Family Calliphoridae

Blowflies, fleece flies, and screwworms in the family Calliphoridae, and in the genera *Calliphora, Chrysomya, Cochliomyia, Lucilia,* and *Phormia,* may parasitize sheep and goats. Other animals may also be affected. The New World screwworm, *Cochliomyia hominivorax,* and the Old World screwworm, *Chrysomya bezziana,* deposit eggs on healthy tissue, while other Calliphorid flies deposit eggs on decomposing carcasses, soiled fleece, or devitalized tissues. Screwworm and primary blowfly (*Lucilia, Phormia,* and *Calliphora*) larvae invade soft tissue (myiasis) with the aid of mouth hooks. The larvae produce proteolytic enzymes that liquefy damaged tissues. Secondary blowflies (*Calliphora, Chrysomya,* and *Cochliomyia macellaria*) only attack areas previously damaged, causing lesions to extend into the body[59]. Bacterial septicemia, toxemia, and liquefaction of tissues occur. Young animals may be killed by invasion of the abdominal cavity by screwworm larvae.

The damage caused by screwworms is further complicated by secondary myiasis because the wound attracts other flies. Affected sheep usually withdraw from the flock, stamp their feet, and smack their lips. The animals become anorexic and depressed. A characteristic foul odor emanates from the lesions. Parting the fleece reveals the maggots in and on the tissues. The portion of the body routinely "struck" or "blown" is where moisture from urine, feces, or excessive rainfall has led to fermentation of the wool (woolrot), which attracts flies, though wool rot is not necessary for screwworm strike.

Infested sheep may be treated by removing the wool from the affected area. Applying topical insecticides with residual activity, such as diazinon, cypermethrin, or deltamethrin, kills the maggots and protects against further strikes. Applying products that contain pine tar blocks the odor of wounds, thereby reducing the attraction for flies.

Regular full body shearing or crutching of areas where moisture is likely to be retained, and selecting animals that have fewer skin folds in areas subject to moisture from feces or urine, lowers the incidence of fly strike, except for that of screwworms. Applying residual insecticides or insect growth regulators to sheep may be essential in some areas[59]. Prompt disposal of carcasses reduces the number of adult flies in the environment. Treating or preventing diarrheal diseases creates a less desirable ovipositing medium. Fly maggots may also infest humans; however, contact with infested sheep or goats are not direct sources of infestation to humans.

Family Ceratopogonidae

Biting gnats of the genus *Culicoides* commonly attack sheep, goats, and other warm-blooded animals. Gnats cause annoyance and in some host species are associated with bite hypersensivity. Bluetongue virus may be transmitted to small ruminants through the feeding activity of *Culicoides*. Because the flies usually feed during crepuscular periods, placing animals in a stable during these times inhibits the feeding activity. Screens must have a very fine mesh because the gnats pass through mosquito netting. Pyrethroids have some insecticidal and repellant activities. *Culicoides* readily feed on humans.

Family Culicidae

Sheep and goats are susceptible to blood feeding by mosquitoes in the genera *Aedes, Anopheles, Culex, Mansonia,* and others. Mosquitoes feed on all mammals, reptiles, and birds. Some hosts may be preferred by certain species but most are opportunistic feeders. In sheep and goats they are nuisance feeders and may cause considerable vexation. They are important vectors of a number of disease agents in some hosts. Taxonomic keys are useful for identifying species of adult or immature mosquitoes. Screening mosquitoes out of buildings and regularly cleaning water troughs prevents mosquitoes from completing the life cycle within the building. Mosquitoes are vectors for several very important human diseases but none are transmitted though feeding on sheep or goats.

Family Hippoboscidae

The sheep ked, *Melophagus ovinus,* is a brown, hairy, wingless fly that measures approximately 5 mm in length. It has a short, broad head and body and six legs, discounting the other common name "sheep tick." The sheep ked is an obligate permanent parasite of sheep. The female deposits a single larva, which pupates on the host immediately. The pupa adheres to wool and the adults emerge in approximately three weeks. Both sexes suck blood. The female only produces a single larva every 10 to 12 days, with a total lifetime production of about 15 larvae. Thus, ked populations increase more slowly than those of other flies. The stercorarian *Trypanosoma melophagum* is transmitted when sheep ingest infested keds. Clinical signs of ked infestation include anemia, loss of condition, and irritation, which causes rubbing and wool loss. Populations of *M. ovinus* build up during the winter, and then decline with spring shearing. Treating with insecticides following shearing is effective. Newly arriving sheep should be treated prior to release into the flock. Sheep keds do not feed on humans.

Family Muscidae

Muscoid flies are common pests of sheep, goats, and other animals. Important species include the housefly *Musca domestica,* the face fly *Musca autumnalis,* the head fly *Hydrotaea irritans,* the stable fly *Stomoxys calcitrans,* the horn fly *Haematobia irritans,* and latrine flies in the genus *Fannia*. Houseflies feed on secretions, especially those emanating from wounds. The face fly prefers nasal and ocular secretions of pastured livestock. The head fly feeds on wounds and ocular secretions of sheep, cattle, and horses in Europe. Stable flies preferentially feed on the ears of dogs and the legs of livestock. Cattle are the preferred hosts of horn flies, but they will feed on other livestock, including sheep and goats.

The principal importance of these flies is as sources of annoyance. However, mechanical transmission of bacteria that cause keratoconjunctivitis may also be important in specific situations. *Hydrotaea* has rasps on the mouthparts, which cause skin irritation that may lead to self-mutilation of the heads of sheep. The bites of stable flies are extremely annoying. Thus, feeding requires several minutes to complete, with frequent interruptions to avoid the defensive behaviors of the host. Widespread mechanical transmission of parasites such as *Trypanosoma* is possible.

Environmental sanitation is the preferred method of control to prevent ovipositing. Composting organic waste and using parasitoids[114], entomopathogenic fungi[115], sodium bisulfate[116], and juvenile hormone analogs[17] may lower the reproductive success of *M. domestica*. Sprays on resting surfaces, traps, and sticky tapes lower the number of adult flies[117]. Sheep and goats can be largely protected from horn flies by separating them from cattle or pastures formerly used by cattle. Pesticide resistance is common among horn flies. *Musca domestica* is the primary annoyance fly for humans throughout the world, though humans are attractive hosts for stable flies as well. Horn flies generally are not attracted to humans, but they may bite on occasion. Muscoid flies serve as mechanical vectors of bacteria, viruses, and protozoa that are infectious to humans.

Family Oestridae

Sheep and goats may be infested with *Oestrus ovis*, the sheep bot fly. The larvae are found in the cranial sinuses and nasal passages. Adult flies rest on vertical surfaces near sites of host congregation. Very little damage is associated with migration of low numbers of larvae in the nasal passages. There may be sneezing and excessive nasal discharge. If the "bot" dies in the sinuses, the breakdown of the larva and subsequent bacterial proliferation may lead to meningitis following lysis of the calvarium. Heavily infested animals may be unthrifty and become uncoordinated[59]. The adult fly activity causes the sheep to stamp their feet and mob up into a circle with their heads down and into the center. Sheep become preoccupied with evading infestation when the flies are active.

Several products kill bot larvae, including nitroxynil, rafoxinide, trichlorfon, and dichlorvos. However, dead bots may become trapped in the nasal cavity or sinuses. Ivermectin is extremely effective in controlling this parasite, which has largely disappeared where the treatment has been used as an anthelmintic. There are reports of humans developing ocular infestations and conjunctivitis. Humans working closely with small ruminants are at greater risk for attack.

Family Psychodidae

Vertebrates, including sheep and goats in semiarid areas of the tropics and subtropics, are susceptible to attack by sand flies. In the Old World, sand flies are in the genus *Phlebotomus*. New World sand flies are in the genus *Lutzomyia*. If the numbers are high enough they can annoy small ruminants. Fine mesh screens and residual insecticides on the walls of buildings where the adult fly rests prevent entry of sand flies into animal facilities. Sand flies transmit *Leishmania* spp. to humans.

Family Sarcophagidae

Flies in the family Sarcophagidae, including those in the genera *Sarcophaga* and *Wohlfartia,* are referred to as "flesh flies." Larvae are deposited on damaged tissues or decaying meat. *Wohlfahrtia magnifica* is a particular problem for sheep in central Europe and Asia[69]. Larvae enter tissue through wounds or mucous membranes. Tissue destruction occurs through the feeding activity of the flies. Insecticides applied locally or systemically kill the larvae. Infestations can be prevented by screening and using fly repellants. Humans may be hosts for larval flesh flies. Handling sheep or goats is not a source of the infestation.

Family Simuliidae

Sheep, goats, and other warm-blooded animals are susceptible to attack by members of the genus *Simulium,* also known as buffalo gnats or blackflies. The bites are vicious and may result in petechial hemorrhages at feeding sites, followed by edema of the face and head, leading to respiratory distress. Insecticides applied to breeding streams may interrupt the mass emergence of flies. Repellants may be of some value. Screens may slow them down, but they must be very fine to exclude blackflies. Humans are a desirable host and *Simulium* spp. transmits important agents such as *Onchocerca volvulus,* the cause of "river blindness" in west central Africa.

Family Tabanidae

The family Tabanidae includes horseflies in the genera *Hybomitra* and *Tabanus,* and deerflies in the genera *Chrysops* and *Haematopota.* Warm-blooded animals, including sheep and goats, are suitable hosts. Larger host species are most attractive and more avidly fed upon than smaller hosts such as rodents. Adult female tabanids fly long distances in search of a blood meal. They feed and lay eggs every three or four days. They cause so much pain when feeding that they are frequently interrupted, but feeding continues until the fly is satiated.

This style of feeding is very effective for the mechanical transmission of several protozoan, bacterial, and viral agents. *Trypanosoma evansi* and *T. vivax* are transmitted efficiently by tabanids. The vexation caused by these flies causes animals to abandon grazing or resting areas or hide in brush if available. Because of the variety of places the flies breed and their ability to fly long distances, control of the immature flies is unlikely. Likewise, treating a host with a repellant or insecticide is unlikely to prevent feeding. Even if the fly dies as a result of its feeding behavior, it has still caused vexation and has not prevented mechanical transmission of agents. Flytraps placed on dark colored panels and/or carbon dioxide attractants may be of some value[59]. Humans are often a preferable host for *Chrysops* and in some areas *Tabanus* also feeds on humans. The bites are painful and the filarid nematode *Loa loa* is transmitted to humans by tabanids in West Africa.

Order Phthiraptera

Suborder Anoplura

Linognathus spp. **Morphology.** Sheep and goats may serve as hosts for several species of *Linognathus*, including *L. africanus*, *L. ovillus*, *L. pedalis*, and *L. stenopsis*. *Linognathus* are dark gray sucking lice with a long, narrow head. The forelegs are smaller than the other two pairs, which are similar in length. All legs possess a single claw. The antennae have five segments. Adult lice measure 2 mm to 3 mm long. There is an expanded post-antennal bulge in *L. africanus,* which is diagnostic for the species.

Hosts. *Linognathus africanus,* the blue louse, infests sheep, goats, and deer. The foot louse, *L. pedalis,* infests the hairy areas on the lower legs of sheep. *Linognathus ovillus,* the face louse or sheep sucking louse, is generally found on the hairy portion of the face of sheep but will move to the rest of the body. The goat sucking louse, *L. stenopsis,* is found on goats but has been reported on sheep as well[118].

Life Cycle. The eggs are attached to a single or several hairs and hatch after an incubation period of one to two weeks. Development through the nymphal instars takes approximately three weeks. The female lays, on average, one egg per day.

Pathologic Effects and Clinical Disease. Sucking lice cause anemia and dermatitis. Populations of the body lice, *L. africanus* and *L. stenopsis,* are more likely to reach clinically significant levels. The face louse may invade other portions of the body but is not often found in sufficient numbers to induce dissemination. Death losses due to exsanguination have been reported with *L. africanus*[119]. Clinical signs of heavy infestation include anemia and pruritus, with wool slipping from the skin due to self-mutilation. In general, infestations of small ruminants with chewing lice are more pathogenic than infestations with sucking lice.

Diagnosis, Treatment, and Prevention. Diagnosis is by identifying lice based on morphologic features. Treatment consists of shearing, followed by treatment with insecticides a few weeks later when adequate wool has regrown. Depending on the insecticide used, treatment may have to be repeated twice at biweekly intervals to expose the lice to insecticides when they are not in the egg. Because of the effectiveness of ivermectin against cattle sucking lice, it is presumed that ivermectin is effective in sheep and goats but treatment must be repeated to affect nymphs hatching after treatment.

Public Health Considerations. Lice are highly host specific. With the exception of *L. africanus,* lice of sheep and goats only survive for short periods when cross-infesting the other host. Lice of sheep and goats do not become established on humans.

Suborder Mallophaga

Bovicola spp. **Morphology.** *Bovicola* spp. are small lice with broad heads and a single claw on the end of the legs. They actively move about on the host. The immature lice are similar to the adults except they are smaller. The eggs (nits) are attached to wool or hair.

Hosts. *Bovicola* (Syn. *Damalinia*) *ovis* is the sheep biting louse or body louse. *Bovicola* (Syn. *Damalinia*) *caprae* is the goat biting louse and occurs on all goats. *Bovicola limbatus* (Syn. *D. limbata*), the Angora goat biting louse, and *B.* (Syn. *Damalinia*) *crassipes,* the yellow louse, are found only on Angora goats.

Life Cycle. Operculated eggs are attached to hair or wool near the skin. Eggs hatch in seven to 14 days. Nymphs feed on skin debris and undergo three molts to the adult stage. The female begins depositing eggs about 35 days after infestation, and produces about one egg a day for a life of about 35 days[118].

Pathologic Effects and Clinical Disease. Heavy louse infestation causes rubbing and disrupts feeding activities of the host. There may be matting of mohair because the nits are attached to several hairs. Both sheep and goats are likely to lose weight. Serum seeps from sites of louse feeding and host rubbing. Both the quality and quantity of wool are diminished due to the effects of *B. ovis.* All chewing lice on Angora goats adversely affect mohair quality. A condition known as "cockle," which is a pelt defect, was shown to be associated with the presence of *B. ovis*[120].

Diagnosis, Treatment, and Prevention. Diagnosis is by identifying the louse. Treatment is similar to that described for sucking lice. Wet wool is an impediment to the lice and the number of lice is minimal under constant moist conditions. Wetting the body of sheep infested by *B. ovis* following shearing had a 95% or greater reduction in louse numbers when compared to conventional insecticides or organic compounds[121].

Public Health Considerations. Lice are extremely host specific and will not establish on humans.

Order Siphonaptera

Ctenocephalides felis

Morphology. Adult *Ctenocephalides felis* is dark brown, move laterally compressed, and rapidly through the host pelage. The hind limbs are much longer than the anterior legs, hence the flea's tremendous ability to jump. *Ctenocephalides* have genal and pronotal combs. The larvae are hairy, maggot-like creatures and the cocoon is wooly with detritus adhered to it.

Hosts. Cats and dogs are the favored hosts but other animals, including kids and lambs, are frequently infested when confined where barn cats or dogs frequent.

Life Cycle. The eggs are laid on the host but usually fall off into the environment, where they hatch in days to weeks. The larva feeds on organic material, including adult flea feces. The larva molts twice, spins a cocoon, and pupates. Development is temperature-dependent and may occur in as little as three weeks under favorable conditions. The flea leaves the puparium in response to vibrations and jumps onto a passing host. The larva remains on the host, feeding intermittently. The female produces an average of 27 eggs per day and may produce eggs for 100 days.

Pathologic Effects and Clinical Disease. Young animals raised in stables where cats are present may be exposed to tremendous numbers of fleas, resulting in infestations heavy enough to cause exsanguination[168]. Because the environment off the host is suitable for larval development and young ruminants are not efficient groomers, the number of fleas can become tremendous. Because the young are most heavily infested they develop the most marked clinical signs. It is unknown whether this is due to the development of a hypersensivity reaction which limits flea feeding or because older animals are more likely to escape severe infestation.

Diagnosis, Treatment, and Prevention. Diagnosis is by identifying dark brown, laterally compressed insects that move rapidly through the host pelage. Pesticides effective against fleas in pets should be effective, but the major emphasis should be placed on removing bedding, using growth regulators, and excluding cats and dogs from the premises.

Public Health Considerations. While humans are not a preferred host, newly emerged fleas will avidly feed on them.

Class Arachnida

Ticks

Family Argasidae
Ornithodoros spp. **Morphology.** *Ornithodoros* are large, soft ticks. The species of importance include *O. coriaceus, O. lahorensis, O. moubata, O. savignyi, O. talaje,* and *O. turicata.*

Hosts. *Ornithodoros* ticks are indiscriminate feeders in the geographic area in which each species is found. They readily feed on sheep and goats. *Ornithodoros coriaceus, O. talaje,* and *O. turicata* are found in North America; *O. lahorensis* and *O. savignyi* are found in Eastern Europe and Asia; and *O. moubata* is found in Africa.

Life Cycle. *Ornithodoros* spp. feed for short time periods, typically at night, and then leave the host and hide in resting areas such as buildings, under trees, etc. All stages feed for 15 to 30 minutes at a time[17,122]. The females deposit eggs after each feeding and may continue feeding and egg deposition for up to two years.

Pathologic Effects and Clinical Disease. *Ornithodoros* are known to transmit *Coxiella burnetti,* the agent of Q fever. *Ornithodoros lahorensis* has been implicated in the transmission of *Theileria ovis* and *Anaplasma ovis* to goats. The genus has also been implicated in tick paralysis and tick worry in sheep[69]. Because the ticks are night feeders and not readily detected, they frequently go undetected as causes of anemia and loss of condition.

Diagnosis, Treatment, and Prevention. Diagnosis is by finding ticks near resting places such as in animal burrows, under rocks or vegetation, or on the walls of buildings that house sheep and goats. Macrolides readily kill *Ornithodoros* ticks. Pyrethroids or amitraz may have some value in preventing the ticks from feeding. Identifying the areas where the ticks rest between meals may allow for area treatment of the environment[123].

Public Health Considerations. *Ornithodoros* ticks are the primary agents for the transmission of relapsing fevers to humans. Handling sheep or goats does not place animal workers directly at risk for disease, but ticks may serve as vectors to infect personnel.

Otobius megnini. **Morphology.** *Otobius megnini,* the spinose ear tick, has a white, teardrop-shaped larval stage measuring 2 mm to 3 mm long, and possesses six tiny legs. The nymphal stages are gray, up to 10 mm in length, with a very spiny cuticle, and the eight legs are easily seen. Only larvae and nymphs are parasitic because the adults live off the host in a protected area where they produce eggs.

Hosts. Mammals, including sheep and goats, are suitable hosts. Some avian species may also become infested. The ticks live deep in the ear canal of animals in North and South America, India, and southern Africa. Sheep are commonly infested in some geographic areas.

Life Cycle. Adult ticks are free living in protected places such as barns and corrals or under stones where livestock rest. The female produces 500 to 600 eggs over a period of up to six months and then dies. The eggs hatch in three to eight weeks and the larvae are infective but may remain unfed for several months. They enter the ear canal and feed on lymph for five to 10 days before molting to the nymphal stage, which feeds intermittently on blood for one to seven months. The nymph drops off the host and seeks shelter for molting and reproduction[69].

Pathologic Effects and Clinical Disease. Development of clinical acariasis depends on parasite numbers. Although they suck blood and cause irritation, secondary bacterial infection is perhaps the most important feature of infestation. Head shaking, ear rubbing, and other signs of otitis externa are seen in heavily infested animals.

Diagnosis, Treatment, and Prevention. Diagnosis is by finding larvae or nymphs in the ear canal. Diagnosis may be aided by the use of an otoscope. Mechanical removal of the ticks and treatment of secondary bacterial infection are effective. Ear tags impregnated with acaricides should help prevent infestation. Instillation of pesticidal eardrops facilitates both treatment and prevention.

Public Health Considerations. *Otobius megnini* will infest human ears. Thus, animal workers should exercise caution when working around potentially infested sheep and goats.

Family Ixodidae
Amblyomma spp. **Morphology, Hosts, and Life Cycle.** *Amblyomma* are ornate ticks with long mouthparts, eyes, and festoons. Species of *Amblyomma* known to infest sheep and goats include *A. americanum, A. cajennense, A. hebraeum, A. maculatum, A. pomposum,* and *A. variegatum.* The species are generally geographically limited, with *A. americanum* restricted to North America, *A. maculatum* and *A. cajennense* in South and North America, and *A. hebraeum* and *A. pomposum* in Africa. *Amblyomma variegatum* was once only found in tropical Africa but has now established in the Caribbean[124].

Pathologic Effects and Clinical Disease. Several *Amblyomma* spp. are the vectors of *Ehrlichia (Cowdria) ruminantium,* the agent of heartwater, which has the capacity to kill most animals fully susceptible to the infection[125]. In addition, *Rickettsia rickettsii* (Rocky Mountain spotted fever), *Borrelia lonestari* (Master's disease), *Dermatophilus congolensis* (lumpy wool disease) and *Franciscella tularensis* (tularemia) are transmitted by *Amblyomma* spp. The bites are vicious and secondary infections and self-trauma may occur. Tick worry caused by these vicious biters may cause sheep and goats to lose weight. Breaking of the ear cartilage may be associated with *A. maculatum.* Dermatophilosis in sheep and goats is often associated with the feeding activities of *Amblyomma* spp. Tick paralysis has been described with *Amblyomma.*

Diagnosis, Treatment, and Prevention. Diagnosis is by identifying the characteristic ticks on the host. Tick sprays and dips may help control infestations on animals. Using ear tags impregnated with an acaracide may control *Amblyomma maculatum,* an ear tick. However, the seasonality of the particular species and the effectiveness of various acaricides may vary considerably. No one program is universally effective. Sheep and goats entering a laboratory animal facility from a tick endemic area should be dipped.

Public Health Considerations. Several agents are transmitted to humans by *Amblyomma* ticks. However, handling sheep and goats should not transmit these agents. Plucking an engorged tick off the body of any host with bare hands may result in contamination of small lesions on the hands with coxal fluids, which may be rich in some infectious agents.

Dermacentor spp. **Morphology, Hosts, and Life Cycle.** Most *Dermacentor* are ornate and have short mouthparts, eyes, and festoons. Ticks in the genus *Dermacentor* are indiscriminate feeders, and readily infest sheep and goats. The larvae tend to feed on smaller hosts while adult ticks prefer larger mammals. *Dermacentor andersoni, D. albipictus, D. occidentalis,* and *D. variablis* are North American species. *Dermacentor reticulatus* and *D. marginatus* are northern European and Asian species. All are three-host ticks except *D. albipictus,* the "winter tick," which is a one-host tick that tends to feed on larger mammals. The life cycle of *Dermacentor* is described in Chapter 6, Biology of Arthropods.

Pathologic Effects and Clinical Disease. Infestation by *Dermacentor* may result in tick paralysis.

Diagnosis, Treatment, and Prevention. Identification of adult ticks is done by the use of keys specific for a geographic region. Tick sprays and dips may help control infestations on animals. However, the seasonality of the particular species and the effectiveness of various acaricides may vary considerably. No one program is universally effective. Sheep and goats entering a laboratory animal facility from a tick endemic area should be dipped.

Public Health Considerations. Several agents are transmitted to humans by *Dermacentor* ticks. However, handling sheep and goats should not transmit these agents. Plucking an engorged tick off the body of any host with bare hands may result in contamination of small lesions on the hands with coxal fluids, which may have agents such as *Rickettsia rickettsii,* the agent of Rocky Mountain Spotted Fever.

Haemaphysalis spp. *Haemaphysalis* spp. are inornate ticks with short mouthparts and festoons, but lack eyes. There are lateral projections on the second segment of the palps. While most *Haemaphysalis* are host specific, some are indiscriminate feeders. *Haemaphysalis punctata* is a parasite of livestock in Europe, Asia, and northern Africa. *Haemaphysalis longicornis* is primarily a cattle tick in eastern Asia and Australia, as is *H. bispinosa* in New Zealand. The life cycle is presented in Chapter 6, Biology of Arthropods. *Haemaphysalis* may cause tick worry when large numbers are present. *Babesia motasi* and *Theileria ovis* are transmitted to sheep by *H. punctata.* Diagnosis, treatment, prevention, and public health considerations are as described for *Dermacentor.*

Hyalomma spp. *Hyalomma* are usually inornate ticks with banded legs, long mouthparts, and eyes. Some species have festoons. The males have adanal shields. Larvae and nymphs usually feed on small mammals and birds and adults feed on larger grazing animals. Sheep and goats are suitable hosts in Asia, southern Europe, and Africa. The life cycle is presented in Chapter 6, Biology of Arthropods. Infestation with *Hyalomma* results in tick toxicosis characterized by mucous membrane hyperemia and moist eczema. Diagnosis, treatment, prevention, and public health considerations are as described for *Dermacentor.*

Ixodes spp. Ticks of the genus *Ixodes* are ornate and possess long mouthparts. A taxonomic key to the genus is a groove that curves in front of the anus. Many *Ixodes* are host specific; others readily feed on sheep and/or goats. *Ixodes ricinus* is commonly found on sheep in northern Europe. A similar species, *I. persulcatus,* occurs in eastern Europe and northern Asia. The North American species include *I. scapularis* and *I. pacificus. Ixodes rubicundus* is found in southern Africa and *I. holocyclus* is found in Australia. The life cycle is presented in Chapter 6, Biology of Arthropods. Heavy infestation with *Ixodes* causes tick worry and anemia. Some species, including *I. holocyclus* and *I. rubicundus,* also cause tick paralysis. *Ixodes* sp. transmits louping ill virus, *Ehrlichia phagocytophillia* is the agent of tick borne fever, and *Staphylococcus aureus* causes tick pyemia in sheep. Diagnosis, treatment, prevention, and public health considerations are as described for *Dermacentor.*

Rhipicephalus spp. *Rhipicephalus* are inornate ticks with short mouthparts, eyes, and festoons. The basis capitulum is hexagonal and coxa I has two long, equal spurs. The male has adanal shields. *Rhipicephalus* are found primarily on grazing animals in sub-Saharan Africa. *Rhipicephalus bursa* is found in southern Europe and Africa. In Africa, *R. sanguineus* feeds on a wide range of hosts but elsewhere it is almost exclusively a dog tick and is perhaps the most widespread tick species. The life cycle is presented in Chapter 6, Biology of Arthropods. *Rhipicephalus* are the vectors of several pathogens, including the viruses causing Nairobi sheep disease and louping ill, as well as *Babesia ovis, Borrelia theileri, Coxiella burnetti, Rickettsia conorii, Theileria ovis,* and others[126]. *Rhipicephalus* often attaches on the ears and under the tail of the host. It may cause tick worry, damage to the pinnae, and tick toxicosis when present in large numbers. The primary importance is its ability to transmit a number of important disease-causing agents. Diagnosis, treatment, prevention, and public health considerations are as described for *Dermacentor.*

Mites

Suborder Astigmata
Chorioptes spp. **Morphology, Hosts, and Life Cycle.** *Chorioptes* are oval mites measuring 250 μ to 600 μ long, with all legs extending beyond the body wall. They have rounded mouthparts with a short pellicle and cup-shaped suckers on the tarsus of the forelegs (Figure. 20.3).

Hosts and Life Cycle. The mites are found on cattle, horses, sheep, and goats. The mites are on the legs but may also infest the scrotum and body of individual animals. Strains of the mite appear to be specific to the host[127]. *Chorioptes* lives and feeds on the skin surface. The development from egg through adult takes approximately 10 days.

Pathologic Effects and Clinical Disease. Scrotal mange can reduce ram fertility[127]. Affected goats develop lameness due to foot mange, and severe scrotal lesions. Clinical signs are seldom seen, even though prevalence may be high.

Diagnosis, Treatment, and Prevention. Diagnosis is by finding the characteristic mite associated with skin

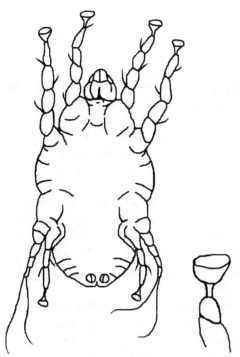

Fig. 20.3 Adult *Chorioptes* spp. (Inset) Tarsus with short pellicle and large, cup-shaped sucker. Courtesy of Catherine G. Wade.

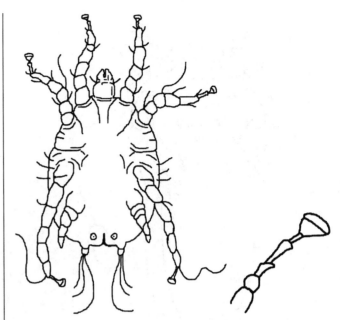

Fig. 20.4 Adult *Psoroptes* spp. (Inset) Tarsus with jointed stalk and small sucker. Courtesy of Catherine G. Wade.

lesions. However, skin scraping is often unrewarding[127]. Doramectin administered at 300 μg/kg is effective against scrotal chorioptic mange[128]. Single-dip treatment with fenvalerate eliminates the infestation[129]. Prophylactic treatment for *Chorioptes* prevents the appearance of chorioptic mange.

Public Health Considerations. *Chorioptes* does not infest humans.

Psoroptes spp. **Morphology, Hosts, and Life Cycle.** *Psoroptes* are oval mites measuring 750 mm long, with all legs extending beyond the body wall. They have pointed mouthparts and jointed bell stalks with suckers on the tarsus of most legs (Figure 20.4). Strains of *Psoroptes* are moderately host-specific. *Psoroptes ovis* occurs on sheep and cattle, while *P. cuniculi* occurs in the ears of rabbits, horses, and goats. The reader is directed to Chapter 15, Parasites of Rabbits, for additional information.

Pathologic Effects and Clinical Disease. *Psoroptes ovis* causes sheep scab. Vesicles form at the sites of mite feeding; these rupture and release serous exudate, then form scabs. Mites may be found at the margins of the inflamed lesions. Affected sheep are intensely pruritic and expend considerable time and energy attempting to relieve pruritus, even at the expense of feeding. Thus, affected animals lose condition. Wool loss may result in hypothermia

in cold environmental conditions. In time, individuals may recover and either completely eliminate the infestation or retain a few mites at sites on the head[130]. Goats infested with *P. cuniculi* shake their heads and scratch their ears. A few individuals may have ear scabs[131].

Diagnosis, Treatment, and Prevention. A tentative diagnosis is based on the onset of clinical signs during colder seasons, and a history of recent introductions of animals into the flock prior to the onset of signs. A superficial scraping at the edge of the lesion reveals the mites. The scabby material may be cleared with 10% potassium hydroxide. Dipping twice with organophosphates or pyrethroids may eliminate the infestation[132]. However, two treatments with injectable ivermectin administered 10 days apart or a single injection of moxidectin[133] or doramectin[134] are also effective. The prophylactic use of moxidectin or plunge dipping in the autumn appears to be effective in controlling sheep scab under field conditions in endemic areas. Treating incoming animals that may be infested before they are introduced to the flock is essential.

Public Health Considerations. *Psoroptes* mites do not survive on humans.

Sarcoptes scabiei. The reader is referred to Chapter 15, Parasites of Rabbits, for information on the biology of *S. scabiei.* Briefly, *S. scabiei* is round and measures 300 μ to 400 μ long. The two front pairs of legs project beyond the body. There are triangular scales on the dorsum and long,

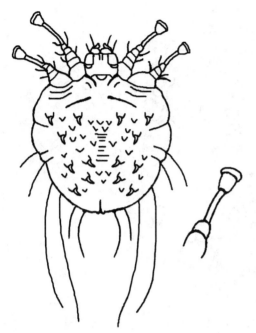

Fig. 20.5 Adult *Sarcoptes scabiei*. (Inset) Tarsus with unjointed stalk and small sucker. Courtesy of Catherine G. Wade.

unjointed bell stalks on the forelimbs (Figure 20.5). *Sarcoptes scabiei* infests most mammalian species, including sheep and goats. Strains are host specific. Sarcoptic mange is intensely pruritic. Infested sheep and goats expend considerable time and energy attempting to relieve pruritus, even at the expense of feeding. Thus, affected animals lose condition. The infestation is found in the wool-free areas of affected sheep. Affected goats develop a thickening of the skin, especially on the face and ears, and the condition causes considerable self-mutilation. Ivermectin and related compounds effectively treat sarcoptic mange when administered twice, one week apart[135]. *Sarcoptes scabei* infests humans, though the strains found on sheep or goats do not persist on people.

Suborder Mesostigmata

Raillietia spp. *Raillietia* are mites measuring 1 mm long. The mouthparts are prominent and the legs are long. *Raillietia* are found deep in the ear canals of goats. *Raillietia caprae* is found in North and South America and *R. manfredi* is found in Australia. *Raillietia auris* normally infests cattle but has been reported in sheep[136]. The female is ovoviviparous. The larvae are active but the nymphal stages are nonfeeding and quickly mature to the adult stage. The mechanisms of transmission remain unknown. *Raillietia* mites are considered commensual on goats and sheep. However, sheep infested with *R. auris* may develop otitis media[122,137]. Diagnosis is by finding mites in the ear canal. Instilling acaricides into the ear canal removes mites. *Raillietia* are not known to infest humans.

Suborder Prostigmata

Demodex spp. **Morphology, Hosts, and Life Cycle.** Information on *Demodex* mites is presented in Chapter 6, Biology of Arthropods, and Chapter 17, Parasites of Dogs. *Demodex* are very host specific. *Demodex ovis* is found in the hair follicles of the face of sheep and *D. caprae* is found in skin nodules on the face and neck, and occasionally elsewhere on the body of goats.

Pathologic Effects and Clinical Disease. Infestations of sheep with *Demodex* are typically asymptomatic. Infested goats develop nodules up to 2 cm in diameter that are filled with mites and debris. Nodule formation does not seem to cause any distress to goats but may result in downgrading of hides.

Diagnosis, Treatment, and Prevention. Diagnosis is by expressing the nodules and recovering mites. *Demodex* mites are considered commensals. Treatment is rarely warranted or effective. *Demodex*-free goats may be produced by cesarean rederivation or removal from the dam at birth.

Public Health Considerations. Humans are not susceptible to infestation with *Demodex* from sheep and goats.

Grain itch mites and Forage mites. Morphology. Grain itch mites (*Pyemotes tritici*) and forage mites (*Acarus farinae* and *Caloglyphus herlesei*) belong to the family Pyemotidae. Grain itch and forage mites are small mites with elongate bodies, reduced mouthparts, and stylet-like chelecerae. Gravid females contain hundreds of eggs that contain developing mites.

Hosts and Life Cycle. Grain itch and forage mites prey on insect larvae. They only contact mammalian hosts when there are large numbers in stored feed and they have no natural hosts to attack. Development from larva to adult occurs in the eggs, which hatch while still within the uterus of the female. Male mites emerge first and mate with the females as they emerge from the genital orifice of the dam. The fertilized females then seek a larval insect on which they feed.

Pathologic Effects and Clinical Disease. The bites produce wheals and papules, which cause intense pruritus, often after the mites have left the host. Lesions are more common on the face and limbs of sheep and goats[138].

Diagnosis, Treatment, and Prevention. Diagnosis is by collection of mites from feed or bedding, using a Berlese funnel. Specimens should be sent to specialists for specific diagnosis. However, pustules or wheals on the face and legs of sheep and goats in confinement are strongly suggestive of infestation by grain itch or forage mites. Removal of infested feed or bedding eliminates the infestation. There is no specific treatment for the bite lesions

Public Health Considerations. Humans may be attacked by forage mites and will exhibit the same signs as livestock. The infestation is acquired by handling the forage.

Psorergates ovis. *Psorergates ovis* is an extremely small, nearly spherical mite, measuring only 170 μ to 190 μ long by 120 μ to 160 μ wide. The legs are separated equally along each side and have two pairs of claws on the tarsus of each leg. Sheep, especially fine wool breeds, are the hosts of *P. ovis.* It has been found in Australia, New Zealand, North and South America, and southern Africa. The mite was eradicated from the United States.

The entire life cycle occurs on the host, with very slow movement of mites over the body. Transmission occurs by direct contact, and only during the period shortly following shearing. From egg, larva, and three nymphal stages to adult, the life cycle is approximately six weeks. Skin irritation and thickening along with fleece derangement due to rubbing are seen with infestations of *P. ovis.* The "itch mite" causes considerable self-mutilation. The fleece may become matted and scurfy[59,139]. Diagnosis is by deep skin scraping along the shorn lateral top line or the bare areas medial to the legs. Other ectoparasites such as lice and other mites, and diseases such as scrapie, must be considered in a differential diagnosis. Amitraz is of some value in the treatment of itch mite[59]. Excluding infested sheep from the flock may prevent infestation of research sheep. Suspect sheep should be scraped carefully to recover mites. The sheep itch mite is not transmissible to humans.

Trombiculids. Trombiculids (chiggers, red bugs, harvest mites) are discussed in Chapter 15, Parasites of Rabbits. Sheep and/or goats are susceptible to attack by *Trombicula* (Syn. *Eutrombicula*) spp., *Leptotrombidium* spp., and *Neotrombicula* (Syn. *Neoschoengastia*) spp. Affected animals become intensely pruritic as a result of the feeding behavior of the mites. A stylostome forms at the feeding site; this is a proliferation of epidermal and inflammatory cells forming a raised wheal with a depressed center. The wheal tends to itch for a week or more following formation. Chigger attacks occur on pastureland or forested areas and are not expected in confinement systems. One species, *Trombicula sarcina,* causes a condition known as "blacksoil" or "leg itch" in sheep in Queensland, Australia. The legs of infested sheep swell and become scabby[69]. Sheep and goats used in research should be housed away from infested grounds. While insecticides may kill the mites, once feeding begins, the reaction to the salivary secretions is inevitable. Therefore, products with residual activity, such as pyrethroids or amitraz, may provide some protection. Chiggers readily feed on humans but tend not to move from host to host.

TABLE 20.1 Parasites of sheep and goats—circulatory and lymphatic systems.

Parasite	Geographic distribution	Hosts	Location in host	Method of infection	Pathologic effects	Zoonosis	Reference
Flagellates							
Trypanosoma evansi	Africa, Asia, South America	Sheep, goats, other mammals	Blood	Mechanical transmission by blood-sucking flies	Lymphadenopathy, splenomegaly, local swelling, edema	Not reported	6, 10
Trypanosoma brucei, T congolense	Central Africa	Sheep, goats, other mammals	Blood	Salivarian transmission by tsetse fly (*Glossina*)	Lymphadenopathy, splenomegaly, myocarditis, myositis, local swelling	*T. brucei* only	2, 10, 69
Trypanosoma melophagium	Americas	Sheep	Blood	Stercorarian transmission by sheep ked (*Melophagus ovinus*)	None	Not reported	10, 170
Trypanosoma theodori	Israel	Goats	Blood	Stercorarian transmission by goat ked (*Lipoptena caprina*)	None	Not reported	10
Trypanosoma vivax	Central Africa, Central and South America	Sheep, goats, other mammals	Blood	Salivarian transmission by tsetse fly (*Glossina*); mechanical transmission by Tabanids	Lymphadenopathy, splenomegaly, myocarditis, myositis, local swelling	Not reported	2, 10, 69
Piroplasmids							
Babesia capreoli, B. motasi, B. ovis	Africa, Asia, Europe	Sheep, goats, deer	Blood	Transmitted by arthropod intermediate host (tick)	Anemia, hemoglobinuria	Not reported	55, 56, 57, 173
Haematoxenus separatus	Africa	Sheep	Blood	Transmitted by arthropod intermediate host (tick)	None	Not reported	190
Theileria hirca	Eastern Europe, Middle East, North Africa	Sheep, goats	Blood, lymph nodes	Transmitted by arthropod intermediate host (tick)	Lymphadenopathy, lymphocytolysis, mucosal hemorrhages, anemia, pulmonary edema	Not reported	173
Theileria ovis	Africa, Asia, Europe	Sheep	Blood, lymph nodes	Transmitted by arthropod intermediate host (tick)	None	Not reported	173
Trematodes							
Schistosoma spp.	Africa, Asia	Sheep, goats, other ruminants, primates	Mesenteric veins, other veins, lung, liver	Skin penetration by cercariae	Enteritis, hepatic fibrosis, vasculitis	Reported	143
Ornithobilharzia turkestanicum	Eurasia	Sheep, goats, other livestock, cats	Mesenteric veins	Ingestion of intermediate host (snail)	Hepatic cirrhosis, intestinal nodules	Not reported	191

Nematodes

Filaroidea

Elaeophora schneideri	Europe, North America	Cervids, sheep	Carotid artery, internal maxillary artery	Transmitted by arthropod intermediate host (tabanid flies)	Dermatitis, ischemic encephalitis	Not reported	165, 166
Onchocerca armillata	Africa, Asia	Sheep, goats, cattle, equids	Aorta	Unknown	Aortic nodules, aneurysms	Not reported	194

Pentastomids

Linguatula serrata	Worldwide	Sheep, goats, rodents, lagomorphs	Mesenteric lymph nodes	Ingestion of eggs in nasal discharge from definitive host (carnivore)	None	Reported	169

TABLE 20.2 Parasites of sheep and goat—enterohepatic system.

Parasite	Geographic distribution	Hosts	Location in host	Method of infection	Pathologic effects	Zoonosis	Reference
Flagellates							
Callimastix frontalis	Unknown	Sheep, goats, cattle	Rumen	Unknown	None	Not reported	10, 202
Chilomastix caprae	Worldwide	Goats	Rumen	Ingestion of cysts passed in feces	None	None	10
Giardia duodenalis	Worldwide	Mammals	Anterior small intestine	Ingestion of cysts in feces	Malabsorption	Possible	13
Moncercomonoides caprae	Unknown	Goats	Rumen	Ingestion of organism passed in feces	None	Not reported	10
Retortamonas ovis	North America	Sheep, cattle	Cecum	Ingestion of cysts in feces	None	Not reported	10, 69
Tetratrichomonas ovis	Worldwide	Sheep	Rumen	Ingestion of trophozoite in feces	None	Not reported	10
Amoebae							
Entamoeba ovis	Worldwide	Sheep	Intestine	Ingestion of cysts in feces	None	Not reported	10
Coccidia							
Cryptosporidium parvum	Worldwide	Sheep, goats, other mammals	Small intestine	Ingestion of sporulated oocyst	Enteritis	Reported	21, 22
Eimeria caprovina	North America	Goats, sheep	Intestine	Ingestion of sporulated oocyst	None	Not reported	28
Eimeria spp.	Worldwide	Goats	Intestine	Ingestion of sporulated oocyst	Enteritis	Not reported	33
Eimeria spp.	Worldwide	Sheep	Intestine	Ingestion of sporulated oocyst	Enteritis	Not reported	29
Ciliates							
Dasytricha ruminantium	Worldwide	Sheep, goats, cattle	Rumen, reticulum	Ingestion	None	Not reported	10
Isotricha spp.	Worldwide	Sheep, goats, cattle	Rumen, reticulum	Ingestion	None	Not reported	10
Ophryoscolex spp.	Worldwide	Sheep, goats, cattle	Rumen, reticulum	Ingestion	None	Not reported	10
Trematodes							
Calicophoron spp.	Australasia, Africa	Sheep, cattle	Rumen, reticulum	Ingestion of metacercariae on vegetation	Immature stages: enteritis, Adult stage: none22	Not reported	69, 175
Ceylonocotyle spp.	Africa, Australasia	Sheep, cattle, antelopes	Rumen, reticulum	Ingestion of metacercariae on vegetation	Immature stages: enteritis, Adult stage: none	Not reported	69, 176
Cotylophoron cotylophorum	Worldwide	Sheep, goats, cattle, other ruminants	Rumen, reticulum	Ingestion of metacercariae on vegetation	Immature stages: enteritis, Adult stage: none	Not reported	69, 177

Species	Geographic distribution	Host	Location	Transmission	Pathology	Prevalence	Ref.
Dicrocoelium dendriticum, D. hospes	Worldwide	Sheep, goats, cattle, deer, lagomorphs, other mammals	Bile ducts	Ingestion of second intermediate host (ant)	Cholangitis, hepatic cirrhosis, fibrosis	Reported	174
Eurytrema pancreaticum	Asia, eastern Europe, South America	Sheep, goats, other ruminants	Pancreatic ducts, bile ducts, duodenum	Ingestion of second intermediate host (grasshopper, cricket)	Ductal inflammation, fibrosis	Reported	192
Explanatum (Gigantocotyle) explanatum	Asia	Water buffalo, cattle, sheep, goats	Bile ducts, gallbladder	Presumed ingestion of metacercariae	Cholangitis	Not reported	140
Fasciola gigantica	Worldwide	Sheep, goats, other ruminants	Bile ducts	Ingestion of metacercariae on vegetation and in water	Cholangitis	Reported	69
Fasciola hepatica	Worldwide	Sheep, goats, other ruminants	Bile ducts	Ingestion of metacercariae on vegetation	Cholangitis	Reported	69
Fascioloides magna	Europe, North America	Deer, other cervids, sheep, goats, cattle, horses	Liver	Ingestion of metacercariae on vegetation	Severe hepatic damage, fibrosis, hemorrhage, peritonitis	Not reported	69, 141
Ogmocotyle indica	India	Cattle, sheep, goats	Rumen, reticulum, abomasum, duodenum	Unknown	None	Not reported	142
Ornithocoelium spp.	Asia	Sheep, cattle	Rumen, reticulum	Ingestion of metacercariae on vegetation	None	Not reported	179
Parafasciolopsis fasciolaemorpha	Europe	Wild goats, elk, deer	Gallbladder	Ingestion of intermediate host (snail)	Unknown	Not reported	69
Paramphistomum cervi	Worldwide	Sheep, goats, other ruminants	Rumen, reticulum	Ingestion of metacercariae on vegetation	Immature stages: enteritis; Adult stage: none	Not reported	178
Paramphistomum ichikawai	Australasia	Sheep, goats, other ruminants	Rumen, reticulum	Ingestion of metacercariae on vegetation	Immature stages: enteritis; Adult stage: none	Not reported	64
Platynosomum ariestes	Brazil	Sheep	Intestine	Unknown	None	Not reported	69
Cestodes							
Larval							
Echinococcus granulosus	Worldwide	Sheep, swine, primates, other mammals	Lung, liver	Ingestion of egg in feces of definitive host (dog)	Hydatid cyst	Common	69
Taenia hydatigena	Worldwide	Sheep, cattle, swine	Liver, peritoneal cavity	Ingestion of egg in canine feces	Hepatitis cysticercosa	Not reported	146

(Continued)

TABLE 20.2 (Continued)

Parasite	Geographic distribution	Hosts	Location in host	Method of infection	Pathologic effects	Zoonosis	Reference
Adult							
Avitellina centripunctata	Africa, Asia, Europe	Sheep	Small intestine	Ingestion of intermediate host (psocid)	None	Not reported	69
Moniezia benedini	Worldwide	Cattle, other ruminants	Small intestine	Ingestion of intermediate host (oribatid mite)	None	Not reported	69
Moniezia expansa	Worldwide	Sheep, goats, deer, antelopes	Small intestine	Ingestion of intermediate host (oribatid mite)	None	Reported	69
Stilesia globipunctata	Africa, Asia, Europe	Sheep, goats, cattle, other ruminants	Small intestine	Ingestion of intermediate host (oribatid mite)	Enteritis, nodule formation	Not reported	144
Stilesia hepatica	Africa, Asia	Sheep, goats, cattle, wild ruminants	Bile ducts	Ingestion of intermediate host (oribatid mite)	Cholangitis	Not reported	145
Thysaniezia (Helictometra) giardi	Africa, Asia, Europe, South America	Sheep, goats, cattle	Small intestine	Ingestion of intermediate host (oribatid mite)	None	Not reported	69
Thysanosoma actinioides	Americas	Sheep, other ruminants	Bile ducts, pancreatic duct, small intestine	Ingestion of intermediate host (oribatid mite)	None	Not reported	69
Nematodes							
Rhabditoidea							
Strongyloides papillosus	Worldwide	Sheep, goats, other ruminants	Small intestine	Skin penetration or transmammary passage by infective larva	Dermatitis, enteritis	Not reported	75
Ascaridoidea							
Ascaris suum	Worldwide	Swine, sheep, cattle, squirrels, dogs	Small intestine	Ingestion of embryonated eggs	Liver spots, pneumonia	Reported	69
Oxyuroidea							
Skrjabinema ovis	Worldwide	Sheep, goats	Colon	Ingestion of embryonated eggs	None	Not reported	180
Skrjabinema caprae	North America	Goats	Colon	Ingestion of embryonated eggs	None	Not reported	193
Strongyloidea							
Bunostomum trigonocephalum	Worldwide	Sheep, goats	Small intestine	Skin penetration or ingestion of infective larva	Local dermatitis, anemia, enteritis	Not reported	69
Chabertia ovina	Worldwide	Sheep, goats, other ruminants	Colon	Ingestion of infective larva	Hemorrhagic enteritis, anemia	Not reported	181

Parasite	Geographic distribution	Hosts	Location	Transmission	Pathology		Reference
Gaigeria pachyscelis	Africa, Asia, South America	Sheep, goats, antelopes	Small intestine	Skin penetration by infective larva	Anemia, hypoproteinemia, emaciation	Not reported	69
Oesophagostomum asperum	Asia, Central America	Goats	Large intestine	Ingestion of infective larva	Unknown	Not reported	69
Oesophagostomum columbianum	Worldwide	Sheep, goats, camelids	Colon	Ingestion of infective larva	Ulcerative nodules, anemia	Not reported	78, 79
Oesophagostomum multifoliatum	Africa	Sheep, goats	Large intestine	Ingestion of infective larva	Unknown	Not reported	148
Oesophagostomum venulosum	Worldwide	Sheep, goats, deer, camelids	Colon	Ingestion of infective larva	None	Not reported	69
Trichostrongyloidea							
Camelostrongylus mentulatus	Worldwide	Sheep, goats, camels, antelopes	Abomasum	Ingestion of infective larva	None	Not reported	155
Cooperia curticei	Australia, Britain, North America	Sheep, goats, cattle, camelids	Small intestine	Ingestion of infective larva	Enteritis	Not reported	161
Cooperia spp.	Worldwide	Cattle, sheep	Small intestine	Ingestion of infective larva	None	Not reported	69
Haemonchus contortus	Worldwide	Sheep, goats, other ruminants	Abomasum	Ingestion of infective larva	Blood loss, anemia	Reported	81
Haemonchus spp.	Worldwide	Cattle, camelids, sheep, goats	Abomasum	Ingestion of infective larva	None	Not reported	69
Marshallagia marshalli	Eurasia, North America	Sheep, goats, wild ruminants	Abomasum, duodenum	Ingestion of infective larva	None	Reported	156
Mecistocirrus digitatus	Asia, Central and South America	Cattle, water buffalo, sheep, goats	Abomasum	Ingestion of infective larva	Abomasitis, anemia	Not reported	159, 160
Nematodirella longispiculata	Eurasia, northern Europe	Wild ruminants, sheep, goats	Small intestine	Ingestion of infective larva	None	Not reported	66
Nematodirus abnormalis	Asia, Eurasia, North America	Sheep, goats, camelids, wild ruminants	Small intestine	Ingestion of infective larva	Enteritis	Not reported	66, 162
Nematodirus battus	North America, northern Europe	Sheep	Small intestine	Ingestion of infective larva	None	Not reported	66, 183
Nematodirus filicollis	Worldwide	Sheep, goats, cattle, cervids	Small intestine	Ingestion of infective larva	None	Not reported	66, 162
Nematodirus helvetianus	Europe, North America	Cattle, sheep	Small intestine	Ingestion of infective larva	None	Not reported	66, 162
Nematodirus spathiger	Worldwide	Sheep, cattle, other ruminants	Small intestine	Ingestion of infective larva	Enteritis	Not reported	66, 162
Ostertagia spp.	Africa, Asia, Europe	Sheep, goats	Abomasum	Ingestion of infective larva	None	Not reported	69, 154
Pseudostertagia bullosa	North America	Sheep, antelopes	Abomasum	Ingestion of infective larva	None	Not reported	157
Skrjabinagia spp.	Europe, Middle East, North Africa	Sheep	Small intestine, abomasum	Ingestion of infective larva	None	Not reported	69

(Continued)

TABLE 20.2 (Continued)

Parasite	Geographic distribution	Hosts	Location in host	Method of infection	Pathologic effects	Zoonosis	Reference
Spiculopteragia spiculoptera	Eurasia	Sheep, cervids	Abomasum	Ingestion of infective larva	None	Not reported	158
Teladorsagia circumcincta	Worldwide	Sheep, goats, camelids, cervids, marmots, lagomorphs	Abomasum	Ingestion of infective larva	Abomasal edema, lymph node enlargement, hypoproteinemia	Not reported	94
Trichostrongylus axei	Worldwide	Sheep, goats, other ruminants, horses, lagomorphs	Abomasum	Ingestion of infective larva	Abomasal edema, hyperplasia	Reported	98
Trichostrongylus capricola	Eurasia, North America	Sheep, goats, cervids, lagomorphs	Small intestine	Ingestion of infective larva	None	Reported	69
Trichostrongylus colubriformis	Worldwide	Sheep, goats, cattle, camels, antelopes, lagomorphs, dogs, swine	Small intestine, abomasum	Ingestion of infective larva	Enteritis	Reported	152
Trichostrongylus longispicularis	Worldwide	Sheep, goats, other ruminants, lagomorphs, swine	Small intestine, abomasum	Ingestion of infective larva	Enteritis	Reported	184
Trichostrongylus probolurus	Africa, Eurasia	Sheep, goats, camels, antelopes	Small intestine	Ingestion of infective larva	None	Not reported	69
Trichostrongylus retortaeformis	Asia, Britain, Europe	Lagomorphs, goats	Small intestine	Ingestion of infective larva	Enteritis	Not reported	152
Trichostrongylus rugatus	Africa, Australia	Sheep, goats	Small intestine	Ingestion of infective larva	None	Not reported	108
Trichostrongylus vitrinus	Worldwide	Sheep, goats, cattle, camels, antelopes, lagomorphs, dogs, swine	Small intestine, abomasum	Ingestion of infective larva	Enteritis	Reported	69
Spiruroidea							
Gongylonema spp.	Worldwide	Sheep, goats, other livestock, lagomorphs	Rumen, esophagus, tongue	Ingestion of arthropod intermediate host (beetle)	Esophagitis	Reported	111
Trichuroidea							
Capillaria bovis, C. longipes	Worldwide	Sheep, goats, other ruminants	Small intestine	Ingestion of embryonated egg	None	Not reported	187
Trichuris spp.	Asia, Americas, Europe	Sheep, goats, other ruminants	Cecum, colon	Ingestion of embryonated egg	Enteritis, blood loss	Not reported	112

TABLE 20.3 Parasites of sheep and goats—skin and connective tissue and musculoskeletal system.

Parasite	Geographic distribution	Hosts	Location in host	Method of infection	Pathologic effects	Zoonosis	Reference
Coccidia							
Besnoitia caprae	Africa	Goats	Skin	Ingestion of sporulated oocysts in feces of definitive host (felid)	Hyperkeratosis	Not reported	18, 19, 172
Sarcocystis capracanis, S. hircicanis	Worldwide	Goats	Muscle	Ingestion of sporocyst in feces of definitive host (canid)	Variable anemia, weight loss, weakness, ataxia, paresis, myositis	Not reported	48
Sarcocystis gigantea, S. moulei	Worldwide	Goats	Muscle	Ingestion of sporocyst in feces of definitive host (felid)	Variable anemia, weight loss, weakness, ataxia, paresis, myositis	Not reported	48
Sarcocystis arieticanis, S. mihoensis	Worldwide	Sheep	Muscle	Ingestion of sporocyst in feces of definitive host (canid)	Variable anemia, weight loss, weakness, ataxia, paresis, myositis	Not reported	48
Sarcocystis tenella	Worldwide	Sheep	Muscle	Ingestion of sporocyst in feces of definitive host (canid)	Anemia, ataxia or paresis, myositis, abortion	Not reported	48
Sarcocystis medusiformis	Worldwide	Sheep	Muscle	Ingestion of sporocyst in feces of definitive host (felid)	Variable anemia, weight loss, weakness, ataxia, paresis, myositis	Not reported	48
Cestodes							
Larval							
Taenia ovis	Worldwide	Sheep	Muscle	Ingestion of egg in canine feces	None	Not reported	146
Nematodes							
Filaroidea							
Onchocerca armillata	Africa, Asia	Sheep, goats, cattle, equids	Skin of withers, neck, umbilical area	Unknown	Dermatitis	Not reported	194
Arthropods							
Diptera (flies)							
Calliphoridae	Worldwide	Sheep, goats, other mammals, birds	Skin wounds	Eggs deposited by female fly	Dermal myiasis, fetid skin wounds	Reported	69

(Continued)

681

TABLE 20.3 (Continued)

Parasite	Geographic distribution	Hosts	Location in host	Method of infection	Pathologic effects	Zoonosis	Reference
Ceratopogonidae (midges)	Worldwide	Sheep, goats, other mammals, birds	Skin	Direct contact	Irritation, pathogen transmission	Common	69
Ctenocephalides felis	Worldwide	Cats, dogs, sheep, goats, other mammals	Skin	Direct contact	Anemia, dermatitis	Common	168
Culicidae (mosquitoes)	Worldwide	Sheep, goats, other terrestrial vertebrates, birds	Skin	Direct contact	Pruritus, local inflammation, pathogen transmission	Common	69
Dermatobia hominis	Worldwide	Humans, sheep, other mammals	Skin	Larva deposited by blood-feeding arthropod	Subcutaneous cysts	Common	69
Hypoderma spp.	North America	Cattle, sheep, horses	Skin	Direct contact	Subcutaneous cysts	Reported	69
Lipotena caprina (ked)	Worldwide	Goats	Skin	Direct contact	Vector of Trypanosoma theodori	Not reported	69
Melophagus ovinus (ked)	Worldwide	Sheep	Skin	Direct contact	Vector of Trypanosoma melophagium	Not reported	69
Muscidae (filth flies)	Worldwide	Sheep, goats, other mammals, birds	Skin	Direct contact	Irritation, pathogen transmission, myiasis	Common	69
Przhevaliskiana silenus	Mediterranean basin	Goats	Skin	Direct contact	Subcutaneous cysts	Not reported	138
Psychodidae (sand flies)	Worldwide	Sheep, goats, other mammals, birds	Skin	Direct contact	Pathogen transmission	Common	69
Sarcophagidae (flesh flies)	Worldwide	Sheep, goats, other mammals, birds	Skin wounds	Larvae deposited by female fly	Dermal myiasis, fetid skin wounds	Reported	69
Simulidae (blackflies)	Worldwide	Sheep, goats, other mammals, birds	Skin	Direct contact	Irritation, pathogen transmission	Common	69
Tabanidae (Horseflies, deerflies)	Worldwide	Sheep, goats, other mammals	Skin	Direct contact	Painful bite, irritation, pathogen transmission	Common	69
Phthiraptera (lice)							
Bovicola (Damalinia) spp.	Africa, Americas, Australia	Sheep, goats	Skin	Direct contact	Debilitation	Not reported	118, 188
Linognathus spp.	Worldwide	Sheep, goats, deer	Skin	Direct contact	Anemia, dermatitis	Not reported	69
Siphonaptera (fleas)							
Ctenocephalides spp.	Worldwide	Cats, dogs, sheep, goats, other mammals	Pelage, skin	Direct contact	Dermatitis, anemia	Common	168

Species	Geographic distribution	Hosts	Location	Transmission	Effects	Occurrence	Reference
Vermipsylla spp.	China, eastern Europe	Sheep, goats, other livestock	Pelage, skin	Direct contact	Unknown	Not reported	69
Ticks (Hard)							
Amblyomma spp.	Africa, Americas	Sheep, goats, other mammals, birds	Skin	Direct contact	Pathogen transmission, secondary bacterial infections	Common	69
Boophilus spp.	Worldwide	Cattle, sheep, goats, other mammals	Skin	Direct contact	Pathogen transmission	Reported	69
Dermacentor spp.	Asia, Europe, North America	Sheep, goats, other mammals	Skin	Direct contact	Pathogen transmission, secondary bacterial infections	Common	69
Haemaphysalis spp.	Europe, Asia, northern Africa	Sheep, goats, other mammals, birds	Skin	Direct contact	Pathogen transmission, tick worry	Reported	69
Hyalomma spp.	Africa, Asia, Europe	Sheep, goats, other mammals, birds	Skin	Direct contact	Tick toxicosis	Reported	69
Ixodes spp.	Worldwide	Sheep, goats, other mammals, birds	Skin	Direct contact	Pathogen transmission, tick worry	Common	69
Rhipicephalus spp.	Africa, Americas, Europe	Sheep, goats, other mammals	Skin	Direct contact	Tick toxicosis, pathogen transmission	Common	69
Ticks (Soft)							
Ornithodoros spp.	Worldwide	Sheep, goats, other mammals	Skin	Direct contact	Anemia, tick paralysis, pathogen transmission	Common	123
Otobius megnini	Africa, Americas, India	Sheep, goats, other mammals	Ears	Direct contact	Otitis externa	Reported	69
Mites							
Astigmates							
Chorioptes spp.	Worldwide	Sheep, goats, cattle, horses	Skin	Direct contact	Mange	Not reported	189
Psoroptes cervinus	US	Wild sheep	Ears	Direct contact	Dermatitis	Not reported	196
Psoroptes cuniculi	Worldwide	Goats, rabbits, horses	Ears	Direct contact	Dermatitis	Not reported	131
Psoroptes ovis	Worldwide	Sheep, cattle	Skin	Direct contact	Dermatitis ("Sheep scab")	Not reported	130
Sarcoptes scabiei var. *ovis*	Worldwide	Sheep, goats, other mammals	Skin	Direct contact	Papular dermatitis, self-inflicted trauma, skin thickening, emaciation, death	Common	195

(Continued)

TABLE 20.3 (Continued)

Parasite	Geographic distribution	Hosts	Location in host	Method of infection	Pathologic effects	Zoonosis	Reference
Mesostigmates							
Raillietia auris	Australia, Europe, North America	Sheep, cattle	Ears	Direct contact	Otitis media	Not reported	136
Raillietia caprae	Americas	Goats	Ears	Direct contact	None	Not reported	197
Raillietia manfredi	Australia	Goats	Ears	Direct contact	None	Not reported	198
Prostigmates							
Demodex spp.	Worldwide	Sheep, goats, other ruminants	Hair follicles, sebaceous glands	Direct contact	Dermatitis	Not reported	199
Grain itch mites and forage mites	Worldwide	Sheep, goats, other mammals	Skin of face, legs	Direct contact with contaminated feed	Wheals, papules	Reported	69
Psorergates ovis	Africa, Americas, Australia, New Zealand	Sheep	Skin	Direct contact	Dermatitis	Not reported	200
Trombiculids	Worldwide	Sheep, goats, other mammals	Skin	Direct contact	Dermatitis	Common	201

684

TABLE 20.4 Parasites of sheep and goats—central nervous, respiratory, and urogenital systems.

Parasite	Geographic distribution	Hosts	Location in host	Method of infection	Pathologic effects	Zoonosis	Reference
Amoebae							
Balamuthia mandrillaris	Asia, Americas	Primates, sheep, dogs	Brain	Inhalation into nasal sinuses	Olfactory tract neuritis, skin ulceration	Reported	16, 171
Coccidia							
Neospora caninum	Worldwide	Sheep, goats, other ruminants other dogs, other mammals	Central nervous system	Ingestion of sporulated oocyst in feces of definitive host (dog), transplacental transmission	Bradyzoite cysts, abortion	Not reported	43, 44
Toxoplasma gondii	Worldwide	Sheep, goats, other mammals	Multiple organs	Ingestion of sporulated oocyst in feces of definitive host (cat)	Abortion	Common	51
Trematodes							
Paragonimus uestermanii	Asia	Goats, other mammals	Lungs, central nervous system	Ingestion of crustacean intermediate host (crab, crayfish)	Focal emphysema, lung cysts	Reported	69
Cestodes							
Larval							
Taenia multiceps	Worldwide	Sheep	Brain, spinal cord	Ingestion of egg in canine feces	Circling, blindness, paraplegia, hyperaesthesia	Not reported	147
Leeches							
Limnatis nilotica	Europe, North Africa	Sheep, other mammals	Pharynx, nasal cavity	Ingestion with contaminated water	Anemia, cranial edema, dyspnea	Reported	69
Nematodes							
Strongyloidea							
Mammomonogamus laryngeus	Asia, South America	Sheep, goats, cattle, cervids	Larynx	Ingestion of infective larva	Laryngeal ulcers	Reported	149
Mammomonogamus nasicola	Africa, Asia, South America	Sheep, goats, cattle, cervids	Nasal cavity	Ingestion of infective larva	Unknown	Not reported	150
Trichostrongyloidea							
Dictyocaulus filaria	Worldwide	Sheep, goats	Trachea, bronchi	Ingestion of infective larva	Bronchitis, pneumonia	Not reported	182

(Continued)

TABLE 20.4 *(Continued)*

Parasite	Geographic distribution	Hosts	Location in host	Method of infection	Pathologic effects	Zoonosis	Reference
Metastrongyloidea							
Cystocaulus nigrescens	Europe, Middle East	Sheep and goats	Lung	Ingestion of intermediate host (snail)	Subpleural nodules	Not reported	69
Muellerius capillaris	Worldwide	Sheep; goats	Lung	Ingestion of intermediate host (snail, slug)	Pulmonary nodules, pneumonia	Not reported	186
Neostrongylus linearis	Europe, Middle East	Sheep; goats	Lung	Ingestion of intermediate host (snail)	None	Not reported	153
Parelaphostrongylus tenuis	North America	Deer, other cervids, sheep, goats	Brain	Ingestion of intermediate host (snail)	Meningitis	Not reported	163, 164
Protostrongylus spp.	Worldwide	Sheep; goats	Lung	Ingestion of intermediate host (snail), transplacental transmission	Bronchiolar occlusion	Not reported	109
Spiculocaulus spp.	Eastern Europe	Sheep; goats	Lung	Ingestion of intermediate host (snail)	Unknown	Not reported	69
Varestrongylus (Bicaulus) spp.	Eastern Europe	Sheep, goats, cervids	Lung	Ingestion of intermediate host (snail)	Unknown	Not reported	69
Spiruroidea							
Thelazia californiensis	Western US	Deer, dogs, sheep, cats	Conjunctival sac	Transmitted by arthropod intermediate host (fly)	None	Reported	69
Thelazia rhodesi	Worldwide	Cattle, sheep, goats	Conjunctival sac	Transmitted by arthropod intermediate host (fly)	None	Not reported	69
Filaroidea							
Setaria digitata	Asia	Horses, sheep, goats	Central nervous system	Transmitted by arthropod intermediate host (mosquito)	Lumbar paralysis due to migrating larvae	Not reported	69
Arthropods							
Diptera (flies)							
Gedoelstia spp.	Africa	Antelopes, sheep	Orbit, nasal passages	Eggs deposited by female fly	Exophthalmus	Reported	167
Oestrus ovis (bot)	Worldwide	Sheep, goats, wild ruminants	Nasal cavity	Larvae deposited by female fly	Sinusitis	Reported	69

REFERENCES

1. Wells, E.A. (1972) The importance of mechanical transmission in the epidemiology of Nagana: A review. *Trop. Anim. Hlth. Prod.* **4**, 74–88.

2. Losos, G.J. and Ikede, B.O. (1972) Review of the pathology of diseases in domestic and laboratory animals caused by *Trypanosoma congolense, T. vivax, T. brucei, T. rhodesiense* and *T. gambiense. Vet. Path.* Supp. **9**, 1–71.

3. Soltys, M.A. and Woo, P.T.K. (1977) Trypanosomes producing disease in livestock in Africa. In: Kreier. J.P. (ed.) *Parasitic Protozoa Vol. I.* Academic Press, New York, NY, 239–296.

4. Anosa, V.O. (1983) Diseases produced by *Trypanosoma vivax* in ruminants, horses and rodents. *Zbl. Vet. Med.* B **30**, 717–741.

5. Mahmoud, M.M. and Gray, A.R. (1980) Trypanosomiasis due to *Trypanosoma evansi* (Steel, 1885) Balbiani, 1888. A review of recent research. *Trop. Animl. Hlth. Prod.* **12**, 35–47.

6. Boid, R., El Amin, E.A., Mahmoud, M.M., and Luckins, A.G. (1981) *Trypanosoma evansi* infections and antibodies in goats, sheep and camels in the Sudan. *Trop. Anim. Hlth. Prod.* **13**, 141–146.

7. Griffin, L. and Allonby, E.W. (1979) Trypanotolerance in breeds of sheep and goats with an experimental infection of *Trypanosoma congolense. Vet. Parasitol.* **5**, 97–105.

8. Mutayoba, B.M., Gombe, S., Waindi, E.N., and Kaaya, G.P. (1989) Comparative trypanotolerance of the small East African breed of goats from different localities to *Trypanosoma congolense* infection. *Vet. Parasitol.* **31**, 95–105.

9. Leeflang, P., Buys, J., and Blotkamp, C. (1978) Studies on *Trypanosoma vivax:* Comparison of parasitological diagnostic methods. *Int. J. Parasitol.* **8**, 15–18.

10. Levine, N.D. (1985) *Veterinary Protozoology.* Iowa State University Press, Ames, IA.

11. Mansfield, J.M. (1977) Nonpathogenic trypanosomes of mammals. In: Kreier, J.P. (ed.) *Parasitic Protozoa Vol. I.* Academic Press, New York, NY, 297–327.

12. Honigberg, B.M. (1978) Trichomonads of veterinary importance. In: Kreier, J.P. (ed.) *Parasitic Protozoa Vol. II.* Academic Press, New York, NY, 163–273.

13. Olson, M.E., McAllister, T.A., Deselliers, L., et al. (1995) Effects of giardiasis on production in a domestic ruminant (lamb) model. *Am. J. Vet. Res.* **56**, 1470–1474.

14. Sutherland, R.J. and Clarkson, A.R. (1984) Giardiasis in intensively reared Saanen kids. *New Zealand Vet. J.* **32**, 34–35.

15. Kulda, J. and Nohynkova, E. (1978) Flagellates of the human intestine and of intestines of other species. In: Kreier, J.P. (ed.) *Parasitic Protozoa Vol. II.* Academic Press, New York, NY, 1–138.

16. Fuentealba, I.C., Wikse, S.E., Read, W.K., Edwards, J.F., and Visvesvara, G.S. (1992) Amebic meningoencephalitis in a sheep. *J. Am. Vet. Med. Assoc.* **200**, 363–365.

17. Marquardt, W.C., Demaree, R.S., and Grieve, R.B. (2000) *Parasitology and Vector Biology.* 2nd ed. Academic Press, New York, NY.

18. Ng'ang'a, C.J. and Kasigazi, S. (1994) Caprine besnoitiosis: studies on the experimental intermediate hosts and the role of the domestic cat in transmission. *Vet. Parasitol.* **52**, 207–210.

19. Cheema, A.H. and Toofanian, F. (1979) Besnoitiosis in wild and domestic goats in Iran. *Cornell Vet.* **69**, 159–168.

20. Bigalke, R.D., Schoeman, J.H., and McCully, R.M. (1974) Immunization against bovine besnoitiosis with a live vaccine prepared from a blue wildebeest strain of *Besnoitia besnoiti* grown in cell cultures. 1. Studies on rabbits. *Onderstepoort J. Vet. Res.* **41**, 1–6.

21. Tzipori, S., Larsen, J., Smith, M., and Leufel, R. (1982) Diarrhea in goat kids attributed to *Cryptosporidium* infection. *Vet. Rec.* **111**, 35–36.

22. Angus, K.W., Appleyard, W.T., Menzies, J.D., Campbell, I., and Sherwood, D. (1982) An outbreak of diarrhea associated with cryptosporidiosis in naturally reared lambs. *Vet. Rec.* **110**, 129–130.

23. Saini, P., Ransom, G., and McNamara, A.M. (2000) Emerging public health concerns regarding cryptosporidiosis. *J. Am. Vet. Med. Assoc.* **217**, 658–663.

24. Muccio, J.L., Grooms, D.L., Mansfield, L.S., Wise, A.G., and Maes, R.K. (2004) Evaluation of two rapid assays for detecting *Cryptosporidium parvum* in calf feces. *J. Am. Vet. Med. Assoc.* **225**, 1090–1092.

25. Egyed, Z., Sreter, T., Szell, A., and Varga, I. (2003) Characterization of *Cryptosporidium* spp, recent developments and future needs. *Vet. Parasitol.* **111**, 103–114.

26. McDougald, L.R. (1979) Attempted cross-transmission of coccidia between sheep and goats and a description of *Eimeria ovinoidalis* sp.n. *J. Protozool.* **26**, 109–113.

27. Levine, N.D. and Ivens, V. (1986) The coccidian parasites (protozoa, apicomplexa) of artiodactyla. *Illinois Biological Monographs* **55** 120–178.

28. Lima, J.D. (1980) *Eimeria caprovina* sp. n. from the domestic goat *Capra hircus,* from the USA. *J. Protozool.* **27**, 153–154.

29. Pout, D.D. (1976) Coccidiosis in sheep: A review. *Vet. Rec.* **98**, 340–341.

30. Gregory, M.W. and Catchpole, J. (1989) Ovine coccidiosis: Pathology of *Eimeria ovinoidalis* infection. *Int. J. Parasitol.* **17**, 1099–1111.

31. Gregory, M.W. and Catchpole, J. (1990) Ovine coccidiosis: The pathology of *Eimeria crandallis* infection. *Int. J. Parasitol.* **20**, 849–860.

32. Coles, G.C. (1997) Control of parasites in goats. *Goat Vet. Soc. J.* **17**, 28–32.

33. Alyousif, M.S., Kasim, A.A., and Al-Shawa, Y.R. (1992) Coccidia of the domestic goat (*Capra hircus*) in Saudi Arabia. *Int. J. Parasitol.* **22**, 807–810.

34. Penzhorn, B.L., Rognile, M.C., Hall, L.L., and Knapp, S.E. (1994) Enteric coccidia of Cashmere goats in southwestern Montana, USA. *Vet. Parasitol.* **55**, 137–142.

35. Gregory M.W., Catchpole, J., Joyner, L.P., and Maund, B.A. (1989) Epidemiology of ovine coccidiosis: Effect of management at lambing. *Vet. Rec.* **124**, 561–562.

36. Catchpole, J., Norton, C.C., and Gregory, M.W. (1993) Immunization of lambs against coccidiosis. *Vet. Rec.* **132**, 56–59.

37. Gregory, M.W. and Catchpole, J. (1989) Ovine coccidiosis: Heavy infection in young lambs increases resistance without causing disease. *Vet. Rec.* **124**, 458–461.

38. Foreyt, W.J. (1986) Epidemiology and control of coccidia in sheep. *Vet. Clinics North Am.: Food Anim. Pract.* **2**, 383–388.

39. Anonymous (1977) *Manual of Veterinary Parasitological Laboratory Techniques Tech Bull 18* 2nd ed. Ministry of Fisheries and Food. Her Majesty's Stationary Office, London, United Kingdom, pp. 129.

40. Foreyt, W.J. (2001) *Veterinary Parasitology: Reference Manual* 5th ed. Iowa State Press, Ames, IA, 235.

41. Craig, T.M. (1986) Epidemiology and control of coccidia in goats. *Vet. Clinics North Am.: Food Anim. Pract.* **2**, 389–395.

42. O'Callaghan, M.G., O'Donoghue, P.J., and Moore, E. (1987) Coccidia of sheep in South Australia. *Vet. Parasitol.* **24**, 175–183.

43. Dubey, J.P. and Lindsay, D.S. (1990) *Neospora caninum* induced abortion in sheep. *J. Vet. Diagnostic Invest.* **2**, 230–233.

44. Dubey, J.P., Morales, J.A., Villalobos, P., Lindsay, D.S., Blagburn, B.L., and Topper, M.J. (1996) Neosporosis-associated abortion in a dairy goat. *J. Am. Vet. Med. Assoc.* **208**, 263–265.

45. Dubey, J.P., Barr, B.C., Barta, J.R., et al. (2002) Redescription of *Neospora caninum* and its differentiation from related coccidia. *Int. J. Parasitol.* **32**, 929–946.

46. Jenkins, M.C., Tuo, W., and Dubey, J.P. (2004) Evaluation of vaccination with *Neospora caninum* protein for prevention of fetal loss associated with experimentally induced neosporosis in sheep. *Am. J. Vet. Res.* **65**, 1404–1408.

47. Odening, K. (1998) The present state of species-systematics in *Sarcocystis* Lankester, 1882 (Protista, Sporozoa, Coccidia). *System. Parasitol.* **41**, 209–233.

48. Dubey, J.P., Speer, C.A., and Fayer, R. (1989) Sarcocystosis in sheep (*Ovis aries*) and Sarcocystosis in goats (*Capra hircus*). In: *Sarcocystosis of Animals and Man.* CRC Press, Boca Raton, FL, 113–125.

49. Caldow, G.L., Gidlow, J.R., and Schock, A. (2000) Clinical, pathological and epidemiological findings in three outbreaks of ovine protozoan myeloencephalitis. *Vet. Rec.* **146**, 7–10.

50. Leek, R.G. and Fayer, R. (1980) Amprolium for prophylaxis of ovine *Sarcocystis. J. Parasitol.* **66**, 100–106.

51. Dubey, J.P. and Beattie, C.P. (1988) Toxoplasmosis in sheep (*Ovis auries*) and Toxoplasmosis in goats (*Capra hircus*). In: *Toxoplasmosis of Animals and Man.* CRC Press. Boca Raton, FL, 61–89.

52. Duncanson, P., Terry, R.S., Smith, J.E., and Hide, G. (2001) High levels of congenital transmission of *Toxoplasma gondii* in a commercial sheep flock. *Int. J. Parasitol.* **31**, 1699–1703.

53. Buxton, D., Thompson, K.M., and Maley, S. (1993) Treatment of ovine toxoplasmosis with a combination of sulphamezathine and pyrimethamine. *Vet. Rec.* **132**, 409–411.

54. Buxton, D., Thompson, K.M., Maley, S., Wright, S., and Bos, H.J. (1993) Experimental challenge of sheep 18 months after vaccination with a live (S48) *Toxoplasma gondii* vaccine. *Vet. Rec.* **133**, 310–312.

55. Kuttler, K.D. (1988) World-wide impact of babesiosis. In: Ristic, M. (ed.) *Babesiosis of Domestic Animals and Man.* CRC Press. Boca Raton, FL, 1–22.

56. Friedhoff, K.T. (1988) Transmission of *Babesia.* In: Ristic, M. (ed.) *Babesiosis of Domestic Animals and Man.* CRC Press. Boca Raton, FL, 23–52.

57. Purnell, R.E., Lewis, D., Holman, M.R., and Young, E.R. (1981) Investigations on a *Babesia* isolated from Scottish sheep. *Parasitol.* **83**, 347–356.

58. Michael, S.A. and El Refaii, A.H. (1982) The effect of imidocarb dipropionate on *Babesia ovis* infection in sheep. *Trop. Anim. Hlth. Prod.* **14**, 1–2.

59. Urquhart, G.M., Armour, J, Duncan, J.L., Dunn, A.M., and Jennings, F.W. (1996) *Veterinary Parasitology* 2nd ed. Blackwell Science, Oxford, United Kingdom, 307.

60. Ogunrinade, A.F. (1984) Infectivity and pathogenicity of *Fasciola gigantica* in west African dwarf sheep and goats. *Trop. Anim. Hlth. Prod.* **16**, 161–166.

61. Reddington, J.J., Leid, R.W., and Wescott, R.B. (1986) The susceptibility of the goat to *Fasciola hepatica* infections. *Vet. Parasitol.* **19**, 145–150.

62. Reichael, M.P. (2002) Performance characteristics of an enzyme-linked immunosorbent assay for the detection of liver fluke (*Fasciola hepatica*) infection in sheep and cattle. *Vet. Parasitol.* **107**, 65–72.

63. Castro-Trejo, L., Garcia-Vasquez, Z., and Casildo-Nieto, J. (1990) The susceptibility of lymnaeid snails to *Paramphistomum cervi* infections in Mexico. *Vet. Parasitol.* **35**, 157–161.

64. Boray, J.C. (1971) The pathogenesis of ovine intestinal paramphistomosis due to *Paramphistomum ichikawai.* In: *Pathology of Parasitic Diseases.* Purdue University Press, West Lafayette, IN, 209–216.

65. Klopfer, U., Neumann, M., Perl, S., Gros, U., and Nobel, T.A. (1977) An outbreak of paramphistomiasis in sheep and concurrently occurring parmphistomiasis and schistosomiasis in cattle. *Refuah. Vet.* **34**, 141–143.

66. Rose, C.H. and Jacobs, D.E. (1990) Epidemiology of *Nematodirus* species infections of sheep in a subarctic climate: development and persistence of larvae on herbage. *Res. Vet. Sci.* **48**, 327–330.

67. Hathaway S.C. and Pullen, M.M. (1990) A risk-assessed evaluation of postmortem meat inspection procedures for ovine thysanosomiasis. *J. Am. Vet. Med. Assoc.* **196**, 860–864.

68. Craig, T.M. and Sheperd, E. (1980) Efficacy of albendazole and levamisole in sheep against *Thysanosoma actinioioides* and *Haemonchus contortus* from the Edwards Plateau, Texas. *Am. J. Vet. Res.* **41**, 425–426.

69. Soulsby, E.J.L. (1982) *Helminths, Arthropods and Protozoa of Domesticated Animals* 7th ed. Lea and Febiger, Philadelphia, PA, 809.

70. Hendrix C.M. and Shealy, P.M. (1991) The changing role of leeches in Veterinary Medicine. *Compendium Cont. Educ.* **13**, 447–455.

71. Levine, N.D. (1968) *Nematode Parasites of Domestic Animals and of Man.* Burgess Publishing Co., Minneapolis, MN, 600.

72. Nwaorgu, O.C. (1983) The development of the free living stages of *Strongyloides papillosus* I. Effect of temperature on the development of the heterogonic and homogonic nematodes in faecal cultures. *Vet. Parasitol.* **13**, 213–223.

73. Nwaorgu, O.C. and Connan, R.M. (1980) The importance of arrested larvae in the maintenance of patent infections of *Strongyloides papillosus* in rabbits and sheep. *Vet. Parasitol.* **7**, 339–346.

74. Cross, R.F. (1978) Influence of environmental factors on transmission of ovine contagious foot rot. *J. Am. Vet. Med. Assoc.* **173**, 1567–1568.

75. Taira, N. and Ura, S. (1991) Sudden death in calves associated with *Strongyloides papillosus* infection. *Vet. Parasitol.* **39**, 313–319.

76. Nakamura, Y., Ooba, C., and Hirose, H. (1998) Recovery from arrhythmias in lambs infected with *Strongyloides papillosus* following worm elimination. *J. Helminthol.* **72**, 43–46.

77. Anderson, R.C. (2000) *Nematode Parasites of Vertebrates. Their Development and Transmission.* 2nd ed. CABI Publishing, New York, NY, 650.

78. Dash, K.M. (1973) The life cycle of *Oesophagostomum columbianum* (Curtice, 1890) in sheep. *Int. J. Parasitol.* **3**, 843–851.

79. Stewart, T.B. and Gasbarre, L.C. (1989) The veterinary importance of nodular worms (*Oesophagostomum* spp). *Parasitol. Today* **5**, 209–213.

80. Ahluwalia, J.S. and Charleston, W.A.G. (1975) Studies on the pathogenicity of *Cooperia curticei* for sheep. *New Zealand Vet. J.* **23**, 197–199.

81. Lichtenfels, J.R., Pilitt, P.A., and Hoberg, E.P. (1994) New morphological characters for identifying individual specimens of *Haemonchus* spp. (Nematoda: Trichostrongyloidea) and a key to species in ruminants of North America. *J. Parasitol.* **80**, 107–119.

82. Zarlenga, D.S., Stringfellow, F., Nobary, M., and Lichtenfels, J.R. (1994) Cloning and characterization of ribosomal RNA genes from three species of *Haemonchus* (Nematoda: Trichostrongyloidea) and identification of PCR primers for rapid differentiation. *Expl. Parasitol.* **78**, 28–36.

83. Conder, G.A., Jen, L.-W., Marbury, K.S., et al. (1990) A novel anthelmintic model utilizing jirds *Meriones unguiculatus,* infected with *Haemonchus contortus. J. Parasitol.* **76**, 168–170.

84. Otsen, M., Hoekstra, R., Plas, M.E., Buntjer, J.B., Lenstra, J.A., and Roos, M.H. (2001) Amplified fragment length polymorphism analysis of genetic diversity of *Haemonchus contortus* during selection for drug resistance. *Int. J. Parasitol.* **31**, 1138–1143.

85. Zajac, A.M. and Gipson, T.A. (2000) Multiple anthelmintic resistance in a goat herd. *Vet. Parasitol.* **87**, 163–172.

86. van Wyk, J.A., Stenson, M.O., van der Merwe, J.S., et al. (1999) Anthelmintic resistance in South Africa; Surveys indicate an extremely serious situation in sheep and goat farming. *Onderstepoort J. Vet. Res.* **66**, 273–284.

87. Hall C.A., Ritchie, L., and McDonell, P.A. (1981) Investigations for anthelmintic resistance in gastrointestinal nematodes from goats. *Res. Vet. Sci.* **31**, 116–119.

88. Coop, R. and Kyriazakis, I. (2001) Influence of host nutrition on the development and consequences of nematode parasitism in ruminants. *Trends Parasitol.* **17**, 325–330.

89. Kates, K.C. (1965) Ecological aspects of helminth transmission in domesticated animals. *Am. Zoologist* **5**, 95–130.

90. Waller, P.J. (2003) Global perspectives on nematode parasite control in ruminant livestock: the need to adopt alternatives to chemotherapy, with emphasis on biological control. *Anim. Hlth. Res. Rev.* **4**, 35–43.

91. Adams D.B. (1984) Infection with *Haemonchus contortus* in sheep and the role of adaptive immunity in selection of the parasite. *Int. J. Parasitol.* **18**, 1071–1075.

92. Gray G.D., Barger, I.A., LeJambre, L.F., and Douch, P.G.C. (1992) Parasitological and immunological responses of genetically resistant Merino sheep on pastures contaminated with parasitic nematodes. *Int. J. Parasitol.* **22**, 417–425.

93. Lancaster, M.B. and Hong, C. (1981) Polymorphism in nematodes. *Syst. Parasitol.* **3**, 29–31.

94. Lichtenfels, J.R. and Hoberg, E.P. (1993) The systematics of nematodes that cause ostertagiasis in domestic and wild ruminants in North America: an update and key to species. *Vet. Parasitol.* **46**, 33–53.

95. Gasnier N., Cabaret, J., and Durette-Desset, M.C. (1997) Sheep and goat lines of *Teladorsagia circumcincta* (nematoda): from allozyme to morphological identification. *J. Parasitol.* **83**, 527–529.

96. Callinan, A.P.L. (1978) The ecology of the free-living stages of *Ostertagia circumcincta*. *Internat. J. Parasitol.* **8**, 233–237.

97. Ross, J.G., Purcell, D.A., and Todd, J.R. (1969) Experimental infection of lambs with *Trichostrongylus axei*. *Res. Vet. Sci.* **10**, 142–150.

98. Abbott, K.A. and McFarland, I.J. (1991) *Trichostrongylus axei* infection as a cause of deaths and loss of weight in sheep. *Aust. Vet. J.* **68**, 368–369.

99. Snider, T.G. III, Williams, J.C., Karns, P.A., Markovits, J.E., and Romaire, T.L. (1988) High concentration of serum gastrin immunoreactivity and abomasal hyperplasia in calves infected with *Ostertagia ostertagi* and/or *Trichostrongylus axei*. *Am. J. Vet. Res.* **49**, 2101–2104.

100. Yamaguchi, T. (1981) *Color Atlas of Clinical Parasitology*. Lea and Febiger. Philadelphia, PA, 293.

101. Wharton, D.A. (1982) The survival of desiccation by the free-living stages of *Trichostrongylus colubriformis* (Nematoda: Trichostrongylidae). *Parasitology* **84**, 455–462.

102. Eysker, M. (1978) Inhibition of the development of *Trichostrongylus* spp. as third stage larvae in sheep. *Vet. Parasitol.* **4**, 29–33.

103. Barker, I.K. (1975) Intestinal pathology associated with *Trichostrongylus colubriformis* infection in sheep: vascular permeability and ultrastructure of the mucosa. *Parasitology.* **70**, 173–180.

104. Sykes, A.R., Coop, R.L., and Angus, K.W. (1975) Experimental production of osteoporosis in growing lambs by continuous dosing with *Trichostrongylus colubriformis* larvae. *J. Comp. Path.* **85**, 549–559.

105. Jones, W.O. and Symons, L.E.A. (1982) Protein synthesis in the whole body, liver, skeletal muscle and kidney cortex of lambs infected by the nematode *Trichostrongylus colubriformis*. *Int. J. Parasitol.* **12**, 295–301.

106. Beveridge, I., Pullman, A.L., Martin, R.R., and Barelds, A. (1989) Effects of temperature and relative humidity on development and survival of the free-living stages of *Trichostrongylus colubriformis*, *T. rugatus* and *T. vitrinus*. *Vet. Parasitol.* **33**, 143–153.

107. Jansen, J. (1982) Justice to *Trichostrongylus longispicularis* Gordon, 1933 (nematoda: Trichostrongylidae). *Syst. Parasitol.* **4**, 141–146.

108. Beveridge, I., Pullman, A.L., Phillips, P.H., Martin, R.R., Barelds, A., and Grimson, R. (1989) Comparison of the effects of infection with *Trichostrongylus colubriformis*, *T. vitrinus* and *T. rugatus* in Merino lambs. *Vet. Parasitol.* **32**, 229–245.

109. Mansfield, L.S., Gamble, H.R., Baker, J.S., and Lichtenfels, J.R. (1993) Lungworm infection in a sheep flock in Maryland. *J. Am. Vet. Med. Assoc.* **202**, 601–606.

110. Hibler, C.P., Lange, R.E., and Metzger, C.J. (1972) Transplacental transmission of *Protostrongylus* spp. in Bighorn sheep. *J. Wildlife Dis.* **8**, 389.

111. Kudo, N., Koneguchi, T., Ikadai, H., and Oyamada, T. (2003) Experimental infection of laboratory animals and sheep with *Gongylonema pulchrum* in Japan. *J. Vet. Med. Sci.* **65**, 921–925.

112. Rickard, L.G. and Bishop, J.K. (1991) Redescription of *Trichuris tenuis* Chandler, 1930, from llamas (*Lama glama*) in Oregon with a key to the species of *Trichuris* present in North American ruminants. *J. Parasitol.* **77**, 70–75.

113. Farleigh, E.A. (1966) Observations on the pathogenic effects of *Trichuris ovis* in sheep under drought conditions. *Aust. Vet. J.* **24**, 462–463.

114. Geden, C.J., Rutz, D.A., Miller, R.W., and Steinkraus, D.C. (1992) Suppression of house flies (Diptera: Muscidae) on New York and Maryland dairies using releases of *Muscidifurax raptor* (Hymenoptera: Pteromalidae) in an integrated management program. *Environ. Ento.* **21**, 1419–1426.

115. Steinkraus, D.C., Geden, C.J., and Rutz, D.A. (1993) Prevalence of *Entomophthora muscae* (Cohn) Fresenius (Zygomycetes: Entomophthoraceae) in house flies (Diptera: Muscidae) on dairy farms in New York and introduction of epizootics. *Biol. Cont.* **3**, 93–100.

116. Sweeney, C.R., Scanlon, T., Russell, G.E., Smith, G., and Boston, R.C. (2000) Effect of daily floor treatment with sodium bisulfate on the fly population of horse stalls. *Am. J. Vet. Res.* **61**, 910–913.

117. Lloyd, J.E. (1985) Arthropod pests of sheep. In: Williams, R.E., Hall, R.D., Broce, A.B., and Scholl, P.J. (eds.) *Livestock Entomology*. John Wiley and Sons. New York, NY, 253–267.

118. Price, M.A. and Graham, O.H. (1997) *Chewing and sucking lice as parasites of mammals and birds*. United States Department Agriculture, ARS Technical Bulletin 1849.

119. McMullin, P.F., Cramer, L.G., Benz, G., Jeromel, P.C., and Gross, S.C. (1989) Control of *Dermatobia hominis* infestation in cattle using an ivermectin slow-release bolus. *Vet. Rec.* **124**, 465.

120. Heath, A.C.G., Cole, D.J.W., Bishop, D.M., Pfeffer, A., Cooper, S.M., and Risdon, P. (1995) Preliminary investigations into the aetiology and treatment of cockle, a sheep pelt defect. *Vet. Parasitol.* **56**, 239–254.

121. Heath A.C.G., Lampkin, N., and Jowett, J.H. (1995) Evaluation of non-conventional treatments for control of the biting louse (*Bovicola ovis*) on sheep. *Med. Vet. Entomol.* **9**, 407–412.

122. Heffner, R.S. and Heffner, H.E. (1983) Effect of cattle ear mite infestation on hearing in a cow. *J. Am. Vet. Med. Assoc.* **182**, 612–614.

123. Hoskins, J.D. and Cupp, E.W. (1988) Ticks of veterinary importance. Part II. The argasidae family: identification, behavior, and associated diseases. *Compend. Cont. Edu. Sm. Anim.* **10**, 699–708.

124. Teel, P.D. (1985) Ticks. In: Williams, R.E., Hall, R.D., Broce, A.B., and Scholl, P.J. (eds.) *Livestock Entomology.* John Wiley and Sons. New York, NY, 129–149.

125. Mebus, C.A. and Logan, L.L. (1988). Heartwater disease of domestic and wild ruminants. *J. Am. Vet. Med. Assoc.* **192**, 950–952.

126. De Vos, A.J. (1981) *Rhipicephalus appendiculatus:* cause and vector of diseases in Africa. *J. So. African Vet. Assoc.* **52**, 315–322.

127. Heath A.D.G., Bishop, D.M., and Tenquist, J.D. (1989) Observations on the potential for natural transfer of *Psoroptes cuniculi* and *Chorioptes bovis* (Acari: Psoroptidae) between goats and sheep. *New Zealand Vet. J.* **37**, 56–58.

128. Sargison, N.D., Scott, P.R., Wilson, D.J., and Bates, P.G. (2000) Chorioptic mange in British Suffolk rams. *Vet. Rec.* **147**, 135–136.

129. Wright, F.C., Guillot, F.S., and George, J.E. (1988) Efficacy of acaricides against chorioptic mange in goats. *Am. J. Vet. Res.* **49**, 903–904.

130. van den Broek, A.H. and Huntley, J.F. (2003) Sheep scab: the disease, pathogenesis and control. *J. Comp. Path.* **128**, 79–91.

131. Williams, J.F. and Williams, C.S.F. (1978) Psoroptic ear mites in dairy goats. *J. Am. Vet. Med. Assoc.* **173**, 1582–1583.

132. Cadiegures, M.-C., Laguerre, C., Roques, M., and Franc, M. (2004) Evaluations of the bioequivalence of two formulations of deltamethrin for treatment of sheep with psoroptic mange. *Am. J. Vet. Res.* **65**, 151–154.

133. O'Brien, D.J., Parker, L.D., Menton, C., Keaveny, C., McCollum, E., and O'Laoide, S. (1996) Treatment and control of psoroptic mange (sheep scab) with moxidectin. *Vet. Rec.* **139**, 437–439.

134. Bates, P.G., Groves, B.A., Courtney, S.A., and Coles, G.C. (1995) Control of sheep scab (*Psoroptes ovis*) on artificially infested sheep with a single injection of doramectin. *Vet. Rec.* **137**, 491–492.

135. Manurung J., Stevenson, P., Beriajaya, and Knox, M.R. (1990) Use of ivermectin to control sarcoptic mange in goats in Indonesia. *Trop. Anim. Health Prod.* **22**, 206–212.

136. Kettle, D.S. (1990) *Medical and Veterinary Entomology.* C.A.B International. Wallingford, United Kingdom, 658.

137. McKee, T.J., Couvillion, C.E., and Randolph, T.C. (1988) Ear mites in cattle: More prevalent than previously thought. *Vet. Med.* **73**, 731–732.

138. Wall, R. and Shearer, D. (2001) *Veterinary Ectoparasites, Biology, Pathology and Control* 2nd ed. Blackwell Science. Oxford, United Kingdom, 262.

139. Johnson, P.W., Plant, J.W., Boray, J.C., Blunt, S.C., and Nicholls, P.J. (1990) The prevalence of itchmite, *Psorergates ovis*, among sheep flocks with a history of fleece derangement. *Aust. Vet. J.* **67**, 117–120.

140. Mazahery, Y., Razmyar, J., and Hoghooghi-Rad, N. (1994) *Explanatum explanatum* (Creplin, 1847) Fukui, 1929, in buffaloes in the Ahwaz area, southwest Iran. *Vet. Parasitol.* **55**, 149–153.

141. Foreyt, W.J. (1990) Domestic sheep as a rare definitive host of the large American liver fluke *Fascioloides magna. J. Parasitol.* **76**, 736–739.

142. Deorani, V.P. (1965) Further contribution to the pathogenesis of *Ogmocotyle indica* (Notocotylidae: Trematoda) infection among hill sheep and goats. *Indian Vet. J.* **42**, 571–576.

143. Ferreras-Estrada, M.C., Garcia-Iglesias, M.J., Perez-Martinez, C., et al. (1998) A pathological study of experimental long-standing *Schistosoma bovis* infection in sheep. *J. Comp. Pathol.* **119**, 479–484.

144. Amjadi, A.R. (1971) Studies on histopathology of *Stilesia globipunctata* infections in Iran. *Vet. Rec.* **8**, 486–488.

145. Nginyi, J.M., Onyango-Abuje, J.A., and Harrison, L.J. (1993) Diagnosis of *Stilesia hepatica* infection in sheep. *Trop. Anim. Health Prod.* **25**, 225–228.

146. Gemmell, M.A. and Lawson, J.R. (1985) The survival in sheep and infectivity to dogs of *Taenia hydatigena* and *T. ovis* in sheep. *Vet. Parasitol.* **17**, 215–218.

147. Edwards, G.T. and Herbert, I.V. (1982) Observations on the course of *Taenia multiceps* infections in sheep: clinical signs and post-mortem findings. *Br. Vet. J.* **138**, 489–500.

148. Fabiyi, J.P. (1978) The occurrence of *Oesophagostomum multifoliatum* Daubney and Hudson, 1932, in Nigerian cattle. *J. Helminthol.* **52**, 335–338.

149. Marques, S.M., Quadros, R.M., and Pilati, C. (2005) *Mammomonogamus laryngeus* (Railliet, 1899) infection in buffaloes in Rio Grande do Sul, Brazil. *Vet. Parasitol.* **30**, 241–243.

150. Opasina, B.A. and Dipeolu, O.O. (1983) Fatal infection of a West African Dwarf sheep with *Mammomonogamus nasicola* (S. *Syngamus nasicola*). *Zentralbl. Veterinarmed. B.* **30**, 313–315.

151. Hart, R.J. and Wagner, A.M. (1971) The pathological physiology of *Gaigeria pachyscelis* infestation. *Onderstepoort J. Vet. Res.* **38**, 111–116.

152. Audebert, F., Cassone, J., Kerboeuf, D., and Durette-Desset, M.C. (2003) Development of *Trichostrongylus colubriformis* and *Trichostrongylus vitrinus,* parasites of ruminants in the rabbit and comparison with *Trichostrongylus retortaeformis. Parasitol. Res.* **90**, 57–63.

153. Castanon Ordonez, L., Cordero del Campillo, M., and Rojo Vazquez, F.A. (1984) Migration and growth of *Neostrongylus linearis* (Marotel, 1913) Gebauer, 1932 in sheep. *Vet. Parasitol.* **15**, 271–284.

154. Sarwar, M.M. (1954) On the occurrence of *Ostertagia pinnata* Daubney, 1933, in association with *Ostertagia trifurcata* Ransom, 1907 in India and Great Britain. *J. Helminthol.* **28**, 150–154.

155. Beveridge, I., Barker, I.K., Rickard, M.D., and Burton, J.D. (1974) Letter: Experimental infection of sheep with *Camelostrongylus mentulatus* and associated gastritis. *Aust. Vet. J.* **50**, 36–37.

156. Sarwar, M.M. (1952) On the synonymy of *Marshallagia orientalis* (Bhalerao, 1932) with *Marshallagia marshalli* and a record of its occurrence from the mountainous region of the Punjab. *Parasitology* **42**, 125.

157. Hoberg, E.P. and Abrams, A. (2005) *Pseudostertagia bullosa* (Nematoda: Trichostrongyloidea) in artiodactyl hosts from North America: redescription and comments on systematics. *J. Parasitol.* **91**, 370–381.

158. Rickard, L.G., Hoberg, E.P., Allen, N.M., Zimmerman, G.L., and Craig, T.M. (1993) *Spiculopteragia spiculoptera* and *S. asymmetrica* (Nematoda: Trichostrongyloidea) from red deer (*Cervus elaphus*) in Texas. *J. Wildl. Dis.* **29**, 512–515.

159. Fernando, S.T. (1965) Morphology, systematics, and geographic distribution of *Mecistocirrus digitatus*, a trichostrongylid parasite of ruminants. *J. Parasitol.* **51**, 149–155.

160. Fernando, S.T. (1965) The life cycle of *Mecistocirrus digitatus,* a trichostrongylid parasite of ruminants. *J. Parasitol.* **51**, 156–163.

161. Ahluwalia, J.S. and Charleston, W.A. (1975) Studies on the pathogenicity of *Cooperia curticei* for sheep. *N.Z. Vet. J.* **23**, 197–199.

162. Becklund, W.W. and Walker, M.L. (1967) *Nematodirus* of domestic sheep, *Ovis aries,* in the United States with a key to the species. *J. Parasitol.* **53**, 777–781.

163. Guthery, F.S., Beasom, S.L., and Jones, L. (1979) Cerebrospinal nematodiasis caused by *Parelaphostrongylus tenuis* in Angora goats in Texas. *J. Wildl. Dis.* **15**, 37–42.

164. Jortner, B.S., Troutt, H.F., Collins, T., and Scarratt, K. (1985) Lesions of spinal cord parelaphostrongylosis in sheep. Sequential changes following intramedullary larval migration. *Vet. Pathol.* **22**, 137–140.

165. Hibler, C.P. and Adcock, J.L. (1968) Redescription of *Elaeophora schneideri* Wehr and Dikmans, 1935 (Nematoda: Filarioidea). *J. Parasitol.* **54**, 1095–1098.

166. Jensen, R. and Seghetti, L. (1955) Elaeophoriasis in sheep. *J. Am. Vet. Med. Assoc.* **127**, 499–505.

167. Bisley, G.G. (1972) A case of intraocular myiasis in man due to the first stage larva of the Oestrid fly *Gedoelstia* spp. *East Afr. Med. J.* **49**, 768–771.

168. Fagbemi, B.O. (1982) Effect of *Ctenocephalides felis strongylus* infestation on the performance of West African dwarf sheep and goats. *Vet. Q.* **4**, 92–95.

169. el-Refaii, A.H. and Michael, S.A. (1988) *Linguatula serrata* Frohlich—a case report of larvae among sheep and goats in Egypt. *J. Egypt. Soc. Parasitol.* **18**, 353–354.

170. Costa, J.O., dos Santos Lima, W., Leite, A.C., Guimaraes, M.P., and Torres, L.D. (1983) *Melophagus ovinus* and *Trypanosoma* (*Megatrypanum*) *melophagium* in ovines in the State of Minas Gerais, Brazil. *Mem. Inst. Oswaldo Cruz.* **78**, 101–103.

171. Deol, I., Robledo, L., Meza, A., Visvesvara, G.S., and Andrews, R.J. (2000) Encephalitis due to a free-living amoeba (*Balamuthia mandrillaris*): case report with literature review. *Surg. Neurol.* **53**, 611–616.

172. Njenga, J.M., Bwangamoi, O., Kangethe, E.K., Mugera, G.M., and Mutiga, E.R. (1995) Comparative ultrastructural studies on *Besnoitia besnoiti* and *Besnoitia caprae*. *Vet. Res. Commun.* **19**, 295–308.

173. Schnittger, L., Yin, H., Gubbels, M.J., et al. (2003) Phylogeny of sheep and goat *Theileria* and *Babesia* parasites. *Parasitol. Res.* **91**, 398–406.

174. Theodoridis, Y., Duncan, J.L., MacLean, J.M., and Himonas, C.A. (1991) Pathophysiological studies on *Dicrocoelium dendriticum* infection in sheep. *Vet. Parasitol.* **39**, 61–66.

175. Jain, P.C. and Kamalapur. S.K. (1970) On the occurrence of *Calicophoron cauliorchis* (Stiles and Goldberger, 1910) Nasmark, 1937 paramphistomidae: trematoda in sheep in India. *Indian Vet. J.* **47**, 307–308.

176. Dinnik, J.A. (1956) On *Ceylonocotyle scoliocoelium* (Fischoeder, 1904) and its intermediate host in Kenya, East Africa. *J. Helminthol.* **30**, 149–156.

177. Varma, A.K. (1961) Observations on the biology and pathogenicity of *Cotylophoron cotylophorum* (Fischoeder, 1901). *J. Helminthol.* **35**, 161–168.

178. Kraneburg, W. and Boch, J. (1978) Biology and pathogenicity of the domestic ruminal fluke *Paramphistomum cervi*. 3. Development in cattle, sheep and deer. *Berl. Munch. Tierarztl. Wochenschr.* **91**, 71–75.

179. Sharma, P.N. and Hanna, R.E. (1988) Ultrastructure and cytochemistry of the tegument of *Orthocoelium scoliocoelium* and *Paramphistomum cervi* (Trematoda: Digenea). *J. Helminthol.* **62**, 331–343.

180. Shahlapoor, A.A. (1965) A note on the identification of *Skrjabinema ovis* (Skrjabin, 1915) and *Trichostrongylus* spp. in sheep and goats in Iran. *J. Helminthol.* **39**, 273–276.

181. Herd, R.P. (1971) The parasitic life cycle of *Chabertia ovina* (Fabricius, 1788) in sheep. *Int. J. Parasitol.* **1**, 189–199.

182. Goldberg, A. (1952) Experimental infection of sheep and goats with the nematode lungworm, *Dictyocaulus filaria*. *Am. J. Vet. Res.* **13**, 531–536.

183. Thomas, R.F. (1959) A comparative study of the life histories of *Nematodirus battus* and *N. filicollis,* nematode parasites of sheep. *Parasitology.* **49**, 374–386.

184. Sommerville, R.I. (1956) A note on the specific identity of *Trichostrongylus longispicularis* Gordon, 1933. *J. Helminthol.* **30**, 21–24.

185. Coop, R.L., Angus, K.W., and Sykes, A.R. (1979) Chronic infection with *Trichostrongylus vitrinus* in sheep. Pathological changes in the small intestine. *Res. Vet. Sci.* **26**, 363–371.

186. Sauerlander, R. (1988) Experimental infection of sheep and goats with *Muellerius capillaris* (Protostrongylidae, Nematoda). *Zentralbl. Veterinarmed. B.* **35**, 525–548.

187. Worley, D.E., Barrett, R.E., and Knapp, S.E. (1980) Hosts and distribution of *Capillaria bovis* (Schnyder, 1906) in domestic and wild ruminants in northwestern United States. *J. Parasitol.* **66**, 695–696.

188. O'Callaghan, M.G., Moore, E., and Langman, M. (1988) *Damalinia caprae* infestations on sheep. *Aust. Vet. J.* **65**, 66.

189. Zahler, M., Hendrikx, W.M., Essig, A., Rinder, H., and Gothe, R. (2001) Taxonomic reconsideration of the genus *Chorioptes* Gervais and van Beneden, 1859 (Acari: Psoroptidae). *Exp. Appl. Acarol.* **25**, 517–523.

190. Young, A.S. and Mchinja, S.F. (1977) Observations on *Haematoxenus separatus* Uilenberg and Andreasen 1974 in the erythrocytes of Kenyan sheep. *Res. Vet. Sci.* **23**, 387–388.

191. Massoud, J. (1971) The pathology of *Ornithobilharzia turkestanicum* and *Schistosoma bovis* in cattle, sheep and goats in Iran. *Trans. R. Soc. Trop. Med. Hyg.* **65**, 431.

192. Graydon, R.J., Carmichael, I.H., Sanchez, M.D., Weidosari, E., and Widjayanti, S. (1992) Mortalities and wasting in Indonesian sheep associated with the trematode *Eurytrema pancreaticum*. *Vet. Rec.* **131**, 443.

193. Lloyd, S. and Soulsby, E.J. (1978) Survey of parasites in dairy goats. *Am. J. Vet. Res.* **39**, 1057–1059.

194. Bain, O. (1975) Redescription of five species of *Onchocerca*. *Ann. Parasitol. Hum. Comp.* **50**, 763–788.

195. Abu-Samra, M.T., Ibrahim, K.E., and Aziz, M.A. (1984) Experimental infection of goats with *Sarcoptes scabiei* var. *ovis*. *Ann. Trop. Med. Parasitol.* **78**, 55–61.

196. Zahler, M., Hendrikx, W.M., Essig, A., Rinder, H., and Gothe, R. (2000) Species of the genus *Psoroptes* (Acari: Psoroptidae): a taxonomic consideration. *Exp. Appl. Acarol.* **24**, 213–225.

197. Friel, J. and Greiner, E.C. (1988) Ear mites from domestic goats in Florida. *Exp. Appl. Acarol.* **4**, 345–351.

198. Cook, R.W. (1981) Ear mites (*Raillietia manfredi* and *Psoroptes cuniculi*) in goats in New South Wales. *Aust. Vet. J.* **57**, 72–74.

199. Bukva, V. (1990) Three species of the hair follicle mites (Acari: Demodicidae) parasitizing the sheep, *Ovis aries* L. *Folia Parasitol* (Praha) **37**, 81–91.

200. Sinclair, A. (1990) The epidermal location and possible feeding site of *Psorergates ovis,* the sheep itch mite. *Aust. Vet. J.* **67**, 59–62.

201. Otto, Q.T. and Jordaan, L.C. (1992) An orf-like condition caused by trombiculid mites on sheep in South Africa. *Onderstepoort J. Vet. Res.* **59**, 335–356.

202. Orpin, C.G. (1974) The rumen flagellate *Callimastix frontalis:* does sequestration occur? *J. Gen. Microbiol.* **84**, 395–398.

CHAPTER
21

Parasites of Non-human Primates

Frank Cogswell, PhD

INTRODUCTION

Increasing numbers of non-human primates (NHP) are being used in biomedical research as models for infectious diseases. Most laboratory primates are Old World species, and include the macaques—rhesus, pigtail, and cynomolgus monkeys—as well as mangabeys and African green monkeys. Chimpanzees are still used for selected studies, although the expense of their keep is often prohibitive. New World species such as squirrel and owl monkeys, but also capuchins and marmosets, are also extensively used animal models. Wild-caught animals frequently bring their parasites with them, and while often not extremely pathogenic, these parasites may represent unwanted research variables. In addition, the federally funded NHP breeding centers may house breeding colonies of NHP outdoors, contributing to the diversity of parasites seen in these animals.

This chapter focuses on parasites found in the most important NHP hosts used in the laboratory. Others[1,2,3] have provided extensive lists of primate parasites by organ system. The interested reader is directed to significant publications covering helminth parasites of NHP[4] and the pathology of primate parasitic diseases[5]. Because many parasites of non-human primates are shared with humans, some may wish to consult an atlas of human parasites[6] to assist in parasite speciation.

PROTOZOA

Phylum Sarcomastigophora

Class Mastigophora (Flagellates)

Hemoflagellates

Trypanosoma cruzi *Trypanosoma cruzi* is an important human pathogen in the Western Hemisphere and has been described in outdoor NHP colonies in Texas, Louisiana, and Georgia. The biology of *T. cruzi* is presented in Chapter 17, Parasites of Dogs. Several species of wild and domestic animals serve as reservoirs for infection of outdoor-housed NHP in the southern United States and Mexico[7]. Among NHP, infections have been described in marmosets, capuchins, squirrel monkeys, spider monkeys and other simian primates in Central and South America[8,9]. In the United States, natural infections with *T. cruzi* have been described in laboratory squirrel monkeys, capuchins, rhesus monkeys, pigtail macaques (*Macaca nemestrina*), and baboons[10].

The infection appears to be clinically silent in rhesus macaques and is usually diagnosed at necropsy (Figure 21.1). Myocarditis and myositis are occasionally seen histologically but clinical correlates are usually not present. Diagnosis is made by finding the circulating parasites in the blood, or after culturing. A dipstick format ELISA (InBios International) test works well in NHP for demonstrating exposure to the organism.

Trypanosoma minasense *Trypanosoma minasense* (Syn. *Trypanosoma advieri*, *T. brirnonti*, *T. devei*, *T. escomeli*, *T. florestali*, *T. manguin-hense*, *T. mycetae*) is a nonpathogenic flagellate found in marmosets, capuchins, squirrel monkeys, spider monkeys, howler monkeys, night monkeys, woolly monkeys, and humans in Central and South America[8]. The trypomastigote form in the blood is sinuous and 29 μ to 46 μ long and the nucleus is usually at, or just anterior to, the middle of the body. The kinetoplast is small and well anterior. The undulating membrane is

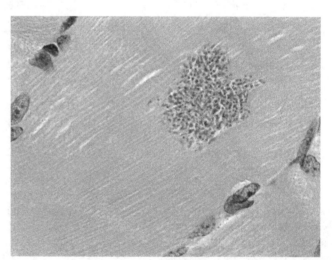

Fig. 21.1 Low power magnification of *Trypanosoma cruzi* in the heart of a monkey. Courtesy of Dr. Peter Didier.

fairly well developed, and the free flagellum is usually one-sixth to one-third of the body length. *Trypanosoma minasense* does not appear to be pathogenic for vertebrates and therefore must be distinguished from the pathogenic *T. cruzi* with which it is sometimes found in mixed infection. It is unlikely to occur in the laboratory except in primates obtained from endemic areas. Microscopic diagnosis is as described for *T. cruzi*.

Trypanosoma rangeli *Trypanosoma rangeli* (Syn. *Trypanosoma ariarii*, *T. cebus*, *T. guatemalense*, *T. saimirii*) occurs in capuchins and humans in Central and South America[8,9,11–13], as well as owl and squirrel monkeys in Colombia, Peru, and Bolivia[14]. Rhesus macaques can be infected experimentally, but natural infections are unlikely to occur in the laboratory. Trypomastigotes are found in the blood and measure 26 μ to 36 μ long with a pointed posterior end, a small, subterminal kinetoplast, and a rippled undulating membrane with a free flagellum[9]. The most common vector is the reduviid bug *Rhodnius prolixus*, but *Triatoma dimidiata* and other reduviids have also been found to be infected. Infection of the vertebrate host is either by bite or by fecal contamination, and is generally asymptomatic[9]. However, it must be distinguished from pathogenic trypanosomes, and especially from *T. cruzi*, with which it is sometimes found in mixed infection. *Trypanosoma rangeli* is larger than *T. cruzi* and has a much smaller kinetoplast. Microscopic diagnosis is as described for *T. cruzi*.

Trypanosoma sanmartini *Trypanosoma sanmartini* was described from squirrel monkeys in Colombia[15]. It greatly resembles *T. cruzi* and may be an aberrant strain or subspecies[8]. Trypomastigotes are curved, often S-shaped, with a large, ovoid kinetoplast at the posterior tip and moderately developed undulating membrane. Trypomastigotes measure 17 μ to 24 μ long, including a free flagellum that is 4 μ to 9 μ long and 2 μ to 3 μ wide. It is unlikely to occur in the laboratory except in squirrel monkeys obtained from endemic areas. Infections are of unknown pathogenicity. Microscopic diagnosis is as described for *T. cruzi*.

Enteric flagellates

Chilomastix mesnili *Chilomastix mesnili* (Syn. *Chilomastix hominis*, *C. suis*) is common in the cecum and colon of rhesus monkeys, cynomolgus monkeys, green monkeys, baboons, capuchins, orangutans, chimpanzees, and others[9]. Trophozoites are piriform with an anterior nucleus, a large cytostomal groove near the anterior end, three anterior flagella, a short fourth flagellum which undulates within the cytostomal groove, and a cytoplasmic fibril along the anterior end and sides of the cytostomal groove[9]. Cysts are usually lemon-shaped and contain one nucleus and the organelles of the trophozoite. Trophozoites measure 6 μ to 24 μ long by 3 μ to 10 μ wide, while cysts measure 6.5 μ to 10 μ long[6]. Infection rates in laboratory colonies are unknown but may be high in wild-caught primates. Infections are typically asymptomatic. Humans are also susceptible to infection. Diagnosis is by finding cysts in fecal smears or floatations.

Enteromonas hominis *Enteromonas hominis* (Syn. *Tricercomonas intestinalis*, *Octomitus hominis*, *Enteromonas bengalensis*) occurs uncommonly in the cecum of the rat, hamster, rhesus monkey, other macaques, and humans throughout the world[9,16]. Trophozoites are spherical or piriform, with three short anterior flagella, one of which is sometimes difficult to see. A fourth flagellum runs along the flattened body surface and extends freely at the posterior end. There is an anterior nucleus and a strand-like funis extending posteriorly from the blepharoplast along the body surface[9]. There is no cytostome. Trophozoites measure 4 μ to 10 μ long by 3 μ to 6 μ wide and have many food vacuoles that contain bacteria. The cysts are ovoid and contain four nuclei when mature.

Giardia lamblia **Morphology.** *Giardia lamblia* (Syn. *Lamblia intestinalis*, *Megastoma entericum*, *Giardia duodenalis*) is morphologically similar to *G. canis*, which is described in Chapter 17, Parasites of Dogs.

Hosts and Life Cycle. *Giardia lamblia* is found in the duodenum, jejunum, and upper ileum of humans, rhesus monkeys, cynomolgus monkeys, chimpanzees, and other primates[17]. Infections are common throughout the world. The life cycle is as described for *G. canis*. Primates become infected via ingestion of feed or water that is contaminated with cysts.

Pathologic Effects and Clinical Disease. Infection with *G. lamblia* causes diarrhea, which may be severe, in captive rhesus macaques and other NHP.

Diagnosis, Treatment, and Prevention. Diagnosis is made by identifying the cysts and occasionally trophozoites in a direct fecal smear, or cysts in $ZnSO_4$ fecal flotation. Commercially available ELISA kits (Remel, Inc. Xpect®) allow detection of an exoantigen in stool samples with a 97% sensitivity and specificity, and do not require microscopic expertise. Treatment consists of oral metronidazole (25 mg/kg twice per day for five days) or oral fenbendazole (50 mg/kg once per day for five days). Infections may be reduced in incidence by strict adherence to sanitation procedures.

Public Health Considerations. *Giardia lamblia* is infectious to animal workers. Infected animals and stool samples should be handled with caution.

Hexamita pitheci

Hexamita pitheci has been reported in the cecum and colon of rhesus monkeys in South America[18]. The incidence of infection is unknown. Trophozoites measure 2.5 μ to 3 μ long by 1.5 μ to 2 μ wide. A similar and perhaps identical species of *Hexamita* has been found in feces of the rhesus monkey and the chimpanzee in North America[19]. In the latter case, trophozoites measured 4 μ to 6 μ long by 2 μ to 4 μ wide.

Pentatrichomonas hominis

Pentatrichomonas hominis is a common inhabitant of the cecum and colon of rhesus monkeys, cynomolgus monkeys, chimpanzees, orangutans, and other primates, including humans, throughout the world[20–22]. Trophozoites have three to five anterior flagella[9] and measure 8 μ to 20 μ long by 3 μ to 14 μ wide. The absence of a cyst stage makes direct fecal smear the diagnostic method of choice. The incidence of this flagellate in laboratory primates is common in specimens obtained from their natural habitat. It is very common in diarrheic stool samples from colony animals but it does not cause diarrhea.

Retortamonas intestinalis

Retortamonas intestinalis (Syn. *Embadomonas intestinalis*) occurs in the cecum of rhesus monkeys, chimpanzees, and other simian primates throughout the world[9]. Trophozoites are piriform or fusiform and are drawn out posteriorly, with an anterior nucleus, large anterior cytostome, anterior flagellum, posteriorly directed trailing flagellum which emerges from the cytostomal groove, and cytostomal fibril around the anterior end and sides of the cytostome[6]. Trophozoites measure 4 μ to 9 μ long by 3 μ to 4 μ wide (Figure 21.2). Cysts are piriform or ovoid, have one or two nuclei, and measure 4 μ to 7 μ long by 3 μ to 5 μ wide. The incidence of infection is unknown.

Trichomonas tenax

Trichomonas tenax is a nonpathogenic trichomonad commonly found in the mouth, especially between the gums and teeth, of rhesus monkeys,

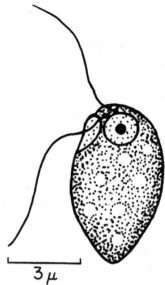

Fig. 21.2 *Retortamonas* trophozoite. Courtesy of N.D. Levine, University of Illinois.

cynomolgus monkeys, baboons, and humans throughout the world[21,23]. Trophozoites measure 4 μ to 16 μ by 2 μ to 15 μ[23,24]. The incidence of infection in laboratory colonies is unknown. Infections may be common in primates obtained from their natural environment.

Class Sarcodina (Amoebae)

Dientamoeba fragilis

Dientamoeba fragilis occurs in the cecum and colon of rhesus and cynomolgus monkeys in Asia and in humans throughout the world[9,21,25]. Although infections have not been observed in feral baboons, an 8% incidence has been noted in captive baboons in the United States[26]. While infected humans sometimes develop mucoid diarrhea, infections in NHP are typically asymptomatic[9]. Trophozoites measure 3 μ to 22 μ in diameter but more typically measure 6 μ to 12 μ[9] (Figure 21.3).

Endolimax nana

Endolimax nana is common in the cecum and colon of rhesus monkeys, cynomolgus monkeys, other macaques, patas monkeys, guenons, mangabeys, baboons, capuchins, chimpanzees, gorillas, and humans throughout the world[9,16,20–,22,27–30]. Trophozoites measure 6 μ to 15 μ in diameter while the cysts measure 5 μ to 14 μ in diameter[9] (Figure 21.3). Infections are common in laboratory primates obtained from the wild. Infections with *E. nana* are nonpathogenic.

Ameba	Trophozoite	Cyst

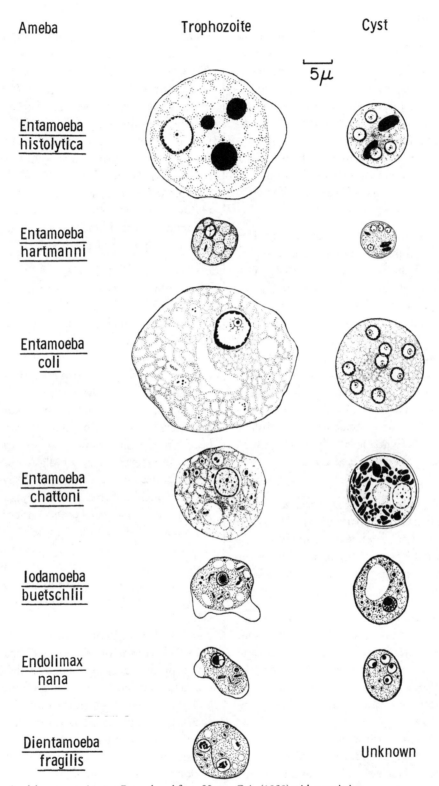

Fig. 21.3 Amebas affecting laboratory primates. Reproduced from Hoare, C.A. (1959) with permission.

Entamoeba chattoni

Entamoeba chattoni (Syn. *Entamoeba polecki*) occurs in the cecum and colon of many primates, including humans[9]. *Entamoeba chattoni* may be more common in monkeys than *E. histolytica*, but most workers have failed to recognize it. It has been reported from laboratory monkeys in the United States and Germany, and probably occurs throughout the world[31]. Trophozoites measure 9 μ to 20 μ long, while cysts measure 6 μ to 18 μ in diameter[9] (Figure 21.3). Infections have been associated with diarrhea in humans[32], but its pathogenicity for laboratory primates is unknown.

Entamoeba coli

Entamoeba coli is the most common amoeba found in humans and is also very common in other primates[9,29,33]. *Entamoeba coli* occurs in the cecum and colon of rhesus monkeys, cynomolgus monkeys, other macaques, green monkeys, baboons, gibbons, orangutans, chimpanzees, gorillas, other nonhuman primates, and pigs throughout the world. It is common in laboratory primates obtained from their natural habitat[16,22,30,34] (Figure 21.3). Like other amoeba, *E. coli* reproduces by binary fission and is transmitted by ingestion of cysts. Trophozoites measure 15 μ to 50 μ in diameter (usually 20 μ to 30 μ) while the cysts measure 10 μ to 33 μ in diameter[9]. Incidence at the Tulane National Primate Research Center is 90% in monkeys with diarrhea, though *E. coli* is not considered a pathogen[35].

Entamoeba dispar

Entamoeba dispar is morphologically identical to *E. histolytica* but differs in that it is nonpathogenic. *Entamoeba dispar* is more prevalent than *E. histolytica*. *Entamoeba dispar* may be differentiated from *E. hartmanni* solely on the basis of size, and can be differentiated from *E. histolytica* on the basis of zymodeme analysis and PCR assay[36].

Entamoeba gingivalis

Entamoeba gingivalis occurs in the mouth of rhesus monkeys, cynomolgus monkeys, baboons, chimpanzees, and humans throughout the world[9]. Trophozoites may be found between the teeth, under the edge of the gums, and in the tartar. Trophozoites measure 5 μ to 35 μ long (usually 10 μ to 20 μ). *Entamoeba gingivalis* thrives on diseased gums and was once thought to cause pyorrhea in humans. Trophozoites feed on leucocytes, epithelial cells, bacteria, and rarely, erythrocytes. There are no cysts, and transmission is generally by oral contact. It is common in primates[17] and is usually associated with diseased gums but is itself considered nonpathogenic.

Entamoeba hartmanni

Entamoeba hartmanni closely resembles *E. histolytica* and has now been accepted as the name for the "small race" *E. histolytica* in the older texts. It is considered nonpathogenic[9] and is differentiated from *E. histolytica* essentially on the basis of its smaller size (Figure 21.3). The incidence and distribution of *E. hartmanni* in laboratory animals are unknown because in the past it has been confused with *E. histolytica*. It has been reported in the cecum and colon of rhesus monkeys and humans in North America, and probably occurs throughout the world. Two types of *Entamoeba* with tetranucleate cysts were seen in one study of naturally infected monkeys[37]. The smaller race was undoubtedly *E. hartmanni*.

Entamoeba histolytica

Morphology. *Entamoeba histolytica* trophozoites measure 12 μ to 15 μ in diameter[9,38] (Figure 21.3). The nucleus is vesicular and contains a small, central endosome with a ring of small, peripheral granules[9]. Cysts measure 10 μ to 20 μ in diameter and have four nuclei when mature. Rod-like chromatoid bodies with rounded ends are often present.

Hosts. *Entamoeba histolytica* (Syn. *Entamoeba caudate*) occurs in the cecum and colon of most primates, including humans, throughout the world[9]. Infections have been reported in a number of species[16,17,39–42], including rhesus monkeys[37,40], cynomolgus monkeys, pigtail monkeys, bonnet monkeys, green monkeys, baboons[29,33], langurs, capuchins, spider monkeys[40], howler monkeys, woolly monkeys, marmosets[8], gibbons, orangutans, and chimpanzees[20,34,42]. This organism is apparently common in Old World monkeys but uncommon or rare in New World monkeys obtained from their natural habitat[17]. Although the infection rate in nature is often low, it can increase rapidly in the laboratory and persist for an extended period[42].

Life Cycle. Reproduction is by binary fission[9]. The amoeba becomes round and small before encysting. A cyst wall is produced, and the nucleus divides twice, producing four small nuclei. Nuclei emerge from the cyst and divide, and the organism separates into eight minute amoebas, each of which grows into a trophozoite. Transmission is by ingestion of cysts passed in the feces of chronic carriers. Hosts with dysentery only pass trophozoites and are not important sources of infection.

Pathologic Effects. Pathologic effects include chronic, mild colitis, characterized by congestion, petechial hemorrhages, and ulcers[37,42,43,44,45]. Trophozoites initially invade

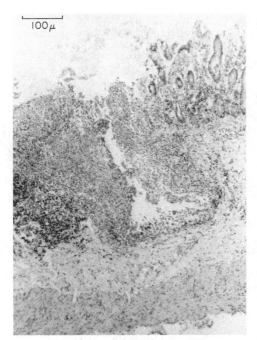

Fig. 21.4 *Entamoeba histolytica* infection in a capuchin. Typical bottle- or flask-shaped intestinal ulcer. Reproduced from Vickers, J.H. (1969) with permission.

the mucosa and form small colonies. These colonies then extend into the submucosa and occasionally the muscularis. They produce typical bottle- or flask-shaped ulcers (Figure 21.4)[46] that range in size from a few millimeters to large, confluent lesions involving wide areas of the colon. Trophozoites are present in and adjacent to the ulcers but tissue reaction is minimal in the absence of secondary bacterial invasion. Trophozoites sometimes enter the lymphatics but are generally filtered out in the lymph nodes. Occasionally trophozoites enter the mesenteric venules and are carried to the liver, lungs, brain, and other organs, where they cause abscesses which may reach several centimeters in diameter.

Clinical Disease. In most cases, infection with *E. histolytica* causes few if any clinical signs of disease. However, strains differ in virulence. Other variables affecting pathogenicity include the species and nutritional status of the host, environmental factors, and the enteric bacterial flora. New World monkeys are more susceptible to developing clinical disease than Old World monkeys[17]. The most common clinical sign is diarrhea, which may be hemorrhagic[9,40,42].

Diagnosis. Diagnosis is made by microscopic identification of the organism in the feces or from ulcers[9]. Commercially available ELISA tests are often the best approach in the absence of trained microscopists[47,48]. For example, the ProspecT© microplate assay kit (Remel, Inc., Lenexa, KS) gives very satisfactory results. Because *E. histolytica* is common and often minimally pathogenic in NHP, other possible causes of enteritis must be considered. It is important to differentiate *E. histolytica* from nonpathogenic amoebae.

Treatment and Prevention. Infections can be treated with metronidazole. Sanitation is important in the prevention of amoebiasis. Trophozoites are readily destroyed with common disinfectants, but cysts are more resistant, and hot water or steam is required to kill them[49,50]. Because *E. histolytica* is common in primates, all animals in a colony should be examined periodically. New animals should be quarantined for at least two months, and they should be examined several times during this period. Infected animals should be treated whether or not they show signs of disease.

Public Health Considerations. *Entamoeba histolytica* causes amoebic dysentery, a serious human disease. Because of the high incidence of *E. histolytica* in nonhuman primates, all NHP should be considered infected and handled with care. Humans have acquired the pathogen from laboratory primates, and animal technicians and caretakers who work with primates obtained from their natural environment are at greater risk of infection.

Iodamoeba butschlii

Iodamoeba butschlii is common in the cecum and colon of rhesus monkeys, cynomolgus monkeys, other macaques, green monkeys, other guenons, mangabeys, mandrills, baboons, capuchins, chimpanzees, gorillas, and humans throughout the world[9,16,20–22]. Infections are also common in laboratory primates obtained from their natural habitat. The incidence of this apparently harmless commensal at the Tulane National Primate Research Center is 6% according to the most recent survey. Trophozoites measure 4 μ to 20 μ long (usually 9 μ to 14 μ) while cysts measure 5 μ to 14 μ long (usually 8 μ to 10 μ) (Figure 21.3).

Phylum Apicomplexa

Class Piroplasmidia

Entopolypoides macaci

Entopolypoides macaci is a *Babesia*-like piroplasm that is found in the erythrocytes of several species of monkeys and baboons[51]. Early forms appear as fine rings with a large vacuole but later stages include appliqué forms and Maltese cross forms similar to *Babesia*. In susceptible animals the parasite produces prolonged and intense parasitemia but does not seem to be pathogenic beyond a mild anemia. Susceptible NHP include guenons, patas monkeys, baboons, and some macaque species. Other macaques, capuchins, owl monkeys, and chimpanzees are refractory to experimental blood inoculation. The vector is unknown. Recent evidence based on rRNA suggests that *Entopolypoides* may be synonymous with *Babesia*[52]. This conclusion is also consistent with the variation seen in the prepatent period and course of infection in different hosts. Treatment with 4 aminoquinolines (chloroquine) is not effective; however primaquine (4 mg/kg for three days) appears to be effective. It is unknown whether humans are susceptible to infection with *E. macaci*.

Class Haemosporidia

Hepatocystis kochi

Hepatocystis kochi is largely confined to arboreal mammals of the Old World tropics and is apparently absent from New World species. *Hepatocystis kochi* is common in African green monkeys, whereas oriental monkeys harbor *H. semnopitheci*. The genus is characterized by having only circulating gametocytes (Figure 21.5) and many assume it is a more primitive ancestor of *Plasmodium*[53]. The liver stage (merocyst) is macroscopic and not easily overlooked at necropsy. When the merozoites burst from the merocyst a portion invade red cells and a small percentage reinvade the liver parenchyma to continue a cycle of pre-erythrocytic schizogony, resulting in multifocal hepatic lesions (Figure 21.6). *Hepatocystis kochi* appears to be nonpathogenic for the NHP host.

The vector is a gnat of the genus *Culicoides*. The prepatent period is two months and erythrocytic rings require four days to mature to gametocytes, which live approximately a month in the peripheral blood. Para-

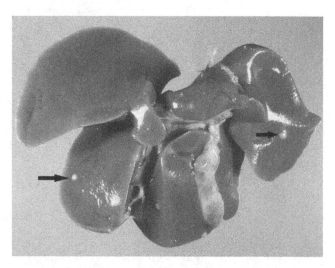

Fig. 21.6   *Hepatocystis kochi* (arrows) in the liver of an African green monkey (*Cercopithecus aethiops*). Courtesy of Dr. Peter Didier.

sitemia may reach high levels (220,000/ml of blood), although animals appear to tolerate the infection well with no signs of disease.

Plasmodium inui

Morphology. *Plasmodium inui* appears as early ring forms (trophozoites) with a single large nucleus. Stippling (similar to Zeimann's stippling) is evident as the trophozoites grow, and band forms, similar to those of *P. malariae,* are often seen. Schizonts appear after 48 hours and the merozoites number up to 18 with 12 being the usual number. The macrogametocyte stains light blue and pigment is evident. The microgametocyte is reddish purple with a prominent nucleus on Giemsa staining. The pre-erythrocytic forms have been described[54].

Hosts. The natural hosts of *P. inui* include macaques, Celebes black apes (*Cynopithecus niger*), and langurs (*Presbytis* sp.). Essentially all primate species normally found in Southeast Asia are susceptible to infection.

Life Cycle. *Plasmodium inui* is a quartan malarial parasite with a 72-hour asexual cycle in the circulating blood. Mosquito species in the United States, including *Anopheles quadrimaculatus,* are suitable intermediate hosts.

Pathologic Effects and Clinical Disease. Pathologic effects are limited to mild anemia. Thus, clinical signs are typically absent, though immunocompromised animals may be more severely affected.

Diagnosis. Parasites may appear in the blood in response to the stress of capture or shipping[55]. Definitive diagnosis is by evaluation of thick and thin Giemsa-stained

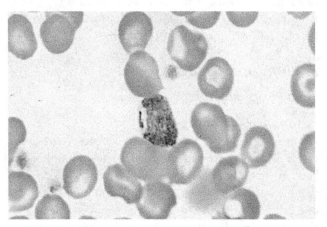

Fig. 21.5   *Hepatocystis kochi* in the blood of a monkey.

blood smears. Dipstick tests that detect circulating antigens may be useful but suffer from cross reactivity with other *Plasmodium* sp. PCR can be used to type isolates and is equivalent in sensitivity to thick blood smears. Nested PCR can also be used if necessary.

Treatment and Prevention. Infected animals should be treated with chloroquine phosphate (7 mg/kg for five days), which can be given orally or intramuscularly. Oral administration of mefloquine is also effective (20 mg/kg, one treatment). Incoming animals should be evaluated prior to release into the animal colony.

Public Health Considerations. Humans may become infected with *P. inui*.

Plasmodium sp.

At least 20 species of *Plasmodium* have been identified in lemurs, monkeys and apes, in addition to the four species which normally parasitize humans (*P. vivax, P. falciparum, P. ovale, P. malariae*) and which have been shown to infect some primate species[56]. Determination of *Plasmodium* species is best accomplished with full color plates and descriptions of each stage of the parasite. Life cycles are similar to those of *Plasmodium* sp. found in non-human primates.

PHYLUM MICROSPORA

Microsporidia are single-celled, obligate intracellular fungi. Fifteen species are known to infect mammals, including NHP. Although they have been recently reclassified as fungi, they are included in this text for historical reasons. *Encephalitozoon cuniculi* and *Enterocytozoon bieneusi* have been reported from NHP[57]. The infections are often clinically silent, and chronic in immunocompetent hosts. *Enterocytozoon bieneusi* primarily infects the gall bladder and biliary tract in rhesus macaques. Lesions include biliary epithelial hyperplasia and periportal fibrosis. The infection may be more disseminated in immunocompromised animals[58]. Diagnosis is by identifying the organism in urine, stool, or respiratory secretions with modified trichrome stains. Treatment options are few. Drugs used to treat human infections include albendazole or fumagillin, an antibiotic and anti-angiogenic derived from *Aspergillus*.

PHYLUM CILIOPHORA

Balantidium coli

Morphology, Hosts, and Life Cycle. The morphology of *Balantidium coli* (Syn. *Balantidium aragaoi, B. cunhamunizi,*

B. philippinensis, B. rhesum, B. simile, B. suis, B. wenrichi) is described in Chapter 19, Parasites of Swine. *Balantidium coli* is common in the cecum and colon of many species of NHP including rhesus monkeys, cynomolgus monkeys, spider monkeys, howler monkeys, capuchins, baboons, orangutans, chimpanzees, and gorillas[3,20–22,34,43]. Infections are common in laboratory primates and incidences as high as 14% and 84% have been reported in captive rhesus monkeys and chimpanzees, respectively[10]. The life cycle is described in Chapter 19, Parasites of Swine.

Pathologic Effects and Clinical Disease. *Balantidium coli* is not normally considered a primary pathogen[59] but may appear as a secondary invader of lesions initiated by pathogenic bacteria or viruses. When *B. coli* serves as a primary pathogen infection is associated with diarrhea and ulcerative enteritis (Figure 21.7). Ulcers may extend to the muscularis mucosae and be accompanied by lymphocytic infiltration and occasionally coagulation necrosis and hemorrhage. Organisms often occur in groups in the tissues or in the capillaries, lymphatics, and regional lymph nodes.

Diagnosis, Treatment, and Prevention. Diagnosis is by identifying the organism in characteristic lesions. The presence of concomitant pathogenic microorganisms must be considered. Treatment consists of oral metronidazole or oxytetracycline. Sanitation prevents infection, and the elimination of starches from the diet controls the infection by removing an important source of nutrients for the organism. Good nutrition and the routine treatment of newly arrived asymptomatic carriers are recommended[17].

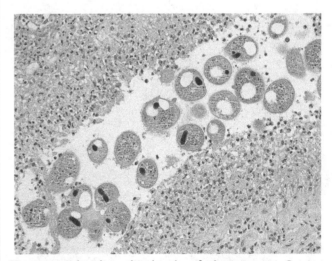

Fig. 21.7 *Balantidium coli* in the colon of a rhesus macaque. Courtesy of Dr. Peter Didier.

Public Health Considerations. Animal workers are susceptible to infection with *B. coli*. Thus, primate care personnel should practice excellent personal hygiene. Immune-compromised people suffer more severe infections, and therefore should not work with infected primates.

Troglodytella abrassarti

Morphology. *Troglodytella abrassarti* trophozoites are ellipsoidal and flattened and measure 145 μ to 174 μ long by 87 μ to 126 μ wide[60,61] (Figure 21.8). Trophozoites possess three zones of membranelles, or cirri, and an adoral zone. The zones of cirri are arranged in incomplete circlets, which give the impression that they would form a spiral if they were continuous. There is a continuous or noncontinuous anterior zone on the ventral surface, a continuous posterior zone on the dorsal surface, and a small zone between them on each side. There are skeletal plates beneath the surface in the anterior region. The macronucleus is L-shaped, and there are about eight contractile vacuoles arranged in two circles or parallel to the bands of cirri.

Hosts and Life Cycle. *Troglodytella abrassarti* occurs in the cecum and colon of the chimpanzee in central Africa and has been reported in laboratory chimps newly imported into the United States[34]. Infections are more common in recently captured chimpanzees than in those maintained in captivity. The life cycle has not been described but is presumed to be direct.

Pathologic Effects and Clinical Disease. *Troglodytella abrassarti* is usually considered nonpathogenic, but it has been cited as a possible cause of colitis in chimpanzees[62].

Diagnosis, Treatment, and Prevention. Tentative diagnosis is made by identifying the organism in the feces or colon in association with colitis. Because T. *abrassarti* is probably nonpathogenic, it is important to investigate other possible causes of colitis. No control or treatment measures have been reported.

Public Health Considerations. *Troglodytella abrassarti* is of no known public health importance.

TREMATODES

Athesmia foxi

Morphology. Adult flukes are long and slender, measuring about 8.5 mm long by 0.7 mm wide (Figure 21.9). The egg is ovoid and golden brown, has a thick shell and operculum, and measures 27 μ to 34 μ long by 17 μ to 21 μ wide[63].

Hosts and Life Cycle. *Athesmia foxi* occurs in the bile duct of capuchins, squirrel monkeys, tamarins, and titi monkeys of northern South America, and in a wild rat (*Rattus argentiventer*) in the Malay Peninsula[63]. Infections are common in laboratory primates obtained from South America. Incidences of 43% in 16 capuchins[64] and 8% in 455 tamarins

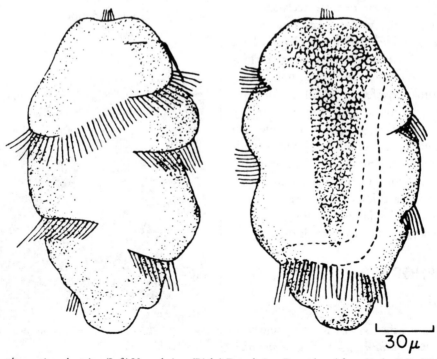

30μ

Fig. 21.8 *Troglodytella abrassarti* trophozoite. (Left) Ventral view. (Right) Dorsal view. Reproduced from Kudo, R.R. (1966) with permission.

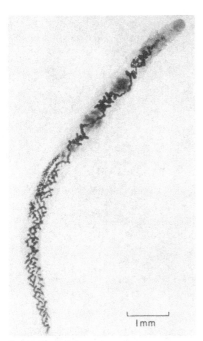

Fig. 21.9 *Athesmia foxi* adult.

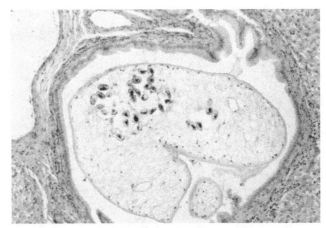

Fig. 21.10 *Athesmia foxi* in the bile duct of a monkey.

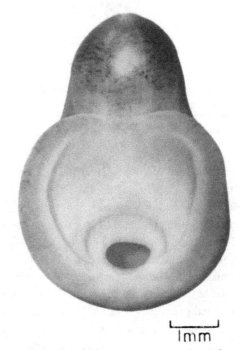

Fig. 21.11 *Gastrodiscoides hominis* adult. Reproduced from Graham, G.L. (1960) with permission.

have been reported[65]. The life cycle is not completely known, but is known to include a mollusk intermediate host.

Pathologic Effects and Clinical Disease. Heavy infections with *A. foxi* occur[17] and cause enlargement and partial obstruction of the bile duct (Figure 21.10). The epithelial lining is inflamed and may become necrotic[64].

Diagnosis, Treatment, and Prevention. Diagnosis is by demonstrating adult flukes in the bile duct at necropsy, or by demonstrating the eggs in the feces. Because of the need for an intermediate host, transmission in the laboratory cannot occur and no special control procedures are required. No treatment is reported.

Public Health Considerations. *Athesmia foxi* has not been reported from humans. Because of the need for an intermediate mollusk host, infected laboratory animals are not a direct hazard to humans.

Gastrodiscoides hominis

Gastrodiscoides hominis occurs in the cecum and colon of cynomolgus monkeys, pigs, and humans in India, Southeast Asia, Indonesia, and the Philippine Islands[66,67]. In the past, infections were common in laboratory monkeys[68]. In one survey, 21.4% of roughly 1,200 cynomolgus monkeys were found to be infected[64]. The adult is a small orange-red fluke (Figure 21.11)[67,68,69,70]. Adult flukes measure 6 mm long by 3 mm wide and have a cuplike discoidal hind body, a cone-shaped anterior end, and a small anterior sucker. The egg is operculated and spindle-shaped, has bluntly rounded ends, measures 150 μ to 152 μ long by 60 μ to 72 μ wide, and is unembryonated when passed[66] (Figure 21.12). *Gastrodiscoides hominis* usually occurs in large numbers in infected animals[66] (Figure 21.13), and causes mucous diarrhea and mild, chronic enteritis[66]. Diagnosis is based on demonstration of the eggs in the feces or adult flukes in the cecum and colon.

Schistosoma sp.

Morphology. Schistosomes typically occur in pairs with the long, slender female residing within the sex canal of the

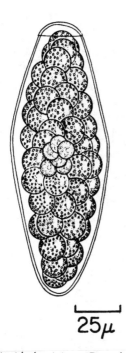

Fig. 21.12 *Gastrodiscoides hominis* egg. Reproduced from Faust, E.C. (1949) with permission.

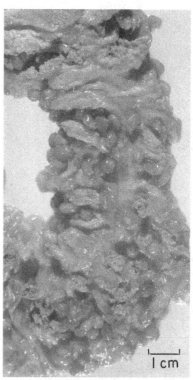

Fig. 21.13 *Gastrodiscoides hominis* adults in the colon of a monkey. Reproduced from Whitney, R.A., Johnson, D.J., and Cole, W.C. (1967) with permission.

short, muscular male[66] (Figure 21.14). The male of *Schistosoma japonicum* measures 12 mm to 20 mm long by 0.5 mm wide. Female flukes measure 15 mm to 30 mm long by 0.1 mm to 0.3 mm wide. The egg is spineless, rotund, 70 μ to 100 μ long by 50 μ to 65 μ wide, and fully embryonated when passed in the feces (Figure 21.15).

The male of *S. mansoni* measures 6.4 mm to 9.9 mm long and the female measures 7.2 mm to 14 mm long. The egg is elongated to ovoid, measures 114 μ to 175 μ long by 45 μ to 68 μ wide, is rounded at both ends, has a lateral spine (Figure 21.15), and is fully embryonated when passed in the feces.

The male of *S. haematobium* measures 10 mm to 15 mm long and about 1 mm in diameter. The female measures 20 mm long by 0.25 mm wide. The egg is elongated to ovoid, measures 112 μ to 117 μ long by 40 μ to 70 μ wide, is rounded at the anterior end, has a posterior terminal spine (Figure 21.15), and is fully embryonated when passed.

Hosts. *Schistosoma mansoni* occurs in the mesenteric veins of squirrel monkeys, guenons, baboons, and humans in the West Indies, South America, and Africa[71-73]. Infections are common in baboons obtained from their natural habitat but rare in squirrel monkeys and guenons.

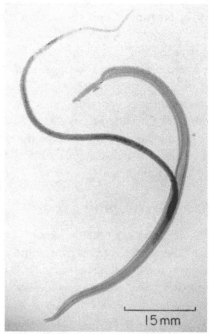

Fig. 21.14 *Schistosoma mansoni* male and female. Courtesy of Marietta Voge, University of California.

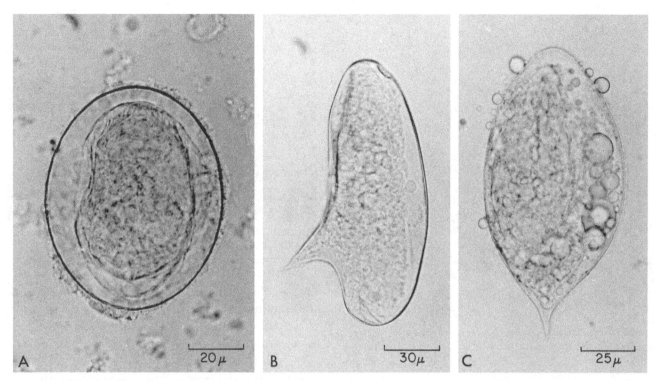

Fig. 21.15 *Schistosoma* eggs. (A) *S. japonicum.* (B) *S. mansoni.* (C) *S. haematobium.* Courtesy of Marietta Voge, University of California.

Schistosoma haematobium occurs in the pelvic and mesenteric veins of guenons, baboons, chimpanzees, and humans in southern Europe, Africa, and western Asia[66,72,74]. Infections are common in baboons obtained from their natural habitat but rare in guenons and chimps. *Schistosoma japonicum* has been reported from *Macaca fasicularis* and *M. fasicularis phillippinensis.* Although all three species of *Schistosoma* are serious pathogens for humans[66], they are of little importance in laboratory animals and are usually observed only at necropsy.

Life Cycle. The life cycles for all three species of *Schistosoma* are similar. Eggs are excreted by the host in the feces (*S. japonicum, S. mansoni*) or in the urine (*S. haematobium*). Eggs hatch in water and the released miracidia penetrate snails, in which they develop into cercariae before emerging into the surrounding water. Infection of the endothermal host occurs by skin penetration of the cercariae and possibly by ingestion of contaminated water. The cercariae develop while migrating through the tissues and eventually reach the mesenteric or pelvic vessels as young worms. The complete life cycle requires eight to 12 weeks; adult worms sometimes live for 20 to 30 years.

Pathologic Effects and Clinical Disease. The principal effects are caused by the eggs[66]. Adult flukes in the mesenteric vessels deposit their eggs in the venules of the intestine; those in the pelvic vessels deposit their eggs in the venules of the urinary bladder[74]. Some eggs escape from the venules, filter through the intestinal and bladder walls, and eventually break through into the lumen. Other eggs enter the circulation as emboli. These become lodged in various tissues where they often cause severe foreign-body reactions. Granulomas also occur in the liver, brain, spleen, and other organs[75] (Figure 21.16). Clinical signs include pyrexia, hemorrhagic diarrhea or hematuria, and ascites.

Diagnosis, Treatment, and Prevention. Diagnosis is by demonstrating eggs in the feces or urine, or adult worms in the blood vessels at necropsy. Kato-Katz fecal smears as well as formalin-ether sedimentation can aid diagnosis of intestinal schistosomes. Syringe filtration methods for urine are less than satisfactory and sedimentation flasks using a volume of urine are preferred. PCR may be of some use, although the number of eggs shed in a given infection usually makes diagnosis relatively straightforward. Natural transmission cannot occur in the laboratory; therefore no special control procedures are required. Treatment consists of oral administration of praziquantel.

Public Health Considerations. Although schistosomiasis is one of the most important diseases of humans,

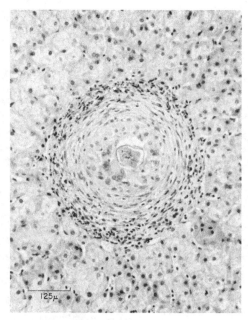

Fig. 21.16 *Schistosoma mansoni* egg in the liver tissue of an experimentally infected chimpanzee. Reproduced from Sadun, E.H., von Lichtenberg, F., Hickman, R.L., Bruce, J.I., Smith, J.H., and Schoenbechler, M.J. (1966) with permission.

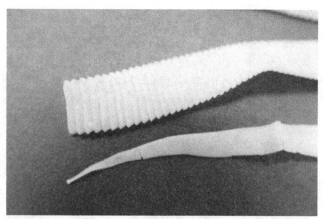

Fig. 21.17 *Bertiella studeri* from a rhesus macaque. Courtesy of Maury Duplantis.

infected laboratory animals are not a direct hazard for animal workers because of the requirement for an intermediate host. However, because of the importance of this disease in humans, excreta from infected animals should be decontaminated before being discarded.

CESTODES

Bertiella studeri

Morphology. Adult *Bertiella studeri* (Syn. *Bertiella cercopitheci, B. conferta, B. satyri, Bertia polyorchis*) measure 10 cm to 30 cm long by 1 cm wide[76]. The scolex is devoid of hooks. The segments are about eight times wider than they are long (Figure 21.17) and contain only one set of male and female reproductive organs. Gravid proglottids are filled with eggs enclosed in a sac-like uterus. Eggs are thin-shelled, measure 38 μ to 45 μ in diameter, and contain an embryo which is surrounded by a pyriform inner shell with a bicornate protrusion.

Hosts and Life Cycle. *Bertiella studeri* is a cyclophyllidean tapeworm known to occur in the small intestine of rhesus monkeys, cynomolgus monkeys, Japanese macaques, guenons, mandrills, baboons, gibbons, chim-

panzees, orangutans, and humans in Africa and Asia. Laboratory primates obtained from the wild are frequently infected. Typical incidences are 3.6% to 14% in the rhesus monkey[77], 1.4% to 5.3% in the cynomolgus monkey[78], 7.1% in the Japanese macaque[79], and 7.7% in baboons[33]. Eggs passed in the feces are ingested by various free-living oribatid mites[76]. The larva develops in the mite, and the vertebrate host becomes infected by accidentally ingesting an infected mite with vegetation.

Pathologic Effects and Clinical Disease. *Bertiella studeri* causes no apparent clinical signs or lesions.

Diagnosis, Treatment, and Prevention. Infections are most often diagnosed by observing worms in the stool. Treatment is generally not warranted. Preventing exposure to intermediate hosts prevents the pathogen from establishing in the animal colony.

Public Health Considerations. *Bertiella studeri* infects humans but should not be a hazard in animal colonies, provided that the intermediate host is excluded.

LEECHES

Dinobdella ferox

Morphology. *Dinobdella ferox* measures 3.5 cm to 6.0 cm long and 0.5 to 0.8 cm wide[80,81] (Figure 21.18). Like other leeches, *D. ferox* has a dorsoventrally flattened body which is dark red when engorged[80,81].

Hosts. This leech is widespread in southern Asia, where it frequently invades the pharynx of ruminants and occasionally the upper respiratory tract of dogs, monkeys, and humans. *Dinobdella ferox* may be a common inhabitant of the nasal cavities of macaques obtained from their

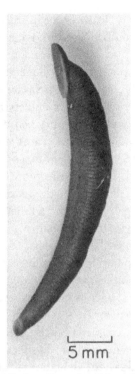

Fig. 21.18 *Dinobdella ferox.* Reproduced from Pryor, W.H., Bergner, J.F. Jr., and Raulston, G.L. (1970) with permission.

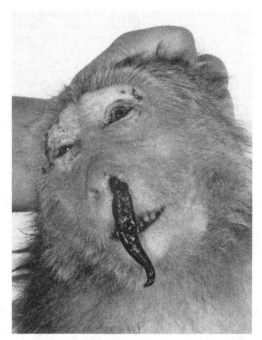

Fig. 21.19 *Dinobdella ferox* extending from the nares of a Formosan macaque. Reproduced from Pryor, W.H., Bergner, J.F. Jr., and Raulston, G.L. (1970) with permission.

natural habitat[80,81]. Incidence rates of 4% to 6% have been observed in laboratory macaques[82]. Laboratory monkeys obtained from endemic areas, particularly Taiwan, are likely to be infected.

Life Cycle. The life cycle is similar to that of *Limnatis nilotica,* which is described in Chapter 17, Parasites of Dogs. Primates often become infected while drinking. Leeches attach to the mucosa of the upper respiratory tract or pharynx, suck blood, and remain attached for weeks[82] or months[80] until mature.

Pathologic Effects and Clinical Disease. Infection with one or two parasites usually produces few signs, but severe infection causes restlessness, epistaxis, anemia, weakness, asphyxiation, and sometimes death[82]. Lesions consist of mild, localized, chronic inflammation of the nasopharyngeal mucosa with increased mucus production.

Diagnosis, Treatment, and Prevention. Diagnosis is based on recognition of the leech. Infection in macaques is most easily detected by examining the host's nares with a flashlight[82]. When the monkey is initially handled, the parasite withdraws from view, but it will reappear if the host is held quietly[82] (Figure 21.19). Newly acquired animals from endemic areas should be examined on arrival and treated if infected. The leech is usually removable by

gentle traction with forceps[82]. If forceps alone are insufficient, spraying the leech lightly with an insecticide is often helpful.

Public Health Considerations. Although *D. ferox* readily feeds upon humans, exposure under laboratory conditions is unlikely. However, care should be taken when removing leeches from affected animals.

NEMATODES

Superfamily Rhabditoidea

Strongyloides cebus

Morphology. The parasitic female worm is filiform, measures 2 mm to 5 mm long by 30 μ to 80 μ wide, and has a short pointed tail, a small buccal capsule, and a narrow cylindrical esophagus that extends a quarter of the length of the worm. The vulva, which is in the posterior third of the body, opens into opposed uteri with reflexed ovaries. Parasitic males have not been observed. The egg measures 40 μ to 70 μ long by 20 μ to 35 μ wide (Figure 21.20). Eggs are thin-shelled, transparent, and embryonated when passed by the female worm, and they hatch while in transit within the intestine. The first-stage rhabditiform larvae

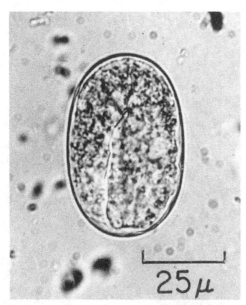

Fig. 21.20 *Strongyloides fülleborni* egg. Reproduced from Tanaka, H., Fukui, M., Yamamoto, H., Hayama, S., and Kodera, S. (1962) with permission.

measure 150 μ to 390 μ long when passed in the feces but grow rapidly to 800 μ long. Larvae have a short, muscular esophagus that ends in a valved bulb preceded by a constriction.

Hosts. *Strongyloides cebus* occurs in monkeys in Central and South America. Infections are common in squirrel monkeys, woolly monkeys, capuchins, and spider monkeys[83].

Life Cycle. Soil-dwelling adults may continue through successive free-living generations before initiating an infective larval stage, which enters a suitable host via penetration of the host's skin or oral mucosa. Larvae migrate through the bloodstream to the heart and lungs, pass up the trachea to the mouth, and are swallowed to establish infection with adult parthenogenic female worms in the duodenum and jejunum. Re-infection by rapidly molting larvae passing through the intestines increases worm burdens significantly (hyperinfection). Modification of this pattern of infection, termed autoinfection, occurs when third-stage infective larvae pass through the anus and penetrate the perianal or perineal skin. Both of the latter routes involve blood-borne migration via the portal system to the liver, heart, and lung, and then air duct passage to the mouth, followed by the intestinal phase.

Pathologic Effects and Clinical Disease. Infection is usually mild or unapparent but sometimes it is severe, especially in debilitated, caged primates. When present,

pathologic effects typically occur in three distinct phases, each with characteristic signs and lesions: the invasion phase, migratory phase, and intestinal phase[84].

The invasion phase occurs when infective larvae penetrate the skin or buccal mucosa. Invasion may be accompanied by local irritation, pruritus, and erythema.

The migratory phase occurs when infective larvae are carried by the venous circulation to the heart and lungs, break into the alveoli, enter the bronchi, and are coughed up and swallowed. In mild infections this phase usually produces only a sporadic cough. In massive infections, especially in young or debilitated animals, larval migration produces an acute local inflammatory reaction around the affected alveoli, as well as occasional bronchopneumonia, pericarditis, pulmonary hemorrhaging, and death[17,85].

During the intestinal phase, worms penetrate the intestinal crypts and burrow into the glandular epithelium. Often the intestinal mucosa is riddled with worms. The intestinal phase is characterized by diarrhea, which may become hemorrhagic and/or chronic[17]. Other clinical signs include listlessness, debilitation, anorexia, emaciation, reduced growth rate, and sometimes prostration and death[17,84]. Lesions observed at necropsy are those of an acute enteritis, sometimes hemorrhagic and necrotic[84], and are occasionally accompanied by secondary peritonitis and eosinophilia and increased lymphoid tissue in the jejunum.

Diagnosis. Diagnosis is based on clinical signs and identification of the eggs or larvae in the feces, using either a direct smear or $ZnSo_4$ flotation. If the fecal specimen is contaminated with soil, one must be careful to differentiate *Strongyloides* larvae from free-living larvae[67]. Adult worms may also be observed at necropsy. They are usually confined to the anterior small intestinal epithelium and are thin, transparent, and difficult to see.

Treatment and Prevention. Sanitation and management are the primary methods of control. Because first-stage larvae passed in the feces can develop into third-stage infective larvae within 48 hours, it is important that feces be removed daily and that food and water be kept free of contamination[34,86]. Particular care must be taken to prevent the free-living stages from reproducing in cages. Because moisture is essential to the survival of larvae, keeping surfaces dry greatly aids in controlling this parasite. Newly acquired primates should be examined on arrival and treated if infected. Infections may be effectively treated with ivermectin (400 μg/kg IM) diluted in sterile propylene glycol. Alternatively, moxidectin (500 μg/kg) can be applied topically and may offer some advantages over ivermectin[87].

Public Health Considerations. *Strongyloides cebus* is not known to infect humans.

Strongyloides fülleborni

Morphology. *Strongyloides fülleborni* is morphologically similar to *S. cebus.*

Hosts. *Strongyloides fülleborni* is found in macaques, guenons, baboons, chimpanzees, and occasionally, humans in Africa and Asia. Infections are common in rhesus monkeys[16,30,43,88], cynomolgus monkeys[16,88,89], chimpanzees[34], and other laboratory primates[17]. At one time, approximately 23% of captive primates housed at Tulane National Primate Research Center were infected with *S. fülleborni*[10].

Life Cycle. The life cycle is as described for *S. cebus.* In addition to larval penetration of the skin or intestinal mucosa, *S. fülleborni* may also be transmitted via placental or colostral transfer. Evidence for prenatal or early post-gestational transmission consists of unpublished reports that 75% of nursing infants at the California National Primate Research Center excreted *S. fülleborni* ova, while only 16% of their mothers were found to be shedding ova in their feces. In fact, the youngest monkeys found positive were only 12 days old. Interestingly, transmission of *S. fülleborni* by mothers' milk has been shown in humans in Africa[90].

Pathologic Effects and Clinical Disease. The pathologic effects and clinical disease are similar to those described for *S. cebus.* In young, debilitated or malnourished primates subject to massive infection and re-infection with *S. fülleborni,* mortality is sometimes high[67].

Diagnosis, Treatment, and Prevention. These aspects are similar to those described for *S. cebus.*

Public Health Considerations. *Strongyloides fülleborni* may be transmitted from monkeys and chimpanzees to humans[17]. Animal care personnel should be alerted to this risk and instructed in proper personal hygiene and safe methods of handling infected animals and excrement.

Superfamily Oxyuroidea

Enterobius vermicularis

Morphology. Adult male *Enterobius vermicularis* measures 2 mm to 5 mm long by 0.1 mm to 0.2 mm wide. Adult female worms measure 8 mm to 13 mm long by 0.3 mm to 0.5 mm wide and are frequently laden with eggs. Eggs are slightly flattened on one side and measure 50 μ to 60 μ long by 20 μ to 30 μ wide[91] (Figure 21.21).

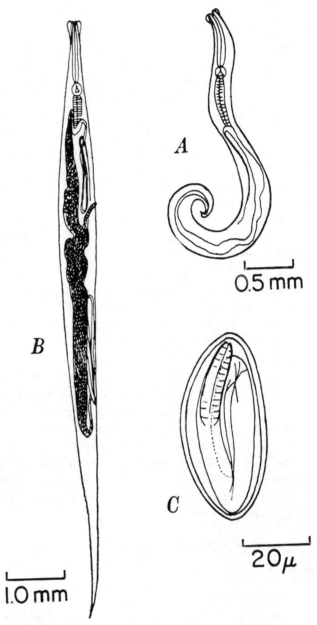

Fig. 21.21 *Enterobius vermicularis* (A) Male. (B) Female. (C) Embryonated egg. Reproduced from Little, M.D.(1966) with permission.

Hosts. *Enterobius vermicularis* is the common pinworm of humans, but also readily infects captive chimpanzees, gibbons, and marmosets[17]. Wild NHP are rarely infected, but may become infected in captivity[17,78]. Cross infection between simian primates and humans occurs readily in captivity[17], but in nature, each genus of primate probably has its own species of parasite[92].

Life Cycle. The life cycle is direct[66]. Eggs are deposited by the adult female in the perianal or perineal region and contain fully developed larvae within six hours. Infection is by ingestion of infective eggs. The eggs hatch in the small intestine and reach maturity in the large intestine. The complete life cycle requires 15 to 28 days. In humans, aberrant migration of worms may result in worms in the appendix or ovary.

Pathologic Effects and Clinical Disease. Infection is associated with perianal pruritus, restlessness, and increased aggressiveness[93]. Enteric pathology is rare, even with heavy infections.

Diagnosis, Treatment, and Prevention. Diagnosis is usually made by demonstrating adult worms emerging from the anus or by identifying eggs recovered from the perianal region[66]. Many biological supply houses (Trend, Inc.) sell sticky paddles for pinworm diagnosis in children and these are similarly useful for sampling NHP. Control is difficult, owing to deposition of large numbers of infective eggs on the host skin and the absence of an immune response which permits repeated autoinfection or cross infection. Control may be accomplished only by extreme measures of sanitation and mass treatment of all animals in a colony at the same time, or by initiating a new colony by Caesarean rederivation. Treatment of simian primates with ivermectin has been reported to be effective.

Public Health Considerations. Not only are naturally infected primates potential sources of human infection, captive primates can acquire *E. vermicularis* from animal workers.

Superfamily Strongyloidea

Oesophagostomum sp.

Morphology. Primates are susceptible to infection with multiple species of *Oesophagostomum,* or "nodular" worms. Adult *O. apiostomum* measure 8 mm to 10.5 mm long by 0.2 mm to 0.3 mm wide[86]. The eggs of *Oesophagostomum* are typical strongyle-type eggs. Eggs of *O. apiostomum* measure 60 μ to 63 μ long by 27 μ to 40 μ wide, while eggs of *O. aculeatum* measure 69 μ to 86 μ long by 35 μ to 55 μ wide (Figure 21.22)[79,86].

Hosts. *Oesophagostomum* is the most common nematode of Old World monkeys and apes[17]. Infections occur in macaques, guenons, mangabeys, baboons, chimpanzees, and gorillas. Humans are also susceptible. Infection with *O. apiostomum* is considered most common[17], but accurate information on incidence rates and geographic distribution

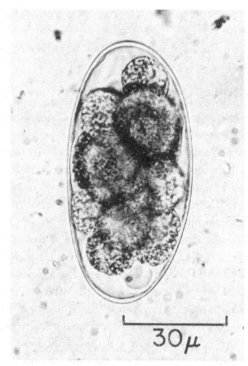

Fig. 21.22 *Oesophagostomum aculeatum* egg. Reproduced from Tanaka, H., Fukui, M., Yamamoto, H., Hayama, S., and Kodera, S. (1962) with permission.

of the various species is lacking because identification often ends at the genus level[66]. *Oesophagostomum bifurcatum* is common in Africa and Asia, and incidence rates of 33% to 55% have been reported in rhesus monkeys recently imported into the United States[67]. *Oesophagostomum aculeatum* has been found in 28% to 62% of Japanese macaques and cynomolgus monkeys[78,79]. An unidentified species was found in 45% of chimpanzees recently imported into the United States from Africa[34], where *O. bifurcatum* and *O. stephanostomum* are common[66].

Life Cycle. Eggs are usually in an early division stage when passed in the feces and, under favorable conditions, hatch in 24 to 48 hours. Infection is by ingestion of an infective larva[66]. The larva passes directly to the colon, penetrates deeply into the mucosa, and induces the development of a large, firm, encapsulated nodule. No visceral migration occurs. The nodule ruptures in five to eight days, and the worm escapes into the lumen and matures.

Pathologic Effects and Clinical Disease. Intestinal nodules measure 2 mm to 4 mm in diameter and may appear white, or black if hemorrhage has occurred within the nodule. Occasionally an ulcer is seen in the intestinal mucosa with an irregular fistulous tract leading to a nodule in the muscularis mucosa[86,88]. Nodules in which the worm is permanently encapsulated because of an immune response by the host have caseous and often calcified centers[86]. Heavy infections may result in formation of fibrous adhesions which may cause obstruction or ascites[17]. Heavily infected animals may develop diarrhea, weight loss, debilitation, and increased mortality[17]. Light infections are usually unapparent.

Diagnosis. A tentative diagnosis is made in the living animal by identification of the eggs in the feces. However, because hookworm and *Oesophagostomum* eggs are similar, a positive identification can be made only by identifying the adult worm in the intestine.

Treatment and Prevention. Sanitation and management, the primary methods of control, rapidly reduce the incidence of infection in a colony[86,94]. Newly acquired primates should be examined on arrival and either treated or eliminated, if infected. Infections may be eliminated with ivermectin (400 μg/kg IM), diluted in sterile propylene glycol. Treatment should be repeated in two weeks.

Public Health Considerations. *Oesophagostomum* sp. has been reported in humans[17,66]. Animal workers should practice excellent personal hygiene when working with infected animals or excreta.

Ternidens diminutus

Ternidens diminutus occurs in the cecum and colon of macaques, guenons, baboons, chimpanzees, gorillas, and humans in Asia and Africa[17,95,96]. Morphologically, the adult worms and eggs resemble those of *Oesophagostomum*[17,79]. The eggs measure 57 μ to 65 μ long by 36 μ to 45 μ wide (Figure 21.23). The life cycle is similar to that of *Oesophagostomum*. Incidences of 60% in green monkeys and 76% in baboons have been reported in southern Africa[97]. Infections are uncommon in laboratory monkeys, with the exception of one older report in which incidence was 21%[67]. Adult worms suck blood and may cause anemia and cystic nodules in the colon wall. Methods of diagnosis and treatment are similar to those of *Oesophagostomum*. Because *T. diminutus* infects humans, animal workers should practice excellent personal hygiene when working with infected animals or excreta.

Superfamily Trichostrongyloidea

Molineus sp.

Morphology. Adult *Molineus* are small, slender, pale red worms[98]. Adult male worms measure 3 mm to 4.8 mm

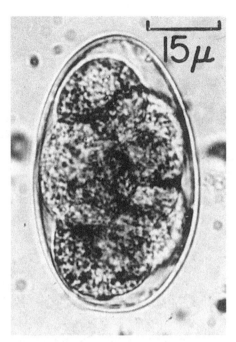

Fig. 21.23 *Ternidens deminutus* egg. Reproduced from Tanaka, H., Fukui, M., Yamamoto, H., Hayama, S., and Kodera, S. (1962) with permission.

long, while adult female worms measure 3.2 mm to 5.3 mm long. The egg is ellipsoidal and measures 40 μ to 52 μ long by 20 μ to 29 μ wide (Figure 21.24).

Hosts and Life Cycle. *Molineus torulosus* occurs in the small intestine of capuchins, squirrel monkeys, and night monkeys in Brazil and *Cebus* spp. from South America[98–101]. Infections are common in capuchins obtained from the wild but absent in those raised in the laboratory. *Molineus vexillarius* occurs in the stomach and small intestine of tamarins in Peru. Infections are common in wild monkeys, with an incidence of 95% reported[65], but absent in laboratory-raised monkeys[102]. *Molineus elegans* occurs in the small intestine of squirrel monkeys and capuchins in Brazil, while *M. vogelianus* is found in pottos (*Perodicticus*) in Africa[98]. The rates of infection with *M. elegans* and *M. vogelianus* are unknown. The life cycle is unknown, but is probably direct, typical of the superfamily. The larvae live and mature in cysts on the small intestine. Adult worms remain permanently encysted. Eggs are laid and make their way to the intestinal lumen through narrow channels.

Pathologic Effects and Clinical Disease. Only *M. torulosus* is pathogenic, causing hemorrhages and necrotic ulcers in the intestinal wall and diverticula[101]. Other *Molineus* spp. are less pathogenic.

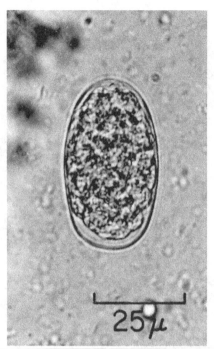

Fig. 21.24 *Molineus vexillarius* egg.

Diagnosis, Treatment, and Prevention. Diagnosis is based on demonstrating eggs in the feces or adult worms in the intestine or stomach at necropsy. Treatment strategies have not been described, but sanitation and good management may be sufficient. Laboratories that have experienced heavy infections in newly acquired specimens report a decline in incidence with time and an absence of the parasite in laboratory-reared specimens[65,102].

Public Health Considerations. *Molineus* is not known to infect humans.

Nochtia nochti

Morphology. Adult *Nochtia nochti* are bright red and filiform[103]. Adult male worms measure 5.7 mm to 6.5 mm long by 100 μ to 140 μ wide, while adult female worms measure 7.6 mm to 9.9 mm long by 150 μ to 170 μ wide. The egg is thin-shelled and ellipsoidal and measures 60 μ to 80 μ long by 35 μ to 42 μ wide.

Hosts. *Nochtia nochti* occurs in the stomach of rhesus, cynomolgus, and stumptail macaques in India, Indonesia, and Thailand[104]. Although frequently unrecognized because of its small size, *N. nochti* was found in 4.9% of 1,200 cynomolgus monkeys[78] and 33% of 48 stumptail macaques[104] examined.

Life Cycle. The life cycle is direct[103]. Eggs laid by the female embryonate in about 12 hours, hatch soon afterward,

and reach the infective larval stage in about five to six days. The method of infection is uncertain but is presumed to be by ingestion of infective larvae.

Pathologic Effects and Clinical Disease. *Nochtia nochti* causes the formation of apparently benign tumors, which appear as hyperemic, cauliflower-like masses protruding from the gastric wall at the junction of the fundus and pylorus (Figure 21.25)[104,105]. Adult worms and eggs may be found deep within each tumor. No worms occur free in the stomach, and no tumors are produced elsewhere.

Diagnosis, Treatment, and Prevention. Diagnosis is based on recognition of gastric tumors containing adult worms. No treatment recommendations are available. It is likely that treatment with avermectins would be curative.

Public Health Considerations. *Nochtia nochti* does not infect humans.

Superfamily Spiruroidea

Streptopharagus sp.

Primates are susceptible to infection with the thelaziid nematodes *Streptopharagus armatus* and *S. pigmentatus*. Adult worms are found in the stomach of monkeys and apes. *Streptopharagus armatus* occurs in macaques, guenons, patas monkeys, baboons, and gibbons in the United States, Japan, and Africa. It is common in the cynomolgus monkey (10.5%) and Japanese macaque (14.3%) but uncommon in the rhesus monkey (0.5%) and other simian primates[79,88]. *Streptopharagus pigmentatus* occurs in macaques, guenons, baboons, and gibbons in the United States, Europe, Africa, and Asia. It is common in

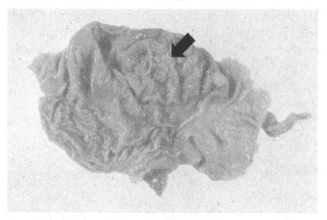

Fig. 21.25 *Nochtia nochti* infection. Cauliflower-like masses (arrow) protruding from the gastric wall of a macaque.

rhesus monkeys (24%) but uncommon in cynomolgus monkeys (3.3%) and other primates[16,67,78]. The eggs are asymmetrical, measure 28 μ to 38 μ long by 17 μ to 22 μ wide, have a thick shell, and are embryonated when passed in the feces (Figure 21.26)[89]. Little is known of the life cycle or pathologic effects of either species.

Superfamily Filaroidea

Morphology. Adult worms are slender and thin in the posterior region and have a smooth or finely striated cuticle[106]. Adult and microfilariae vary in size based on species. Adult male *Dipetalonema marmosetae* measure 39 mm long while *D. gracile* measures 84 mm long. Adult female worms measure 87 mm to 199 mm long. Microfilariae of *D. gracile* measure 130 μ long while those of *D. tamarinae* measure 406 μ to 430 μ long.

Hosts. Several species of filarids may be found in primates. Commonly found species include *Dipetalonema barbascalensis*, *D. caudispina*, *D. gracile*, *D. marmosetae*, and *D. tamarinae*. Adults of these filarial nematodes are frequently found in the peritoneal cavity of Central and South American primates[107]. *Dipetalonema barbascalensis* has been reported from *Aotus*[108]. *Dipetalonema caudispina*

infects capuchins and squirrel monkeys. *Dipetalonema gracile* occurs in capuchins, spider monkeys, woolly monkeys, squirrel monkeys, and marmosets. *Dipetalonema marmosetae* is found in capuchins, spider monkeys, squirrel monkeys, and marmosets. Finally, *D. tamarinae* infects marmosets. All of these parasites are common in laboratory monkeys obtained from the wild[65,102,106,109].

Life Cycle. The life cycles for each of these filarids are indirect. Microfilariae occur in the blood. Development to the infective stage occurs in arthropods, typically mosquitoes. Transmission to the primate definitive host occurs when a mosquito takes a blood meal.

Pathologic Effects and Clinical Disease. The adult worms are usually found lying free in the peritoneal cavity (Figure 21.27)[109,110]. While peritoneal adhesions have been reported in heavy infections, the worms usually cause little or no pathology. Thus, clinical signs are uncommon.

Diagnosis, Treatment, Prevention. Diagnosis is based on demonstration of adult worms in the peritoneal cavity or microfilariae in the blood. Adult worms are typically discovered at necropsy. Transmission in the laboratory is unlikely, and no special control procedures are necessary other than eliminating possible arthropod vectors.

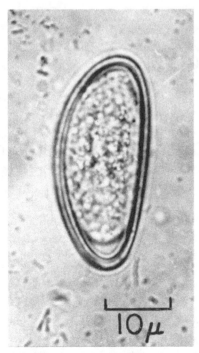

Fig. 21.26 *Streptopharagus armatus* egg. Reproduced from Tanaka, H., Fukui, M., Yamamoto, H., Hayama, S., and Kodera, S. (1962) with permission.

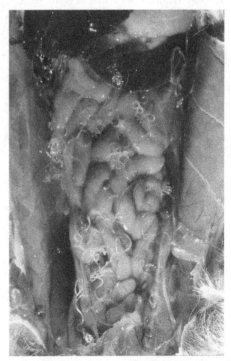

Fig. 21.27 *Dipetalonema* adults in the peritoneal cavity of a squirrel monkey. Reproduced from Whitney, R.A., Johnson, D.J., and Cole, W.C. (1967) with permission.

Public Health Considerations. The *Dipetalonema* found in NHP are not known to infect humans.

Superfamily Trichuroidea

Anatrichosoma cutaneum

Morphology. Adult male *Anatrichosoma cutaneum* have not been described. Adult female worms measure 22 mm to 25 mm long. Eggs are elliptical with bipolar plugs, and measure 56 μ to 70 μ long by 38 μ to 48 μ wide (Figure 21.28).

Hosts and Life Cycle. *Anatrichosoma cutaneum* has been encountered in the nasal mucosa and skin of rhesus monkeys[16,111]. Although reported only from the United States[111], it undoubtedly occurs in the wild. Infection in the skin is rare and has been reported only once[17]. The life cycle is unknown but is probably direct. Eggs in the nasal mucosa are embryonated when laid[111].

Pathologic Effects and Clinical Disease. The presence of *A. cutaneum* in the nasal passages is usually unapparent. Infection results in hyperplasia and parakeratosis of the nasal mucosa but only mild to moderate inflammation (Figure 21.29)[111]. In the skin, the parasite may cause a subcutaneous foreign body reaction but epithelial hyperplasia and parakeratosis are mild.

Diagnosis, Treatment, and Prevention. Diagnosis is made by demonstrating the characteristic eggs on a nasal swab. Treatment regimens have not been described. It is possible that anthelmintics that are effective against other trichurids would also be effective against *A. cutaneum*.

Public Health Considerations. Humans are susceptible to infection with *A. cutaneum* and develop a form of

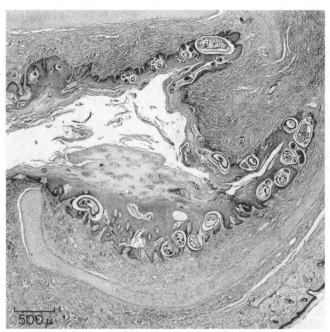

Fig. 21.29 *Anatrichosoma cutaneum.* Section from the nasal passage of a monkey. Reproduced from Allen, A.M. (1960) with permission.

creeping eruption. Thus, animal care workers should handle infected animals with caution.

Calodium hepaticum

The morphology, host range, and life cycle of *Calodium hepaticum* (Syn. *Capillaria hepatica, Hepaticola hepatica*) are described in Chapter 11, Parasites of Rats and Mice. Infections have occasionally been reported in feral primates, including rhesus monkeys, capuchins, spider monkeys, and chimpanzees[88]. Worms develop to maturity in the liver. The liver surface of infected animals contains white or yellow patches or nodules, which contain the adult worms and eggs. Heavy accumulations of eggs cause localized liver damage and cirrhosis, which may progress to fatal hepatitis in primates[67]. Diagnosis is by demonstrating parasites and eggs in histologic sections of liver. Treatment regimens have not been described. Natural transmission in the laboratory is unlikely, and no special control procedures are required. Humans are susceptible to infection with *C. hepaticum,* but cases of human infection are rare.

Trichuris trichiura

Morphology. Adult *Trichuris trichiura* resemble those of *T. vulpis* of dogs. Male worms measure 30 mm to 45 mm long, while females measure 35 mm to 50 mm long. The egg is oval, has bipolar plugs, measures 50 μ long by 22 μ wide, and is unsegmented when passed in the feces (Figure 21.30).

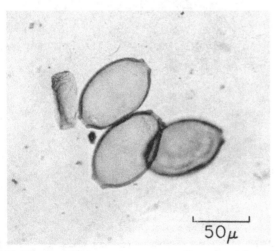

Fig. 21.28 *Anatrichosoma cutaneum* eggs. Reproduced from Allen, A.M. (1960) with permission.

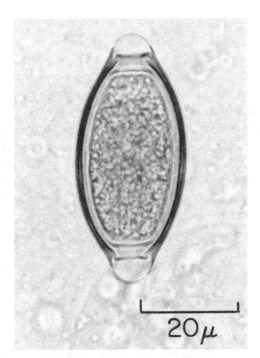

Fig. 21.30 *Trichuris trichiura* egg. Courtesy of Technical Sergeant R.R. Estes, U.S. Air Force School of Aerospace Medicine.

Hosts. *Trichuris trichiura* occurs in the large intestine of humans and many simian primates throughout the world. It is most prevalent in the tropics and subtropics. Affected laboratory primates[16] include macaques[30,78], green monkeys, baboons[33], and chimpanzees[67,79], where incidence rates may reach nearly 100%.

Life Cycle. The life cycle is direct and infection is by ingestion of embryonated eggs. The eggs are unembryonated when passed in the feces and require 10 days in the soil to reach the infective stage. After ingestion, the egg shell is digested away and the larvae pass to the cecum, where they embed their anterior ends into the mucosa.

Pathologic Effects and Clinical Disease. Light infections with *T. trichiura* produce few pathologic effects or clinical disease[67]. Heavy infections may result in severe enteritis, with anorexia, mucoid diarrhea, and occasionally death[67,112].

Diagnosis, Treatment, and Prevention. Diagnosis is made by finding characteristic eggs in the stool. Once housing areas are contaminated, control is challenging. Trichurid eggs are notoriously long-lived in the environment, making complete eradication difficult. Control may be facilitated by sanitation, elimination of conditions favorable to egg development, and regular treatment of infected animals. Newly acquired animals should be exam-ined on arrival and treated if infected. Effective anthelmintics are as described for *T. vulpis* infections in dogs.

Public Health Considerations. *Trichuris trichiura* infecting NHP is similar, if not identical to, isolates recovered from humans. Thus, animal workers should exercise excellent personal hygiene when working around infected NHP and their waste.

ACANTHOCEPHALA

Prosthenorchis spp.

Morphology. Adult *Prosthenorchis* are cylindrical, curved ventrally or spirally, and irregularly wrinkled transversely. Adult male worms measure 20 mm to 30 mm long and female worms measure 30 mm to 50 mm long[113]. The proboscis is globular and has five to seven rows of hooks. The eggs are large and measure 42 μ to 53 μ long by 65 μ to 81 μ wide, and contain an embryo (acanthor) with hooks (Figure 21.31)[114].

Hosts. *Prosthenorchis* is the most important intestinal parasite of Central and South American monkeys[64,102,115–118]. *Prosthenorchis elegans* is the most common

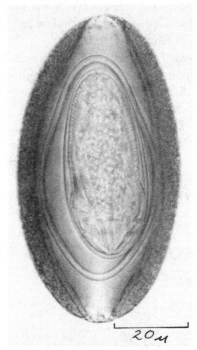

Fig. 21.31 *Prosthenorchis elegans* egg. Reproduced from Worms, M.J. (1967) with permission.

species; *P. spirula* less common. Both species are native to South America but are now found wherever New World primates are kept in captivity[119]. Although marmosets, tamarins, squirrel monkeys, spider monkeys, and capuchins are the natural hosts, infections may be transmitted to macaques, chimpanzees, gibbons, lemurs, and pottos (*Perodicticus*)[119].

Life Cycle. Eggs passed in primate feces are ingested by a cockroach intermediate host[120]. The primate host is infected by ingesting an infected cockroach. Use of the cockroach as intermediate host facilitates establishment of this parasite in primate facilities, where cockroaches may be abundant.

Pathologic Effects and Clinical Disease. Adult worms attach to the intestinal wall by deeply embedding the spiny proboscis into the mucosa[116]. The terminal portion of the ileum is the most common site of attachment, but worms may also attach in the cecum and colon[64,116]. Inflammation, necrosis, and ulceration occur at attachment sites[116-118]. Intussusception or complete obstruction of the intestine in the region of the ileocecal valve sometimes occurs[102,119]. Occasionally the parasite penetrates the gut wall and enters the peritoneal cavity, causing peritonitis[116,119]. Grossly observed lesions include abscesses and granulomata at the attachment sites. Lesions appear on the serosal surface of the intestine as firm white nodules, several millimeters in diameter[64,115,116]. Clinical signs vary with parasite burden, and may include diarrhea, anorexia, debilitation, and death[102,116-118].

Diagnosis, Treatment, and Prevention. Diagnosis is by identification of eggs in the feces or adult worms in the intestine[102]. Sanitation and cockroach control interrupt the life cycle and prevent infection within the research colony. No effective treatment has been reported.

Public Health Considerations. Human infections have not been reported with *Prosthenorchis*. Although human infections seem possible because of the broad host spectrum of *Prosthenorchis,* human infection would require ingestion of an infected cockroach.

ARTHROPODS

Class Insecta

Order Phthiraptera

Pedicinus eurygaster
Morphology. *Pedicinus eurygaster* is a slender louse, measuring 1 mm to 3 mm long, with a long head and two to

three lateral abdominal plates[121]. The head has a pair of distinct eyes. The abdomen is membranous, except for the usual terminal and genital plates, and has several rows of minute hairs on both sides[121]. The egg is oval and operculated, and measures 0.6 mm to 0.9 mm long by 0.3 mm to 0.5 mm in diameter.

Hosts and Life Cycle. *Pedicinus eurygaster* is found on macaques of tropical Asia. *Pedicinus obtusus* (Figure 21.32) occurs on langurs or leaf monkeys, green monkeys, other guenons, and sometimes macaques and baboons of southeastern Asia and Africa. *Pedicinus patas* is found on guenons and colobus monkeys of India and Africa. *P. miobergi* occurs on howler monkeys of South America[96,121-123]. Although Old World laboratory primates obtained from the wild are only occasionally infested with these lice[43,124], infestation of wild New World specimens is common[123]. The complete life cycle is unknown. Transmission is presumably by direct contact.

Pathologic Effects and Clinical Disease. Infestations with *Pedicinus* are considered asymptomatic[124].

Diagnosis, Treatment, and Prevention. Diagnosis is based on demonstration of lice. Newly acquired monkeys should be examined and, if infested, isolated and treated. A dust containing 5% carbaryl, 0.1% pyrethrins, 2%

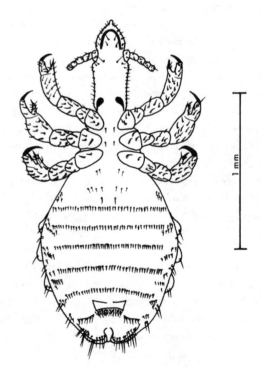

Fig. 21.32 *Pedicinus obtusus* female, ventral view. Courtesy of K.C. Kim, Pennsylvania State University.

dichlorophen, and 1% piperonyl butoxide (Diryl, Pitman-Moore), applied topically, has proven effective[43]. Treated animals should be placed in clean, disinfected cages. Treatment should be repeated at weekly intervals for two to three weeks.

Public Health Considerations. Humans are not susceptible to infestation with *Pedicinus* sp.

Order Siphonaptera

Morphology. The male *Tunga penetrans* (sand flea, jigger flea) is small, measuring only 0.5 mm long. The female is larger than the male, measuring 1 mm long. The thorax is short; the three thoracic terga collectively are shorter than the first abdominal tergite. The metathoracic coxae lack patches of spiniform bristles, and females lack spiracles on the second and third abdominal segments. The head has an acute frontal angle and lacks both a genal ctenidium and large setae.

Hosts and Life Cycle. *Tunga penetrans* is distributed throughout tropical regions of the Americas and Africa. It attacks a wide variety of hosts, especially humans and pigs[125–127]. Laboratory guenons and baboons obtained from the wild are frequently infested. The female flea embeds its mouthparts in the skin and becomes firmly attached to the host. The male flea does not embed. The dermis of the host proliferates and encapsulates the entire body of the flea, except for the terminal abdominal segments which protrude through a small pore. Copulation occurs after encapsulation. The female increases in size to about 5 mm to 7 mm. Eggs are expelled through the dermal pore, drop to the ground, and hatch in a few days under ideal conditions. Larvae feed on the feces of the adults. The entire life cycle requires about 17 days[128].

Pathologic Effects and Clinical Disease. Implanted female fleas cause intense local irritation and pruritus. In guenons and baboons, *T. penetrans* often invades the hard skin pads on the buttocks, resulting in secondary bacterial infection.

Diagnosis, Treatment, and Prevention. Diagnosis is based on identifying the parasite in the dermal lesions. *Tunga penetrans* infestations are only common in primates obtained from the wild. Standard treatment consists of surgical removal of female fleas and sterilization of the wound. It is unknown whether broad-spectrum acaricides such as ivermectin would effectively eliminate an infestation.

Public Health Considerations. Humans are commonly affected in endemic areas[126]. Animal workers should use caution when working with infested monkeys.

Class Arachnida

Mites

Pneumonyssus simicola

Morphology. *Pneumonyssus simicola* (Syn. *Pneumonyssus foxi, P. griffithi, P. macaci*), the lung mite of monkeys, is yellow-white, elongate, and ovoid (Figure 21.33)[129]. Female mites measure 700 μ to 850 μ long, while males measure 500 μ long. Both sexes have a single small dorsal plate. The female sternal plate is longer than it is wide and has three pairs of setae. An epigynial plate is absent, and the female genital opening is a transverse slit between the fourth set of coxae. Palps are composed of four free segments. Chelicerae are short with opposed chelae; the movable chela is more developed than the fixed chela. Legs are long and have small setae and terminal claws. The egg is glistening white and spherical, and measures 250 μ to 450 μ in diameter[130].

Hosts. Prior to the routine use of ivermectin in primate colonies, *P. simicola* was extremely common in newly

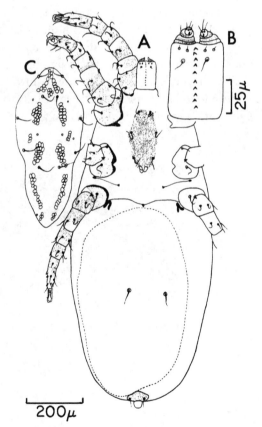

Fig. 21.33 *Pneumonyssus simicola* female. (A) Ventral view. (B) Gnathosoma (enlarged). (C) Dorsal shield. Reproduced from Fain, A. (1961) with permission.

acquired rhesus macaques, with prevalence rates of up to 100% frequently reported. Infections have also been reported from the silvered leaf monkey[131] and from several additional macaque species[132–135]. There is a single report of *P. simicola* from a baboon[136]. With the possible exception of the baboon, *P. simicola* is restricted to members of the genus *Macaca* originating in Asia and the Philippine Islands. Mites found in the respiratory tract of African primates, such as guenons, baboons, chimpanzees, and gorillas, are probably different species of *Pneumonyssus*[132,137]. Current incidence rates of infection in laboratory macaques are unknown, but are likely very low in monkeys that are routinely medicated with ivermectin or related compounds.

Life Cycle. The complete life cycle is unknown but it has been suggested that all stages are found in the lungs[138]. Eggs presumably hatch within the female, and fully developed larvae are deposited. Larvae occur in pulmonary nodules and also in the bronchi. They are the only stage commonly found free in the bronchi and are presumed to be the infective stage[139]. The protonymph and deutonymph stages are brief and have been seen only under experimental conditions[140]. Adults are found in pulmonary lesions that usually open into a bronchiole. There is evidence that the mites suck blood[138], but they have also been reported to feed on lymph and pulmonary epithelium cells[141]. The mode of transmission is unknown. Mites have not been found in monkeys delivered by cesarean section or in those born naturally in the laboratory that are

removed from their mothers at birth[142–144]. It seems that larval mites are transferred from the bronchi through direct contact, coughing, or sneezing[139].

Pathologic Effects. Gross lesions range in appearance from minute, pale spots to discreet yellowish foci a few millimeters in diameter (Figure 21.34)[138,145]. Lesions may number from a few to hundreds, and occur in the lung parenchyma near the surface of the lung and elevated above it, or deeper within the lobes[139]. Superficially, mite lesions resemble tubercles but are less firm. Rarely is there any hemorrhage near the mites. When magnified, lesions appear as pale, white, jelly-like masses which sometimes have a minute slit or opening in the center[145]. The lesions and surrounding tissue contain a characteristic golden brown to black pigment. One to 20 mites, predominantly females but sometimes eggs, larvae, or males, are easily teased from the lesion (Figure 21.35)[139,146].

Histopathologic lesions are characterized by the presence of the mite in association with localized bronchiolitis and peribronchiolitis, or focal pneumonitis in which eosinophils are prominent, and sometimes by bronchiolectasis. Pigments and double refractile needles are found in or near the mites or their associated lesions. Pigment is not seen in the lungs of normal monkeys and does not contain carbon or melanin but does contain iron, and may result from the digestion and excretion of host blood proteins[138].

Clinical Disease. Clinical signs are usually absent[138,147]. Paroxysmal coughing and sneezing may occur but are

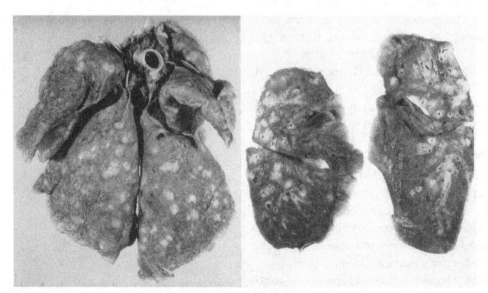

Fig. 21.34   Gross lesions of *Pneumonyssus simicola* infection in preserved lung specimens from a monkey. Note the numerous pale foci beneath pleura (left) and on cut surface (right). Courtesy of J.R.M. Innes, Bionetics Research Laboratories.

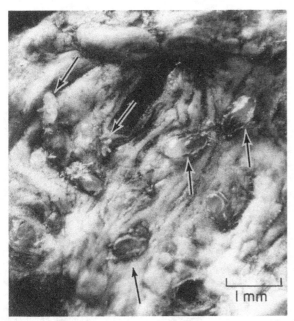

Fig. 21.35 Magnification of gross lesions of *Pneumonyssus simicola* infection in the lung of a monkey. Note the mites (arrows) teased from typical lesions. Courtesy of J.R.M. Innes, Bionetics Research Laboratories.

uncommon and may be due to other causes of respiratory disease. Although earlier workers attributed fatalities to this mite, it is probably the direct cause of death only in massive infections[145].

Diagnosis. Diagnosis of *P. simicola* infection in live monkeys is difficult. Routine radiographic or hematologic examinations have no value[138,147]. Sometimes larvae can be demonstrated in tracheobronchial washings, but a negative finding does not exclude the possibility of infection[139]. Gross lesions produced by the mite must be differentiated from those of tuberculosis. The finding of mites or the characteristic pigment and crystals associated with them in histologic sections is diagnostic of lung mite infection, but not necessarily of *P. simicola* infection. Although *P. simicola* is the usual lung mite affecting the rhesus monkey, *Rhinophaga dinolti* is sometimes found[148]. Differentiation

is based primarily on morphology of the tarsal claws. The claws on the first leg of females of *R. dinolti* are much less developed than those on the third leg, whereas all tarsal claws of *P. simicola* are subequal in size. All lung mites of simian primates are morphologically similar and therefore are not easily identified in cross section. Identification is a matter for the medical entomologist, who should be supplied with whole mites (as opposed to sections) whenever possible.

Treatment and Prevention. Affected macaques should be treated with ivermectin (200 µg/kg) every three weeks. Because rates of infection have declined dramatically with the routine use of ivermectin, infections are only occasionally discovered at necropsy. Animals obtained from the wild should be treated before release into the colony.

Public Health Considerations. Lung mites of macaques do not infect humans. Despite reports to the contrary, mites recovered from human cases of pulmonary acariasis are unrelated to lung mites of monkeys.

Class Pentastomida

Porocephalus spp.

The definitive hosts of *Porocephalus* are snakes, while the intermediate hosts are monkeys. The infection requires a predator-prey relationship to become established or maintained. *Porocephalus clavatus* occurs in squirrel monkeys in South America, and is apparently common in tamarins obtained from the wild[149]. *Porocephalus crotali* occurs in marmosets[150] and tamarins (*Sanguinus nigricollis*) in North and South America[65,116]. A pentastomid nymph thought to be *P. stilesi* was recovered from the meninges of a *Saimiri* monkey, where it was encapsulated by connective tissue[151]. *Porocephalus subulifer* has been found in a guenon[150] and in a galago[152] and is confined to tropical Africa[150]. *Porocephalus* nymphs are occasionally found in the viscera of laboratory monkeys, and are relatively benign parasites.

TABLE 21.1 Parasites of non-human primates—circulatory and lymphatic systems.

Parasite	Geographic distribution	Hosts	Location in host	Method of infection	Pathologic effects	Zoonosis	Reference
Flagellates							
Trypanosoma minasense	Central and South America	New World monkeys	Blood	Wound contamination with feces of reduviid bug	None	Reported	168
Trypanosoma primatum	West Africa	Guenons, apes	Blood	Unknown	None	Not reported	169
Piroplasmids							
Babesia pitheci	Africa, Europe	Old World monkeys	Erythrocytes	Transmitted by arthropod intermediate host (tick)	None	Not reported	170
Entopolypoides macaci	Africa, Indonesia	Guenons, patas monkeys, baboons, some macaques	Erythrocytes	Transmitted by arthropod intermediate host (tick)	Anemia	Not reported	51
Haemosporids							
Hepatocystis kochi	Central Africa	Old World monkeys	Erythrocytes	Transmitted by arthropod intermediate host (midge)	Focal hepatitis	Not reported	171
Hepatocystis semnopitheci	Asia	Old World monkeys	Erythrocytes	Transmitted by arthropod intermediate host (midge)	Unknown	Not reported	172
Hepatocystis taiwanensis	Taiwan	Macaques	Erythrocytes	Transmitted by arthropod (midge) intermediate host	Unknown	Not reported	173
Plasmodium brasilianum	Americas	New World monkeys	Erythrocytes	Transmitted by arthropod intermediate host (mosquito)	Quartan malaria	Reported	174
Plasmodium coatneyi	Malaysia	Macaques, other monkeys	Erythrocytes	Transmitted by arthropod intermediate host (mosquito)	Tertian malaria	Reported	175
Plasmodium cynomolgi	Asia	Old World monkeys	Erythrocytes	Transmitted by arthropod intermediate host (mosquito)	Splenomegaly, hepatic congestion	Reported	154

Species	Geographic distribution	Host	Site of infection	Transmission	Disease		
Plasmodium eylesi	Malaysia	Gibbons	Erythrocytes	Transmitted by arthropod intermediate host (mosquito)	Tertian malaria	Not reported	176
Plasmodium fieldi	Malaysia	Pigtail macaques	Erythrocytes	Transmitted by arthropod (mosquito) intermediate host	Tertian malaria	Not reported	177
Plasmodium fragile	India, Ceylon	Macaques	Erythrocytes	Transmitted by arthropod (mosquito) intermediate host	Tertian malaria	Not reported	178
Plasmodium girardi	Madagascar	Lemurs	Erythrocytes	Transmitted by arthropod intermediate host (mosquito)	Quartan malaria	Not reported	179
Plasmodium gonderi	West central Africa	Mangabeys, mandrills	Erythrocytes	Transmitted by arthropod (mosquito) intermediate host	Tertian malaria	Not reported	180
Plasmodium hylobati	Indonesia	Gibbons	Erythrocytes	Transmitted by arthropod intermediate host (mosquito)	Quartan malaria	Not reported	181
Plasmodium jefferyi	Malaysia	Gibbons	Erythrocytes	Transmitted by arthropod intermediate host (mosquito)	Tertian malaria	Not reported	182
Plasmodium inui	Asia	Macaques	Erythrocytes	Transmitted by arthropod intermediate host (mosquito)	Quartan malaria	Reported	183
Plasmodium knowlesi	Asia	Old World monkeys	Erythrocytes	Transmitted by arthropod intermediate host (mosquito)	Quotidian malaria	Reported	184
Plasmodium lemuris	Madagascar	Lemurs	Erythrocytes	Transmitted by arthropod intermediate host (mosquito)	Unknown	Not reported	185
Plasmodium malariae	Africa	Chimpanzees	Erythrocytes	Transmitted by arthropod intermediate host (mosquito)	Quartan malaria	Reported	186

(Continued)

TABLE 21.1 (Continued)

Parasite	Geographic distribution	Hosts	Location in host	Method of infection	Pathologic effects	Zoonosis	Reference
Plasmodium pitheci	Indonesia	Orangutans	Erythrocytes	Transmitted by arthropod intermediate host (mosquito)	Tertian malaria	Not reported	187
Plasmodium reichenowi	Africa	Apes	Erythrocytes	Transmitted by arthropod intermediate host (mosquito)	Tertian malaria	Not reported	188
Plasmodium schwetzi	Africa	Chimpanzees, gorillas	Erythrocytes	Transmitted by arthropod intermediate host (mosquito)	Tertian malaria	Reported	189
Plasmodium simiovale	Ceylon	Toque macaques (*Macaca sinica*)	Erythrocytes	Transmitted by arthropod intermediate host (mosquito)	Tertian malaria	Not reported	190
Plasmodium simium	Brazil	New World monkeys	Erythrocytes	Transmitted by arthropod intermediate host (mosquito)	Tertian malaria	Reported	191
Plasmodium youngi	Malaysia	Gibbons	Erythrocytes	Transmitted by arthropod intermediate host (mosquito)	Severe tertian malaria	Not reported	192
Trematodes							
Digenetic							
Schistosoma haematobium	Africa, Asia, Europe	Old World monkeys, chimpanzees	Pelvic vein, mesenteric veins	Skin penetration by cercaria; possibly ingestion of cercaria	Cystitis	Common	193
Schistosoma mansoni	Africa, South America, West Indies	Primates	Mesenteric veins	Skin penetration by cercaria; possibly ingestion of cercaria	Granulomas in various organs	Common	194
Nematodes							
Filaroidea							
Brugia malayi	Asia	Macaques, langurs	Lymphatics	Bite of mosquito	Lymphangitis	Reported	165

TABLE 21.2 Parasites of non-human primates—enterohepatic system.

Parasite	Geographic distribution	Hosts	Location in host	Method of infection	Pathologic effects	Zoonosis	Reference
Flagellates							
Chilomastix mesnili	Worldwide	Swine, primates	Cecum, colon	Ingestion of organism passed in feces	None	Reported	9
Giardia lamblia	Worldwide	Primates	Anterior small intestine	Ingestion of organism passed in feces	Enteritis	Common	9
Retortamonas intestinalis	Worldwide	Primates	Cecum	Ingestion of organism passed in feces	None	Reported	9
Spironucleus pitheci	South America	Rhesus monkeys	Cecum, colon	Ingestion of organism passed in feces	None	Not reported	9
Trichomonas tenax	Worldwide	Primates	Mouth	Oral contact	None	Common	9
Amoebae							
Dientamoeba fragilis	Worldwide	Old World monkeys	Cecum, colon	Ingestion of cysts passed in feces	Unknown	Common	26
Endolimax nana	Worldwide	Swine, primates	Cecum, colon	Ingestion of cysts passed in feces	None	Common	16
Entamoeba chattoni	Worldwide	Primates	Cecum, colon	Ingestion of cysts passed in feces	None	Reported	196
Entamoeba coli	Worldwide	Swine, primates	Cecum, colon	Ingestion of cysts passed in feces	None	Reported	16
Entamoeba gingivalis	Worldwide	Dogs, cats, primates	Mouth	Oral contact	None	Common	9
Entamoeba histolytica	Worldwide	Primates, swine, dogs, cats	Large intestine, liver, brain, spleen	Ingestion of cysts passed in feces	Enteritis, hepatitis	Common	197
Iodamoeba buetschlii	Worldwide	Primates, swine	Cecum, colon	Ingestion of cysts passed in feces	None	Not reported	198

(Continued)

723

TABLE 21.2 (Continued)

Parasite	Geographic distribution	Hosts	Location in host	Method of infection	Pathologic effects	Zoonosis	Reference
Coccidia							
Eimeria galago, E. lemuris, E. otolicni	Africa	Galagos	Intestine	Ingestion of sporulated oocyst	Unknown	Not reported	199
Isospora arctopitheci	South America	New World primates	Intestine	Ingestion of sporulated oocyst	Unknown	Not reported	200
Ciliates							
Balantidium coli	Worldwide	Swine, primates, rats, hamsters, dogs	Cecum, colon	Ingestion of cysts or trophozoites passed in feces	Enteritis	Common	201
Troglodytella abrassarti	Worldwide	Chimpanzees	Cecum, colon	Ingestion of organism passed in feces	Colitis	Not reported	202
Troglodytella gorillae	Worldwide	Gorillas	Cecum, colon	Presumably by ingestion of organisms passed in feces	Unknown	None known	203
Trematodes							
Artyfechinostomum sp.	Asia	Macaques, swine, other vertebrates	Intestine	Unknown	Enteritis	Reported	204
Athesmia foxi	Asia, South America	New World monkeys, wild rats (*Rattus argentiventer*)	Bile duct	Unknown	Cholangio-hepatitis	Not reported	63
Brodenia laciniata	Africa	Baboons	Pancreas	Unknown	Unknown	Not reported	204
Brodenia serrata	Africa	Mangabeys	Pancreas	Unknown	Unknown	Not reported	204
Controrchis biliophilus	Central America	New World monkeys	Gallbladder, intestine	Unknown	Unknown	Not reported	205
Dicrocoelium colobusicola	Central Africa	Colobus monkeys	Bile duct	Ingestion of second intermediate host	Unknown	Not reported	204
Eurytrema brumpti	Central Africa	Chimpanzees, gorillas	Bile duct, pancreas	Ingestion of second intermediate host	Cholangitis	Not reported	206

Species	Geographic distribution	Host	Location in host	Mode of infection	Pathology	Prevalence	Ref.
Fasciolopsis buski	Asia	Rhesus monkeys, swine	Duodenum, stomach	Ingestion of metacercaria encysted on vegetation	None	Reported	207
Gastrodiscoides hominis	Asia	Macaques, swine	Cecum, colon	Ingestion of metacercaria encysted on vegetation	Enteritis	Common	68
Haplorchis yokogawai	Asia	Macaques	Small intestine	Ingestion of metacercaria encysted in fish	Unknown	Not reported	208
Leipertrema reuelli	Africa	Orangutans	Pancreas	Unknown	Unknown	Not reported	204
Neodiplostomum tamarini	South America	Tamarins	Small intestine	Unknown	Unknown	Not reported	65
Ogmocotyle ailuri	Asia	Macaques	Intestine	Unknown	Unknown	Not reported	209
Phaneropsolus oviformis	Asia	Macaques, slow loris	Intestine	Unknown	Unknown	Not reported	210
Phaneropsolus orbicularis	South America	New world monkeys	Intestine	Unknown	Unknown	Not reported	211
Platynosomum amazonensis, P. marmoseti	South America	Tamarins	Gallbladder, bile duct	Unknown	Unknown	Not reported	65
Primatotrema macacae	Asia	Macaques	Intestine	Unknown	Unknown	Not reported	210
Reptilotrema primata	Asia	Macaques	Intestine	Unknown	Unknown	Not reported	204
Watsonius macaci	Asia	Cynomolgus monkey	Intestine	Ingestion of metacercaria on vegetation	Enteritis	Reported	78
Watsonius sp.	Western Africa	Guenons, baboons	Intestine	Ingestion of metacercaria on vegetation	Enteritis	Reported	66, 96
Cestodes							
Cyclophyllidea							
Atriotaenia (Oochoristica) megastoma	Central and South America	New World monkeys	Small intestine	Probably by ingestion of infected insect	None known	Not reported	65
Bertiella sp.	Africa, Asia	Old World primates	Small intestine	Probably by ingestion of free-living mites	None known	Reported	212
Hymenolepis cebidarum	Central and South America	Marmosets, titi monkeys	Intestine	Unknown	Unknown	Not reported	116
Hymenolepis diminuta	South America	Owl monkeys	Intestine	Ingestion of arthropod intermediate host	None	Reported	155

(Continued)

TABLE 21.2 *(Continued)*

Parasite	Geographic distribution	Hosts	Location in host	Method of infection	Pathologic effects	Zoonosis	Reference
Moniezia rugosa	South America	Capuchins, howler monkeys, spider monkeys	Small intestine	Probably by ingestion of infected mites	None known	Not reported	213
Paratriotaenia oedipomidatis	South America	Marmosets	Small intestine	Probably by ingestion of infected insect	None known	Not reported	214
Raillietina sp.	Central and South America	Howler monkeys	Intestine	Unknown	Unknown	Reported	119
Rodentolepis nana	Worldwide	Primates	Intestine	Ingestion of arthropod intermediate host	Catarrhal enteritis	Reported	156
Cestodes							
Larval							
Echinococcus granulosus	Worldwide	Sheep, swine, primates, other mammals	Liver, lung, heart	Ingestion of egg in feces of definitive host (dog)	Hydatid cyst	Common	159
Taenia hydatigena	Worldwide	Primates, ruminants, swine	Liver, peritoneal cavity	Ingestion of embryonated egg passed by definitive host (dog)	Liver damage, peritonitis	Reported	215
Nematodes							
Rhabditoidea							
Strongyloides cebus	Central and South America	New World monkeys	Duodenum, jejunum, lung (larvae)	Ingestion of infective larva or penetration of skin or buccal mucosa by larva	Broncho-pneumonia enteritis	Not reported	65, 83
Strongyloides fuelleborni	Africa, Asia	Old World monkeys, chimpanzees	Duodenum, jejunum, lung (larvae)	Ingestion of infective larva or penetration of skin or buccal mucosa by larva	Broncho-pneumonia, enteritis	Reported	83
Strongyloides stercoralis	Worldwide	Apes	Duodenum, jejunum, lung (larvae)	Ingestion of infective larva or penetration of skin or buccal mucosa by larva	Broncho-pneumonia, enteritis	Common	161

Parasite	Distribution	Host	Location	Transmission	Pathology	Prevalence	Reference
Ascaridoidea							
Ascaris lumbricoides	Worldwide	Primates	Small intestine	Ingestion of embryonated egg	Hepatic abscesses	Common	216
Subuluroidea							
Subulura distans	Africa, Asia	Old World primates	Stomach, small intestine, colon	Ingestion of intermediate host (cockroaches)	Unknown	Not reported	96
Subulura jacchi	Americas	Marmosets, tamarins	Small intestine	Ingestion of intermediate host (cockroaches)	Unknown	Not reported	218
Subulura malayensis	Malay Peninsula	Macaques	Colon	Unknown	Unknown	Not reported	219
Oxyuroidea							
Enterobius anthropopitheci	Africa	Chimpanzees	Large intestine	Ingestion of embryonated egg	Perianal pruritus	Not reported	220
Enterobius bipapillatus	Africa	Rhesus monkeys, chimpanzees	Large intestine	Ingestion of embryonated egg	Perianal pruritus	Not reported	221
Enterobius brevicauda	Africa	Baboons	Large intestine	Ingestion of embryonated egg	Perianal pruritus	Not reported	221
Enterobius buckleyi	Borneo	Orangutans	Large intestine	Ingestion of embryonated egg	Perianal pruritus	Not reported	221
Enterobius interlabiatus, E. microon	South America	Night monkeys	Large intestine	Ingestion of embryonated egg	Perianal pruritus	Not reported	221
Enterobius lerouxi	Africa	Gorillas	Large intestine	Ingestion of embryonated egg	Perianal pruritus	Not reported	221
Enterobius vermicularis	Worldwide	Marmosets, gibbons, chimpanzees	Large intestine	Ingestion of embryonated egg	Perianal pruritus	Common	222
Lobatorobius scleratus	Central and South America	Squirrel monkeys	Cecum, colon	Ingestion of embryonated egg	Unknown	Not reported	221
Oxyuronema atelophorum	Central America	Spider monkeys	Large intestine	Ingestion of embryonated egg	Hemorrhagic enteritis	Not reported	221
Trypanoxyuris sp.	South America	New World monkeys	Colon	Ingestion of embryonated egg	Unknown	Not reported	65, 217
Strongylida							
Ancylostoma duodenale	Worldwide	Primates	Small intestine	Ingestion of infective larva or skin penetration	Anemia	Common	43
Characostomum asimilium	Africa, Asia	Macaques, guenons, slow loris	Small intestine	Probably ingestion of embryonated egg	Unknown	Not reported	221
Globocephalus simiae	Malay Peninsula, Indonesia	Rhesus monkeys	Small intestine	Probably ingestion of embryonated egg	Anemia	Not reported	223

(*Continued*)

TABLE 21.2 (*Continued*)

Parasite	Geographic distribution	Hosts	Location in host	Method of effects	Pathologic Zoonosis	Reference
Necator americanus	Worldwide	Primates	Small intestine	Larval penetration of skin	Anemia	Common	162
Oesophagostomum aculeatum	Asia	Macaques	Colon	Ingestion of infective larva	Nodules in wall of colon	Reported	224
Oesophagostomum apiostomum	Africa, Asia	Macaques	Colon, rarely omentum	Ingestion of infective larva	Nodules in wall of colon	Reported	225
Oesophagostomum bifurcum	Africa, Asia	Old World monkeys	Colon	Ingestion of infective larva	Nodules in wall f colon	Reported (may be different strain)	226
Oesophagostomum stephanostomum	Africa	Baboons, chimpanzee, gorilla	Colon	Ingestion of infective larva	Nodules in wall of colon	Reported	227
Ternidens deminutus	Africa, Asia	Old World monkeys, chimpanzees, gorillas	Cecum, colon	Ingestion of infective larva	Anemia, nodules in wall of colon	Reported	228

Trichostrongyloidea

Parasite	Geographic distribution	Hosts	Location in host	Method of effects	Pathologic Zoonosis	Reference
Graphidioides berlai	Brazil	New World monkeys	Intestine	Probably ingestion of larva	Unknown	Not reported	221
Longistriata dubia	South America	New World monkeys	Small intestine	Probably ingestion of larva or skin penetration	Unknown	Not reported	65
Molineus torulosus	Brazil	New World monkeys	Small intestine	Probably ingestion of larva	Hemorrhagic enteritis	Not reported	229
Molineus vexillarius	Peru	Tamarins	Small intestine, stomach	Probably ingestion of larva	None	Not reported	230
Molineus vogelianus	Africa	Pottos (*Perodicticus*)	Small intestine	Probably ingestion of larva	Unknown	Not reported	231
Nematodirus weinbergi	Africa	Chimpanzees	Small intestine	Ingestion of larva	Unknown	Not reported	221
Nochtia nochti	Asia	Macaques	Stomach	Probably ingestion of larva	Gastric tumors	Not reported	104
Pithecostrongylus alatus	Malaysia	Guenons, orangutans	Intestine	Unknown	Unknown	Not reported	221
Trichostrongylus colubriformis	Worldwide	Ruminants, Old World monkeys, apes, lagomorphs, other mammals	Small intestine	Ingestion of larva	Mild enteritis	Reported	144

728

Spiruroidea

Species	Distribution	Hosts	Location	Transmission	Pathology	Human infection	Ref.
Chituwoodspirura serrata	Central America	Chimpanzees, gorillas	Stomach, small intestine	Ingestion of intermediate host (insects)	Unknown	Reported	221
Gongylonema macrogubernaculum	Worldwide	Macaques	Esophagus, stomach	Ingestion of intermediate host (insects)	Esophagitis	Not reported	278
Gongylonema pulchrum	Worldwide	Primates, wild carnivores, ruminants, swine	Tongue, oral cavity, esophagus, stomach	Ingestion of intermediate host (cockroaches, dung beetles)	None	Reported	232
Physaloptera caucasica	Africa, Eurasia	Old World monkeys, orangutans	Esophagus, stomach, duodenum	Ingestion of intermediate host (beetles)	Esophagitis, gastritis, enteritis	Reported	233
Physaloptera dilatata	South America	New World monkeys	Stomach	Ingestion of intermediate host (insects)	Gastritis	Not reported	102
Physaloptera tumefaciens	Asia	Macaques	Stomach	Ingestion of intermediate host (insects)	Hemorrhagic gastritis	Not reported	234
Physaloptera poicilometra	Africa	Mangabeys, guenons	Stomach	Ingestion of intermediate host (insects)	Mild gastritis	Not reported	235
Rictularia alphi	Eurasia	Monkeys	Small intestine	Ingestion of intermediate host (arthropods)	Unknown	Not reported	219
Spirura guianensis	South America	Tamarins, marsupials, armadillos	Esophagus	Unknown	Esophagus	Reported	221
Streptopharagus armatus	Africa, Japan	Old World monkeys, gibbons	Stomach	Ingestion of intermediate host (arthropods)	Unknown	Not reported	96
Streptopharagus pigmentatus	Africa, Asia	Old World monkeys, gibbons	Stomach	Ingestion of intermediate host (arthropods)	Unknown	Not reported	236
Trichospirura leptostoma	Americas	New World primates	Pancreas	Ingestion of arthropod intermediate host (cockroaches)	Pancreatitis	Not reported	163

Trichuroidea

Species	Distribution	Hosts	Location	Transmission	Pathology	Human infection	Ref.
Trichuris trichiura	Worldwide	Primates	Cecum, colon	Ingestion of embryonated egg	Enteritis	Common	237

729

(Continued)

TABLE 21.2 (Continued)

Parasite	Geographic distribution	Hosts	Location in host	Method of infection	Pathologic effects	Zoonosis	Reference
Acanthocephala							
Prosthenorchis elegans	Worldwide	Primates	Ileum, cecum, colon	Ingestion of intermediate host (cockroaches)	Colitis	Not reported	238
Prosthenorchis spirula	Worldwide	Monkeys, chimpanzee, lemurs, pottos (*Perodicticus*)	Ileum, cecum, colon	Ingestion of intermediate host (cockroaches)	Enteritis	Not reported	84
Pentastomids							
Porocephalus clavatus	South America	Tamarins, marmosets	Liver, lungs, peritoneum, meninges, other tissues	Ingestion of eggs passed by definitive host (snakes)	Cysts in liver, lungs, peritoneum, meninges, other tissues	Not reported	239
Porocephalus subulifer	Africa	Guenons, galagos	Viscera	Ingestion of eggs passed by definitive host (snakes)	Cysts in viscera	Not reported	152

TABLE 21.3 Parasites of non-human primates—musculoskeletal system, skin, and connective tissue.

Parasite	Geographic distribution	Hosts	Location in host	Method of infection	Pathologic effects	Zoonosis	Reference
Protozoa							
Coccidia							
Sarcocystis kortei	Worldwide	Rhesus monkeys	Striated muscle, smooth muscle	Ingestion of organism in muscle or oocysts passed in feces	Cysts in muscle	Not reported	240
Sarcocystis nesbitti	India	Rhesus monkeys	Striated muscle	Ingestion of organism in muscle or oocysts passed in feces	Cysts in muscle	Not reported	240, 241
Sarcocystis sp.	Africa, Asia	Baboons, macaques	Striated muscle	Ingestion of organism in muscle or oocysts passed in feces	Cysts in muscle	Reported	242
Sarcocystis sp.	South America	New World monkeys	Striated muscle, smooth muscle	Ingestion of organism in muscle or oocysts passed in feces	Cysts in muscle	Reported	116
Cestodes							
Larval							
Mesocestoides sp.	Africa, Asia, Europe	Old World monkeys	Larva: peritoneal cavity	Presumably by ingestion of first intermediate host	Cysts in abdominal organs	Not reported	243
Spirometra reptans	South America	Marmosets, squirrel monkeys	Adult: small intestine Larva: connective tissue	Ingestion of intermediate host (crustaceans)	Cysts in connective tissue	Reported	244
Spirometra sp.	Africa	Green monkeys	Abdominal cavity	Probably ingestion of unknown intermediate host	Cysts in abdominal cavity	Not reported	245
Taenia saginata	Asia	Macaques	Abdominal cavity, viscera	Ingestion of egg	Cysticerci	Common	157
Filaroidea							
Dipetalonema atelense	Central America	Spider monkeys	Connective tissue	Bite of arthropod	None	Not reported	221
Dipetalonema caudispina	South America	Capuchins, squirrel monkeys	Abdominal cavity	Bite of arthropod	None	Not reported	246
Dipetalonema digitatum	India	Macaques, gibbons	Abdominal cavity	Bite of arthropod	Unknown	Not reported	247

(Continued)

TABLE 21.3 (Continued)

Parasite	Geographic distribution	Hosts	Location in host	Method of infection	Pathologic effects	Zoonosis	Reference
Dipetalonema gracile	Central and South America	New World monkeys	Abdominal cavity	Bite of arthropod	Abdominal adhesions	Not reported	248
Dipetalonema marmosetae	Central America	New World monkeys	Subcutis, body cavity	Bite of arthropod	Unknown	Not reported	249
Dipetalonema obtusa	Central and South America	Capuchins, squirrel monkeys	Esophageal connective tissue	Bite of arthropod	Unknown	Not reported	250
Dipetalonema perstans	Africa	Apes	Subcutis, body cavity	Bite of arthropod (flies, ticks, mosquitoes)	Vascular occlusion	Reported	251
Dipetalonema rodhaini	Central Africa	Chimpanzees	Subcutis, body cavity	Bite of arthropod	Unknown	Not reported	221
Dipetalonema streptocerca	Central Africa	Apes	Subcutis, abdominal cavity	Bite of midge	Unknown	Reported	252
Dipetalonema tamarinae	South America	Marmosets	Abdominal cavity	Bite of arthropod	Unknown	Not reported	102
Dipetalonema tenue	Argentina	Capuchins	Subcutis, body cavity	Bite of unknown invertebrate	Unknown	Not reported	221
Dipetalonema vanhoofi	Africa	Baboons, chimpanzees	Abdominal cavity	Bite of arthropod	Abdominal nodules	Not reported	253
Dirofilaria corynodes	Africa	Guenons, mangabeys, langurs, apes	Subcutis	Bite of mosquito	Unknown	Not reported	164
Dirofilaria magnilarvatum	Asia	Macaques	Subcutis, peritoneal membranes	Bite of mosquito	Unknown	Not reported	254
Dirofilaria pongoi	Indonesia	Gibbons, orangutans	Subcutis	Bite of mosquito	Unknown	Not reported	255
Edesonfilaria malayensis	Southeastern Asia	Cynomolgus monkeys	Abdominal cavity	Unknown	Unknown	Not reported	256
Loa loa	Africa	Old World monkeys	Subcutis, mesenteries, eyes	Bite of tabanid fly	Subcutaneous swelling	Reported (probably different strains)	257
Macacanema formosana	Taiwan	Macaques	Peritracheal connective tissue	Possibly bite of midge	Unknown	Reported	258

Arthropods

Diptera (flies)

Cordylobia anthropophaga	Africa, Europe	Rats, other mammals	Subcutis	Eggs deposited by adult fly	Dermal myiasis	Reported	166
Dermatobia hominis	Central and South America	Rodents, other mammals, some birds	Subcutis	Eggs deposited by adult fly	Dermal myiasis	Reported	167

Phthiraptera (lice)

Pedicinus eurygaster	Asia	Macaques	Pelage	Direct contact	None known	Not reported	259
Pedicinus hamadryas	Africa	Baboons	Pelage	Direct contact	None known	Not reported	96
Pedicinus mjobergi	South America	Howler monkeys	Pelage	Direct contact	None known	Not reported	260
Pedicinus obtusus	Africa, southeastern Asia	Old World monkeys	Pelage	Direct contact	None known	Not reported	259
Pedicinus patas	India, Africa	Guenons, colobus monkeys	Pelage	Direct contact	None known	Not reported	261
Pediculus schaeffi	Africa	Chimpanzees	Pelage	Direct contact	None known	Not reported	262

Siphonaptera (fleas)

Pulex irritans	Worldwide	Primates, rats, rabbits, dogs, cats, swine	Skin, pelage	Direct contact	Intermediate host for *Dipylidium caninum*	Reported	263
Tunga penetrans	Tropical areas of Western Hemisphere and Africa	Guenons, baboons, swine	Embedded in skin of host, usually in buttocks of laboratory primates	Direct contact	Dermal cysts	Reported	264

Arachnida

Mites

Astigmates

Alouattalges corbeti	South America	Howler monkeys, night monkeys	Skin	Direct contact	Unknown	Not reported	265
Audycoptes sp.	South America	Squirrel monkeys	Hair follicles	Direct contact	Unknown	Not reported	266
Cosarcoptes scanloni	Southeastern Asia	Cynomolgus monkeys	Skin	Direct contact	Unknown	Not reported	267
Fonsecalges saimirii	South America	Squirrel monkeys, tamarins	Skin	Direct contact	Possibly dermatitis	Not reported	268

(Continued)

TABLE 21.3 (*Continued*)

Parasite	Geographic distribution	Hosts	Location in host	Method of infection	Pathologic effects	Zoonosis	Reference
Lemurnyssus galagoensis	Africa	Galagos	Nasal cavities	Direct contact	Unknown	Not reported	269
Listrocarpus sp.	South America	New World monkeys	Skin	Direct contact	Unknown	Not reported	270
Notoedres galagoensis	Central Africa	Galagos	Skin	Direct contact	Unknown	Not reported	266
Pangorillages pani	Africa	Chimpanzees	Skin	Direct contact	Unknown	Not reported	271
Paracoroptes gordoni	Africa	Guenons	Skin of body, ears	Direct contact	Dermatitis	Not reported	272
Pithesarcoptes talapoini	Africa, Europe	Guenons	Skin	Direct contact	Scabby dermatitis, alopecia	Not reported	273
Prosarcoptes pitheci	Africa, Europe	Monkeys	Skin	Direct contact	Dermatitis	Not reported	273
Rhyncoptes anastosi	South America	Marmosets, tamarins	Skin	Direct contact	Unknown	Not reported	274
Rhyncoptes cebi	South America	Capuchins	Skin	Direct contact	Unknown	Not reported	275
Rhyncoptes cercopitheci	Africa	Guenons	Skin	Direct contact	Unknown	Not reported	275
Saimirioptes paradoxus	South America	Squirrel monkeys	Skin	Direct contact	Unknown	Not reported	266
Prostigmates							
Psorergates cercopitheci	Africa	Guenons, mangabeys	Skin	Direct contact	Dermatitis	Not reported	276
Pentastomids							
Gigliolella brumpti	Madagascar	Fat-tailed dwarf lemurs (*Cheirogaleus medius*)	Mesentery	Presumably by ingestion of eggs passed by definitive host	Benign mesenteric cysts	Not reported	277

TABLE 21.4. Parasites of non-human primates—nervous, respiratory, and urogenital systems.

Parasite	Geographic distribution	Hosts	Location in host	Method of infection	Pathologic effects	Zoonosis	Reference
Protozoal							
Flagellates							
Tetratrichomonas macovaginae	North America	Macaques	Vagina	Venereal contact	Unknown	Not reported	94, 153
Cestodes							
Larval							
Multiceps serialis	Africa	Baboons, macaques	Brain	Ingestion of egg	Coenurus	Reported	17, 158
Spirometra sp.	Asia	Macaques	Lungs, subcutaneous tissues	Ingestion of infected intermediate host	Sparganosis	Common	160
Nematodes							
Metastrongyloidea							
Filariopsis arator	South America	Capuchins	Lungs	Unknown	Unknown	Not reported	221
Filaroides barretoi	South America	Marmosets	Lungs	Unknown	Pulmonary atelectasis	Not reported	28
Filaroides gordius	South America	Squirrel monkeys	Lungs	Unknown	Pulmonary atelectasis	Not reported	28
Filaroides sp.	Americas	Tamarins	Lungs	Unknown	Unknown	Not reported	65
Spirurida							
Metathelazia ascaroides	Unknown	Guenons	Lungs	Unknown	Unknown	Not reported	221
Trichuroidea							
Anatrichosoma cutaneum	Asia	Macaques	Nasal mucosa	Ingestion of egg	Rhinitis	Reported	279
Anatrichosoma cynomolgi	Asia	Cynomolgus monkeys	Nasal mucosa	Ingestion of egg	Rhinitis	Not reported	279
Leeches							
Dinobdella ferox	Southern Asia	Macaques, dogs, cats, ruminants	Nasal cavities, pharynx	Invasion of mouth or nares while drinking	Anemia, asphyxiation, sometimes death	Reported	82

(Continued)

735

TABLE 21.4. Parasites of non-human primates—nervous, respiratory, and urogenital systems.

Parasite	Geographic distribution	Hosts	Location in host	Method of infection	Pathologic effects	Zoonosis	Reference
Arachnida							
Mites							
Astigmates							
Mortelmansia sp.	South America	Squirrel monkeys, marmosets	Nasal cavities	Direct contact	Unknown	Not reported	28
Mesostigmates							
Pneumonyssus simicola	Asia	Macaques	Lungs	Direct contact	Focal pneumonia	Not reported	138
Pneumonyssus duttoni	Africa	Guenons	Trachea	Direct contact	Tracheitis	Not reported	132
Pneumonyssus santos-diasi	Africa	Baboons, guenons	Lungs	Direct contact	Unknown	Not reported	280
Pneumonyssus longus	Africa	Guenons, chimpanzees	Lungs	Direct contact	Unknown	Not reported	132
Pneumonyssus oudemansi	Africa	Guenons, apes	Lungs	Direct contact	Unknown	Not reported	132
Pneumonyssus africanus	Africa	Guenons	Bronchi	Direct contact	Unknown	Not reported	132
Pneumonyssus mossambicencis	Africa	Baboons	Lungs	Direct contact	Unknown	Not reported	281
Pneumonyssus congoensis	Africa	Baboons	Lungs	Direct contact	Unknown	Not reported	96
Rhinophaga dinolti	Asia	Rhesus macaques	Lungs	Direct contact	Unknown	Not reported	282
Rhinophaga papionis	Africa	Baboons	Lungs	Direct contact	Chronic pneumonitis	Not reported	96
Pneumonyssoides stammeri	South America	Woolly monkeys	Nasal cavities, sinuses	Direct contact	Unknown	Not reported	129

REFERENCES

1. Bowman, D.D. (1999) *Georgi's Parasitology for Veterinarians,* 7th ed. W.B. Saunders Co., Philadelphia, PA.

2. Caminiti, B. (1984) Parasites of the digestive system of non-human primates and Tupaiidae: a bibliography, 1970–1984, *Primate Information Center, University of Washington.*

3. Kuntz, R.E. and Myers, B.J. (1969) A checklist of parasites and commensals reported for the Taiwan macaque (*Macaca cyclopis* Swinhoe, 1862). *Primates* **10,** 71–80.

4. Orihel, T.C. (1970) The helminth parasites of nonhuman primates and man. *Lab. Anim. Care* **20,** 395–401.

5. Orihel, T.C. and Siebold, H.R. (1972) Nematodes of the bowel and tissues. In: Fiennes, R.N. (ed), *Pathology of Simian Primates.* Karger Publishing, London, UK.

6. Ash, L.R. and Orihel, T.C. (1997) *Atlas of Human Parasitology,* 4th ed. American Society Clinical Pathologists, Chicago, IL.

7. Dorn, P., Daigle, M., and Cogswell, F. (2005) Chagas transmission in a primate colony in Louisiana. American Society of Tropical Medicine and Hygiene 54th Annual Meeting, Washington, D.C., December 11, 2005.

8. Dunn, F.L., Lambrecht, F.L., and duPlessis, R. (1963) Trypanosomes of South American monkeys and marmosets. *Am. J. Trop. Med. Hyg.* **12,** 524–534.

9. Levine, N.D. (1985) *Veterinary Protozoology.* Iowa State University Press, Ames, IA.

10. Cogswell, F.B. (2007) Enzootic parasites in an outdoor rhesus colony. *J. Med. Primatol.* Submitted for publication.

11. D'Alessandro, A., Eberjard, M., de Hincapie, O., and Halstead, S. (1986) *Trypanosoma cruzi* and *Trypanosoma rangeli* in *Saimiri sciureus* from Brazil and *Sanguinus mistax* from Brazil. *Am. J. Trop. Med. Hyg.* **35,** 285–289.

12. Groot, H. (1951) Nuevo foco de trypanosomiasis humana en Colombia. *Anales Soc. Biol. Bogota* **4,** 220–221.

13. Groot, H., Renjifo, S., and Uribe, C. (1951) *Trypanosoma ariarii,* N. sp., from man found in Colombia. *Am. J. Trop. Med. Hyg.* **31,** 673–691.

14. Sullivan, J., Steurer, F., Benavides, G., Tarleton, R.L., Eberhard, M.L., and Landry, S. (1993) Trypanosomes and microfilariae in feral owl and squirrel monkeys maintained in research colonies. *Am. J. Trop. Med. Hyg.* **49,** 254–259.

15. Garnham, P. and Gonzales-Mugaburu, L. (1962) A new trypanosome in *Saimiri* monkeys from Colombia. *Rev. Inst. Med. Trop. Sao Paulo* **4,** 79–84.

16. Reardon, L.V. and Rininger, B.F. (1968) A survey of parasites in laboratory primates. *Lab. Anim. Care* **18,** 577–580.

17. Ruch, T.C. (1959). *Diseases of Laboratory Primates.* W.B. Saunders Company, Philadelphia, PA.

18. daCunha, A. and Muniz, J. (1929) Nota sobre os parasitas intestinaes do Macacus rhesus com descripcao de uma nova especie de *Octomitus. Mem. Institute Oswaldo Cruz* **5,** 34–35.

19. Wenrich, D.H. (1933) A species of *Hexamita* (Protozoa, Flagellata) from the intestine of a monkey (*Macacus rhesus*). *J. Parasitol.* **33,** 177–188.

20. Hegner, R.W. (1934) Intestinal protozoa of chimpanzees. *Am. J. Hyg.* **19,** 480–501.

21. Hegner, R.W. and Chu, H.J. (1930) A survey of protozoa parasitic in plants and animals of the Philippine Islands. *Philippine J. Sci.* **43,** 451–482.

22. Poindexter, H.A. (1942) A study of the intestinal parasites of the monkeys of the Santiago Island primate colony. *Puerto Rico J. Pub. Health Trop. Med.* **18,** 175–191.

23. Wenrich, D.H. (1947) The species of *Trichomonas* in man. *J. Parasitol.* **33,** 177–188.

24. Honigberg, B.M. and Lee, J.J. (1959) Structure and division of *Trichomonas tenax* (O.F. Muller). *Am. J. Hyg.* **69,** 177–201.

25. Knowles, R. and Das Gupta, B.M. (1936) Some observations on the intestinal protozoa of macaques. *Indian J. Med. Res.* **24,** 547–556.

26. Kuntz, R.E. and Myers, B.J. (1967). *Microbiological Parameters of the Baboon (Papio sp.): Parasitology.* University of Texas Press, Austin, TX, 741–755.

27. Hoare, C.A. (1959) Amoebic infections in animals. *Vet. Rev. Annot.* **5,** 91–102.

28. Dunn, F.L. (1968). *The Parasites of Saimiri in the Context of Platyrrhine Parasitism.* Academic Press, London, UK.

29. Kuntz, R.E., Myers, B.J., and Vice, T.E. (1967). Intestinal protozoans and parasites of the gelada baboon (*Theropithecus gelada* Ruppel, 1835). *Proc. Helminthol. Soc. Washington, D.C.* **34,** 65–66.

30. Rowland, E. and Vandenbergh, J.G. (1965) A survey of intestinal parasites in a new colony of rhesus monkeys. *J. Parasitol.* **51,** 294–295.

31. Kessel, J.F. and Johnstone, H.G. (1949) The occurrence of *Endamoeba polecki* Prowazek 1912 in *Macaca mulatta* and in man. *Am. J. Trop. Med.* **29,** 311–317.

32. Burrows, R.B. and Klink, G.E. (1955) *Endamoeba polecki* infections in man. *Am. J. Hyg.* **62,** 155–167.

33. Kuntz, R.E. and Myers, B.J. (1966) Parasites of baboons (*Papio doguera* Pucheran 1856) captured in Kenya and Tanzania, East Africa. *Primates* **7,** 27–32.

34. Van Riper, O.C., Day, J.W., Fineg, J., and Prine, J.R. (1966). Intestinal parasites of recently imported chimpanzees. *Lab. Anim. Care* **16,** 360–363.

35. Sestak, K., Merit, C.K., Borda, J., Saylor, E., Schwamberger, S., Cogswell, F., et al. (2003) Infectious agent and immune response characteristics of chronic enterocolitis in captive rhesus macaques. *Infect. Immun.* **71,** 4079–4086.

36. Sanuki, J., Asai, T., Okuzawa, E., Kobayashi, S., and Takeuchi, T. (1997) Identification of *Entamoeba histolytica* and *E. dispar* cysts in stool by polymerase chain reaction. *Parasitol. Res.* **83,** 96–98.

37. Bond, V.P., Bostick, W., Hansen, E.L., and Anderson, H.H. (1946) Pathologic study of natural amebic infection in macaques. *Am. J. Trop. Med.* **26,** 625–629.

38. Hoare, C.A. (1958) The enigma of host-parasite relations in amebiasis. *Rice Institute Pamphlet* **45,** 23–35.

39. Bourova, L.F. (1946) Etude experimentale des amibes du type *histolytica* chez les singes inferieurs. *Ann. Parasitol. Hum. Comp.* **21,** 97–118.

40. Johnson, C.M. (1941) Observations on natural infections of *Entamoeba histolytica* in *Ateles* and rhesus monkeys. *Am. J. Trop. Med.* **21,** 49–61.

41. Kessel, J.F. (1928) Intestinal protozoa of monkeys. *Univ. Calif. (Berkeley) Publ. Zool.* **31,** 275–306.

42. Miller, M.J. and Bray, R.S. (1966) *Entamoeba histolytica* infections in the chimpanzee (*Pan satyrus*). *J. Parasitol.* **52,** 386–388.

43. Young, R.J., Fremming, B.D., Benson, R.E., and Harris, M.D. (1957) Care and management of a *Macaca mulatta* monkey colony. *Proc. Anim. Care Panel* **7,** 67–82.

44. Bostrom, R.E., Ferrell, J.F., and Martin, J.E. (1968) Simian amebiasis with lesions simulating human amebic dysentery. *19th Annual Meeting Am. Assoc. Lab Anim. Sci., Las Vegas* **Abstract 51.**

45. Fremming, B.D., Vogel, F.S., Benson, R.E, and Young, R.J. (1955) A fatal case of amebiasis with liver abscesses and ulcerative colitis in a chimpanzee. *J. Am. Vet. Med. Assoc.* **126**, 406–407.

46. Vickers, J.H. (1969) Diseases of primates affecting the choice of species for toxicologic studies. *Ann. N.Y. Acad. Sci.* **162**, 659–672.

47. Grundy, M., Voller, A, and Warhurst, D. (1987) An enzyme linked immunosorbent assay for the detection of *Entamoeba histolytica* antigens in fecal material. *Trans. R. Soc. Trop. Med. Hyg.* **81**, 627–632.

48. Ungar, B., Yolken, R.H., and Quinn, T.C. (1985) Use of a monoclonal antibody in an enzyme linked immunoassay for the detection of *Entamoeba histolytica* in fecal specimens. *Am. J. Trop. Med. Hyg.* **34**, 465–472.

49. Beaver, P.C. and Deschamps, G. (1949) The viability of *E. histolytica* cysts in soil. *Am. J. Trop. Med.* **29**, 189–191.

50. Halpern, B. and Dolkart, R.E. (1954) The effect of cold temperatures on the viability of cysts of *Entamoeba histolytica*. *Am. J. Trop. Med. Hyg.* **3**, 276–282.

51. Hawking, F. (1972) *Entopolypoides macaci,* a *Babesia*-like parasite in *Cercopithecus* monkeys. *Parasitology* **65**, 89–109.

52. Bronsdon, M.A., Homer, M.J., Magera, J.M.H., Harrison, C., Andrews, R.G., Bielitzki, J.T., et al. (1999) Detection of enzootic Babesiosis in baboons (*Papio cynocephalus*) and phylogenetic evidence supporting synonymy of the genera *Entopolypoides* and *Babesia. J. Clin. Microbiol.* **37**, 1548–1553.

53. Garnham, P.C.C. (1966) *Malaria Parasites and Other Haemosporidia.* Blackwell Scientific Publications, Oxford, UK.

54. Sullivan, J.S., Nace, D., Williams, T., Guarner, J., Noland, G.S., and Collins, W.E. (2003) The development of exoerythrocytic stages of *Plasmodium inui shortti* in New World monkeys. *J. Parasitol.* **89**, 637–639.

55. Cogswell, F.B. (2000) Malaria and piroplasms of non-human primates. In: Bowman, D.D. (ed.) *Companion and Exotic Animal Parasitology,* International Veterinary Information Service. Ithaca, NY.

56. Garnham, P.C.C. (1963) Distribution of Simian Malaria Parasites in Various Hosts. *J. Parasitol.* **49**, 905– 911.

57. Didier, E.S., Didier, P.J., Snowden, K.F., and Shadduck, J.A. (2000) Microsporidiosis in mammals. *Microbes Infect.* **2**, 709–720.

58. Green, L.C., Didier, P.J., Bowers, L.C., and Didier, E.S. (2004) Natural and experimental infection of immunocompromised rhesus macaques (*Macaca mulatta*) with the microsporidian *Enterocytozoon bieneusi* genotype D. *Microbes Infect.* **6**, 996–1002.

59. Yidi, H. (1989) Investigation of infected state of *Balantidium coli* in rhesus monkey groups. *Zool. Res.* **10**, 151–155.

60. Brumpt, E. and Joyeux, C. (1912) Sur un infusoire nouveau parasite du chimpanze *Troglodytella abrassarti,* N.g. n. sp. *Bull Soc. Pathol. Exotique* **5**, 499–503.

61. Kudo, R.R. (1966) *Protozoology.* 5th ed. Charles C. Thomas, Springfield, IL.

62. Curasson, G.C.M. (1929) *Troglodytella abrassarti,* infusoire pathogene du chimpanze. *Ann. Parasitol. Hum. Comp.* **7**, 465–468.

63. Faust. E.C. (1967) *Athesmia* (Trematoda: Dicrocoeliidae) Odhner, 1911 liver fluke of monkeys from Colombia, South America, and other mammalian hosts. *Trans. Am. Microscop. Soc.* **86**, 113–119.

64. Garner, E., Hemrick, F., and Rudiger, H. (1967) Multiple helminth infections in cinnamon-ringtail monkeys (*Cebus albifrons*). *Lab. Anim. Care* **17**, 310–315.

65. Cosgrove, G.E., Nelson, B., and Gengozian, N. (1968) Helminth parasites of the tamarin, *Sanguinus fuscicollis. Lab. Anim. Care* **18**, 654–656.

66. Beaver, P.C., Jung, R.C., and Cupp, E.W. (1984) *Clinical Parasitology,* 9th ed. Lea and Febiger, Philadelphia, PA.

67. Graham, G.L. (1960) Parasitism in monkeys. *Ann. NY Acad. Sci.* **85**, 735–992.

68. Herman, L.H. (1967) *Gastrodiscus hominis* infestation in two monkeys. *Vet. Med.* **62**, 355–356.

69. Faust, E.C. (1949) *Human Helminthology.* 3rd ed. Lea and Febiger, Philadelphia, PA.

70. Whitney, R.A., Johnson, D.J., and Cole, W.C. (1967) *The Subhuman Primate: A Guide to the Veterinarian.* Edgewood Arsenal, Maryland, 100–126.

71. Lapage, G. (1968). *Veterinary Parasitology.* Oliver and Boyd, Edinburgh, Scotland.

72. Purvis, A.J., Ellison, I.R., and Husting, E.L. (1965) A short note on the findings of Schistosomes in baboons (*Papio rhodesiae*). *Cent. Afr. J. Med.* **11**, 368.

73. Swellengrebel, N.H. and Rijpstra, A.C. (1965) Lateral spined schistosome ova in the intestine of a squirrel monkey from Surinam. *Trop. Geograph. Med.* **17**, 80–84.

74. DePaoli, A. (1965) *Schistosoma haematobium* in the chimpanzee—a natural infection. *Am. J. Trop,. Med. Hyg.* **14**, 561–565.

75. Sadun, E.H., von Lichtenberg, F., Hickman, R.L., Bruce, J.I., Smith, J.H., and Schoenbechler, M.J. (1966) *Schistosoma mansoni* in the chimpanzee: Parasitologic, clinical, serologic, pathologic and radiologic observations. *Am. J. Trop. Med. Hyg.* **15**, 496–506.

76. Stunkard, H.W. (1940) The morphology and life history of the cestode, *Bertiella studeri. Am. J. Trop. Med. Hyg.* **20**, 305–333.

77. Eberhard, M.L. (1981) Intestinal parasitism in an outdoor breeding colony of *Macaca mulatta. Lab. Anim. Sci.* **31**, 282–285.

78. Hashimoto, I. and Honjo, S. (1966) Survey of helminth parasites in cynomolgus monkeys (*Macaca irus*). *Jpn. J. Med. Sci. Biol.* **19**, 218.

79. Tanaka, H., Fukui, M., Yamamoto, H., Hayama, S., and Kodera, S. (1962) Studies on the identification of common intestinal parasites of primates. *Bull. Exp. Animals* **11**, 111– 116.

80. Bywater, J.E.C. and Mann, K.H. (1960) Infestation of a monkey with a leech *Dinobdella ferox. Vet. Record* **72**, 955.

81. Fox, J.G. and Ediger, R.D. (1970) Nasal leech infestation in the rhesus monkey. *Lab. Anim. Care* **20**, 1137–1138.

82. Pryor, W.H., Bergner, J.F. Jr., and Raulston, G.L. (1970) Leech (*Dinobdella ferox*) infection of a Taiwan monkey (*Macaca cyclopis*). *J. Am. Vet. Med. Assoc.* **157**, 1926–1927.

83. Little, M.D.(1966) Comparative morphology of six species of *Strongyloides* (Nematoda) and redefinition of the genus. *J. Parasitol.* **52**, 69–84.

84. Soulsby, E.J.L. (1982) *Helminths, Arthropods and Protozoa of Domesticated Animals.* 7th ed. Lea and Febiger, Philadelphia, PA.

85. Liebegott, G. (1962) Pericarditis verminosa (*Strongyloides*) beim Schimpanzsen. *Virchows Arch. Pathol. Anat. Physiol. Klin. Med.* **335**, 211–225.

86. Habermann, R.T. and Williams, F.P. Jr. (1958) The identification and control of helminths in laboratory animals. *J. Natl. Cancer. Inst.* **20**, 979–1009.

87. Dufour, J., Bohm, R., Cogswell, F., and Falkenstein, S. (2006) Comparison of efficacy of moxidectin and ivermectin in treatment of *Strongyloides fülleborni* infection in rhesus macaques. *J. Med. Primatol.* **35** 172–176.

88. Habermann, R.T. and Williams, F.P. Jr. (1957) Diseases seen at necropsy of 708 *Macaca mulatta* (rhesus monkey) and *Macaca philippinensis* (cynomolgus monkey). *Am. J. Vet. Res.* **18**, 419–426.

89. Sasa, M., Tanaka, H., Fukui, M., and Takata, A. (1962) Internal parasites of laboratory animals. In: Harris, R.J.C. (ed), *The Problems of Laboratory Animal Disease.* Academic Press, London, UK.

90. Brown, R.C. and Girardeau, M.H.F. (1976) Transmammary passage of *Strongyloides* sp. larvae in the human host. *Am. J. Trop. Med. Hyg.* **26,** 215–219.

91. Faust, E.C. and Russell, P.F. (1964) *Craig and Faust's Clinical Parasitology.* 7th ed. Lea and Febiger, Philadelphia, PA.

92. Inglis, W.G. (1961) The oxyurid parasites (Nematoda) of primates. *Proc. Zool. Soc. London* **136,** 103–122.

93. Christensen, L.T. (1964) Chimp and owners share worm infestation. *Vet. Med.* **59,** 801–803.

94. Ratcliffe, H.L. (1945) Infectious diseases of laboratory animals. *Ann. NY Acad. Sci.* **46,** 77–96.

95. Amberson, E.M. and Schwarz, E. (1952) *Ternidens deminutus* Railliet and Henry, a nematode parasite of man and primates. *Ann. Trop. Med. Parasitol.* **46,** 227–237.

96. Myers, B.J. and Kuntz, R.E. (1965) A checklist of parasites reported for the baboon. *Primates* **6,** 137–194.

97. Nelson, G.S. (1965) The parasitic helminths of baboons with particular reference to species transmissible to man. In: Vagtborg, H. (ed), *The Baboon in Medical Research.* University of Texas Press, Austin, TX, 441–470.

98. Dunn, F.L. (1961) *Molineus vexillarius* sp. n. (Nematoda: Trichostrongylidae) from a Peruvian primate, *Tamarinus nigricollis* (Spix, 1823). *J. Parasitol.* **47,** 953–956.

99. Durette-Desset, M., Fribourg Blanc, L.A., and Vuong, P.N. (2001) *Molineus torulosus* (Nematoda Trichostrongylina, Molineoidea) a parasite of Neotropical primates: new morphological and histological data. *Parasite* **8,** 53–60.

100. Brack, M., Myers, B.J., and Kuntz, R.E. (1973) Pathogenic properties of *Molineus torulosus* in capuchin monkeys, *Cebus apella. Lab. Anim. Sci.* **23,** 360–365.

101. Durette-Desset, M.C., Fribourg Blanc, L.A., and Vuong, P.N. (2001) *Molineus torulosus* (Nematoda, Trichostrongylina, Molineoidea) a parasite of Neotropical primates: new morphological and histological data. *Parasite* **8,** 53–60.

102. Deinhardt, F., Holmes, A.W., Devine, J., and Deinhardt, J. (1967) Marmosets as laboratory animals IV. The microbiology of laboratory kept marmosets. *Lab. Anim. Care* **17,** 48– 70.

103. Bonne, C. and Sandground, J.H. (1939) On the production of gastric tumors bordering on malignancy in Javanese monkeys through the agency of *Nochtia nochti,* a parasitic nematode. *Am. J. Cancer* **37,** 173–185.

104. Smetana, H.F. and Orihel, T.C. (1969) Gastric papillomata in *Macaca speciosa* induced by *Nochtia nochti* (Nematoda: Trichostrongyloidea). *J. Parasitol.* **55,** 349–351.

105. Abbott, D.P. and Majeed, S.K. (1984) A survey of parasitic lesions in wild-caught, laboratory-maintained primates: (rhesus, cynomolgus, and baboon). *Vet. Pathol.* **21,** 198–207.

106. Dunn, F.L. and Lambrecht, F. (1963) On some filarial parasites of South American primates with a description of *Tetrapetalonema tamarinae* n.sp. from Peruvian Tamarin Marmoset, *Tamarinus nigricollis* (Spix, 1823). *J. Helminthol.* **37,** 261–286.

107. Webber, W.A. and Hawking, F. (1955) The filarial worms *Dipetalonema digitatum* and *D. gracile* in monkeys. *Parasitology* 45, 401–408.

108. Esslinger, J.H. and Gardiner, C.H. (1974) *Dipetalonema barbascalensis* sp. N. (Nematoda: Filaroidea) from the owl monkey, *Aotus trivirga-*

tus, with a consideration of the status of *Parlitomosa zakii* Nagaty, 1935. *J. Parasitol.* **60,** 1001–1005.

109. Garner, E. (1967) *Dipetalonema gracile* infections in squirrel monkeys (*Saimiri sciureus*). *Lab. Anim. Digest* **3,** 16–17.

110. Witney, R.A., Johnson, D.J., and Cole, W.C. (1967) *The Subhuman Primate: A Guide for the Veterinarian.* Edgewood Arsenal, MD.

111. Allen, A.M. (1960) Occurrence of the nematode, *Anatrichosoma cutaneum,* in the nasal mucosae of *Macaca mulatta* monkeys. *Am. J. Vet. Res.* **21,** 389–392.

112. Thienpont, D., Mortelmans, J., and Vercruysse, J. (1962) Contribution a l'etude de la Trichuriose du chimpanze et de son traitement avec la methyridine. *Ann. Soc. Belge. Med. Trop.* **2,** 211–218.

113. Machado Filho, D.A. (1950) Revisao do genero Prosthenorchis Travassos, 1915 (Acanthocephala). *Mem. Institute Oswaldo Cruz* **48,** 495–544.

114. Worms, M.J. (1967) Parasites of newly imported animals. *J. Inst. Anim. Technicians* **18,** 39–47.

115. Middleton, C.C., Clarkson, T.B., and Garner, F.M. (1964) Parasites of squirrel monkeys (*Saimiri sciureus*). *Lab. Anim. Care* **14,** 335.

116. Nelson, B., Cosgrove, G.E., and Genozian, N. (1966) Diseases of an imported primate *Tamarinus nigricollis. Lab. Anim. Care* **16,** 255–275.

117. Richart, R. and Benirschke, K.B. (1963). Causes of death in a colony of marmoset monkeys. *J. Pathol. Bacteriol.* **86,** 221–223.

118. Takos, M.J. and Thomas, J. (1958) The pathology and pathogenesis of fatal infections due to an acanthocephalid parasite of marmoset monkeys. *Am. J. Trop. Med. Hyg.* **7,** 90–94.

119. Dunn, F.L. (1963) Acanthocephalans and cestodes of South American monkeys and marmosets. *J. Parasitol.* **49,** 717–722.

120. Brumpt, E. and Urbain, A. (1938) Epizootie vermineuse por Acanthocephales (*Prosthenorchis*) yant sevi a la singerie due Museum de Paris. *Ann. Parasitol. Hum. Comp.* **16,** 289–300.

121. Kuhn, H.-J. and Ludwig, H.W. (1967) Die affenlause deer gattung Pedicinus. *Z. Zool. Syst. Evolutionsforsch* **5,** 144–256.

122. Hopkins, G.H.E. (1949) The host associations of the lice of mammals. *Proc. Zool. Soc. London* **119,** 387–604.

123. Pope, B.L. (1966) Some parasites of the howler monkey of northern Argentina. *J. Parasitol.* **52,** 166–168.

124. Luck, C.R. (1957) The vervet monkey (*Cercopithecus aethiops*), numerous varieties. In: Worden, A.N. and Lane-Petter, W.L. (eds.), *The UFAW Handbook on the Care and Management of Laboratory Animals.* The Universities Federation for Animal Welfare, Blackwell Science Ltd., Edinburgh, Scotland.

125. Hopkins, G.H.E. and Rothschild, M. (1953) *An Illustrated Catalog of the Rothschild Collection of Fleas (Siphonaptera) in the British Museum (Nat. History): Vol I. Tungidae and Pulicidae.* British Museum (Nat. History). London, UK and Ames, IA.

126. Matheson, R. (1950) *Medical Entomology,* 2nd ed. Comstock Publishing, Ithaca, NY.

127. Tipton, V.J. and Mendez, E. (1966) The fleas (Siphonaptera) of Panama. In: Wenzel, R.L. and Tipton, V.J. (eds.), *The Ectoparasites of Panama,* Field Museum of Natural History, Chicago, IL.

128. Hicks, E.P. (1930) The early stages of the jigger, *Tunga penetrans. Ann. Trop. Med. Parasitol.* **24,** 575– 586.

129. Fain, A. (1961) Sur le statut de deux especes d'acariens de genre Pneumonyssus Banks. Designation d'un neotype pour *Pneumonyssus simicola* Banks, 1901 (Mesostigmata: Halarachnidae). *Z. Parasitenk.* **21,** 141–150.

130. Grinker, J.A., Karlin, D.A. and Manalo Estrella, P. (1962). Lung mites: Pulmonary acariasis in the primate. *Aerosp. Med.* **33**, 841–845.

131. Stiller, D., Sirimanne, R.A., Roberts, C.R., and Eluthesen, K. (1974) The silvered leaf monkey as a natural host of the lung mite, *Pneumonyssus simicola* Banks, (Acarina: Halarachnidae) in Malaysia: a preliminary report. *Southeast Asian J. Trop. Med. Public Health* **5**, 458.

132. Fain, A. (1959) Les acariens de genre *Pneumonyssus* Banks, parasites endopulmonaires des singes au Congo Belge (Halarchnidae: Mesostigmata). *Ann. Parasitol. Hum. Comp.* **34**, 126–148.

133. Honjo, S.K.M., Fujiwara, T., Suzuki, Y., and Imaizumi, K. (1963) Statistical survey of internal parasites in cynomolgus monkeys (*Macaca irus*). *Jpn. J. Med. Sci. Biol.* **16**, 217–224.

134. Banks, N. (1901) A new genus of endoparasitic acarians. *Geneesk. Tijdschr. Nederl.-Indie.* **41**, 334–336.

135. Strandtmann, R.W. and Wharton, G.W. (1958) *A Manual of Mesostigmatid Mites Parasitic on Vertebrates.* University of Maryland, College Park, MD.

136. Vitzthum, H. (1930) *Pneumonyssus stammeri* ein neuer Lungenparasit. *Z. Parasitenk.* **2**, 595–615.

137. Ewing, H.E. (1929). Notes on the lung mites of primates (Acarina: Dermanyssidae), including the description of a new species. *Proc. Entomol. Soc. Wash D.C.* **31**, 126–130.

138. Innes, J.R.M., Colton, M.W., Yevich, P.P., and Smith, C.L. (1954) Pulmonary Acariasis as an enzootic disease caused by *Pneumonyssus simicola* in imported monkeys. *Am. J. Pathol.* **30**, 813–835.

139. Baker, E.W., Evans, T.M., Gold, D.J., Hull, W.B., and Keegan, H.L. (1956) *A Manual of Parasitic Mites of Medical or Economic Importance. Tech. Publ. Natl. Pest Control. Assoc., Inc.*

140. Hull, W.B. (1956) The nymphal stages of *Pneumonyssus simicola* Banks, 1901 (Acarina: Halarachnidae). *J. Parasitol.* **42**, 653–656.

141. Hughes, T.E. (1959) *Mites, or the Acari.* Athlone Press, London, UK.

142. Fremming, B.D., Harris, M.D. Jr., Young, R.J., and Benson, R.E. (1957) Preliminary investigation into the life cycle of the monkey lung mite (*Pneumonyssus foxi*). *Am. J. Vet. Res.* **18**, 427–428.

143. Knezevich, A.L. and McNulty, W.P. Jr. (1970) Pulmonary acariasis (*Pneumonyssus simicola*) in colony-bred *Macaca mulatta*. *Lab. Anim. Care* **20**, 693–696.

144. Valerio, D.A., Miller, R.L., Innes, J.R.M., Courtney, K.D., Pallota, A.J., and Guttmacher, R.M. (1969) *Macaca mulatta: Management of a Breeding Colony.* Academic Press, New York, NY.

145. Stone, W.B. and Hughes, J.A. (1969) Massive pulmonary acariasis in the pig-tailed macaque. *Bull. Wildlife Dis. Assoc.* **5**, 20–22.

146. Lee, R.E., Williams, R.B. Jr., Hull, W.B., and Stein, S.N. (1954) Significance of pulmonary acariasis in rhesus monkeys (*Macaca mulatta*). *Federation Proc.* **13**, 85– 86.

147. Furman, D., Bonash, H., Springsteen, R., Stiller, D., and Rahlmann, D.F. (1974) Studies on the biology of the lung mite *Pneumonyssus simicola* Banks (Acarina: Halarachnidae) and diagnosis of infestation in macaques. *Lab. Anim. Sci.* **24**, 622–629.

148. Furman, D.P. (1954) A revision of the genus *Pneumonyssus* (Acarina: Halarachnidae). *J. Parasitol.* **40**, 31–42.

149. Self, J.T. and Cosgrove, J.C. (1968). Pentastome larvae in laboratory primates. *J. Parasitol* **34**, 21–23.

150. Heymons, R. (1935) Pentastomida. In: Bronn, H.G. (ed.), *Klassen und Ordnungen des Tierreichs,* Akademische Verlagsgesellschaft M.B.H, 1–268.

151. Fredrickson, R., Haines, D.E., and Hall, J.E. (1985) Pentastomid nymph from the brain of a squirrel monkey (*Saimiri sciureus*). II. Morphology of the host response. *J. Med. Primatol.* **14**, 209–223.

152. Fain, A. (1961) Les pentastomides de l'Afrique Centrale. *Ann. Musee. Roy. Afrique Centrale Ser 8, Sci. Zool.* **92**, 1–115.

153. Hegner, R.W. and Ratcliffe, H. (1927) Trichomonads from the vagina of the monkey, from the mouth of the cat and man, and from intestine of the monkey, opossum and prairie-dog. *J. Parasitol.* **14**, 27–35.

154. Collins, W.E., Warren, M., Sullivan, J.S., Galland, G.G., Nace, D., Williams, A., et al. (2005) Studies on two strains of *Plasmodium cynomolgi* in New World and Old World monkeys and mosquitoes. *J. Parasitol.* **91**, 280–283.

155. Michaud, C., Tantalean, M., Ique, C., Montoya, E., and Gozalo, A. (2003) A survey for helminth parasites in feral New World non-human primate populations and its comparison with parasitological data from man in the region. *J. Med. Primatol.* **32**, 341–345.

156. Nasher, A.K. (1988) Zoonotic parasite infections of the Arabian sacred baboon *Papio hamadryas arabicus* Thomas in Asir Province, Saudi Arabia. *Ann. Parasitol. Hum. Comp.* **63**, 448–454.

157. Chung, W.C., Lin, C.Y., and Fan, P.C. (1996) Ectopic locations of *Taenia saginata asiatica* cysticerci in the abdominal cavity of domestic pig and monkey. *J. Parasitol.* **82**, 1032–1034.

158. Sandground, J.H. (1937) On the coenurus from the brain of a monkey. *J. Parasitol.* **23**, 482–490.

159. Plesker, R., Bauer, C., Tackmann, K., and Dinkel, A. (2001) Hydatid echinococcosis (*Echinococcus granulosus*) in a laboratory colony of pig-tailed macaques (*Macaca nemestrina*). *J. Vet. Med. B Infect. Dis. Vet. Public Health.* **48**, 367–372.

160. Opuni, E.K. and Muller, R.L. (1975) Studies on *Spirometra theileri* (Baer, 1925) n. comb. 2. Pathology of experimental plerocercoid infections. *J. Helminthol.* **49**, 121–127.

161. Desportes, C. (1945) Sur *Strongyloides stercoralis* (Bavay 1876) et sur les strongyloides de primates. *Ann. Parasitol. Humaine Comparee* **20**, 160–190.

162. Benson, R.E., Fremming, B.D., and Young, R.J. (1955) *Care and Management of Chimpanzees at the Radiobiological Laboratory of the University of Texas and the United States Air Force.* School of Aviation Medicine, U.S. Air Force Report, 48–55.

163. Hawkins, J.V., Clapp, N.K., Carson, R.L., Henke, M.A., McCracken, M.D., Faulkner, C.T., and Patton, S. (1997) Diagnosis and treatment of *Trichospirura leptostoma* infection in common marmosets (*Callithrix jacchus*). *Contemp. Top. Lab. Anim. Sci.* **36**, 52–55.

164. Orihel, T.C. (1969) *Dirofilaria corynodes* (Von Linstow, 1899): morphology and life history. *J. Parasitol.* **55**, 94–103.

165. Mak, J.W., Choong, M.F., Suresh, K., and Lam, P.L. (1990) Experimental infection of the leaf-monkey, *Presbytis cristata,* with subperiodic *Brugia malayi. Parasitol. Res.* **76**, 689–691.

166. Curtis, S.J., Edwards, C., Athulathmuda, C., and Paul, J. (2006) Case of the month: Cutaneous myiasis in a returning traveler from the Algarve: first report of tumbu maggots, *Cordylobia anthropophaga,* acquired in Portugal. *Emerg. Med. J.* **23**, 236–237.

167. Sampson, C.E., MaGuire, J., and Eriksson, E. (2001) Botfly myiasis: case report and brief review. *Ann. Plast. Surg.* **46**, 150–152.

168. de Resende, D.M., Pereira, L.H., and Lobo, A. (1994) Long-term patency of blood parasitism by *Trypanosoma minasense* and Microfilariae in *Callithrix penicillata* marmosets (Primates, Callitrichidae), caught at the wild and maintained in captivity. *Mem. Inst. Oswaldo Cruz.* **89**, 127–128.

169. Reichenow, E. (1917) Parásitos de la sangre y del intestino de los monos antropomorfos africanos. *Bol. Real Soc. Espan. Hist. Nat. Secc. Biol.* **17**, 312–332.

170. Hill, W.C.O. (1954) Report of the Society's prosector for the year 1953. *Proc. Zool. Soc. London.* **124**, 303–311.

171. Zeiss, C.J. and Shomer, N. (2001) Hepatocystosis in a baboon (*Papio anubis*). *Contemp. Top. Lab. Anim. Sci.* **40**, 41–42.

172. Garnham, P.C. and Rajapaksa, N. (1973) Malaria parasites in *Presbytis aygula*. New host record of *Hepatocystis semnopitheci*. *Trans. R. Soc. Trop. Med. Hyg.* **67**, 2.

173. Takenaka, T., Hashimoto, K., Gotou, H., Matsumoto, S., and Nishikawa, T. (1990) Studies on Hepatocystis sp. in rhesus monkeys from Yunnan, China. *Jikken Dobutsu* **39**, 273– 279.

174. Lourenco-de-Oliveira, R. and Deane, L.M. (1995) Simian malaria at two sites in the Brazilian Amazon. I. The infection rates of *Plasmodium brasilianum* in non-human primates. *Mem. Inst. Oswaldo Cruz.* **90**, 331–339.

175. Sullivan, J.S., Bounngaseng, A., Stewart, A., Sullivan, J.J., Galland, G.G., Fleetwood, H., et al. (2005) Infection of *Saimiri boliviensis* monkeys with *Plasmodium coatneyi*. *J. Parasitol.* **91**, 479–481.

176. Warren, Mc.W., Bennett, G.F., Sandosham, A.A., and Coatney, G.R. (1965) *Plasmodium eylesi* sp. nov., a tertian malaria parasite from the white-handed gibbon, *Hylobates lar*. *Ann. Trop. Med. Parasitol.* **59**, 500–508.

177. Eyles, D.E., Laing, A.B., and Fong. Y.L. (1962) *Plasmodium fieldi* sp. nov., a new species of malaria parasite from the pigtailed macaque in Malaya. *Ann. Trop. Med. Parasitol.* **56**, 242–247.

178. Puri, S.K. and Dutta, G.P. (1994) *Presbytis entellus*, a new experimental host for *Plasmodium fragile*. *J. Parasitol.* **80**, 156–158.

179. Buck, G., Coudurier, J., and Quesnel, J.J. (1952) Two new Plasmodia observed in a splenectomized lemur of Madagascar. *Arch. Inst. Pasteur Alger.* **30**, 240–243.

180. Sullivan, J.S., Jennings, V.M., Guarner, J., Noland, G.S., Kendall, J., and Collins, W.E. (2002) Infection of *Aotus* and *Saimiri* monkeys with *Plasmodium gonderi*. *J. Parasitol.* **88**, 422–425.

181. Collins, W.E., Contacos, P.G., Garnham, P.C., Warren, M., and Skinner, J.C. (1972) *Plasmodium hylobati*: a malaria parasite of the gibbon. *J. Parasitol.* **58**, 123–128.

182. Coatney, G.R., Orihel, T.C., and Warren, M. (1969) *Plasmodium jefferyi*: a redescription. *J. Parasitol.* **55**, 1235–1239.

183. Collins, W.E. and Warren, M. (1998) Studies on infections with two strains of *Plasmodium inui* from Taiwan in rhesus monkeys and different anopheline mosquitoes. *J. Parasitol.* **84**, 547–551.

184. Chen, L., Li, G., Lu, Y., and Luo, Z. (2001) Histopathological changes of *Macaca mulatta* infected with *Plasmodium knowlesi*. *Chin. Med. J.* **114**, 1073–1077.

185. Huff, C.G. and Hoogstraal, H. (1963) *Plasmodium lemuris* n. sp. from *Lemur collaris* E. Geoffroy. *J. Inf. Dis.* **112**, 233–236.

186. Bray, R.S. (1960) Studies on malaria in chimpanzees: VIII. The experimental transmission and pre-erythrocytic phase of *Plasmodium malariae*, with a note on the host-range of the parasite. *Am. J. Trop. Med. Hyg.* **9**, 455–465.

187. Peters, W. (1976) Malaria of the orangutan (*Pongo pygmaeus*) in Borneo. *Philos. Trans. R. Soc. Lond. B Biol. Sci.* **28**, 439–482.

188. Bray, R.S. (1956) Studies on malaria in chimpanzees. I. The erythrocytic forms of *Plasmodium reichenowi*. *J. Parasitol.* **42**, 588–592.

189. Contacos, P.G., Coatney, G.R., Orihel, T.C., Collins, W.E., Chin, W., and Jeter, M.H. (1970) Transmission of *Plasmodium schwetzi* from the chimpanzee to man by mosquito bite. *Am. J. Trop. Med. Hyg.* **19**, 190–195.

190. Collins, W.E. and Contacos, P.G. (1979) Infection and transmission studies with *Plasmodium simiovale* in the *Macaca mulatta* monkey. *J. Parasitol.* **65**, 609–612.

191. Collins, W.E., Contacos, P.G., Guinn, E.G., and Skinner, J.C. (1973) *Plasmodium simium* in the *Aotus trivirgatus* monkey. *J. Parasitol.* **59**, 49–51.

192. Eyles, D.E., Fong, Y.L., Dunn, F.L., Guinn, E., Warren, M., and Sandosham, A.A. (1964) *Plasmodium youngi* n. sp., a malaria parasite of the Malayan gibbon, *Hylobates lar lar*. *Am. J. Trop. Med. Hyg.* **13**, 248–255.

193. Soliman, L.A., Cheever, A.W., Kuntz, R.E., and Myers, B.J. (1974) Lesions of bladder muscle in baboons and monkeys infected with *Schistosoma haematobium*. *Tropenmed. Parasitol.* **25**, 327–333.

194. Kuntz, R.E., Huang, T., and Moore, J.A. (1977) Patas monkey (*Erythrocebus patas*) naturally infected with *Schistosoma mansoni*. *J. Parasitol.* **63**, 166– 167.

195. Vickers, J.H. and Penner, L.R. (1968) Cysticercosis in four rhesus brains. *J. Am. Vet. Med. Assoc.* **153**, 868– 871.

196. Vogel, P., Zaucha, G., Goodwin, S.D., Kuehl, K., and Fritz, D. (1996) Rapid postmortem invasion of cecal mucosa of macaques by nonpathogenic *Entamoeba chattoni*. *Am. J. Trop. Med. Hyg.* **55**, 595–602.

197. Takano, J., Narita, T., Tachibana, H., Shimizu, T., Komatsubara, H., Terao, K., et al. (2005) *Entamoeba histolytica* and *Entamoeba dispar* infections in cynomolgus monkeys imported into Japan for research. *Parasitol. Res.* **97**, 255–257.

198. Westphal, A. (1973) *Iodamoeba buetschlii*. *Dtsch. Med. Wochenschr.* **16**, 581.

199. Poelma, F.G. (1966) *Eimeria lemuris* n. sp., *E. galago* n. sp. and *E. otolicni* n. sp. from a galago *Galago senegalensis*. *J. Protozool.* **13**, 547– 549.

200. Hendricks, L.D. (1977) Host range characteristics of the primate coccidian, *Isospora arctopitheci* Rodhain 1933 (Protozoa: Eimeriidae). *J. Parasitol.* **63**, 32–35.

201. Yang, Y., Zeng, L., Li, M., and Zhou, J. (1995) Diarrhoea in piglets and monkeys experimentally infected with *Balantidium coli* isolated from human faeces. *J. Trop. Med. Hyg.* **98**, 69–72.

202. O'Donoghue, P.J., Gasser, R.B., and Tribe, A. (1993) New host record for the entodiniomorphid ciliate, *Troglodytella abrassarti*, from siamangs (*Hylobates syndactylus*). *Int. J. Parasitol.* **23**, 415–418.

203. Reichenow, E. (1920) Den Wiederkäuer-Infusorien verwandt Formen aus Gorilla und Schimpanse. *Arch. Protistenk.* **41**, 1–33.

204. Cosgrove, G.E. (1966) The trematodes of laboratory primates. *Lab. Anim. Care* **16**, 23–39.

205. Stuart, M.D., Greenspan, L.L., Glander, K.E., and Clarke, M.R. (1990) A coprological survey of parasites of wild mantled howling monkeys, *Alouatta palliata palliata*. *J. Wildl. Dis.* **26**, 547–549.

206. Stunkard, H.W. and Goss, L.J. (1950) *Eurytrema brumpti* railliet, Henry and Joyeux, 1912 (Trematoda: Dicrocoeliidae), from the pancreas and liver of African anthropoid apes. *J. Parasitol.* **36**, 574–581.

207. Hartman, H.A. (1961) The intestinal fluke (*Fasciolopsis buski*) in a monkey. *Am. J. Vet. Res.* **22**, 1123– 1126.

208. Scholz, T., Ditrich, O., Tuma, M., and Giboda, M. (1991) Study of the body surface of *Haplorchis yokogawai* (Katsuta, 1932) and *H. taichui* (Nishigori, 1924) (Trematoda: Heterophyidae). *Southeast Asian J. Trop. Med. Public Health.* **22**, 443–448.

209. Yoshimura, K., Hishinuma, Y., and Sato, M. (1969) *Ogmocotyle ailuri* (Price, 1954) in the Taiwanese monkey, *Macaca cyclopis* (Swinhoe, 1862). *J. Parasitol.* **55**, 460.

210. Premvati, G. (1958) *Primatotrema macacae* gen. nov., sp. nov. from Macaque Rhesus monkeys, and a redescription of *Phaneropsolus oviforme* Poirier (1886) Looss. 1899 (Lecithodendriidae). *J. Parasitol.* **44**, 639–642.

211. Knudsen, D.E. (1994) The lecithodendriid trematode *Phaneropsolus orbicularis* from the duodenum of an owl monkey. *Lab. Anim. Sci.* **44**, 549–550.

212. Gillespie, T.R., Greiner, E.C., and Chapman, C.A. (2005) Gastrointestinal parasites of the colobus monkeys of Uganda. *J. Parasitol.* **91**, 569–573.

213. Stuart, M., Pendergast, V., Rumfelt, S., Pierberg, S., Greenspan, L., Glander, K., et al. (1998) Parasites of wild howlers (*Alouatta* spp.). *Int. J. Primatol.* **19,** 493–512.

214. Stunkard, H.W. (1965) *Paratriotaenia oedipomidatis* gen. et sp. n. (Cestoda), from a marmoset. *J. Parasitol.* **51,** 545–551.

215. Hobbs, T.R., Colgin, L.M., Maginnis, G.M., and Lewis, A.D. (2003) Abdominal cysticercosis in a rhesus macaque (*Macaca mulatta*). *Comp. Med.* **53,** 545–547.

216. Michaud, C., Tantalean, M., Ique, C., Montoya, E., and Gozalo, A. (2003) A survey for helminth parasites in feral New World non-human primate populations and its comparison with parasitological data from man in the region. *J. Med. Primatol.* **32,** 341–345.

217. Hugot, J.P., Gardner, S.L., and Morand, S. (1996) The Enterobiinae subfam. Nov. (Nematoda, Oxyurida) pinworm parasites of primates and rodents. *Int. J. Parasitol.* **26,** 147–159.

218. Chaubaud, A.G. and Lariviere, M. (1955) Life cycle of an ascarid *Subulura jacchi* from the cockroach *Blabera fusca,* parasitic upon primates. *C.R. Seances Soc. Biol. Fil.* **149,** 1416–1419.

219. Yamashita, J. (1963) Ecological relationships between parasites and primates. *Primates* **4,** 1–96.

220. Hasegawa, H., Ikeda, Y., Fujisaki, A., Moscovice, L.R., Petrzelkova, K.J., Kaur, T., et al. (2005) Morphology of chimpanzee pinworms, *Enterobius* (*Enterobius*) *anthropopitheci* (Gedoelst, 1916) (Nematoda: Oxyuridae), collected from chimpanzees, *Pan troglodytes,* on Rubondo Island, Tanzania. *J. Parasitol.* **91,** 1314–1317.

221. Yamaguti, S. (1961) The nematodes of vertebrates. In: *Systema Helminthum.* Interscience Publishers, Inc., New York, NY.

222. Munene, E., Otsyula, M., Mbaabu, D.A., Mutahi, W.T., Muriuki, S.M., and Muchemi, G.M. (1998) Helminth and protozoan gastrointestinal tract parasites in captive and wild-trapped African non-human primates. *Vet. Parasitol.* **78,** 195–201.

223. Yamaguti, S. (1954) Studies of helminth fauna of Japan: Part 51. Mammalian nematodes. V. *Acta Med. Okayama* **9,** 105–121.

224. Horii, Y., Ishii, A., Owhashi, M., Miyoshi, M., and Usui, M. (1985) Neutrophilic nodules in the intestinal walls of Japanese monkeys associated with the neutrophil chemotactic activity of larval extracts and secretions of *Oesophagostomum aculeatum. Res. Vet. Sci.* **38,** 115–119.

225. Siang, T.K. and Joe, L.K. (1953) Redescription of *Oesophagostomum apiostomum* (Willach, 1891, Railliet and Henry, 1905) from man and monkeys in Indonesia. *Doc. Med. Geogr. Trop.* **5,** 123–127.

226. Eberhard, M.L., Kovacs-Nace, E., Blotkamp, J., Verwij, J.J., Asigri, V.A., and Polderman, A.M. (2001) Experimental *Oesophagostomum bifurcum* in monkeys. *J. Helminthol.* **75,** 51–56.

227. Gasser, R.B., Woods, W.G., Huffman, M.A., Blotkamp, J., and Polderman, A.M. (1999) Molecular separation of *Oesophagostomum stephanostomum* and *Oesophagostomum bifurcum* (Nematoda: Strongyloidea) from non-human primates. *Int. J. Parasitol.* **29,** 1087–1091.

228. Goldsmid, J.M. (1971) Studies on the life cycle and biology of *Ternidens deminutus* (Railliet and Henry, 1905), (Nematoda: Strongylidae). *J. Helminthol.* **45,** 341–352.

229. Durette-Desset, M.C., Fribourg Blanc, L.A., and Vuong, P.N. (2001) *Molineus torulosus* (Nematoda, Trichostrongylina, Molineoidea) a parasite of Neotropical primates: new morphological and histological data. *Parasite* **8,** 53–60.

230. Dunn, F.L. (1961) *Molineus vexillarius* sp. n. (Nematoda: Trichostrongylidae) from a Peruvian primate, *Tamarinus nigricollis* (Spix, 1823). *J. Parasitol.* **47,** 953–956.

231. Durette-Desset, M.C. and Chabaud, A.G. (1981) Molineinae parasites of mammals. *Ann. Parasitol. Hum. Comp.* **56,** 489–502.

232. Sato, H., Une, Y., and Takada, M. (2005) High incidence of the gullet worm, *Gongylonema pulchrum,* in a squirrel monkey colony in a zoological garden in Japan. *Vet. Parasitol.* **20,** 131–137.

233. Brede, H.D. and Burger, P.J. (1977) *Physaloptera caucasica* (= *Abbreviata caucasica*) in the South African baboon (*Papio ursinus*). *Arb. Paul Ehrlich Inst. Georg Speyer Haus Ferdinand Blum Inst. Frankf. A M.* **71,** 119–122.

234. Windle, D.W., Reigel, D.H., and Heckman, M.G. (1970) *Physaloptera tumefaciens* in the stump-tailed macaque (*Macaca arctoides*). *Lab. Anim. Care* **20,** 763– 767.

235. Slaughter, L.J. and Bostrom, R.E. (1969) Physalopterid (*Abbreviata poicilometra*) infection in a sooty mangabey monkey. *Lab. Anim. Care* **19,** 235–236.

236. Pettifer, H.L. (1984) The helminth fauna of the digestive tracts of chacma baboons, *Papio ursinus,* from different localities in the Transvaal. *Onderstepoort J. Vet. Res.* **51,** 161–170.

237. Ooi, H.K., Tenora, F., Itoh, K., and Kamiya, M. (1993) Comparative study of *Trichuris trichiura* from non-human primates and from man, and their difference with *T. suis. J. Vet. Med. Sci.* **55,** 363–366.

238. Chen, P.H., Miller, G.F., and Powell, D.A. (2000) Colitis in a female tamarin (*Saguinus mystax*). *Contemp. Top. Lab. Anim. Sci.* **39,** 47–49.

239. Fox, J.G., Diaz, J.R., and Barth, R.A. (1972) Nymphal *Porocephalus clavatus* in the brain of a squirrel monkey, *Saimiri sciureus. Lab. Anim. Sci.* **22,** 908– 910.

240. Mandour, A.M. (1969) *Sarcocystis nesbitti* n. sp. from the rhesus monkey. *J. Protozool.* **16,** 353–354.

241. Yang, Z.Q., Wei, C.G., Zen, J.S., Song, J.L., Zuo, Y.X., He, Y.S., et al. (2005) A taxonomic re-appraisal of *Sarcocystis nesbitti* (Protozoa: Sarcocystidae) from the monkey *Macaca fascicularis* in Yunnan, PR China. *Parasitol. Int.* **54,** 75–81.

242. Mehlhorn, H., Heydorn, A.O., and Janitschke, K. (1977) Light and electron microscopical study on sarcocysts from muscles of the rhesus monkey (*Macaca mulatta*), Baboon (*Papio cynocephalus*) and Tamarin (*Saguinus*(=*Oedipomidas*) *oedipus*). *Z Parasitenkd.* **51,** 165–178.

243. Reid, W.A. and Reardon, M.J. (1976) *Mesocestoides* in the baboon and its development in laboratory animals. *J. Med. Primatol.* **5,** 345–352.

244. Corkum, K.G. (1966) Sparganosis in some vertebrates of Louisiana and observations on a human infection. *J. Parasitol.* **52,** 444–448.

245. Morton, H.L. 1969. Sparganosis in African green monkeys (*Cercopithecus aethiops*). *Lab. Anim. Care* **19,** 253–255.

246. Sullivan, J.J., Steurer, F., Benavides, G., Tarleton, R.L., Eberhard, M.L., and Landry, S. (1993) Trypanosomes and microfilariae in feral owl and squirrel monkeys maintained in research colonies. *Am. J. Trop. Med. Hyg.* **49,** 254– 259.

247. Mak, J.W., Inder-Singh, K., Yen, P.K., and Yap, L.F. (1980) *Dipetalonema digitatum* (Chandler 1929) infection in the leaf monkey, *Presbytis obscura* (Reid). *Southeast Asian J. Trop. Med. Public Health.* **11,** 141.

248. Baker, D.G. and Babcock, R.E. Jr. (1996) Diagnostic exercise: Abdominal parasites in a spider monkey. *Lab. Anim. Sci.* **46,** 338–340.

249. Werner, H. and Lange, W. (1968) Infection of marmoset-pinche monkeys of the species *Saguinus* (*Oedipomidas*) *oedipus* with microfilariae of the species *Dipetalonema marmosetae* Faust 1935. *Zentralbl. Bakteriol.* **208,** 568–578.

250. Esslinger, J.H. (1966) *Dipetalonema obtusa* (McCoy, 1936) comb. n. (Filarioidea: Onchocercidae) in Colombian primates, with a description of the adult. *J. Parasitol.* **52,** 498–502.

251. Habermann, R.T. and Menges, R.W. (1968) Filariasis (*Acanthocheilonema perstans*) in a gorilla (a case history). *Vet. Med. Small Anim. Clin.* **63,** 1040– 1043.

252. Neafie, R.C., Connor, D.H., and Meyers, W.M. (1975) *Dipetalonema streptocerca* (Macfie and Corson, 1922): description of the adult female. *Am. J. Trop. Med. Hyg.* **24**, 264–267.

253. Moysan, F., van Hoegaerden, M., Cooper, R.W., Bhatia, S.C., Poltera, A.A., Striebel, H.P., et al. (1988) Antifilarial activity of CGP 20,376 in chimpanzees (*Pan t. troglodytes*) naturally infected with *Dipetalonema vanhoofi. Trop. Med. Parasitol.* **39**, 35–39.

254. Price, D.L. (1959) *Dirofilaria magnilarvatum* n. sp. (Nematoda: Filarioidea) from *Macaca irus* Cuvier. I. Description of the adult filarial worms. *J. Parasitol.* **45**, 499–504.

255. Canestri Trotti, G., Pampiglione, S., and Rivasi, F. (1997) The species of the genus *Dirofilaria*, Railliet and Henry, 1911. *Parassitologia* **39**, 369–374.

256. Nonoyama, T., Sugitani, T., Orita, S., and Miyajima, H. (1984) A pathological study in cynomolgus monkeys infected with *Edesonfilaria malayensis. Lab. Anim. Sci.* **34**, 604–609.

257. Orihel, T.C. and Eberhard, M.L. (1985) *Loa loa*: development and course of patency in experimentally-infected primates. *Trop. Med. Parasitol.* **36**, 215–224.

258. Lau, L.I., Lee, F.L., Hsu, W.M., Pampiglione, S., Fioravanti, M.L., and Orihel, T.C. (2002) Human subconjunctival infection of *Macacanema formosana*: the first case of human infection reported worldwide. *Arch. Ophthalmol.* **120**, 643–647.

259. Zamma, K. (2002) Grooming site preferences determined by lice infection among Japanese macaques in Arashiyama. *Primates* **43**, 41–49.

260. Pope, B.L. (1966) Some parasites of the howler monkey of northern Argentina. *J. Parasitol.* **52**, 166–168.

261. Kuhn, H.J. and Ludwig, H.W. (1967) Die Affenläuse der Gattung *Pedicinus. Z. Zool. Syst. Evolutionsforsch.* **5**, 144–256.

262. Kim, K.C. and Emerson, K.C. (1968) Descriptions of two species of Pediculidae (Anoplura) from great apes (Primates, Pongidae). *J. Parasitol.* **54**, 690–695.

263. Rolain, J.M., Bourry, O., Davoust, B., and Raoult, D. (2005) *Bartonella quintana* and *Rickettsia felis* in Gabon. *Emerg. Infect. Dis.* **11**, 1742–1744.

264. Pampiglione, S., Trentini, M., Fioravanti, M.L., and Gustinelli, A. (2004) Differential diagnosis between *Tunga penetrans* (L., 1758) and *T. trimamillata* Pampiglione et al., 2002 (Insecta, Siphonaptera), the two species of the genus *Tunga* parasitic in man. *Parasite* **11**, 51–57.

265. Fain, A. (1966) Les acariens producteurs de gale chez les lémuriens et les singes: II. Nouvelles observations avec description d'une espèce nouvelle. *Acarologia* **8**, 94–114.

266. Fain, A. (1968). Notes sur trois acariens remarquables (Sarcoptiformes). *Acarologia* **10**, 276–291.

267. O'Connor, B.M. (1982) Evolutionary ecology of Astigmatid mites. *Ann. Rev. Entomol.* **27**, 385–409.

268. Flatt, R.E. and Patton, N.M. (1969) A mite infestation in squirrel monkeys (*Saimiri sciureus*). *J. Am. Vet. Med. Assoc.* **155**, 1233–1235.

269. Fain, A. (1964). Les Lemurnyssidae parasites nasicoles des Lorisidae africanis et des Cebidae sud-américains. Description d'une espèce nouvelle (Acarina: Sarcoptiformes). *Ann. Soc. Belg. Med. Trop.* **44**, 453–458.

270. Fain, A. (1967) Diagnoses d'Acariens Sarcoptiformes nouveaux. *Rev. Zool. Bot. Afr.* **65**, 378–382.

271. Fain, A. (1962) *Pangorillages pani* g. n., sp. n. Acarien psorique du Chimpanzé (Psoralgidae: Sarcoptiformes). *Rev. Zool. Bot. Afr.* **66**, 283–290.

272. Fain, A. (1963) Les acariens producteurs de gale chez les lemuriens et les singes avec une étude des Psoroptidae (Sarcoptiformes). *Bull. Inst. Roy. Sci. Nat. Belg.* **39**, 1–125.

273. Fain, A. (1968). Étude de la variabilite de *Sarcoptes scabiei* avec une revision des Sarcoptidae. *Acta Zool. Pathol. Antverpiensia* **47**, 3–196.

274. Wilson, N., Dietz, J.M., and Whitaker, J.O. Jr. (1989) Ectoparasitic acari found on golden lion tamarins (*Leontopithecus rosalia rosalia*) from Brazil. *J. Wildl. Dis.* **25**, 433–435.

275. Fain, A. (1965). A review of the family Rhyncoptidae Lawrence parasitic on porcupines and monkeys (Acarina: Sarcoptiformes), In: Naegele, J.A. (ed.) *Advances in Acarology*. Vol. II, Cornell University Press, Ithaca, NY. 135–159.

276. Seier, J.V.(1985) Psorergatic acariasis in vervet monkeys. *Lab. Anim.* **19**, 236–239.

277. Chabaud, A.G. and Choquet, M.-T. (1954) Nymphes du Pentastome *Gigliolella* (n. gen.) *brumpti* (Giglioli 1922) chez un Lemurien. *Riv. Parassitologia* **15**, 331–336.

278. Craig, L.E., Kinsella, J.M., Lodwick, L.J., Cranfield, M.R., and Strandberg, J.D. (1998) *Gongylonema macrogubernaculum* in captive African squirrels (*Funisciurus substriatus* and *Xerus erythropus*) and lion-tailed macaques (*Macaca silenus*). *J. Zoo Wildl. Med.* **29**, 331–337.

279. Allen, A.M. (1960) Occurrence of the nematode, *Anatrichosoma cutaneum*, in the nasal mucosae of *Macaca mulatta* monkeys. *Am. J. Vet. Res.* **21**, 389–392.

280. Kim, J.C. (1976) Scanning electron microscopic studies of simian lung mites (*Pneumonyssus santos-diasi*, Zumpt and Till, 1954). *J. Med. Primatol.* **5**, 3–12.

281. Kim, J.C. and Kalterm S.S. (1975) Pathology of pulmonary acariasis in Baboons (*Papio* sp.). *J. Med. Primatol.* **4**, 70–82.

282. Fain, A. (1955) Deux nouveaux acariens de la famille Halarachnidae Oudemans, parasites des fosses nasals des singes au Congo Belge et au Ruanda-Urandi. *Rev. Zool. Bot. Afr.* **51**, 307–324.

APPENDIX

Cynthia Lang, DVM, MS; and Stephanie D. Lewis, DVM

Albendazole

Activity: Broad spectrum against a variety of nematodes, cestodes, and protozoa. Used in dogs for *Filaroides* species, *Capillaria plica,* and Leishmaniasis. Used in dogs and cats for *Paragonimus kellicotti* and *Giardia*.

    MOA: The precise biochemical mechanism of action is not clear. It appears to cause selective degeneration of cytoplasmic microtubules in intestinal and tegmental cells of intestinal helminths and their tissue-dwelling larvae.

Dogs

For Filaroides hirthi:
- 50 mg/kg PO q12h for 5 days, repeat in 21 days. During therapy symptoms may suddenly worsen, presumably due to worm death[1].
- 25 mg/kg PO q12h for 5 days, repeat in 2 weeks[2].

For Filaroides osleri:
- 9.5 mg/kg for 55 days or 25 mg/kg PO bid for 5 days. Repeat therapy in 2 weeks[3].
- 25 mg/kg PO q12h for 5 days, repeat in 2 weeks[2].

For Capillaria plica:
- 50 mg/kg q12h for 10–14 days. May cause anorexia[4].

For Paragonimus kellicotti:
- 50 mg/kg PO per day for 21 days[5].
- 30 mg/kg PO once daily for 12 days[3].
- 25 mg/kg PO q12 h for 14 days[2].

For Giardia:
- 25 mg/kg PO q12h for 4 doses[6].

- 25 mg/kg PO q12h for 5 days[7].
- 25 mg/kg PO q12h for 2–5 days[8].

For Leishmaniasis:
- 10 mg/kg PO once daily for 30 days or 5 mg/kg PO q6h for 60 days[9].

Cats

For Paragonimus kellicotti:
- 50 mg/kg PO per day for 21 days[5].
- 25 mg/kg PO q12h for 10–21 days[1].
- 30 mg/kg once daily for 6 days[3].
- 25 mg/kg PO q12h for 14 days[2].

For Giardia:
- 25 mg/kg PO q12h for 5 days[7].

For treatment of liver flukes (Platynosomum or Opisthorchiidae families):
- 50 mg/kg PO once daily until ova are gone[10].

Rabbits

For Encephalitozoon phacoclastic uveitis:
- 30 mg/kg PO once daily for 30 days, then 15 mg/kg PO once daily for 30 days[11].
- 7.5–20 mg/kg PO q24h for 3–14 days[12].

Chinchillas

For Giardia:
- 50–100 mg/kg PO once daily for 3 days[13].
- 25 mg/kg PO q12h for 2 days[14].

Reptiles

- Most species: 50 mg/kg PO for ascarids[15].

Birds

Ratites:

- Using the suspension: 1 ml/22 kg of body weight twice daily for 3 days; repeat in 2 weeks[16].
- 5.2 mg/kg PO q12h for 3 days, repeat in 14 days[17].
- Has efficacy against tapeworms and flagellate parasites.

Poultry:

- 10 mg/kg PO once[18].

Ramphastids:

- 15–20 mg/kg PO once[19].

Doves and rock partridges:

- 25–50 mg/kg PO q24h for 3–4 days[20].

Amazon parrots:

- 50 mg/kg PO q24h for 5 days for microsporidian ketatoconjunctivitis[21].

Sheep and Goats

For susceptible parasites:

- 7.5 mg/kg PO; 15 mg/kg PO for adult liver flukes[5].

For adult liver flukes in sheep:

- 7.6 mg/kg[22].

Swine

For susceptible parasites:

- 5–10 mg/kg PO[5].

Primates

For treatment of Filaroides:

- 25 mg/kg PO q12h for 5 days[23].

For treatment of nematode infections in prosimians:

- 10 mg/kg PO[24].

For treatment of red ruffed lemurs with Subcutaneous cysticercosis:

- 28.5 mg/animal PO q12h for 10 days for 3 treatments with a 10-day interval[25].

REFERENCES

1. Hawkins, E.C., Ettinger, S.J., and Suter, P.F. (1989) Diseases of the Lower Respiratory Tract (lung) and Pulmonary Edema. In: Ettinger, S.J. (ed.) *Textbook of Veterinary Internal Medicine,* W.B. Saunders, Philadelphia, 816–866.

2. Reinemeyer, C. (1995) Parasites of the respiratory system. In: Bonagura, J. (ed.) *Kirk's Current Veterinary Therapy: XII,* W.B. Saunders, Philadelphia, 895–898.

3. Todd, K.S., Paul, A.J., and DiPietro, J.A. (1985) Parasitic Diseases. In: Davis, L.E. (ed.) *Handbook of Small Animal Therapeutics,* Churchill Livingstone, New York, 89–126.

4. Brown, S.A. and Barsanti, J.A. (1989) Diseases of the Bladder and Urethra. In: S.J. Ettinger (ed.) *Textbook of Veterinary Medicine,* W.B. Saunders, Philadelphia, 2108–2141.

5. Roberson, E.L. (1988) Antinematodal Agents. In: Booth, N.H. and McDonald, L.E. (eds.) *Veterinary Pharmacology and Therapeutics,* Iowa State University Press, Ames, IA, 882–927.

6. Barr, S., Bowman, D., Heller, R., and Erb, H. Efficacy of albendazole against Giardia species in dogs and cats—Abstract. 38th Annual Meeting—AAVP. Edited by American Association of Veterinary Practitioners.

7. Barr, S. and Bowman, D. (1994) Giardiasis in Dogs and Cats. *Comp. CE* **16,** 603–610.

8. Lappin, M. (2000) Protozoal and Miscellaneous Infections. In: Ettinger, S. and Feldman, E. (eds.) *Textbook of Veterinary Internal Medicine: Diseases of the Dog and Cat,* W.B. Saunders, Philadelphia, 408–417.

9. Greene, C. and Watson, A. (1998) Antimicrobial Drug Formulary. In: Greene, C. (ed.) *Infectious Diseases of the Dog and Cat,* W.B. Saunders, Philadelphia, 790–919.

10. Taboada, J. (1999) Feline Liver Diseases. The North American Veterinary Conference, Orlando, FL.

11. Ivey, E. and Morrisey, J. (2000) Therapeutics for Rabbits. *Vet. Clin. N. Am: Exotic Animal Pract.* **3,** 183–213.

12. Harcourt-Brown, F. (2002) *Textbook of Rabbit Medicine,* Butterworth-Heinemann, Oxford, 94–120.

13. Hayes, P. (2000) Diseases of Chinchillas. In: Bonagura, J. (ed.) *Kirk's Current Veterinary Therapy: XIII Small Animal Practice,* W.B. Saunders, Philadelphia, 1152–1157.

14. Donnelly, T. M. (2004) Disease Problems of Chinchillas. In: Queensberry, K.E. and Carpenter, J.W. (eds.) Ferrets, *Rabbits, and Rodents: Clinical Medicine and Surgery,* 2nd ed. W.B. Saunders, St. Louis, MO, 255–265.

15. Stein, G. (1996) Reptile and amphibian formulary. In: Mander, D.R. (ed.) *Reptile Medicine and Surgery,* W.B. Saunders, Philadelphia, 465–472.

16. Jenson, J. (1998) Current Ratite Therapy. *Vet. Clin. N. Am: Food Anim. Pract.* **16,** 3.

17. Tully, T.N. (1996) Therapeutics. In: Tully, T.N. and Shane, S.M. (eds.) *Ratite Management, Medicine, and Surgery,* Krieger, Malabar, FL, 155–163.

18. Csikó, G.Y., Banhidi G.Y., Semjén, G., et al. (1996) Metabolism and pharmacokinetics of albendazole after oral administration to chickens. *J. Vet. Pharmacol. Ther.* **19,** 322–325.

19. Cornelissen, H. (1993) Behavior, anatomy, feeding and medical problems of toucans in captivity. *Proc. Euro. Conf. Avian Med. Surg.* pp. 446–453.

20. Stalis, I.H., Rideout, B.A., Allen, J.L., et al. (1995) Possible albendazole toxicity in birds. *Proc. Joint Conf. Am. Assoc. Zoo Vet.* pp. 190–191.

21. Canny, C.J., Ward, D.A., Patton, S., et al. (1999) Microsporidian keratoconjunctivitis in a double yellow-headed Amazon parrot (*Amazona ochocephala oratrix*). *J. Avian Med. Surg.* **13,** 279–286.

22. Paul, J.W. (1986) Anthelmintic Therapy. In: Howard, J.W. (ed.) *Current Veterinary Therapy: Food Animal Practice 2*, W.B. Saunders, Philadelphia, 39–44.

23. Wolf, P.L. (1993) Parasites of the New World Primates. In: Fowler, M.D. (ed.) *Zoo and Wild Animal Medicine: Current Therapy 3*, W.B. Saunders, Philadelphia, 378–389.

24. Junge, R.E. (2003) *Zoo and Wild Animal Medicine*, Fowler, M.E. and Miller, R.E. (eds.) W.B. Saunders, Philadelphia, 334–336.

25. Young, L.A., Morris, P.J., Keener, L,. et al. (2000) Subcutaneous *Taenia crassiceps* cysticercosis in a red ruffed lemur (*Varecia variegata rubra*). *Proc. Am. Assoc. Zoo Vet.* 251–252.

Amitraz

Activity: Used primarily for the treatment of generalized demodicosis, also other mites.

    MOA: Poorly understood. It possesses α-2 adrenergic activity.

Dogs

For generalized Demodicosis:

- 250 ppm (one 10.6 ml bottle of Mitaban in 2 gallons of warm water) topically every 14 days for 3–6 treatments. Do not rinse or towel dry (Package Insert; Mitaban®—Upjohn).
- For dogs only chronically managed by the above therapy, higher doses may be tried to achieve a cure. However, owners must be informed of the risk involved with the treatment. Initially, try the 250-ppm solution once weekly for 4 weeks. If a positive response is seen, continue treatment until a negative skin scraping is achieved and then for an additional 30 days. If the weekly 250-ppm application fails, a solution of 500 ppm may be tried (1 bottle in 1 gallon of water) weekly as above. If the 500-ppm treatment does not provide a positive response, a 1,000-ppm solution may be tried, but the risk for toxicity is extremely high and it is unlikely that the dog will be cured using amitraz[1].
- For dogs unresponsive to conventional therapy (labeled), prepare a 0.125% solution by diluting 1 ml of the 12.5% commercially available large animal product (Taktic®) in 100 ml of water. Using a sponge, rub the diluted solution(0.125%) daily onto one-half of the dog's body, alternating sides on a daily basis. Let the solution air dry. The dog should be hospitalized for the first week of treatment to observe for any adverse effects. Therapy should be continued for 2 weeks after multiple negative skin scrapings.
- Dogs can also receive otic therapy with a diluted solution of amitraz (1 ml of Taktic in 8.5 ml of mineral oil) every 3–7 days unless irritation develops. One researcher also treats pododermatitis with the 0.125% solution. Reported adverse effects are mild and low in frequency. It is important that owners are well-informed and adequately trained before treatment with this unapproved therapy[2].

For treatment of scabies in older puppies and adult dogs:

- Dilute and treat per label recommendation 250 ppm (one 10.6 ml bottle of Mitaban in 2 gallons of warm water) topically every 14 days for 3–6 treatments. Do not rinse or towel dry[3].

Cats

For Demodicosis:

- Dilute amitraz to 125 ppm and apply every 7–14 days[4].

Mice, Rats, Gerbils, Hamsters, and Chinchillas

- 1.4 ml per liter topically every 2 weeks for 3–6 treatments. Not recommended in young animals[5].

Rabbits

- Not recommended.

Ferrets

- Apply topically to affected areas at full concentration every 7–14 days for 3–6 treatments[6,7].

Guinea Pigs

- 1.4 ml per liter topically (apply with cotton ball or brush) every 2 weeks for 3–6 treatments. Not recommended in young animals[5].
- 0.3% solution topically once a week[6].

Goats

For Demodectic mange:

- 10.6 ml of amitraz solution (19.9% Mitaban®) in 2 gallons of water. Use a whole-body dip; repeat every 14 days for 2–3 treatments[8].

Primates

- 250-ppm solution. Dip for 2–5 minutes duration every 2 weeks for 4 treatments or until resolution of skin lesions. Treatment dose was used in tamarins for demodectic manage. No bathing or hair coat clipping was performed, dip was not rinsed from animals, and they were dried with a hot-air dryer. Transient ataxia developed for 72 hours after the first treatment[9].

REFERENCES

1. Miller, W. (1992) Follicular Disorders of the Doberman Pinscher. In: Kirk, R. and Bonagura, J. (eds.) *Current Veterinary Therapy XI: Small Animal Practice,* W.B. Saunders Company, Philadelphia, 515–518.

2. Mundell, A. (1994) Demodicosis. In: Birchard, S. and Sherding, R. (eds.) *Saunders Manual of Small Animal Practice,* W.B. Saunders Company, Philadelphia, 290–294.

3. Moriello, K. (1992) Treatment of Sarcoptes and *Cheyletiella* Infestations. In: Kirk, R. and Bonagura, J. (eds.) *Current Veterinary XI: Small Animal Practice,* W.B. Saunders Company, Philadelphia.

4. White, S. (2000) Veterinary Dermatology: New Treatments, "New" Diseases, The North American Veterinary Conference, Orlando, FL.

5. Adamcak, A. and Otten, B. (2000) Rodent Therapeutics. *Vet. Clin. N. Am: Exotic Anim. Pract.* **3,** 221–240.

6. Morrisey, J.K. and Carpenter, J.W. (2004) Formulary. In: Quesenberry, K.E. and Carpenter, J.W. (eds.) *Ferrets, Rabbits, and Rodents: Clinical Medicine and Surgery,* 2nd ed. W.B. Saunders, St. Louis, 436–444.

7. Smith, D.A. and Burgmann, P.M. (1997) Formulary. In: Hillyer, E.V. and Quesenberry, K.E. (eds.) *Ferrets, Rabbits, and Rodents: Clinical Medicine and Surgery,* W.B. Saunders, Philadelphia, 394–395.

8. Rosser, E. (1993) Parasitic Dermatoses. In: Howard, J. (ed.) *Current Veterinary Therapy 3: Food Animal Practice,* W.B. Saunders, Philadelphia, 882–890.

9. James, S.B. and Raphael, B L. (2000) Demodicosis in red-haired tamarins (*Sanguinus midas*). *J. Zoo. Wildl. Med.* **31,** 251–254.

Amprolium

Activity: Anticoccidial. In poultry it is used as a therapeutic and has good activity against *Eimeria tenella* and *E. acervulina*. It has fair to weak activity *against E. maxima, E. mivati, E. necatrix,* and *E. brunetti*.

MOA: Thiamine analog that competitively inhibits thiamine use by the coccidian. Seems to primarily prevent differentiation of the first generation schizont into metrozoites.

Dogs

For Coccidiosis:
- For pups <10 kg, give 100-mg total dose using the 20% powder in a gelatin capsule PO once daily for 7–12 days[1].
- For pups ≥10 kg, give 200 mg total dose using the 20% powder in a gelatin capsule PO once daily for 7–12 days[1].
- For pups or bitches, give 250–300 mg total dose using the 20% powder in food once daily for 7–12 days[1].
- For pups or bitches, give 30 ml of the 9.6% solution in one gallon of water, no other water provided, for 7–10 days[1].

As a Prophylaxis:
- 1.25 grams of 20% powder in food to feed 4 pups daily. Do not give with medicated water[2].
- 30 ml of 9.6% solution in 1 gallon (3.8 L) of drinking water. Give as the sole source of water for 7 days prior to shipping. Do not give with medicated food. Bitches may be given medicated water for 10 days prior to whelping[2].

Cats

For Coccidiosis:
- 300–400 mg/kg in food once daily for 5 days[1].
- 110–220 mg/kg in water once daily for 7–12 days, or 1.5 teaspoons in one gallon of water once daily for 7–12 days[1].
- 110–220 mg/kg PO[1].
- 60–100 mg PO once daily for 7 days for *Cystoisospora* spp[3].

Mice, Rats, Gerbils, and Hamsters

- 10–20 mg/kg total daily dose divided q8-24h SC or IM[4].

Rabbits

- 0.5 ml/pint of drinking water using the 9.6% solution for 10 days[5,6].
- 1 ml/7kg of body weight once daily in the drinking water using the 9.6% solution for 5 days[7].
- 0.5 ml/500ml of drinking water using the 9.6% solution for 10 days[7].
- 5 ml/gallon of drinking water using the 9.6% solution for 21 days[8].

Ferrets

- 19 mg/kg PO q24h[9].

Chinchillas

- 10–15 mg/kg per day divided q8-24h SQ, IM, or IV[4].

Birds

Most species, including parakeets and finches:
- 50–100 mg/L of drinking water for 5–7 days[10,11,12].

Pet birds:
- 2 ml/gallon of drinking water using the 9.6% solution for 5 days or longer. Supplement the diet with vitamin B. Some strains are resistant in toucans and mynahs[13].

Pigeons:
- 25 mg/kg/day PO[14].
- 1/4 tsp/L of drinking water using the 20% powder for 3–5 days[15,16].
- 200 mg/L of drinking water for flock treatment[15].

Poultry:
- 115–235 mg/kg in feed[17].
- 575 mg/L in drinking water using the 9.6% solution[18].
- 1/4 tsp/L of drinking water using the 20% powder for 3–5 days[14,15].

Chickens:
- 13–26 mg/kg PO[19].

Psittacines (keas):
- 250 mg/L of drinking water for 7 days for *Sarcocystis*. Use in combination with pyrimethamine and primaquine[20].

Raptors:
- 30 mg/kg PO q24h for 5 days[21].

Sheep and Goats

- For lambs, give 55 mg/kg PO daily for 19 days[22].

Swine

- 25–65 mg/kg PO once or twice daily for 3–4 days[22].
- 100 mg/kg/day in food or water[23].

REFERENCES

1. Greene, C.E. and Watson, A.D.J. (1998) Antimicrobial drug formulary. In: Greene, C. (ed.) *Infectious Diseases of the Dog and Cat,* 2nd ed. W.B. Saunders, Philadelphia, 807.
2. USPC. (1989) Veterinary information—appendix V. In: *Drug Information for the Health Professional,* United States Pharmacopeial Convention, Rockville, 2811–2860.
3. Lappin, M. (2000) Protozoal and miscellaneous infections. In: Ettinger, S. and Feldman, E. (eds.) *Textbook of Veterinary Internal Medicine: Diseases of the Dog and Cat,* W.B. Saunders, Philadelphia, 408–417.
4. Adamcak, A. and Otten, B. (2000) Rodent therapeutics *Vet. Clin. N. Am: Exotic Anim. Pract.* **3,** 221–240.
5. Harkness, J.E. and Wagner, J.E. (1995) *The Biology and Medicine of Rabbits and Rodents,* 4th ed. Williams and Wilkins, Philadelphia.
6. Hillyer, E.V. (1994) Pet rabbits. *Vet. Clin. N. Am: Small Anim. Pract.* **24,** 25–65.
7. Ivey, E. and Morrisey, J. (2000) Therapeutics in rabbits. *Vet Clin. N. Am: Exotic Anim. Pract.* **3,** 183–213.
8. Quesenberry, K.E. (2002) Rabbits. In: Birchard, S.J. and Sherding, R.G. (eds.) *Saunders Manual of Small Animal Practice,* W.B. Saunders, Philadelphia, 1345–1362.
9. Brown, S.A. (1999) Ferret Drug Dosages. In: Antinoff, N., Bauck, L. and Boyer, T.H., et al. (eds.) *Exotic Formulary,* 2nd ed. American Animal Hospital Association. Lakewood, CO, 43–61.
10. Marshall, R. (1993) Avian anthelmintics and antiprotozoals. *Semin. Avian Exotic Pet Med.* **2,** 33–41.
11. Moore, D.M. and Rice, R.L. (1998) Exotic animal formulary In: Holt, K.M., Boothe, D.M. and Gaumnitz, J., et al. (eds.) *Veterinary values,* 5th ed. Veterinary Medicine Publishing Group. Lenexa, KS, 159–245.
12. Samour, J. (2000) Pharmaceutics commonly used in avian medicine. In: Samour, J. (ed.) *Avian Medicine,* Mosby, Philadelphia, 388–418.
13. Clubb, S.L. (1986) Therapeutics: individual and flock treatment regimens. In: Harrison, G.J. and Harrison, L.R. (eds.) *Clinical Avian Medicine and Surgery,* W.B. Saunders, Philadelphia, 327–355.
14. Harper, F.D.W. (1996) Poor performance and weight loss. In: Beynon, P.H., Forbes, N.A. and Harcourt-Brown, N.A. (eds.) *BSAVA Manual of Raptors, Pigeons and Waterfowl,* Iowa State University Press, Ames, IA, 272–278.
15. Harlin, R.W. (1994) Pigeons. In: *Vet. Clin. N. Am: Small Anim. Pract.* **24,** 157–173.
16. Harlin, R.W. (1995) Backyard poultry. *Proc. Mid-Atlantic States Assoc. Avian Vet. Conf.* 65–68.
17. Stadler, C. and Carpenter, J.W. (1996) Parasites of backyard game birds. *Semin. Avian Exotic Pet Med.* **5,** 85–96.
18. Carpenter, N.A. (2000) Anseriform and galliform therapeutics. *Vet. Clin. N. Am: Exotic Anim. Pract.* **3,** 1–17.
19. Hamamoto, K., Koike, R., and Machida, Y. (2000) Bioavailability of amprolium in fasting and nonfasting chickens after intravenous and oral administration. *J. Vet. Pharmacol. Ther.* **23,** 9–14.
20. Weston, H.S. (1996) The successful treatment of sarcocystosis in two keas (*Nestor nobilis*) at the Franklin Park Zoo. *Proc. Am. Assoc. Zoo Vet.* pp. 186–191.
21. Heidenreich, M. (1997) *Birds of Prey, Medicine and Management.* Blackwell Science, Malden, MA.
22. Howard, J.L. (1986) *Current Veterinary Therapy 2, Food Animal Practice,* W.B. Saunders, Philadelphia.
23. Todd, K.S., Paul, A.J., and DiPietro, J.A. (1985) Parasitic diseases. In: Davis, L.E. (ed.) *Handbook of Small Animal Therapeutics,* Churchill Livingstone, New York, 89–126.

Clorsulon

Activity: Used for the treatment of adult liver flukes (*Fasciola hepatica*) and immature liver flukes greater than 8 weeks old. Also effective against *Fasciola gigantica.*

MOA: Clorsulon inhibits the glycolic pathway of the fluke, depriving it of its primary metabolic energy source.

Birds

For treatment of trematodes in psittacines:
- 20 mg/kg PO q14 for 3 treatments[1,2].

For treatment of cestodes and trematodes in waterfowl and raptors:
- 20 mg/kg PO three times a week for 14 days[3,4].

Sheep

- 7.0 mg/kg PO[5].

REFERENCES

1. Clyde, V.L. and Patton, S. (1996) Diagnosis, treatment, and control of common parasites in companion and aviary birds. *Semin. Avian Exotic Pet Med.* **5,** 75–84.
2. Ritchie, B.W. and Harrison, G.J. (1994) Formulary. In: Ritchie, B.W., Harrison, G.L. and Harrison, L.R. (eds.) *Avian Medicine: Principles and Application,* Wingers, Lake Worth, FL, 457–478.
3. Beynon, P.H., Forbes, N.A, and Harcourt-Brown, N.H. (1996) *BSAVA Manual of Raptors, Pigeons, and Waterfowl,* Iowa State University Press, Ames, IA, 202–215.
4. Brown, M.J. and Cromie, R.L. (1996) Weight loss and enteritis. In: Beynon, P.H., Forbes, N.A. and Harcourt-Brown, N.H. (eds.) *BSAVA Manual of Raptors, Pigeons, and Waterfowl,* Iowa State University Press, Ames, Iowa, 322–329.
5. Roberson, E.L. (1988) Anticestodal and Antitrematodal drugs. In: Booth, N.H. and McDonald, L.E. (eds.) *Veterinary Pharmacology and Therapeutics,* Iowa State University Press, Ames, IA, 928–949.

Copper Sulfate

Activity: Used to treat trematode ectoparasites and protozoan in fish. Toxic to invertebrates, plants, and gill tissue. Copper can be removed by activated carbon.

   MOA: Copper sulfate causes inactivation of enzyme systems in susceptible parasites.

Fish

Susceptible parasites:

- 100 mg/L for a 1–5 min. bath. Prepare a stock solution of 1 mg/ml (1 g $CuSO_4 \times 5\ H_2O$ in 250 mL distilled water)[1].
- 0.1–0.2 mg/L; use higher dose in hard water[2].
- Maintain free-ion levels at 0.15–0.2 mg/L tank water until therapeutic effect[3].
- Maintain copper levels at 0.2 mg/L tank water for 14–21 days[4].
- Citrated copper sulfate; prepare 1 mg/ml (3 g $CuSO_4 \times 5\ H_2O$ and 2 g citric acid monohydrate in 750 ml distilled water[5].
- Maintain free-ion levels at 0.25–1.0 mg/L for 24–48 hr bath[5].

REFERENCES

1. Callahan, H.A. and Noga, E.J. (2002) Tricaine dramatically reduces the ability to diagnose protozoan ectoparasites (*Ichthyobodo necator)* infections. *J. Fish Dis.* **25,** 433–437.
2. Treves-Brown, K.M. (2000) *Applied Fish Pharmacology,* Kluwer Academic Publishers, Dodrecht, The Netherlands.
3. Noga, E.J. (2000) *Fish Disease: Diagnosis and Treatment,* Iowa State University Press, Ames, IA.
4. Whitaker, B.R. (1999) Preventable medicine programs for fish. In: Fowler, M.E. and Miller, R.E. (eds.) *Zoo and Wild Animal Medicine: Current Therapy 4,* W.B. Saunders, Philadelphia, 163–181.
5. Harms, C.A. (1996) Treatments for parasitic diseases of aquarium and ornamental fish. *Semin. Avian Exotic Pet Med.* **5,** 54–63.

Cythioate

Activity: Use for flea and tick control and the treatment of demodectic mites.

   MOA: Cythioate is an oral organophosphate drug which inhibits acetylcholinesterase in fleas, ticks, and mites, inhibiting neuromuscular transmission.

Dogs

For flea control:

- 1 ml of liquid (16 mg) PO for every 10 lbs of body weight once every third day or twice a week. Apply to food and mix thoroughly. The first week of therapy will kill 95% of fleas. Additional treatments for several weeks may be necessary to remove fleas due to re-infestation (Package insert; Proban®—Miles).
- 1 30-mg tablet for each 20 lbs of body weight once every third day or twice a week (Package insert; Proban®—Bayer).

Decoquinate

Activity: Coccidiostat. Used in goats for the prevention of *Eimeria christenseni* and *E. ninakohlyakimoviae.* In broilers it is used for the prevention *Eimeria tenella, E. brunetti, E. necatrix, E. mivati, E. maxima,* and *E. acervulina.*

   MOA: A 4-hydroxy quinolone that disrupts the electron transport in the mitochondrial cytochrome system of the sporozoite stage.

Dogs

Prophylaxis for Coccidiosis:
- 50 mg/kg PO once daily[1].

Rabbits

- 62.5 ppm in feed for coccidiosis[2].

Birds

Chickens:
- 30 mg/kg of feed for coccida[3] (not approved for laying chickens).

Goats

Prophylaxis for Coccidiosis:
• 0.5 mg/kg per day in feed[4].

REFERENCES

1. Matz, M. (1995) Gastrointestinal ulcer therapy. In: Bonagura, J. (ed.) *Kirk's Current Veterinary Therapy: XII,* W.B. Saunders, Philadelphia, 706–710.
2. Harkness, J.E. and Wagner, J.E. (1995) *The Biology and Medicine of Rabbits and Rodents,* 4th ed. Williams and Wilkins, Philadelphia.
3. Tanner, A.C. (2000) Antimicrobial drug use in poultry. In: Prescott, J. and Baggot, J. (eds.) *Antimicrobial Therapy in Veterinary Medicine,* 3rd ed. Iowa State University Press, Ames, IA, 637–655.
4. Bretzlaff, K. (1993) Production medicine and health programs in goats. In: Howard, J. (ed.) *Current Veterinary Therapy 3: Food Animal Practice,* W.B. Saunders, Philadelphia, 162–167.

Dichlorvos

Activity: Used in dogs and cats for the treatment of roundworms. It is also used for ectoparasite prevention in birds and pocket pets.

MOA: An organophosphate drug which inhibits acetylcholinesterase in susceptible parasites, inhibiting neuromuscular transmission.

Dogs

• 26.4–33 mg/kg PO[1].
• Adults: 27–33 mg/kg PO; puppies: 11 mg/kg PO[2].

Cats

• 11 mg/kg PO[1,2].

Mice, Rats, Gerbils, Hamsters, Guinea Pigs, and Chinchillas

• Hang 5 cm of a dichlorvos strip 6 inches above the cage for 24 hours, twice a week, for 3 weeks[3,4].
• Hang a strip in the room for 24 hours once a week for 6 weeks or lay a 1-inch square on the cage for 24 hours once a week for 6 weeks[4].
• Hang a strip 15 cm above the cage for 24 hours, then twice a week for 3 weeks[3].

Miniature Pigs

For Ascaris, Trichuris, Ascarops strongylina, and Oesophagostomum species:
• 20 mg/kg PO[5].

Primates

For Gastrointestinal nematodes:
• 10–15 mg/kg PO q24 hours for 2–3 days[6].

REFERENCES

1. Papich, M. (1992) Table of Common Drugs: Appropriate Dosages. In: Kirk, R. and Bonagura, J. (eds.) *Current Veterinary Therapy XI: Small Animal Practice,* W.B. Saunders, Philadelphia, 1233–1249.
2. Sherding, R. and Johnson, S. (1994) Diseases of the Intestines. In: Birchard, S.J. and Sherding, R.J. (eds.) *Saunders Manual of Small Animal Practice,* W.B. Saunders, Philadelphia, 687–714.
3. Anderson, N.L. (1994) Basic husbandry and medicine of pocket pets. In: Birchard, S.J. and Sherding, R.J. (eds.) *Saunders Manual of Small Animal Practice,* W.B. Saunders, Philadelphia, 1363–1389.
4. Amdack, A. and Otten, B. (2000) Rodent Therapeutics. *Vet. Clin. N. Am: Exotic Anim. Pract.* **3,** 221–237.
5. Boldrick, L. (1993) *Veterinary Care of Pot-Bellied Pet Pigs,* All Publishing, Orange, CA.
6. Holmes, D.D. (1984) *Clinical Laboratory Animal Medicine,* Iowa State University Press, Ames, IA.

Diethylcarbamazine Citrate

Activity: Used for heartworm prevention (*Dirofilaria immitis*) in susceptible animals and the treatment of ascariasis in dogs.

MOA: The exact mechanism of action of this piperazine-derivative is poorly understood. It is suspected that the drug acts on the parasite's nervous system, resulting in paralysis.

Dogs

For heartworm prevention:
• 6.6 mg/kg PO once daily preceding infection and for 60 days following last exposure to mosquitoes[1].
• 6.6 mg/kg PO once daily from the beginning of mosquito season and for two months thereafter. Should be given year-round where mosquitoes are active throughout the year[2].
• 2.5–3 mg/kg PO daily; begin prior to mosquito season[3].
• 5–7 mg/kg PO daily. Begin before mosquito season and continue for 60 days after. Year-round treatment is needed where mosquitoes are active throughout the year[4].

For treatment of other susceptible parasites (do not use in Microfilaria-positive patients):

For ascarids:
• Treatment: 55–110 mg/kg PO[2].
• Prevention: 6.6 mg/kg PO per day[2].

For lungworms (Crenosoma vulpis):
- 80 mg/kg PO q12h for 3 days[2].

Cats

For ascarids:
- 55–110 mg/kg PO[2].

Ferrets

For heartworm prevention:
- 5.5 mg/kg PO once a day[5].
- 5–11 mg/kg PO once a day[6,7].

Primates

For owl monkeys with Filariasis (dipetalonema):
- 6–20 mg/kg PO once a day for 6–15 days[8,9].
- 20–40 mg/kg PO once a day for 7–21 days[10].

For squirrel monkeys with Filariasis (effective against Microfilaria and adults):
- 50 mg/kg PO once a day for 10 days[11].

REFERENCES

1. Knight, D.H. (1988) Heartworm Disease. In: Morgan, R.V. (ed.) *Handbook of Small Animal Practice,* Churchill Livingstone, New York, 139–148.
2. Todd, K.S., Paul, A.J. and DiPietro, J.A. (1985) Parasitic Diseases. In: Davis, L.E. (ed.) *Handbook of Small Animal Therapeutics,* Churchill Livingstone, New York, 89–126.
3. Rawlings, C.A. and Calvert, C.A. (1989) Heartworm Disease. In: Ettinger, S.J. (ed.) *Textbook of Veterinary Internal Medicine,* W.B. Saunders, Philadelphia, 1163–1184.
4. Calvert, C.A. and Rawlings, C.A. (1986) Therapy of Canine Heartworm Disease. In: Kirk, R.W. (ed.) *Current Veterinary Therapy IX: Small Animal Practice,* W.B. Saunders, Philadelphia, 406–419.
5. Randolph, R.W. (1986) Preventative Medical Care for the Pet Ferret. In: Kirk, R.W. (ed.) *Current Veterinary Therapy IX: Small Animal Practice,* W.B. Saunders, Philadelphia, 772–774.
6. Besch-Williford, C.L. (1987) Biology and Medicine of the Ferret. *Vet. Clin. N. Am: Small Anim. Prac.* **17,** 1155–1183.
7. Hillyer, E.V. and Brown, S.A. (2000) Ferrets. In: Birchard, S.J. and Sherding, R.G. (eds.) *Saunders Manual of Small Animal Practice,* W.B. Saunders, Philadelphia, 1464–1492.
8. Tantaléan, M. and Gozalo, A. (1994) Parasites of the *Aotus* monkey. In: Baer, J.F., Weller, R.E. and Kakoma, I. (eds.) *Aotus: the Owl Monkey,* Academic Press, San Diego, CA, 353–374.
9. Wolff, P.L. (1993) Parasites of the new world primates. In: Fowler, M.E. (ed.) *Zoo and Wild Animal Medicine: Current Therapy 3,* W.B. Saunders, Philadelphia, 378–389.
10. Johnson-Delaney, C.A. (1994) Primates. *Vet Clin. N. Am: Small Anim. Pract.* **24,** 121–156.
11. Eberhard, M.L. (1982) Chemotherapy of filariasis in squirrel monkeys (*Saimiri sciureus*). *Lab Animal Sci.* **32,** 397–400.

Epsiprantel

Activity: Oral cestocide for dogs (*Dipylidium caninum* and *Taenia pisiformis*) and cats (*Dipylidium caninum* and *Taenia taeniaeformis*) greater than 7 weeks old.

MOA: The exact mechanism of action is unknown. Calcium regulation appears to be altered in the tapeworm, which may interfere with worm attachment to the host or aid in digestion of the parasite.

Dogs

- 5.5 mg/kg PO once (Package insert; Cestex®—Pfizer).

Cats

- 2.75 mg/kg PO once (Package insert; Cestex®—Pfizer).

Febantel

Activity: Used in combination with praziquantel to treat dogs and puppies for hookworms, whipworms, roundworms, and tapeworms. Used in combination with praziquantel to treat cats and kittens for hookworms, roundworms, and tapeworms.

MOA: The exact mechanism of action is unknown. It is suspected that glucose uptake is inhibited, thereby blocking the parasite's metabolic energy source.

Dogs

For use in combination with praziquantel (Vercom®) for labeled parasites:
- Older than 6 months of age: 10 mg/kg (febantel)/1 mg/kg (praziquantel) PO for 3 days.
- For puppies: 15 mg/kg (febantel)/1.5 mg/kg (praziquantel) PO for 3 days (Package Insert; Vercom®—Paste—Miles).

Cats

For use in combination with praziquantel (Vercom®) for labeled parasites:
- Older than 6 months of age: 10 mg/kg (febantel)/1 mg/kg (praziquantel) PO for 3 days.
- For kittens: 15 mg/kg (febantel)/1.5 mg/kg (praziquantel) PO for 3 days (Package Insert; Vercom®—Paste—Miles).

Fenbendazole

Activity: Used to treat ascarids, hookworms, whipworms, and tapeworms in dogs. Although not approved, it is also used to treat ascarids, hookworms, *Strongyloides,* and tapeworms (*Taenia* only) in cats and susceptible parasites in sheep, goats, swine, birds, amphibians, reptiles, rodents, rabbits, ferrets, fish, and primates.

MOA: The precise biochemical mechanism of action is not clear. It appears to cause selective degeneration of cytoplasmic microtubules in intestinal and tegmental cells of intestinal helminths and their tissue-dwelling larvae.

Dogs

For treatment of susceptible ascarids, hookworms, whipworms, and tapeworms (Taenia spp. only):
- 50 mg/kg PO for 3 consecutive days (Package insert; Panacur®—Hoechst).
- 55 mg/kg PO for 3 days (5 days for *Taenia*)[1,2].

For Capillaria plica:
- 50 mg/kg once daily for 3 days; repeat a single 50 mg/kg dose 3 weeks later[3].
- 50 mg/kg PO once daily for 3–10 days[4].

For Capillaria aerophila:
- 25–50 mg/kg q12 h for 10–14 days[5].
- 50 mg/kg once daily for 10–14 days[6].

For Filaroides hirthi:
- 50 mg/kg PO once daily for 14 days[5].
- 50 mg/kg once daily for 10–14 days[6].

For Trichuris colitis/Typhlitis:
- 50 mg/kg PO once daily for 3 consecutive days; repeat in 2–3 weeks and again in 2 months[7].

For Crenosoma vulpis:
- 50 m/kg PO once daily for 3 days[6].

For Eucoleus boehmi:
- 50 mg/kg PO once daily for 10–14 days[6].

For Giardia:
- 50 mg/kg PO once daily for 3 days[8,9].
- 25 mg/kg PO q12h for 3–7 days[10].

Cats

For susceptible ascarids, hookworms, strongyloides, and tapeworms (Taenia spp. only):
- 50 mg/kg PO for 5 days[11].

For lungworms (Aelurostrongylus abstrusus):
- 25–50 mg/kg PO q12 h for 10–14 days[5].
- 50 mg/kg PO for 10 days[12].
- 20 mg/kg PO once daily for 5 days; repeat in 5 days[6].

For lungworms (Capillaria aerophila):
- 50 mg/kg PO for 10 days[12].
- 50 mg/kg PO once daily for 10–14 days[6].

For Capillaria feliscati:
- 25 mg/kg q12h PO for 3–10 days[4].
- 25 mg/kg q12h for 10 days[13].

For Paragonimus kellicotti:
- 25–50 mg/kg PO twice daily for 10–14 days[14].
- 50 mg/kg PO once daily for 10–14 days[6].

For Pancreatic flukes (Eurytrema procyonis):
- 30 mg/kg PO daily for 6 days[15].

For Giardia:
- In young kittens: 50 mg/kg PO (using the suspension) once a day for 3–5 days[16].

Mice, Rats, Hamsters, Gerbils, and Guinea Pigs

For susceptible infections:
- 20 mg/kg PO q24h for 5 days[17].

For pinworms:
- 50 mg/kg PO once[18].
- 0.3% feed for 14 days (clinical trial for cestodes and pinworms in mice)[19].

For Giardia:
- 20–50 mg/kg PO once daily for 5 days[20,21].

Rabbits

For susceptible infections:
- 5 mg/kg PO[22].
- 10 mg/kg PO, repeat in 14 days as needed[23].
- 50 ppm in feed for 2–6 weeks[22].

For pinworms:
- 50 mg/kg PO once[18].

For Encephalitozoonosis prevention:
- 20 mg/kg PO q24h for 7 days before and 2 days after mixing rabbits[24].

For treatment of Encephalitozoonosis:
- 20 mg/kg PO q24h for 28 days (if failed to clear all parasites)[24].

Ferrets

For susceptible infections:
- 20 mg/kg PO q24h for 5 days[25].

Chinchillas

For Giardia:
- 25 mg/kg PO once daily for 3 days[26].
- 25–50 mg/kg PO once daily for 5 days[20].

Amphibians

For gastrointestinal nematodes:
- 30–50 mg/kg PO[27].
- 100 mg/kg PO, repeat in 14 days[28].
- 50–100 mg/kg PO, repeat in 2–3 weeks as needed[29].
- 50 mg/kg PO q24h for 3–5 days, repeat in 14–21 days (for resistant infections)[30].
- 100 mg/kg PO on day 1 of fenbendazole, then 0.2 mg/kg ivermectin PO on days 2 and 11[28].

For gastrointestinal nematodes with concurrent protozoal infection:
- 100 mg/kg PO of fenbendazole, repeat in 10–14 days with 10 mg/kg metronidazole PO q24h for 5 days[28].

Reptiles

For susceptible infections:
- 50–100 mg/kg PO once; repeat in 2–3 weeks as needed[31,32,33,34,35].
- 25 mg/kg PO q7d for up to 4 treatments[36].
- 50 mg/kg PO q24h for 3–5 days[37].

For nematodes in chameleons:
- 50 mg/kg PO q24h for 3 days every 7–10 days[38].

For flagellates, nematodes, and Giardia in chameleons:
- 50 mg/kg PO q24h for 3–5 days[38].

For tortoises:
- 50 mg/kg PO q24h for 3 days or 100 mg/kg PO q14–21d[39].

For turtles:
- 100 mg/kg PO q48h for 3 treatments, repeat the 3 treatments in 21 days[40,41].

Fish

For susceptible infections:
- 0.2% in feed for 3 days, repeat in 14–21 days[42].
- 2.5 mg/g in feed for 2–3 days, repeat in 14 days[43].
- 50 mg/kg PO q24h for 2 days, repeat in 14 days[43].

For non-encysted gastrointestinal nematodes:
- 2 mg/L tank water q7d for 3 treatments[44].

For treatment of Bothriocephalus acheilognathi in carp:
- 40 mg/kg in feed q4d for 2 treatments[45].

For medicated brine shrimp:
- Place live brine shrimp in 400 mg fenbendazole per 100 ml water for 15–20 minutes immediately before feeding fish. Feed for 2 consecutive days and repeat in 14 days[43].

Birds

For Ascaridia in most species:
- Do not use during molting or nesting.
- 10–50 mg/kg PO once; repeat in 10 days[46].
- 25 mg/kg PO, repeat in 14 days[47,48].

For flukes or microfilaria in most species:
- 10–50 mg/kg PO once daily for 5 days.
- Ineffective against gizzard worms in finches[46].

For nematodes and some trematodes in most species:
- Do not use during molting or nesting.
- 10–50 mg/kg PO once daily for 3–5 days.
- 20–100 mg/kg oral single dose range.
- 125 mg/L of drinking water for 5 days (50–100 mg/L for 5 days in finches).
- 100 mg/kg of feed for 5 days[49].
- 50 mg/kg PO q24 for 3 days[47,50].

For Capillaria in most species:
- 50 mg/kg PO q24 for 5 days[47].

For susceptible infections in ratites:
- 15 mg/kg PO once daily for 3 days[51].

For treatment of Capillaria in chickens:
- 1.5–3.9 mg/kg PO q24h for 3 days[52].
- 80 mg/kg feed[52].

For treatment of nematodes in pigeons:
- 10–12 mg/kg PO q24h for 3 days[53].

For treatment of Heterakis and ascarids in pheasants:
- 10–40 mg/kg PO[54].

For treatment of Syngamus, Heterakis, and Ascaridia in partridges and pheasants:
- 12 mg/kg PO[55].

For treatment of nematodes and trematodes in game birds:
- 53 mg/kg feed for 5–7 days[56].

For treatment of nematodes and trematodes in raptors:
- 10–50 mg/kg PO, repeat in 14 days[57].

For treatment of Capillaria in raptors:
- 20 mg/kg PO q24 for 5 days[58].
- 25–50 mg/kg PO q24h for 5 days, repeat in 10–14 days[57].
- 100 mg/kg PO once, repeat in 10–14 days[57].

For treatment of filarids in raptors:
- 20 mg/kg PO q24h for 14 days[58].

For susceptible infections in waterfowl:
- 5–15 mg/kg PO q24h for 5 days[59].

For susceptible infections in psittacines:
- 15 mg/kg PO q24h for 5 days[60].

For treatment of ascarids in psittacines:
- 20–50 mg/kg PO q24h, repeat in 10 days[60,61].

For treatment of trematodes and Microfilaria in psittacines:
- 20–50 mg/kg PO q24h for 3 days[61].

For treatment of Capillaria in psittacines:
- 20–50 mg/kg PO q24h for 5 days[61].

Sheep and Goats

For susceptible parasites:
- 5 mg/kg in feed for 3 days[62].

Swine

For susceptible parasites:
- 5 mg/kg PO.
- 3 mg/kg in feed for 3 days.
- 10 mg/kg for ascarids[62].

For whipworm in potbellied pigs:
- 10 mg/kg PO q24h for 3 days[63].

Primates

For susceptible infections in lemurs:
- 50 mg/kg PO q24h for 3 days[64].

For Filaroides:
- 50 mg/kg PO q24h for 14 days[65].

REFERENCES

1. Chiapella, A.M. (1988) Diseases of the Small Intestine. In: Morgan, R.V. (ed.) *Handbook of Small Animal Practice,* Churchill Livingstone, New York, 395–420.
2. Reinemeyer, C.R. (1985) Strategies for Management of Gastrointestinal Parasitism of Small Animals. In: *Eighth Annual Kal Kan Symposium for the Treatment of Small Animal Diseases,* Vernon, Kal Kan Foods, Inc., 25–32.
3. Todd, K.S., Paul, A.J. and DiPietro, J.A. (1985) Parasitic Diseases. In: Davis, L.E. (ed.) *Handbook of Small Animal Therapeutics,* Churchill Livingstone, New York, 89–126.
4. Brown, S.A. and Prestwood. A.K. (1986) Parasites of the Urinary Tract. In: Kirk, R.W. (ed.) *Current Veterinary Therapy IX, Small Animal Practice,* W.B. Saunders, Philadelphia, 1153–1155.
5. Hawkins, E.C., Ettinger, S.J. and Suter, P.F. (1989) Diseases of the lower respiratory tract (lung) and pulmonary edema. In: Ettinger, S.J. (ed.) *Textbook of Veterinary Internal Medicine,* W.B. Saunders, Philadelphia, 816–866.
6. Reinemeyer, C. (1995) Parasites of the respiratory system. In: Bonagura, J. (ed.) *Kirk's Current Veterinary Therapy: XII,* W.B. Saunders, Philadelphia, 895–898.
7. DeNovo, R.C. (1988) Diseases of the Large Bowel. In: Morgan, R.V. (ed.) *Handbook of Small Animal Practice,* Churchill Livingstone, New York, 421–439.
8. Barr, S. and Bowman, D. (1994) Giardiasis in Dogs and Cats. *Comp. CE* **16,** 603–610.
9. Greene, C. and Watson, A. (1998) Antimicrobial drug formulary. In: Greene, C. (ed.) *Infectious Diseases of the Dog and Cat,* W.B. Saunders, Philadelphia, 790–919.
10. Lappin, M. (2000) Protozoal and Miscellaneous Infections. In: Ettinger, S. and Feldman, E. (eds.) *Textbook of Veterinary Internal Medicine: Diseases of the Dog and Cat,* W.B. Saunders, Philadelphia, 408–417.
11. Dimski, D.S. (1989) Helminth and Noncoccidial Protozoan Parasites of the Gastrointestinal Tract. In: Sherding. R.G. (ed.) *The Cat: Diseases and Clinical Management,* Churchill Livingstone, New York, 459–477.
12. Pechman, R.D. (1989) Respiratory parasites. In: Sherding, R.G. (ed.) *The Cat: Diseases and Clinical Management,* Churchill Livingstone, New York, 484–494.
13. Brown, S.A. and Barsanti, J.A. (1989) Diseases of the Bladder and Urethra. In: Ettinger, S.L. (ed.) *Textbook of Veterinary Medicine,* W.B. Saunders, Philadelphia, 2108–2141.
14. Hawkins, E. (2000) Pulmonary Parenchymal Diseases. In: Ettinger, S. and Feldman, E. (eds.) *Textbook of Veterinary Internal Medicine: Diseases of the Dog and Cat,* W.B. Saunders, Philadelphia, 1061–1091.
15. Steiner, J. and Williams, D. (2000) Feline Exocrine Pancreatic Disease. In: Bonagura, J. (ed.) *Kirk's Current Veterinary Therapy: XIII Small Animal Practice,* W.B. Saunders, Philadelphia, 701–705.
16. Tams, T. (1999) *Acute Diarrheal Diseases of the Dog and Cat.* The North American Veterinary Conference, Orlando, FL.
17. Allen, D.G., Pringle, J.K., and Smith, D.A. (eds.) (1993) *Handbook of Veterinary Drugs,* J.B. Lippincott, Philadelphia.
18. Burke, T. (1999) *Husbandry and Medicine of Rodents and Lagomorphs.* Central Veterinary Conference, Kansas City, MO.
19. Taffs, L.F. (1976) Further studies on the efficacy of thiabendazole given in the diet of mice infected with *H. nana, S. obvelata,* and *A. tetraptera. Vet. Rec.* **99,** 143–144.
20. Adamcak, A. and Otten, B. (2000) Rodent Therapeutics. *Vet. Clin. N. Am: Exotic Anim. Pract.* **3,** 221–240.

21. Burke, T.J. (1995) "Wet tail" in hamsters and other diarrheas of small rodents. In: Bonagura, J.D. (ed.) *Kirk's Current Veterinary Therapy XII: Small Animal Practice*, W.B. Saunders, Philadelphia, 1336–1339.

22. Okerman, L. (1994) *Diseases of Domestic Rabbits*, 2nd ed. Blackwell Scientific, Oxford.

23. Hillyer, E.V. (1994) Pet rabbits. *Vet. Clin. N. Am: Small Anim. Pract.* **24,** 25–65.

24. Suter, C., Muller-Doblies, U.U., Hatt, J.M., et al. (2001) Prevention and treatment of *Encephalitozoon cuniculi* infection in rabbits with fenbendazole. *Vet. Rec.* **148,** 478–480.

25. Morrisey, J.K. (1999) Parasites of ferrets, rabbits and rodents. *Semin. Avian Exotic Pet Med.* **5,** 106–114.

26. Hayes, P. (2000) Diseases of chinchillas. In: Bonagura, J. (ed.) *Kirk's Current Veterinary Therapy: XIII Small Animal Practice*, W.B. Saunders, Philadelphia, 1152–1157.

27. Crawshaw, G.J. (1993) Amphibian Medicine. In: Fowler, M.E. (ed.) *Zoo and Wild Animal Medicine: Current Therapy 3*, W.B. Saunders, Philadelphia, 131–139.

28. Whitaker, B.R. (1997) Developing an effective quarantine program for amphibians. *Proc. North Am: Vet Conf.* 764–765.

29. Poynton, S.L. and Whitaker, B.R. (1994) Protozoa in poison dart frogs (*Dendrobatidae*): clinical assessment and identification. *J. Zoo Wildl. Med.* **25,** 29–39.

30. Wright, K.M. and Whitaker, B.R. (2001) Pharmacotherapeutics. In: Wright, K.M. and Whitaker, B.R. (eds.) *Amphibian Medicine and Captive Husbandry*, Krieger Publishing, Malabar, FL, 309–330.

31. Gauvin, J. (1993) Drug Therapy in reptiles. *Seminars in Avian and Exotic Med.* **2,** 48–59.

32. Barten, S.L. (1993) The medical care of iguanas and other pet lizards. *Vet. Clin. N. Am: Small Anim. Pract.* **23,** 1213–1249.

33. Jacobson, E.R. (1988) Use of chemotherapeutics in reptile medicine. In: Jacobson, E.R. and Kollias, G.V. (eds.) *Exotic Animals*, Churchill Livingstone, New York, 35–48.

34. Jacobson, E.R. (1993) Snakes. *Vet. Clin. N. Am: Small Anim. Pract.* **23,** 1179–1212.

35. Marks, S.K. and Cinto, S.B. (1990) Hematology and serum chemistry of the radiated tortoise (*Testudo radiata*). *J. Zoo Wildl. Med.* **21,** 342–344.

36. Klingenberg, R.J. (1996) Parasitology for the practitioner. *Proc. North Am. Vet. Conf.* pp. 826–827.

37. Gillespie, D. (1994) Reptiles. In: Birchard, S.J. and Sherding, R.G. (eds.) *Saunders Manual of Small Animal Practice*, W.B. Saunders, Philadelphia, 1390–1411.

38. Klingenberg, R.J. (2000) Diagnosing parasites of old world chameleons. *Exotic DVM.* **1,** 17–21.

39. Wright, K.M. (1997) Common medical problems of tortoises. *Proc. North Am. Vet. Conf.* 769–771.

40. Boyer, T.H. (1992) Common problems in box turtles (*Terrapene* spp.) in captivity. *Bull. Assoc. Rept. Amph. Vet.* **2,** 9–14.

41. Messonnier, S. (1996) Formulary for exotic pets. *Vet. Forum* **Aug,** 46–49.

42. Lewbart, G.A. (1998) Emergency and critical care of fish. *Vet. Clin. N. Am: Exotic Anim. Pract.* **1,** 233–249.

43. Whitaker, B.R. (1999) Preventable medicine programs for fish. In: Fowler, M.E. and Miller, R.E. (eds.) *Zoo and Wild Animal Medicine: Current Therapy 4*, W.B. Saunders, Philadelphia, 163–181.

44. Noga, E.J. (2000) *Fish Disease: Diagnosis and Treatment*, Iowa State University Press, Ames, Iowa.

45. Treves-Brown, K.M. (2000) *Applied Fish Pharmacology*, Kluwer Academic Publishers, Dodrecht, The Netherlands.

46. Clubb, S.L. (1986) Therapeutics: Individual and Flock Treatment Regimens. In: Harrison, G.J. and Harrison, L.R. (eds.) *Clinical Avian Medicine and Surgery*, W.B. Saunders, Philadelphia, 327–355.

47. Clyde, V.L. and Patton, S. (1996) Diagnosis, treatment, and control of common parasites in companion and aviary birds. *Semin. Avian Exotic Pet. Med.* **5,** 75–84.

48. Smith, S.A. (1993) Diagnosis and treatment of helminthes in birds of prey. In: Redig, P.T., Cooper, J.E., and Remple, J.D., et al. (eds.) *Raptor Biomedicine*, University of Minnesota, Minneapolis, MN, 21–27.

49. Marshall, R. (1993) Avian anthelmintics and antiprotozoals. *Semin. Avian and Exotic Med.* **2,** 33–41.

50. Rupiper, D.J. and Ehrenberg, M. (1994) Introduction to pigeon practice. *Proc. Annu. Conf. Assoc. Avian Vet.* 203–211.

51. Jenson, J. (1998) Current ratite therapy. *Vet. Clin. N. Am: Food Anim. Pract.* **16,** 3.

52. Taylor, S.M., Kenny, J., Houston, A., et al. (1993) Efficacy, pharmacokinetics, and effect on egg-laying and hatchability of two dose rates of in-feed fenbendazole for the treatment of *Capillaria* species infections in chickens. *Vet. Rec.* **133,** 519–521.

53. Harlin, R.W. (2000) Pigeon therapeutics. *Vet. Clin. N. Am: Exotic Anim. Pract.* **3,** 19–34.

54. Carpenter, N.A. (2000) Anseriform and galliform therapeutics. *Vet. Clin. N. Am: Exotic Anim. Pract.* **3,** 1–17.

55. Byrne, R.F., Davis, C., and Lister, S.A., et al. (2001) Prescribing for birds. In: Bishop, Y. (ed.) *The Veterinary Formulary*, 5th ed. Pharmaceutical Press, London, 43–56.

56. Stadler, C. and Carpenter, J.W. (1996) Parasites of backyard game birds. *Semin. Avian Exotic Pet Med.* **5,** 85–96.

57. Huckabee, J.R. (2000) Raptor therapeutics. *Vet. Clin. N. Am: Exotic Anim. Pract.* **3,** 91–116.

58. Beynon, P.H., Forbes, N.A., and Harcourt-Brown, N.H. (1996) *BSAVA Manual of Raptors, Pigeons and Waterfowl*, Iowa State University Press, Ames, IA.

59. Ritchie, B.W. and Harrison, G.J. (1994) Formulary. In: Ritchie, B.W., Harrison, G.J., and Harrison, L.R. (eds.) *Avian Medicine: Principle and Application*, Wingers, Lake Worth, FL, 227–253.

60. Samour, J. (2000) Pharmaceutics commonly used in avian medicine. In: Samour, J. (ed.) *Avian Medicine*, Mosby, Philadelphia, 388–418.

61. Tully, T.N. (2000) Psittacine therapeutics. *Vet. Clin. N. Am: Exotic Anim. Pract.* **3,** 59–90.

62. Roberson, E.L. (1988) Antinematodal Agents. In: Booth, N.H. and McDonald, L.E. (eds.) *Veterinary Pharmacology and Therapeutics*, Iowa State University Press, Ames, IA, 882–927.

63. Braun, W.F. Jr. and Casteel, S.W. (1993) Potbellied Pigs—miniature porcine pets. *Vet. Clin. N. Am: Small Anim. Pract.* **23,** 1149–1177.

64. Feeser, P. and White, F. (1992) Medical management of *Lemur catta, Varecia variegate,* and *Propithecus verreauxi* in natural habitat enclosures. *Proc. Am. Assoc. Zoo Vet/Am. Assoc. Wildl. Vet.* pp. 320–323.

65. Wolff, P.L. (1993) Parasites of the new world primates. In: Fowler, M.E. (ed.) *Zoo and Wild Animal Medicine: Current Therapy 3*, W.B. Saunders, Philadelphia, 378–389.

Fenthion

Activity: Used to treat susceptible ectoparasites in dogs (fleas) and swine (lice).

MOA: Fenthion is a topical organophosphate drug that inhibits acetylcholinesterase in susceptible ectoparasites, inhibiting neuromuscular transmission.

Dogs

For treatment of fleas:

- 4–8 mg/kg topically, not more frequently than once every 2 weeks (Package Insert; Pro-spot®—Miles).

Swine

- 1/2 fl oz/100 lbs body weight of 3% topical fenthion (Package Insert; Tiguvon®—Miles).
- Slaughter withdraw: 14 days.

Fipronil

Activity: Used to prevent and treat fleas and ticks in dogs and cats. Off-label use in: reptiles, birds, rodents, and ferrets. Fipronil is contraindicated in rabbits.

MOA: Fipronil interferes with gamma-aminobutyric acid (GABA) regulated chloride channels which results in the disruption of CNS activity.

Dogs

- Frontline® Top Spot may be applied once a month to dogs with severe flea allergy dermatitis or in high risk areas. Dogs without severe flea allergies and ticks are not a threat.
- Frontline® Top Spot may be applied once ever 2–3 months. (Label information; Frontline® Top Spot—Merial).
- Frontline® Topical Spray (0.29%) may be applied at the intervals mentioned above at the rate of 1.5–3 ml per lb of body weight (1–2 pumps/lb. using the 250 ml bottle and 3–6 pumps/lb. using the 100 ml bottle). Dogs with long hair or thick coats should receive the higher dose rate.

Cats

- Apply Frontline® Top Spot once a month for flea and tick control (Label information; Frontline® Top Spot—Merial).
- Frontline® Topical Spray (0.29%) may be applied at the intervals mentioned above at the rate of 1.5–3 ml per lb of body weight (1–2 pumps/lb. using the 250 ml bottle and 3–6 pumps/lb. using the 100 ml bottle). Cats with long hair or thick coats should receive the higher dose rate.

Mice, Hamsters, and Chipmunks

For treatment of adult fleas:

- 7.5 mg/kg topically q30–60 days[1].

Rabbits

- Fipronil is contraindicated in rabbits[2].

Ferrets

For treatment of adult fleas:

- Topical Spray (0.29%) may be applied at the rate of 1 pump of spray or 1/5–1/2 of cat pipette topical q60 days[2].
- 0.2–0.4 ml topically q30d[3].

Reptiles

For susceptible infections:

- Topical Spray (0.29%) may be sprayed or wiped on q7–10 days[4].

Birds

For susceptible infections:

- Topical Spray (0.29%) may be sprayed on skin once, then repeated in 30 days as needed[5].

REFERENCES

1. Richardson, V.C.G. (1997) *Diseases of Small Domestic Rodents,* Blackwell Scientific, Oxford.
2. Morrisey, J.K. (1998) Ectoparasites of small mammals. *Proc. North Am. Vet. Conf.* 844–845.
3. Williams, B.H. (2000) Therapeutics in ferrets. *Vet. Clin. N. Am: Exotic Anim. Pract.* **3,** 131–153.
4. Divers, S.J. (1999) Clinical evaluation of reptiles. *Vet. Clin. N. Am: Exotic Anim. Pract.* **2,** 291–331.
5. Beynon, P.H., Forbes, N.A., and Harcourt-Brown N.H. (1996) *BSAVA Manual of Raptors, Pigeons and Waterfowl,* Iowa State University Press, Ames, IA.

Formalin

Activity: Used to treat protozoa, trematodes, and crustacean ectoparasites in fish. Formalin is a carcinogen and toxic to plants.

MOA: Formalin denatures peptides, resulting in the death of susceptible parasites.

Fish

- All doses are based on volumes of 100% formalin.
- Some fish are very sensitive to formalin; therefore it is recommended to test on a smaller number of fish first.

For Ichthyophthirius:

- 0.025 ml/L tank water q48h for 3 treatments; change up to 50% of water on alternating days[1].

- 0.025 ml/L of formalin combined with 0.1 mg/L malachite green in tank water every 48 hours for 3 treatments; change 50% of tank water on alternating days[1].

For susceptible parasites:
- 0.015–0.025 ml/L tank water[1].
- 0.125–0.25 ml/L for up to 60 min. bath, repeat q24h for 2–3 days as needed; only treat every 3 days if using maximum dose[1].
- 0.4 ml/L for up to 60 min. bath every 3 days, up to 3 treatments (soft water)[2].
- 0.5 ml/L for up to 60 min. bath every 3 days, up to 3 treatments (hard water)[2].
- 25 mg/L water in ponds; <250 mg/L water for 1 hr. in tanks and raceways[3].
- 10 ppm in bath indefinitely (hybrid striped bass and other sensitive species)[4].
- 15–25 ppm in bath indefinitely or repeated every 3 days with 70%–90% water changes[4].
- 250 ppm for 5–10 min. dip[4].
- 400 ppm in soft water for up to 1 hr. bath every 3 days for 3 treatments[4].
- 500 ppm in hard water for up to 1 hr. bath every 3 days for 3 treatments[4].

REFERENCES

1. Noga, E.J. (2000) *Fish Disease: Diagnosis and Treatment,* Iowa State University Press, Ames, IA.
2. Stoskopf, M.K. (1993) Appendix V: Chemotherapeutics. In: Stoskopf, M.K. (ed.) *Fish Medicine,* W.B. Saunders, Philadelphia, 832–839.
3. Klesius, P. and Rogers, W. (1995) Parasitisms of catfish and other farm-raised food fish. *J. Am. Vet. Med. Assoc.* **207,** 1473–1478.
4. Harms, C.A. (1996) Treatments for parasitic diseases of aquarium and ornamental fish. *Semin. Exotic Pet Med.* **5(2),** 54–63.

Furazolidone

Activity: Used in dogs, cats, and primates primarily for the treatment of *Giardia.* Furazolidone also has antiparasitic effects against *Trichomonas* and coccidiosis.

MOA: The mechanism of action of furazolidone against protozoa is poorly understood.

Dogs

For Amebic Colitis:
- 2.2 mg/kg PO q8h for 7 days[1].

For Coccidiosis:
- 8–20 mg/kg PO for 1 week[1].

For Giardia:
- 4 mg/kg PO q12h for 7 days[2].

For Cystoisospora spp.:
- 8–20 mg/kg PO q12–24h for 5 days[2].

For Amebiasis:
- 2.2 mg/kg PO q8h for 7 days[3].

Cats

For Giardia:
- 4 mg/kg PO q12h for 7–10 days; if re-treatment is needed, dose may be increased or treatment time lengthened[4].
- 4 mg/kg PO q12h for 5 days[1].
- 4 mg/kg PO q12h for 7 days[2].
- 4 mg/kg PO q12h for 5–10 days[3].

For Amebic Colitis:
- 2.2 mg/kg PO q8h for 7 days[1,3].

For Coccidiosis:
- 8–20 mg/kg PO for 1 week[1,3].

For Cystoisospora spp.:
- 8–20 mg/kg PO q12–24h for 5 days[2].

Primates

For treatment of Giardia in great apes:
- 5 mg/kg PO q6h for 7 days (juvenile great apes)[5].
- 100 mg/animal PO for 7 days (adult great apes)[5].

REFERENCES

1. Sherding, R. and Johnson, S. (1994) Diseases of the intestines. In: Rirchard, S. and Sherding, R. (eds.) *Saunders Manual of Small Animal Practice,* W.B. Saunders, Philadelphia, 687–714.
2. Lappin, M. (2000) Protozoal and Miscellaneous Infections. In: Ettinger, S. and Feldman, E. (eds.) *Textbook of Veterinary Internal Medicine: Diseases of the Dog and Cat,* W.B. Saunders, Philadelphia, 408–417.
3. Greene, C. and Watson, A. (1998) Antimicrobial Drug Formulary. In: Greene, C. (ed.) *Infectious Diseases of the Dog and Cat,* W.B. Saunders, Philadelphia, 790–919.
4. Reinemeyer, C. (1992) Feline gastrointestinal parasites. In: Kirk, R. and Bonagura, J. (eds.) *Current Veterinary Therapy XI: Small Animal Practice,* W.B. Saunders, Philadelphia, 626–630.
5. Swenson, R.B. (1993) Protozoal parasites of great apes. In: Fowler, M.E. (ed.) *Zoo and Wild Animal Medicine: Current Therapy 3,* W.B. Saunders, Philadelphia, 352–355.

Imidacloprid

Activity: Used topically to treat and prevent fleas (adult and larval) in dogs and cats. Also used off label in ferrets and rabbits.

MOA: Imidacloprid acts on nicotinic acetylcholine receptors resulting in CNS impairment and death in susceptible parasites.

Dogs and Cats

For fleas:

- Apply as directed once a month; do not re-treat more than once weekly. (Package instructions; Advantage®—Bayer).

Rabbits

For fleas:

- Use feline dose; place in 2–3 areas along dorsum[1].
- 10–16 mg/kg (single 0.4 ml dose, 10% solution) as a single topical application[2,3].

Prairie Dogs

- 1/2 kitten dose topically[4].

Ferrets

- 1 cat dose divided into 2–3 spots along dorsum once a month[5].
- 0.1 ml topically once a month[6].
- 0.4 ml topically once a month[7].

REFERENCES

1. Ivey, E. and Morrisey, J. (2000) Therapeutics for Rabbits. *Vet. Clin. N. Am: Exotic Anim Pract* **3**, 183–213.
2. Harcourt-Brown, F. (2002) *Textbook of Rabbit Medicine,* Butterworth-Heinemann, Oxford, 94–120.
3. Hutchinson, M., Jacobs, D., Bell G., et al. (2001) Evaluation of imidacloprid for the treatment and prevention of cat flea (*Ctenocephalides felis*) infestations on rabbits. *Vet. Rec.* **148**, 695–696.
4. Morrisey, J.K. and Carpenter, J.W. (2004) Formulary. In: Quesenberry, K.E. and Carpenter, J.W. (eds.) *Ferrets, Rabbits, and Rodents: Clinical Medicine and Surgery,* 2nd ed. W.B. Saunders, St. Louis, MO, 436–444.
5. Morrisey, J.K. (1998) Ectoparasites of ferrets and rabbits. *Proc. North Am. Vet. Conf.* 844–845.
6. Williams, B.H. (2000) Therapeutics in ferrets. *Vet. Clin. N. Am: Exotic Anim. Pract.* **3**, 131–153.
7. Lewington, J.H. (2000) *Ferret Husbandry, Medicine, and Surgery,* Butterworth-Heinemann, Oxford, 273–282.

Imidocarb

Activity: Used to treat *Babesia* and related parasites in dogs, cats, and sheep.

MOA: Imidocarb is thought to act on protozoa by inhibiting DNA replication and repair by combining with nucleic acids.

Dogs

For Babesiosis:

- 6.6 mg/kg IM or SC; repeat dose in 2 weeks (Package Insert; Imizol®—Schering).
- 5–6.6 mg/kg IM or SC; repeat in 14 days or 7.5 mg/kg IM or SC once[1].

For Ehrlichiosis:

- 5 mg/kg IM or SC; repeat in 14–21 days or 5 mg/kg IM repeat in 84 days[1].

For Hepatozoonosis:

- 5 mg/kg IM or SC every 14 days until parasitemia clears. 1–2 injections are usually sufficient[2].

Cats

For Cytauxzoon felis:

- 5 mg/kg IM every 2 weeks[3].

Sheep

For Babesiosis:

- 1.2 mg/kg IM; repeat in 10–14 days[4].

REFERENCES

1. Greene, C. and Watson, A. (1998) Antimicrobial drug formulary. In: Greene, C. (ed.) *Infectious Diseases of the Dog and Cat,* W.B. Saunders, Philadelphia, 790–919.
2. Macintire, D. (1999) *Canine Hepatozoonosis.* American College of Veterinary Internal Medicine: 17th Annual Veterinary Medical Forum, Chicago, IL.
3. Lappin, M. (2000) Protozoal and miscellaneous infections. In: Ettinger, S. and Feldman, E. (eds.) *Textbook of Veterinary Internal Medicine: Diseases of the Dog and Cat,* W.B. Saunders, Philadelphia, 408–417.
4. McHardy, N., Woolon, R., and Clampitt, R. (1986) Efficacy, toxicity, and metabolism of imidocarb dipropionate in the treatment of *Babesia ovis* infection in sheep. *Res. Vet. Sci.* **41**, 14–20.

Ivermectin

Activity: Used in a variety of species as a parasiticide. Contraindicated in collies and fish.

MOA: Ivermectin stimulates the release of gamma-aminobutyric acid (GABA) at presynaptic neurons, resulting in paralysis and death of the parasite. Ivermectin is ineffective against parasites that do not utilize GABA, such as tapeworms and liver flukes.

Dogs

For heartworm prevention:

- 0.006 mg/kg (6mcg/kg) PO once monthly[1].

- 6–12 mcg/kg PO once monthly[2].
- Minimum dosage of 5.98 mcg/kg (0.00598 mg/kg) PO per month[3].
- Minimum dosage of 6 mcg/kg (0.006 mg/kg) PO every 30 days.
- Three tablet sizes are available (0–25 lbs, 26–50 lbs, and 51–100 lbs.). Dogs weighing more than 100 lbs should receive additional drug so that the minimum dosage is covered (Package insert; Heartgard 30®—MSD).

As a microfilaricide:

- Administer 0.05 mg/kg 3–4 weeks after adulticide therapy. (Dilute 10 mg/ml solution—Ivomec®—to a 1:10 solution with propylene glycol.) Admit the dog to hospital and monitor for symptoms of toxicity (depression, mydriasis, ataxia, vomiting, diarrhea, and shock) throughout the day. Treat any toxicity symptoms (seen <5% of the time) with fluids and corticosteroids. If signs of toxicity are absent, the dog may be sent home in the afternoon. Have dog return in 3 weeks to test for concentration of microfilaria. If microfilaria test is negative, begin prophylaxis therapy; if positive, re-check in one week. If microfilaria persist 4 weeks after treatment, reevaluate for adult heartworms. For more information, see the complete reference[1].
- 50–200 mcg/kg (0.05–0.2 mg/kg) as a single dose; contraindicated in collies[4]. 4 weeks after adulticidal therapy, give 50 mcg/kg PO in the morning. (Dilute 10 mg/ml solution—Ivomec®— to a 1:10 solution with propylene glycol.) Monitor for symptoms of toxicity throughout the day. If none are observed, the dog may be sent home in the afternoon. Contraindicated in collies and collie-mix breeds[3].

As an ectoparasiticide (miticide):
for Sarcoptes scabiei or Otodectes cynotis:

- 300 mcg/kg (0.3 mg/kg) SC or PO; repeat in 14 days[5].

For Demodicosis:

- 400–600 mcg/kg PO daily. Consider using the test dose method: Begin at 100mcg/kg PO and increase by 100 mcg/day until the target dose is reached. Discontinue if toxicity is seen.
- Do not use in collies, Shelties, Old English Sheepdogs, and other herding dogs[6].

As an endoparasiticide:

For Capillaria spp.(lungworm):

- 0.2 mg/kg PO once[7].

For Filaroides osleri:

- 0.4 mg/kg SC once[8].

For Eucoleus boehmi:

- 0.2 mg/kg PO once[8].

For Pneumonyssoides caninum:

- 0.2 mg/kg SC once[8].

Cats

For heartworm prevention:

- Minimum effective dosage: 24 mcg/kg (0.024 mg/kg) PO every 30–45 days. Hookworms are also controlled at this dosage[9].

For Aelurostrongylus abstrusus:

- 0.4 mg/kg SC once[8,10].

Mice, Rats, Gerbils, Guinea Pigs, and Chinchillas

For sarcoptid and some fur mites:

- 200–250 mcg/kg SC. Cages cleaned and disinfected[11].
- 200 mcg/kg SC or PO every 7 days for 3 weeks[12].
- 0.2–0.4 mg/kg SC q7–14d; preferred dose appears to be 0.4 mg/kg q7d[13].

For mite control in mice:

- Spray animals with 1% ivermectin diluted 1:100 with 1:1 propylene glycol/water (0.1 mg/ml) or apply topically behind ear 4–5 times a year[14,15].

For guinea pigs with sarcoptid mites:

- 0.5 mg/kg SC; repeat q14d[16].

For pinworms in mice:

- 8 mg/L drinking water for 4 days/week for 5 weeks[17].

For pinworms in rats:

- 25 mg/L drinking water for 4 days/week for 5 weeks[17].

For sarcoptid and some fur mites in hamsters:

- 200–500 mcg/kg SC or PO every 14 days for 3 weeks[12].
- 0.2–0.4 mg/kg SC q7–14d; preferred dose appears to be 0.4 mg/kg q7d[13].

Rabbits

For Sarcoptes scabiei and Notoedres cati:

- 0.3–0.4 mg/kg SC; repeat in 14 days[18].
- 0.2–0.4 mg/kg SC q10–14d[13].
- 0.4 mg/kg PO, SC q7–14d[19].
- 0.4 mg/kg SC q7d for 2–3 weeks[20].
- 0.6 mg/kg SC q14d[21].

For ear mites (Psoroptes):
- 0.2–0.44 mg/kg PO or SC; repeat in 8–18 days[18].
- 200 mcg/kg SC; repeat in 2 weeks. All rabbits in colony should be treated and cages cleaned and disinfected[11].
- 0.1–0.2 mg/kg SC; repeat in 14 days[22].

Ferrets

For heartworm prevention:
- 0.02 mg/kg PO monthly[23].
- 0.05 mg/kg PO q30d; administer 1 month before and continue 2 months past possible mosquito exposure[24,25].
- 0.055 mg/ferret PO q30d (Heartgard®—Merial); use small cat dose[24].

As a microfilaricide:
- 0.05 mg/kg PO or SC; use 3–4 weeks postadulticide treatment[24,25].

For Sarcoptic mange:
- 0.2–0.5 mg/kg SC; repeat q14d for 3 treatments[24].
- 0.4 mg/kg PO or SC; repeat in 14–28 days[24,26].

For ear mites:
- 0.5–1.0 mg/kg in ears (half dose in each ear); repeat in 14 days; treat cats and dogs in house concurrently[24,27].

Amphibians

For nematodes (including lungworms) and mites:
- 0.2–0.4 mg/kg PO or SC; repeat q14d as needed[28].
- 10 mg/L as 60 min bath, repeat q14d as needed for mites[29].
- 2 mg/kg topically; repeat in 2–3 weeks[30].

Reptiles

- **Note:** Ivermectin is toxic to chelonians; use of Ivermectin on colored skin may result in discoloration.

For most nematodes, ectoparasites (mites):
- For lizards (except skinks), snakes (except indigos)[31], and alligators: 200 mcg/kg (0.2 mg/kg) IM, SC, or PO once; repeat in 2 weeks[32,33,34,35].
- For lizards (except skinks) and snakes (except indigos): 5–10 mg/L water topical q4–5d up to 28 days, spray on skin and in cage[36,37].

Birds

For ascarids, Capillaria, and other intestinal worms, Knemidocoptes pilae (scaly face and leg mites):
- Dilute to a 2 mg/ml concentration, and use immediately after diluting.

For most birds:
- Inject 220 mcg/kg IM[38].

Parakeets:
- 0.02 mg/30 g (2000 mcg/30 g) IM[38].

Parrots:
- 0.1 mg IM[38].

Macaws:
- 0.2 mg IM[38].

Finches:
- 0.02 mg IM[38].

Raptors:
- 0.4 mg/kg SC once[39].

Pigeons:
- 0.5–1.0 mg/kg PO, IM once[40].

Canaries:
- 0.8–1.0 mg/L of drinking water[41].

For ascarids, Coccidia, and other intestinal nematodes, Knemidocoptes pilae (scaly face and leg mites), Oxyspirura, gapeworms:
- Dilute bovine preparation (10 mg/ml) 1:4 with propylene glycol.
- For most species: 200 mcg/kg IM or PO; repeat in 10–14 days[42].
- For budgerigars: 0.01 ml of diluted product (see above) IM or PO[42].

For treatment of susceptible parasites in most species:
- 200 mcg/kg (0.2 mg/kg) SC; dilute using propylene glycol[43].
- 0.2 mg/kg PO, SQ, or IM. Can dilute with water or saline for immediate use or propylene glycol for extended use[44,45,46,47].

For treatment of susceptible parasites in ratites:
- 200 mcg/kg (0.2 mg/kg) SC, PO, or IM[48].

For quill mites in canaries:
- 0.2 mg/kg SC, or topical on skin. Repeat in 4 days if live mites are still present[49].

Sheep

For susceptible parasites:
- 200 mcg/kg for nasal bite infection[50].
- 200 mcg/kg SC for one dose[51].

Goats

For susceptible parasites:
- 200 mcg/kg SC for one dose[51].

Swine

For susceptible parasites:
- 300 mcg/kg (0.3 mg/kg) SC in the neck behind the ear (Product Information; Ivomec® Inj. For Swine 1%— MSD).
- 300 mcg/kg (0.3 mg/kg) SC or IM once for internal parasites and repeated in 10–14 days for external parasites in potbellied pigs[52].
- 0.3 mg/kg PO, SC, or IM in miniature pigs; repeat in 10–14 days for sarcoptic mange[53].

Primates

For susceptible parasites:
- 0.2 mg/kg PO, SC, or IM; may repeat in 10–14 days[54,55,56].

REFERENCES

1. Hribernik, T.N. (1989) Canine and Feline Heartworm Disease. In: Kirk, R.W. (ed.) *Current Veterinary Therapy X: Small Animal Practice,* W.B. Saunders, Philadelphia, 263–270.

2. Knight, D. (2000) CVT update: heartworm testing and prevention in dogs. In: Bonagura, J. (ed.) *Kirk's Current Veterinary Therapy: XIII Small Animal Practice,* W.B. Saunders, Philadelphia, 777–782.

3. Rawlings, C.A. and Calvert, C.A. (1989) Heartworm disease. In: Ettinger, S.J. (ed.) *Textbook of Veterinary Internal Medicine,* W.B. Saunders, Philadelphia, 1163–1184.

4. Knight, D.H. (1988) Heartworm disease. In: Morgan, R.V. (ed.) *Handbook of Small Animal Practice,* Churchill Livingstone, New York, 139–148.

5. Paradis, M. (1989) Ivermectin in small animal dermatology. In: Kirk, R.W. (ed.) *Current Veterinary Therapy X: Small Animal Practice,* W.B. Saunders, Philadelphia, 560–563.

6. DeManuelle, T. (2000) *Current treatment of canine demodicosis.* The North American Veterinary Conference, Orlando, FL.

7. Bauer, T.G. (1988) Diseases of the Lower Airway. In: Morgan, R.V. (ed.) *Handbook of Small Animal Practice,* Churchill Livingstone, New York, 185–193.

8. Reinemeyer, C. (1995) Parasites of the respiratory system. In: Bonagura, J. (ed.) *Kirk's Current Veterinary Therapy: XII,* W.B. Saunders, Philadelphia, 895–898.

9. Knight, D. (1995) Guidelines for diagnosis and management of heartworm (*Dirofilaria immitis*) infection. In: Bonagura, J. (ed.) *Kirk's Current Veterinary Therapy XII,* W.B. Saunders, Philadelphia, 879–887.

10. Hawkins, E. (2000) Pulmonary Parenchymal Diseases. In: Ettinger, S. and Feldman, E. (eds.) *Textbook of Veterinary Internal Medicine: Diseases of the Dog and Cat,* W.B. Saunders, Philadelphia, 1061–1091.

11. Burke, T. (1999) *Husbandry and Medicine of Rodents and Lagomorphs.* Central Veterinary Conference, Kansas City, MO.

12. Adamcak, A. and Otten, B. (2000) Rodent Therapeutics. *Vet. Clin. N. Am: Exotic Anim. Pract.* **3,** 221–240.

13. Morrisey, J.K. and Carpenter, J.W. (2004) Formulary. In: Quesenberry, K.E. and Carpenter, J.W. (eds.) *Ferrets, Rabbits, and Rodents: Clinical Medicine and Surgery,* 2nd ed. W.B. Saunders, St. Louis, MO, 436–444.

14. Baumans, V., Havenaar, R., Van Herck, H., et al. (1988) The effectiveness of Ivomec and Neguvon on the control of murine mites. *Lab Anim.* **22,** 243–245.

15. Harkness, J.E. and Wagner, J.E. (1995) *The Biology and Medicine of Rabbits and Rodents,* 4th ed. Williams and Wilkins, Philadelphia.

16. Quesenberry, K.E. (1997) Medical Management of gerbils, hamsters, and guinea pigs. Proc. 21st Annu. Waltham/OSU Symp. 51–55.

17. Klement, P., Augustine, J.M., Delaney, K.M., et al. (1996) An oral ivermectin regimen that eradicates pinworms (*Syphacia* sp.) in rats and mice. *Lab. Anim. Sci.* **46,** 286–290.

18. Ivey, E. and Morrisey, J. (2000) Therapeutics for Rabbits. *Vet. Clin. N. Am: Exotic Anim. Pract.* **3,** 183–213.

19. Hillyer, E.V. (1994) Pet rabbits. *Vet. Clin. N. Am: Small Anim. Pract.* **24,** 25–65.

20. Quesenberry, K.E (1994) Rabbits. In: Birchard, S.J. and Sherding, R.G. (eds.) *Saunders Manual of Small Animal Practice,* W.B. Saunders, Philadelphia, 1345–1362.

21. Morrisey, J.K. (1988) Ectoparasites of ferrets and rabbits. *Proc. North Am. Vet. Conf.* pp. 844–845.

22. Bowman, D.D., Fogelson, M.L., and Carbone L.G. (1992) Effect of ivermectin on the control of ear mites (*Psoroptes cuniculi*) in naturally infested rabbits. *Am. J. Vet. Res.* **53,** 105–109.

23. Hoeffer, H. (2000) Heart disease in ferrets. In: Bonagura, J. (ed.) *Kirk's Current Veterinary Therapy: XIII Small Animal Practice,* W.B. Saunders, Philadelphia, 1144–1148.

24. Hillyer, E.V. and Brown, S.A. (2000) Ferrets. In: Birchard, S.J. and Sherding, R.G. (eds.) *Saunders Manual of Small Animal Practice,* W.B. Saunders, Philadelphia, 1464–1492.

25. Supakornde, J.P., McCall, J.W., Lewis, R.E., et al. (1992) Biology, diagnosis, and prevention of heartworm infection in ferrets. *Proc. Heartworm Symp.* pp. 59–69.

26. Rosenthal, K. (1994) Ferrets. *Vet. Clin. N. Am. Small Anim. Pract.* **24,** 1–23.

27. Brown, S.A. (1999) Ferret drug doses. In: Antinoff, N., Bauck, L. and Boyer, T.H., et al. (eds.) *Exotic Formulary,* 2nd ed. American Animal Hospital Association, Lakewood, CO, 43–61.

28. Crawshaw, G.J. (1993) Amphibian Medicine. In: Fowler, M.E. (ed.) *Zoo and Wild Animal Medicine: Current Therapy 3,* W.B. Saunders, Philadelphia, 131–139.

29. Wright, K.M. and Whitaker, B.R. (2001) Pharmacotherapeutics. In: Wright, K.M. and Whitaker, B.R. (eds.) *Amphibian Medicine and Captive Husbandry,* Krieger Publishing, Malabar, FL, 309–330.

30. Letcher, J. and Glade, M. (1992) Efficacy of ivermectin as an anthelmintic in leopard frogs. *J. Am. Vet. Med. Assoc.* **200,** 537–538.

31. Boyer, T.H. (1998) *Essentials of Reptiles: A Guide for Practitioners,* AAHA Press, Lakewood, CO.

32. Gauvin, J. (1993) Drug therapy in reptiles. *Seminars in Avian and Exotic Med.* **2,** 48–59.

33. Barten, S.L. (1993) The medical care of iguanas and other common pet lizards. *Vet Clin. N. Am. Small Anim. Pract.* **23,** 1213–1249.

34. Jacobson, E.R. (1988) Use of chemotherapeutics in reptile medicine. In: Jacobson, E.R. and Kollias, G.V. (eds.) *Exotic Animals,* Churchill Livingstone, New York, 35–48.

35. Wilson, S.C. and Carpenter, J.W. (1996) Endoparasitic diseases of reptiles. *Semin. Avian Exotic Pet Med.* **5,** 64–74.

36. Allen, D.G., Pringle, J.K., and Smith, D. (1993) *Handbook of Veterinary Drugs,* J.B. Lippincott, Philadelphia, 534–567.

37. Klingenberg, R.J. (1996) Parasitology for the practitioner. *Proc. North Am. Vet. Conf.* pp. 826–827.

38. Stunkard, J.M. (1984) *Diagnosis, Treatment, and Husbandry of Pet Birds,* Stunkard Publishing, Edgewater, MD.

39. Marshall, R. (1993) Avian anthelmintics and antiprotozoals. *Semin. Avian Exotic Pet Med.* **2,** 22–41.

40. Harlin, R.W. (1995) *Backyard Poultry.* Proc. Mid-Atlantic States Assoc. Avian Vet. Conf. 65–68.

41. Dorrestein, G.M. (1995) Infectious diseases and their therapy in Passeriformes. In: *Antimicrobial Therapy in Caged Birds and Exotic Pets,* Veterinary Learning Systems, Trenton, NJ, 11–27.

42. Clubb, S.L. (1986) Therapeutics: Individual and Flock Treatment Regimens. In: Harrison, G.L. and Harrison, L.R. (eds.) *Clinical Avian Medicine and Surgery,* W.B. Saunders, Philadelphia, 327–355.

43. Sikarskie, J.G. (1986) The use of ivermectin in birds, reptiles, and small mammals. In: Kirk, R.W. (ed.) *Current Veterinary Therapy IX: Small Animal Practice,* W.B. Saunders, Philadelphia, 743–745.

44. Bishop, Y. (ed.) (2001) *The Veterinary Formulary,* 5th ed. Pharmaceutical Press, London.

45. Brown, M.J. and Cromie, R.L. (1996) Weight loss and enteritis. In: Beynon, P.H., Forbes, N.A. and Harcourt-Brown, N.H. (eds.) BSAVA *Manual of Raptors, Pigeons, and Waterfowl,* Iowa State University Press, Ames, IA, 322–329.

46. Hogan, H.L., Joseph, B., Hendrickson, R., et al. (1984) Efficacy and safety of ivermectin treatment for scaly leg mite infestation in parakeets. *Proc. Am. Assoc. Zoo Vet.* 156.

47. Stadler, C. and Carpenter, J.W. (1996) Parasites of backyard game birds. *Semin. Avian Exotic Pet. Med.* **5,** 85–96.

48. Jenson, J. (1998) Current ratite therapy. *Vet. Clin. N. Am: Food Animal Pract.* **16,** 3.

49. Dorrestein, G.M., Van Der Horst, H.H.A., Cremers, H.J., et al. (1997) Quill mite (*Dermoglyphus passerinus*) infestation of canaries (*Serinus canaria*): diagnosis and treatment. *Avian. Pathol.* **26,** 195–199.

50. Bennet, D.G. (1986) Parasites of the Respiratory System. In: Howard, J.L. (ed.) *Current Veterinary Therapy: Food Animal Practice 2,* W.B. Saunders, Philadelphia, 684–687.

51. Upson, D.W. (1988) *Handbook of Clinical Veterinary Pharmacology.* 3rd ed. Dan Epson Enterprises, Manhattan.

52. Braun, W. (1995) Potbellied pigs: General medical care. In: Bonagura, J. (ed.) *Kirk's Current Veterinary Therapy: XII,* W.B. Saunders, Philadelphia, 1388–1389.

53. Braun, W.F. Jr. and Casteel, S.W. (1993) Potbellied pigs—miniature porcine pets. *Vet. Clin. N. Am: Small Anim. Pract.* **23,** 1149–1177.

54. Feeser, P. and White, F. (1992) Medical management of *Lemur catta, Varecia variegate,* and *Propithecus verreauxi* in natural habitat enclosures. *Proc. Am. Assoc. Zoo Vet/Am. Assoc. Wildl. Vet.* 320–323.

55. Johnson-Delaney, C.A. (1994) Primates. *Vet. Clin .N. Am: Small Anim. Pract.* **24,** 121–156.

56. Wolff, P.L. (1993) Parasites of the new world primates. In: Fowler, M.E. (ed.) *Zoo and Wild Animal Medicine: Current Therapy 3,* W.B. Saunders, Philadelphia, 378–389.

Levamisole

Activity: Levamisole is an antinematodal parasiticide used to treat susceptible parasites in multiple species. It is also used as an immune stimulant.

MOA: Levamisole stimulates the sympathetic and parasympathetic ganglia in susceptible parasites, resulting in paralysis and expulsion.

Dogs

As a microfilaricide:

- 10 mg/kg PO once a day for 6–10 days[1].
- 11 mg/kg PO once a day for 6–12 days; examine blood on the 6th day, discontinue when the microfilaria are negative. Possible side effects: the risk of toxicity increases with the duration of the treatment[2].
- 11 mg/kg PO once a day for 6–12 days; examine blood within 7–10 days and at weekly intervals. Avoid giving on an empty stomach. A "conditioning" dose of 5 mg/kg PO once a day may be necessary. Discontinue if abnormal behavior or ataxia develops[3].

For lungworms:

- 7.5 mg/kg PO bid or 25 mg/kg PO every other day for 10 days[4].

For Crenosoma vulpis:

- 8 mg/kg once[2].

For Capillaria:

- 7–12 mg/kg once daily PO for 3–7 days[5].
- 10 mg/kg PO once daily for 5 days; repeat in 9 days (for *C. aerophila*)[6].

For Filaroides osleri:

- 7–12 mg/kg once daily PO for 20–45 days[5].

Cats

As a microfilaricide:

- 10 mg/kg PO once a day for 7 days[7].

For treatment of Ollulanus tricuspis:

- 5 mg/kg SC[2].

For lungworms:

- 20–40 mg/kg PO every other day for 5–6 treatments[1].
- 25 mg/kg every other day for 10–14 days[5].

For Aelurostrongylus abstrusus:

- 100 mg PO daily every other day for 5 treatments; give atropine (0.5 mg SC 15 minutes before administering)[2].
- 15 mg/kg PO every other day for 3 treatments, then 3 days later give 30 mg/kg PO, then 2 days later give 60 mg/kg[2].

For Capillaria aerophila:

- 4.4 mg/kg SC for 2 days, then 8.8 mg/kg once 2 weeks later[2].

- 5 mg/kg PO once daily for 5 days, followed by 9 days of no therapy; repeat two times[2].
- 10 mg/kg PO once daily for 5 days; repeat in 9 days[6].

Rabbits

For nematodes:
- 12.5–20 mg/kg PO (for gastric nematodes) or SC (for extragastric nematodes)[8].

Amphibians

For susceptible nematodes (including lungworms):
- 10 mg/kg topically[9] or IM[10] or intracoelomic[11]; repeat in 2 weeks.
- 100 mg/L for > 72h bath (resistant nematodes)[9].
- 100–300 mg/L for 24h bath; repeat in 1–2 weeks[9].

For cutaneous nematodes in african clawed frogs:
- 12 mg/L bath for 4 days; use > 4.2 L of tank water/frog[12].

Reptiles

For susceptible nematodes (including lungworms):
- Has a narrow margin of safety (do not use in debilitated animals or concurrently with chloramphenicol)
- 5–10 mg/kg SC, ICe; repeat in 14 days[13].
- 10–20 mg/kg SC, IM, or ICe[14].
- 5 mg/kg in chelonians[15].
- 10 mg/kg in lizards[16] and snakes[17].

Fish

For intestinal nematodes:
- 1–2 mg/L for 24h bath[18].
- 10 mg/kg PO q7d for 3 treatments[18].
- 11 mg/kg IM q7d for 2 treatments[18].

For external trematodes:
- 50 mg/L for 2h bath[18].
- 4 g/kg feed q7d for 3 treatments[18].

Birds

For intestinal nematodes:
For most species:
- 5–15 ml/gallon (using 13.65% injectable) of drinking water for 1–2 days; repeat in 10 days. If birds refuse to drink, withhold water prior to treating[19].
- 10–20 mg/kg SC once[20].

- Parenteral use: 4–8 mg/kg IM or SC; repeat in 14 days. May cause vomiting, ataxia, or death. Do not use in debilitated birds[19].
- 264–396 mg/L drinking water for 3 days[21].

For pigeons, raptors, and psittacines:
- 20 mg/kg PO once in psittacines, pigeons, and raptors[20].
- 15 mg/kg (using 13.65% injectable) for gavage in Australian parakeets or desert birds that that will not drink; repeat in 10 days[19].
- 10–20 mg/kg PO q24h for 2 days in raptors[22].
- 375 mg/L drinking water as sole water source for 24 hr, repeat in 7 days for pigeons[23].
- 100–200 mg/L drinking water for 3 days for psittacines and raptors[21].

For game birds and waterfowl:
- 20–25 mg/kg SC in game birds[24].
- 20–50 mg/kg PO once for waterfowl[23,25].
- 265–525 mg/L drinking water for 1 day, repeat in 7–14 days for game birds[24,26].

For poultry and ratites:
- 30 mg/kg PO q10d for poultry[24] and ratites[27].
- 18–36 mg/kg PO in poultry[28].
- 265–525 mg/L drinking water for 1 day; repeat in 7–14 days for poultry[24,26].

For finches:
- 80 mg/L drinking water for 3 days[25].

For Capillaria infections:
- 15–30 mg/kg orally as a single bolus or through a crop tube[29].
- 2.25 mg/gallon of drinking water for 4–5 days; repeat treatment in 10–14 days[29].
- 40 mg/kg PO once in psittacines, pigeons, and raptors[20,30].

For Libyostrongylus douglassii in ratites:
- 30 mg/kg PO or IM at one month of age, then once a month for 7 treatments, then 4 times yearly[31].

Sheep and Goats

For susceptible nematodes:
- Refer to specific label direction for approved products.
- 7.5 mg/kg PO[28].

For removal of Dictyocaulus viviparus:
- 8 mg/kg PO[32].

Swine

For susceptible nematodes:
- Refer to specific label direction for approved products.
- 8 mg/kg PO in feed or water[33].
- 7.5 mg/kg PO[28].
- 10 mg/kg PO[34].

For Metastrongylus (mature and immature):
- 8 mg/kg PO in feed or water[32].

Primates

For susceptible infections:
- 5 mg/kg PO; repeat in 21 days[35].
- 10 mg/kg PO (Strongyloides, Filaroides, and Trichuris)[36].

For the treatment of Physaloptera in prosimians:
- 2.5 mg/kg PO q24h for 14 days[37].

For the treatment of oral Spiruridiasis in saki monkeys:
- 4–5 mg/kg PO q24h for 6 days[38].

REFERENCES

1. Kirk, R.W. (1989) *Current Veterinary Therapy X, Small Animal Practice,* W.B. Saunders, Philadelphia.
2. Todd, K.S., Paul, A.J., and DiPietro, J.A. (1985) Parasitic diseases. In: Davis, L.E. (ed.) *Handbook of Small Animal Therapeutics,* Churchill Livingstone, New York, 89–126.
3. Knight, D.H. (1988) Heartworm disease. In: Morgan, R.V. (ed.) *Handbook of Small Animal Practice,* Churchill Livingstone, New York, 139–148.
4. Bauer, T G. (1988) Diseases of the lower airway. In: Morgan, R.V. (ed.) *Handbook of Small Animal Practice,* Churchill Livingstone, New York, 185–193.
5. Roudebush, P. (1985) Respiratory diseases. In: Davis, L.E. (ed.) *Handbook of Small Animal Therapeutics,* Churchill Livingstone, New York, 287–332.
6. Reinemeyer, C. (1995) Parasites of the respiratory system. In: Bonagura, J. (ed.) *Kirk's Current Veterinary Therapy: XII,* W.B. Saunders, Philadelphia, 895–898.
7. Dillon, R. (1986) Feline Heartworm Disease. In: Kirk, R.W. (ed.) *Current Veterinary Therapy IX: Small Animal Practice,* W.B. Saunders, Philadelphia, 420–425.
8. Ivey, E. and Morrisey, J. (2000) Therapeutics for rabbits. *Vet. Clin. N. Am. Exotic Anim. Pract.* 3, 183–213.
9. Wright, K.M. and Whitaker, B.R. (2001b) Pharmacotherapeutics. In: Wright, K.M. and Whitaker, B.R. (eds.) *Amphibian Medicine and Captive Husbandry,* Krieger Publishing, Malabar, FL, 309–330.
10. Crawshaw, G.J. (1992) Amphibian Medicine. In: Kirk, R.W. and Bonagura, J.D. (eds.) *Kirk's Current Veterinary Therapy XI. Small Animal Practice,* W.B. Saunders, Philadelphia, 1219–1230.
11. Wright, K.M. (2001a) Trauma. In: Wright, K.M. and Whitaker, B.R. (eds.) *Amphibian Medicine and Captive Husbandry,* Krieger Publishing, Malabar, FL, 233–238.
12. Iglauer, F., Willmann, F., Hilken, G., et al. (1997) Anthelmintic treatment to eradicate cutaneous capillariasis in a colony of South African clawed frogs (*Xenopus laevis*). *Lab Anim. Sci.* 47, 477–482.
13. Klingenberg, R.J. (1996) Therapeutics. In: Mader, D.R. (ed.) *Reptile Medicine and Surgery,* W.B. Saunders, Philadelphia, 299–321.
14. Jenkins, J.R. (1991) A formulary for reptile and amphibian medicine. Proc. Fourth Annu. Avian/Exotic Anim. Med. Symp. University of California, Davis, CA, 24–27.
15. Mautino, M. and Page, C.D. (1993) Biology and medicine of turtles and tortoises. *Vet. Clin. N. Am.: Small Anim. Pract.* **23**, 1251–1270.
16. Barten, S.L. (1993) The medical care of iguanas and other common pet lizards. *Vet. Clin. N. Am. Small Anim. Pract.* **23**, 1213–1249.
17. Jacobson, E.R. (1988) Use of chemotherapeutics in reptile medicine. In: Jacobson, E.R. and Kollias, G.V. (eds.) *Exotic Animals,* Churchill Livingstone, New York, 35–48.
18. Harms, C.A. (1996) Treatments for parasitic diseases of aquarium and ornamental fish. *Semin. Avian Exotic Pet. Med.* **5**, 54–63.
19. Clubb, S.L. (1986) Therapeutics: Individual and Flock Treatment Regimens. In: Harrison, G.J. and Harrison, L.R. (eds.) *Clinical Avian Medicine and Surgery,* W.B. Saunders, Philadelphia, 327–355.
20. Marshall, R. (1993) Avian anthelmintics and antiprotozoals. *Semin. Avian Exotic Pet Med.* **2**, 22–41.
21. Coles, B.H. (2001) Prescribing for exotic birds. In: Bishop, Y. (ed.) *The Veterinary Formulary,* 5th ed. Pharmaceutical Press, London, 99–105.
22. Huckabee, J.R. (2000) Raptor therapeutics. *Vet. Clin. N. Am. Exotic Anim. Pract.* **3**, 91–116.
23. Samour, J. (2000) Pharmaceuticals commonly used in avian medicine. In: Samour, J. (ed.) *Avian Medicine,* Mosby, Philadelphia, 388–418.
24. Stadler, C. and Carpenter, J.W. (1996) Parasites of backyard game birds. *Semin. Avian Exotic Pet. Med.* **5**, 85–96.
25. Ritchie, B.W. and Harrison, G.J. (1997) Formulary. In: Ritchie, B.W. and Harrison, G.J. (eds.) *Avian Medicine: Principles and Application,* Abridged Edition. Wingers, Lake Worth, FL, 227–253.
26. Wigle, W.L. (2000) Respiratory diseases of gallinaceous birds. *Vet. Clin. N. Am: Exotic Anim. Pract.* **3**, 403–421.
27. Tully, T.N. (1996) Therapeutics. In: Tully, T.N. and Shane, S.M. (eds.) *Ratite Management, Medicine, and Surgery,* Krieger, Malabar, FL, 155–163.
28. Brander, C.G., Pugh, D.M., and Bywater, R.J. (1982) *Veterinary Applied Pharmacology and Therapeutics,* 4th ed. London: Ballière Tindall.
29. Flammer, K. (1986) Oropharyngeal Diseases in Caged Birds. In: Kirk, R.W. (ed.) *Current Veterinary Therapy XI: Small Animal Practice,* W.B. Saunders, Philadelphia, 699–702.
30. Harlin, R.W. (1994) Pigeons. *Vet. Clin. N. Am. Small Anim. Pract.* **24**, 157–173.
31. Jenson, J. (1998) Current ratite therapy. *Vet. Clinics N. Am. Food Anim. Pract.* **16**, 3.
32. Bennet, D.G. (1986) Parasites of the respiratory system. In: Howard, J.L. (ed.) *Current Veterinary Therapy: Food Animal Practice 2,* W.B. Saunders, Philadelphia, 684–687.
33. Howard, J.L. (1986) *Current Veterinary Therapy 2, Food Animals Practice,* W.B. Saunders, Philadelphia.
34. Boldrick, L. (1993) *Veterinary Care of Pot-Bellied Pet Pigs,* All Publishing, Orange, CA.
35. Holmes, D.D. (1984) *Clinical Laboratory Animal Medicine,* Iowa State University Press, Ames, IA.
36. Wolff, P.L. (1993) Parasites of the new world primates. In: Fowler, M.E. (ed.) *Zoo and Wild Animal Medicine: Current Therapy 3,* W.B. Saunders, Philadelphia, 378–389.

37. Junge, R.E. (1999) Diseases of prosimians. In: Fowler, M.E. and Miller, R.E. (eds.) *Zoo and Wild Animal Medicine: Current Therapy 4,* W.B. Saunders, Philadelphia, 365–368.
38. Montali, R.J. and Bush, M. (1999) Diseases of callitrichidae. In: Fowler, M.E. (ed.) *Zoo and Wild Animal Medicine: Current Therapy 4,* W.B. Saunders, Philadelphia, 369–376.

Lufenuron

Activity: Flea control.

　MOA: Inhibits chitin synthesis. Flea eggs are prevented from developing into adults.

Dogs

- Program flavor tabs and tablets are recommended at 10 mg/kg PO once monthly to pups 6 weeks of age and older.
- Program (lufenuron) flavor tabs and tablets: for dogs up to 10 lbs give 1 45-mg tablet; 11–20 lbs give 1 90-mg tablet; 21–45 lbs give 1 204.9-mg tablet, 46–90 lbs give 1 409.8-mg tablet; dogs over 90 lbs should receive the appropriate combination of tablets (Program® Flavor Tabs and Tablets—Novartis).
- Sentinel flavor tabs are recommended once monthly, given orally, at the minimum dosage rate of 0.23 mg of milbemycin oxime per pound (0.5 mg/kg) and 4.55 mg of lufenuron per pound (10 mg/kg) to pups 4 weeks of age or greater and 2 pounds of body weight or greater.
- Milbemycin/Lufenuron tablets: 2–10 lbs give 1 2.3 mg/46.0-mg tablet; 11–25 lbs give 1 5.75 mg/115-mg tablet; 26–50 lbs give 1 11.5 mg/230-mg tablet; 51–100 lbs give 1 23.0 mg/460-mg tablet; provide the appropriate combination of tablets to dogs over 100 pounds (Package Insert; Sentinel®—Novartis).
- See description of milbemycin oxime.

Cats

- 30 mg/kg PO once monthly or 10 mg/kg SC once every 6 months for kittens 6 weeks of age and older. (Package Insert; Program®—Novartis).
- Program (lufenuron) oral tablets: for cats up to 6 lbs give 1 90-mg tablet; 7–15 lbs give 1 204.9-mg tablet; for cats over 15 lbs provide the appropriate combination of tablets (Program® Flavor Tab—Novartis).
- Program (lufenuron) oral suspension (in tube packs): for cats up to 10 lbs give 135 mg; 11–20 lbs give 270 mg, for cats over 20 lbs provide the appropriate combination of tube packs (Program® Suspension—Novartis).
- Program (lufenuron) 6-month injectable: 100 mg/ml in 10 syringe packages. For cats up to 8.8 lbs give 0.4 ml (40 mg) prefilled syringe; 8.9–17.6 lbs give 0.8 ml (80 mg) prefilled syringe (Program® 6-Month Injectable—Novartis).

Rabbits

- 30 mg/kg PO once monthly[1].

Ferrets

- 30–45 mg/kg PO once monthly[2].

REFERENCES

1. Ivey, E. and Morrisey, J. (2000) Therapeutics in rabbits. *Vet Clin. N. Am: Exotic Anim. Pract* **3,** 183–213.
2. Morrisey, J.K. (1998) Ectoparasites of ferrets and rodents. *Proc. N. Am: Vet. Conf.* 844–845.

Malachite Green

Activity: For use in freshwater fish and amphibians for protozoan ectoparasites. Toxic to some fish species and fry, also mutagenic and teratogenic. Increased toxicity at higher temperatures and lower pH. Toxic to plants.

　MOA: Malachite green is a protein-binding dye which permeates the cellular membrane resulting in cell damage and death of susceptible parasites.

Amphibians

For protozoa:

- 0.15 mg/L for 1 hr bath every 24 hr to effect[1].

Fish

For protozoal ectoparasites in freshwater fish:

- Prepare stock solution 3.7 mg/ml (1.4 g malachite green in 380 ml water).
- 100 mg/L topical to skin lesions[2].
- 0.1 mg/L tank water q3d for 3 treatments[2].
- 0–60 mg/L for 10–30 sec. bath[2].
- 1 mg/L for 30–60 min. bath; use 2 mg/L if pH is high[2].
- See formalin for combination.

REFERENCES

1. Raphael, B.L. (1993) Amphibians. *Vet. Clin. N. Am: Small. Anim. Pract.* **23,** 1271–1286.
2. Noga, E.J. (2000) *Fish Disease: Diagnosis and Treatment,* Iowa State University Press, Ames, IA.

Melarsomine

Activity: Heartworm treatment of stabilized class I, II, and III heartworm disease caused by stage L_5 larvae to mature adult infections by *Dirofilaria immitis*.

    MOA: Exact mechanism is not known.

Dogs

- Consult manufacturers' worksheets to determine the classification and recommended needle size.
- Class I: 2.5 mg/kg deep IM as directed (lumbar epaxial muscles: L3–L5) twice 24 hours apart and rest. Use alternating sides with each administration. The regimen may be repeated in 4 months (Package Insert; Immiticide®—Merial).
- Class II: 2.5 mg/kg deep IM as directed (lumbar epaxial muscles: L3–L5) twice 24 hours apart and rest; give symptomatic treatment as required. Use alternating sides with each administration. The regimen may be repeated in 4 months(Package Insert; Immiticide®—Merial).
- Class III: 2.5 mg/kg deep IM as directed (lumbar epaxial muscles: L3–L5). Strict rest and give all necessary systemic treatment. One month later, give 2.5 mg/kg deep IM as directed (lumbar epaxial muscles: L3–L5) twice 24 hours apart (Package Insert; Immiticide®—Merial).

Ferrets

- 2.5 mg/kg IM once; repeat in 30 days with two treatments 24 hours apart. After treatment use prednisone at 1 mg/kg q24h for 4 months[1].

REFERENCE

1. Brown, S.A. (1999) Ferret drug dosages. In: Antinoff, N.L., Bauck, T.H. and Boyer, N., et al. (eds.) *Exotic Animal Formulary*, 2nd ed. American Hospital Association, Lakewood, CO, 43–61.

Metronidazole

Activity: Parasiticidal: *Giardia, Trichomonas, Balantidium coli,* and *Entamoeba histolytica*.

    MOA: Poorly understood. Trichomonacidal and amebicidal; it acts as a direct amebicide.

Dogs

For treatment of Giardia:
- 25 mg/kg PO q12h for 8 days[1].
- 44 mg/kg PO initially, then 22 mg/kg PO q8h for 5 days[2].
- 25–65 mg/kg PO once daily for 5 days[3].
- 30–60 mg/kg PO once daily for 5–7 days (also for trichomoniasis)[4].
- 25 mg/kg PO q12h for 8 days for *Entamoeba histolytica* or *Pentatrichomonas hominis*[1].

Cats

For treatment of Giardia:
- 25 mg/kg PO q12h daily for 8 days[1].
- 8–10 mg/kg PO q12h daily for 10 days (also for trichomoniasis)[4].

For other protozoal infections: Entamoeba histolytica or Pentatrichomonas hominis:
- 25 mg/kg PO q12h for 8 days[1].

Mice

- 3.5 mg/ml of drinking water for 5 days[5].
- 2.5 mg/ml of drinking water for 5 days[5].

Rats

- 20–60 mg/kg PO q8–12h[5].
- 2.5 mg/ml in water for 5 days[5].

Gerbils and Hamsters

- 7.5 mg/70–90 grams of body weight PO q8h[5].

Ferrets

For susceptible infections:
- 10–30 mg/kg PO once to twice daily[6].
- 15–20 mg/kg PO q12h for 2 weeks for gastrointestinal protozoa[7].

Chinchillas

- 50–60 mg/kg PO twice daily for 5 days as an parasiticide for *Giardia*. Use with caution[8].

Guinea Pigs

- 10–40 mg/kg PO once daily[5].
- 25 mg/kg PO q12h[9].

Amphibians

- 10 mg/kg PO q24h for 5–10 days for protozoa[10,11].
- 50 mg/kg PO q24h for 3–5 days for confirmed cases of amoebiasis and flagellate overload[11].

- 100 mg/kg PO q3d for protozoa[12].
- 100–150 mg/kg PO; repeat in 2–3 weeks or as needed for protozoa such as *Entamoeba, Hexamita, Opalina*[13].
- 500 mg/100 g of feed for 3–4 treatments for ciliates[13,14].

For aquatic amphibians:
- 50 mg/L of water for 24h for protozoa[11,15].

Reptiles

For amoebae and flagellates in most species:
- 100–275 mg/kg PO; repeat in 1–2 weeks.

For Drymarchon spp., Lampropeltis pyromelana, and Lampropeltis zonata:
- 40 mg/kg PO once; repeat in 2 weeks[16].

Most species:
- 25–40 mg/kg PO on days 1 and 3 or q24h for up to 7 days[17].
- 100 mg/kg PO q3d for 14–28 days[18].

Most species (except uracoan rattlers, milk snakes, tricolor king snakes, and indigo snakes):
- 100 mg/kg PO; repeat in 14 days[19,20,21,22].

Uracoan rattlers, milk snakes, tricolor king snakes, and indigo snakes:
- 40 mg/kg PO; repeat in 14 days[21].

Corn snakes:
- 50 mg/kg PO q48h[23].

Chameleons:
- 40–60 mg/kg PO q7–14d for 2–3 treatments[24].
- 50 mg/kg PO q24h for 2–5d when accompanied by increased gastrointestinal symptoms[25].

Chelonians:
- 50 mg/kg PO q24h for 3–5 days or 100 mg/kg PO q14–21d[26].

Fish
- 6.6 mg/L of water q24h for 3 days or 25 mg/L of water q48h for 3 treatments for *Spironucleus* and other internal and external flagellates[27].
- 25 mg/kg q24h in feed for 5–10 days or 100 mg/kg q24h for 3 days[27].
- 6.25–18 mg/g of feed for 5 days[28].
- 50 mg/kg PO q24h for 5 days[29].

Birds

Most species:
- 20–35 mg/kg IM q24h for 2 days[30].
- 25–50 mg/kg PO q12–24h for 5–10 days[31].

Psittacines:
- 30 mg/kg PO q12h for 10 days[32].
- 10–20 mg/kg IM q24h for 2 days[31].
- 10–30 mg/kg PO or IM q12h for 10 days[33,34].

Psittacine neonates:
- 25 mg/kg PO q12h for 2–10 days[35].

Canaries:
- 100 mg/L of drinking water or 100 mg/kg of soft feed[36].

Budgerigars:
- 40 mg/kg PO q24h for 7 days[37].

Finches:
- 30 mg/kg once by gavage or 40 mg/L of water for treatment of *Cochlosoma*[38].

Gouldian finches:
- 30 mg/kg PO q12h for 6 days for *Trichomonas*[39].

Pigeons:
- 10–20 mg/kg IM q24h for 2 days[40].
- 50 mg/kg PO q12h for 5 days[41].
- 4 g/gal of drinking water[42].

Poultry:
- 110 mg/kg PO q12h for *Histomonas*[43].
- 30 mg/kg PO q12h[44].

Raptors:
- 30 mg/kg PO q12h for 5–7 days[45].

Raptors, for trichomonas:
- 50 mg/kg PO q24h for 5 days[46] or 100 mg/kg PO q24h for 3 days[47].

Game birds:
- 1.5 g/gal of drinking water for 5–15 days[48].
- 400 mg/L of drinking water for 5–15 days for protozoal sinusitis[49].

Ratites:
- 20–25 mg/kg PO q12h[50].
- 1250 mg/L of drinking water for 7–10 days[51].

Rheas:
- 40 mg/kg PO q24h [52].

Miniature pigs

- 66 mg/kg PO q24h[53].

Primates

- 17.5–25 mg/kg PO q12h for 10 days for enteric flagellates and amoebas[54].
- 30–50 mg/kg PO q12h for 5–10 days for *Balantidium coli*[54,55].

REFERENCES

1. Lappin, M. (2000) Protozoal and miscellaneous infections. In: Ettinger, S. and Feldman, E. (eds.) *Textbook of Veterinary Medicine: Diseases of the Dog and Cat*, W.B. Saunders Co., Philadelphia, 408–417.
2. Todd, K.S., Paul, A.J., and DiPietro, J.A. (1985) Parasitic disease. In: Davis, L.E. (ed.) *Handbook of Small Animal Therapeutics*, Churchill Livingstone, New York, 89–126.
3. Longhofer, S.L. (1988) Chemotherapy of rickettsial, protozoal, and chlamydial diseases. *Vet Clin. N. Am: Small Anim. Pract.* **18**, 1183–1196.
4. Chiapella, A.M. (1988) Diseases of the small intestine. In: Morgan, R.V. (ed.) *Handbook of Small Animal Practice*, Churchill Livingstone, New York, 395–420.
5. Adamcak, A. and Otten, B. (2000) Rodent therapeutics In: *Vet Clin. N. Am. Exotic Anim. Pract.* **3**, 221–240.
6. Williams, B. (2000) Therapeutics in ferrets. *Vet Clin. N. Am. Exotic Anim. Pract.* **3**, 131–153.
7. Brown, S.A. (1993) Ferrets. In: Jerkins, J.R. and Brown, S.A. (eds.) *A Practitioner's Guide to Rabbits and Ferrets*, American Hospital Association, Lakewood, CO, 43–111.
8. Harkness, J.E. (1993) *A practitioner's guide to domestic rodents*, American Hospital Association, Lakewood, CO.
9. Morrisey, J.K. and Carpenter, J.W. (2004) Formulary. In: Quesenberry, K.E. and Carpenter, J.W. (eds.) *Ferrets, Rabbits, and Rodents: Clinical Medicine and Surgery*, 2nd ed. W.B. Saunders, St. Louis, MO, 436–444.
10. Whitaker, B.R. (1997) Developing an effective quarantine program for amphibians. *Proc. N. Am. Vet. Conf.* 764–765.
11. Wright, K.M. (1997b) Treating parasites in amphibians. *Proc. N. Am. Vet. Conf.* 772.
12. G.J. (1998) Amphibian emergency and critical care. *Vet. Clin. N. Am: Exotic Anim. Pract.* **1**, 207–231.
13. Raphael, B.L. (1993) Amphibians. *Vet. Clin. N. Am: Small Anim. Pract.* **23**, 1271–1286.
14. Crawshaw, G.J. (1989) Medical care of amphibians. *Proc. Am. Assoc. Zoo. Vet.* 155–165.
15. Stein, G. (1996) Reptile and amphibian formulary. In: Mader, D.R. (ed.) *Reptile Medicine and Surgery*, W.B. Saunders, Philadelphia, 465–472.
16. Gauvin, J. (1993) Drug therapy in reptiles. *Seminar in Avian and Exotic Medicine.* **2**, 48–59.
17. Klingenberg, R.J. (1996) Parasitology for the practitioner. *Proc. North Am: Vet. Conf.* 826–827.
18. Bauck, L., Boyer, T.H., Brown, S.A., et al. (1995) *Exotic Animal Formulary*, American Animal Hospital Association, Lakewood, CO. 19–36.
19. Barten, S.L. (1993) The medical care of iguanas and other common pet lizards. *Vet. Clin. N. Am: Small Anim. Pract.* **23**, 1213–1249.
20. Jacobson, E.R. (1993a) Antimicrobial drug use in reptiles. In: Prescott, J.F. Baggot, J.D. (eds.) *Antimicrobial Therapy in Veterinary Medicine*, Iowa State University Press, Ames, IA.
21. Jacobson, E.R. (1993b) Snakes. *Vet. Clin. N. Am. Small Anim. Pract.* **23**, 1179–1212.
22. Jacobson, E.R. (1995) Use of antimicrobial therapy in reptiles. In: *Antimicrobial Therapy in Caged Birds and Exotic Pets*, Veterinary Learning Systems, Trenton, NJ, 28–37.
23. Bodri, M.S., Rambo, T.M., Wagner, R.A., et al. (2001) Pharmacokinetics of metronidazole administered as a single oral bolus to corn snakes, *Elaphe guttata*. *Proc. Assoc. Rept. Amph. Vet.* 121–122.
24. Stahl, S.J. (1998) Common medical problems of Old World chameleons. *Proc. N. Am. Vet. Conf.* 814–817.
25. Klingenberg, R.J. (2000) Diagnosing parasites of Old World chameleons. *Exotic DVM* **1**, 17–21.
26. Wright, K.M. (1997a) Common medical problems of tortoises. *Proc. N. Am. Vet. Conf.* 769–771.
27. Noga, E.J. (2000) *Fish Diseases: Diagnosis and Treatment*, Iowa State University Press, Ames, IA.
28. Whitaker, B.R. (1999) Preventative medicine programs for fish. In: Fowler, M.E. and Miller, R.E. (eds.) *Zoo and Wild Animal Medicine: Current Therapy 4*, WB Saunders, Philadelphia, 163–181.
29. Harms, C.A. (1996) Treatment for parasitic diseases of aquarium and ornamental fish. *Semin. Avian Exotic Pet Med.* **5**, 54–63.
30. Ritchie, B.W. (1990) Avian therapeutics. *Proc Annu. Conf. Assoc. Avian Vet.* 415–431.
31. Hoppes, S. (1998) Common parasites in companion birds. *Proc. Annu. Conf. Assoc. Avian Vet.* 213–216.
32. Murphy, J. (1992) Psittacine trichomoniasis. *Proc. Annu. Conf. Assoc. Avian Vet.* 165–170.
33. Samour, J. (2000) Pharmaceutics commonly used in avian medicine. In: Samour, J. (ed.) *Avian Medicine*, Mosby, Philadelphia, 388–418.
34. Tully, T.N. (2000) Psittacine therapeutics. *Vet. Clin. N. Am: Exotic Anim. Pract.* **3**, 59–90.
35. Joyner, K.L. (1991) Pediatric therapeutics. *Proc. Annu. Conf. Assoc. Avian Vet.* 188–199.
36. Dorrestein, G.M. (1995) Infectious diseases and their therapy in Passeriformes. In: *Antimicrobial therapy in caged birds and exotic pets*, Veterinary Learning Systems Co., Trenton, NJ, 11–27.
37. Ramsay, E.C., Drew, M.L., and Johnson, B. (1990) Trichomoniasis in a flock of budgerigars. *Proc. Annu. Conf. Assoc. Avian Vet.* 309–311.
38. Filippich, L.J. and O'Donoghue, P.J. (1997) Cochlosoma infections in finches. *Aust. Vet. J.* **75**, 561–563.
39. Bauck, L. and Brash, M. (1999) Survey of diseases of Lady Gouldian finch. *Proc. Annu. Conf. Assoc. Avian Vet.* 204–212.
40. Marshall, R. (1993) Avian anthelmintics and antiprotozoals. *Semin. Avian Exotic Pet Med.* **2**, 33–41.
41. Rupiper, D.J. and Ehrenberg, M. (1994) Introduction to pigeon practice. *Proc. Annu. Conf. Assoc. Avian Vet.* 203–211.
42. Harlin, R.W. (1994) Pigeons. *Vet. Clin. N. Am: Small Anim. Pract.* **24**, 157–173.
43. Harlin, R.W. (1995) Backyard poultry. *Proc. Mid-Atlantic States Assoc. Avian Vet Conf.* 65–68.
44. Cybulski, W., Larsson, P., Tjälve, H., et al. (1996) Disposition of metronidazole in hens (*Gallus gallus*) and quails (*Coturnix coturnix japonica*): pharmacokinetics and whole-body autoradiography. *J. Vet. Pharmacol. Therap.* **19**, 352–358.
45. Redig, P.T. (1992) Health management of raptors trained for falconry. *Proc. Annu. Conf. Assoc. Avian Vet.* 258–264.

46. Huckabee, J.R. (2000) Raptor therapeutics. *Vet. Clin. N. Am: Exotic Anim. Pract.* **3,** 91–116.

47. Samour, J.H. and Naldo, J. (2001) Serratospiculiasis in captive falcons in the Middle East: a review. *J. Avian Med. Surg.* **15,** 2–9.

48. Stadler, C. and Carpenter, J.W. (1996) Parasites of backyard game birds. *Semin. Avian Exotic Pet Med.* **5,** 85–96.

49. St. Leger, J., Read, D.H., and Shivaprasad, H.L. (1998) Passerine protozoal sinusitis: an infection you should know about. *Proc. Annu. Assoc. Avian Vet.* 157–160.

50. Tully, T.N. and Shane, S.M. (1996) Ratite formulary. In: Tully, T.N. and Shane, S.M. (eds.) *Ratite Management, Medicine, and Surgery.* Krieger Publishing, Malabar, FL, 158–163.

51. Moore, D.M. and Rice, R.L. (1998) Exotic animal formulary In: Holt, K.M., Boothe, D.M., and Gaumnitz, J. et al. (eds.) *Veterinary values* 5th ed. Veterinary Medicine Publishing Group. Lenexa, KS, 159–249.

52. Randolf, K. (1995) Equine encephalitis virus in ratites. *Proc. Annu. Conf. Assoc. Avian Vet.* 249–252.

53. Swindle, M.M. (1993) Minipigs as pets. *Proc. North Am. Vet. Conf.* 648–649.

54. Wolf, P.L. (1993) Parasites of the new world primates. In: Fowler M.E. (ed.) *Zoo and Wild Animal Medicine: Current Therapy 3,* WB Saunders Co, Philadelphia, 378–389.

55. Marks, S.K. (1994) Disease review: balantidiasis. *A report of the American Association of Zoo Veterinarians Infectious Disease Committee,* Philadelphia.

Milbemycin Oxime

Activity: Heartworm prophylaxis, Microfilaricide, Demodicosis treatment. In dogs Sentinel is indicated for use in the prevention of heartworm disease caused by *Dirofilaria immitis,* control of the adult hookworm *Ancylostoma caninum,* and removal and control of the adult roundworms *Toxocara canis* and *Toxascaris leonina* and the adult whipworm *Trichuris vulpis.* Sentinel also contains lufenuron, which prevents the development of flea eggs, but does not kill adult fleas. (Package Insert; Sentinel®—Novartis). In cats, Interceptor is indicated for use in the prevention of heartworm disease caused by *Dirofilaria immitis* and removal of the adult hookworm *Ancylostoma tubaeforme* and the adult roundworm *Toxocara cati* (Package Insert; Interceptor®—Novartis).

See the description for lufenuron.

MOA: Gamma-aminobutyric acid (GABA) inhibitor of invertebrates.

Dogs

- 0.5–2 mg/kg PO once daily for generalized demodicosis[1].
- 1 mg/kg PO daily for one month past the point of negative skin scrapings for generalized demodicosis[2].
- 2 mg/kg PO every 7 days for 3 doses or 0.75 mg/kg once daily for 30 days for treatment of sarcoptic mange[3].

- 2 mg/kg PO every 7 days for 3 doses for treatment of cheyletiellosis[3].
- Interceptor flavor tabs are recommended once monthly, given orally, at the minimum dosage rate of 0.23 mg of milbemycin oxime per pound of body weight to pups 4 weeks of age or greater and 2 pounds of body weight or greater.
- Milbemycin tablets: 2–10 lbs give one 2.3-mg tablet, 11–25 lbs give one 5.75-mg tablet, 26–50 lbs give one 11.5-mg tablet, 51–100 lbs give one 23-mg tablet; provide the appropriate combination of tablets to dogs over 100 pounds (Package Insert; Interceptor®—Novartis).
- Sentinel flavor tabs are recommended once monthly, given orally, at the minimum dosage rate of 0.23 mg of milbemycin oxime per pound (0.5 mg/kg) and 4.55 mg of lufenuron per pound (10 mg/kg) to pups 4 weeks of age or greater and 2 pounds of body weight or greater. For dogs 2–10 lbs give one 2.3-mg/46-mg tablet, 11–25 lbs give one 5.75 mg/115-mg tablet, 26–50 lbs give one 11.5 mg/230-mg tablet, 51–100 lbs give one 23 mg/460-mg tablet; provide the appropriate combination of tablets to dogs over 100 pounds (Package Insert; Sentinel®—Novartis).

Cats

- Interceptor flavor tabs are recommended once monthly, given orally, at the minimum dosage rate of 0.9 mg of milbemycin oxime per pound of body weight to kittens 6 weeks of age or greater and 1.5 pounds of body weight or greater.
- 1.5–6 lbs give one 5.75-mg tablet, 6.1–12 lbs give one 11.5-mg tablet, 12.1–25 lbs give one 23-mg tablet; provide the appropriate combination of tablets to cats over 25 pounds (Package Insert; Interceptor®—Novartis).

Ferrets

- Interceptor at 1.15–2.33 mg/kg PO q30d for heartworm prevention[4].

Birds

Turkeys:
- Interceptor at 0.2 mg/kg PO q28d for nematodes[5].

Galliformes:
- Interceptor at 2 mg/kg PO; repeat in 28 days for nematodes[6].

REFERENCES

1. DeManuelle, T. (2000) Current treatment of canine demodicosis. *The North American Veterinary Conference.* Orlando, FL.
2. Mundell, A. (1994) Demodicosis. In: Birchard, S. and Sherding, R. (eds.) *Saunders Manual of Small Animal Practice,* W.B. Saunders, Philadelphia, 290–294.
3. White, S. (2000) Veterinary Dermatology: New Treatments, "New" Diseases. *The North American Veterinary Conference.* Orlando, FL.
4. Smith, D.A. and Burgmann, P.M. (1997) In: Hillyer, E.V. and Quesenberry, K.E. (eds.) *Ferrets, Rabbits, and Rodents: Clinical Medicine and Surgery,* W.B. Saunders, Philadelphia, 394–395.
5. Carpenter, N.A. (2000) Anseriform and galliform therapeutics. *Vet. Clin. N. Am: Exotic Anim. Pract.* **3,** 1–17.
6. Hedberg, G.E. and Bennett, R.A. (1994) Preliminary studies on the use of milbemycin oxime in galliforms. *Proc. Annu. Conf. Assoc. Avian Vet.* 261–264.

Morantel Tartrate

Activity: In cattle it is labeled for the removal of the adult forms of *Haemonchus* spp., *Ostertagia* spp, *Trichostrongylus* spp., *Nematodirus* spp., *Cooperia* spp., and *Oesophagostomum radiatum.*

MOA: Acts as a depolarizing neuromuscular blocking agent, similar to acetylcholine, which paralyzes susceptible parasites. In *Haemonchus* species it also acts as an inhibitor of fumarate reductase.

Sheep

* 10 mg/kg PO[1].

REFERENCE

1. Roberson, E.L. (1988) Antimicrobial agents. In: Booth, N.H. and McDonald, L.E. (eds.) *Veterinary Pharmacology and Therapeutics,* Iowa State University Press, Ames, IA, 882–927.

Moxidectin

Proheart®6 is currently off the market.

Activity: In dogs moxidectin (Proheart®6) is labeled for heartworm prevention and hookworm treatment.

MOA: Affects chloride ion channels and enhances the release of gamma-aminobutyric acid (GABA) at presynaptic neurons.

Dogs

* 3 mcg/kg PO once monthly for heartworm prevention. (Package Insert; Proheart®6—Fort Dodge).
* 0.05 ml/kg (0.17 mg/kg) of the constituted product SC (left or right side of dorsum of the neck cranial to the scapula) every 6 months for heartworm prevention. May not be effective for treatment of hookworms for the entire 6 months (Package Insert; Proheart®6—Fort Dodge).
* 0.2–0.4 mg/kg PO once daily for generalized demodicosis. Clinical cure averages 75 days and parasitic cure averages 112 days[1].

Rabbits

* 0.2 mg/kg PO; repeat in 10 days for Psoroptic mange[2].

Amphibians

* 200 ug/kg SC every 4 months for nematodes[3].

Birds

Ramphastids:

* 0.2 mg/kg IM once[4].

Raptors and red-crested cardinals:

* 0.2 mg/kg PO[5].

REFERENCES

1. Merchant, S. (2000) New therapies in veterinary dermatology. *American Animal Hospital Association 67th Annual Meeting,* Toronto.
2. Wagner, R. and Wendlberger, U. (2000) Field efficacy of moxidectin in dogs and rabbits naturally infested with *Sarcoptes* spp., *Demodex* spp., and *Psoroptes* spp. Mites. *Vet. Parasitol.* **93,** 149–158.
3. Shilton, C.M., Smith, D.A., Crawshaw, G.J., et al. (2001) Corneal lipid deposition in Cuban tree frogs (*Osteopilus septentrionalis*) and its relationship to serum lipids: an experimental study. *J. Zoo Wildl. Med.* **32,** 305–319.
4. Cubas, Z.S. (2001) Medicine: family Rhamphastidae (toucans). In: Fowler, M.E. and Cubas, Z.S. (eds.) *Biology, Medicine, and Surgery of South American Wild Animals,* Iowa State University Press, Ames, IA, 188–199.
5. Samour, J.H. and Naldo, J. (2001) Serratospiculiasis in captive falcons in the Middle East: a review. *J. Avian Med. Surg.* **15,** 2–9.

Oxfendazole

Activity: In horses it is labeled for the removal of large roundworms (*Parascaris equorum*), large strongyles (*Strongylus edentatus, S. equinus,* and *S. vulgaris*), small strongyles, and pinworms (*Oxyuris equi*).

MOA: Interferes with polymerization of microtubules; causes death by starvation.

Amphibians

* 5 mg/kg PO[1].

Reptiles

Most species:
• 68 mg/kg; repeat in 14–28 days as needed[2].

Birds

Most species (includes finches):
• 10–40 mg/kg PO once[3,4].

Raptors:
• 20 mg/kg PO once[5].

Ramphastids:
• 15–25 mg/kg PO; repeat in 15 days if needed[6].

Sheep

• 5 mg/kg PO[7,8].

Goats

• 7.5 mg/kg PO[7].

Swine

• 3–4.5 mg/kg PO[7].

REFERENCES

1. Williams, D.L. (1991) Amphibians. In: Beyon, P.H. and Cooper, J.E. (eds.) *Manual of Exotic Pets,* British Small Animal Veterinary Association, Gloucestershire, England, 261–271.
2. Divers, S.J. (1999) Clinical evaluation of reptiles. *Vet. Clin. N. Am. Exotic Anim. Pract.* **2,** 291–331.
3. Marshall, R. (1993) Avian anthelmintics and antiprotozoals. *Semin. Avian Exotic Pet. Med.* **2** 33–41.
4. Steinhort, L.A. Diagnosis and treatment of common diseases of finches. In: Bonagura, J.D. (ed.) *Kirk's Current Veterinary Therapy XIII,* W.B. Saunders, Philadelphia, 119–1123.
5. Heidenreich, M. (1997) *Birds of Prey, Medicine and Management,* Blackwell Science, Malden, MA.
6. Cubas, Z.S. (2001) Medicine: family Rhamphastidae (toucans). In: Fowler, M.E. and Cubas, Z.S. (eds.) *Biology, Medicine, and Surgery of South American Wild Animals,* Iowa State University Press, Ames, IA, 188–199.
7. Roberson, E.L. (1988) Antimicrobial agents. In: Booth, N.H. and McDonald, L.E. (eds.) *Veterinary Pharmacology and Therapeutics,* Iowa State University Press, Ames, IA, 882–927.
8. Brander, C.G., Pugh, D.M., and Bywater, R.J. (1982) *Veterinary Applied Pharmacology and Therapeutics,* 4th ed. Balliére Tindall, London.

Oxibendazole

Activity: In horses it is labeled for the removal of large roundworms (*Parascaris equorum*), large strongyles (*Strongylus edentatus, S. equinus,* and *S. vulgaris*), small strongyles, threadworms, and pinworms (*Oxyuris equi*).

MOA: Interferes with polymerization of microtubules; causes death by starvation.

Sheep

• 10–20 mg/kg PO[1].

Swine

• 15 mg/kg PO[2].

References

1. Brander, C.G., Pugh, D.M., and Bywater, R.J. (1982) *Veterinary Applied Pharmacology and Therapeutics,* 4th ed. Balliére Tindall, London.
2. Roberson, E.L. (1988) Antimicrobial agents. In: Booth, N.H. and McDonald, L.E. (eds.) *Veterinary Pharmacology and Therapeutics,* Iowa State University Press, Ames, IA, 882–927.

Piperazine

Activity: Labeled for the treatment of ascarids in dogs, cats, horses, poultry, and swine.

MOA: Believed to block acetylcholine at the neuromuscular junctions, thus paralyzing the ascarids.

Dogs and Cats

• 45–65 mg of base/kg PO. 150 mg maximum for cats and puppies less than 2.5 kg[1,2].
• 110 mg/kg PO; repeat in 21 days[3].
• 20–30 mg/kg PO once[4].

Rodents

Citrate formulation:
• 2–5 mg/ml of drinking water for 7 days, then discontinued for 7 days, followed by another 7 days PO for the treatment of pinworms[5].

Mice and Rats

• Adipate formulation: 4–7 mg/ml of drinking water for 3–10 days[6].
• Citrate formulation: 4–5 mg/ml of drinking water for 7 days, then discontinued for 7 days, followed by another 7 days[6].
• Citrate formulation: 3 grams/L of drinking water for 2 weeks for the treatment of pinworms[7].
• Citrate formulation: 2–5 mg/ml of drinking water for 7 days, then discontinued for 7 days, followed by another 7 days for the treatment of pinworms and tapeworms[8].

Rats

• Adipate formulation: 200 mg/kg PO q24h for 7 days, then discontinued for 7 days, followed by another

7 days for the treatment of pinworms; or 0.5 mg/ml of drinking water for 21 days for the treatment of pinworms[5].

Gerbils

- Adipate formulation: 200–600 mg/kg PO q24h for 7 days, then discontinued for 7 days, followed by another 7 days[5].
- Citrate formulation: 3 grams/L of drinking water for 2 weeks for the treatment of pinworms[7].
- Citrate formulation: 2–5 mg/ml of drinking water for 7 days, then discontinued for 7 days, followed by another 7 days for the treatment of pinworms and tapeworms[8].

Hamsters

- Adipate formulation: 3–5 mg/ml of drinking water for 7 days, then discontinued for 7 days, followed by another 7 days[6].
- Citrate formulation: 10 mg/ml of drinking water for 7 days, then discontinued for 7 days, followed by another 7 days[6].
- Citrate formulation: 3 grams/L of drinking water for 2 weeks for the treatment of pinworms[7].
- Citrate formulation: 2–5 mg/ml of drinking water for 7 days, then discontinued for 7 days, followed by another 7 days for the treatment of pinworms and tapeworms[8].

Rabbits

- Adipate formulation: 500 mg/kg PO for 2 days[9].
- Adipate formulation: For adult rabbits 200–500 mg/kg PO q24h for 2 days; for young rabbits 750 mg/kg PO q24h for 2 days for the treatment of pinworms[10].
- Citrate formulation: 200 mg/kg PO; repeat in 14–21 days[11,12].
- Citrate formulation: 3 grams/L of drinking water for 2 weeks for the treatment of pinworms[7].
- Citrate formulation: 100 mg/kg PO q24h for 2 days for the treatment of pinworms[10].

Ferrets

- 50–100 mg/kg PO for 14 days[13].

Chinchillas

- Adipate formulation: 500 mg/kg PO q24h[6].
- Citrate formulation: 100 mg/kg PO q24h for 2 days[6].
- Citrate formulation: 2–5 mg/ml of drinking water for 7 days, then discontinued for 7 days, followed by

another 7 days for the treatment of pinworms and tapeworms[8].

Guinea Pigs

- Adipate formulation: 4–7 mg/ml of drinking water for 3–10 days[6].
- Citrate formulation: 10 mg ml of drinking water for 7 days, then discontinued for 7 days, followed by another 7 days[6].
- Citrate formulation: 2–5 mg/ml of drinking water for 7 days, then discontinued for 7 days, followed by another 7 days for the treatment of pinworms and tapeworms[8].

Amphibians

- 50 mg/kg PO; repeat in 2 weeks[14].

Reptiles

Most species:
- 40–60 mg/kg PO; repeat in 14 days[15].

Crocodilians:
- 50 mg/kg PO; repeat in 14 days[14].

Fish

- 10 mg/kg q24h for 3 days for nonencysted gastrointestinal nematodes[16].

Birds

Pigeons:
- 35 mg/kg PO q24h for 2 days for ascarids or 79 mg/L of water for 2 days for ascarids[17].
- 250 mg/kg PO once[18,19].
- 1000 mg/L of drinking water for 3 days[18,19].
- 1000–2000 mg/L of drinking water for 1–2 days[20,21].

Chickens:
- 50–100 mg/kg PO once[21,22].

Turkeys:
- 100–400 mg per bird PO[21].

Poultry:
- 100–500 mg/kg PO once; repeat in 10–14 days for ascarids[23].

Game birds:
- 100–500 mg/kg PO once; repeat in 10–14 days[21].
- 1000–2000 mg/L of drinking water for 1–2 days[20,21].
- 2000–4000 mg/kg of feed[21].

Waterfowl:

- 45–200 mg/kg PO once for *Tetrameres* and *Capillaria*[24].
- 1600–2600 mg/L of drinking water for *Tetrameres* and *Capillaria*[25].

Psittacines:

- 250 mg/kg PO once[18,19].

Raptors:

- 100 mg/kg PO; repeat in 14 days[19,26].
- 1000 mg/L of drinking water for 3 days[18,19].

Parakeets and canaries:

- Citrate formulation at 0.5 mg/kg[27].

Swine

- 110 mg/kg (as base). Citrate salt usually used in feed as a one day treatment, and hexahydrate in drinking water. Dose must be consumed in 8–12 hours[2].

Miniature pigs:

- 200 mg/kg PO[28].

Primates

- 65 mg/kg PO q24h for 10 days[29].

REFERENCES

1. Cornelius, L.M. and Roberson. E.L. (1986) Treatment of gastrointestinal parasitism. In: Kirk, R.W. (ed.) *Current Veterinary Therapy: IX: Small Animal Practice,* W.B. Saunders, Philadelphia.
2. Roberson, E.L. (1988) Antimicrobial agents. In: Booth, N.H. and McDonald, L.E. (eds.) *Veterinary Pharmacology and Therapeutics,* Iowa State University Press, Ames, IA, 882–927.
3. Kirk, R.W. (1986) Current Veterinary Therapy IX: Small Animal Practice, W.B. Saunders, Philadelphia.
4. Davis, L.E. (1985) *Handbook of Small Animal Therapeutics,* Churchill Livingstone, New York.
5. Anderson, N.L. (1994) Basic husbandry and medicine of pocket pets. In: Birchard, S.J. and Sherding, R.G. (eds.) *Saunders Manual of Small Animal Practice,* W.B. Saunders, Philadelphia, 1363–1389.
6. Morrisey, J.K. and Carpenter, J.W. (2004) Formulary. In: Quesenberry, K.E. and Carpenter, J.W. (eds.) *Ferrets, Rabbits, and Rodents: Clinical Medicine and Surgery,* 2nd ed. W.B. Saunders, St. Louis, MO, 436–444.
7. Burke, T. (1999) Husbandry and Medicine of Rodents and Lagomorphs. *Central Veterinary Conference,* Kansas City, MO.
8. Adamcak, A. and Otten, B. (2000) *Rodent therapeutics. Vet. Clin. N. Am: Exotic Anim. Pract.* **3,** 221–240
9. Krus, A.L., Wesbroth, S.H., Flatt, R.E., et al. (1984) Biology and Diseases of Rabbits. In: Fox J.G., Cohen, B.J. and Loew, F.M. (eds.) *Laboratory Animal Medicine,* Academic Press, Orlando, FL, 207–240.
10. Ivey, E. and Morrisey, J. (2000) Therapeutics for rabbits. *Vet. Clin. N. Am: Exotic Anim. Pract.* **3,** 183–213.
11. Hillyer, E.V. (1994) Pet rabbits. *Vet. Clin. N. Am: Small Anim. Pract.* **24,** 25–65.
12. Quesenberry, K.E. (1994) Rabbits. In: Birchard, S.J. and Sherding, R.G. (eds.) *Saunders Manual of Small Animal Practice,* W.B. Saunders, Philadelphia, 1345–1362.
13. Brown, S.A. (1999) Ferret Drug Dosages. In: Antinoff, N., Bauck, L. and Boyer, T.H., et al. (eds.) *Exotic Formulary,* 2nd ed. American Animal Hospital Association, Lakewood, CO, 43–61.
14. Jacobson, E., Kollias, G.V., and Peters, L.J. (1983) Dosages for antibiotics and parasiticides used in exotic animals. *Compend. Contin. Educ. Pract. Vet.* **5.** 315–324.
15. Allen, D.G., Pringle, J.K., and Smith, D. (1993) *Handbook of Veterinary Drugs,* J.B. Lippincott, Philadelphia, 534–567.
16. Noga, E.J. (2000) Fish Diseases: Diagnosis and Treatment. Iowa State University Press, Ames, IA.
17. Harlin, R.W. (2000) Pigeon Therapeutics. *Vet. Clin. N. Am: Exotic Anim. Pract.* **3,** 19–34.
18. Beynon, P.H., Forbes, N.A., and Harcourt-Brown, N.H. (1996) *BSAVA Manual of Raptors, Pigeons and Waterfowl,* Iowa State University Press, Ames, IA.
19. Marshall, R. (1993) Avian anthelmintics and antiprotozoals. *Semin. Avian Exotic Pet Med.* **2,** 33–41.
20. Byrne, R.F., Davis, C., Lister, S.A., et al. (2001) Prescribing for birds. In: Bishop, Y. (ed.) *The Veterinary Formulary,* 5th ed. Pharmaceutical Press, London, 43–56.
21. Stadler, C. and Carpenter, J.W. (1996) Parasites of backyard game birds. *Semin. Avian Exotic Pet Med.* **5,** 85–96.
22. Moore, D.M. and Rice, L.R. (1998) Exotic animal formulary. In: Holt, K.M., Booth, D.M. and Gaumnitz, J., et al. (eds.) *Veterinary Values,* 5th ed. Veterinary Medicine Publishing Group, Lenexa, KS, 159–245.
23. Clubb, S.L. (1986) Therapeutics: Individual and flock treatment regimens. In: Harrison, G.J. and Harrison, L.R. (eds.) *Clinical Avian Medicine and Surgery,* W.B. Saunders, Philadelphia, 327–355.
24. Ritchie, B.W. and Harrison, G.L. (1994) Formulary. In: Ritchie, B.W., Harrison, G.L., and Harrison, L.R. (eds.) *Avian Medicine: Principles and Application,* Wingers, Lake Worth, FL, 457–478.
25. Carpenter, N.A. (2000) Anseriform and galliform therapeutics. *Vet. Clin. N. Am: Exotic Anim. Pract.* **3,** 1–17.
26. Joseph, V. (1995) Preventative health programs for falconry birds. *Proc. Annu. Conf. Assoc. Avian Vet.* 171–178.
27. Stunkard, J.M. (1984) *Diagnosis, Treatment and Husbandry of Pet Birds,* Stunkard Publishing, Edgewater, MD.
28. Boldrick, L. (1993) *Veterinary Care of Pot-Bellied Pet Pigs,* All Publishing, Orange, CA.
29. Holmes D.D. (1984) *Clinical Laboratory Animal Medicine,* Iowa State University Press, Ames, IA.

Praziquantel

Activity: In dogs it is labeled for the treatment of *Dipylidium caninum, Taenia pisiformis,* and *Echinococcus granulosus.* In cats it is labeled for the treatment of *Dipylidium caninum* and *Taenia taeniaeformis.*

  MOA: The exact mechanism has not been completely determined. At low concentrations it appears to impair the worm's sucker function and increases its motility. At higher concentrations it increases the contraction of the worm's strobila (proglottid chain). At very high concentrations the contractions are irreversible. At specific sites on the cestode integument it causes vacuolization with subsequent disintegration.

Dogs

- IM or SC using the 56.8 mg/ml injectable product: 5 lbs or less administer 17 mg (0.3 ml), 6–10 lbs administer 28.4 mg (0.5 ml), 11–25 lbs administer 56.8 mg (1.0 ml), over 25 lbs administer 0.2 ml/5 lb body weight, maximum of 3 ml (Package insert; Droncit® Injectable and Tablets—Miles).
- Oral using the 34-mg canine tablet: 5 lbs or less administer 17 mg (1/2 tablet), 6–10 lbs administer 34 mg (1 tablet), 11–15 lbs administer 51 mg (1.5 tablets), 16–30 lbs administer 68 mg (2 tablets), 31–45 lbs administer 102 mg (3 tablets), 46–60 lbs administer 136 mg (4 tablets), over 60 lbs administer 170 mg (5 tablets maximum) (Package insert; Droncit® Injectable and Tablets—Miles).
- 10 mg/kg for *Echinococcus granulosis*[1].
- 7.5 mg/kg PO once for *Diphyllobothrium* sp.[2].
- 7.5 mg/kg PO q24h for 2 days for *Spirometra mansonoides* and *Diphyllobothrium erinacei*[3].
- 23–25 mg/kg PO q8h for 3 days for *Paragonimus kellicotti*[4,5].
- 20–40 mg/kg once daily for 3–10 days for liver flukes of *Platynosomum* and Opisthorchiidae[6].

Cats

- IM or SQ using the 56.8 mg/ml injectable product: under 5 lbs administer 11.4 mg (0.2 ml), 5–10 lbs administer 22.7 mg (0.4 ml), 10 lb and over administer 34.1 mg (0.6 ml maximum) (Package insert; Droncit® Injectable and Tablets—Miles).
- Oral using the 23 mg feline tablet: 4 lbs and under administer 11.5 mg (1/2 tablet), 5–11 lbs administer 23 mg (1 tablet), Over 11 lbs administer 34.5 mg (1.5 tablets) (Package insert; Droncit® Injectable and Tablets—Miles).
- 23–25 mg/kg PO q8h for 3 days for *Paragonimus kellicotti*[4,5].

Rodents

All species:

- 6–10 mg/kg PO or SQ; repeat in 10 days for cestodes[7,8].

Gerbils, Mice, and Rats

- 30 mg/kg PO q14d for 3 treatments[9].
- 30 mg/kg PO once for cestodes[10].
- 6–10 mg/kg PO for cestodes[11].

Hamsters

- 30 mg/kg PO once for cestodes[10].
- 6–10 mg/kg PO for cestodes[11].

Rabbits

- 5–10 mg/kg SQ, PO, or IM; repeat in 10 days[12].

Ferrets

- 5–10 mg/kg PO or SC; repeat in 10–14 days for cestodes[8,13].

Chinchillas

- 6–10 mg/kg PO[14].
- 6–10 mg/kg PO for cestodes[11].

Guinea Pigs

- 6–10 mg/kg PO for cestodes[11].

Amphibians

- 8–24 m/kg topical, PO, SQ, or intracoelomic; repeat q14d for trematodes and cestodes[15].
- 10 mg/L of water for 3 hrs, repeat q7–21d for trematodes and cestodes[15].

Reptiles

Most species:

- 8 mg/kg PO, SC, or IM; repeat in 14 days for trematodes and cestodes[16,17,18].

Chameleons:

- 5–10 mg/kg PO q14d for flukes[19].

Loggerhead sea turtles:

- 25 mg/kg PO q3h for 3 treatments[20].

Fish

- 5–10 mg/L of water for 3–6 hrs; repeat in 7 days for Monogenean trematodes and cestodes. Some marine fish are sensitive and may be toxic to *Corydoras* catfish[21].
- 2 mg/L or water for 2–4 hrs for metacercaria[22].
- 5 mg/kg PO q24h for 3 treatments[23].
- 2–10 mg/L of water for up to 4 hrs. Monitor for lethargy, incoordination, and loss of equilibrium[24].

- 5–12 mg/g of feed for 3 days[24].
- 5 mg/kg PO in feed q7d for up to 3 treatments[25].
- 5 mg/kg PO or intracoelomic; repeat in 14–21 days for cestodes, some internal digenean trematodes[21].
- 50 mg/kg PO once via gavage or give 0.5% in feed at 1% of body weight per day for adult cestodes[26].

Birds

Most species including pigeons:
- 10–20 mg/kg PO; repeat in 10–14 days[27].

Most species except finches:
- 7.5 mg/kg SC or IM; repeat in 2–4 weeks[28].
- 1/4 of 1 23-mg tablet/kg PO in food or via gavage; repeat in 10–14 days for cestodes; injectable form is toxic to finches[29].

Finches:
- 12-mg crushed tablet baked into a 9" × 9" × 2" cake. Withhold regular food and preexpose to a nonmedicated cake[30].

Chickens:
- 8.5 mg/kg IM; 10 mg/kg PO; 11 mg/kg SQ once[12].

Psittacines:
- 5–10 mg/kg PO; repeat in 2–4 weeks[28].
- 9 mg/kg IM; repeat in 10 days for cestodes[31].
- 9 mg/kg IM q24h for 3 days, then PO q24h for 11 days for trematodes[32].

Passerines:
- 5–10 mg/kg PO; repeat in 2–4 weeks[28].

Raptors:
- 30–50 mg/kg PO, SC, or IM; repeat in 14 days for cestodes[33,34].
- 9 mg/kg IM q24h for 3 days, then PO q24h for 11 days for trematodes[33].
- 5–10 mg/kg PO or SC q24h for 14 days for trematodes[33,35,36].

Waterfowl:
- 10–20 mg/kg SC or IM, repeat in 10 days for cestodes[37].
- 5–10 mg/kg PO or SC q24h for 14 days for trematodes[35,36].
- 10 mg/kg PO, SC, or IM q24h for 14 days for trematodes[10].

Toucans:
- 10 mg/kg IM q24h for 3 days, then PO q24h for 11 days[10].

- 10 mg/kg PO, SC, or IM q24h for 14 days for trematodes[10]; this can be followed with 6 mg/kg PO q24h for 14 days[38].

Sheep and Goats

- 10–15 mg/kg for all species of *Moniezia, Stilesia,* and *Avitellina*[3].

Primates

- 15–20 mg/kg PO or IM for some cestodes[39].
- 40 mg/kg PO or IM for trematodes[39].

Red ruffed lemurs:
- 23 mg PO q10d for 3 treatments. Administer with albendazole.
- 28.5 mg PO q12h for 10 days for 3 treatments with a 10-day interval for subcutaneous cysticercosis[40].

REFERENCES

1. Sherding, R.G. (1989) Diseases of the Small Bowel. In: Ettinger, S.J. (ed.) *Textbook of Veterinary Medicine,* W.B. Saunders, Philadelphia, 1323–1296.
2. Kirkpatrick, C.E., Knochenhauer, A.W., and Jacobsen, S.L. (1987) Use of praziquantel for treatment of *Diphyllobothrium* sp. in a dog. *JAVMA* **190,** 557–558.
3. Roberson, E.L. (1988) Anticestodal and Antitrematodal Drugs. In: Booth, N.H. and McDonald, L.E. (eds.) *Veterinary Pharmacology and Therapeutics,* Iowa State University Press, Ames, IA, 928–949.
4. Reinemeyer, C. (1995) Parasites of the Respiratory System. In: Bonagura, J. (ed.) *Kirk's Current Veterinary Therapy: XII,* W.B. Saunders, Philadelphia, 895–898.
5. Hawkins, E. (2000) Pulmonary Parenchymal Diseases. In: Ettinger, S. and Feldman, E. (eds.) *Textbook of Veterinary Internal Medicine: Diseases of the Dog and Cat,* W.B. Saunders, Philadelphia, 1061–1091.
6. Taboada, J. (1999) Feline liver diseases. The North American Veterinary Conference, Orlando, FL.
7. Harkness, J.E. and Wagner, J.E. (1995) *The Biology and Medicine of Rabbits and Rodents,* 4th ed. Williams and Wilkins, Philadelphia.
8. Morrisey, J.K. and Carpenter, J.W. (2004) Formulary. In: Quesenberry, K.E. and Carpenter, J.W. (eds.) *Ferrets, Rabbits, and Rodents: Clinical Medicine and* Surgery, 2nd ed. W.B. Saunders, St. Louis, MO, 436–444.
9. Burke, T.J. (1995) "Wet tail" in hamsters and other diarrheas of small rodents. In: Bonagura, J.D. (ed.) *Kirk's Current Veterinary Therapy XII: Small Animal Practice,* W.B. Saunders, Philadelphia, 1336–1339.
10. Burke, T. (1999) Husbandry and Medicine of Rodents and Lagomorphs. Central Veterinary Conference, Kansas City, MO.
11. Adamcak, A. and Otten, B. (2000) Rodent therapeutics. *Vet. Clin. N. Am: Exotic Anim. Pract.* **3,** 221–240.
12. Allen, D.G., Pringle, J.K., and Smith, D.A. (1993) *Handbook of Veterinary Drugs,* J.B. Lippincott, Philadelphia.
13. Brown, S.A. (1993) Ferrets. In: Jerkins, J.R. and Brown, S.A. (eds.) *A Practitioner's Guide to Rabbits and Ferrets.* American Hospital Association, Lakewood, CO, 43–111.
14. Hayes, P. (2000) Diseases of chinchillas. In: Bonagura, J. (ed.) *Kirk's Current Veterinary Therapy: XIII Small Animal Practice,* W.B. Saunders, Philadelphia, 1152–1157.

15. Wright, K.M. and Whitaker, B.R. (2001) Pharmacotherapeutics. In: Wright, K.M. and Whitaker, B.R. (eds.) *Amphibian Medicine and Captive Husbandry*, Krieger Publishing, Malabar, FL, 309–330.

16. Barten, S.L. (1993) The medical care of iguanas and other common pet lizards. *Vet. Clin. N. Am: Small Anim. Pract.* **23**, 1213–1249.

17. Jacobson, E.R. (1993) Snakes. *Vet. Clin. N. Am: Small Anim. Pract.* **23**, 1179–1212.

18. Jenkins, J.R. (1992) Husbandry and diseases of Old World chameleons. *J. Sm. Exotic Anim. Med.* **1**, 145–192.

19. Klingenberg, R.J. (2000) Diagnosing parasites of Old World chameleons. *Exotic DVM.* **1**, 17–21.

20. Jacobson, E.R., Harman, G., Laille, E., et al. (2002) Plasma concentrations of praziquantel in loggerhead sea turtles, *Caretta caretta*, following oral administration of single and multiple doses. *Proc. Assoc. Rept. Amph. Vet.* 37–39.

21. Lewbart, G.A. (1998) Emergency and critical care of fish. *Vet. Clin. N. Am: Exotic. Anim. Pract.* **1**, 233–249.

22. Plumb, J.A. and Rogers, W.A. (1990) Effect of Droncit (praziquantel) on yellow grubs *Clinostomum marginatum* and eye flukes *Diplostomum spathaceum* in channel catfish. *J. Aquat. Anim. Health* **2**, 204–206.

23. Treves-Brown, K.M. (2000) *Applied Fish Pharmacology*, Kluwer Academic Publishers, Dodrecht, The Netherlands.

24. Whitaker, B.R. (1999) Preventative medicine programs for fish. In: Fowler, M.E. and Miller, R.E. (eds.) *Zoo and Wild Animal Medicine: Current Therapy 4*, W.B. Saunders, Philadelphia, 163–181.

25. Stoskopf, M.K. (1999) Fish pharmacotherapeutics. In: Fowler, M.E. and Miller, R.E. (eds.) *Zoo and Wild Animal Medicine: Current Therapy 4*, W.B. Saunders Co., Philadelphia, 182–189.

26. Noga, E.J. (2000) *Fish Disease: Diagnosis and Treatment*, Iowa State University Press, Ames, IA.

27. Lung, N.P. and Romagnano, A. (1995) Current approaches to feather picking. In: Bonagura, J.D. (ed.) *Kirk's Current Veterinary Therapy XII: Small Animal Practice*, W.B. Saunders, Philadelphia, 1303–1307.

28. Coles, B.H. (2001) Prescribing for exotic birds. In: Bishop, Y. (ed.) *The Veterinary Formulary*, 5th ed. *Pharmaceutical Press*, London, 99–105.

29. Clubb, S.L. (1986) Therapeutics: individual and flock treatment regimens. In: Harrison, G.J. and Harrison, L.R. (eds.) *Clinical Avian Medicine and Surgery*, W.B. Saunders, Philadelphia, 327–355.

30. Marshall, R. (1993) Avian anthelmintics and antiprotozoals. *Semin. Avian Exotic Pet Med.* **2**, 33–41.

31. Beynon, P.H., Forbes N.A., and Lawton, M.P.C. (1996) *Manual of Psittacine Birds*, Iowa State University Press, Ames, IA.

32. Tully, T.N. (2000) Psittacine therapeutics. *Vet Clin. N. Am: Exotic Anim. Pract.* **3**, 59–90.

33. Huckabee, J.R. (2000) Raptor therapeutics. *Vet. Clin. N. Am: Exotic Anim. Pract.* **3**, 91–116.

34. Joseph, V. (1995) Preventative health programs for falconry birds. *Proc. Annu. Conf. Assoc. Avian Vet.* 171–178.

35. Beynon, P.H., Forbes, N.A., and Harcourt-Brown, N.H. (1996) *BSAVA Manual of Raptors, Pigeons, and Waterfowl*, Iowa State University Press, Ames, IA.

36. Carpenter, N.A. (2000) Anseriform and galliform therapeutics. *Vet. Clin. N. Am: Small Anim. Pract.* **3**, 1–17.

37. Brown, M.J. and Cromie, R.L. (1996) Weight loss and enteritis. In: Beynon, P.H., Forbes, N.A., and Harcourt-Brown, N.H. (eds.) *BSAVA Manual of Raptors, Pigeons, and Waterfowl*, Iowa State University Press, Ames, IA, 322–329.

38. Ritchie, B.W. and Harrison, G.J. (1997) Formulary. In: Ritchie, B. W., Harrison, G.J., and Harrison, L.R. (eds.). *Avian Medicine: Principles and Application, Abridged Edition*, Wingers, Lake Worth, Fl, 227–253.

39. Wolff, P.L. (1993) Parasites of the New World primates. In: Fowler, M.E. (ed.) *Zoo and Wild Animal Medicine: Current Therapy 3*, W.B. Saunders, Philadelphia, 378–389.

40. Young, L.A., Morris, P.J., Keene, L., et al. (2000) Subcutaneous *Taenia crassiceps* cysticercosis in a red ruffed lemur (*Varecia variegata rubra*). *Proc. Am. Assoc. Zoo Vet.* 251–252.

Pyrantel

Activity: In dogs it is labeled for removal of ascarids (*Toxocara canis, Toxascaris leonina*), hookworms (*Ancylostoma caninum, Uncinaria stenocephala*), and stomach worms (*Physaloptera*). In swine tartate formulation is labeled for prevention and removal of large roundworms (*Ascaris suum*) and *Oesophagostomum* spp. It also has activity against the stomach worm (*Hyostrongylus rubidus*).

MOA: Pyrantel paralyzes the parasite. It is a depolarizing neuromuscular blocking agent that possesses nicotine-like abilities and acts similarly to acetylcholine; it also inhibits cholinesterase.

Dogs

- 10 mg/kg (as base) PO for dogs weighing less than 5 lbs, 5 mg/kg (as base) PO for dogs weighing more than 5 lbs.
- Treat puppies at 2, 3, 4, 6, 8, and 10 weeks of age.
- Treat lactating bitches 2–3 weeks after whelping.
- Do follow-up fecal examination 2–4 weeks after treating to determine need for retreatment. (Label directions; Nemex® Tabs—Pfizer).

Cats

Ascarids, hookworms, Physaloptera:

- 5 mg/kg PO once for *Physaloptera;* repeat in two weeks for ascarids and hookworms[1].
- 10 mg/kg; repeat in 3 weeks[2].

Rodents

- Pamoate formulation: 50 mg/kg PO for nematodiasis[3].

Rabbits

- Pamoate formulation: 5–10 mg/kg PO, SQ, or IM; repeat in 10 days[4].
- Pamoate formulation: 5–10 mg/kg PO; repeat in 14–21 days[5].

Ferrets

- Pamoate formulation: 4.4 mg/kg PO; repeat in 14 days[6].

Reptiles

- Pamoate formulation: 5 mg/kg PO; repeat in 14 days for nematodes[7].

Fish

- Pamoate formulation: 10 mg/kg in feed once for gastric nematodes[8].

Birds

Most species:

- Pamoate formulation at 7 mg/kg PO; repeat in 14 days[9].
- 4.5 mg/kg PO once; repeat in 14 days for nematodes[10].

Psittacines and passerines:

- 100 mg/kg PO once for nematodes[11].

Pigeons:

- Pamoate formulation at 20–25 mg/kg PO[12].

Raptors:

- Pamoate formulation at 7–20 mg/kg PO; repeat in 14 days[13] or 20 mg/kg PO once[14].

Ramphastids:

- Pamoate formulation at 70 mg/kg PO once; repeat if necessary[15].

Sheep and Goats

- Tartrate formulation: 25 mg/kg PO[16].

Swine

- Tartrate formulation: 22 mg/kg PO or in feed at a rate of 800 g/ton as a single treatment for removal of *Ascaris suum* or *Oesophagostomum* spp.
- 2.6 mg/kg PO or in feed at a rate of 96 g/ton for 3 days for *Ascaris suum* only[17].
- Tartrate formulation: 22 mg/kg PO with a maximum of 2 grams per animal[16].
- 6.6 mg/kg PO for ascarids and nodular worms in pot-bellied pigs[18].

Primates

Prosimians:

- Pamoate formulation at 5–10 mg/kg PO for 3 days for nematodes[19].

Lemurs:

- Pamoate formulation at 6 mg/kg PO[20].
- 11 mg/kg PO once for hookworms (*Necator* spp.) and pinworms[21].

REFERENCES

1. Dimski, D.S. (1989) Helminth and noncoccidial protozoan parasites of the gastrointestinal tract. In: Sherding, R.G. (ed.) *The Cat: Diseases and Clinical Management,* Churchill Livingstone, New York, 459–477.
2. Kirk, R.W. (1989) *Current Veterinary Therapy X, Small Animal Practice,* W.B. Saunders, Philadelphia.
3. Adamcak, A. and Otten, B. (2000) Rodent therapeutics. *Vet. Clin. N. Am: Exotic Anim. Pract.* **3,** 221–240.
4. Morrisey, J.K. and Carpenter, J.W. (2004) Formulary. In: Quesenberry, K.E. and Carpenter, J.W. (eds.) *Ferrets, Rabbits, and Rodents: Clinical Medicine and Surgery,* 2nd ed. W.B. Saunders, St. Louis, MO, 436–444.
5. Quesenberry, K.E. (1994) Rabbits. In: Birchard, S.J. and Sherding, R.G. (eds.) *Saunders Manual of Small Animal Practice,* W.B. Saunders, Philadelphia, 1345–1362.
6. Brown, S.A. (1999) Ferret Drug Dosages. In: Antinoff, N., Bauck, L., Boyer, T.H., et al. (eds.) *Exotic Formulary* 2nd ed. American Animal Hospital Association. Lakewood, CO, 43–61.
7. Frye, F.L. (1994) *Reptile Clinician's Handbook. Krieger Publishing,* Malabar, FL.
8. Stoskopf, M.K. (1999) Fish pharmacotherapeutics. In: Fowler, M.E. and Miller, R.E. (eds.) *Zoo and Wild Animal Medicine: Current Therapy 4,* W.B. Saunders, Philadelphia, 182–189.
9. Clyde, V.L. (1996) Diagnosis, treatment and control of common parasites in companion and aviary birds. *Semin. Avian Exotic Pet Med.* **5,** 75–84.
10. Clubb, S.L. (1986) Therapeutics: individual and flock treatment regimens. In: Harrison, G.J. and Harrison, L.R. (eds.) *Clinical Avian Medicine and Surgery,* W.B. Saunders, Philadelphia, 327–355.
11. Marshall, R. (1993) Avian anthelmintics and antiprotozoals. *Semin. Avian Exotic Pet Med.* **2,** 33–41.
12. Harlin, R.W. (1995) Backyard poultry. *Proc. Mid-Atlantic States Assoc. Avian Vet. Conf.* 65–68.
13. Huckabee, J.R. (2000) Raptor therapeutics. *Vet Clin. N. Am: Exotic Anim. Pract.* **3,** 91–116.
14. Beynon, P.H., Forbes, N.A., and Harcourt-Brown, N.H. (1996) *BSAVA Manual of Raptors, Pigeons, and Waterfowl,* Iowa State University Press, Ames, IA.
15. Cubas, Z.S. (2001) Medicine: family Rhamphastidae (toucans). In: Fowler, M.E. and Cubas, Z.S. (eds.) *Biology, Medicine, and Surgery of South American Wild Animals,* Iowa State University Press, Ames, IA, 188–199.
16. Roberson, E.L. (1988) Antinematodal agents. In: Booth, N.H. and McDonald, L.E. (eds.) *Veterinary Pharmacology and Therapeutics,* Iowa State University Press, Ames, IA, 882–927.
17. Paul, J.W. (1986) Anthelmintic therapy. In: Howard, J.L. (ed.) *Current Veterinary Therapy: Food Animal Practice 2,* W.B. Saunders, Philadelphia, 39–44.
18. Braun, W. (1995) Potbellied pigs: general medical care. In: Bonagura, J. (ed.) *Kirk's Current Veterinary Therapy: XII,* W.B. Saunders, Philadelphia, 1388–1389.

19. Junge, R.E. (2003) Prosimians. In: Fowler, M.E. and Miller, R.E. (eds.) *Zoo and Wild Animal Medicine*, W.B. Saunders, Philadelphia, 334–346.
20. Feeser, P. and White, F. (1992) Medical management of *Lemur catta*, *Varecia variegata*, *Propithecus verreauxi* in natural habitat enclosures. *Proc. Am. Assoc. Zoo Vet./Am. Assoc. Wildl. Vet.* 320–323.
21. Wolff, P.L. (1993) Parasites of the New World primates. In: Fowler, M.E. (ed.) *Zoo and Wild Animal Medicine: Current Therapy 3*, W.B. Saunders, Philadelphia, 378–389.

Pyrimethamine

Activity: Used to treat toxoplasmosis. Often used in combination with sulfonamides.

MOA: Folic acid antagonist that inhibits the enzyme dihydrofolate reductase.

Dogs

- 0.5–1 mg/kg PO once daily for two days, then 0.25 mg/kg PO once daily for 2 weeks for toxoplasmosis. Give with sulfadiazine at 30–50 mg/kg PO divided bid-qid for 1–2 weeks[1].
- 0.25–0.5 mg/kg once daily for 28 days for toxoplasmosis[2].
- 1 mg/kg once daily for 28 days for *Neospora*. Give with trimethoprim sulfa[2].
- 0.25–0.5 mg/kg once daily for 2–4 weeks for *Hepatozoon canis*. Give with trimethoprim sulfa and clindamycin[2].

Birds

Most species:
- 0.5 mg/kg PO q12h for 14–28 days or 100 mg/kg feed[3].
- 0.5–1.0 mg/kg PO q12h for 2–4 days, then 0.25 mg/kg PO q12h for 30 days for *Sarcocystis*. Give with trimethoprim sulfa at 5 mg/kg IM q12h or 30–100 mg/kg PO q12h for 7 days[4].

Psittacines (keas):
- 0.5 mg/kg PO q12h for 45 days for *Sarcocystis*. Give with amprolium and primaquine[5].

Game birds:
- 1 mg/kg of feed[6].

Raptors:
- 0.25–0.5 mg/kg PO q12h for 30 days[7].

Waterfowl:
- 0.5 mg/kg PO q12h for 30 days for *Sarcocystis*[8].
- 0.25–0.5 mg/kg PO q12h for 30 days[7].

Eclectus and amazon parrots:
- 0.5–1.0 mg/kg PO q12h for 30 days[9].

Primates

- 10 mg/kg q24h for *Plasmodium*[10].

Great apes:

- 2.0 mg/kg q24h for 3 days then 1.0 mg/kg q 24h for 28 days for *Toxoplasma*. Maximum dosages of 100 mg/animal q24h for days 1–3 and 25 mg/animal q24h for 28 days. Treat concurrently with sulfadiazine and supplement with folic acid[11,12].

REFERENCES

1. Murtaugh, R.J. (1988) Protozoal diseases. In: Morgan, R.V. (ed.) *Handbook of Small Animal Practice*, Churchill Livingstone, New York, 1009–1028.
2. Swango, L.J., Bankemper, K.W., and Kong, L.I. (1989) Bacterial, rickettsial, protozoal, and miscellaneous infections. In: Ettinger, S.J. (ed.) *Textbook of Veterinary Internal Medicine*, W.B. Saunders, Philadelphia, 265–297.
3. Clyde, V.L. and Patton, S. (1996) Diagnosis, treatment and control of common parasites in companion and aviary birds. *Semin. Avian Exotic Pet Med.* **5,** 75–84.
4. Hoppes, S. (1998) Common parasites in companion birds. *Proc. Annu. Conf. Assoc. Avian Vet.* 213–216.
5. Weston, H.S. (1996) The successful treatment of sarcocystosis in two keas (*Nestor nobilis*) at the Franklin Park Zoo. *Proc. Am. Assoc. Zoo Vet.* 186–191.
6. Stadler, C. and Carpenter, J.W. (1996) Parasites of backyard game birds. *Semin. Avian Exotic Pet Med.* **5,** 85–96.
7. Beynon, P.H., Forbes, N.A., and Harcourt-Brown, N.H. (1996) *BSAVA Manual of Raptors, Pigeons, and Waterfowl*, Iowa State University Press, Ames, IA.
8. Brown, M.J. and Cromie, R.L. (1996) Weight loss and enteritis. In: Beynon, P.H., Forbes, N.A., and Harcourt-Brown, N.H. (eds.) *BSAVA Manual of Raptors, Pigeons, and Waterfowl*, Iowa State University Press, Ames, IA, 322–329.
9. Page, D.C., Schmidt, R.E., English, J.H., et al. (1992) Antemortem diagnosis and treatment of sarcocystosis in two species of psittacines. *J. Zoo Wildl. Med.* **23,** 77–85.
10. Puri, S.K. and Singh, N. (2000) Azithromycin: antimalarial profile against blood-and-sporozoite-induced infections in mice and monkeys. *Exp. Parasitol.* **94,** 8–14.
11. Swenson, R.B. (1993) Protozoal parasites of great apes. In: Fowler, M.E. (ed.) *Zoo and Wild Animal Medicine: Current Therapy 3*, W.B. Saunders, Philadelphia, 352–355.
12. Wolff, P.L. (1993) Parasites of the New World primates. In: Fowler, M.E. (ed.) *Zoo and Wild Animal Medicine: Current Therapy 3*, W.B. Saunders, Philadelphia, 378–389.

Quinacrine

Activity: Primarily used against *Giardia*, *Trichomonas*, and *Leishmania*.

MOA: Not completely understood. Against *Giardia* it binds to DNA by intercalation to adjacent base pair, inhibiting RNA transcription and translocation. Interferes with electron transport. Inhibits succinate oxidation and cholinesterase.

Dogs

- 6.6 mg/kg PO q12h for 5 days[1,2].
- 50–100 mg per dog PO q12h for 3 days, skip 3 days, then repeat for 3 more days[3].

Cats

- 11 mg/kg PO once daily for 5 days[1].
- 6.6 mg/kg PO twice daily for 5 days[4].
- 10 mg/kg PO once daily for 5 days for coccidiosis[3].

Rodents

- 75 mg/kg q8h[5].

Chinchillas

- 75 mg/kg q8h for giardiasis[5].

Reptiles

Most species:
- 19–100 mg/kg PO q48h for 14–21 days for some hematozoa[6].

Birds

Most species:
- 7.5 mg/kg PO q24h for 10 days for *Atoxoplasma*[7].
- 5–10 mg/kg PO q24h for 7–10 days; use higher doses for *Lankesterella* and *Plasmodium*[7,8].

Pigeons:
- 26–79 mg/L of drinking water for 10–21 days[9].

Primates

Great apes:
- 2 mg/kg PO q8h for 7 days for *Giardia;* maximum dose of 300 mg/day[10].

REFERENCES

1. Papich, M. (1992) Table of common drugs: approximate dosages. In: Kirk, R. and Bonagura, J. (eds.) *Current Veterinary Therapy: XIII Small Animal Practice*, W.B. Saunders, Philadelphia, 1233–1249.
2. Sherding, R. and Johnson, S. (1994) Diseases of the intestines. In: Birchard, S. and Sherding, R. (eds.) *Saunders Manual of Small Animal Practice*, W.B. Saunders, Philadelphia, 777–792.
3. Greene, C.E. and Watson, A.D.J. (1998) Antimicrobial drug formulary. In: Greene, C. (ed.) *Infectious Diseases of the Dog and Cat*, 2nd ed. W.B. Saunders, Philadelphia, 790–919.
4. Barr, M. and Bowman, D. (1994) Giardiasis in dogs and cats. *Comp. CE.* **16**, 603–610.
5. Adamcak, A. and Otten, B. (2000) Rodent therapeutics. *Vet. Clin. N. Am: Exotic Anim. Pract.* 3, 221–237.
6. Willette-Frahm, M., Wright, K.M., and Thode, B.C. (1995) Select protozoal diseases in amphibians and reptiles: a report for the Infectious Diseases Committee, American Association of Zoo Veterinarians. *Bull. Assoc. Rept. Amph. Vet.* **5**, 19–29.
7. Marshall, R. (1993) Avian anthelmintics and antiprotozoals. *Semin. Avian Exotic Pet Med.* **2**, 33– 41.
8. Ritchie, B.W. and Harrison, G.J. (1994) Formulary. In: Ritchie, B.W., Harrison, G.J., and Harrison, L.R. (eds.) *Avian Medicine: Principles and Application*, Wingers, Lake Worth, Fl, 457–478.
9. LaBonde, J. (1995) Toxicity in pet avian patients. *Semin. Avian Exotic Pet Med.* **4**, 23–31.
10. Swenson, R.B. (1993) Protozoal parasites of great apes. In: Fowler, M.E. (ed.) *Zoo and Wild Animal Medicine: Current Therapy 3*, W.B. Saunders, Philadelphia, 352–355.

Selamectin

Activity: Control and prevention of flea infestation by *Ctenocephalides felis* in dogs and cats (Package Insert; Revolution®—Pfizer). Prevention of heartworm disease by *Dirofilaria immitis* in dogs and cats (Package Insert; Revolution®—Pfizer). Treatment and control of ear mite infestation by *Otodectes cynotis* in dogs and cats (Package Insert; Revolution®—Pfizer). Treatment and control of sarcoptic mange by *Sarcoptes scabiei* in dogs only (Package Insert; Revolution®—Pfizer). Control of the American Dog Tick, *Dermacentor variabilis,* in dogs only (Package Insert; Revolution®—Pfizer). Treatment and control of the roundworm *Toxocara cati* and the hookworm *Ancylostoma tubaeforme* in cats only (Package Insert; Revolution®—Pfizer).

MOA: Believed to enhance chloride permeability and the release of gamma-aminobutyric acid (GABA) at presynaptic neurons. Thus, it causes parasite paralysis.

Dogs

- The recommended dose of selamectin is 2.7 mg/lb or 6 mg/kg of body weight for dogs 6 weeks of age and older, administered topically (Package Insert; Revolution®—Pfizer). See package insert for further details on how to apply Revolution topically.

For dogs up to 5 lbs:
- 15 mg per tube; 0.25 ml administered volume (Package Insert; Revolution®—Pfizer).

For dogs 5.1–10 lbs:
- 30 mg per tube; 0.25 administered volume (Package Insert; Revolution®—Pfizer).

For dogs 10.1–20 lbs:
- 60 mg per tube; 0.5 administered volume (Package Insert; Revolution®—Pfizer).

For dogs 20.1–40 lbs:
- 120 mg per tube; 1.0 administered volume (Package Insert; Revolution®—Pfizer).

for dogs 40.1–85 lbs:
- 240 mg per tube; 2.0 administered volume (Package Insert; Revolution®—Pfizer).

For dogs 85.1–130 lbs:
- Use two tubes (120 mg per tube + 240 mg per tube); 3.0 administered volume (Package Insert; Revolution®—Pfizer).

Cats

- The recommended dose of selamectin is 2.7 mg/lb or 6 mg/kg of body weight for cats 8 weeks of age and older (Package Insert; Revolution®—Pfizer).

For cats up to 5 lbs:
- 15 mg per tube; 0.25 ml administered volume (Package Insert; Revolution®—Pfizer).

For cats 5.1–15 lbs:
- 45 mg per tube; 0.75 administered volume (Package Insert; Revolution®—Pfizer).

Rabbits

- Revolution topically at 6–10 mg/kg[1].

Guinea Pigs

- 6 mg/kg topically[1].

REFERENCE

1. Morrisey, J.K. and Carpenter, J.W. (2004) Formulary. In: Quesenberry, K.E. and Carpenter, J.W. (eds.) *Ferrets, Rabbits, and Rodents: Clinical Medicine and Surgery,* 2nd ed. W.B. Saunders, St. Louis, MO, 436–444.

Sodium Chloride

Activity: Used in freshwater fish for the treatment of protozoan and trematode ectoparasites and in amphibians for the treatment of ectoparasitic protozoa.

MOA: Lowers energy expenditure and increases slime coat production, resulting in sloughing of parasites.

Amphibians

For ectoparasites:
- 4–6 g/L bath[1].
- 6 g/L for 5–10 min. bath every 24h for 3–5 days[2].
- 25 g/L for 10 min. or less bath[3].

Fish

- Artificial sea salts preferred, sea water is normally 30–35 g/L.
- Species sensitivity is highly variable (catfish).
- Toxic to some plants.

For ectoparasites:
- 1–5 g/L tank water indefinitely[4].
- 10–30 g/L for up to 30 min. bath; use low dose for salt-sensitive fish[4].
- 30 g/L for 10 min.; for fish over 100 g only[5].
- 30–35 g/L for 4–5 min. bath; safe for most goldfish and koi[6].
- 0.5–1% in water for an indefinite period; 3% in water for 30 sec. to 10 min. (dip); 1% for 10 min. to 2 hr. (dip)[7].

REFERENCES

1. Raphael, B.L. (1993) Amphibians. *Vet. Clin. N. Am: Small Anim. Pract.* **23,** 1271–1286.
2. Willette-Frahm, M., Wright, K.M., and Thode, B.C. (1995) Select protozoan diseases in amphibians and reptiles. *Bull. Assoc. Rept. Amph. Vet.* **5,** 19–29.
3. Crawshaw, G.J. (1998) Amphibian emergency and critical care. *Vet. Clin. N. Am: Exotic Anim. Pract.* **1,** 207–231.
4. Noga, E.J. (2000) *Fish Disease: Diagnosis and Treatment,* Iowa State University Press, Ames, Iowa.
5. Treves-Brown, K.M. (2000) *Applied Fish Pharmacology,* Kluwer Academic Publishers, Dodrecht, The Netherlands.
6. Lewbart, G.A. (1998) Emergency and critical care of fish. *Vet. Clin. N. Am: Exotic Anim. Pract.* **1,** 233–249.
7. Klesius, P. and Rogers, W. (1995) Parasitisms of catfish and other farm-raised food fish. *J. Am. Vet. Med. Assoc.* **207,** 1473–1478.

Thiabendazole

Activity: An anthelmintic that also has antifungal activity. In sheep and goats it is labeled for the removal of *Haemonchus* spp., *Ostertagia* spp., *Trichostrongylus* spp., *Nematodirus* spp., *Cooperia* spp., *Chabertia* spp., *Bunostomum* spp., and *Oesophagostomum* spp. In swine it is labeled for the prevention of large roundworms (*Ascaris suum*) and in baby pigs it is labeled for the removal of *Strongyloides ransomi*. In dogs it has been used for the removal of *Toxocara canis, Toxascaris leonina, Strongyloides stercoralis,* and *Filaroides*. It is also used to treat nasal aspergillosis and penicillinosis.

MOA: Thiabendazole yields benzimidazoles after biotransformation. The mechanism of action is not clearly understood. Benzimidazoles seem to interfere with microtubular function and inhibit the helminth-specific mitochondrial fumarate reductase system. Thiabendazole may perform both of these actions. The rumen acts as a slow release site. It may be more effective in ruminants than other species.

Dogs

- 50–60 mg/kg PO for treatment of *Strongyloides stercoralis*[1].
- 35 mg/kg PO twice daily for 5 days, then 70 mg/kg PO twice daily for 21 days for *Filaroides*. Also, give 0.55 mg/kg PO of prednisone twice daily every other day[2].

Rats, Mice, Gerbils, Hamsters, and Guinea Pigs

- 100 mg/kg PO q24h for 5 days[3].

Rabbits

- 25–50 mg/kg PO[4].
- 50 mg/kg PO once[5].
- 50–100 mg/kg PO q24h for 5 days[3].
- 50–100 mg/kg PO for 5 days for pinworms[6].
- 50 mg/kg PO; repeat in 3 weeks for pinworms[6].

Chinchillas

- 50–100 mg/kg PO q24h for 5 days[7].

Amphibians

- 50–100 mg/kg PO; repeat in 2 weeks as needed for gastrointestinal nematodes[8].
- 100 mg/L of bath water; repeat in 2 weeks for verminous dermatitis[9].

Reptiles

- 50–100 mg/kg PO; repeat in 14 days for nematodes[10,11].

Fish

- 10–25 mg/kg in feed; repeat in 10 days or 66 mg/kg PO once for gastric nematodes. Anorexia may be seen at the high dose, which usually resolves in 2–4 days[12].

Birds

Most species:
- 40–100 mg/kg PO q24h for 7 days or 100–500 mg/kg PO once[13].
- 250–500 mg/kg PO once; repeat in 10–14 days for ascarids[14].
- 100 mg/kg PO once daily for 7–10 days for *Syngamus trachea*[14].

- 100 mg/kg PO q24h for 7–10 days for gapeworms and ascarids[15,16].
- 250–500 mg/kg PO; repeat in 10–14 days for ascarids and *Syngamus*[16,17].

Chickens, pheasants, turkeys, and pigeons:
- Mix 0.5% in feed for 10 days or administer orally at 44 mg/kg as a single dose for ascarids, gapeworms, and *Capillaria*[18].

Psittacines:
- 44 mg/kg PO; do not exceed this dose for ascarids, gapeworms, and *Capillaria*[18].

Falcons:
- 100 mg/kg PO once for ascarids, gapeworms, and *Capillaria*[18].

Raptors:
- 100 mg/kg PO once; repeat in 10–14 days[19].
- 250 mg/lb for thorny headed worms[18].

Waterfowl:
- 250 mg/lb for thorny headed worms[18].

Sheep and Goats

For sheep:
- 50–100 mg/kg PO[20].

For goats:
- 44 mg/kg PO or 66 mg/kg PO for severe infections[21].

Swine

- For baby pigs give 62–83 mg/kg PO for *Strongyloides ransomi*, retreat in 5–7 days if necessary. For *Ascaris suum* prevention feed at 0.05–0.1% per ton of feed for 2 weeks, then 0.005–0.02% per ton for 8–14 weeks[21].
- 75 mg/kg PO[22].
- 50 mg/kg PO[20].

Primates

- 50 mg/kg PO q24h for 2 days for *Strongyloides* and hookworms (*Necator* spp.)[23].
- 75–100 mg/kg PO; repeat in 21 days[24].

REFERENCES

1. Todd, K S., Paul, A.J., and DiPietro, J.A. (1985) Parasitic disease. In: Davis, L.E. (ed.) *Handbook of Small Animal Therapeutics*, Churchill Livingstone, New York, 89–126.
2. Ettinger, S., Kantrowitz, B., et al. (2000) Diseases of the trachea. Ettinger, S. and Feldman, E. (eds.) In: *Textbook of Internal Medicine: Diseases of the Dog and Cat*, W.B. Saunders Philadelphia, **2**, 1040–1055.

3. Allen, D.G., Pringe, J.K., and Smith, D.A. *Handbook of Veterinary Drugs,* J.B. Lippincott, Philadelphia.

4. Gillett, C.S. (1994) Selected drug dosages and clinical reference data. In: Manning, P.J., Ringler, D.H., and Newcomer, C.E. (eds.) *The Biology of the Laboratory* Rabbit, 2nd ed. Academic Press, San Diego, CA, 467–472.

5. Burke, T. (1999) *Husbandry and Medicine of Rodents and Lagomorphs.* Central Veterinary Conference, Kansas City, MO.

6. Ivey, E. and Morrisey, J. (2000) Therapeutics in rabbits. *Vet Clin. N. Am: Exotic Anim. Pract.* **3,** 183–213.

7. Adamcak, A. and Otten, B. (2000) Rodent therapeutics. *Vet. Clin. N. Am: Exotic Anim. Pract.* **3,** 221–240.

8. Jacobson, E., Kollias, G.V., and Peters, L.J. (1983) Dosages for antibiotics and parasiticides used in exotic animals. *Compend. Contin. Educ. Pract. Vet.* **5,** 315–324.

9. Williams, D.L. (1995) Amphibian dermatology. In: Bonagura J.D. (ed.) *Kirk's Current Veterinary Therapy XII: Small Animal Practice,* W.B. Saunders, Philadelphia, 1375–1379.

10. Frye, F.L. (1994) *Reptile Clinician's Handbook,* Krieger Publishing, Malabar, FL.

11. Jacobson, E.R. (1993) Snakes. *Vet. Clin. N. Am: Small Anim. Pract.* **23,** 1179–1212.

12. Stoskopf, M.K. (1999) Fish pharmacotherapeutics. In: Fowler, M.E. and Miller, R.E. (eds.) *Zoo and Wild Animal Medicine: Current Therapy 4,* W.B. Saunders, Philadelphia, 182–189.

13. Marshall, R. (1993) Avian anthelmintics and antiprotozoals. *Semin. Avian Exotic Pet Med.* **2,** 33–41.

14. Clubb, S.L. (1986) Therapeutics: individual and flock treatment regimens. In: Harrison, G.J. and Harrison, L.R. (eds.) *Clinical Avian Medicine and Surgery,* W.B. Saunders, Philadelphia, 327–355.

15. Johnson-Delaney, C.A. and Harrison, L.R. (1996) In: Johnson-Delaney, C.A. and Harrison, L.R.(eds.) *Exotic Companion Medicine Handbook of Veterinarians,* Wingers, Lake Worth, FL.

16. Samour, J. (2000) Pharmaceutics commonly used in avian medicine. In: Samour, J. (ed.) *Avian Medicine,* Mosby, Philadelphia, 388–418.

17. Tully, T.N. (2000) Psittacine therapeutics. *Vet. Clin. N. Am: Exotic Anim. Pract.* **3,** 59–90.

18. Stunkard, J.M. (1984) *Diagnosis, Treatment and Husbandry of Pet Birds,* Stunkard Publishing, Edgewater, MD.

19. Smith, S.A. (1996) Parasites of birds of prey: their diagnosis and treatment. *Semin. Avian Exotic Pet Med.* **5,** 97–105.

20. Brander, C.G., Pugh, D.M., and Bywater, R.J. (1982) *Veterinary Applied Pharmacology and Therapeutics,* 4th ed. Balliére Tindall, London.

21. Paul, J.W. (1986) Anthelmintic therapy. In: Howard, J.L. (ed.) *Current Veterinary Therapy: Food Animal Practice 2,* W.B. Saunders, Philadelphia, 39–44.

22. Roberson, E.L. (1988) Antinematodal agents. In: Booth, N.H. and McDonald, L.E. (eds.) *Veterinary Pharmacology and Therapeutics,* Iowa State University Press, Ames, IA, 882–927.

23. Wolff, P.L. (1993) Parasites of the New World primates. In: Fowler, M.E. (ed.) *Zoo and Wild Animal Medicine: Current Therapy 3,* W.B. Saunders, Philadelphia, 378–389.

24. Holmes, D.D. (1984) *Clinical Laboratory Animal Medicine,* Iowa State University Press, Ames, IA.

Trichlorfon (dimethyl phosphonate)

Activity: For the treatment of oviparous monogeneans in freshwater and marine fish. Also for the treatment of ectoparasites in crustaceans. Trichlorfon is neurotoxic; avoid inhalation and skin contact.

MOA: Trichlorfon is an organophosphate which inhibits acetylcholinesterase in susceptible parasites, resulting in inhibition of neuromuscular transmission.

Fish

For freshwater fish:
- 0.25 mg/L tank water
- Use 0.5 mg/L tank water if > 27°C (80°F) and treat q3d for 2 treatments for *Dactylogyrus* and other oviparous monogeneans.
- Treat q7d for 4 treatments for anchor worms; single treatments are adequate for copepods, other monogeneans, *Argulus,* and leeches[1].

For marine fish:
- 0.5–1.0 mg/L tank water.
- Treat q3d for 2 treatments for oviparous monogeneans; use 1 mg/L q48h for 3 treatments for turbellarians; single treatments are adequate for copepods (except sea lice), other monogeneans, *Argulus,* and leeches[1].

For Crustacean ectoparasites:
- 0.5 mg/L tank water q10d for 3 treatments[2].

REFERENCES

1. Noga, E.J. (2000) *Fish Disease: Diagnosis and Treatment.* Iowa State University Press, Ames, IA.

2. Lewbart, G.A. (1998) Emergency and critical care of fish. *Vet. Clin. N. Am: Exotic Anim. Pract.* **1,** 233–249.

APPENDIX TABLE I. Antiparasitic agents.

Drugs							Species											
	Dog	Cat	Mouse	Rat	Gerbil	Hamster	Guinea pig	Chinchilla	Ferret	Rabbit	Amphibian	Reptile	Fish	Bird	Sheep	Goat	Swine	Primate
Albendazole	X	X					X	X		X		X	X	X	X	X	X	
Amitraz	X	X	X	X	X	X		X	X	X				X	X			
Amprolium	X	X	X	X	X	X	X	X	X	X			X	X	X	X		
Chlorsulon													X	X				
Copper Sulfate													X					
Cythioate	X																	
Decoquinate	X									X				X		X	X	X
Dichlorvos	X	X	X	X	X	X	X	X							X			
Diethylcarbamazine Citrate	X	X																X
Epsiprantel	X	X																
Febantel	X	X																
Fenbendazole	X	X	X	X	X	X	X	X	X	X	X	X	X	X	X	X	X	X
Fenthion	X	X	X							X								X
Fipronil	X	X	X			X			X			X						X
Formalin	X	X																X
Furazolidone	X	X	X															
Imidacloprid	X	X							X	X								X
Imidocarb	X	X																
Ivermectin	X	X	X	X	X		X	X	X	X	X	X		X	X	X	X	X
Levamisole	X	X									X	X	X	X	X	X	X	X
Lufenuron	X	X								X	X							X
Malachite Green											X		X					X
Melarsomine	X								X									
Metronidazole	X	X	X	X	X	X	X	X	X		X	X	X					
Milbemycin Oxime	X	X							X		X	X		X	X	X		X
Morantel Tartrate																		
Moxidectin	X									X	X							X
Oxfendazole	X											X	X			X		X
Oxibendazole	X										X	X	X	X	X		X	X
Piperazine	X	X	X	X	X	X	X	X	X	X	X	X	X	X	X	X	X	X
Praziquantel	X	X	X	X	X	X	X	X	X	X	X	X	X	X	X	X	X	X
Pyrantel	X	X	X	X	X	X			X	X		X	X	X	X	X	X	X
Pyrimethamine	X	X																
Quinacrine	X	X	X	X	X	X	X			X	X		X					
Selamectin	X	X					X			X								
Sodium Chloride																X	X	
Thiabendazole	X	X	X	X	X	X	X	X		X	X	X	X	X	X	X	X	X
Trichlorfon	X	X	X	X	X							X			X		X	X

GLOSSARY

Adhesive disk: The ventral sucking disk of *Giardia* species. It attaches the parasite to the intestinal surface.

Amastigote: Developmental stage found in some flagellate parasites including *Leishmania* and *Trypanosoma cruzi*. Amastigotes are spherical and contain a nucleus, a kinetoplast, and rudimentary internal flagella. Amastigotes are in the intermediate host.

Ametabolous: Undergoing slight or no metamorphosis.

Anamorphosis: Arthropod development in which segments are added to the body after each molt, gradually transforming the young into an adult.

Anchoring disk: Present in the anterior end of spores of microsporidia. The anchoring disk is used to stabilize the polar tube.

Anterior station (salivarian) development: Development of protozoan parasites in the anterior portion of the insect digestive tract.

Apical complex: Present in apicomplexan parasites (Coccidia), it is an anterior complex composed of polar rings, a conoid, rhoptries, micronemes, dense granules, and subpellicular microtubules. It is involved in host cell penetration.

Apterous: Having no wings.

Axostyle: A tube-like structure in some flagellated protozoans that extends from the area of the blepharoplast to the posterior end, from which it may protrude.

Binary fission: Asexual division that produces two similar organisms.

Blepharoplast: A cytoplasmic mass of chromatin located at the base of the flagellum.

Bradyzoite: A slowly dividing stage of *Toxoplasma, Neospora,* or *Sarcocystis* parasites that is found in tissue cysts.

Chitin: High-molecular-weight polymer of N-acetyl glucosamine. Makes up the bulk of the arthropod procuticle.

Coelom: Body cavity lined by cells from the embryonic mesoderm; much reduced in arthropods.

Conoid: Present in most apicomplexan parasites, it is a hollow truncated cone composed of spirally arranged microfibrillar elements. It is part of the apical complex.

Coprozoic: Living in feces.

Ctenidium: A row of stout, peg-like spines on the head or first tergite of many fleas.

Cyst: Infective stage of protozoan parasites that are found in the environment. A cyst encloses infective stages. There are many types of cysts.

Dense granules: Special organelles found in apicomplexan parasites. They are involved predominantly in modifying the host cell after invasion.

Dioecious: Separate sexes; males and females are separate individuals.

Ecdysis: Molting of rigid portions of the arthropod cuticle, thereby allowing for growth of the arthropod body before the newly secreted cuticle hardens.

Endodyogeny: Specialized type of binary fission that produces daughter cells.

Endopodite: The medial branch of a biramous appendage of an arthropod.

Enteroepithelial cycle: The intestinal developmental cycle of *T. gondii* in cat enterocytes that results in the production of sexual stages and oocysts. The enteroepithelial cycle is initiated only by bradyzoites.

Epicuticle: Thinner outer layer of the arthropod cuticle. Primarily made up of sclerotized proteins.

Excystation: The process by which infective stages are released from the cyst.

Exopodite: The lateral branch of a biramous appendage of an arthropod.

Gamont: A sexual stage. A macrogamont is a female sexual stage. A microgamont is a male sexual stage.

Haustellum: A portion of the proboscis adapted as a sucking organ.

Hemimetabolous: Metamorphosis involving a larva (in this case called a nymph) and adult.

Hemocoel: Main body cavity of arthropods between organs and through which the blood, lymph, and interstitial fluid (hemolymph) circulate.

Hemolymph: Blood, lymph, and interstitial fluid; circulates in the hemocoel of arthropods.

Histozoic: Living within the tissues of a host.

Holometabolous: Metamorphosis involving a larva, pupa, and adult.

Holotrichous: Possessing cilia over the entire surface.

Intralecithal cleavage: Nuclei undergo multiple divisions within the yolk mass without concurrent cytokinesis.

Kala-azar: Disease caused by *Leishmania donovani,* visceral leishmaniasis.

Karyokinesis: Nuclear division.

Kinetoplast: Darkly staining structure found in *Leishmania, Trypanosoma,* and other kinetoplastid flagellates. It represents a specialized portion of the mitochondrion that contains a high concentration of mtDNA.

Kinetosomes: Basal granules making up the blepharoplast.

Macrogamont: A uninucleate female gamete (ovum, egg). After fertilization a macrogamont produces an oocyst wall and becomes an oocyst.

Macronuleus: A large darkly staining nucleus found in ciliates. The macronuleus regulates metabolism of the ciliate.

Malpighian tubules: A series of excretory ducts leading from the posterior portion of the alimentary canal of arthropods.

Median bodies: Dark-staining structures located in *Giardia* trophozoites and cysts.

Meront (Coccidia): See schizont.

Meront (Microsporidia): Major proliferative stage of microsporidia life cycle. Undergoes several rounds of division by binary fission or multiple fission (schizogony).

Merozoite: A uninucleate motile asexual stage of Apicomplexan parasites. Merozoites are produced by schizonts.

Mesothorax: The middle of three divisions of the thorax of an insect; bears the middle pair of legs and first pair (or only functional pair) of wings.

Metamere: Also referred to as a "somite." One of the body segments of an arthropod. Each metamere contains identical or similar representatives of specific organ systems.

Metathorax: The posterior of three divisions of the thorax of an insect; bears the third pair of legs and second pair of wings.

Microgamete: A biflagellated sexual stage (sperm) that is actively motile and fertilizes a macrogamont.

Microgamont: A male sexual stage that undergoes multiple karyokinesis and produces biflagellated microgametes that are actively motile and fertilize the macrogamonts.

Micronemes: Special organelles found in apicomplexan parasites. They are osmiophilic, electron-dense, rod-like bodies that are most numerous in the anterior one-half of the parasite. They are involved in host cell attachment by invasive stages.

Micronucleus: A small nucleus found in ciliates. It is primarily involved in sexual recombination and genetics of ciliates.

Oocyst: Stage of apicomplexan parasites that produces sporozoites. Oocysts of coccidial parasites are excreted in the feces and usually must sporulate in the environment.

Opisthaptor: The posterior attachment organ of the monogenetic trematodes.

Parabasal body: A cytoplasmic body (Golgi apparatus) closely associated with the kinetoplast.

Patent period: The length of time that parasite cysts or ova are excreted by an infected host.

Parasitophorous vacuole: A host-cell-derived vacuole in which stages of parasites live inside of host cells.

Pelta: A small "shield-like" structure in the anterior of the flagellate trophozoite that overlaps the capitulum of the axostyle.

Peritrichous: Having a band of cilia around the mouth.

Plasmodia: A mass of cells formed by the aggregation of many amoeboid cells.

Pleurite: Lateral sclerite of a metamere on the side of an arthropod.

Polar tube: Organelle unique to microsporidian spores; used to infect new host cells. The polar tube is extruded and penetrates a new host cell, allowing sporoplasm to pass through.

Polaroplast: A lamellar organelle in the anterior end of spores of members of the Phylum Microspora. This organelle is unique to microsporidian spores and may act like a Golgi apparatus.

Posterior station (stercorarian) development: Development of protozoan parasites in the posterior portion of the insect digestive tract.

Prepatent period: The length of time it takes from inoculation of parasite stages into the host until new parasite stages are excreted by the host.

Procuticle: Thicker layer beneath the arthropod epicuticle; provides rigidity. Primarily made up of chitin.

Prohaptor: A structure at the anterior end of monogenetic trematodes; composed of adhesive and feeding organs.

Promastigote: The insect stage of *Leishmania* species. It is elongate and contains a nucleus, kinetoplast, and flagellum.

Refractile bodies: Special organelles found in apicomplexan parasites. They are osmiophilic, electron-dense, homogenous structures, and are present in the sporozoites of many *Eimeria* species.

Romana's sign: Swollen, reddened eye caused by inflammation due to rubbing infective *T. cruzi* trypomastigotes into the eye.

Rhoptries: Special organelles found in apicomplexan parasites. They are osmiophilic, electron-dense, club-shaped structures that originate in the conoidal end of sporozoites and merozoites. Rhoptry proteins are involved in parasitophorous vacuole formation.

Sarcocyst: A muscle cyst of *Sarcocystis* species.

Schizont: An asexual stage that is multinucleate.

Schizocoely: Development of the coelom from a split in the mesoderm.

Schizogony: The process of merozoite formation in coccidial parasites.

Sclerites: Inflexible plates or sections of arthropod cuticle bound by suture lines or flexible, membranous portions of cuticle.

Spore: Infective stage of microsporidia passed in urine or feces. Spores are immediately infective and environmentally resistant.

Sporoblast (Coccidia): During sporogony, sporoblast produces sporocysts that contain sporozoites.

Sporoblast (Microsporidia): Stage of microsporidian life cycle that synthesizes spore organelles to create mature infective spores.

Sporogony (Coccidia): Development of the unsporulated noninfectious oocyst into the sporulated infectious oocyst. Sporogony usually occurs in the environment.

Sporogony (Microsporidia): Production of infective spores by sporoblasts.

Sporont (Coccidia): Central cell in unsporulated oocysts. A sporont produces sporoblasts.

Sporont (Microsporidia): Intermediate stage of the microsporidian life cycle. May divide by binary fission, or may immediately convert to sporoblast.

Sporoplasm: Contents of the mature microsporidial spore that are passed into a new host cell.

Sporocyst: A sporocyst encloses sporozoites. A sporocyst is usually enclosed inside an oocyst.

Sporozoite: Infective asexual stage that is in the oocyst of Apicomplexan parasites.

Sternite: Main sclerite of a metamere on the ventrum of an arthropod.

Subpellicular microtubule cytoskeleton: The "skeleton" of many protozoa. Provides support and can be involved in locomotion.

Synanthropic: Living in or around human dwellings.

Tachyzoite: A rapidly dividing zoite which causes tissue lesions and disseminates the infection. Present during the acute phase and relapsing phases of toxoplasmosis and neosporosis.

Tagmata (singular "tagma"): Groups of adjacent metameres into distinct body regions, each serving a particular function.

Tergite: Main sclerite of a metamere on the dorsum of an arthropod.

Trypomastigote: Elongate bloodstream form of the genus *Trypanosoma;* also the infective stage in the insect vector.

Wall-forming bodies: Specialized structures found in the macrogamonts of coccidial parasites. They are eosinophilic in hematoxylin and eosin sections. Wall-forming bodies produce the environmentally resistant oocyst wall.

Xenoma: A symbiotic structure composed of hypertrophied host cells and intracellular parasites, such as microsporidia.

Zoite: A collective term for infective stages of apicomplexan parasites.

INDEX

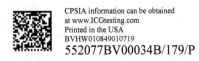

CPSIA information can be obtained
at www.ICGtesting.com
Printed in the USA
BVHW010849010719

552077BV00034B/179/P

9 780813 812021